EDITION

UNIVERSITY OF IOWA

THE FAMILY MEDICINE HANDBOOK

MARK A. GRABER, MD

Professor, Departments of Family Medicine
and Emergency Medicine
University of Iowa Carver College of Medicine
Iowa City, Iowa

JENNIFER L. JONES, MD

Former Chief Resident
Department of Family Medicine
University of Iowa Carver College of Medicine
Iowa City, Iowa
Attending Physician,
Superior Health Medical Group,
Duluth, Minnesota

JASON K. WILBUR, MD

Assistant Professor, Department of Family Medicine
University of Iowa Carver College of Medicine
Iowa City, Iowa

SAUNDERS

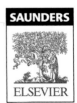

ELSEVIER

SAUNDERS
ELSEVIER

1600 John F. Kennedy Blvd.
Ste 1800
Philadelphia, PA 19103-2899

THE FAMILY MEDICINE HANDBOOK   ISBN-13: 978-0-323-03949-9
Copyright © 2006, 2001, 1997,   ISBN-10: 0-323-03949-9
1994, 1990 by Mosby, Inc., an affiliate of Elsevier Inc.

Library of Congress Cataloging-in-Publication Data

University of Iowa the family medicine handbook/ [edited by] Mark A. Graber, Jennifer Jones, and Jason Wilbur. -- 5th ed.
    p.; cm.
  Rev. ed. of: Family practice handbook. 4th ed. 2001
  Includes bibliographical references and index.
  ISBN 0-323-03949-9
    1. Family medicine--Handbooks, manuals, etc. I. Graber, Mark A., MD. II. Jones, Jennifer L. III. Wilbur, Jason K. IV. University of Iowa. V. Family practice handbook. VI. Title: Family medicine handbook.
  [DNLM: 1. Family Practice--Handbooks. WB 39 U58 2006]
RC55.F25 2006
616--dc22

2006043846

Acquisitions Editor: Joanne Husovski
Developmental Editors: Jerisha Parker, Nicole Mercurio
Publishing Services Manager: Frank Polizzano
Project Manager: Joan Nikelsky
Design Direction: Gene Harris

Printed in the United States of America

Last digit is the print number: 9 8 7 6 5 4 3 2 1

Notice

Knowledge and best practice in this field are constantly changing. As new research and experience broaden our knowledge, changes in practice, treatment, and drug therapy may become necessary or appropriate. Readers are advised to check the most current information provided (i) on procedures featured or (ii) by the manufacturer of each product to be administered, to verify the recommended dose or formula, the method and duration of administration, and contraindications. It is the responsibility of the practitioner, relying on their own experience and knowledge of the patient, to make diagnoses, to determine dosages and the best treatment for each individual patient, and to take all appropriate safety precautions. To the fullest extent of the law, neither the Publisher nor the Editors assume any liability for any injury and/or damage to persons or property arising out of or related to any use of the material contained in this book.

The Publisher

Contributors

All authors and editors were at the University of Iowa during the writing of this book.

Editors

Mark A. Graber, MD
Professor, Departments of Family Medicine and Emergency Medicine, University of Iowa Carver College of Medicine, Iowa City, Iowa

Jennifer L. Jones, MD
Former Chief Resident, Department of Family Medicine, University of Iowa Carver College of Medicine, Iowa City, Iowa; Attending Physician, Superior Health Medical Group, Duluth, Minnesota

Jason K. Wilbur, MD
Assistant Professor, Department of Family Medicine, University of Iowa Carver College of Medicine, Iowa City, Iowa

Authors

Alison C. Abreu, MD
Associate, Departments of Family Medicine and Psychiatry, University of Iowa Carver College of Medicine, Iowa City, Iowa

Jatinder P. S. Ahluwalia, MD
Associate Professor of Medicine, Division of Gastroenterology and Hepatology, Southern Illinois University School of Medicine, Springfield, Illinois

Antoine Azar, MD
Fellow, Infectious Diseases and Allergy/Immunology, Department of Internal Medicine, University of Iowa Carver College of Medicine, Iowa City, Iowa

David A. Bedell, MD
Associate Professor, Department of Family Medicine, University of Iowa Carver College of Medicine, Iowa City, Iowa

James Bonucchi, MD
Resident, Department of Internal Medicine, University of Iowa Carver College of Medicine, Iowa City, Iowa

Dana Collaguazo, MD
Assistant Professor, Department of Emergency Medicine, University of Iowa Carver College of Medicine, Iowa City, Iowa

Kevin C. Doerschug, MD
Assistant Professor, Pulmonary and Critical Care Medicine, Department of Internal Medicine, University of Iowa Carver College of Medicine, Iowa City, Iowa

Devang R. Doshi, MD, FAAP
Staff Physician, Pediatric Pulmonology, Allergy/Immunology, Department of Pediatrics and Internal Medicine, William Beaumont Hospital, Royal Oak, Michigan

Wissam El Atrouni
Fellow, Infectious Disease, Mayo Clinic, Rochester, Minnesota

Michael E. Ernst, PharmD
Associate Professor, Division of Clinical and Administrative Pharmacy, College of Pharmacy, and Department of Family Medicine, University of Iowa, Carver College of Medicine, Iowa City, Iowa

Scott Frisbie, PA-C
Private Practice, Steindler Orthopedics, Iowa City, Iowa

M. Brian Hartz, MD
Fellow, Pulmonary and Critical Care Medicine, Department of Internal Medicine, University of Iowa Carver College of Medicine, Iowa City, Iowa

Ali J. Husain, MD
Fellow, Division of Gastroenterology, Department of Internal Medicine, University of Iowa Carver College of Medicine, Iowa City, Iowa

Oladipo Kukoyi, MD
Associate, Departments of Family Medicine and Psychiatry, University of Iowa Carver College of Medicine, Iowa City, Iowa

Barcey T. Levy, PhD, MD
Professor, Department of Family Medicine, University of Iowa Carver College of Medicine, Iowa City, Iowa

Lauri Lopp, MD
Associate, Department of Family Medicine, University of Iowa Carver College of Medicine, Iowa City, Iowa

Deepak Madhavan, MD
Epilepsy Fellow, New York University Comprehensive Epilepsy Center, New York, New York

Coleman O. Martin, MD
Fellow Associate, Interventional Neurology, Department of Neurology, University of Iowa Carver College of Medicine, Iowa City, Iowa

Bobby Peters, MD
Assistant Professor, Department of Emergency Medicine, University of Iowa Carver College of Medicine, Iowa City, Iowa

Philip M. Polgreen, MD
Associate, Division of Infectious Disease, Department of Internal Medicine, University of Iowa Carver College of Medicine, Iowa City, Iowa

Christopher C. Russi, DO
Assistant Professor, Department of Emergency Medicine, University of Iowa Carver College of Medicine, Iowa City, Iowa

Tracy Shaw, MD
Former Chief Resident, Department of Pediatrics, University of Iowa Carver College of Medicine; Private Practice in Pediatrics, Iowa City, Iowa

Wendy Shen, MD
Associate, Department of Family Medicine, University of Iowa Carver College of Medicine, Iowa City, Iowa

Rogelio G. Silva, MD
Fellow, Division of Gastroenterology, Department of Internal Medicine, University of Iowa Carver College of Medicine, Iowa City, Iowa

Kelly Skelly, MD
Assistant Professor, Department of Family Medicine, University of Iowa Carver College of Medicine, Iowa City, Iowa

Jennifer J. G. Steffensmeier, PharmD
Assistant Professor, Division of Clinical and Administrative Pharmacy, University of Iowa College of Pharmacy; Department of Pharmacy, Veterans Affairs Medical Center, Iowa City, Iowa

Deborah Wilbur, MD
Fellow, Division of Hematology and Oncology, Department of Internal Medicine, University of Iowa Carver College of Medicine, Iowa City, Iowa

CONTRIBUTORS

Preface

This is my 12th year as lead editor of the *University of Iowa Family Practice Handbook*, now retitled *Family Medicine Handbook* to reflect the evolving emphasis in this dynamic field.

A lot has changed in the practice of family medicine in 12 years. We have gone from being physicians to gatekeepers and back again. Evidence-based medicine became a religion and has finally reached an equilibrium that recognizes the role of clinical judgment. One thing that has never changed, however, is the need for concise, easy-to-read, up-to-date information on a broad range of topics. This is the approach that I have taken with this handbook since the beginning. Although no one book can serve as a sole reference in any field of study, the authors, the other editors, and I have tried to include information not only about common illnesses but also about illnesses that might be seen only once or twice in a career.

As with previous editions, this fifth edition should prove useful as a reference for physicians, medical students, physician assistants, physician assistant students, nurse practitioners, and other health care professionals at various stages of practice. We hope you enjoy using this text and find it of assistance in your day-to-day practice. Feel free to give us feedback. We take it seriously and try to incorporate as many of your suggestions as possible in each edition, as space allows. You can reach me at mark-graber@uiowa.edu. Or you can reach Dr. Wilbur at jason-wilbur@uiowa.edu. Dr. Jones is off to new and exciting things ....

Mark A. Graber, MD

Acknowledgments

The editors would like to express their appreciation to all of the contributing authors—and to the laser printers that sacrificed their all-too-brief existence selflessly cranking out page after page of copy. We would offer to give them an appropriate burial, but they are considered toxic waste (the printers, not the authors). So it is an unceremonious trip to the recycling center for them! Perhaps part of them will find reincarnation as a cardiac stent or the like, improving their lot in life during their next cycle.

Mark would like to thank Jen and Jason for their exquisite editing abilities. **Special thanks** to Anna Mackenzie Jones, who selflessly put off being born *until the very day* this book was finished and we gave her the secret "it's OK to come out now" signal. He also would like to thank Hetty, Rachel, and Abe (as always) for their patience and support. Finally, thanks to Buckethead, Bjork, and Praxis for providing the late-night music that formed the soundtrack leading to the completion of this project.

Jennifer would like to thank Mark Graber for giving her the opportunity to be a part of this project and for his patience throughout; Paul Jones for his constant support, both emotionally and technologically; and Chris Bell for the casserole.

Jason would like to thank his mentors in geriatric medicine, particularly Gerald Jogerst, Margo Schilling, Richard Dobyns, Gretchen Schmuch, and Sherry McKay. Of course he thanks his family, Deb, Kenny, and Teddy, who occasionally gave him some peace and quiet to work on editing. Finally, he thanks the coffee cartel and roasters of fine coffee everywhere, without whom there would be no fuel for such endeavors.

No electrons were destroyed in the preparation of this book (but some may have been "neutralized").

Contents

CONTENTS

CONTENTS

Abbreviations

AAA	abdominal aortic aneurysm
A-a	alveolar–arterial oxygen gradient
ABCs	airway, breathing, circulation
ABG	arterial blood gas
ABPA	allergic bronchopulmonary aspergillosis
ac	before meals (ante cibum)
AC	acromioclavicular
ACE	angiotensin-converting enzyme
aCL	anticardiolipin (antibody)
ACLS	advanced cardiac life support
ACOG	American College of Obstetrics and Gynecology
ACS	acute coronary syndrome
ACTH	adrenocorticotropic hormone
AD	Alzheimer's dementia or disease
ADA	American Dietetic Association
AED	antiepileptic drug
A fib	atrial fibrillation
AFB	acid-fast bacilli
AFP	alpha fetoprotein
AFV	amniotic fluid volume
AGCUS	atypical glandular cells of undetermined significance
AI	amnioinfusion
AIDS	acquired immunodeficiency syndrome
ALS	amyotrophic lateral sclerosis
ALT	alanine aminotransferase
ANA	antinuclear antibody
ANCA	antineutrophil cytoplasmic antibody
AP	anteroposterior
APACHE	Acute Physiology and Chronic Health Evaluation
APS	antiphospholipid syndrome
APSAC	anistreplase, anisoylated plasminogen-streptokinase activator complex
aPTT	activated partial thromboplastin time
ARB	angiotensin-receptor blocker
ARC	AIDS-related complex
ARDS	acute respiratory distress syndrome
ARF	acute renal failure
ASA	acetylsalicylic acid
ASAP	as soon as possible
ASC-H	atypical squamous cells, cannot exclude high-grade lesion

ASCUS	atypical squamous cells of undetermined signifcance
ASO	antistreptolysin O antibody
AST	aspartate aminotransferase
Atg	anti-human thymocyte globulin
ATN	acute tubular necrosis
ATS	American Thoracic Society
AV	arteriovenous; atrioventricular
AVM	arteriovenous malformation
AZT	zidovudine (Azidothymidine)
B$_6$	vitamin B$_6$
B$_{12}$	vitamin B$_{12}$
BAER	brain stem auditory evoked response
BBT	basal body temperature
BCG	bacille Calmette-Guérin
BCP	birth control pill
BHCG	β-human chorionic gonadotropin
bid	twice a day (bis in die)
BiPAP	bilevel positive airway pressure
BOOP	bronchiolitis obliterans–organizing pneumonia
BP	blood pressure
BPAD	bipolar affective disorder
BPH	benign prostatic hypertrophy
bpm	beats per minute
BPP	biophysical profile
BPPV	benign paroxysmal positional vertigo
BPSD	behavioral and psychological symptoms of dementia
BSA	body surface area
BUN	blood urea nitrogen
BV	bacterial vaginosis
BVM	bag-valve-mask
C&S	culture and sensitivity
C-peptide	insulin chain C-peptide
C-section	cesarean section
C-spine	cervical spine
CABG	coronary artery bypass graft
CACl$_2$	calcium chloride
CAD	coronary artery disease
cap	capsule
c-ANCA	central antineutrophil cytoplasmic antibody
CBC	complete blood cell count
cc	cubic centimeter (gases only)
CD4+	helper T cell (cluster of differentiation no. 4+)
CDC	Centers for Disease Control and Prevention
CEA	carcinoembryonic antigen

CF	cystic fibrosis
CFU	colony-forming unit
CHF	congestive heart failure
chol	cholesterol
CIN	cervical intraepithelial neoplasia (1 to 3: mild to severe)
CIS	carcinoma in situ
CK	creatine kinase
CLL	chronic lymphocytic leukemia
cm	centimeter
CMV	cytomegalovirus
CNS	central nervous system
CO_2	carbon dioxide
COPD	chronic obstructive pulmonary disease
CPAP	continuous positive airway pressure
CP/CPPS	chronic prostatitis/chronic pelvic pain syndrome
CPD	cephalopelvic disproportion
CPK	creatine phosphokinase
CPK-MB	creatine phosphokinase, myocardial bands
CPPD	calcium pyrophosphate dihydratae (crystals) (pseudogout)
CPR	cardiopulmonary resuscitation
Cr	creatinine
CR	controlled release
CRF	chronic renal failure
CRP	C-reactive protein
CSF	cerebrospinal fluid
CST	contraction stress fluid
CT	computed tomography
CVA	cerebrovascular accident
CVAT	costovertebral-angle tenderness
CVD	cerebrovascular disease
CVN	central venous nutrition
CVP	central venous pressure
CVS	cardiovascular system
c/w	consistent with
CXR	chest x-ray film or radiograph
D&C	dilation and curettage
DBP	diastolic blood pressure
DDAVP	1-deamino-8-D-arginine vasopressin
ddC	dideoxycytidine, zalcitabine (Hivid)
ddI	dideoxyinosine, didanosine
D_5W, $D_{10}W$	5% dextrose in water, 10% dextrose in water
DES	diethylstilbestrol
DFA	direct fluorescent antibody
D4T	stavudine
DHE	dihydroergotamine

DHT	dihydrotestosterone
DIC	disseminated intravascular coagulation
DIP	distal interphalangeal joint
DKA	diabetic ketoacidosis
dL	deciliter
DLCO	diffusing capacity of lung for carbon monoxide
DM	diabetes mellitus
DMSO	dimethyl sulfoxide
DPL	diagnostic peritoneal lavage
DPT	diphtheria–pertussis–tetanus (vaccine)
DS	double strength
dsDNA	double-stranded deoxyribonucleic acid
DSM-IV	*Diagnostic and Statistical Manual of Mental Disorders*, 4th edition
DTR	deep tendon reflexes
DTs	delirium tremens
DVT	deep venous thrombosis
D/W	dextrose in water
EBV	Epstein–Barr virus
ECF	extracellular fluid
ECG	electrocardiogram
ECMO	extracorporeal membrane oxygenation
ED	emergency department
EDC	estimated date of confinement
EEG	electroencephalogram
EES	erythromycin ethylsuccinate
EF	ejection fraction
EGD	esophagogastroduodenoscopy
EIA	enzyme immunoassay
ELISA	enzyme-linked immunosorbent assay
EM	erythema multiforme
EMG	electromyogram
ENG	electronystagmography
ENT	ear, nose, throat
ERCP	endoscopic retrograde cholangiopancreatography
ESR	erythrocyte sedimentation rate
ET	endotracheal tube
Fab	antibody fragment
FAST	focused assessment with sonography for trauma
FB	foreign body
FDA	U.S. Food and Drug Administration
Fe	iron
FE$_{Na}$	fractional excretion of sodium
FEF	forced expiratory flow

FEF$_{25-75\%}$	forced expiratory flow, midexpiratory phase
FEV$_1$	forced expiratory volume in 1 second
FFP	fresh frozen plasma
FGR	fetal growth restriction
FH	family history
F$_{IO_2}$	fraction of inspired oxygen
fL	femtoliter
FSH	follicle-stimulating hormone
FTA	fluorescent treponemal antibody
FTA-ABS	fluorescent treponemal antibody absorption (test)
5-FU	5-fluorouracil
F/U	follow-up (study, exam, text, care)
FUO	fever of unknown origin
FVC	forced vital capacity
G	gauge
g	gram
G6PD	glucose-6-phosphate dehydrogenase
GAG	glycosaminoglycan
GBS	group B streptococci; Guillain–Barré syndrome
GC	gram-negative intracellular diplococci
GCS	Glasgow Coma Scale
G-CSF	granulocyte colony-stimulating factor
GCT	glucose challenge test
GDM	gestational diabetes mellitus
GE	gastroesophageal
GERD	gastroesophageal reflux disease
GFR	glomerular filtration rate
GHB	gamma hydroxybutyrate
GI	gastrointestinal
GM-CSF	granulocyte-macrophage colony-stimulating factor
GN	glomerulonephritis
GnRH	gonadotropin-releasing hormone
GODM	gestational-onset diabetes mellitus
Gp IIB/IIIA	glycoprotein IIB/IIIA
gt, gtt	drop, drops (gutta, guttae)
GTT	glucose tolerance test
GU	genitourinary
GXT	graded exercise stress test
GYN	gynecologic
h	hour
H$_1$**, H**$_2$	histamine type 1, histamine type 2 receptors
H&P	history and physical examination
HAART	highly active antiretroviral therapy
HAV	hepatitis A virus

ABBREVIATIONS

Hb	hemoglobin
HBO	hyperbaric oxygen
HBV	hepatitis B virus
HC/AC	head circumference–to–abdominal circumference ratio
HCG	human chorionic gonadotropin
Hct	hematocrit
HCTZ	hydrochlorothiazide
HCV	hepatitis C virus
HDL	high-density lipoprotein
HDV	hepatitis D virus
HELLP	hemolysis, elevated liver enzymes, and low platelet count (syndrome)
HepBsAg	hepatitis B surface antigen
HEV	hepatitis E virus
HGE	human granulocytic ehrlichiosis
HIDA	hydroxy iminodiacetic acid
HIV	human immunodeficiency virus
HMG CoA	3-hydroxy-3-methylglutaryl coenzyme A
HME	human monocytic ehrlichiosis
h/o	history of
HPF	high-power field
HPV	human papillomavirus
HRT	hormone replacement therapy
hs	at bedtime (hora somni)
HSV	herpes simplex virus
ht	height
HTN	hypertension
HUS	hemolytic uremic syndrome
HZV	herpes zoster virus
I&D	incision and drainage
IBS	irritable bowel syndrome
ICF	intracellular fluid
ICP	intracranial pressure
ICU	intensive care unit
ID	infectious disease
IDDM	insulin-dependent diabetes mellitus (now T1DM)
IFA	immunofluorescence assay
IFN α-2a	interferon alfa-2a
IGF	insulin-like growth factor
IHC	immunohistochemistry
IHSS	idiopathic hypertrophic aortic stenosis
IL	interleukin (e.g., IL-2)
IM	intramuscular
IMV	intermittent mandatory ventilation
in	inch

IN	intranasally
INH	isoniazid, isonicotinic acid hydrazide
INR	International Normalized Ratio
IO	intraosseous
IPPV	intermittent positive-pressure ventilation
ISA	intrinsic stimulating activity
ITP	idiopathic thrombocytopenia purpura
IU	International Unit
IUD	intrauterine device
IUFD	intrauterine fetal demise
IUGR	intrauterine growth restriction
IUP	intrauterine pregnancy
IV	intravenous
IVC	inferior vena cava
IVDA	intravenous drug abuser
IVP	intravenous pyelogram
JNC 7	Seventh Report of the Joint National Committee on Prevention, Detection, Evaluation, and Treatment of High Blood Pressure
JRA	juvenile rheumatoid arthritis
JVD	jugular venous distention
kg	kilogram
K, K⁺	potassium
KOH	potassium hydroxide
KS	Kaposi's sarcoma
LA	lupus anticoagulant
LAT	preparation of lidocaine, epinephrine (adrenaline), tetracaine
lb	pound
LBBB	left bundle branch block
LDH	lactate dehydrogenase
LDL	low-density lipoprotein
LE	lupus erythematosus
LES	lower esophageal sphincter
LFT	liver function test
LGI	lower gastrointestinal
LH	luteinizing hormone
LLQ	left lower quadrant
LMP	last menstrual period
LMW	low molecular weight
LOC	loss of consciousness
LP	lumbar puncture
LR	lactated Ringer's solution
L/S	lectin-to-sphingomyelin ratio

ABBREVIATIONS

LSIL	low-grade squamous intraepithelial lesion
LTBI	latent tuberculosis infection
LTC	long-term care
LTCF	long-term care facility
LUQ	left upper quadrant
LV	left ventricular
LVH	left ventricular hypertrophy
MAI/MAC	*Mycobacterium avium-intracellulare/M. avium* complex
MAO	monoamine oxidase
MAOI	monoamine oxidase inhibitor
MAST	military antishock trousers
MCP	metacarpophalangeal
MCV	mean corpuscular volume
MDD	major depressive disorder
MDI	metered dose inhaler
MEE	middle ear effusion
mEq	milliequivalent
mg	milligram
µg	microgram
MGUS	monoclonal gammopathy of undetermined significance
MI	myocardial infarction
MIC	minimum inhibitory concentration
min	minute
mm Hg	millimeters of mercury
mmol	millimole
MMPI	Minnesota Multiphasic Personality Inventory
MMR	measles, mumps, and rubella (vaccine)
MMSE	Mini-Mental State Examination
mOsm	milliosmole
MR	measles and rubella (vaccine)
MRI	magnetic resonance imaging
MRSA	methicillin-resistant *Staphylococcus aureus*
MS	multiple sclerosis
MTP	metatarsophalangeal joint
MVA	motor vehicle accident
MVP	mitral valve prolapse
N&V	nausea and vomiting
NCV	nerve conduction velocity
NG	nasogastric
NHL	non-Hodgkin's lymphoma
NIDDM	non–insulin-dependent diabetes mellitus (now T2DM)
NIH	National Institutes of Health
NNH	number needed to harm
NNT	number needed to treat

NPH	neutral protamine Hagedorn
NPO	nothing by mouth (nulla per os)
NS	normal saline solution
NSAID	nonsteroidal antiinflammatory drug
NSR	normal sinus rhythm
NST	nonstress test
NSVD	normal spontaneous vaginal delivery
NTD	neural tube defect
NTG	nitroglycerin
NYHA	New York Heart Association
O&P	ova and parasites
OA	osteoarthritis
OCD	obsessive–compulsive disorder
OCP	oral contraceptive pill
OD	overdose
17-OHS	17-hydroxysteroid (17-hydroxycorticosteroid)
OM	otitis media
OPV	oral poliovirus vaccine
OR	operating room
ORS	oral rehydration solution
OSA	obstructive sleep apnea
Osm	osmole, osmolality
OTC	over the counter
PA	posteroanterior
PAC	premature atrial contraction
PALS	pediatric advanced life support
2-PAM	pralidoxime
PaO$_2$	partial pressure of arterial oxygen
PAO$_2$	partial pressure of alveolar oxygen
Pap	Papanicolaou test or smear
PAS	para-aminosalicylic acid
PCA	patient-controlled analgesia
PCN	penicillin
PCO$_2$	partial pressure of carbon dioxide
PCOD	polycystic ovarian disease
PCP	*Pneumocystis carinii* pneumonia
PCR	polymerase chain reaction
PCWP	pulmonary capillary wedge pressure
PD	Parkinson's disease
PDA	patent ductus arteriosus
PDA	personal data assistant
PE	physical examination
PE	pulmonary embolism
PEA	pulseless electrical activity

PEEP	positive end-expiratory pressure
PEFR	peak expiratory flow rate
PEP	postexposure prophylaxis
PET	positron emission tomography
PFT	pulmonary function test
PG	phosphatidylglycerol
PGE	prostaglandin E (PGE$_1$, PGE$_2$)
pH	hydrogen-ion concentration
PID	pelvic inflammatory disease
PIH	pregnancy-induced hypertension
PIP	proximal interphalangeal joint
plt	platelet
PMDD	premenstrual dysphoric disorder
PMN	polymorphonuclear lymphocyte
PMR	polymyalgia rheumatica
PMS	premenstrual syndrome
PO	by mouth (per os)
PO$_2$	partial pressure of oxygen
POD	postoperative day
PPD	purified protein derivative
PR	per rectum
prn	as needed (pro re nata)
PROM	premature rupture of membranes
PRSP	penicillin-resistant *Streptococcus pneumoniae*
PSA	prostate-specific antigen
PSVT	paroxysmal supraventricular tachycardia
PT	prothrombin time
PTCA	percutaneous transluminal coronary angioplasty
PTL	premature labor
PTSD	post-traumatic stress disorder
PTT	partial thromboplastin time
PTU	propylthiouracil
PUD	peptic ulcer disease
PVC	premature ventricular contraction
qac	before meals (quaque ante cibum)
qd	every day (quaque die)
qhs	at bedtime (quaque hora somni)
qid	four times per day (quater in die)
qod	every other day (quaque altera die)
RA	rheumatoid arthritis
RBC	red blood cell
RCA	right coronary artery
REM	rapid eye movement
RF	renal failure

RFI	renal failure index
RIA	radioimmunoassay
RIND	reversible ischemic neurologic deficit
RLQ	right lower quadrant
RLS	restless legs syndrome
RMSF	Rocky Mountain spotted fever
r/o	rule out
ROM	range of motion; rupture of membranes
RPR	rapid plasma reagin
RSI	rapid sequence intubation
RSV	respiratory syncytial virus
rt-PA	recombinant tissue type plasminogen activator (recombinant Alteplase)
RUQ	right upper quadrant
RV	residual volume
RVMI	right ventricular myocardial infarction
SAARD	slow-acting antirheumatic drug
SAH	subarachnoid hemorrhage
SARS	severe acute respiratory syndrome
SBP	systolic blood pressure
SC	subcutaneous
SCIWORA	spinal cord injury without radiologic abnormality
SGA	small for gestational age
SGOT	serum glutamic oxaloacetic transaminate (aspartate aminotransferase)
SGPT	serum glutamic pyruvic transaminase (alanine aminotransferase)
SIADH	syndrome of inappropriate antidiuretic hormone secretion
SIDS	sudden infant death syndrome
SIL	squamous intraepithelial lesions
SIRS	systemic inflammatory response syndrome
SK	streptokinase
SL	sublingual
SLE	systemic lupus erythematosus
SLR	straight-leg raising (test)
SNRI	serotonin and norepinephrine reuptake inhibitor
SOB	shortness of breath
sp gr	specific gravity
SPECT	single-photon emission computed tomography
SPEP	serum protein electrophoresis
SQ	subcutaneous
SR	slow release
SROM	spontaneous rupture of membrane
SS	single strength
SSKI	saturated solution of potassium iodide

SSRI	selective serotonin reuptake inhibitor
STD	sexually transmitted disease
T$_3$	triiodothyronine
T$_4$	thyroxine
TAC	preparation of tetracycline, epinephrine (adrenaline), and cocaine
TB	tuberculosis
TBG	thyroxine-binding globulin
TBSA	total body surface area
TBW	total body water
3TC	lamivudine
TCA	tricyclic antidepressant
TEDS	thromboembolic disease support (stockings, hose)
TEE	transesophageal echocardiography
TENS	transcutaneous electrical nerve stimulation
TFT	thyroid function test
TG	triglyceride(s)
TIA	transient ischemic attack
tid	three times a day (ter in die)
tiw	three times a week (ter in "week")
TIBC	total iron-binding capacity
TIPS	transjugular intrahepatic portosystemic shunt
TLC	total lung capacity
TM	tympanic membrane
TMJ	temporomandibular joint
TMP-SMX	trimethoprim-sulfamethoxazole
TORCHS	toxoplasmosis, rubella, cytomegalovirus, herpes simplex, syphilis (infection)
tPA	tissue plasminogen activator
TPN	total parenteral nutrition
TRH	thyrotropin-releasing hormone
TSB	total serum bilirubin
TSH	thyroid-stimulating hormone
TSS	toxic shock syndrome
TTP	thrombotic thrombocytopenic purpura
TURP	transurethral prostatectomy
TWAR	Taiwan acute respiratory disease
U	unit
UA	urinalysis
UC	ulcerative colitis
UGI	upper gastrointestinal
U/P	urine-to-plasma ratio
URI	upper respiratory infection
US	ultrasonography, ultrasound

UTI	urinary tract infection
UV	ultraviolet (radiation)
UVA	ultraviolet A
UVB	ultraviolet B
V fib	ventricular fibrillation
V tach	ventricular tachycardia
VBAC	vaginal birth after cesarean section
VC	vital capacity
VCUG	voiding cystourethrogram
VDRL	Venereal Disease Research Laboratories
V̇/Q̇	ventilation–perfusion ratio
VSD	ventricular septal defect
VT	tidal volume
VT	vestibular training
vWF	von Willebrand factor
VZIG	varicella-zoster immune globulin
WBC	white blood cell
WHO	World Health Organization
wt	weight

Resuscitation, Airway Management, and Acute Arrhythmias

Christopher C. Russi and Mark A. Graber

KEY TO ADULT AND PEDIATRIC CARDIAC RESUSCITATION ALGORITHMS AND DRUG DOSE TABLES

Adult Cardiac Resuscitation Based on 2005 AHA Guidelines

Pediatric Cardiac Resuscitation

Neonatal Cardiac Resuscitation

AIRWAY MANAGEMENT AND RAPID SEQUENCE INTUBATION

I. Airway Management.

A. Adequate anesthesia is critical for intubation in the awake patient.

1. If you have time, lidocaine 4%, 5 mL by hand-held nebulizer, facilitates intubation by blocking the gag reflex and providing excellent topical anesthesia.

2. In nasal intubation, cetacaine/lidocaine spray and lidocaine jelly are helpful.

RESUSCITATION, AIRWAY MANAGEMENT, AND ACUTE ARRHYTHMIAS

B. Nasal intubation

1. This is a blind and challenging technique. Putting 5 cc of air in the ET balloon once it is in the posterior pharynx can facilitate a difficult intubation.

2. Nasal intubation is contraindicated in apnea, in bleeding disorders, after fibrinolytic administration, and in patients with a basilar skull fracture or midface trauma.

3. The patient must be breathing to receive this technique.

4. Almost all patients intubated nasally develop a sinusitis and should be given antibiotics if prolonged intubation is required.

II. RSI (Box 1-1 and Table 1-1).

Before you try this technique, be sure you are able to control the airway, because the patient will be paralyzed and unable to breathe. Always assess tube placement by auscultation, radiograph, oxygen saturation, and end-tidal CO_2 (which will be low in esophageal intubation).

A. Indications: respiratory failure, acute intracranial lesions, some overdoses, status epilepticus, combative trauma patients whose behavior threatens life, possible cervical spine fracture where immobilization is not possible secondary to delirium, etc.

BOX 1-1

RAPID SEQUENCE INTUBATION

Patient will not be able to maintain an airway or breathe after paralysis. Use this technique only if you are comfortable performing intubation.

BEFORE PARALYSIS

- Preoxygenate, IV lines, monitor, oximetry, equipment including that for emergency surgical airway control
- Lidocaine 1 mg/kg (100 mg*)[1]
- Atropine 0.01 mg/kg (0.5 mg*)[2]
- Vecuronium 0.01 mg/kg (1 mg*)[3] prevents fasciculation *if* using succinylcholine (no need with rocuronium or vecuronium).
- Begin Sellick maneuver (cricothyroid pressure to prevent vomiting and aspiration).

PARALYSIS

- Midazolam 0.1 mg/kg (7 mg*)[4] *or* etomidate 0.3 mg/kg IV (duration 3-5 min)
- Succinylcholine 1.5 mg/kg (100 mg*)[5] *or* rocuronium 0.6-1.2 mg/kg IV *or* vecuronium 0.10 mg/kg (10 mg*)

INTUBATION WHEN RELAXED

- Assess tube placement
- Check patient's temperature 8 min after intubation if succinylcholine is used

---

*Usual adult dosage.

[1]May be omitted in patients without head injury. *Efficacy in protecting against ICP rise in closed head injury is questionable.*

[2]May be omitted in adults with no preexistent bradycardia.

[3]May use pancuronium (same dose). This step is optional.

[4]May use thiopental 3-5 mg/kg (300 mg*). *Caution: Thiopental causes hypotension and should be avoided in patients with marginal blood pressure.*

[5]Dose in children is 1.5-2 mg/kg.

TABLE 1-1

ENDOTRACHEAL TUBE SIZES FOR CHILDREN

Age	Endotracheal Tube Size
Premature	2.5, 3.0 uncuffed
Newborn	3.0, 3.5 uncuffed
6 mo	3.5 uncuffed
12-18 mo	4.0, 4.5 uncuffed
2 y	4.5, 5.0 uncuffed
4 y	5.0, 5.5 uncuffed
6 y	5.5 uncuffed
8 y	6.0 cuffed or uncuffed
10 y	6.5 cuffed
12 y	7.0 cuffed
>12 y	7.0-8.0 cuffed

To calculate: Approximate tube size = (age/4) + 4 (If >1 year of age.)

B. Drugs

1. Succinylcholine.
   a. Contraindicated in penetrating ocular trauma and hyperkalemia.
   b. Can cause bradycardia, increased intraocular and intracranial pressure, increased gastric pressure, and emesis.
   c. Rarely causes malignant hyperthermia.
   d. Can cause fatal hyperkalemia in those with risk factors in particular time frames:
      i. Burns 24 hours to 2 years after burn.
      ii. Denervation (e.g., stroke, spinal cord injury) 1 week to 6 months after injury and always in MS and ALS.
      iii. Crushed muscle 7 d to 90 days after injury. **Do not use succinylcholine in these patients.**
2. Vecuronium: Rapid onset (1 min, max 3-5 min, duration 25-40 min), nondepolarizing, no cardiac toxicity.
3. Rocuronium: Rapid onset (<2 min, max 3 min, duration 31 min average), nondepolarizing, no cardiac toxicity.
C. **Procedure.** See Box 1-1.

ADVANCED CARDIAC LIFE SUPPORT

I. **General.** The ABCs common to all emergency situations:
A. Airway, including relieving obstruction and positioning.
B. Breathing, including 100% O_2 by BVM or (preferably) intubation.
C. Circulation, CPR.
D. Drugs (Table 1-2): **Lidocaine, atropine, naloxone, and epinephrine may be given via endotracheal tube.** Give 10 mL sterile water (best) or saline after drug. Efficacy by ET tube questionable. IO preferable even in adults!
II. **Specific Rhythms and Their Treatment** (Figs. 1-1 to 1-7).

Text continued on p. 12

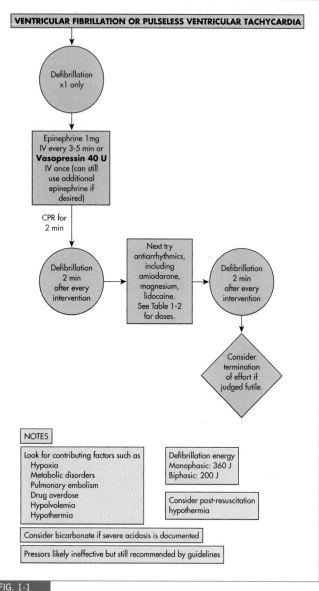

FIG. 1-1

Ventricular fibrillation or pulseless ventricular tachycardia.

Torsade de pointes (polymorphic ventricular tachycardia)

Caused by digitalis toxicity, erythromycin, lidocaine, tricyclic antidepressants, quinidine, procainamide, mexiletine, tocainide, amiodarone, nifedipine, cisapride, antipsychotics, and others. Also, hypothermia and toxins, including arsenic and organophosphate poisoning. Other causes include hypocalcemia, hypomagnesemia, hypokalemia, and neurologic processes, including stroke and subarachnoid bleeding.

Avoid drugs that could prolong the QT interval further such as quinidine, lidocaine, and disopyramide.

TREATMENT

Treat like pulseless V-tach

Magnesium is probably the best pharmacologic approach, although V-fib or V-tach can recur. Give 2 g bolus of $MgSO_4$ (10 mL of a 20% solution) over 1 to 2 min (can push if not perfusing). May follow with a second or third bolus if necessary at 5 to 15 min. Infusions of 3 to 20 mg/min for 7 to 48 h or until the QT interval has decreased to < 0.50 sec. Magnesium toxicity is heralded by areflexia, bradycardia, coma, respiratory depression; it should not be a problem in doses noted above. Magnesium is relatively contraindicated in renal failure.

Temporary overdrive pacing at 90-120 beats per minute.

Amiodarone or lidocaine can be tried.

FIG. 1-1—cont'd

TABLE 1-2

ADULT CARDIAC DRUG DOSES*

Drug	Dose
Adenosine	6 mg IV bolus followed by 12 mg IV
	Follow with 30 mL saline flush
Amiodarone	Pulseless V tach/V fib: 300 mg IV push; may repeat with 150 mg
	Perfusing rhythm: 150 mg IV slowly
Atropine	0.5-1 mg IV; total 0.04 mg/kg
Diltiazem	0.25 mg/kg IV over 2 min followed by 0.35 mg/kg
	Drip at 5-15 mg/h (see verapamil)
Epinephrine	1 mg IV push q3-5min (max 0.02 mg/kg, but high dose is of questionable benefit and may increase risk of mortality)
Isoproterenol	2-8 µg/min for overdrive pacing of torsades (no longer available in United States)
Lidocaine	Pulseless V-tach/V-fib: 1.5 mg/kg IV push, repeat in 3-5 min to total of 3 mg/kg
	Perfusing rhythm: 1-1.5 mg/kg slowly, then 0.5-0.75 mg/kg IV in 5-10 min to total of 3 mg/kg
	Drip: 2-4 mg/min
Magnesium	1-2 g IV push
Metoprolol	5 mg IV slowly with 5 mg q5min to total of 15 mg. May titrate to effect
Procainamide	17 mg/kg IV, max rate 30 mg/min
	Drip: 1-4 mg/min
Sodium bicarbonate	1 mEq/kg
Sotalol	1.0-1.5 mg/kg infused at 10 mg/min (not approved in United States)
Vasopressin	40 U IV, single dose only
Verapamil	2.5-5 mg IV; repeat with 5-10 mg; max 20 mg
	May pretreat with 3.3 mL CaCl to mitigate hypotension
	Drip: 5-10 mg/h

*See also specific algorithms.

RESUSCITATION, AIRWAY MANAGEMENT, AND ACUTE ARRHYTHMIAS   1

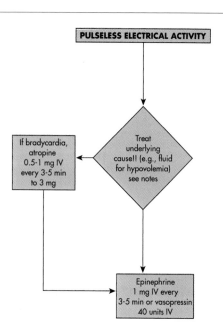

PULSELESS ELECTRICAL ACTIVITY

If bradycardia, atropine 0.5-1 mg IV every 3-5 min to 3 mg

Treat underlying cause!! (e.g., fluid for hypovolemia) see notes

Epinephrine 1 mg IV every 3-5 min or vasopressin 40 units IV

NOTES

PEA is absence of a pulse despite organized complexes at an adequate rate.

Consider underlying causes including hypothermia, hypovolemia, cardiac tamponade, pulmonary embolism, hypoxia, tension pneumothorax, acidosis, massive infarction, hyperkalemia, hypokalemia, overdose (β-blockers, calcium channel blockers, etc.)

If you are sure there is massive pulmonary embolism, you may try thrombolytics if other measures fail (see Chapter 4)

FIG. 1-2

Pulseless electrical activity.

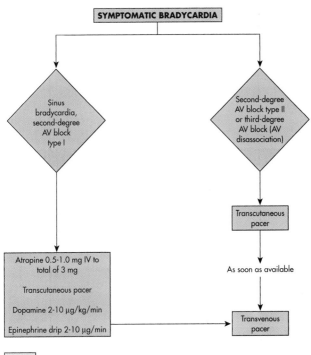

SYMPTOMATIC BRADYCARDIA

Sinus bradycardia, second-degree AV block type I

Second-degree AV block type II or third-degree AV block (AV disassociation)

Transcutaneous pacer

Atropine 0.5-1.0 mg IV to total of 3 mg

Transcutaneous pacer

Dopamine 2-10 μg/kg/min

Epinephrine drip 2-10 μg/min

As soon as available

Transvenous pacer

NOTES

Bradycardia is a pulse <60 or a pulse that is lower than expected for the clinical situation (e.g., a pulse of 70 in a patient with hypovolemia)

Symptomatic = hypotension, poor perfusion (e.g., CNS changes), weakness, etc.

Types of heart block:
  I. First-degree AV block with fixed PR interval >0.20 sec.
  II. Second-degree AV block.
      a. Mobitz type I (Wenckebach): progressive prolongation of PR interval until there is a nonconducted P wave.
      b. Mobitz type II: fixed PR interval with dropped beats (may require a pacer).
  III. Third-degree AV block: no consistent relationship between P waves and QRS complexes.

For calcium channel blocker overdose, use calcium chloride 0.5-1 g IV slow push.
For β-blocker overdose, consider glucogon 5-10 mg IV followed by a drip of 1-5 mg/h.

FIG. 1-3

Symptomatic bradycardia.

RESUSCITATION, AIRWAY MANAGEMENT, AND ACUTE ARRHYTHMIAS   1

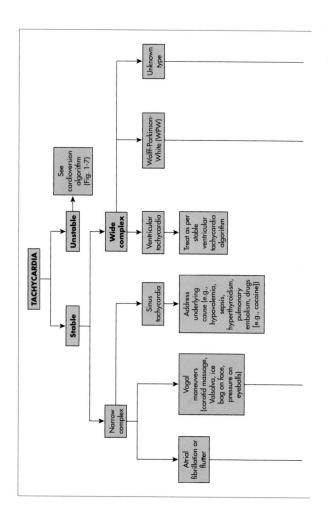

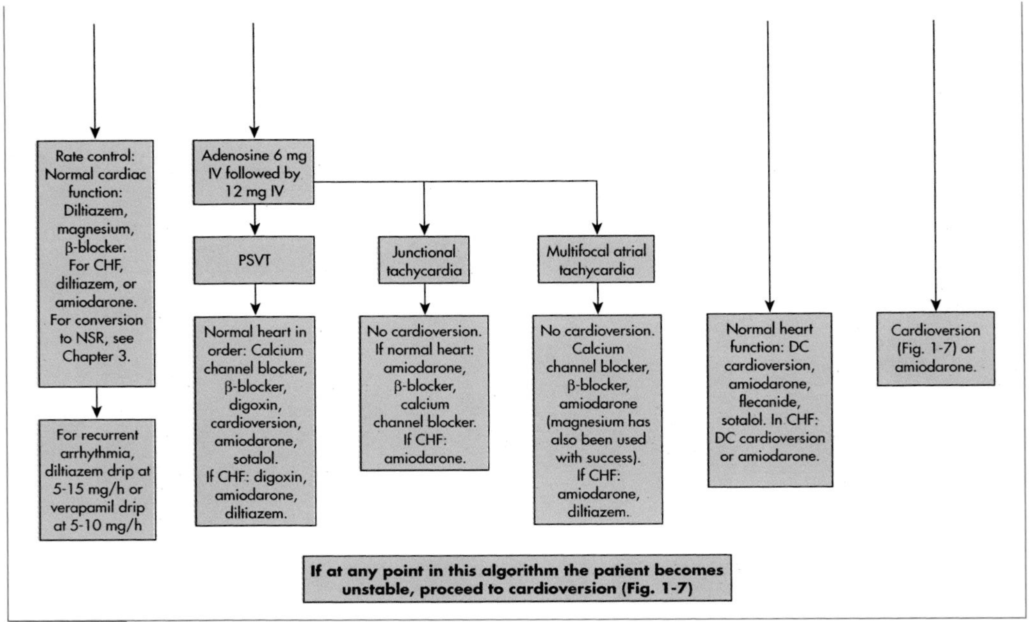
Rate control: Normal cardiac function: Diltiazem, magnesium, β-blocker. For CHF, diltiazem, or amiodarone. For conversion to NSR, see Chapter 3.
For recurrent arrhythmia, diltiazem drip at 5-15 mg/h or verapamil drip at 5-10 mg/h
Adenosine 6 mg IV followed by 12 mg IV
PSVT
Normal heart in order: Calcium channel blocker, β-blocker, digoxin, cardioversion, amiodarone, sotalol. If CHF: digoxin, amiodarone, diltiazem.
Junctional tachycardia
No cardioversion. If normal heart: amiodarone, β-blocker, calcium channel blocker. If CHF: amiodarone.
Multifocal atrial tachycardia
No cardioversion. Calcium channel blocker, β-blocker, amiodarone (magnesium has also been used with success). If CHF: amiodarone, diltiazem.
Normal heart function: DC cardioversion, amiodarone, flecanide, sotalol. In CHF: DC cardioversion or amiodarone.
Cardioversion (Fig. 1-7) or amiodarone.
If at any point in this algorithm the patient becomes unstable, proceed to cardioversion (Fig. 1-7)

FIG. 1-4

Stable and unstable tachycardia.

(Continued)

NOTES

CHF for purposes of this algorithm means clinical CHF or EF <40%.
Unstable means hypotension, poor perfusion, cardiac ischemia, etc., related to rate.
Stable means good perfusion, no cardiac, ischemia, stable, adequate blood pressure, etc.
No DC cardioversion or narrow complex tachycardia with EF <40% or CHF unless patient becomes unstable.
Can pretreat with calcium chloride, 3.3 mL IV before using calcium channel blockers. This mitigates hypotension without affecting antiarrhythmic properties.
Digoxin will not convert A fib but may facilitate conversion by improving cardiac function. 50% will spontaneously convert to NSR.
Carotid massage has <0.28% complication rate and most of these are transitory (e.g., TIA).
Start appropriate oral medications as indicated (e.g., verapamil to prevent recurrent PSVT).

FIG. 1-4—cont'd

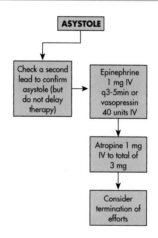

ASYSTOLE
Check a second lead to confirm asystole (but do not delay therapy)
Epinephrine 1 mg IV q3-5min or vasopressin 40 units IV
Atropine 1 mg IV to total of 3 mg
Consider termination of efforts

NOTES

Recovery from true asystole is rare.

Consider defibrillation if fine V fib is a possibility (about 9%) but not routinely recommended.

Aminophylline 250 mg IV has been successful in **uncontrolled** human trials but showed no benefit in swine trials. It is not standard of care but can be tried if conventional therapy has failed.

Transcutaneous pacing no longer recommended.

FIG. 1-5
Asystole.

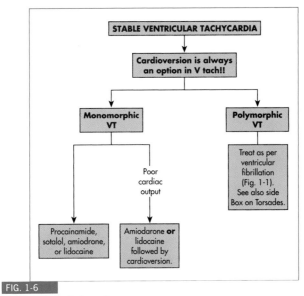

FIG. 1-6

Stable ventricular tachycardia.

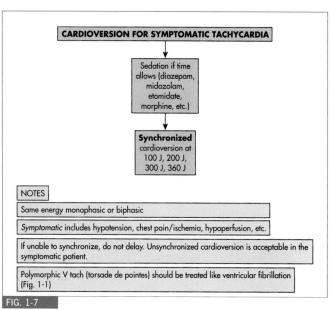

FIG. 1-7

Cardioversion for symptomatic tachycardia.

CRITICAL PEDIATRIC LIFE SUPPORT

I. Pediatric Advanced Life Support.

A. Breathing. Remember positioning, suctioning, airway.

1. Pediatric cardiac arrest is almost always secondary to respiratory insult.

2. Immediately treat any signs of respiratory distress such as tachypnea, retractions, or stridor. (See Tables 2-1 and 12-9 for differentials.)

3. Immediately provide humidified oxygen in the highest concentration possible. Treat the underlying cause!

4. For suspected epiglottitis, do not move the patient or apply oxygen. Any agitation to the child can precipitate airway obstruction. See Chapter 12 for a discussion of epiglottitis.

5. Aspiration of a foreign body is especially prevalent in children <5 years old.

a. **Presentation.** Sudden-onset dyspnea, stridor, gagging.

b. **Treatment.** Observe as long as the child is moving air well and coughing. If there is increased respiratory difficulty or cough is ineffective, try the Heimlich maneuver or direct visualization of cords and removal of foreign body, if necessary.

c. **BVM with 100% O_2 is usually adequate, even in situations such as epiglottitis**. If you must intubate, see Box 1-1 for RSI and Table 1-1 for ET tube size. **Use extreme caution** and be certain you can manage the airway.

B. Cardiac assessment (Figs. 1-8 to 1-11)

1. Tachycardia is the usual response to stress.
2. Bradycardia is evidence of impending cardiac arrest.
3. Blood pressure might remain normal until cardiopulmonary arrest.
4. Observe level of consciousness, urine output, capillary refill, and color as gauge of end-organ perfusion.
5. IV fluid resuscitation: 20 mL/kg IV bolus NS. May repeat twice or even more if needed.
6. Efficacy of high-dose epinephrine (0.1 mg/kg) is unclear. It likely worsens outcome.
7. Drugs for pediatric resuscitation are shown in **Table 1-3**.

II. Neonatal Resuscitation (Fig. 1-12).

A. One-minute Apgar score <5 indicates intrapartum asphyxia, 5 to 7 indicates mild asphyxia, and >7 is normal. Reassess every 5 minutes until score is >7.

B. Medications for neonatal resuscitation are shown in **Table 1-4**.

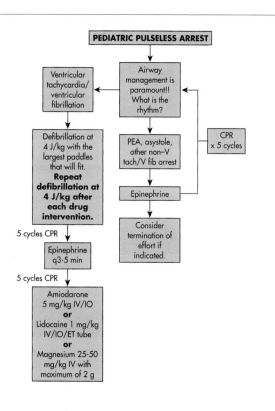

PEDIATRIC PULSELESS ARREST

Airway management is paramount!! What is the rhythm?

Ventricular tachycardia/ ventricular fibrillation

CPR x 5 cycles

PEA, asystole, other non–V tach/V fib arrest

Defibrillation at 4 J/kg with the largest paddles that will fit. **Repeat defibrillation at 4 J/kg after each drug intervention.**

Epinephrine

Consider termination of effort if indicated.

5 cycles CPR

Epinephrine q3-5 min

5 cycles CPR

Amiodarone 5 mg/kg IV/IO **or** Lidocaine 1 mg/kg IV/IO/ET tube **or** Magnesium 25-50 mg/kg IV with maximum of 2 g

NOTES

Same energy monophasic or biphasic

Most pediatric cardiac arrest is a primary pulmonary event. Airway management and oxygenation is crucial.

Consider underlying causes, including hypothermia, hypovolemia, cardiac tamponade, pulmonary embolism, hypoxia, tension pneumothorax, acidosis, massive infarction, hyperkalemia, hypokalemia, overdose (e.g., β-blockers, calcium channel blockers), etc.

Epinephrine dose: IV/IO 0.01 mg/kg (1:10,000, 0.1 mL/kg)
By ET tube: 0.1 mg/kg (1:1000, 0.1 mL/kg)

IV pressors (e.g., dopamine) as needed. Bicarbonate as needed for documented acidosis.

FIG. 1-8

Pediatric pulseless arrest.

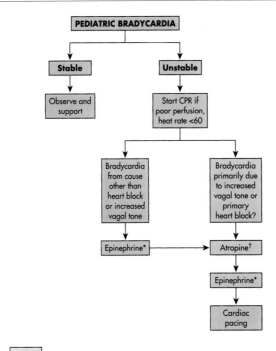

PEDIATRIC BRADYCARDIA

Stable → Observe and support

Unstable → Start CPR if poor perfusion, heat rate <60

- Bradycardia from cause other than heart block or increased vagal tone → Epinephrine*
- Bradycardia primarily due to increased vagal tone or primary heart block? → Atropine† → Epinephrine* → Cardiac pacing

NOTES

Unstable is defined as poor perfusion, hypotension, mental status changes, etc., secondary to cardiac status.

*Epinephrine dose: IV/IO 0.01 mg/kg (1:10,000, 0.1 mL/kg)
By ET tube: 0.1 mg/kg (1:1000, 0.1 mL/kg). Repeat every 3-5 min.

†Atropine dose 0.02 mg/kg with minimum of 0.1 mg. Maximum total dose 1mg.

Consider underlying causes, including hypothermia, hypovolemia, cardiac tamponade, hypoxia, head injury, overdose (e.g., β-blockers, calcium channel blockers, digoxin), head injury, etc.

FIG. 1-9

Pediatric bradycardia.

RESUSCITATION, AIRWAY MANAGEMENT, AND ACUTE ARRHYTHMIAS   1

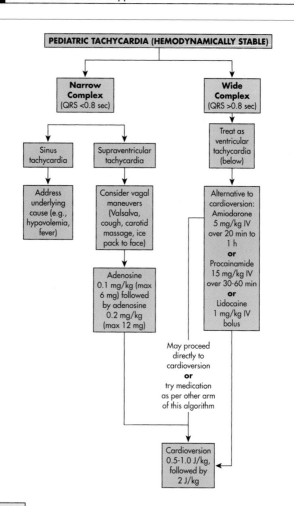

PEDIATRIC TACHYCARDIA (HEMODYNAMICALLY STABLE)

Narrow Complex (QRS <0.8 sec)

Wide Complex (QRS >0.8 sec)

Treat as ventricular tachycardia (below)

Sinus tachycardia

Supraventricular tachycardia

Address underlying cause (e.g., hypovolemia, fever)

Consider vagal maneuvers (Valsalva, cough, carotid massage, ice pack to face)

Adenosine 0.1 mg/kg (max 6 mg) followed by adenosine 0.2 mg/kg (max 12 mg)

Alternative to cardioversion: Amiodarone 5 mg/kg IV over 20 min to 1 h **or** Procainamide 15 mg/kg IV over 30-60 min **or** Lidocaine 1 mg/kg IV bolus

May proceed directly to cardioversion **or** try medication as per other arm of this algorithm

Cardioversion 0.5-1.0 J/kg, followed by 2 J/kg

NOTES

Stable means no signs or symptoms of hypoperfusion such as mental status changes, cyanosis, hypotension.

Consider underlying causes including hypothermia, hypovolemia, cardiac tamponade, pulmonary embolism, hypoxia, tension pneumothorax, acidosis, massive infarction, hyperkalemia, hypokalemia, overdose (e.g., β-blockers, calcium channel blockers), etc.

Consultation with pediatric cardiology is suggested before cardioversion.

FIG. 1-10

Hemodynamically stable pediatric tachycardia.

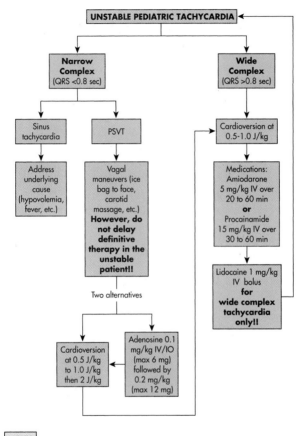

FIG. 1-11

Unstable pediatric tachycardia.

TABLE 1-3

DOSES FOR PEDIATRIC RESUSCITATION

Treatment	Dose	Comments
Adenosine	0.1-0.2 mg/kg	Rapid IV bolus
		Max single dose: 12 mg
Atropine sulfate	0.02 mg/kg/dose	Min dose: 0.1 mg
		Max total dose in child: 1 mg
Bretylium tosylate	5 mg/kg; may increase to 10 mg/kg/dose	Rapid IV
Calcium chloride 10%	20 mg/kg/dose	Give slowly
Defibrillation	2 J/kg	
	If this is not effective, use 4 J/kg	
Dobutamine HCl*†	2-20 mg/kg/min	Titrate to desired effect
Dopamine HCl*†	2-20 µg/kg/min	Adrenergic action dominates at ≥15-20 µg/kg/min
Epinephrine for bradycardia	IV/IO: 0.01 mg/kg (1:10,000) = 0.1 mL/kg 1:10,000	Be aware of effective dose of preservatives administered (if preservatives are present in epinephrine preparation) when high doses are used.
	ET: 0.1 mg/kg (1:10,000) = 0.1 mL/kg 1:10,000	

Drug	Dose	Comments
Epinephrine for asystolic or pulseless arrest	First dose: IV/IO: 0.01 mg/kg (1:10,000) = 0.1 mL/kg of 1:10,000 ET: 0.1 mg/kg (1:1000) = 0.1 mL/kg of 1:1000 Doses as high as 0.2 mg/kg may be effective Subsequent doses: IV/IO/ET: 0.1 mg/kg (1:1000) = 0.1 mL/kg of 1:1000 Doses as high as 0.2 mg/kg may be effective	Be aware of effective dose of preservatives administered (if preservatives are present in epinephrine preparation) when high doses are used
Epinephrine infusion	Initial dose: 0.1 μg/kg/min Higher infusion dose used if asystole is present	Titrate to desired effect (0.1-0.1 μg/kg/min)
Lidocaine	1 mg/kg/dose	
Lidocaine infusion	20-50 μg/kg/min	
Sodium bicarbonate	1 mEq/kg/dose or 0.3 × kg × base deficit	Infuse slowly and only if ventilation is adequate

*Run these drugs in rapidly at first to clean the line and ensure drug delivery. When you note a clinical response (increase in heart rate, BP), decrease drip rate to desired infusion rate.
†Dilutions: 6 × body weight (kg) = mg in 100 mL D_5W; then 1 mL/h = 1.0 μg/kg/min.
Adapted from Emergency Cardiac Care Committee and Subcommittees, American Heart Association: *JAMA* 268(16):2171-2183, 1992.

RESUSCITATION, AIRWAY MANAGEMENT, AND ACUTE ARRHYTHMIAS　1

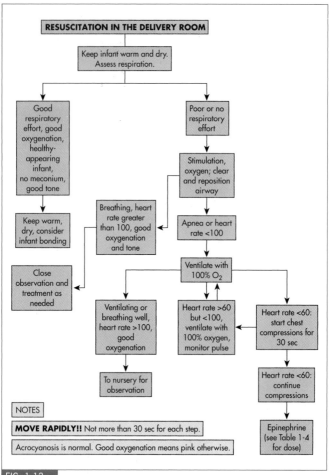

RESUSCITATION IN THE DELIVERY ROOM

Keep infant warm and dry.
Assess respiration.

Good respiratory effort, good oxygenation, healthy-appearing infant, no meconium, good tone

Poor or no respiratory effort

Stimulation, oxygen; clear and reposition airway

Keep warm, dry, consider infant bonding

Breathing, heart rate greater than 100, good oxygenation and tone

Apnea or heart rate <100

Close observation and treatment as needed

Ventilate with 100% O_2

Ventilating or breathing well, heart rate >100, good oxygenation

Heart rate >60 but <100, ventilate with 100% oxygen, monitor pulse

Heart rate <60: start chest compressions for 30 sec

To nursery for observation

Heart rate <60: continue compressions

NOTES

MOVE RAPIDLY!! Not more than 30 sec for each step.

Acrocyanosis is normal. Good oxygenation means pink otherwise.

Epinephrine (see Table 1-4 for dose)

FIG. 1-12

Resuscitation in the delivery room.

TABLE 1-4
MEDICATIONS FOR NEONATAL RESUSCITATION

Medication	Concentration to Administer	Preparation	Dosage and Route	Total Dose/Infant Weight	Total mL	Rate and Precautions
Epinephrine	1:10 000	1 mL	0.1-0.3 mL/kg IV or ET	1 kg	0.1-0.3	Give rapidly
				2 kg	0.2-0.6	May dilute with normal saline to
				3 kg	0.3-0.9	1-2 mL if giving ET
				4 kg	0.4-1.2	
Volume expanders	Whole blood, 5% albumin–saline, normal saline, lactated Ringer's	40 mL	10 mL/kg IV	1 kg	10	Give over 5-10 min
				2 kg	20	
				3 kg	30	
				4 kg	40	

| | | | | Total Dose/Infant | | |
Medication	Concentration to Administer	Preparation	Dosage and Route	Weight	Total Dose	Total mL	Rate and Precautions
Sodium bicarbonate	0.5 mEq/mL (4.2% solution)	20 mL or two 10-mL prefilled syringes	2 mEq/kg IV	1 kg	2 mEq	4	Give slowly, over ≥2 min
				2 kg	4 mEq	8	Give only if infant is being effectively ventilated
				3 kg	6 mEq	12	
				4 kg	8 mEq	16	

(Continued)

RESUSCITATION, AIRWAY MANAGEMENT, AND ACUTE ARRHYTHMIAS 1

TABLE 1-4
MEDICATIONS FOR NEONATAL RESUSCITATION—cont'd

Medication	Concentration to Administer	Preparation	Dosage and Route	Total Dose/Infant			Rate and Precautions
				Weight	Total Dose	Total mL	
Naloxone hydrochloride	0.4 mg/mL	1 mL	0.1 mg/kg (0.25 mL/kg) IV, ET, IM, SQ	1 kg	0.1 mg	0.25	Give rapidly IV, ET preferred IM, SQ acceptable
				2 kg	0.2 mg	0.50	
				3 kg	0.3 mg	0.75	
				4 kg	0.4 mg	1	
	1.0 mg/mL	1 mL	0.1 mL/kg (0.1 mL/kg) IV, ET, IM, SQ	1 kg	0.1 mg	0.1	
				2 kg	0.2 mg	0.2	
				3 kg	0.3 mg	0.3	
				4 kg	0.4 mg	0.4	

Medication			Dosage and Route	Total Dose/Infant		Rate and Precautions
				Weight	Total µg/min	
Dopamine			Begin at 5 µg/min (may increase to 20 µg/min if necessary) IV	1 kg	5-20	Give as continuous infusion using an infusion pump Monitor heart rate and blood pressure closely Seek consultation
				2 kg	10-40	
				3 kg	15-60	
				4 kg	20-80	

Dosage Calculation

[6 × wt (kg) × dose (µg/min)]/desired fluid (mL/min) = mg dopamine per 100 mL solution

From Bloom RS, Cropley C, for the AHA/AAP Neonatal Resuscitation Program Steering Committee: *Textbook of Neonatal Resuscitation*. Dallas: American Heart Association, 1994.

Emergency Medicine

Dana Collaguazo, Bobby Peters, and Mark A. Graber

MANAGEMENT OF ACUTE CHEST PAIN IN THE EMERGENCY DEPARTMENT SETTING

I. **Approach to Acute Chest Pain.**

A. **See** Table 2-1 for a partial differential diagnosis of chest pain. **Box 2-1** shows the characteristics of chest pain and likelihood ratio of coronary artery disease.

B. **Obtain** an ECG, CXR, CBC, cardiac enzymes (e.g., CPK, CPK-MB, troponin T or I, or myoglobin, depending on your institutional standard), coagulation studies, and electrolytes as indicated. A systemic cause for angina (e.g., increased metabolic demand) might be found, such as anemia or pneumonia. Do not withhold treatment until laboratory results are available.

C. **The character of the pain might help you decide if the patient has cardiac disease, but cannot absolutely rule out cardiac disease** (see Table 2-1). Age, smoking, family history of cardiac disease, and hypertension poor predictors of who has cardiac disease and should not influence your decision making. They can change prior probability, but even "low-risk" patients might have cardiac disease.

D. **Response to NTG does not predict cardiac disease.** Patients who respond to NTG are **less likely to have cardiac disease.**

II. **For cardiac pain**, administer oxygen to all patients with potential cardiac-related chest pain. **If the patient's blood pressure will tolerate either nitrates or a β-blocker, the β-blocker is preferable.** β-Blockers have unequivocally been shown to reduce infarct size in hemodynamically stable patients.

A. **Nitrates,** either SL NTG 0.4 mg or IV NTG 10 to 300 μg/min, should be administered. Start IV NTG at 20 μg/min and increase by 20 μg/min q5min until pain is relieved or the blood pressure begins to be unacceptably low. Occasionally a patient becomes hypotensive after the SL administration of NTG, so prior establishment of an IV dose is prudent although not mandatory. Hypotension related to nitrate use responds to fluids and is self-limited. **This is not a contraindication to the judicious use of IV NTG.** Prolonged or severe hypotension related to the use of nitrates is suggestive of a right ventricular infarction, which is often associated with an inferior wall MI and can be diagnosed by the use of right chest leads (see Chapter 3). Other processes that affect right ventricular function (e.g., pulmonary embolism, pericardial tamponade) can also cause nitrate-related hypotension. Tolerance to nitrates can develop within 24 hours. **Inquiry about recent sildenafil citrate (Viagra), vardenafil (Levitra), and tadalafil (Cialis) use is imperative because refractory hypotension can result and their use is a contraindication to the use of nitrates.**

TABLE 2-1

PARTIAL DIFFERENTIAL DIAGNOSIS OF ACUTE CHEST PAIN

Diagnosis	Cardinal Symptoms	Diagnosed By	Treated By	Commonly Mistaken For	Pitfalls and Comments
Angina-acute MI	Substantial pressure with radiation to arms, neck, jaw; dyspnea; diaphoresis; occurs with exertion	History and ECG may show evidence of ischemia but may be normal in up to 50% with angina-acute MI	See text	Multiple illnesses, including gastric pain, musculoskeletal pain	Pain may be of any type, and sharp or burning pain does not exclude cardiac ischemia (Box 2-1) Diabetic patients and elderly often have atypical presentation with only dyspnea or epigastric pain May have right-sided chest pain, etc.
Anxiety and hyperventilation	May feel chest pain, SOB, feeling of impending death May have associated circumoral and acral paresthesias	Diagnosis of exclusion Generally have increased stress, history of similar episodes	Reassurance, diazepam IV	Cardiac disease	May have syncope secondary to CNS vasospasm May be associated carpal and pedal spasms
Esophageal spasm	May mimic MI or angina May respond to nitrates or calcium channel blockers	Barium swallow or manometry	See Chapter 5, Gastroenterology and Hepatology	Cardiac disease	Need to r/o cardiac causes, since can mimic well

Gastritis/ esophagitis	Burning chest pain	Endoscopy, upper GI series, clinically	See text	May be relieved by "GI cocktail" (e.g., Maalox 30 mL, lidocaine 2% 15 mL), but not diagnostic because some of those with cardiac disease will also have pain relief
Musculoskeletal, including costochondritis, muscle strain, intercostal strain, rib fracture	Usually tender over specific point that reproduces pain May be history of injury; may be respirophasic (pleuritic in nature)	History, physical Pain may be increased on motion	Cardiac disease and vice versa	Presence of musculoskeletal disease does not r/o other causes of chest pain
Pericarditis	Pleuritic, radiates to shoulder, worse when lying down, better sitting up May have a rub	ECG shows diffuse ST elevation and PR depression, but 20% are false negative	See Chapter 3, Cardiology	May be viral, associated with renal failure, TB, or may be carcinomatous from breast or lung cancer
Pleurisy	Respirophasic (pleuritic) chest pain, usually sharp	Diagnosis of exclusion	Anti-inflammatory such as indomethacin	May be viral or associated with pulmonary embolism, pericarditis, pneumonia, etc. Must r/o serious cause
Pneumonia	Generally have associated cough, fever	CXR, CBC, clinical picture	Antibiotics (see Chapter 4, Pulmonary Medicine)	May have associated abdominal pain, N&V

(Continued)

EMERGENCY MEDICINE 2

TABLE 2-1
PARTIAL DIFFERENTIAL DIAGNOSIS OF ACUTE CHEST PAIN—cont'd

Diagnosis	Cardinal Symptoms	Diagnosed By	Treated By	Commonly Mistaken For	Pitfalls and Comments
Pulmonary embolism	Sudden onset, respirophasic (pleuritic in nature), dyspnea (see Chapter 4, Pulmonary Medicine)	Tachycardia, hypoxia, tachypnea May have normal O_2, however Need $\dot{V}/\dot{Q}$ scan, angiogram, or spiral CT	See Chapter 4, Pulmonary Medicine		Keep high clinical suspicion because any symptom or sign may be absent (see Chapter 4, Pulmonary Medicine)
Spontaneous pneumomediastinum	Sudden onset, severe pleuritic pain	CXR	Observation		May occur with Valsalva maneuver, especially with smoking crack, marijuana from bong (water pipe)
Spontaneous pneumothorax	Sudden-onset severe pain (pleuritic in nature), dyspnea	CXR (expiratory)	Chest tube (see text) Oxygen may hasten resolution	Pulmonary embolism, substernal catch, pneumonia	May be spontaneous to bleb rupture or secondary to trauma
Thoracic aortic aneurysm	Sudden-onset tearing pain radiating to back, arms, jaw, neck	Angiography, CT, or TEE	See text	MI, gastritis, esophageal spasm, etc.	May have unequal pulses and BP in upper extremities, but this may be absent

> **BOX 2-1**
>
> **CHARACTERISTICS OF CHEST PAIN AND LIKELIHOOD RATIO OF CORONARY ARTERY DISEASE**
>
> Chest pain radiation to left: LR 2
> Chest pain radiation to right: LR 3
> Chest pain radiation to both: LR 7
> Pressure, squeezing, aching: LR <2
> Pleuritic, sharp, stabbing, positional, reproducible pain on palpation: LR 0.2-0.4
> Normal ECG: LR 0.1-0.3
> Hypotension: LR 3
> Chest pain: Squeezing, pressure: LR 1 (does not help differentiate cardiac from noncardiac disease)

LR, likelihood ratio.

2

EMERGENCY MEDICINE

B. Aspirin 325 mg (not enteric coated) should be administered to any patient with possible angina who does not have a contraindication such as active bleeding. **Patients on warfarin should still receive aspirin.** Patients with a true allergy to aspirin should receive clopidogrel (Plavix) at a loading dose of 300 mg instead of aspirin.

C. β-Blockers, such as metoprolol 15 mg IV in 5-mg aliquots q5min, can be helpful in patients without failure and a hyperdynamic state. Contraindications include heart block, bradycardia, uncontrolled CHF, and hypotension, among others. β-Blockers can generally be used safely in those with COPD and asthma. Use clinical judgment.

D. Morphine given in 2- to 4-mg aliquots IV can be helpful in relieving chest pain and cardiac ischemia. The total dose usually should not exceed 12 to 14 mg. It may increase mortality.

E. Heparin is helpful in the patient with unstable angina and can be used in addition to aspirin in the patient without contraindications. Weight-based dosing is preferred for heparin. See Chapter 6 for dosing. Enoxaparin (1 mg/kg SQ q12h) and other LMW heparins might be **marginally** superior to standard heparin in this setting, but guidelines suggest the use of unfractionated heparin. (See Chapter 6 for anticoagulation guidelines.)

F. Calcium channel blockers. Diltiazem: Recent evidence indicates that IV diltiazem 25 mg × 2 min followed by a drip at 5 mg/h can be useful for refractory angina; **this is not standard of care, however.** IV diltiazem should be used cautiously in combination with IV β-blockers because the combination can cause AV conduction disturbances.

G. Glycoprotein IIb/IIIa inhibitors. In patients being managed **interventionally** (e.g., by PTCA and/or stent), Gp IIb/IIIa inhibitors are clearly useful. In noninterventional settings, they might still be appropriate for the care of high-risk patients (e.g., continued ischemia, elevated troponin); however, local practices can differ widely and thus it is best to discuss with your cardiologist.

    H. Thrombolytics might be indicated in the event of an MI. See section on myocardial infarction in Chapter 3 for management details.

    I. If anemic, consider transfusions as necessary.

III. Disposition. Patients should be admitted for unstable angina as well as to rule out or confirm actual MI. The decision should be based on the history and a clinical gestalt because the initial ECG might not reflect an acute MI in 50% of those with an acute MI. Enzymes are also not helpful in deciding who to admit because the CPK and troponin T might not be elevated for up to 6 hours after an infarction. (CPK is more sensitive than troponin at 4 to 8 hours (84% vs. 74%) and at 8 to 12 hours (94% vs. 88%). Troponin is essentially 100% at 12 hours, whereas the CPK sensitivity falls off.

SEIZURES

  I. Febrile Seizures.

A. Salient features.

1. Generalized, nonfocal seizure with an autosomal dominant transmission. Patients are usually 6 months to 5 years of age.

2. **Always self-limited,** generally after 4 to 5 minutes but can last up to 15 minutes.

3. **Little postictal phase** with prompt return of baseline mental status. If postictal, drowsy, or more than one seizure, see grand mal (later).

4. **A chronic seizure disorder will develop in 2% to 5%.** Forty-eight percent under 15 months of age will have a recurrent febrile seizure in the future, as will 30% of those over 15 months and 45% of those with a first-degree relative with h/o febrile seizures.

5. The American Academy of Pediatrics recommends against routine CT scanning, blood work, or EEG of patients with febrile seizures. Consider an LP for children under 18 months of age, and perform LP on those under 12 months of age.

6. **Admission and work-up (CT/MRI or EEG) are indicated if** there are focal signs or altered mental status because by definition these patients do not have simple febrile seizures. **A metabolic work-up and work-up for meningitis should be done if appropriate.** A finger-stick glucose should be obtained unless the patient is clinically normal.

B. Therapy.

1. **No specific therapy for seizure** (but see grand mal [later] if seizure is protracted); treat underlying cause of fever. Always evaluate patient clinically for meningitis or other bacterial infection. It is not necessary to do a lumbar puncture in simple febrile seizures unless otherwise indicated.

2. The American Academy of Pediatrics does not recommend seizure prophylaxis for patients with one or more febrile seizures.

3. **Long-term treatment.** Chronic phenobarbital therapy prevents recurrence but can adversely affect learning. Valproic acid is as effective as phenobarbital with fewer behavioral effects (but with other drawbacks such as liver toxicity). Neither carbamazepine nor phenytoin is effective in preventing recurrent febrile seizures.

4. **Prevention. Acetaminophen and ibuprofen at the onset of a fever do not prevent febrile seizures.** Diazepam 0.33 mg/kg PR q8h starting at onset of fever and continuing for 24 hours after the fever reduced febrile seizures by 82% in those treated (intention-to-treat analysis equaled decrease of 44%). Oral diazepam may also be used.

II. **Grand Mal Seizures and Status Epilepticus**.

A. **Salient features.**

1. **Grand mal seizure:** generalized motor activity with tonic-clonic jerking, LOC.

2. **Status epilepticus:** prolonged seizure of >15 minutes (if still seizing when ED is reached, by definition the patient has status epilepticus if transport time is included).

3. **Postictal state:** might have focal signs or symptoms and a prolonged postictal state with confusion, headache, deep sleep with gradual awakening.

4. Fever may be present, but this is not a simple febrile seizure.

B. **Etiology.**

1. **Metabolic.** Check electrolytes, glucose, Ca, Mg, CBC.

2. **Toxins.** Look for pinpoint pupils, dilated pupils, excess salivation, etc. (See section on overdosage and toxidromes, later). Get drug (prescription and illegal usage) history from family or drug screen.

3. **Hypoxia.** Check respiratory status.

4. **Infection.** If clinically indicated, perform LP.

5. **Space-occupying lesions** (e.g., subdural hematoma, subarachnoid bleed, tumor). Evaluate with noncontrast CT.

6. **Poor compliance with medications.**

7. **Sleep deprivation, alcohol use.**

8. Do a CT to rule out mass lesion (abscess) before doing LP in those with HIV infection (because of risk of toxoplasmosis) and those with localizing signs/symptoms, **but do not withhold antibiotics to do a CT.**

C. **Target the work-up as indicated by history.** It is not necessary to repeat all labs on a patient with a known seizure disorder with a simple exacerbation caused by poor compliance. Watch for a change in type or frequency of seizure to guide your work-up. Drug levels are indicated in any patient using antiepileptics, theophylline, or another seizure-inducing agent.

D. **Treatment.** Because of the short half-life of benzodiazepines, patients usually need a longer-acting agent (e.g., phenytoin or phenobarbital) once the initial seizure resolves. Be sure to get levels in those already taking drugs.

1. **Be prepared to manage the airway.** Seizures can cause hypoxia and treatment (benzodiazepines, phenobarbital) can cause apnea.
2. **Correct the underlying metabolic problem if one is present.**

Step 1: Medications for Treating Ongoing Seizures

3. **Lorazepam** (Ativan): Adults: 0.03 to 0.05 mg/kg IV (2 to 4 mg, 1- to 2-mg aliquots); children: 0.05 to 0.1 mg/kg IV (maximum 4 mg); or double this rectally if IV access not possible. **Advantage over diazepam** is longer clinical half-life (hours of seizure suppression vs. minutes) with less respiratory depression and need for intubation.
4. **Alternative is diazepam** (Valium) 0.1 to 0.3 mg/kg IV (5-10 mg in adult but might need 20 to 30 mg), or double this rectally if no IV access. If these do not work, try the following medications.

Step 2: Medications for Treating Ongoing Seizures

5. **Phenobarbital** 15 to 20 mg/kg IV (maximum 25-30 mg/kg) at 25 to 50 mg/min. May give IM. **Respiratory depression is additive to that of benzodiazepines so patient might need intubation.**
6. **Phenytoin** (Dilantin) 15 mg/kg IV (1 mg/kg per minute IV, not to exceed 50 mg/min). Do not exceed 1 g in adults; mix with NS (50 mL/500 mg in adults); use in-line filter.
   a. **Monitor for QT prolongation** and stop infusion if increases by >50% (risk of torsades de pointes).
   b. An alternative to phenytoin is fosphenytoin (Cerebyx), a prodrug that requires metabolism to the active form. **There is little advantage to fosphenytoin; cardiotoxicity, local irritation, etc., are comparable.** The primary advantage is its absorption IM, and it can be administered rapidly. The major disadvantage is cost. Fosphenytoin should be infused at 100 to 150 mg/min; subtherapeutic levels can occur if infused slowly. Therapeutic blood levels occur in 30 minutes if drug is rapidly infused. Dosing is the same as for phenytoin. The fosphenytoin dose is expressed as the phenytoin equivalent. **Use in those with hepatic and renal disease is problematic because of slower-than-normal metabolism to active drug, and should be avoided.**

Step 3: Medications for Treating Ongoing Seizures

If the preceding does not work (lidocaine and midazolam are not approved for these indications, but are well tested):
7. **Lidocaine** 1.5 to 2 mg/kg IV × 2 min and repeated in 5 minutes if necessary with a drip at 3 to 4 mg/min. Same class of drugs as phenytoin and an excellent membrane stabilizer.

8. **Midazolam** has been found to be useful in those unresponsive to full loading doses of lorazepam, phenobarbital, and phenytoin. Give midazolam bolus of 0.2 mg/kg IV followed by infusion of 0.75 to 11 µg/kg per minute. Can also give IM 0.07 to 0.3 mg/kg. This might control seizures a bit faster but cannot titrate dose.

Step 4: Medications for Treating Ongoing Seizures

9. **Barbiturate coma or propofol.**

Special Situations

10. **Pyridoxine.** A very rare patient (generally children or those with an INH overdose) responds to pyridoxine, and if no other measures work, consider pyridoxine (vitamin B_6) 100 mg IV. **If you suspect INH overdose,** give 4 g IV and then 1 g IV q30min until equal to amount INH ingested; may give by IV push if patient is seizing. For children with INH overdose, give 40 mg/kg IV. Most vitamin B_6-responsive seizures occur in infants, but they have rarely been reported de novo in older children.

11. **Magnesium.** Remember the use of magnesium sulfate in women who might have eclampsia (even up to 2-3 weeks after delivery). Give 2- to 4-g bolus over 1 to 2 minutes. Repeat q15min to maximum of 6 g. **These loading doses should be fine in patients with renal failure**. Drip at 1 to 3 g/h if needed **and no renal failure.**

E. **Disposition.** Neurology consultation (but not necessarily admission) should be considered in patients with new-onset seizures, a focal neurologic exam, a change in seizure pattern, or poorly controlled seizures. Admission criteria include persistent decreased mental status, CNS infection, new intracranial lesion, acute head trauma, status epilepticus, eclampsia, or underlying correctable medical problems (e.g., hypoxia, hypoglycemia, hyponatremia, dysrhythmia, significant ethanol withdrawal). **Whether to start anticonvulsants after a first seizure is controversial.** Approximately 50% of patients with one seizure will have another within 2 years if not treated long term, as will 24% of those treated. An EEG should be performed 3 weeks after the initial seizure (it will be abnormal immediately after a seizure and therefore does not give any information on an underlying seizure focus).

III. **Neonatal Seizures.**

A. **Can be atypical in physical presentation because of CNS immaturity.**

1. **Grand mal** can manifest with sequential clonic-tonic movements of extremities or only focal symptoms.

2. **Autonomic seizures** are noted by changes in respirations, heart rate, and pupils.

3. **Myoclonic seizures** consist of single clonic motions throughout day.

B. **It is important to pursue a cause because frequently there is a specific treatment available.**
1. **In ED, check** electrolytes, calcium, glucose, magnesium, CBC, blood culture, and LP.
2. Obtain EEG, CT, skull radiograph, long bone radiograph as indicated.
3. Measure bilirubin, ABG, urine amino acids as indicated.
C. **Treatment for neonatal seizures in this order and in absence of known correctable cause:**
1. **Glucose** 2 mL/kg of D25.
2. **Pyridoxine** (vitamin B_6) 50 to 100 mg IV push.
3. **Calcium gluconate** (10%) 30 to 60 mg/kg (1-2 mL/kg of 10% solution, maximum 10 mL), slow IV on monitor.
4. **Magnesium sulfate** 50% solution, 0.2 mL/kg IM or IV
5. **Phenobarbital.** Premature infant, 10 to 20 mg/kg IM or IV; term infant, 10 to 15 mg/kg IM or IV. Infuse no faster than 30 mg/min.
6. **Phenytoin** 10 to 15 mg/kg IV. Infuse no faster than 1 mg/kg per minute.
7. **Lorazepam** 0.05 to 0.15 mg/kg IV.
8. **Diazepam** 0.2 mg/kg, repeat twice. Maximum dose 5 mg age <5 years, 10 mg age >10 years. **Diazepam and lorazepam increase hyperbilirubinemia by uncoupling albumin-bilirubin complex; therefore, be careful in children with jaundice.**

ASTHMA/COPD/DYSPNEA (SEE ALSO CHAPTER 4)

I. **Upper airway disease/obstruction/foreign body aspiration. As a general rule: Inspiratory stridor is above the cords, inspiratory and expiratory stridor is in the trachea, wheezing is below the trachea** (see appropriate chapters for in-depth discussions).
A. **Foreign body aspiration.** Diagnosis is made preoperatively only 60% of the time.
1. **Clinical presentation.** Most patients are 3 months to 6 years of age, and have a triphasic history:
a. With initial aspiration, there is cough, choking, gagging, stridor, and wheeze.
b. FB then passes into smaller airways, initiating silent phase.
c. Recurrent pneumonia, wheezing, abscess, and bronchiectasis then develop.
d. One third of aspirations are not witnessed or not remembered by caregiver.
2. **Radiographs** can show air trapping on exhalation, but one fourth have negative radiograph. Radiography is only 50% specific. Do CXR with patient lying on affected side. Dependent lung will not deflate normally if there is FB obstruction.
3. **Bronchoscopy** is the diagnostic procedure of choice if there is any question.

4. **Treatment.**
a. **Without respiratory distress.** Refer for removal by rigid bronchoscopy.
b. **With respiratory distress.**
   (1) **If the patient is breathing,** do not interfere; allow the child's efforts to attempt to clear the foreign body.
   (2) **If not moving air,** American Heart Association obstructed airway maneuvers should be used. For infants, use five interscapular back blows with the child's head lower than the chest, alternating with five chest compressions. In older children, use Heimlich maneuver. Advanced cardiac life support protocol should be initiated if necessary.
   (3) **BVM ventilations can convert a total obstruction to a partial one** by pushing FB into a main bronchus.
   (4) Immediate direct laryngoscopy and removal with Magill forceps should be performed.
   (5) If unsuccessful, cricothyrotomy or intubation if needed. Use the endotracheal tube to push the foreign body to the carina or into one of the mainstem bronchi.

5. **Prevention.** Infants and young children should not eat nuts, popcorn, hot dogs, uncooked carrots, whole grapes, or hard candies. Balloons and surgical gloves are especially dangerous for young children. Dice food. Avoid small toys. Educate parents.

6. **In those with stridor, think of epiglottitis** (in adults as well), croup, retropharyngeal abscess, angioedema. See the section on stridor in Chapter 12.

B. **Pneumothorax** (see chest trauma section, later).

C. **CHF, "cardiac asthma."** Look for basilar rales, peripheral edema, JVD, frothy sputum (see Chapter 3).

D. **Pulmonary embolism** (see Chapter 4).

E. **Pneumonia.** Fever, chills, purulent sputum, infiltrate or localized rales (see Chapter 4).

F. **COPD.** Usually have prior history (see Chapter 4).

G. **Central hyperventilation and metabolic acidosis.** Lungs clear, ABG reflects metabolic acidosis or primary respiratory alkalosis. (See Chapter 6 for a discussion of acid-base disturbance.)

H. **Anemia** (see Chapter 6).

I. **Wegener's** and other connective tissue disorders (see Chapter 4).

J. **Hypersensitivity pneumonitis** (see Chapter 4).

II. **Acute Asthma**

A. **Diagnose by history and physical examination.**

1. **History.** Important elements of the history are onset; trigger of current exacerbation; severity of symptoms, including limitation of exercise tolerance, interference with sleep, medications, prior hospitalizations and ED visits; severe exacerbations in past requiring ICU admissions or intubation; any other chronic medical conditions.

2. **Physical examination.**

2

EMERGENCY MEDICINE

a. **Document severity** of respiratory compromise: speech difficulty, use of accessory muscles of respiration, inability to lie supine, pulsus paradoxus (>12 mm Hg fall in systolic BP during inspiration—see section on cardiac tamponade for procedure to determine pulsus paradoxus), tachycardia, tachypnea, cyanosis, level of alertness, air movement, wheezing.

b. **Complications** of severe asthma include pneumothorax, pneumomediastinum, and respiratory failure.

c. **Wheezing** can be an unreliable guide to the degree of obstruction; severe obstruction can be associated with a "silent chest" because of little or no air movement.

d. **Functional assessment.** Monitor peak flow (see Tables 23-9 and 23-10 for normal range) or FEV_1. Check pulse oximetry. Infants become hypoxemic earlier than adults, and physical assessment of respiratory status in children is less reliable. Check O_2 saturations on all infants and children by pulse oximetry. Room air saturation should be >95%. A room air saturation <93% in infants usually is predictive of the need for hospitalization. Check an arterial or capillary blood gas level on infants with O_2 saturation <90% or as needed.

e. **Beware if patient seems too calm. This can represent CO_2 retention and narcosis.**

B. **Lab tests.** Do not withhold oxygen or delay treatment waiting for lab tests and radiographs. After initial stabilization, consider the following:

1. CBC if patient has fever or purulent sputum.

2. Obtain CXR if you suspect complication such as pneumonia or pneumothorax or if patient does not respond to treatment; **there is no need for CXR in routine asthma exacerbations.**

3. Serum theophylline concentration in all patients taking theophylline.

4. Consider ABG in patients with severe distress, poor response to treatment, or abnormal pulse oximetry.

C. **High-risk patients.** Those at high risk of asthma-related death or life-threatening deterioration include **infants** <1 year of age and those with:

1. **Prior intubation** for asthma or prior ICU admission, two or more hospitalizations for asthma in past year, three or more ED visits in past year, hospitalization or ED visit in past month.

2. **Use of or withdrawal from systemic corticosteroids,** h/o syncope or seizure related to hypoxia from asthma, poor social situation, or psychiatric disease.

3. **Less than 10% improvement in PEFR** or FEV_1 in ED; PEFR or FEV_1 <25% predicted.

4. **Pco_2 40 mm Hg or higher. A normal Pco_2 is abnormal in the setting of asthma exacerbations where the patient should be hyperventilating, resulting in a low Pco_2. A normal Pco_2 can herald impending respiratory failure.**

III. **Treatment for Asthma or COPD.**

A. Oxygen might be needed to support the patient and should not be withheld even to do an ABG. **Do not withhold oxygen from a hypoxic patient with COPD.** The oxygen saturation should be kept above 90%. If oxygen causes respiratory depression, the patient can be intubated.

B. Hydration is without benefit if the patient is euvolemic, and aggressive IV hydration can precipitate CHF.

C. If asthma is severe, consider cardiac monitoring.

D. β-Agonists are the mainstay of treatment. Albuterol is generally more effective in asthma, whereas ipratropium is generally more effective in COPD.

1. **Albuterol,** 2.5 mg in 3 mL of NS by nebulizer (adults). May give up to four treatments per hour. Some studies suggest that continuously nebulized albuterol works better. IV albuterol has been used but has little advantage over inhaled.

a. In children, can use albuterol 0.15 to 0.3 mg/kg by nebulizer every hour (ideally divided q20min or given continuously × 1 h). The 0.3 mg/kg dosing is significantly better in moderate to severe asthma. Can use nebulized albuterol continuously if needed in children as well.

b. Tachycardia does not increase after first several doses, and because tachycardia is usually hypoxia driven, the pulse rate can drop with treatment.

c. Albuterol can cause hypokalemia by shifting potassium intracellularly, but this is "never" clinically significant.

d. Metered-dose inhaler used with a spacer is as effective as a nebulizer if six to eight activations by spacer are used, which is equal to one nebulized treatment.

2. **Epinephrine,** 1:1000, 0.01 mg/kg SQ, maximum 0.3 to 0.4 mg can be used in those too sick to use a nebulizer (use 0.1 mL/10 kg). For those facing intubation, IV epinephrine may be used (but reserve for these patients with severe disease!). The dose is 2 to 10 mL of a 1:10,000 solution (0.1 mL/kg of a 1:10,000 solution, maximum 1 mg) administered over 5 minutes. This can be repeated with an infusion at 1 to 20 μg/min if there is improvement.

E. Steroids reduce return visits and admission rates. Steroids are more effective in asthma than in COPD, but do help in acute COPD exacerbations. Steroids should be used in most patients: always in those already receiving steroids and in most of those who fail to clear after one nebulizer treatment.

1. **In the ED:** For adults, methylprednisolone 125 mg IV or prednisone 60 mg PO. For children, methylprednisolone 1 to 2 mg/kg IV or prednisone 2 mg/kg PO.

2. **In the hospital:** For adults, methylprednisolone 60 mg IV q6h or prednisone 60 mg PO depending on patient severity. For children, 2 mg/kg per day divided q6h, or prednisone 2 mg/kg PO.

2

EMERGENCY MEDICINE

3. **On discharge from the ED:** For adults, prednisone 40 to 60 mg PO for 5 to 7 days. For children, prednisone or prednisolone 1 mg/kg per day for 5 to 7 days. An alternative for adults is methylprednisolone 160 mg IM as a single dose.

a. All evidence indicates that steroids given PO are just as effective as IV in acute exacerbations of asthma.

b. There is no need for a steroid taper in those not previously receiving steroids if only for a 5- to 7-day course. There is no increase in relapse without taper and no adrenal suppression with a 1-week course.

c. Although the dose of prednisone in children has traditionally been 2 mg/kg, recent data suggest this is no better than 1 mg/kg and is associated with significantly more side effects.

d. **Remember that patients who are on chronic steroids always require a burst of steroids with an acute exacerbation and do need a taper because they are adrenally suppressed.**

F. **Anticholinergics work better in COPD** than asthma but do have some bronchodilating effect and are effective in those with moderate or severe disease. They do not add anything to β-agonists in those with mild disease, however. Both can be mixed in the same nebulizer with albuterol.

1. **Ipratropium** can be used by metered-dose inhaler or nebulizer. The dose is 0.5 mg by nebulizer and can be given twice in the first hour of therapy. This is preferred over atropine because there is little systemic effect.

2. **Atropine** 0.4 to 2 mg (adult, 0.025 mg/kg) is given by nebulizer if ipratropium not available. Can increase heart rate and cause pupils to dilate from contact with mist.

G. **Theophylline-aminophylline. There no evidence that adding theophylline-aminophylline to maximized β-adrenergic therapy is helpful in the treatment of acute asthma.** It is arrhythmogenic and has as a very low therapeutic index; always check a drug level if you believe it is necessary to use this drug.

1. Although frequent, optimal doses of β-agonists are more effective, if you choose to use aminophylline, use a 6 mg/kg loading dose to maximum of 350 mg over 30 to 45 minutes, followed by a drip at 0.6 mg/kg per hour, not to exceed 50 to 60 mg/h. Levels should be checked. Maintenance dose depends on patient's smoking status, presence of cor pulmonale, and age.

H. **Magnesium sulfate** can produce transient improvement in asthma for 60 to 90 minutes.

1. Reasonable if patient has failed conventional therapy; less toxic than theophylline.

2. **Dose:** In adults, 2 g IV over 15 to 20 minutes (may mix in 50 mL NS). Very safe, but do not use in renal failure. Might produce flushing and transient hypotension, but these are rare.

3. Magnesium sulfate has been successfully used in children. The dose is 25 mg/kg.

I. **Heliox** (helium/oxygen mixture) can help in the patient with severe disease. Intubation and nasal CPAP are a last resort and might not work well in the asthmatic patient.

IV. **Disposition.** Admit if there is persistent respiratory distress; O_2 saturation <94% after treatment (children); PEFR <60% of predicated value in children or failure to increase by 15% above baseline or absolute value of 200 L/min in adults; failure of FEV_1 to increase by 500 mL or produce a total of <1.6 L (adults); hypercapnia (retaining CO_2 over baseline value); or pneumothorax. In addition, clinical judgment is important. If the patient does not look well or still feels dyspneic, consider admission to hospital.

COMA

I. **Coma Can Be Caused Only By:**
   - Bilateral cortical disease.
   - Reticular activating system compromise.
II. **What To Do First in Coma.**
A. **ABCs, including cervical spine immobilization** if any possibility of trauma.
1. If patient has hypertension with associated bradycardia, consider increased ICP.
2. Intubate to protect airway if no gag reflex or if otherwise indicated.
B. **Check finger-stick glucose** (if available) and rapidly administer:
1. **Thiamine** 100 mg IV prevents Wernicke-Korsakoff encephalopathy.
a. Do not withhold glucose if thiamine not available. A single dose of glucose will not induce Wernicke-Korsakoff encephalopathy.
2. **Glucose** 25 to 50 g IV treats hypoglycemia.
3. **Naloxone** 2 to 4 ampules of 0.4 mg treats narcotic overdose.
a. Some start with 2 mg and then 4 mg if no response.
b. Be sure to restrain the patient if you suspect naloxone will precipitate narcotic withdrawal.
4. **If benzodiazepine overdose is suspected** (diazepam, alprazolam, and others), give flumazenil (Romazicon) 0.2 mg up to 5 mg IV. **Do not use flumazenil if you suspect any other overdose, concurrent TCA overdose, or chronic benzodiazepine use.** It can precipitate status epilepticus and is contraindicated! It should not be routinely administered to the unconscious patient unless there is a clear indication and no contraindication. Intubation and supportive care are generally preferred for benzodiazepine overdose.
III. **Differential Diagnosis of Coma.**
A. **Coma with no localizing CNS signs can be caused by the following, among others:**
1. **Metabolic insults,** including hypoglycemia, uremia, nonketotic hyperosmolar coma, Addison's disease, diabetic ketoacidosis, hypothyroidism, and hepatic coma (increased ammonia).

2

EMERGENCY MEDICINE

a. Children and young adults often develop spontaneous hypoglycemia after a fast and also can present with hypoglycemic coma after ingestion of alcohol, including mouthwash.

2. **Respiratory factors,** including hypoxia, hypercapnia.

3. **Intoxication,** including barbiturates, alcohol, opiates, carbon monoxide poisoning, and benzodiazepines.

4. **Infections** (severe systemic), including sepsis, pneumonia, typhoid fever.

5. **Shock,** including hypovolemic, cardiogenic, septic, and anaphylactic.

6. **Epilepsy,** including atonic seizures (no obvious abnormal motor activity).

7. **Hypertensive encephalopathy.**

8. **Environmental factors,** including hyperthermia (heat stroke), hypothermia.

B. Coma with meningeal irritation without localizing signs can be caused by meningitis, subarachnoid hemorrhage from ruptured aneurysm, AV malformation.

C. If focal brain stem or lateralizing signs, consider pontine hemorrhage, CVA, brain abscess, subdural-epidural hemorrhage.

D. If patient appears awake but is unresponsive:

1. **Abulic state.** Because frontal lobe function is depressed, it can take several minutes for the patient to answer a question.

2. **Locked-in syndrome.** Destruction of pontine motor tracts; upward gaze is preserved.

3. **Psychogenic state.** Consider psychiatric disease.

IV. To Differentiate between Cortical and Brain Stem Lesions.

A. Use calorics—ice water in each ear. *Nystagmus* refers to the fast return phase. **Four possible responses:**

1. Both eyes deviate toward side cold water instilled and have good nystagmus (e.g., eyes return to center). Patient not comatose.

2. Both eyes deviate toward cold water; no fast return phase. Brain stem function intact. Coma is caused by bilateral cortical problem.

3. No eye movement despite cold stimuli to both sides. No brain stem function (same as absent oculocephalic reflex, or "doll's eyes"). Not necessarily a permanent lesion; can be caused by severe hypothermia or drug overdose.

4. Movement of only one eye ipsilateral to stimulus indicates an intranuclear lesion, which almost always indicates brain stem damage and demands rapid evaluation to determine if a correctable lesion is present.

B. Pupils.

1. Generally resistant to metabolic insult.

2. Remember that a dilated eye might be secondary to topical or systemic drugs.

3. A dilated pupil in an alert person is not secondary to impending herniation; herniating patients are always unconscious. **However, a unilateral dilated pupil in an unconscious patient can herald imminent uncal herniation.**

4. Propoxyphene (Darvon and others) can cause coma without pinpoint pupils.

5. Eyes deviate toward side of physiologically inactive lesion (CVA) and away from an active lesion (seizure).

6. Five percent of the normal population have anisocoria (asymmetric pupils).

V. Laboratory Work-up of Coma.

A. CBC, electrolytes, BUN, creatinine, glucose, calcium, magnesium, arterial blood gas, toxic screen, carboxyhemoglobin, liver enzymes, serum ammonia, etc., as indicated by clinical presentation.

B. CT scan and LP. **If you suspect meningitis, do not withhold antibiotics while waiting to do an LP. Antibiotics should** be started before the patient goes to the CT scanner. Your culture results will not be affected.

HEAD TRAUMA

See also evaluation of coma.

I. Glasgow Coma Scale (Table 2-2). Useful in a general sense, but 18% of those with a GCS score of 15 have an abnormal CT scan, and 5% of those with a GCS score of 15 require neurosurgical intervention. The GCS score is especially unreliable in children. Interrater reliability of the GCS is very poor. **A GCS of 8 or less mandates intubation!**

II. Classification of Head Injuries and Treatment.

A. Frequently associated with other severe trauma.

1. **ABCs take priority.** Saving only the head will not save the patient.

2. **Hypotension in adults can be caused by head injury** (Mahoney et al., 2003), but this is a diagnosis of exclusion. Look for other injuries, including cord injuries and hemorrhage first!

3. **Physical exam** includes complete neurologic exam as well as inspection for evidence of basilar skull fracture (e.g., CSF rhinorrhea, Battle's sign, raccoon eyes, hemotympanum).

B. Criteria for CT scan in head trauma (Box 2-2).

C. Classification of injuries.

1. **Low-risk injuries.**

a. **Criteria.**

(1) Minor trauma, scalp wounds.

(2) No signs of intracranial injury, no LOC or LOC for less than 1 minute, no amnesia. Could have up to three episodes of vomiting; GCS 15.

(3) Patient has returned to baseline functioning.

b. **Treatment.** Observation for any sign or symptom of brain injury. Must discharge to a reliable observer who will continue observation at home.

2. **Moderate-risk injuries.**

a. **Criteria.** Symptoms consistent with intracranial injury, including protracted vomiting (more than three episodes), LOC for >1 minute, severe headache, post-traumatic seizures, amnesia, evidence of basilar skull fracture (CSF rhinorrhea, Battle's sign, raccoon eyes, hemotympanum). Nonfocal neurologic exam results.

b. **Treatment.** Admit for observation, monitoring, and "neuro checks."

TABLE 2-2
GLASGOW COMA SCALE

Parameter	Response	Score
Eye opening	Spontaneous	4
	To voice	3
	To pain	2
	None	1
Verbal response	Oriented	5
	Confused	4
	Inappropriate	3
	Incomprehensible sounds	2
	None	1
Motor response	Obeys verbal commands	6
	Localizes pain	5
	Withdraws to pain	4
	Flexion response to pain	3
	Extension response to pain	2
	None	1

3. **High-risk injuries.**
   a. **Criteria.** Depressed level of consciousness, focal neurologic signs, penetrating injury of skull or palpable depressed skull fractures.
   b. **Approach.** Immediate CT, neurosurgical consultation.
   c. **Support and treat increased ICP** while awaiting definitive neurosurgical care. **There is little evidence to support most of these measures, but**

BOX 2-2

CRITERIA FOR OBTAINING CT SCAN IN TRAUMA

ADULTS

- Headache
- Vomiting
- Age >60 y
- Patient has used drugs or alcohol
- Memory deficit
- Seizure

CHILDREN

Age >2 y

- LOC
- Amnesia
- Seizure
- Headache
- Persistent vomiting (number?)
- Irritability
- Behavior changes

Age <2 y but >3 mo

- Any of the above *or*
- Any unusual behavior
- Large scalp hematoma

Age <3 mo

- Any of the above *or*
- Any scalp hematoma
- Any significant mechanism

Note: These criteria are based on the best available evidence. Studies are under way to refine these criteria.

they are still the standard of care. **Use only in those with increased ICP. Prophylactic hyperventilation, mannitol, etc., in those without increased ICP are contraindicated and can worsen outcomes.**
Small-scale studies suggest that there is a good relationship between intraocular pressure and ICP. Measuring the intraocular pressure could help you decide if the patient has an elevated ICP.

(1) **Intubation.** Pretreatment with lidocaine 1 mg/kg IV can prevent rise in ICP. See also sections on RSI and resuscitation in Chapter 1.
(2) **Hyperventilation** is used to maintain Po_2 >90 torr, Pco_2 25 to 30 torr.
   (a) PEEP is relatively contraindicated because it reduces cerebral blood flow.
   (b) Avoid tight cervical collars. Any pressure on the external jugular veins will increase ICP.
   (c) Hyperventilation can actually increase ischemia in at-risk brain tissue if the Pco_2 is <25 torr by causing excessive vasoconstriction and is falling out of favor. **Prophylactic hyperventilation for those without increased ICP is contraindicated and worsens outcomes.**
(3) **Maintain normal cardiac output.**
   (a) If hypotensive from other cause such as multiple trauma, treat shock as usual. NS is preferred over LR because LR is slightly hypotonic. Hypertonic saline (3% or 7.5%; see section on shock, later) can be used, but there is no clear evidence that it improves neurologic outcome.
   (b) If markedly hypertensive, consider labetalol or nitroprusside. A vasodilator, such as nitroprusside, increases cerebral blood flow and ICP (see section on hypertensive emergencies for dosing). See neurology chapter for BP guidelines.
(4) **Mannitol** 1 g/kg IV × 20 min induces osmotic diuresis. (Controversial if patient not herniating. Consult your neurosurgeon.) Avoid if hypotensive or have CHF/renal failure.
(5) **Furosemide** (Lasix and others) 20 mg IV is recommended by some authors. Avoid if hypotensive.
(6) **Elevation of the head** has not been shown to be of any benefit.
(7) **Steroids are ineffective** in controlling ICP in the trauma setting.
(8) **Seizure prophylaxis.** Phenytoin will reduce seizures in the first week (number needed to treat [NNT] = 10) after injury, but does not change the overall outcome.

D. Skull radiographs.

1. Not indicated in adults unless you suspect depressed fracture and cannot palpate skull because of hematoma **and** cannot get head CT with bone windows.
2. Plain radiographs might be useful in those up to 7 years of age because a skull fracture can lead to nonunion due to rapid head growth, and for documentation of abuse. Use clinical judgment as to severity of injury.

2

EMERGENCY MEDICINE

III. **Concussion:** Box 2-3 summarizes recommendations for returning to sports activities after concussion.

IV. **Postconcussive syndrome.**
  A. Can occur with minor trauma and is characterized by headache, depression, memory difficulty, attention deficit, personality changes, vertigo and light-headedness, and a negative CT (could represent disruption of axonal support structures, axonal stretching). MRI might show microhemorrhages.

BOX 2-3

RETURNING TO SPORTS ACTIVITIES AFTER CONCUSSION

SUMMARY OF RECOMMENDATIONS FOR MANAGEMENT OF CONCUSSION IN SPORTS

A concussion is defined as head trauma–induced alteration in mental status that might or might not involve LOC. Concussions are graded in three categories. Definitions and treatment recommendations for each category are presented below.

Grade 1 Concussion

Definition: Transient confusion, no LOC, and a duration of mental status abnormalities of <15 min.

Management: The athlete should be removed from sports activity, examined immediately and at 5-min intervals, and allowed to return that day to the sports activity only if postconcussive symptoms resolve within 15 min. Any athlete who incurs a second grade 1 concussion on the same day should be removed from sports activity until asymptomatic for 1 wk.

Grade 2 Concussion

Definition: Transient confusion, no LOC, and a duration of mental status abnormalities of >15 min.

Management: The athlete should be removed from sports activity and examined frequently to assess the evolution of symptoms, with more extensive diagnostic evaluation if the symptoms worsen or persist for >1 wk. The athlete should return to sports activity only after asymptomatic for 1 full week. Any athlete who incurs a grade 2 concussion subsequent to a grade 1 concussion on the same day should be removed from sports activity until asymptomatic for 2 wk.

Grade 3 Concussion

Definition: LOC, either brief (seconds) or prolonged (minutes or longer).

Management: The athlete should be removed from sports activity for 1 full week without symptoms if the LOC is brief or 2 full weeks without symptoms if the LOC is prolonged. If still unconscious or if abnormal neurologic signs are present at the time of initial evaluation, the athlete should be transported by ambulance to the nearest hospital ED. An athlete who suffers a second grade 3 concussion should be removed from sports activity until asymptomatic for 1 mo. Any athlete with an abnormality on CT or MRI brain scan consistent with brain swelling, contusion, or other intracranial lesion should be removed from sports activities for the season and discouraged from future return to participation in contact sports.

Source: Quality Standards Subcommittee, American Academy of Neurology.
(From Centers for Disease Control and Prevention: Sports-related recurrent brain injuries— United States. MMWR Morb Mortal Wkly Rep 46:224-227, 1997.)

B. Patients might have abnormal findings on formal neuropsychological testing. Fifteen percent still have symptoms at 1 year even after minor brain injury.

C. Treat headache with non-narcotic analgesics (e.g., NSAIDs) and TCAs. Treat depression as indicated in Chapter 18.

TRAUMA

Multiple Trauma and General Principles

Use clinical judgment. Not every trauma victim needs every test.
I. Stabilization and Primary Survey.
   Remember ABCDE: Airway, Breathing, Circulation, Drugs/Disability/ Allergies, Eating/Exposure. **Keep patient warm! Hypothermia contributes to mortality.**

A. Airway. If the patient has depressed level of consciousness or upper airway bleeding, intubate **without moving neck.**

1. Intubation is safe even with neck fracture, but avoid Sellick maneuver.

2. Confirm ET placement with a radiograph and by auscultation, oxygen saturation, and end-tidal CO_2 (low in esophageal intubation).

B. Breathing. Ventilate with 100% O_2. Check breath sounds and place chest tubes as needed for hemothorax, pneumothorax, or tension pneumothorax.

C. Circulation. For "all" multiple trauma victims:

1. Stop obvious bleeding with pressure. Consider the chest and abdomen to be sites of potential blood loss in the hypotensive patient.

2. Place two large-bore peripheral IV lines (14-16 gauge). The short catheters allow more rapid volume replacement than longer central lines.

3. Run NS or LR wide open if tachycardic or hypotensive. Using warmed fluids decreases mortality and helps preserve hemostatic mechanisms.

a. **As a rule of thumb, if more than 2 L of isotonic fluid is needed in the trauma setting, the patient will need blood.**

b. Can also use 3% or 7.5% NS (250 mL × 1-5 min) if unable to infuse large volumes.

c. For children, use NS 20 mL/kg IV as a bolus and repeat to a total of 60 mL/kg. Consider blood at this point if the child is still hypotensive from hypovolemia.

d. There is no advantage to colloids in this setting.

e. Not all people in shock have tachycardia, and hypotension can be a late finding. This is especially true in children. Use clinical judgment.

f. Hypotension can be caused by head trauma, but this is a diagnosis of exclusion.

D. Drugs, disability, allergies. Document functional status for a baseline examination.

E. Eating and exposure. Document time of last meal. Uncover the patient, including visualizing the back.

2

EMERGENCY MEDICINE

F. A Foley catheter should be inserted after ruling out GU tract trauma (see section on urologic trauma). Urine output is a good indication of adequate perfusion. Try to maintain output at 30 to 60 mL/h in adults or 0.5 to 1 mL/kg per hour in children.

II. Laboratory and X-ray Evaluation of the Multiple Trauma Patient.

A. CBC, electrolytes, BUN, creatinine, glucose, coagulation studies, liver enzymes, amylase, lipase, UA, pregnancy test, ABG. Not all patients need all tests; use clinical judgment. (CBC often indicates an anemia with acute blood loss, but the CBC might not reflect the true magnitude of the problem until blood equilibrates with infused fluids—generally 15 minutes.)

B. If patient known to be hypotensive in the field, get two units of type O-negative blood ready.

C. Radiographs. C-spine (AP, lateral, odontoid), CXR, AP pelvis. C-spine films should be done in the radiology suite as long as patient is maintained in immobilization. Cross table films are frequently inadequate. CT is another option for clearing the C-spine and is replacing plain films in many centers.

D. Remember antibiotics, tetanus prophylaxis, and CT scan as indicated. Obtain a full spine series when the patient is stable.

III. Secondary Survey To Set Further Priorities.

A. Stabilize patient first.

B. Perform complete head-to-toe examination.

C. Pass NG tube if no contraindication such as basilar skull fracture or midface trauma. An orogastric tube can be passed if there is midface trauma, etc.

D. Identify possible internal injuries (see specific sections later). Any head-injured, unconscious, multitrauma patient should have the abdomen evaluated by CT, focused assessment with sonography for trauma (FAST), or DPL because of an inability to report pain accurately.

E. Splint bones and attend to other obvious injuries.

F. A comment on MAST (military antishock trousers, pneumatic antishock garment): They are contraindicated in penetrating cardiac trauma, cardiogenic shock, impaled objects/evisceration, and diaphragmatic injury. Head injury is not a contraindication. They could help stem intra-abdominal bleeding from the spleen and aorta. Overall benefit is probably less than previously believed; MAST are falling out of favor. They are useful when stabilizing pelvic and femur fractures.

Neck Trauma

I. General.

A. Initial treatment. Must immobilize neck **and restrain chest** to immobilize C-spine. If C-spine injury is strongly suspected and unable to restrain patient, consider paralysis (see section on RSI, Chapter 1).

1. **Neutral position** differs in adults and children: Children <8 years of age might require elevation of shoulders and back to approximate a neutral position. Adults and older children might require padding under the head to approximate a neutral position. **Most important, however, is maintaining immobilization.**

2. Prolonged Immobilization (even <30 minutes) on a backboard will cause most patients to have occipital headache and lumbosacral pain regardless of underlying trauma.

B. Blunt trauma to the neck should make one think about possible vascular injury (carotid, basilar arteries).

II. **Clearing the Cervical Spine.**

A. **To clear the C-spine clinically, all of the criteria in** Box 2-4 **must be met. These criteria have not been adequately tested in children. All other patients require clearance of the C-spine by radiograph.**

B. **X-ray approach.**

1. Three views are needed, including lateral film showing all seven cervical vertebrae and the C7-T1 interspace, and a PA and an odontoid view to rule out a C-spine fracture. **The most common cause of missed C-spine injuries is an inadequate C-spine series.** If radiographs are inadequate or there is a questionable fracture, CT scanning might be helpful.

2. **Flexion/extension films** can be done to rule out ligamentous injury in the patient with persistent neck pain once C-spine fractures have been ruled out by radiography. Do not force flexion or extension; let the patient control head movement

3. **Those with one spinal fracture have about a 10% chance of having another, noncontiguous, spinal fracture and should have a full spine series.**

C. **Parameters of normal C-spines and types of fractures** (Table 2-3).

D. Table 2-4 lists **common C-spine injuries.**

III. **Cord Injuries: Transection.**

A. **Look for** paralysis and other signs of cord injury, including priapism, urinary retention, fecal incontinence, paralytic ileus, and immediate loss of all sensation and reflex activity below the level of the injury.

2

EMERGENCY MEDICINE

BOX 2-4
CRITERIA FOR RULING OUT C-SPINE FRACTURES ON A CLINICAL BASIS
Patient does not complain of neck pain when asked *and*
Patient does not have neck tenderness on palpation *and*
Patient does not have any h/o LOC *and*
Patient does not have any mental status changes resulting from trauma, alcohol, drugs, etc., *and*
Patient has no symptoms referable to a neck injury, such as paralysis or sensory changes (including transitory symptoms now resolved) *and*
Patient has no other distracting, painful injuries, such as fractured ankle or ribs.

MEASURABLE PARAMETERS OF NORMAL C-SPINES

Parameter	Adults	Children
Predental space	3 mm	4-5 mm
C2/C3 pseudosubluxation	3 mm	4-5 mm
Retropharyngeal space	<7 mm (5 mm by some sources)	1/2-2/3 vertebral body distance AP
Cord dimension	10-13 mm	Adult size, age 6 y

Note: Forty percent of children <7 y of age and 20% of those 16 y of age have anterior displacement of C2 on C3; 14% of children ≤8 y of age have C3/C4 subluxation; 60%-70% of fractures in children occur in C1/C2; 16% of adult fractures occur at C1/C2; 20% of young children have increased space between dens and anterior arch of C1.

B. Spinal neurogenic shock leads to vasomotor instability from loss of autonomic tone and can lead to hypotension or temperature instability. This will respond to adrenergic agents (e.g., dopamine).

C. If the injury is above C5, the patient **might develop hypoxia** and hypoventilation: consider intubation.

D. SCIWORA syndrome. Neurologic symptoms frequently occur in children without associated C-spine fractures (SCIWORA syndrome). This could be responsible for up to 70% of cord injuries in children and is especially common in children younger than 8 years. Presentation of the neurologic deficit can be delayed up to 4 days. MRI can demonstrate the cord injury. Those with delayed presentation and an intact cord generally recover function. SCIWORA syndrome can also occur in adults.

E. Any person with a spinal cord injury (including SCIWORA syndrome) should receive methylprednisolone 30 mg/kg × 1 h followed by 5.4 mg/kg per hour IV over the next 23 hours. This should be started within 8 hours of the injury. The benefit is marginal and there are downsides, such as infection. Many centers are no longer using this treatment. Check with your institution.

IV. Penetrating Neck Trauma.

A. Although management still controversial, "all" should be explored in the OR if there is penetration of the platysma.

B. Do *not* remove foreign body until patient is in OR.

C. Consider CT/angiography if foreign body is close to arterial blood supply.

V. Airway Injuries.

A. Clinical signs include stridor, hoarseness, dyspnea, and subcutaneous emphysema.

B. Management: ENT consult, early oral intubation if possible and indicated. Expanding hematoma can rapidly compromise the airway and make intubation progressively more difficult. Avoid causing further trauma.

TABLE 2-4
COMMON C-SPINE INJURIES

Name	Stable or Unstable	Mechanism/Clinical Setting	Radiologic Findings
C1			
Jefferson fracture	Moderately unstable	Burst fracture occurs with axial load or vertebral compression	Displaced lateral aspects of C1 on odontoid view, predental space >3 mm
Atlantoaxial subluxation	Highly unstable	Found in Down syndrome, RA, other destructive processes	Asymmetric lateral bodies on odontoid view, increased predental space
C2			
Odontoid fracture	Highly unstable	Mechanism poorly understood	May be difficult to see on plain film; High clinical suspicion requires CT
Hangman's fracture	Unstable	Occurs with sudden deceleration (hanging) and with hyperextension as in MVA	Bilateral pedicle fracture of C2 with or without anterior subluxation; look on lateral film
ANY LEVEL			
Flexion teardrop injury	Highly unstable	Sudden and forceful flexion	Large wedge off anterior aspect of effected vertebra; Ligamentous instability causes alignment abnormalities
Bilateral facet dislocations	Highly unstable	Flexion or combined flexion/rotation	Anterior displacement of 50% or more of one cervical vertebrae on lateral view
Unilateral facet dislocations	Unstable	Flexion or combined flexion/rotation	Anterior dislocation 25%-33% of one cervical vertebra on lateral view; An abrupt transition in rotation so that lateral view of effected vertebra rotated; Lateral displacement of spinous process on AP view
LOWER CERVICAL OR UPPER THORACIC			
Clay shoveler's fracture	Very stable	Flexion such as when picking up and throwing heavy loads (e.g., snow or clay)	Avulsion of posterior aspect of spinous process; frequently an incidental finding

EMERGENCY MEDICINE 2

Chest Trauma

I. Types of Injury and Treatment.

A. Flail chest. Paradoxical chest wall motion secondary to multiple fractured ribs.

1. **Treatment** is by intubation if respiration is compromised. Positive-pressure ventilation can lead to a tension pneumothorax. Prophylactic placement of a chest tube should be considered.

B. Tension pneumothorax. Air under pressure in the pleural space.

1. **Features** are decreased breath sounds, shifted heart sounds, dyspnea, trachea shift from midline, hyper-resonance on percussion, distended neck veins, chest pain, hypotension.

2. **Treatment** is by needle thoracostomy in the second intercostal space, midclavicular line, followed by a chest tube at fourth or fifth interspace in the midaxillary line.

C. Simple pneumothorax-hemothorax from deceleration or penetrating trauma (pneumothorax can also occur spontaneously).

1. **Symptoms** as for tension pneumothorax, but without midline shift; might have hypotension from blood loss in hemothorax.

2. Expiratory films are more sensitive than a standard CXR. CT scanning is more sensitive, but the clinical significance of pneumothorax-hemothorax found only on CT scan is unknown. Some suggest placement of a chest tube if the patient has rib fractures and is going to have positive-pressure ventilation.

3. **Treatment** is by tube thoracostomy (chest tube; see Chapter 21). If small pneumothorax (<15%), observe and administer oxygen, which will hasten resolution of pneumothorax fourfold.

D. Cardiac tamponade.

1. **Clinically:** The patient will have hypotension, JVD, muffled heart sounds, pulsus paradoxus.

a. **Pulsus paradoxus.** Normally, systolic pressure drops less than 10 mm Hg on inspiration. Measure systolic pressure when patient has exhaled. Next, have the patient inhale and determine the difference between the two systolic pressures. If this number is >10, pulsus paradoxus is present.

2. **Treatment** is rapid fluid infusion, pericardiocentesis.

E. Myocardial contusion defined as blunt trauma to the heart.

1. ECG abnormalities are seen in 33% to 88%. Many have a normal CPK-MB level, and there is no correlation between the CPK-MB and the degree of injury. Best diagnostic tests are echocardiography and first-pass biventricular angiography.

2. Best approach is simply to monitor the hemodynamically stable patient. Specific intervention is seldom needed, and the stable patient does not require diagnostic imaging studies to "prove" the presence of cardiac contusion. Usually the only clinical problem is episodes of PSVT or self-limited ventricular tachycardia. In the patient with preexisting cardiac disease, myocardial contusion can be manifest as CHF.

F. Aortic disruption from deceleration injury.

1. **Look for** widened mediastinum (75% sensitive) on chest radiograph. Blurred and enlarged aortic knob, esophageal deviation to right (look at NG tube), apical cap (blood collected at the upper apex of the lungs) are present in less than 25% of aortic injuries. Thus, absence of radiographic signs does not guarantee an intact aorta. Definitive diagnosis is by CT, TEE, or angiography, depending on your institution's protocol. Many patients with aortic injury have associated cardiac injury, including tamponade.

2. **Open emergency thoracotomy is not indicated for blunt chest trauma.** It is almost never successful. A stab wound to the heart or aorta might be amenable to ED intervention. Do this only if trained in the technique and with the blessing of the surgeon who will manage the case in the OR unless the patient obviously will die if not treated immediately.

Abdominal Trauma in the Major Trauma Victim (Including Assault and Abuse in Children)

I. **Diagnosis. Possible intra-abdominal injury indicated by:**

A. Systolic blood pressure <100 mm Hg or hematocrit <29. No criterion is absolute, and physical examination is only about 65% accurate; use clinical judgment.

B. "Lap-belt ecchymosis" in children is associated with hollow organ injury, lumbar spine fracture, solid organ (liver/spleen) injury. Could portend severe injury in adults as well.

C. Elevated ALT and AST might indicate liver injury.

D. Patients with severe chest injuries or pelvic fractures are more likely to have intra-abdominal injury.

II. **Penetrating Trauma of Abdomen.**

A. Requires exploration if penetrates the peritoneum.

B. Some centers are doing CT only, but this is not yet universally accepted as the standard of care.

III. **Blunt Trauma of the Abdomen.**

A. If the patient is hemodynamically unstable and has an acute abdomen, laparotomy is necessary. Do not wait for CT, US, or DPL before consulting surgery.

B. If the patient is hemodynamically stable and complains of abdominal pain or is intoxicated or has head injury, proceed with CT, US, or DPL. Both CT and DPL have strengths and weaknesses. US is rapidly available at the bedside; however, it is less sensitive than CT.

Extremity Trauma

See Chapter 16 for fracture and dislocation management. These are the lowest-priority injuries early on unless there is a threat to a limb.

2

EMERGENCY MEDICINE

I. **Arterial Injury.**

A. Can be caused by blunt or sharp injury. Blunt can be more dangerous because less obvious.

B. **Absolute indications for arteriogram.** Pain, pallor, paralysis, paresthesia, pulselessness, hemorrhage, expanding hematoma, bruits. **Twenty percent of arterial injuries have a palpable pulse distal to the injury.**

C. **Penetrating trauma** near a vessel is not necessarily an indication for arteriography.

1. **Arterial pressure index** (arterial pressure in injured limb divided by arterial pressure in unaffected limb): If >0.90, can safely observe in the absence of other indications for arteriography.

2. Shotgun injuries are a high-risk category and should be studied with arteriography.

II. **Compartment Syndrome.**

A. **Caused especially by** crush injuries, electrical burns, circumferential scars, tight casts, hematoma in compartment, snake bites, and anything else that can increase pressure in a compartment.

B. **Can result in** muscle, nerve, and vessel necrosis from hypoperfusion.

C. **Clinical presentation.**

1. Severe, constant pain in affected limb, pain on muscle palpation, passive stretch, and active contraction, paresthesia, and loss of distal pulses are late signs and herald poor outcome.

2. Compartment might be tense, but normal turgor does not rule out compartment syndrome. Can diagnose by manometry:

a. Normal tissue pressure is <10 mm Hg.

b. Capillary blood flow compromised at 20 mm Hg.

c. At risk for ischemic necrosis above 30 mm Hg.

D. **Treatment** is by fasciotomy and requires immediate surgical consultation.

III. **Amputations.** Control bleeding with direct pressure. Avoid clamping vessels. Place severed part in saline-soaked gauze, place in plastic bag, and put in cooler with ice. Avoid freezing part. Refer to plastic or orthopedic surgery.

Urologic Trauma

I. **Kidney Trauma.**

A. **Blunt.**

1. **If <30 RBC/HPF.** Serious injury is rare **(but does occur)** if the patient has microscopic hematuria with <30 RBC/HPF and if the patient is hemodynamically stable and there are no other significant intra-abdominal injuries. IVP or CT is not required in these patients unless they have other another indication (e.g., multiple trauma) or indications of urologic trauma, such as pelvic fractures, lower rib fractures, or localized hematoma, because a surgically correctable lesion is unlikely. **Management** consists of frequent monitoring of vital signs and repeat UA at about 4 hours.

2. **In those with >30 RBC/HPF, gross hematuria, or <30 RBC/HPF and shock or intra-abdominal injury,** IVP or CT is indicated.

a. CT scanning has replaced IVP in evaluating renal injury in most settings because it can also help define other intra-abdominal trauma.

b. IVP has a 30% false-negative rate in those with renal pedicle injuries, which represent 2% of all renal injuries. Thirty-six percent of those with pedicle injuries do not have hematuria. However, they usually have a deceleration mechanism suggestive of this injury and other associated injuries. IVP will show a nonfunctioning kidney.

c. Most renal contusions, tears, and hematomas can be managed conservatively.

d. Renal pelvis rupture is rare and manifests with high fever and increasing abdominal pain and tenderness over days. It is diagnosed by retrograde pyelography.

B. Penetrating. All penetrating trauma to the kidney warrants investigation, including IVP or CT. Some would argue for surgical exploration in all of these patients.

II. Urethral Trauma. Heralded by blood at the meatus, a high-riding prostate in men. This requires retrograde urethrography before catheterization or other manipulation of the urethra. Obtain urology consultation. In an emergency, a temporary urostomy can be preformed by using the Seldinger technique and placing a central line into the distended bladder transabdominally.

III. Bladder Trauma. Bladder trauma is usually related to pelvic fracture. A cystogram shows extravasation of urine into abdomen. Exploration of the abdomen and surgical repair are indicated.

HYPERTENSIVE CRISIS

I. Hypertensive Emergency. Clinically, a hypertensive emergency (also termed *malignant hypertension*) is defined by presence of end-organ damage or dysfunction, including CHF, renal failure, hypertensive encephalopathy, hematuria, and retinal hemorrhage. It is not based on the absolute level of BP. Some patients with a diastolic BP of 130 mm Hg might be asymptomatic, whereas some with a diastolic BP of 100 mm Hg could have acute end-organ injury.

A. Goal is to reduce BP by 30% in 30 minutes. Patients with chronic hypertension might not tolerate a "normal" BP, so be judicious when lowering BP.

B. Drugs.

1. **Nitroprusside.** Mix 50 mg of nitroprusside in 500 mL D_5W (100 mg/mL) and start infusion at 0.5 µg/kg per minute. Titrate until desired BP reduction is obtained. Average dose is 0.5 to 3 µg/kg per minute (maximum dose, 10 µg/kg per minute).

a. Very potent arterial and venous dilator.
b. Can be used in all hypertensive emergencies, although it is not the drug of choice for preeclampsia (see Chapter 14, Obstetrics).
c. Avoid use with clonidine; there is a risk of MI.
2. **Nitroglycerin.** Mix 25 mg in 250 mL and start infusion at 10 μg/min (6 mL/h). Titrate by 10 to 20 μg/min until desired effect is obtained. Nitroglycerin is a venous and arterial dilator with maximum affect on capacitance vessels.
3. **Labetalol** (Normodyne, Trandate). Give by bolus, 20 to 40 mg IV. May repeat in 10 minutes. Usual effective dose is 50 to 200 mg. May also administer as a continuous infusion of 2 mg/min (mix 200 mg in 160 mL D_5W = 200 mL = 2 mL/min). Stop the infusion when blood pressure control is achieved. Could combine by giving initial bolus and then infusion.
a. Labetalol is a combined α-blocker and β-blocker, although primarily a β-blocker. It does not change cerebral blood flow and is probably the drug of choice in hypertension secondary to increased ICP.
b. It is especially useful in catecholamine-mediated hypertension such as a pheochromocytoma or after discontinuation of clonidine, and avoids the reflex tachycardia seen with nitroglycerin and nitroprusside.
c. The onset is in 5 minutes, maximum response in 10 minutes. Duration is about 8 hours.
Note: The use of oral or sublingual medications in hypertensive emergencies is not indicated.
II. **Hypertensive Urgency includes diastolic pressure >115 mm Hg without evidence of end-organ damage.**
A. **Goal** is to reduce blood pressure to "normal" within 24 to 48 hours. If possible, start the patient on a drug that he or she will be able to continue to use as part of an antihypertensive regimen.
B. **There is no evidence that an elevated diastolic pressure of 115 mm Hg or less is a risk factor for an acute event (stroke, MI) unless there is evidence of end-organ damage (see earlier).** It is clearly a long-term risk factor and requires follow-up care, but does not require emergency treatment.
C. **Never** make the diagnosis of new-onset, mild hypertension in an ED setting. The BP elevation might be attributable to pain or could be situational.
D. **Treatment.**
1. In most patients, simple observation and time are as effective as pharmacologic intervention.
2. Some options for treatment include:
a. **Captopril** 25 mg PO or SL. It is absorbed in 30 minutes SL with peak effect at 50 to 90 minutes.
b. **Labetalol** 200 mg PO.
c. Another antihypertensive of your choice.
d. **Avoid SL nifedipine.** Although rare, it can cause complications such as stroke or MI.

AORTIC DISSECTION (THORACIC)

I. **Characteristics:** Severe, tearing pain in the chest, back, epigastrium, and flanks. Have a high index of suspicion in those with unexplainable chest pain. Pain is generally of short duration and very intense. Pain can migrate from the chest downward as the dissection progresses.

II. **Clinical Findings:** Only 16% have loss of peripheral pulses and only 50% have unequal upper extremity pulses. Only 50% have a new aortic regurgitation murmur. Up to 40% have ECG changes suggestive of ischemia. Rarely, DIC or microangiopathic changes on blood smear are seen.

III. **Diagnosis.**

A. No finding on a plain radiograph is sensitive enough to rule out aortic dissection by its absence. Radiograph might demonstrate a wide mediastinum, blurred and enlarged aortic knob, esophageal deviation to right (look at NG tube), apical cap (blood collected at the upper apex of the lungs). There could be extension of blood beyond the calcific boarder of the aortic wall. However, none of these might be present on the plain radiograph of a patient with aortic dissection.

B. Suspicion requires testing. CT is the most frequently used test but an aortogram remains the gold standard. Transesophageal US is another option but is generally more difficult to obtain acutely.

IV. **Treatment.**

A. **Control blood pressure with a combination of:**

1. **Nitroprusside** (see previous section, Hypertensive Crisis, for dose) and a β-blocker to prevent shear forces caused by reflex tachycardia.

2. **Propranolol** (Inderal): 0.5 to 1 mg IV q2-5min (maximum, 15 mg) to control heart rate (60-80 bpm).
   or

3. **Esmolol:** Mix 5 mg in 500 mL to give concentration of 10 μg/mL. Give loading dose of 500 μg/kg (0.5 mg/kg) × 1 min and start infusion of 50 μg/kg per minute × 4 min. If no response, reinfuse bolus and increase drip to 100 μg/kg per minute × 4 min. Continue this procedure, increasing the drip by 50 μg/kg per minute until you have achieved desired results or get a total of 200 μg/kg per minute, after which there is no added benefit. Esmolol has the advantage of a short, 9-minute, half-life.
   or

4. **Metoprolol:** 5 mg IV q5min for a total of 15 mg or more to control pulse.
   or

5. **Labetalol:** See section on Hypertensive Crisis (earlier) for dosing.

B. **Surgical consultation** is mandatory for consideration of repair. Recently, stents have been used as a temporizing measure. This will vary depending on your institution.

2

EMERGENCY MEDICINE

ABDOMINAL AORTIC ANEURYSM

I. **Characterized by** colicky or constant, severe abdominal or back pain that can radiate to groin, hips, or lower extremities. Can mimic urolithiasis, including hematuria and vomiting.

II. **Exam** might show a pulsatile mass (sensitivity, 44% to 97%), but exam is not adequate to rule out AAA. Might also have a tender and possibly distended abdomen, and signs of shock depending on how much hemorrhage has occurred. Distal pulses are often maintained and are an unreliable sign!

III. **Immediate imaging is indicated,** preferably by bedside US if the patient is unstable, or CT if stable. Treatment as per thoracic dissection (see earlier). Stents are being used for unruptured aneurysms, but, surprisingly, there is no difference in perioperative mortality or complications (although one study suggests that with experienced operators there might be a benefit to stents). In addition, the grafts tend to migrate over time (1-3 years out).

IV. **Appropriate follow-up of the patient with an asymptomatic AAA found on routine exam:**

A. Risk of rupture is essentially 0% for aneurysms <4 cm, 1% annually for aneurysms 4 to 5.0 cm, and 11% for those >5.0 cm. The surgical mortality rate is higher than the risk of rupture in those with AAAs <5.0 to 5.5 cm, and outcome in those with <5.0 cm is the same at 6 years with observation as it is with surgery.

B. **The best strategy** is annual US of those aneurysms <4 cm and twice-yearly US of those >4 cm, with repair at 5.0 to 5.5 cm.

SHOCK

I. **Characterized by** inadequate tissue perfusion and cellular hypofunction/hypoxia.

II. **Classified by Etiology.**

A. **Hypovolemic** shock from volume loss (e.g., dehydration, blood loss, burns).

B. **Distributive** shock based on loss of vascular tone (e.g., anaphylactic, septic, toxic shock).

C. **Cardiogenic** shock based on pump failure.

D. **Dissociative** shock based on inability of RBCs to deliver oxygen (e.g., methemoglobinemia, carbon monoxide poisoning).

III. **Diagnosis.**

A. **Hypotension.** BP drop is a late finding. Orthostatic vital signs could be normal in hypovolemic patients, or normal persons can exhibit orthostatic changes, so use clinical judgment and base treatment on symptoms. In addition, alcohol ingestion, a meal, increased age, antihypertensives, etc., can cause orthostatic changes in BP and pulse in the absence of hypovolemia.

1. Take orthostatic vital signs recumbent and after standing for 1 to 2 minutes.
2. An orthostatic systolic decrease of 10 to 20 mm Hg or increase in pulse of 15 bpm is considered "significant."
3. Four percent of normovolemic patients will have a 30-bpm increase in pulse.
4. Pulse increase of 30 bpm or *severe* postural dizziness has a sensitivity for moderate blood loss of 22% but is 97% sensitive for large blood loss. Moderate dizziness is poorly predictive of volume status.
B. **Tachycardia** is usually present but might not be, especially in the presence of diaphragmatic irritation, which causes vagal stimulation.
C. **Hypoperfusion.** Signs include decreased urine output, decreased mentation, cool extremities, and mottling.
IV. **Treatment.**
   Remember to keep patient warm and in Trendelenburg position if appropriate (contraindicated in CHF, however). Remember the ABCs. Goal of resuscitation is to maintain urine output between 30 and 60 mL/h.
A. **Hypovolemic shock.** See trauma section (earlier).
B. **Septic shock.** See Chapter 10.
C. **Anaphylactic shock** (applies also to acute urticaria).
1. Systemic allergic reaction characterized by urticaria, itching, angioedema, dyspnea/cough/wheezing, and hypotension/syncope. Might have vomiting or diarrhea, diffuse erythroderma. Caused by IgE-mediated hypersensitivity.
2. Anaphylactic shock has an approximately 3% mortality rate.
3. Common causes include foods (especially peanuts and shellfish), insect venoms (especially Hymenoptera stings), drugs, including aspirin and penicillins, and radiocontrast materials (about 5% of patients are allergic).
4. **Seafood allergy is protein related and not related to iodine. Therefore, these patients can have IVP dye. Penicillin-allergic patients can almost always tolerate third-generation cephalosporins.**
5. **Differentiate from scombroid fish poisoning,** which occurs after eating dark meat fish such as tuna (including canned), mackerel, and swordfish. Fish might taste metallic, peppery, or bitter. Onset in 20 to 30 minutes of skin flushing, vomiting, urticaria, wheezing, dyspnea, headache, and palpitations. It is caused by histamine and is self-limited (usually <3 hours). Treat like anaphylaxis.
6. **Management of anaphylaxis.**
a. **Epinephrine.**
   (1) If stable: Epinephrine 0.3 to 0.5 mL of 1:1000 subcutaneous (0.01 mL/kg in children). May repeat q10-15min × 3.
   (2) If hypotensive or unstable: Epinephrine 0.1 to 0.5 mg IV in boluses or can infuse at 1 to 4 μg/min (in adults) or 0.1 μg/kg per minute in children.

2

EMERGENCY MEDICINE

All patients should also get:

b. **Diphenhydramine** 25 to 50 mg PO for mild or up to 2 mg/kg IV for serious reactions (1-1.5 mg/kg per dose in children q6h). This is an H_1 blocker.
and

c. **Cimetidine** 300 mg IV (5-10 mg/kg q6-12h in children, maximum 300 mg/dose), or ranitidine 50 mg IV (0.33-0.66 mg/kg IV q8h in children, maximum 50 mg/dose).

   (1) H_2 blockers have been shown to be more effective than diphenhydramine with less sedation and should be used concurrently with diphenhydramine.

d. **Corticosteroids** will not help stabilize the patient with anaphylactic shock. They are useful in preventing recurrences and in blocking late-phase reactants. Administer hydrocortisone succinate 100 mg IV to block late-phase reactants. Other options are methylprednisolone 60 to 125 mg IV (1-2 mg/kg in children) or PO prednisone.

e. **For wheezing:** Nebulized albuterol ± epinephrine (SQ/IV) as per asthma section, depending on clinical picture.

f. **For discharge:** Because anaphylaxis can be biphasic with recurrence within 48 hours, continue diphenhydramine or hydroxyzine 25 to 50 mg PO q6h and cimetidine 400 mg bid or ranitidine 150 mg PO bid × 48-72 h. Can also continue on prednisone 40 mg qd if desired for 5 to 7 days. This will reduce itching and urticaria.

D. Staphylococcal and streptococcal TSS (see CDC, 1997). See also Chapter 10.

1. **Staphylococcal TSS case definition** includes fever 102°F (38.9°C), diffuse macular rash, desquamation 1 to 2 weeks after onset of illness, hypotension, multisystem involvement, including myalgia (elevated CPK), mucous membrane hyperemia, and renal, hepatic, CNS, or hematologic abnormality (plt <100,000). Differentiate from Kawasaki's disease (see Chapter 12), RMSF, etc.

2. **Streptococcal TSS case definition** includes hypotension, multiorgan involvement, including renal, hematologic (DIC or plt <100,000), liver, or respiratory, generalized erythematous rash, or soft tissue necrosis (e.g., necrotizing fasciitis, myositis, gangrene).

3. Toxic shock is associated with tampon use, but 20% are related to other staphylococcal infections, including postoperative infections, ingrown nails, and abrasions. Streptococcal TSS often is due to skin infection (e.g., after varicella).

4. **Treatment includes** antibiotics (a β-lactamase–resistant penicillin, such as nafcillin or a first-generation cephalosporin, or vancomycin or clindamycin), fluids, and pressors, as noted in discussion of septic shock (see Chapter 10).

E. Cardiogenic shock. See Chapter 3, section on acute pulmonary edema.

OVERDOSE AND TOXIDROMES

I. General Approach.

A. Remember ABCs.

B. Remember to decontaminate gut, clothing, skin, and environment.

C. If patient is unconscious, remember glucose, thiamine, naloxone.

D. Determine to the best of your ability what was ingested. All overdose patients should have serum acetaminophen and salicylate levels drawn (see acetaminophen, later).

E. Contact your closest poison control center for further information about the particular toxin in question.

F. Poisoning (especially recurrent) in a child might indicate neglect but can also be associated with pica and lead toxicity.

II. Gut Decontamination.

A. Ipecac is not useful, is fraught with untoward effects (e.g., delayed charcoal administration, aspiration, prolonged vomiting), and can no longer be recommended.

B. Gastric lavage.

1. **Lavage has fallen out of favor and is not generally effective or recommended beyond 1 to 1.5 hours after ingestion,** but might want to try in severely ill patients. Lavage alone is not adequate and must be combined with charcoal.

2. Use orogastric tube or largest NG tube available.

3. **Patient should have airway protection (patient should be alert or intubated).** Many complications of overdose therapy are related to gastric lavage.

4. Instill 300-mL aliquots of saline and remove until clear or have irrigated with 5 L of fluid.

C. Activated charcoal.

1. Treatment of choice in most ingestions. Best if used within the first hour postingestion of overdose. Does not work for iron, lithium, petroleum distillates, volatiles, and caustics. Not effective if over 2 h since ingestion.

2. Administer activated charcoal 10 to 25 g in children, 50 to 100 g in adults (1 g/kg). A sorbitol mixture reduces transit times but should be used only with the first dose if multiple doses of charcoal are going to be used. There is no evidence that cathartics reduce absorption or toxicity, however.

3. Have the patient drink the charcoal or administer it by NG tube; 30% will vomit the charcoal, but you can readminister it if needed.

4. Multiple-dose charcoal is still controversial. It might be indicated for theophylline, TCAs, phenobarbital, phenytoin, and digitalis.

5. A charcoal-deferoxamine slurry of 3:1 (8 g deferoxamine to 25 g charcoal) by weight will reduce absorption of iron. For lithium, cation exchange resins such as sodium polystyrene sulfonate (Kayexalate) can reduce lithium absorption.

D. Whole-bowel irrigation.

1. Might be useful after the ingestion of enteric-coated and timed-release medications (e.g., verapamil). Might also be useful in "body packers," etc. Reduces bowel transit time. Use in other ingestions might be helpful, but data are sparse. Do not delay charcoal administration to use whole-bowel irrigation.
2. Use polyethylene glycol (GoLYTELY) 1 to 2 L/h in adults, 500 mL/h in children, to a total of 3 to 8 L.

III. Toxidromes are symptom complexes associated with toxins. The most common toxidromes are listed in Table 2-5.

A. Cholinergics. Table 2-5 gives descriptions of toxicity.

1. Affects mostly farmers and other industrial workers.
2. Serum cholinesterase activity can be assayed if there is a question of cholinergic toxicity.
3. Death usually occurs from respiratory muscle depression and excessive secretions or bronchospasm.
4. **Treatment.**
   a. **Decontaminate.** Decontamination includes washing the skin with alkaline soap and then ethanol. Decontaminate GI tract if needed with lavage and multiple-dose charcoal.
   b. **Atropine** 2 mg IV q5min to dry secretions and can require up to 200 to 500 mg (yes, this is not a typo) in first hour; end point is drying of secretions or signs of toxicity. For children, use dose of 0.05 mg/kg. Atropine will treat the muscarinic effects only. Overabundant secretions are a cause of early mortality. Watch for ileus secondary to atropine.
   c. **Pralidoxime** (2-PAM). Adults, 1 to 2 g IV × 15-20 min; children, 20 to 40 mg/kg × 15-20 min. Can repeat in 1 to 2 hours. Follow serum cholinesterase levels.
      (1) 2-PAM regenerates acetylcholine esterase. Should be reserved for those who are symptomatic. Needs to be used early because the organophosphate-enzyme complex becomes irreversible after 24 to 36 hours.
   d. **Morphine and aminophylline are contraindicated.**
5. **Sequelae.**
   a. An intermediate syndrome occurs 24 to 96 hours after treatment of initial insult and manifests with rapidly developing respiratory failure, cranial nerve palsy, and proximal upper limb girdle weakness. Treatment is supportive only, and the condition does not respond to pharmacologic therapy.
   b. Long-term sequelae include impairment of auditory attention, visual memory, visuomotor speed, sequencing, problem solving, motor steadiness, reaction time, and dexterity. No increase in depression, other psychological problems.
   c. Might also have a delayed peripheral neuropathy starting at 1 to 5 weeks that can progress for 3 months but eventually resolves.

B. Anticholinergics. See **Table 2-5** for description of toxicity. Use activated charcoal if indicated. Treat seizures with lorazepam; treat

TABLE 2-5
TOXIDROMES

Toxidrome	Symptoms	Examples	Mnemonic/Notes
Anticholinergic	Tachycardia, mydriasis, warm, flushed skin, urinary retention, confusion	Atropine, scopolamine, belladonna alkaloids, antihistamines (e.g., diphenhydramine), antipsychotics, plants (Jimsonweed, moonflower, and others), tricyclics, mushrooms (*Amanita* species)	Dry as a bone, red as a beet, blind as a bat, mad as a hatter
Cholinergic	Organophosphates, carbamates, pilocarpine, and some mushrooms	Lacrimation, salivation, sweating, diarrhea, headache, defecation, urination, mental status changes, fatigue, convulsions, muscle weakness, miosis cardiovascular collapse, pulmonary secretions, bronchospasm	Blind as a mole, moist as a slug, weak as a kitten
Gamma-hydroxybutyrate	Alternating coma with agitation, hypopnea while comatose, bradycardia while comatose, and myoclonus	GHB, liquid ecstasy	
Opiate	Pinpoint pupils, hypotension, hypopnea, coma, hypothermia	Morphine, heroin, codeine, oxycodone, clonidine, propoxyphene, diphenoxylate (e.g., Lomotil)	Propoxyphene and others may not cause miosis
Sympathomimetic	Tachycardia, HTN, elevated temperature, mydriasis	Cocaine, ecstasy, methamphetamine	

EMERGENCY MEDICINE   **2**

arrhythmias, hyperpyrexia, and hypertension as in any other patient (but avoid class la antiarrhythmic agents). Treat agitation with benzodiazepines (avoid phenothiazines, which have anticholinergic properties). Physostigmine 0.5 to 2 mg IV in adults and 0.02 mg/kg in children may be used if there are severe symptoms that cannot be controlled otherwise (e.g., malignant hypertension, coma with respiratory depression, seizures unresponsive to conventional therapy). Reserve for severe problems: can induce seizures and arrhythmias.
Do not use physostigmine in TCA overdose!

C. Opiate poisoning. See Table 2-5 for description of toxicity.

1. Treatment.

a. **Naloxone** 0.4 to 2 mg in adults up to 10 mg and may repeat if needed. Short acting; half-life is 1.1 hours. Might have recurrent narcotization when naloxone wears off.

b. **Nalmefene.** Long acting, half-life is 10.8 hours. However, the patient should still be observed until there is no possibility of recurrent sedation. Methadone has a longer half-life. For non–opiate-dependent patients, start with 0.5 mg/70 kg and follow with another 1.0 mg/70 kg in 2 to 5 minutes. If total dose of 1.5 mg/70 kg does not work, no further drug is indicated. For opiate-dependent patients, use a test dose of 0.1 mg/70 kg, and if there is no withdrawal in 3 to 5 minutes, follow preceding guidelines.

c. **Use these drugs with caution in those who are narcotic addicts.** You could precipitate acute opiate withdrawal. You can intubate and support until narcotic wears off if this is a concern. Always observe the patient until there is no chance of further respiratory depression. This is especially important with naloxone, which has a relatively short half-life.

IV. Specific Ingestions: Read general guidelines for decontamination first.

A. Petroleum distillates (gasoline, fuel oil, airplane glue).

1. Main toxicity is pulmonary from inhalation.

2. Do not perform lavage or induce vomiting if swallowed.

3. Evaluation includes CXR (ARDS, infiltrates), ABG, and follow clinical course.

4. If no symptoms within 6 hours, no need for further observation.

B. Tricyclic antidepressants.

1. Main toxicity. Cardiac arrhythmias, anticholinergic effects (see toxidrome, earlier), vomiting, hypotension, confusion, seizures.

2. Avoid emesis! The patient might aspirate if he or she seizes or has decreased mental status. Charcoal/lavage (see earlier) is mainstay of decontamination.

3. The patient might appear fine but then rapidly deteriorate, so admit to a monitored unit. Be prepared to intubate the patient. If the patient is totally asymptomatic 6 hours after ingestion, no need to admit to monitored bed, but might require psychiatric admission.

4. **Cardiac complications.** Prolonged QRS, QT interval, torsades de pointes, other arrhythmias.

a. **Sodium bicarbonate** is administered to maintain blood pH >7.45 (1 to 2 mEq/kg bolus until QRS narrows to <100 msec, QT shortens, 2 ampules in 1 L of D_5W as a drip to maintain alkalinization). Helps prevent the development of arrhythmias. Recent data indicate that hyperventilation and saline might also be effective, but are not standard of care.

b. **IV magnesium sulfate** can be used to control torsades de pointes or a prolonged QT interval: 2 g of magnesium sulfate IV × 5-10 min, depending on acuity (see Chapter 1, Resuscitation, Airway Management, and Acute Arrhythmias).

c. **Lidocaine** can be used for arrhythmias as well. Avoid class IA and IC antiarrhythmics, β-blockers, calcium channel blockers, phenytoin.

5. **Neurologic complications:** Agitation, seizures.

a. **Diazepam** 5 to 10 mg or lorazepam 1 to 2 mg IV, titrating to control agitation.

b. Seizures are usually brief and self-limited. Treat as per seizure section (see earlier), with first-line drug being lorazepam 1 to 2 mg IV. Avoid phenytoin!

6. **Hypotension.** Treat initially with fluids and sodium bicarbonate IV (see earlier). Norepinephrine is the vasopressor of choice. Dopamine might produce paradoxical hypotension.

7. Physostigmine, the mainstay of therapy of TCA overdose in the past, is now controversial, might increase mortality, and should not be used for TCA overdose.

C. **Salicylates** (aspirin).

1. **Main toxicity.** Tinnitus, N&V, combined respiratory alkalosis (from central hyperventilation) and metabolic acidosis, fever, hypokalemia, hypoglycemia, seizures, and coma.

a. **Many ingestions are misdiagnosed as sepsis or gastroenteritis on initial presentation (e.g., fever, acidosis, vomiting).** This misdiagnosis is particularly common in the elderly.

2. **Toxic dose:** 150 mg/kg, with 300 mg/kg being very toxic. **The Done nomogram is not accurate and should not be used.**

3. **Treatment.**

a. IV normal saline to maintain BP.

b. Multidose charcoal might be useful.

c. Urine alkalinization (promotes excretion of salicylates). Use IV sodium bicarbonate (1-2 mEq/kg bolus, 2 ampules in 1 L of D_5W as drip). Must have adequate serum potassium; otherwise, potassium will be reabsorbed in exchange for hydrogen ions, and the urine will not be alkalinized.

d. Hemodialysis is indicated for severe toxicity.

4. Follow clinically and with serum salicylate levels.

D. **Acetaminophen** (Tylenol and others).

1. **Main toxicity** is hepatic, which occurs 24 to 72 hours after ingestion. Can also manifest with N&V.

2. **If patient is vomiting and unable to keep down charcoal,** consider metoclopramide. Ondansetron has also been particularly effective. Toxic ingestion is 140 mg/kg or 10 g in adults. In alcoholic patients, the toxic dose is often much less, even as little as 4 g/d.

3. Check **acetaminophen level** at least 4 hours after ingestion. **For extended-release acetaminophen or if there is a coingestion (including food), recheck level at 8 to 12 hours unless acetaminophen is undetectable at 4 hours. Just checking a 4-hour level does not guarantee patient safety.**

4. **Compare to Rumack-Matthew nomogram** to determine risk **(Fig. 2-1).**

5. **If in toxic range,** treat with N-acetylcysteine 140 mg/kg PO or by NG tube, and then 17 doses of 70 mg/kg q4h. IV use is now FDA approved in the United States and is safe and effective. Dosing is N-acetylcysteine 150 mg/kg loading dose in 200 mL $D_5W \times 15$ min, 50 mg/kg in 500 mL $D_5W \times 4$ h, then 100 mg/kg in 1 L $D_5W \times 16$ h. IV use can be associated with an anaphylactoid-type reaction that responds to diphenhydramine and inhaled albuterol (for wheezing). This generally does not preclude further IV use of N-acetylcysteine. Wait 1 hour and if patient is asymptomatic, it is safe to restart the infusion at a slower rate.

6. **Repeat any doses vomited within 1 hour of administration.** Do not withhold N-acetylcysteine even if 24 to 26 hours from ingestion. Late N-acetylcysteine, although not as effective as early, still reduces mortality.

7. **Charcoal** use is indicated in acetaminophen overdose and only minimally interferes with N-acetylcysteine. In addition, charcoal should be given early and N-acetylcysteine at least 4 hours after ingestion. If there is any question, the N-acetylcysteine can be given IV.

E. **Caustic ingestions** include alkalis (drain cleaner), industrial bleach, and battery acid. Household bleach is relatively nontoxic (unless inhaled) and rarely causes any difficulties when ingested.

1. **Main toxicity.** Local tissue necrosis of esophagus is seen with alkalis, and of stomach with acids; respiratory distress. There may be obvious facial-oral burns and emesis. Hoarseness and stridor reflect epiglottic edema; this is especially true with acids. Dyspnea and infiltrates are common if the agent is inhaled, and could progress to ARDS.

2. **Treatment.** Do not induce emesis or lavage patient. Charcoal is not indicated. If there are visible burns, there is a 50% chance of lower burns of significance. However, the absence of visible lesions does not rule out significant injury (10%-30% will have burns beyond the mucosa), and all ingestions need to have EGD. For household bleach: If the patient is asymptomatic, no further treatment or work-up is required. For dyspnea, administer oxygen, obtain CXR and ABG as indicated.

F. **Digoxin.**

1. **Main toxicity.** Any cardiac arrhythmia is possible with digoxin intoxication. Hypokalemia predisposes to digoxin toxicity (but digoxin toxicity causes hyperkalemia).

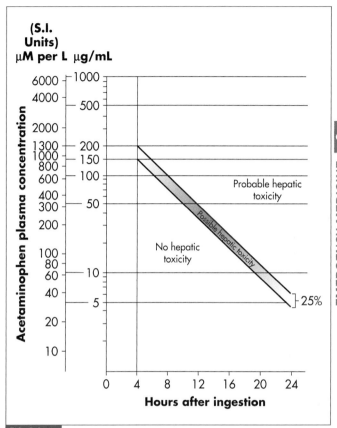

EMERGENCY MEDICINE

2

FIG. 2-1
Rumack-Matthew nomogram for the single acute acetaminophen poisoning: semilogarithmic plot of plasma acetaminophen levels versus time. Cautions for use of this chart include the time coordinates refer to time of ingestion; serum levels drawn before 4 h might not represent peak levels; the graph should be used only in relation to a single acute ingestion; and the lower solid line 25% below the standard nomogram is included to allow for possible errors in acetaminophen plasma assays and estimated time from ingestion of an overdose. *(Adapted from Rumack BH, Matthew H: Acetaminophen poisoning and toxicity. Pediatrics 55:871-876, 1975.)*

2. **Symptoms include** anorexia, N&V, diarrhea, confusion, blurred vision, altered color perception (yellow tinge, but occurs only in a minority).
3. **Laboratory.** Hyperkalemia, elevated serum digoxin level.
4. **Treatment.**
a. Treat arrhythmias as in Chapter 1, Resuscitation, Airway Management, and Acute Arrhythmias (magnesium sulfate is particularly effective for digoxin-induced arrhythmias).
b. Treat hyperkalemia. Avoid calcium because it increases digoxin binding to the heart.
c. Digoxin-specific antibody fragments (Digibind) indicated for:
   (1) Adults: Serum potassium 5 to 5.5 mg/dL, life-threatening arrhythmias; ingestion of 10 mg with signs of toxicity.
   (2) Children: Ingestion of 0.1 mg/kg; serum level 5 mg/dL with signs of toxicity; serum potassium >6.0 mg/dL.
   (3) To treat: Calculate Fab dose: 1 vial of Fab (40 mg) will bind 0.6 mg of digoxin. Calculate total-body digoxin load: Total-body dose digoxin = (serum digoxin level x 5.6 L/kg x weight in kg)/1000 x 0.8 (bioavailability). Vials Fab needed = total-body digoxin/0.6. **If dose unknown** and cannot get digoxin level, give 10 to 20 vials. If more likely a chronic toxicity, give 4 or 5 vials to start.
   (4) Serum digoxin levels are useless after digoxin Fab is given because they will measure both bound and unbound digoxin. Serum digoxin level can increase 10- to 20-fold after digoxin Fab. Watch for hypokalemia from reversing digoxin-induced hyperkalemia.

G. Carbon monoxide.
1. **Main toxicity.** CNS, including confusion, coma, seizures, headache, fatigue, nausea. Might have arrhythmias, cardiac ischemia, and rhabdomyolysis. Consider carbon monoxide poisoning in a cluster of flulike illnesses in the wrong season (e.g., fatigue, muscle aches, nausea).
2. **Diagnosis** is by clinical background, including a clustering of cases, exposure to furnace or car exhaust (especially in children in the back of pickup trucks, etc.), carboxyhemoglobin level. A venous carboxyhemoglobin level is just as good as arterial. Pulse oximetry will generally be normal even in severe carbon monoxide poisoning. Obtain ECG and serum CPK levels.
3. **Treatment.** Administer 100% oxygen (displaces carbon monoxide from hemoglobin). HBO is recommended for any patient with evidence of myocardial ischemia, carboxyhemoglobin level of 30% (some say >18%) at exposure time zero, or any impairment of CNS function. All pregnant women should have HBO. Recent data question the effectiveness of HBO. However, it is still the standard of care.

H. Cocaine and methamphetamines. See Table 2-5 for toxidromes.
1. **Major toxicity.** Seizures, hypertension, tachycardia, paranoid behavior or other alteration in mentation, rhabdomyolysis, myocardial infarction, CVA.

2. **Treatment.** Cocaine has a relatively short half-life, so most symptoms are self-limited. Methamphetamines have a longer half-life and might require treatment.

a. **β-Blockade (esmolol, propranolol, others) is contraindicated in the treatment of cocaine- and methamphetamine-induced hypertension, tachycardia, and coronary spasm unless an α-blocker already has been given. Unopposed α-adrenergic affects can worsen problems.**

b. For coronary vasospasm, hypertension, or tachycardia, observation is probably adequate because cocaine has short half-life. For amphetamines, treatment might be required.

c. If treatment is urgent, phentolamine 5 to 10 mg IV is the drug of choice. Once α-blockade is obtained, β-blockers can be used gently to control arrhythmias.

   (1) Treat as would any MI; thrombolytics are safe. MI and CVA can occur up to 72 hours after cocaine use. Concurrent use of alcohol increases the likelihood of cardiac vasospasm with cocaine use. All chest pain is not MI. Think of pneumomediastinum in crack use, bronchospasm.

d. **Seizures.** Usually self-limited but will respond to normal seizure treatment (see section on seizures, earlier).

e. **CNS symptoms** such as agitation and paranoia can be treated by diazepam or lorazepam.

BITES

I. Mammalian Bites. The main morbidity from animal bites is infection or scarring. Rabies must be considered in any warm-blooded animal bite but is almost nonexistent in the domestic animal population of the United States. It is present in the wild, mainly in bats, raccoons, skunks, or dogs from Mexico or Latin America, Asia, or Africa. Rabies is very rarely found in rodents (e.g., squirrels, rats, mice) and almost never in lagomorphs (rabbits).

A. Gather data on what species of animal was involved and whether it has a current vaccination, whether the attack was provoked or unprovoked, the extent of wounds, and whether the animal is available for examination.

B. Management.

1. Cleanse the wounds thoroughly with soap and water.

2. Contact the local police. Domestic, unvaccinated animals should be observed by a veterinarian for 10 days or killed and the heads refrigerated and sent to an appropriate lab for testing, usually the state lab. All wild animals captured or killed should have the head sent for testing.

3. Check tetanus status and give booster if >5 years have elapsed since immunization.

2

EMERGENCY MEDICINE

4. Treat wound like any other wound, with irrigation and débridement. Do not close puncture wounds or human bites because of high incidence of infection. Consider consultation for extensive damage or facial wound. Dog bites especially cause a lot of soft tissue damage, with pain and surrounding bruising.

5. **Antibiotics for bites:**

a. **Human bites.** Antibiotics should be given prophylactically for all human bites: amoxicillin/clavulanate 20 to 40 mg/kg per day divided tid × 7 d; cefixime is an alternative. Consider IV antibiotics if infection has already occurred, especially on the hand. If a joint might be involved (e.g., MCP joint after an altercation), surgical exploration is indicated.

b. **Cat bites.** Antibiotics are routinely given for cat bites. The drug of choice is amoxicillin/clavulanate 20 to 40 mg/kg per day divided tid × 7 d. Doxycycline and ceftriaxone are acceptable alternatives.

c. **Dog bites.** Only 5% become infected (the same rate as most wounds), and routine prophylaxis is not recommended unless bite is on hands or feet. If need to treat, amoxicillin-clavulanate is the drug of choice with clindamycin, plus a fluoroquinolone or TMP-SMX, being good alternatives. Wounds can be closed if not extensive and not a lot of tissue crushed.

6. **Rabies prophylaxis** should be instituted for all wild carnivore bites (e.g., skunk, fox, raccoon, cat, dog, bat) unless animal is available for study.

a. Administer rabies immunoglobulin 20 IU/kg in persons not previously immunized. It should all be infiltrated around the wound if feasible. Otherwise, give as much as possible infiltrated around the wound and the rest IM.

b. Give human diploid cell rabies vaccine, 1.0 mL IM on days 0, 3, 7, 14, and 28.

c. **For bats:** Transmission without a bite is exceedingly rare. The CDC (1999) recommends, "Postexposure prophylaxis should be considered when direct contact between a human and a bat has occurred, unless the exposed person can be certain a bite, scratch, or mucous membrane exposure did not occur. In instances in which a bat is found indoors and there is no history of bat-human contact, the likely effectiveness of postexposure prophylaxis must be balanced against the low risk such exposures appear to present. In this setting, postexposure prophylaxis can be considered for persons who were in the same room as the bat and who might be unaware that a bite or direct contact had occurred (e.g., a sleeping person awakens to find a bat in the room or an adult witnesses a bat in the room with a previously unattended child, mentally disabled person, or intoxicated person) **and** rabies cannot be ruled out by testing the bat. Postexposure prophylaxis would not be warranted for other household members" (pp 1-21).

II. **Tick Bites and Tick-Related Illness.** See Chapter 10.

III. **Spider Bites.** Spider bites are usually not serious unless there is an allergic reaction. Treatment with ice, cleansing, and acetaminophen is usually adequate. Black widow and brown recluse spiders can cause more severe reactions and occasionally death. Antivenom is available for black widow spider bites but should be used only if the reaction is severe and cannot be controlled with opiates and benzodiazepines. Specific discussion is beyond the scope of this manual.

ENVIRONMENTAL ILLNESS AND BURNS

I. **Sunburn** occurs after exposure to sun and manifests within 24 hours of exposure. Generally peaks at 72 hours and can have erythema, blistering, and pain.

A. Best therapy is prevention by wearing of clothing or sun block and avoiding sun exposure at peak day (10:00 AM to 3:00 PM). Cool compresses and pain medications can give symptomatic relief. Topical steroids (e.g., betamethasone) and oral NSAIDs (e.g., indomethacin) might be beneficial and seem to be additive. Oral prednisone 20 to 30 mg/d in adults can decrease symptoms.

II. **Hyperthermia** results from an imbalance in heat production and dissipation. Predisposing factors include dehydration, chronic illness, old age, alcohol, alteration in skin function (e.g., scleroderma), and drugs, including anticholinergics, phenothiazines, TCAs, MAOIs, amphetamines, and succinylcholine. Think also of thyroid storm.

A. **Malignant hyperthermia.**

1. **Causes.** Occurs in 1 in 20,000 in response to a muscle-relaxing agent (e.g., succinylcholine) or an inhaled anesthetic (e.g., halothane). It is hereditary; it might also be secondary to physical or emotional stress.

2. **Characteristics.** Hyperthermia, muscle rigidity, tachycardia, acidosis, shock, coma, rhabdomyolysis.

3. **Treatment** includes dantrolene 1 to 10 mg/kg IV titrated to effect, management of acidosis and shock, peripheral cooling (see management of heat stroke, later).

B. **Neuroleptic malignant syndrome.**

1. **Cause.** Neuroleptics (e.g., phenothiazines).

2. **Characteristics.** Same symptoms as malignant hyperthermia but generally develops over days instead of minutes.

3. **Treatment.** As per malignant hyperthermia, stop offending drug, use bromocriptine 2.5 mg PO or NG q 6h up to 40 mg/day. Continue for 10 days and titrate down.

C. **Serotonin syndrome.**

1. **Cause.** Serotonin excess. Generally secondary to combination of MAO and SSRI, meperidine plus an SSRI, dextromethorphan, tramadol, or, rarely, excess SSRI ingestion.

2. **Characteristics.** Rapid development of fever, hypertension, muscle rigidity, decreased mental status. Has a much more rapid onset than neuroleptic malignant syndrome.

3. **Treatment.** Treat like malignant hyperthermia (see earlier). Cyproheptadine, a serotonin antagonist, 4 to 12 mg (max 32 mg/24h), might be effective as may propranolol; both these drugs block

serotonin receptors. Use diazepam in 5-mg aliquots IV for muscle spasm, intubate as needed, use cooling blankets, give acetaminophen. Treat hypertension as per malignant hypertension. Olanzapine and chlorpromazine have also been used.

D. Heat cramps.

1. **Cause.** Strenuous physical activity.
2. **Characteristics.** Skeletal muscle cramps, profuse sweating, hyponatremia secondary to free water intake, normal body temperature.
3. **Treatment.** Rest, oral or IV rehydration.

E. Heat exhaustion.

1. **Cause.** Secondary to sweating, volume depletion, tissue hypoperfusion.
2. **Characteristics.** Fatigue, light-headedness, N&V, headache, tachycardia, hyperventilation, hypotension, normal or slightly elevated temperature, profuse sweating.
3. **Treatment.** Rest, rapid IV fluid replacement (1-2 L or more of NS).

F. Heat stroke.

1. **Cause.** Volume depletion, sweating, etc.
2. **Characteristics.** Hyperpyrexia (often >40°C [106°F]). Patient might be sweating or dry and have LOC or alteration in mental status (hallucinations, bizarre behavior, status epilepticus, other neurologic symptoms).
3. **Treatment.** This is a true emergency. Check and follow labs, including electrolytes, CBC twice a day, liver enzymes, CPK (might develop rhabdomyolysis), and clotting studies. Remove clothing; apply water to skin and fan to promote evaporative heat loss. (Avoid inducing shivering and peripheral vasoconstriction with ice. Shivering can be controlled with diazepam IV or chlorpromazine or meperidine.) Treat with fluids (but many do not have significant fluid deficits; be cautious), cooling blankets.

Burns, Cold, and Thermal Injury

I. Assessment of Burns.

A. Surface area (Fig. 2-2).

B. Depth. It is frequently impossible to tell the true depth of a burn at the initial evaluation. All burns should be serially examined over days and followed closely.

1. **Superficial.** Epidermis only, painful and erythematous (previously *first degree*).
2. **Superficial partial thickness.** Epidermis and outer half of dermis with sparing of hairs.
3. **Deep partial thickness.** Epidermis and destruction of reticular dermis. Can easily convert to full thickness in presence of secondary infection, mechanical trauma, or progressive thrombosis (previously *second degree*).
4. **Full thickness.** Appears dry, pearly white, charred, and leathery. Heals by epithelial migration from the periphery and by contracture. Can involve adipose, fascia, muscle, or bone (previously *third degree*).

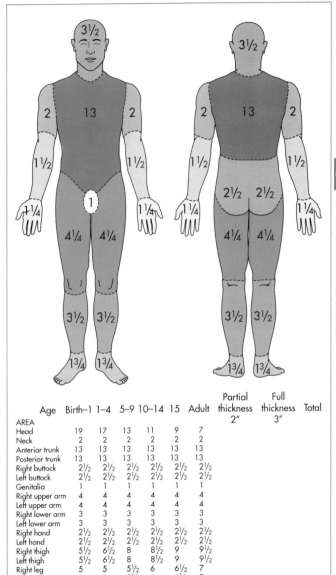

Age	Birth–1	1–4	5–9	10–14	15	Adult	Partial thickness 2″	Full thickness 3″	Total
AREA									
Head	19	17	13	11	9	7			
Neck	2	2	2	2	2	2			
Anterior trunk	13	13	13	13	13	13			
Posterior trunk	13	13	13	13	13	13			
Right buttock	2½	2½	2½	2½	2½	2½			
Left buttock	2½	2½	2½	2½	2½	2½			
Genitalia	1	1	1	1	1	1			
Right upper arm	4	4	4	4	4	4			
Left upper arm	4	4	4	4	4	4			
Right lower arm	3	3	3	3	3	3			
Left lower arm	3	3	3	3	3	3			
Right hand	2½	2½	2½	2½	2½	2½			
Left hand	2½	2½	2½	2½	2½	2½			
Right thigh	5½	6½	8	8½	9	9½			
Left thigh	5½	6½	8	8½	9	9½			
Right leg	5	5	5½	6	6½	7			
Left leg	5	5	5½	6	6½	8			
Right foot	3½	3½	3½	3½	3½	3½			
Left foot	3½	3½	3½	3½	3½	3½			

FIG. 2-2

Estimating surface area in burns. *(Adapted from Nussbaum MS, Berry S [eds]: The Mont Reid Surgical Handbook. St. Louis, Mosby, 1987.)*

C. Severity.
1. **Minor burn** is defined as first-degree and partial-thickness <15% BSA in adults and <10% BSA in children <6 years of age; full-thickness burns >2% BSA in adults.
2. **Moderate burn** defined as partial-thickness 15% to 25% BSA in adults and 10% to 20% in children; full-thickness burns 10% BSA.
3. **Major burn** (requiring burn unit or burn center care) defined as partial-thickness >20% to 25% BSA in adults and >20% in children; full-thickness burns >10% BSA; burns of hands, face, eyes, ears, feet, perineum; inhalation burns; electrical burns; burns complicated by fracture or major trauma; all burns in infants or elderly, and patients at poor risk secondary to prior medical conditions.

D. Causes of burns.
1. **Thermal.**
a. Burns caused by flame, especially with clothing, tend to be full thickness.
b. Molten metal, tars, or melted synthetics lead to prolonged skin contact and should be cooled as rapidly as possible. See later for tar removal.
c. Liquid burns should be cooled rapidly and any clothing in contact with the area rapidly removed to decrease the contact time.
2. **Electrical.** Similar to crush injuries, electrical burns may cause muscle necrosis, rhabdomyolysis, and myoglobinuria.
a. Watch for cardiac arrhythmias. Cardiac monitoring is essential for 24 hours if there is LOC, abnormal initial ECG, or dysrhythmias. It is suggested for all others with significant exposure.
b. Place patient in cervical collar; look for long bone fractures secondary to muscle contraction.
c. In children with lip burns from electrical cords, watch for bleeding from the labial artery 3 or 4 days after injury.
d. Follow CBC, electrolytes, ECG, urine myoglobin, CPK, cardiac enzymes, ABG.
e. Can cause thrombosis of any vessel in the body. Injury usually much greater than is visible on the skin. Be cautious and observe these patients closely. Consider admission.
3. **Chemical agents.**
a. Strong acids are quickly neutralized or quickly absorbed. Rinse off skin and call Poison Control Center for specific instructions.
b. Alkalis cause liquefaction necrosis and can penetrate deeply, leading to progressive necrosis up to several hours after contact.
4. **Radiation.**
a. Radiation burns initially appear hyperemic and can later resemble full-thickness burns. Changes can extend deeply into the tissue.
b. Sunburns are of this type and involve moderate superficial pain.

II. Treatment of Burns.
Always watch for renal failure from rhabdomyolysis and sepsis in severe burns. Remove all jewelry from injured extremities and remove clothes.

A. **ED, including thermal burns.** Cover wounds with NS-soaked gauze (which will help the pain to some degree) and use IV narcotics for pain. Tetanus immunization status should be checked and the patient treated accordingly.

1. **Clean** with bland soap and water. Débride loose and foreign material. May leave blister intact if relatively small and patient is reliable. Rinse well with normal saline.

2. **Wound dressing choices:**

a. A nonadherent inner layer of porous material is followed by soft, bulky, absorbent gauze and covered with a semielastic outer layer.

b. Topical antibacterial agents such as 1% silver sulfadiazine or bacitracin are applied and then covered with gauze pads. See manufacturer's insert for contraindications.

3. **Fluids.** Initiate if burns cover 15% to 20% BSA in adults, >10% in children (see Fig. 2-2).

   - Fluids in first 24 hours = 4 mL/kg per percentage of BSA burned (Parkland formula), plus maintenance IV fluids in children.
   - Give one half in first 8 hours and one half in next 16 hours. Colloids are not indicated in this setting. Goal is to maintain urine output at 1 mL/kg per hour in children, 30 to 60 mL/h in adults.
   - Place Foley catheter to monitor fluid status.

4. **Heterograft, allograft, or xenograft** dressings can be used on an inpatient basis for partial-thickness wounds.

5. **Chemical burns** should be washed with tap water for at least 15 and preferably 30 minutes after powders are removed by brushing. This should be started at the scene if possible. Alkali burns should be irrigated for 1 to 2 hours after injury. Chemical binding might be required for certain burns.

6. **Tar burns** need cooling, gentle cleaning, and application of a petrolatum-based antibacterial ointment. Petroleum-based products, household shortening, or butter can be used to soften the tar for removal. Avoid chemical solvents, which can cause additional burns. After 24 hours the tar can be washed away and the injury treated as a thermal burn.

B. **Follow-up care.**

1. **Daily to twice-daily dressing changes** should be performed. Mild soap can be used for cleaning. Necrotic debris and eschar require débridement, which can be facilitated by tub soaks or whirlpool treatments. Absolute sterility is not mandatory (at home); however, cleanliness and thorough cleaning of hands, sinks, tubs, and any instruments used must be emphasized. Acetic acid 0.25% can be applied for pseudomonal prophylaxis.

2. **Contractures** might not be apparent for weeks to months. Therefore, ROM exercises should be started during the early healing period. If the hands are involved extensively, early excision and autografting can

decrease the scarring of deep partial-thickness and full-thickness burns. Splinting and prolonged physical therapy can be required for rehabilitation. If the patient is prone to keloids, special garments may be used to reduce this scarring.

3. **Analgesics** should be given as needed and especially before dressing changes. Codeine or hydrocodone are normally adequate after the initial ED visit. If the dose is taken a half hour before the dressing change, it will facilitate cleaning and debridement.

4. **All burns should be seen within 24 hours of initial treatment,** and if any signs of infection develop, cultures should be performed and hospitalization considered.

5. **Prophylactic antibiotics should rarely be required** but may be considered for immunocompromised hosts, patients at high risk of endocarditis, or patients with artificial joints. Broad-spectrum coverage with first-generation cephalosporin or with a penicillinase-resistant penicillin plus an aminoglycoside may be used if necessary. Vancomycin might be needed depending on your institution.

6. **In circumferential burns, extensive extremity burns, or electrical burns, watch for vascular or neurologic compromise, indicating a developing compartment syndrome. Immediate escharotomy is then required.** Extremities should be elevated to minimize swelling.

7. **Nutritional support is extremely important in extensive burns.** Metabolic rate can be increased 100% to 200% above normal. IV hyperalimentation might be required until the GI tract is functioning. An NG tube is indicated for paralytic ileus.

8. **β-Blockers early; retrospective evidence** suggests a major decrease in mortality when patients with significant burns are on β-blockers. The idea is that β-blockers attenuate the hypermetabolic state (Arbabi et al., 2004).

III. **Cold Injury.**

   A. **Without tissue freezing.**

   1. **Chilblain.** Peripheral cold injury without freezing of tissue.

   a. **Cause.** Prolonged dry exposure at temperatures above freezing.

   b. **Clinically.** Affected areas are pruritic, reddish-blue, possibly swollen; might have blisters or superficial ulcerations.

   c. **Treatment.** Rewarm as for frostbite (see later).

   d. Areas might be more temperature sensitive in future; there is no permanent injury. Pain medication should be provided.

   2. **Trench foot and immersion injury.**

   a. **Cause.** Prolonged wet exposure at temperatures above freezing.

   b. **Clinically.** Might have tissue destruction resembling partial-thickness burns, including blisters, pain, hypersensitivity to cold. Temperature sensitivity might be permanent.

   c. **Treatment.** Rewarm as for frostbite (see later).

   B. **With tissue freezing: frostbite.**

   1. **Cause.** Freezing of the tissue with ice crystal formation.

2. **Classification.**
a. **Frostnip.** Superficial, skin changes reversible.
   (1) **Clinically.** Skin blanched with loss of sensation.
   (2) **Treatment.** See later.
b. **Superficial frostbite.** Tissue below skin pliable, soft.
   (1) **Clinically**. Blisters in 24 to 48 hours, fluid resorbs, develops hard, blackened eschar, generally superficial, remains sensitive to heat, cold.
   (2) **Treatment.** See later. Treat conservatively. Generally resolves without surgical intervention in 3 to 4 weeks.
c. **Deep frostbite.** Feels woody under skin; affects muscles, tendons, etc.
   (1) **Clinically.** Extremity cool, deep purple or red, with dark, hemorrhagic blisters and loss of distal function. Can take several months to determine extent of injury. Frozen tissue will eventually slough.
   (2) **Treatment.** Rapidly rewarm the part by immersing it in 42°C (108°F) water. Do not rub. Slow rewarming is not as good! If in the field, do not thaw extremity until assured it will not refreeze.
      (a) Pruritus and burning sensation increase with rewarming. Might require narcotic analgesia for severe injury. NSAIDs and topical aloe can help minimize tissue injury.
      (b) Débride clear blisters.
      (c) Use local wound care, whirlpools, topical antibiotics, and débridement as indicated (see section on burns, earlier). Delay surgical intervention. It often looks much worse than it is.

IV. **Hypothermia.**
A. **Defined as** core temperature <35°C (95°F). Need to use a hypothermia thermometer to diagnose because most thermometers will not read low enough.
B. **Predisposing risks.** Chronic illness, altered state of consciousness, elderly, neonates, drugs such as alcohol and barbiturates. Endocrinologic illness (Addison's disease, hypothyroidism, hypopituitarism, hypoglycemia), CNS dysfunction, sepsis.
C. **Causes.** Exposure to cold, metabolic abnormalities.
D. **Clinically.** All changes are progressive and more pronounced with a greater degree of hypothermia.
1. **Presentation** is of progressive decrease in mental status, including confusion, lethargy, coma with areflexia, shivering (or could have loss of shivering reflex), bradycardia, hypotension; cold diuresis; might be hypovolemic.
2. **Cardiac irritability.** Usually progresses from bradycardia to V fib. Do not roughly handle the hypothermic patient; this can induce arrhythmias. ECG might show J wave (Osborne wave).
E. **Treatment.**
1. Remove wet clothing and move to a warm environment.

2. Examine the patient for a full minute (or have on monitor) before beginning CPR because pulse might be very difficult to detect in the bradycardic or hypothermic patient.
3. **For rewarming: If temperature <30°C (86°F), the patient will not generate enough endogenous heat to rewarm himself/herself.** Thus, active rewarming is mandatory.
a. **Passive rewarming.** Use blankets, etc.
b. **Active rewarming.** Use warm water immersion, radiant heat, heated IV fluids, warm, humidified oxygen, external rewarming devices such as hot air external rewarmers. For severe hypothermia, use peritoneal or pleural lavage, mediastinal irrigation, heated hemodialysis or cardiopulmonary bypass. **Although traditionally used, methods such as heated gastric and colonic lavage and heated bladder irrigation do not work and can induce electrolyte abnormalities.**
4. **Peripheral rewarming can be associated with shock, acidosis, and hyperkalemia when cold, acidotic peripheral blood is returned centrally. Central body rewarming is preferred with the extremities left for last.**
F. **No one is dead unless that person is warm and dead.**
1. **If there is V fib,** defibrillate twice and then continue CPR and rewarm to 30°C (86°F). The heart is relatively resistant to drug therapy when cold. Try defibrillation periodically during rewarming.
2. Based on the clinical situation, consider administration of thiamine 100 mg IV, glucose 50 mL of D_{50}, hydrocortisone succinate 100 mg IV, thyroid hormone replacement.

V. Cold Water Drowning
Diving reflex is protective, and a person might survive intact after 40 minutes of cold water drowning. However, this is the exception rather than the rule. Warm patient to at least 86°F or 90°F before abandoning resuscitation.

RHABDOMYOLYSIS

Rhabdomyolysis refers to the breakdown of muscle tissue leading to systemic problems, including renal failure. Renal failure can progress over a number of days, so BUN and creatinine should be checked daily for 72 hours if rhabdomyolysis is suspected. Also watch for developing hyperkalemia (see section on hyperkalemia in Chapter 6 for treatment).
 I. Causes of Rhabdomyolysis Include:
A. Environmental factors, including heat stroke and severe frostbite, some snake bites and scorpion bites.
B. Injuries, including burns and electrical burns, crush injuries, repetitive muscle injury (bongo drumming), compartment syndrome, muscle infarction from ischemia.
C. Toxins, including cocaine, narcotics, amphetamines, gemfibrozil plus an HMG-CoA reductase inhibitor (very rare), amphotericin B, statins, alcohol, carbon monoxide, theophylline.

D. **Overexertion/exercise/metabolic** abnormalities, including prolonged seizures, malignant hyperthermia, neuroleptic malignant syndrome, serotonin syndrome, thyroid storm, hypokalemia, inherited disorders of fatty acid metabolism, diabetic ketoacidosis, glycogen storage diseases, poliomyelitis, dermatomyositis.

E. **Infections** such as influenza, EBV, sepsis, malaria, Legionnaires' disease.

II. **Signs, Symptoms, Systemic Effects.** Muscle aches and cramps, dark/smoky-colored urine from myoglobin, renal failure.

A. **Laboratory/diagnosis.** Myoglobin in urine (positive dipstick for hemoglobin with a negative microscopic exam). Elevated serum CPK (even >100,000 IU/L), myoglobin, aldolase, serum potassium; elevated creatinine and BUN from secondary renal failure. Common lab abnormalities also include hyperphosphatemia and hypocalcemia, followed later in the course by hypercalcemia.

III. **Treatment** is aimed at maintaining a good urine output (200-300 mL/h) and correcting the underlying abnormality.

A. Treat with NS or LR as soon as possible. Maintain urine output at 200 to 300 mL/h. Could require up to 20 L/d. Check electrolytes frequently.

B. One approach is to use mannitol to maintain urine output. Generally give about 12.5 to 25 g (0.5-2.5 g/kg) repeated in one-half hour if there is no diuresis. Maintain urine output with repeated boluses of mannitol and saline as needed. However, if there is no response to the first two boluses, do not give more. Mannitol will cause plasma volume expansion and can precipitate CHF.

C. Others have used a solution of sodium chloride and sodium bicarbonate (sodium 110 mmol/L; chloride 70 mmol/L; bicarbonate 40 mmol/L) in 5% glucose solution to which 10 g of mannitol per liter is added. This is administered at a rate of approximately 12 L/d (in a young, 75-kg adult) to maintain urine output in normal range. IV calcium and vitamin D are indicated if the patient is hypocalcemic.

D. **Alkalinization** of the urine is also important to prevent myoglobin from precipitating in the kidney (see salicylate toxicity section, earlier, for technique).

E. **Dialysis** is used in renal failure.

F. **Fasciotomy** must be performed if there is compartment syndrome.

NECROTIZING FASCIITIS

I. **Definition.** An infection of skin, subcutaneous tissue, and fascia that can also invade underlying muscle, causing myonecrosis. Fournier's gangrene is a subset of this disease localized to the perineal area.

II. **Etiology.** The condition can be caused by multiple bacteria, including gram-positive cocci (*Streptococcus, Staphylococcus*), gram-negative bacilli (*Enterobacter, Proteus, Pseudomonas*), and anaerobes (*Clostridium*). It usually occurs in people with a predisposition because

2

EMERGENCY MEDICINE

of diabetes, peripheral vascular disease, trauma (even minor), or recent surgery.

III. Presentation. Early diagnosis is difficult because symptoms are subtle. Fever and tenderness develop first, followed by swelling and erythema as in cellulitis. It rapidly progresses (1-2 days) to massive SQ edema with blebs, crepitus, and blue, maroon, or black areas of necrosis. Most people present with moderate to severe systemic toxicity, including high fever, tachycardia, delirium, and often shock. Hemolysis and DIC can occur, as can hypocalcemia owing to the necrosis of SQ fat.

IV. Treatment. Treatment includes fluid resuscitation, IV antibiotics, and early incision and drainage with wide débridement of devitalized tissue in the OR. Antibiotics should be broad spectrum to cover mixed aerobe/anaerobe infections (e.g., cefotaxime + either metronidazole or clindamycin). Alternatives include imipenem, piperacillin-tazobactam (Zosyn), or ticarcillin-clavulanate. Calcium and blood products might also be needed because of hypocalcemia and hemolysis.

BIBLIOGRAPHY

American College of Emergency Physicians Clinical Policies Committee and Clinical Policies Subcommittee on Seizure: Clinical policy: Critical issues in the evaluation and management of adult patients presenting to the emergency department with seizures. *Ann Emerg Med* 43:605-625, 2004.

Arbabi S, Ahrns KS, Wahl WL, et al: Beta-blocker use is associated with improved outcomes in adult burn patients. *J Trauma* 56:265-269, 2004.

Baraff LJ, Schriger DL: Orthostatic vital signs: Variation with age, specificity, and sensitivity in detecting a 450 mL blood loss. *Am J Emerg Med* 10:99-103, 1992.

Bizovi K, Aks SE, Paloucek F, et al: Late increase in acetaminophen concentration after overdose of Tylenol Extended Relief. *Ann Emerg Med* 28:549-551, 1996.

Brown MD: Evidence-based emergency medicine: The use of low-molecular weight heparins in acute coronary syndromes [systematic review abstract]. *Ann Emerg Med* 44:76-78, 2004.

Centers for Disease Control and Prevention: Case definitions for infectious conditions under public health surveillance. *MMWR Morb Mortal Wkly Rep* 46(RR-10): 1-55, 1997.

Centers for Disease Control and Prevention: Human rabies prevention—United States, 1999: Recommendations of the Advisory Committee on Immunization Practices (ACIP). *MMWR Morb Mortal Wkly Rep* 48(RR-1):1-21, 1999.

Haude M, Erbel R, Steffen W, et al: Sublingual administration of captopril inpatients with acute myocardial ischemia. *Clin Cardiol* 14:463-468, 1991.

Henry JA, Hoffman JR: Continuing controversy on gut decontamination. *Lancet* 352:420-421, 1998.

Lederle FA, Simel DL: The rational clinical examination: Does this patient have abdominal aortic aneurysm? *JAMA* 281:77-82, 1999.

Mahoney EJ, Biffl WL, Harrington DT, Cioffi WG: Isolated brain injury as a cause of hypotension in the blunt trauma patient. *J Trauma* 55:1065-1069, 2003.

Moore WS, Kashyap VS, Vescera CL, Quinones-Baldrich WJ: Abdominal aortic aneurysm: A 6-year comparison of endovascular versus transabdominal repair. *Ann Surg* 230:298-308, 1999.

Nypaver M, Treloar D: Neutral cervical spine positioning in children. *Ann Emerg Med* 23:208-211, 1994.

Panju AA, Hemmelgarn BR, Guyatt GH, Simel DL: The rational clinical examination: Is this patient having a myocardial infarction? *JAMA* 280:1256-1263, 1998.

Perry HE, Shannon MW: Efficacy of oral versus intravenous *N*-acetylcysteine in acetaminophen overdose: Results of an open-label clinical trial. *J Pediatr* 132:149-152, 1998.

Pollack CV Jr, Roe MT, Peterson ED: 2002 update to the ACC/AHA Guidelines for the management of patients with unstable angina and non-ST-segment elevation MI: Implications for emergency department practice. *Ann Emerg Med* 41:355-369, 2003.

Tenenbein M, Shannon M: The poisoned patient: Is gastrointestinal decontamination all washed up? Two responses. *Pediatr Emerg Care* 14:380-381, 1998.

The UK Small Aneurysm Trial Participants: Mortality results for randomised controlled trial of early elective surgery or ultrasonographic surveillance for small abdominal aortic aneurysms. *Lancet* 352:1649-1655, 1998.

Tintinalli JE, Kelen GD, Stapczynski JS (eds): *Emergency Medicine: A Comprehensive Study Guide*, 5th ed. New York, McGraw-Hill, 1999.

Touger M, Gallagher EJ, Tyrell J: Relationship between venous and arterial carboxyhemoglobin levels in patients with suspected carbon monoxide poisoning. *Ann Emerg Med* 25:481-483, 1995.

Verbeek PR, Geerts WH: Nontapering versus tapering prednisone in acute exacerbations of asthma: A pilot trial. *J Emerg Med* 13:715-719, 1995.

Cardiology

Mark A. Graber

ANGINA

I. Etiology. Angina pectoris is the symptom of myocardial ischemia caused by an imbalance between myocardial oxygen supply and demand.

A. Coronary artery disease (95% of patients).

B. Decreased oxygen supply from anemia, hypotension, vasospasm, myocarditis, embolism, severe hypertrophy (with or without outflow obstruction), or arrhythmias.

C. Increased oxygen demand from exercise, emotional stress, CHF, hypertension, tachycardia, sepsis, etc.

D. Ischemia can occur in patients with normal coronary arteries in the setting of LV hypertrophy, aortic stenosis or insufficiency, hypertrophic cardiomyopathy, coronary vasospasm, myocarditis, embolism, or cocaine abuse.

II. Types.

A. Stable. Intensity, character, and frequency of episodes can be predicted, and angina occurs in response to a known amount of exercise or other stress.

B. Unstable. Intensity, frequency, or duration of episodes is variable or changed and cannot be predicted. Pain is precipitated by less exercise or has longer duration. This includes angina at rest and new-onset angina. **Unstable angina implies coronary artery plaque instability and is classified as an acute coronary syndrome,** as discussed later.

C. Variant. Pain, which can occur at rest, is secondary to vasospasm of coronary arteries and is associated with **ST-segment elevation** that resolves with nitroglycerin or calcium channel blockers.

III. Diagnosis.

A. History. Angina is classically described as substernal chest pressure or heaviness radiating to the left shoulder and arm, neck, or jaw. It is associated with nausea, diaphoresis, and/or shortness of breath. It is usually brought on and exacerbated by exercise or stress and alleviated with rest or sublingual nitroglycerin. Typically, the pain lasts 2 to 10 minutes and rarely 30 minutes.

1. **Atypical presentations** include epigastric pain, indigestion, right arm pain, light-headedness, nausea, and shortness of breath.

2. **Elderly patients might present with** confusion, pallor, syncope, fatigue, or dyspnea.

3. **At least 25% of ischemic episodes are silent, even in patients with a history of typical angina.**

B. Physical exam. An S_4 gallop might be present during an episode. The patient might have dyspnea or diaphoresis or could have a new heart murmur. High-risk features of angina include heart failure and hypotension.

C. Evaluation of patients with chest pain and presumed stable angina. **Which test?** If possible, exercise stress is preferred over pharmacologic stress because it provides prognostic and functional information. **Table 3-1** contains a summary of the test characteristics of various noninvasive tests.

1. **ECG.** During an episode of pain, the ECG might show ST-segment depression or T-wave inversions, or it might be normal. **The absence of ECG changes during an episode of angina does not rule out cardiac ischemia** because the circumflex and posterolateral distributions can be electrically silent.

2. **GXT or treadmill test.** The predictive value of a positive test depends on the prevalence of disease in the population being tested (Bayes' theorem). Specificity is high in particular groups of symptomatic patients but is generally <50% in asymptomatic persons. Compared with men, women (especially young women) have higher rates of false-positive GXT. Overall, the GXT is less sensitive for CAD than is a nuclear study or stress echocardiogram. An early positive GXT might indicate left main disease or three-vessel disease. **Absolute contraindications to GXT** include acute CHF, acute MI, active myocarditis, ongoing unstable angina, recent embolism, dissecting aneurysm, acute illness, thrombophlebitis, moderate to severe aortic stenosis, and an ECG that cannot be interpreted (e.g., LBBB). **Relative contraindications include** severe hypertension, mild to moderate aortic stenosis, hypertrophic obstructive cardiomyopathy, frequent ectopy, and many other conditions that can increase the risk of morbidity in a patient taking a GXT.

3. **Nuclear (thallium or technetium) chemical or exercise stress tests.** Nuclear scans can be useful for patients who cannot tolerate the physical demands of the GXT or in whom the diagnosis will be pursued even in the light of a negative GXT (e.g., those considered to have a high clinical risk of disease). During the test, tracer is taken up by viable, well-perfused myocardium. Areas of myocardial infarction are indicated by fixed perfusion defects with no uptake during rest

TABLE 3-1

SENSITIVITY AND SPECIFICITY OF NONINVASIVE TESTS IN SYMPTOMATIC PATIENTS AND NO WORK-UP BIAS

Test	Sensitivity	Specificity
Exercise stress testing	45%-68%	77%
Thallium stress testing (SPECT)	86%	77%[†]
Stress echocardiography*	76%-86%	88%[†]

*Stress echocardiography is more operator dependent than other tests.
[†]These numbers are an overall approximation based on ranges found in multiple studies.

or exercise. During the nuclear GXT, areas that are hypoperfused (i.e., ischemic) demonstrate thallium uptake only during the postexercise "resting" images. Adenosine, dipyridamole, and dobutamine may be used to augment the perfusion of normal myocardium and shunt blood flow away from areas of relative ischemia. These agents are used in patients who have a contraindication to exercise or are unlikely to attain target heart rates.

4. **Echocardiography.** Allows evaluation of LV function, valvular disease, and wall motion. Images are acquired during peak stress (i.e., during a GXT or with dobutamine) and compared with those at rest. Regional wall-motion abnormalities with stress indicate areas of hypoperfusion or ischemia. Echocardiography is now used more commonly to assess CAD in women because of their high false-positive rate on GXT. It is also gaining increased use among patients with an abnormal baseline ECG, in those receiving digoxin, and after CABG or PTCA. **LBBB and RBBB complicate interpretation** because there is some wall motion abnormality as a result of the depolarization pattern with bundle branch blocks. **LV function and valvular disease are better determined with nonstress echo than with stress echo** because greater attention is paid to valve function with nonstress echo.

5. **MRI/PET scanning.** Cardiac MRI (static, adenosine, dipyridamole, and dobutamine) and PET scanning is a rapidly evolving field with tremendous promise. Many consider MRI with gadolinium to be the gold standard for myocardial viability because the delayed-contrast hyperenhanced images reveal infarcts with unsurpassed spatial resolution (they correlate nearly perfectly with histology) and because nuclear modalities often miss smaller infarcts. For example, myocarditis can mimic acute MI and should be considered when angiography is normal despite chest pain and ST elevation. MRI can define myocardial inflammation and pericardial effusion, and it can reveal accurate and useful information for a variety of other cardiomyopathies.

6. **Coronary angiography** is used to identify foci of coronary disease. It is the evaluation of choice in patients with angina that is poorly responsive to medication or is unstable. It is also indicated in patients whose test results are consistent with a high risk for CAD.

7. **CRP (ultrasensitive-CRP). Generally not recommended.** An elevated CRP is associated with an increased risk of cardiovascular disease. However, the role of CRP levels in risk stratification is not well defined. It clearly has no role in patients with obvious CAD and in those with very low risk. Its best use, if it is to be used at all, is in patients who are at moderate risk for CAD (10-year CAD risk 10%-20%.) **(Fig. 3-1).** An elevated CRP in this group could argue for more intensive risk modification. It is not clear if lowering the CRP per se will reduce cardiac risk.

8. **Homocysteine.** Studies suggest that homocysteine levels correlate with risk of CAD, although specific causal effect is debated. Treatment of elevated levels of homocysteine with B vitamins has not been shown to

3

CARDIOLOGY

ESTIMATE OF 10-YEAR RISK FOR MEN
(Framingham point scores)

Age	Points
20–34	−9
35–39	−4
40–44	0
45–49	3
50–54	6
55–59	8
60–64	10
65–69	11
70–74	12
75–79	13

| Total | Points | | | | |
cholesterol	Age 20–39	Age 40–49	Age 50–59	Age 60–69	Age 70–79
<160	0	0	0	0	0
160–199	4	3	2	1	0
200–239	7	5	3	1	0
240–279	9	6	4	2	1
≥280	11	8	5	3	1

| | Points | | | | |
	Age 20–39	Age 40–49	Age 50–59	Age 60–69	Age 70–79
Nonsmoker	0	0	0	0	0
Smoker	8	5	3	1	1

HDL (mg/dL)	Points
≥60	−1
50–59	0
40–49	1
<40	2

Systolic BP (mmHg)	If untreated	If treated
<120	0	0
120–129	0	1
130–139	1	2
140–159	1	2
≥160	2	3

Point total	10-Year risk %
<0	<1
0	1
1	1
2	1
3	1
4	1
5	2
6	2
7	3
8	4
9	5
10	6
11	8
12	10
13	12
14	16
15	20
16	25
≥17	≥30

10-Year risk _____%

ESTIMATE OF 10-YEAR RISK FOR WOMEN
(Framingham point scores)

Age	Points
20–34	−7
35–39	−3
40–44	0
45–49	3
50–54	6
55–59	8
60–64	10
65–69	12
70–74	14
75–79	16

| Total | Points | | | | |
cholesterol	Age 20–39	Age 40–49	Age 50–59	Age 60–69	Age 70–79
<160	0	0	0	0	0
160–199	4	3	2	1	1
200–239	8	6	4	2	1
240–279	11	8	5	3	2
≥280	13	10	7	4	2

| | Points | | | | |
	Age 20–39	Age 40–49	Age 50–59	Age 60–69	Age 70–79
Nonsmoker	0	0	0	0	0
Smoker	9	7	4	2	1

HDL (mg/dL)	Points
≥60	−1
50–59	0
40–49	1
<40	2

Systolic BP (mmHg)	If untreated	If treated
<120	0	0
120–129	1	3
130–139	2	4
140–159	3	5
≥160	4	6

Point total	10-Year risk %
<9	<1
9	1
10	1
11	1
12	1
13	2
14	2
15	3
16	4
17	5
18	6
19	8
20	11
21	14
22	17
23	22
24	27
≥25	≥30

10-Year risk _____%

FIG. 3-1

Estimation of cardiac risk over 10 years. (*From National Cholesterol Education Program: Third Report of the Expert Panel on Detection, Evaluation, and Treatment of High Blood Cholesterol in Adults [Adult Treatment Panel III]: ATP III at-a-Glance: Quick Desk Reference. Available online at http://www.nhlbi.nih.gov/guidelines/cholesterol/atglance.htm [accessed December 16, 2005].*)

improve outcomes or decrease risk, and likely worsens outcomes. Treatment with folate, B_{12}, and B_6 has actually been shown to increase the rate of restenosis after angioplasty, compared with placebo (FACIT study). Further study is needed before we know how to approach homocysteine levels.

IV. Outpatient Treatment of Stable Angina (also see Guidelines at www.acc.org).

A. Risk assessment addressing blood pressure, glycemic control, and lipids is critical. Patients with CHD risk equivalent (e.g., DM, chronic kidney disease, or 10-year risk >20% as calculated by Framingham equations) should receive intervention as intensive as patients with clinically apparent CHD receive. See Figure 3-1 for risk assessment.

B. Medical management of *stable* angina

1. Aspirin or clopidogrel. Daily aspirin (81-162 mg) inhibits platelet aggregation, reduces death and nonfatal MI, and should be given to all patients unless contraindicated. For those intolerant of or allergic to aspirin, an alternative is clopidogrel (75 mg/d).

2. β-Blockers without intrinsic sympathomimetic activity (e.g., metoprolol) lower myocardial oxygen demand by increasing myocardial perfusion time (prolonging diastole) and by decreasing heart rate, systolic blood pressure, and contractility.

a. Improve survival and prevent adverse events after an MI and in patients with HTN.

b. Especially useful in patients whose angina is regularly provoked by exercise and in patients with DM or *stable* CHF (but might limit exercise tolerance).

c. Patients with asthma and COPD usually tolerate selective β-blockers.

d. Abrupt discontinuation of β-blockers can precipitate rebound tachycardia.

e. Avoid in vasospastic angina.

f. **Contraindications.** See section on ST elevation MI under "Acute Coronary Syndromes."

3. ACE inhibitors are not used as a primary therapy for angina. However, they are indicated in many angina patients because of coexisting DM, HTN, LVH, CHF, etc. They should be used in *all* patients with prior history of MI. Angiotensin receptor blockers (e.g., ARBs, valsartan, candesartan) can be substituted for ACE inhibitors in patients who are intolerant (cough, angioedema). ARBs may not decrease the risk of MI's however.

4. Calcium channel blockers (verapamil, diltiazem, amlodipine, felodipine). Calcium channel blockers (verapamil and diltiazem preferred if patient tolerates them and has no CHF) relieve angina symptoms with efficacy similar to β-blockers. Calcium channel blockers decrease coronary vasospasm and improve collateral flow.

a. Efficacy at preventing adverse outcomes has *not* been established beyond simple lowering of BP.

b. Avoid short-acting nifedipine, which increases adverse events.

   c. Verapamil and diltiazem have negative chronotropic and inotropic effects, which can lead to CHF in patients with impaired LV function.

   d. **Adverse effects.** Heart block or asystole can develop in patients with AV node or sinus node disease. Other common side effects of calcium channel blockers include headache, ankle swelling, GI upset, and constipation. Diltiazem and verapamil are contraindicated after MI in those with CHF or impaired systolic function.

5. **Nitrates** (e.g., nitropaste, nitroglycerin patches, isosorbide dinitrate). Effects include venous and arteriolar vasodilation, which decreases oxygen demand. Tolerance can develop but can be overcome by providing an 8-hour nitrate-free interval each day. Preparations include oral, transdermal patches, ointment, sublingual tablets, or spray. A common side effect is headache, which usually responds to aspirin or acetaminophen and tends to improve with continued use. Sublingual nitroglycerin tablets (0.4 mg prn) or spray are used for acute episodes of angina and may be repeated at 5-minute intervals for up to three doses. *Patients should be instructed to go to the ED immediately if angina is not relieved after one dose of nitroglycerin.*

6. **Enhanced external counterpulsation** involves intermittent compression of the legs and can improve angina in refractory cases. However, additional study is needed.

7. **Other important targets of therapy.** Smoking cessation, exercise, and control of DM and HTN are essential components of prevention. Proper diet, weight management, and exercise are important parts of therapeutic lifestyle changes that in turn affect control of HTN and DM. Regular exercise increases myocardial perfusion and slows disease progression. The importance of exercise was demonstrated in a **small randomized, controlled trial of exercise versus angioplasty in stable patients with preserved systolic function. This trial showed better event-free survival and exercise capacity in the exercise group than the angioplasty group.**

V. **Revascularization in the Angina Patient.**

A. **Indications for CABG in angina patients** (Box 3-1)

1. **CABG is not indicated** for patients with stable angina who have borderline coronary stenoses (50%-60% diameter in locations other than the left main coronary artery) and no demonstrable ischemia on noninvasive testing.

2. Advanced age alone is not a contraindication to CABG. Coronary arteries must be anatomically amenable to bypass.

B. **Intracoronary stenting**

1. PCI confers survival advantage *only* in the setting of acute myocardial infarction. Outside of this setting, PCI has not been shown to prolong survival, and its primary indication is to alleviate symptoms and improve quality of life.

2. **PCI has less associated morbidity than CABG, but patients might require reintervention** (CABG or repeat PCI). Drug-eluting stents appear to dramatically reduce the risk of restenosis; studies defining their role

> **BOX 3-1**
>
> **INDICATIONS FOR CABG IN PATIENTS WITH ANGINA**
>
> INDICATIONS FOR CABG
>
> **Survival Advantage if**
> - Left main disease (>50% luminal narrowing)
> - >70% stenosis in both the proximal LAD and circumflex arteries ("left main equivalent")
> - Three-vessel CAD (>50% stenosis), especially with LV dysfunction (ejection fraction <50%) or large areas of demonstrably ischemic myocardium
>
> OTHER INDICATIONS
>
> **Stable Angina with**
> - Proximal two-vessel disease that includes the LAD and either EF <50% or demonstrable ischemia on noninvasive testing
> - Any one- or two-vessel disease with high-risk criteria on noninvasive testing and a large area of viable myocardium or disabling angina despite maximal noninvasive therapy

are ongoing. PCI can lower (but not always eliminate) the need for antianginal medication.

3. Diabetic patients and women have had less-favorable outcomes with PCI than have nondiabetic patients and men. Consider CABG in these patients.

4. For required anticoagulation and other aspects of treatment, see the section on ST elevation MI under "Acute Coronary Syndromes."

5. **Transmyocardial revascularization** uses a laser to create channels through the myocardium. It can reduce anginal pain, but the effect might be mediated by nerve destruction (i.e., the patient can no longer feel anginal pain) or because of revascularization. There are no long-term outcome studies, and this treatment is currently considered experimental.

ACUTE CORONARY SYNDROMES

I. **General information.**

A. **Terminology**

1. **Acute ST elevation MI** (STEMI [preferred term]; also called "Q-wave MI" and "transmural infarction").

2. **Acute non-ST elevation MI** (preferred term; also called "non-Q wave MI" or "subendocardial MI"). There is **minimal prognostic difference** between STEMI and non-ST elevation MI.

3. **Unstable angina** shows no evidence of myocardial necrosis (e.g., normal troponins), but implies unstable, vulnerable plaque that can be potentially life threatening.

B. **Treatment of acute chest pain** (see Chapter 2 for ED management). Inpatient treatment is indicated for unstable angina, prolonged anginal episode (which might represent an infarction) and MI.

C. **The decision to admit is based on the history, because 50% of patients with acute MI have an initially nondiagnostic ECG** and cardiac enzymes will not be positive for up to 6 hours after an infarction. If ECG changes indicate MI, or if enzymes are positive, treat as per MI section (later).

D. **The presence or absence of traditional risk factors for coronary disease** (e.g., diabetes, hypertension, smoking, family history of premature disease, dyslipidemia) **should *not* be used to determine whether a syndrome represents an acute coronary syndrome (ACS).**

II. **Unstable Angina.**

A. **Unstable angina has three main manifestations: rest angina** (angina occurring at rest and prolonged, usually >20 min), **new-onset angina,** and **increasing angina** (frequent, longer in duration, or occurring with less physical stress).

B. **Management** of unstable angina

1. **Admit to monitored bed.** Confine to bed rest with bedside commode, continuous ECG monitoring, oxygen, and IV access. Obtain screening lab tests, including cardiac enzymes, CBC, glucose, BUN, creatinine, UA, serum electrolytes (including sodium, potassium, chloride, CO_2, and magnesium), and PT, PTT, and INR if planning to anticoagulate.

2. **Obtain serial cardiac enzyme levels.** Cardiac troponin I and T are proteins that are highly sensitive and specific for myocardial injury. These are now considered the standard markers. An alternative is creatine phosphokinase (CPK). Obtain an MB isoenzyme level if the total CPK is elevated because CPK can be the result of both cardiac and other muscle breakdown. The CPK-MB is more sensitive than the troponin at hours 4 through 8 (84% versus 74%) and at 8 to 12 hours (94% versus 88%). The troponin is essentially 100% sensitive at 12 hours. The troponin can remain elevated for 4 to 7 days. Either troponin or CPK levels should be checked q8h × 3 (although if the CPK and troponin are negative at 12 hours after pain resolves, an MI is effectively ruled out). Myoglobin is also being used as a marker and becomes positive earlier after an MI but has no benefit over troponin. **Causes of a false positive troponin** include warfarin, pericarditis, pulmonary embolism, myocarditis, sepsis/critical illness/shock, circulating rheumatoid factor (e.g., in patients with rheumatoid arthritis), heterophilic antibodies (e.g., monoclonal antibodies, or secondary to microbial antigens or foreign proteins), renal failure.

3. **Serial ECGs** with intervals depending on circumstances.

4. **Antiplatelet agents** include aspirin 325 mg, if there is no contraindication, or clopidogrel 300 mg if aspirin is contraindicated. Continue clopidogrel 75 mg/day for 1 to 9 months *with* aspirin if patient is not a candidate for intervention (PTCA, CABG). **Clopidogrel should not be given 5 to 7 days before CABG.** The greatest benefit is within the first month.

5. **Anticoagulation.** For ongoing pain, start heparin, either LMW or weight-based dosing of unfractionated heparin (preferred in patients going for

catheterization or possible CABG). See Chapter 6 for dosing and monitoring strategies.

6. **Glycoprotein inhibitors** (IIB/IIIA inhibitors, e.g., eptifibatide, tirofiban, or abciximab) should be used in patients receiving PCI. Their use in other patients is controversial and the best data suggest at most a small benefit or perhaps even worse outcomes in those not going for intervention.

7. **Increase antianginals.** Topical, oral, IV, or SL **nitrates, β-blockers, calcium channel blockers.** Morphine (2-5 mg q10-20 min) may be given for analgesia, preload reduction, and anxiety. See stable angina section for details on each drug class.

8. **ACE inhibitors** are desirable in settings of frank MI (especially anterior), LV systolic dysfunction, pulmonary edema,or refractory hypertension in the absence of contraindications. Use in unstable angina is less well established. Avoid with SBP <100 mm Hg or if BP is more than 30 mm lower than baseline. ACE inhibitors do have some anti-ischemic effect and might be helpful on this basis.

9. **Other medications.** Sedation might be beneficial in certain patients. Acetaminophen and a stool softener may be given for headache and to prevent the need to strain, respectively.

C. **High-risk angina patients likely will benefit from early intervention if they have the following signs:**

1. **Recurrent angina/ischemia at rest or with low-level activities** despite intensive anti-ischemic therapy.

2. **Elevated troponin; new or presumably new ST-segment depression.**

3. **Recurrent angina/ischemia with CHF symptoms,** an S_3 gallop, pulmonary edema, worsening rales, or new or worsening MR.

4. **High-risk findings on noninvasive stress testing;** depressed LV systolic function (EF <40%); hemodynamic instability; sustained ventricular tachycardia; PCI within past 6 months or any prior CABG.

D. If a patient does not meet high-risk criteria, noninvasive stress testing should be considered. Assessment of LV function is important for prognostication and clarifying therapeutic strategy.

E. **On discharge** optimize therapy for angina and address modification of risk factors (see previous section).

III. **ST Elevation MI (STEMI)**

A. **Infarct location. Table 3-2** shows correlation of ECG changes with location of infarct.

B. Continue and intensify treatment as for ACS. See earlier discussion and Chapter 2.

C. **Reperfusion is the hallmark of STEMI therapy.**

1. **Fibrinolysis versus primary PCI.**

a. **Indications for primary PCI** are shown in Box 3-2. See www.acc.org for class II and III recommendations.

b. **Indications and contraindication for fibrinolysis** are shown in Box 3-3 and Box 3-4.

3

CARDIOLOGY

TABLE 3-2

INFARCT LOCATION BY ECG

ECG Changes	Location of Injury	Coronary Artery Involved
II, III, aV_F, V_{R4}, V_{R5}, V_{R6}*	Inferior wall	RCA or dominant distal left circumflex
V_{1-3}	Anteroseptal	LAD
V_{3-5}	Anterior wall	LAD
V_6, I, aV_L	Lateral	Marginal branch off circumflex or diagonal off LAD
V_8, V_9 elevation; V_1-V_3 depression	Posterior MI	RCA

*Right-sided chest leads (R), now a Class 1 recommendation in suspected inferior wall MI.

2. **Any change in neurologic status after fibrinolysis is considered to represent intracranial hemorrhage until proven otherwise and warrants immediate withholding of all antithrombotic therapy. Brain imaging should be pursued on an emergent basis.** Use reverse coagulopathy with cryoprecipitate, fresh frozen plasma, activated factor VIIa, protamine, and platelets as indicated.
3. **Indications for coronary angiography in those receiving fibrinolysis** are persistent hemodynamic or electrical instability; shock, if the patient is a candidate for revascularization; and mechanical complications from STEMI, such as VSD or severe MR, if the patient is a surgical candidate.
4. **The following suggest successful reperfusion:** relief of symptoms, maintenance or restoration of hemodynamic and/or electrical stability, and a reduction of at least 50% of the initial ST-segment elevation injury pattern on a follow-up ECG 60 to 90 minutes after initiation of therapy.

BOX 3-2

AMERICAN HEART ASSOCIATION CLASS I INDICATIONS FOR PRIMARY PCI IN PATIENTS WITH STEMI

- Symptom onset within last 12 hours, goal of <90 minutes to PCI *and* either
  - ST elevation (>0.1 mV) in two contiguous leads
  - New left bundle branch block (LBBB)
  - Severe CHF and/or pulmonary edema (Killip class 3)
- Age less than 75 years in shock within the first 36 hours of STEMI if PCI can be performed within 18 hours of development of shock
- Recurrent MI
- Other
  - If pain duration is <3 h and PCI will be delayed for >1 h, thrombolytics are preferred.
  - CABG may be preferable in those >75 years of age.
  - PCI is preferred if there is a contraindication to thrombolytics such as bleeding risk.

BOX 3-3

AMERICAN HEART ASSOCIATION RECOMMENDATIONS FOR THROMBOLYTIC USE IN MYOCARDIAL INFARCTION

CLASS 1 RECOMMENDATIONS FOR THE USE OF THROMBOLYTICS IN MYOCARDIAL INFARCTION

- At least 1 mm of ST-segment elevation in at least two adjacent limb leads *or*
- At least 1-2 mm of ST-segment elevation in at least two adjacent precordial leads *or*
- Presence of a new complete bundle branch block that obscures the ST-segment analysis

plus

- History suggestive of myocardial infarction
- <12 hours since the onset of pain
- Age <75 years (although many physicians treat the elderly with thrombolytics)

CLASS 2 RECOMMENDATIONS FOR THE USE OF THROMBOLYTICS IN MYOCARDIAL INFARCTION

- The above ST elevations and age >75 years
- The above ST elevations and 12-24 h after onset of infarction
- Blood pressure of >180 systolic and >100 diastolic in a patient with a "high-risk" myocardial infarction (e.g., the high risk of the MI mitigates the warning about thrombolytic use in uncontrolled hypertension)

---

5. **Thrombolytic regimens include:**
a. **Streptokinase** 1.5 million IU given IV over 30 minutes to 1 hour. Give concurrent heparin.
b. **Alteplase** (recombinant tPA) based on weight: Bolus 15 mg, infusion 0.75 mg/kg over 30 minutes (maximum 50 mg), then 0.5 mg/kg not to exceed 35 mg over the next 60 minutes to an overall maximum of 100 mg. Concurrent heparin infusion is used in most studies.

BOX 3-4

AMERICAN HEART ASSOCIATION CONTRAINDICATIONS TO THE USE OF THROMBOLYTICS IN MYOCARDIAL INFARCTION

ABSOLUTE CONTRAINDICATIONS TO THE USE OF THROMBOLYTIC THERAPY IN MI

Previous hemorrhagic stroke at any time, or stroke within the last 12 months

Known intracranial neoplasm

Active internal bleeding (but not menstrual bleeding)

Suspected aortic dissection

RELATIVE CONTRAINDICATIONS TO THE USE OF THROMBOLYTIC THERAPY IN MI

Uncontrolled hypertension (>180/110) at time of presentation

History of bleeding diathesis, ongoing anticoagulation (INR >2-3)

Trauma, including traumatic CPR within 2-4 wk, major surgery within 3 wk

Noncompressible vascular punctures (e.g., subclavian line)

Internal bleeding within the last 2-4 wk

Pregnancy

Peptic ulcer disease (bleeding or not)

Severe chronic hypertension

c. **Reteplase** (recombinant PA) 10 units over 2 minutes; repeat in 30 minutes. Give concurrent heparin infusion.

d. **Tenecteplase** as a bolus with amount based on weight: 30 mg for weight <60 kg; 35 mg for 60 to 69 kg; 40 mg for 70 to 79 mg; 45 mg for 80 to 89 kg; 50 mg for 90 kg or more. Use concurrent heparin.

6. **Heparin. Low-molecular-weight heparin (LMWH) has no established role with thrombolytics.**

a. Unfractionated heparin should be given to all STEMI patients receiving primary PCI, CABG, or alteplase, reteplase, or tenecteplase. See Chapter 6 for dosing and details of anticoagulation.

b. Patients treated with **nonselective fibrinolytic agents** (streptokinase, anistreplase, urokinase) have less compelling need for unfractionated heparin unless they are at high risk for systemic emboli (large or anterior MI, A Fib), previous embolus, or known LV thrombus. Routine unfractionated heparin for streptokinase is a Class IIB recommendation. However, it is generally given.

c. Platelet counts require daily monitoring.

d. Unfractionated heparin probably should be given for at least 48 hours or until the patient is ambulatory.

e. Discontinuing heparin after 72 hours or so can result in rebound angina because of a relatively hypercoagulable state from antithrombin III deficiency.

D. Other medications in STEMI

1. **Daily aspirin (noncoated; initial dose of 325 mg orally *and chewed*; maintenance dose of 81 to 162 mg) reduces mortality** and should be given indefinitely after STEMI to all patients without a true aspirin allergy.

2. **Clopidogrel** (with aspirin)

a. For 1 month after bare metal stent implantation.

b. For several months after drug-eluting stent implantation (3 mo for sirolimus, 6 mo for paclitaxel), and up to 12 months in patients who are not at high risk for bleeding.

c. Clopidogrel should be withheld for at least 5 days, and preferably for 7 days, before CABG unless the urgency for revascularization outweighs the risks of excess bleeding.

d. Clopidogrel is probably indicated in patients receiving fibrinolytic therapy who are unable to take aspirin because of hypersensitivity or major gastrointestinal intolerance.

e. **If the patient is going to be managed noninvasively, add clopidogrel 75 mg/day to aspirin for 1 to 9 months after STEMI.**

3. **Intravenous nitroglycerin** (NTG)

a. **Indications** include ongoing ischemic discomfort, control of hypertension, or management of pulmonary congestion. **There is little evidence that NTG affects mortality. Thus, intravenous nitroglycerin should not preclude therapy with other proven mortality-reducing interventions such as β-blockers or ACE inhibitors.** So if the blood pressure is marginal, choose a β-blocker rather than NTG.

b. **Contraindications** include systolic blood pressure <90 mm Hg or ≥30 mm Hg below baseline, severe bradycardia (<50 bpm), tachycardia (>100 bpm), or suspected RV infarction (use cautiously!). Nitrates should not be administered to patients who have received a phosphodiesterase inhibitor for erectile dysfunction within the last 24 hours (48 h for tadalafil).

4. **β-Blockers** (e.g., metoprolol 5-mg IV aliquots, titrate to pulse and BP)

a. **β-Blockers reduce mortality and should be administered promptly to patients who are hemodynamically stable and have no contraindication, irrespective of concomitant fibrinolytic therapy or performance of primary PCI.**

b. **Absolute contraindications** include severe bradycardia, sick sinus syndrome, preexisting high degree of AV block, and severe, *unstable* LV systolic failure.

c. **Relative contraindications.** Lengthening of the PR interval 0.24 seconds, second- or third-degree AV block, bradycardia with pulse <50, SBP <90 mm Hg, pulmonary artery wedge pressure greater than 20 to 24 mm Hg, rales audible in greater than one-third of the lung fields, wheezing or history of asthma or bronchospasm, and recent use of IV calcium channel blockers.

5. **ACE inhibitors** should be considered for all STEMI patients (acutely and long term) as long as there is no hypotension (SBP <100 or <30 mm Hg below baseline). ACE inhibitors should be administered orally and carefully titrated within the first 24 hours of STEMI, especially to patients with anterior infarction, pulmonary congestion, radiographic evidence of CHF or LVEF <0.40, in the absence of hypotension or known contraindications to the class of medications. ARBs (valsartan and candesartan) are an alternative.

6. **Aldosterone blockers.** Spironolactone (25-50 mg) added to ACE inhibitor therapy given **during convalescence** decreases long-term mortality and is indicated in patients who have CHF or EF <40% on Day 3 to 14 after an MI and in diabetic patients. Eplerenone (25-50 mg daily) is a more expensive alternative with more drug interactions. There is a serious risk of hyperkalemia with these drugs, requiring vigilant monitoring of serum potassium (e.g., after 48 hours, 1 week, 4 weeks, and then monthly after starting treatment). **Aldosterone blockers are contraindicated in** men with serum creatinine >2.5, women with serum creatinine >2.0, and patients with hyperkalemia or taking other potassium-sparing diuretics.

7. **Prophylactic antiarrhythmic therapy (beyond β-blockers) is not indicated and can be harmful,** but treat arrhythmias as per protocols in Chapter 1.

8. **Insulin** infusion to normalize blood glucose is recommended for patients with STEMI and diabetes, especially if the course is complicated.

9. **Warfarin** can be given to

a. Anyone with another indication for warfarin (e.g., DVT, A Fib).

b. **Aspirin allergic patients with**

(1) No stent: INR 2.5 to 3.5.

(2) Stent: INR 2.0 to 3.0 *plus* clopidogrel.

  c. Patients with LV thrombus for 3 months and indefinitely if at low risk for bleeding.

10. Oxygen. Supplemental oxygen should be administered to patients with arterial oxygen desaturation (Sao_2 <90%). It is reasonable to administer supplemental oxygen to all patients with uncomplicated STEMI during the first 6 hours.

11. Morphine sulfate (2-4 mg IV, with increments of 2-8 mg IV repeated at 5- to 15-min intervals) is the analgesic of choice for management of pain associated with STEMI. May increase mortality; no good randomized trials.

12. Other considerations. Hypotensive patients without clinical evidence of volume overload should receive rapid volume loading with an intravenous infusion. Vasopressor support should be administered for hypotension that does not resolve after volume loading. Smoking cessation should be documented; it is a commonly scrutinized *quality indicator* used by external entities to measure performance. Other quality indicators are aspirin and β-blocker on admission and discharge, time to reperfusion, and ACE inhibitor at discharge for systolic dysfunction.

E. Dysrhythmias (see Chapter 1 for acute treatment of dysrhythmias). **Implantable cardioverter defibrillators (ICD) are indicated for:**

1. V fib or hemodynamically significant sustained V Tach more than 2 days after STEMI, provided the arrhythmia is not judged due to transient or reversible ischemia or reinfarction (level 1A recommendation).

2. Patients more than 1 month after STEMI with LVEF between 0.31 and 0.40, who demonstrate additional evidence of electrical instability (e.g., nonsustained V tach), and have inducible V Fib or sustained V Tach on electrophysiologic testing (level IB recommendation).

3. See CHF section for indications for ICD in CHF.

F. Types of heart block and indications for a pacemaker in patients with STEMI are shown in **Boxes 3-5 and 3-6.**

BOX 3-5
HEART BLOCKS BY MI LOCATION
ANTERIOR MYOCARDIAL INFARCTION
Bundle branch blocks
Mobitz type II second-degree heart block
INFERIOR MYOCARDIAL INFARCTION
Bradycardia from
Mobitz type I second-degree heart block
Third-degree heart block

> **BOX 3-6**
>
> **CLASS I INDICATIONS FOR PACEMAKER IN PATIENTS WITH AN ACUTE MYOCARDIAL INFARCTION**
>
> New left bundle branch block plus first-degree AV block
>
> New right bundle branch block plus left anterior fascicular block plus first-degree AV block
>
> Mobitz type II heart block
>
> Third-degree heart block

3

CARDIOLOGY

COMPLICATIONS OF ACUTE MYOCARDIAL INFARCTION

I. **Left Ventricular Dysfunction (see section on congestive failure for long-term management of CHF).**

A. **The extent of LV dysfunction in the days after an acute MI provides prognostic information** and should be measured in all STEMI patients (e.g., by echocardiogram or radionuclide study).

B. Catheterization should be considered for patients with an LVEF <0.40.

C. Patients with LVEF >0.40 should undergo exercise testing either in the hospital or early after discharge.

1. Patients with baseline abnormalities that compromise ECG interpretation should have echocardiography or myocardial perfusion imaging.

2. Exercise testing should not be performed within 2 to 3 days of STEMI in patients who have not undergone successful reperfusion.

3. Exercise testing should not be performed to evaluate patients with STEMI who have unstable postinfarction angina, decompensated CHF, life-threatening cardiac arrhythmias, noncardiac conditions that severely limit their ability to exercise, or other absolute contraindications to exercise testing.

II. **Right Ventricular Dysfunction and Infarction.**

A. **RV dysfunction is especially common with an inferior wall MI.** Pronounced hypotension in response to nitrates strongly suggests the diagnosis.

B. **The triad of clear lung fields, hypotension, and jugular venous distention in a patient with an inferior infarction is highly suggestive of an RV infarction.** Jugular venous distention has a sensitivity of 88% and a specificity of 69% for RV infarction. Kussmaul's venous sign (distention of the jugular vein during inspiration) is also highly suggestive. There might also be tricuspid regurgitation, RV gallops, and AV dissociation.

C. **An ECG with right-sided chest leads can confirm RV MI.** A 1-mm ST-segment elevation in the right precordial lead (CR_{4R}) is highly predictive for an RV MI (sensitivity, 70%; specificity, 100%). Other ECG findings include right bundle branch block and complete heart block.

D. Echocardiography can reveal RV wall dyskinesia and dilation. There might be abnormal interventricular septal motion because of a reversal in the transseptal pressure gradient secondary to increased RV end-diastolic pressure.

E. In addition to conduction deficits, patients with RV MI can develop RV mural thrombi (placing them at high risk for pulmonary embolism), tricuspid regurgitation, and pericarditis.

F. Treat RV infarction/failure as follows:

1. **Maintain RV preload with volume loading as indicated.** An infusion of IV normal saline often corrects hypotension and increases cardiac output. Nitrates, diuretics, and morphine sulfate are all relatively contraindicated, because these medications decrease preload.

2. **Reduce RV afterload if there is concomitant LV dysfunction by treating left-sided CHF.**

3. **Initiate inotropic support with dobutamine if the patient is not stabilized with a saline infusion.**

4. **Begin sequential atrioventricular pacing if the patient develops complete heart block.**

5. **Initiate thrombolytic therapy or perform angioplasty as indicated.**

G. Among patients who survive a right ventricular infarction, RV function returns to nearly normal levels over time. After infarction that leads to clinically significant RV dysfunction, it is reasonable to delay CABG surgery for 4 weeks to allow recovery of contractile performance.

III. Arrhythmias Complicating Acute MI.

A. Premature ventricular complexes are common in the first 72 hours after an MI. Treatment of isolated ventricular premature beats, couplets, and nonsustained VT is *not* recommended unless they lead to hemodynamic compromise. Antiarrhythmic therapy is not indicated for accelerated idioventricular rhythm. Antiarrhythmic therapy is not indicated for accelerated junctional rhythm.

B. Ventricular tachycardia or fibrillation is treated using the protocol in Figure 1-1.

C. Supraventricular tachycardias including PSVT, A Fib, and atrial flutter are discussed in Chapter 1.

1. Tachycardia increases O_2 demand; treat promptly.

2. Rule out reversible underlying causes (e.g., hypokalemia, hypomagnesemia, and hypoxia).

IV. Atrioventricular Blocks.

A. See Box 3-6 for pacemaker indications.

B. Second-degree Mobitz I (Wenckebach) block is common in acute inferior infarction. See the ACLS protocol in Figure 1-3. Permanent pacemaker is rarely required, because Wenckebach block usually resolves within days.

C. Second-degree Mobitz II block usually occurs in patients with acute anterior MI. A permanent pacemaker should be placed if the block persists.

D. Third-degree AV block is often transient in the setting of an acute inferior MI. When associated with an anterior MI, it often represents necrosis of the conducting tissue below the AV node and could be permanent, requiring permanent pacemaker implantation.

E. Bundle branch block

1. LBBB is the most common bundle branch block seen with an MI. The combination of RBBB and a left anterior hemiblock is also often seen.

2. When a bundle branch block occurs, the site of the infarction is usually anteroseptal, and the infarct is often large.

3. If the patient is known to have an old bundle branch or fascicular block, a temporary pacemaker is not necessarily indicated unless dictated by the patient's symptoms and hemodynamic status.

V. Left Ventricular Aneurysm.

A. Incidence is 7% to 15%. LV aneurysm is suggested by persistent ST elevations weeks to months after an MI.

B. It can lead to CHF, systemic emboli (caused by mural thrombus formation), and recurrent arrhythmias.

C. It can be demonstrated on echocardiogram or radionuclide ventriculogram.

D. Indications for surgery include symptomatic CHF, angina, malignant ventricular arrhythmias, and systemic embolism.

E. Some authors recommend long-term anticoagulation to reduce the risk of embolization.

VI. Recurrent Chest Pain; differential and treatment.

A. Extension of MI

1. Occurs in 10% to 15%.

2. Is characterized by re-elevation of cardiac enzymes and additional ECG changes.

3. Has a higher risk in the 12 months after an MI in patients with non–Q wave infarcts than in patients with transmural infarcts.

B. Angina (for treatment and diagnosis, see previous section). If post-MI angina is refractory to medical therapy, cardiac catheterization might be indicated to define anatomy and suitability for revascularization or to perform PTCA.

C. Pericarditis can occur after an MI or as the result of a viral infection (especially Coxsackievirus) or secondary to uremia. In the setting of an infarction, pericarditis usually occurs after a large transmural infarct.

1. **Physical exam** could reveal an audible friction rub.

2. **Symptoms:** Pleuritic pain might be present and is exacerbated by lying supine and relieved by sitting forward. It tends to radiate to the shoulder and be worse on inspiration.

3. **ECG might show diffuse ST-segment elevations and PR depression,** and echocardiogram often reveals the presence of a pericardial effusion. However, the ECG is falsely negative in up to 20%, and absence of pericardial fluid does not rule out pericarditis.

3

CARDIOLOGY

4. **Treatment of pericarditis**

a. **After STEMI,** aspirin is recommended for treatment of pericarditis. Doses as high as 650 mg orally (enteric coated) every 4 to 6 hours might be needed. Colchicine 0.6 mg PO q12h has also been used. Avoid other NSAIDS in the peri-infarction period due to lack of adequate platelet inhibition. Anticoagulation should be immediately discontinued if pericardial effusion develops or increases. Steroids can be used as a last resort but should otherwise be avoided.

b. **If viral/inflammatory such as from lupus,** treat with NSAIDs, especially indomethacin. Consider colchicine 0.6 mg PO q12h. Steroids may be used for viral pericarditis.

D. **Pulmonary embolism** (see section in Chapter 4).

E. **Pneumonia.**

F. **Dressler's Syndrome.**

1. **Cause** is pleuropericarditis occurring usually 2 to 4 weeks after an MI. It possibly represents an autoimmune inflammatory reaction. It can also occur after cardiac surgery.

2. **Symptoms** are pericardial and pleural pain.

3. **Signs** are fever, pericardial friction rub (might be intermittent), and perhaps decreased breath sounds at lung bases and a pleural rub. Chest radiograph might show enlarged cardiac silhouette because of pericardial effusion. ECG might show diffuse ST-segment elevations, decreased R-wave voltage, and occasionally electrical alternans. An echocardiogram might show pericardial effusion.

4. **Treatment.** Dressler's syndrome is usually self-limited. Aspirin is the drug of choice. NSAIDS (e.g., indomethacin or ibuprofen) are second line; prednisone 60 mg daily is third line. Taper prednisone as soon as possible. Avoid anticoagulation to prevent pericardial bleeding and tamponade.

CARDIAC ARRHYTHMIAS

For outpatient assessment, an event monitor worn for a prolonged period and activated when the patient has symptoms is more sensitive than a 24- to 48-hour Holter monitor and is the preferred modality for intermittent or sporadic arrhythmias.

I. **Atrial Fibrillation.** A Fib results in the loss of atrial contraction and an irregular ventricular rate. It is clinically recognized by an irregularly irregular heart rate. Some causes include HTN, hyperthyroidism, acute pulmonary embolism, CHF, structural and valvular disease (especially mitral valve), acute alcohol use ("holiday heart"), and postoperative state, especially thoracotomy. Incidence increases with age.

A. See the protocol in Figure 1-5 for acute management of A Fib with a rapid ventricular response.

B. **Rhythm versus rate control.** The AFFIRM trial (Wyse et al, 2002) showed no benefit of "rhythm control" (defibrillation and antiarrhythmic therapy) over "rate control," but the study population had relatively preserved systolic function. Although the results might not extend to those with systolic dysfunction, those with a rate-control strategy had fewer side effects from medications and fewer hospital admissions.

C. **Drugs for rate control.** Use agents that increase the refractory period of the AV node (digoxin, verapamil, diltiazem, or β-blockers). The ventricular rate should be decreased to a range of 60 to100 bpm. **Generally, β-blockers are the drugs of choice followed by calcium channel blockers. The use of digoxin is discouraged because it is proarrhythmic and less effective than other drugs.** Digoxin is useful in rate control in those who are at bed rest; it does not control heart rate during exercise.

D. **Anticoagulation in atrial fibrillation**

1. **Anticoagulation with warfarin to a target INR of 2.0 to 3.0 is indicated in** patients with prior thromboembolism, TIA, systolic dysfunction, heart failure, older age (>75 years), diabetes, hypertension, and mitral stenosis. Aspirin can be used but is less effective.

2. **Aspirin (325 mg) or warfarin is indicated in** patients 65 to 75 years of age with none of the above risks ("lone A Fib").

3. **Aspirin (325 mg) is indicated in** patients younger than 65 years of age without the above risk factors.

4. **Patients experiencing A Fib after cardiac surgery** should be anticoagulated for at least several weeks after sinus rhythm returns, especially if risk factors for stroke are present.

5. **Atrial flutter.** Some would anticoagulate those with atrial flutter, but the evidence is not as compelling as for A Fib.

E. **Many patients with A Fib convert back to sinus rhythm spontaneously** (50% or so in first 24 h). You may attempt to convert back to a sinus rhythm with either class III drugs (amiodarone or sotalol) or class I drugs (quinidine or procainamide), flecainide, or electrical cardioversion. However, these **patients should be anticoagulated for 3 weeks before cardioversion if A Fib has been present for more than 48 hours.** Anticoagulation should be continued for 2 weeks after conversion. Ibutilide is out of favor.

F. **Flecainide and propafenone** can be used PRN in selected outpatients to convert A Fib. See Alboni et al, 2004, for details.

G. **Ablation procedures** can cure both A Fib and atrial flutter. A Fib ablation has a lower success rate than atrial flutter ablation and is technically more difficult.

II. **Paroxysmal Supraventricular Tachycardia.** PSVT is most commonly caused by atrioventricular node reentry with 1:1 atrioventricular conduction, although it can also be caused by sinus node reentry,

3

CARDIOLOGY

atrial ectopy, or an accessory pathway. It may be associated with Wolff–Parkinson–White syndrome.

A. PSVT must be distinguished from a ventricular tachycardia.

B. See the protocol in Figure 1-5 for acute management.

C. PSVT may be chronically suppressed with calcium channel blockers (verapamil and diltiazem). However, radioablation of the accessory pathway is both safe and effective.

III. Ventricular Tachycardia. V Tach is a ventricular rate generally 150 to 180 bpm. Rhythm tends to be regular. By definition, it is characterized by three or more consecutive complexes arising inferior to the bifurcation of the bundle of His at a rate that exceeds 100 bpm.

A. V Tach can be caused by heart disease, electrolyte imbalances, hypoxia, or drug toxicity. The most frequent cause of sustained ventricular tachycardia is reentry along the margin of old infarcted myocardium.

B. See the protocol in Figures 1-1 and 1-6 for acute treatment.

C. Because recurrence rates are high, long-term antiarrhythmic therapy or implantation of a cardioverter–defibrillator may be indicated for those with sustained or symptomatic ventricular tachycardia. **Overall, implantable defibrillators have the best outcomes.** Traditional antiarrhythmic agents (e.g., flecainide/encainide) actually increase mortality two- to threefold. Sotalol and amiodarone might be helpful but are less effective than an ICD. β-Blockers (such as metoprolol or propranolol) also can be useful. Generally, a cardiology consult should be obtained to determine the best treatment approach for this arrhythmia.

IV. Sick Sinus Syndrome.

A. Sick sinus syndrome consists of episodes of bradycardia interspersed with episodic tachycardia from sinus tachycardia or atrial fibrillation. It can cause syncope.

B. It is generally a disease of the elderly.

C. Treatment generally requires a pacemaker to prevent bradycardia as well as medications such as verapamil to control tachycardia.

VALVULAR HEART DISEASE

I. General. Valvular heart disease can manifest with a spectrum of symptoms based on the valve involved and whether the disease is stenosis or regurgitation, right or left sided, and single valve or multivalve. An echocardiogram is the study of choice in a patient with a heart murmur to determine if the murmur is the result of a valvular lesion. **Table 3-3** summarizes the approach to valvular heart disease.

II. Mitral Valve Prolapse.

A. MVP can result from leaflet billowing, progressive expansion of the mitral annulus, or valve-leaflet myxomatous degeneration. Most patients with MVP are asymptomatic and have a benign clinical course.

TABLE 3-3
COMMON VALVULAR LESIONS AND THEIR MANAGEMENT

Lesion	Etiology	Symptoms	Complications	Treatment	Endocarditis Prophylaxis?	Follow-up and Notes
Mitral stenosis	Rheumatic heart disease	CHF, dyspnea often precipitated by pregnancy or A Fib	A Fib, pulmonary hypertension with cor pulmonale, pulmonary fibrosis or edema	Repair or replacement before symptoms are severe	Yes	Periodic (1-2 y) echo
Mitral regurgitation	CAD, endocarditis, connective tissue disorder, dilated cardiomyopathy	CHF, respiratory distress	A Fib	Treat for CHF, replace valve if EF < 60% or chamber begins to dilate	Yes	Periodic echo (1-2 y); avoid vasodilators in asymptomatic patients
Mitral valve prolapse	See text	See text	See text	See text	See text	See text
Aortic stenosis	Congenital bicuspid valve, rheumatic heart disease, age-related valve sclerosis	Angina, syncope, CHF		Repair or replace valve as soon as possible. If CHF, patients survive <2 y; 75% mortality in 3 y if symptomatic.	Yes	Any symptomatic patient should have cardiac cath and consideration for valve replacement. If asymptomatic, echo every 12 mo. Statins can delay progression.

(Continued)

CARDIOLOGY   3

TABLE 3-3

COMMON VALVULAR LESIONS AND THEIR MANAGEMENT—cont'd

Lesion	Etiology	Symptoms	Complications	Treatment	Endocarditis Prophylaxis?	Follow-up and Notes
Aortic regurgitation (chronic)	Rheumatic fever, myxomatous degeneration, Marfan's syndrome, syphilis, Reiter's disease, ankylosing spondylitis	CHF, PND, palpitations; chest, neck, back pain		Echo every 6 mo to 1 y, with valve replacement while EF is not <55%	Yes	
Aortic regurgitation (acute)	Trauma, endocarditis, acute rheumatic fever, dissection	Sudden onset dyspnea, tachycardia, tachypnea, shock				

cath, catheterization; echo, echocardiography.

B. Symptoms can include palpitations, fatigue, dyspnea, syncope, atypical chest pain, and episodes of supraventricular tachycardia. **However, these symptoms are as common in the general population as in those with MVP, and many patients with MVP that is found incidentally on echocardiography do not have these symptoms.**

C. A small fraction of patients experience strokes, TIAs, seizures, or episodes of amaurosis fugax, but whether this is related to the MVP is questionable (Freed et al, 1999). Patients with severe myxomatous change and thickened leaflets are at greatest risk for embolic events.

D. Examination. MVP is associated with a midsystolic click, which might be intermittent. If there is mitral regurgitation, the aforementioned click will be followed by a midsystolic to late systolic murmur.

E. Management and treatment. Diagnosis can be confirmed with echocardiography. Antibiotic prophylaxis should be given to patients with MVP who have regurgitation or are symptomatic from their illness.

CONGESTIVE HEART FAILURE

I. Causes. Two-thirds of cases are caused by CAD. The second most common cause is dilated cardiomyopathy, which can be idiopathic or can result from toxins (alcohol, cocaine, doxorubicin), infection (often viral), or collagen vascular disease. Other causes include chronic HTN (diastolic dysfunction), valvular heart disease, hypertrophic cardiomyopathy, and restrictive cardiomyopathy (amyloidosis, sarcoidosis, and hemochromatosis). Causes of primary right-sided failure include sleep apnea and chronic pulmonary embolism.

II. Evaluation.

A. History. Typical symptoms include fatigue, dyspnea, orthopnea, paroxysmal nocturnal dyspnea, nocturia, or chronic cough.

B. Physical exam. Signs include JVD, hepatojugular reflux, S_3 gallop, rales, and peripheral edema. However, these are not present in all patients with CHF.

C. Studies include baseline CXR and ECG. An echocardiogram should always be done to evaluate LV and RV ejection fractions, movement of chamber walls and valves, and chamber sizes and to differentiate systolic from diastolic dysfunction. In systolic dysfunction, ejection fraction is decreased. Check electrolytes, BUN, creatinine, ABG, CBC, and serum digoxin level if indicated. Patients should also be evaluated for obstructive sleep apnea, which can lead to CHF (see Chapter 4).

D. New York Heart Association Classification

1. NYHA class I: Symptoms at a similar level of exertion as a normal patient.

2. NYHA class II: Symptoms with ordinary exertion (e.g., climbing steps, walking outside).

3. NYHA class III: Symptoms with less than ordinary exertion (moving about the house).
4. NYHA class IV: Symptoms at rest.
III. Diagnosis and Treatment of *Acute* CHF Secondary to Systolic Dysfunction.
A. Precipitators of acute pulmonary edema (in a previously compensated patient) include poor compliance with medical or diet therapy, increased metabolic demands (infection [especially pneumonia], pregnancy, anemia, hyperthyroidism), progression of underlying heart disease (ischemia or valvular disease), arrhythmias (e.g., tachycardia), drug effect (β-blockers, calcium channel blockers, other negative inotropes, NSAIDS, glitazones), silent MI, and pulmonary embolism.
B. Diagnosis of pulmonary edema is usually made initially by physical exam and confirmed by CXR. Treatment might have to be started before one obtains a detailed history, etc. However, once the patient is stable, a careful work-up should be undertaken to determine underlying causes and precipitating factors.
1. **History** includes past history of cardiac and pulmonary disease or hypertension and history of shortness of breath, orthopnea, dyspnea on exertion, faintness, or chest pain. Other features of the history include recent weight gain, edema, infection, exposure to toxic inhalants, smoke, and possible aspiration. Note current medication regimen, compliance with diet and medications, and use of NSAIDs. Paroxysmal nocturnal dyspnea and orthopnea are *not* specific for CHF.
2. **Physical exam** finds tachypnea and tachycardia; often BP is elevated. If the patient has fever, suspect concurrent infection, which can increase metabolic demand and lead to CHF. Cyanosis, diaphoresis, retractions, use of accessory muscles of respiration, wheezing ("cardiac asthma"), and rales on lung auscultation are often present. Cough can be productive of pink, frothy sputum. Listen for S_3 gallop or murmurs. Peripheral edema and positive hepatojugular reflux are suggestive of CHF; bruits might be a clue to underlying vascular disease.
C. Diagnostic tests
1. **Lab tests:** Electrolytes, BUN, creatinine, cardiac enzymes, serum protein and albumin, urinalysis, differential CBC count, and ABG (if indicated).
2. **Brain natriuretic peptide (BNP)** is useful in the acute situation in patients in whom the diagnosis is not clear. A BNP of >100 pg/mL is 90% sensitive and 76% specific and has an 83% positive predictive value for CHF. Overall, a BNP between 100 pg/mL and 500 pg/mL is considered indiscriminant; <100 pg/mL effectively rules out CHF and >500 pg/mL effectively rules in CHF. **An elevated BNP does not exclude the presence of other disease.** Higher levels are less sensitive but more specific. **Baseline levels are critical to interpretation of the BNP. Some patients are asymptomatic with a BNP of 500 pg/mL and others are highly symptomatic at a BNP of 120 pg/mL.** Higher BNP is associated with a worse overall outcome. BNP can be followed

serially to determine the effectiveness of an intervention (useful when trying to maximize therapy for an outpatient). **Causes of a false positive BNP include anything that can cause right atrial stretching including** PE, renal failure, MI, angina, COPD, or cor pulmonale or other cause of pulmonary hypertension. However, these elevations are generally less than 400-500 pg/mL.

3. **CXR** initially shows interstitial edema as well as thickening and loss of definition of the shadows of pulmonary vasculature. Fluid in septal planes and interlobular fissures cause the characteristic appearance of Kerley A and B lines. Eventually, pleural effusions and perihilar alveolar edema can develop in the classic butterfly pattern. CXR findings can lag behind the clinical presentation by up to 12 hours and can take 4 days to clear after clinical improvement in the patient.

4. **ECG.** Evaluate for evidence of MI and arrhythmia. The sudden onset of atrial fibrillation or PSVT can cause acute decompensation in previously stable chronic CHF. LVH can signal underlying aortic stenosis, hypertension, or cardiomyopathy (the sensitivity of ECG for LVH is only in the 30%-60% range with a specificity of 80%.)

5. **Echocardiography** is not imperative immediately. In the work-up for an underlying cause, it is useful to evaluate for valvular disease, valvular vegetations, wall-motion abnormalities, LV function, and cardiomyopathy.

D. Treatment of acute CHF

1. **Oxygen** can be given by nasal cannula or mask. The patient may require endotracheal intubation if unable to adequately oxygenate despite use of 100% oxygen by nonrebreather mask. Mask CPAP has been shown to reduce the need for intubation and is an excellent alternative.

2. **Other general measures** include elevating the head of the bed. A Swan-Ganz catheter for hemodynamic monitoring might be necessary if the patient becomes hypotensive. **However, Swan-Ganz catheters likely have an adverse effect on mortality and should be used only after careful consideration.** If indicated, place a Foley catheter for fluid management.

3. **Medications**

a. **Nitroglycerin (preferred) and other vasodilators are considered the first drug of choice in acute CHF** and act by decreasing preload and afterload, thereby decreasing LV work. They can also reverse myocardial ischemia. IV nitroglycerin is commonly used, especially if there is concern that ischemia is an underlying or precipitating factor. Start at 10 to 20 mg/min and increase by increments of 10 to 20 mg/min q5min until the desired effect is achieved. Sublingual nitroglycerin 0.4 mg repeated q5min prn can also be used acutely, as can topical nitrates. However, topical nitrates might not be effective acutely because maximal effect occurs at 120 minutes. Nitroprusside is an alternative (start at 0.5 mg/kg/ min and increase by 0.5 mg/kg/min q5min). Most patients respond to less than 10 mg/kg per minute, but titrate to effect. Nitroprusside is more likely to cause hypotension than is IV nitroglycerin.

CARDIOLOGY 3

A fluid bolus might help to reverse nitrate-induced hypotension but should be used judiciously in those with CHF.

b. **Furosemide and other diuretics.** If the patient has never been treated with furosemide, you may start with 20 mg IV and observe the response. Titrate dose upward until adequate diuresis is established. If the patient is receiving long-term furosemide, give 1 to 2 times the usual daily dose by slow IV bolus. Larger doses (up to 1 g) might be needed in patients receiving large baseline doses or with a history of renal disease. Alternatively, a furosemide drip can be established for higher doses. Give 20% of the dose (200 mg) as a bolus and infuse the rest over 8 hours. This has a greater efficacy than a single large bolus does. Up to 2 g has been safely administered in this fashion. Ethacrynic acid (25-100 mg IV) might be needed if the patient does not respond to furosemide. Bumetanide (0.5-1.0 mg IV) can also be used. Adding metolazone (5-20 mg PO) or chlorothiazide (500 mg IV) to furosemide can generate additional diuresis. Some authors consider phlebotomy if diuretics are ineffective and the patient has a high Hct, but this is a high-risk procedure.

c. **Morphine** acts as a venodilator and decreases anxiety. Start with 1 to 2 mg IV. Titrate carefully in COPD and CHF, because narcotics can decrease respiratory drive.

d. **ACE inhibitors can be used acutely in the management of CHF** but are more common as chronic therapy. Captopril is given 12.5 to 25 mg SL or IV at 0.16 mg/min increased by 0.08 mg/min q5min until it has the desired effect. IV enalapril is also available. This is safe and effective and can be used in patients unresponsive to oxygen, nitrates, and diuretics.

e. **Dobutamine (2.5-15 mg/kg/min) or dopamine (2-20 mg/kg/min)** may be needed for pressure support or as a positive inotrope. These drugs are effective immediately; "renal dose" dopamine is not effective at increasing GFR or urine output. Dopamine increases peripheral resistance and blood pressure; dobutamine is primarily a positive inotrope and chronotrope and decreases peripheral resistance.

f. **Nesiritide, a recombinant BNP analogue is not recommended.** It is no more effective than optimal nitrate therapy, is associated with more prolonged hypotension, and increases renal failure and likely mortality. It is very expensive and interferes with BNP determination.

g. **Digoxin** might help to improve symptoms but is arrhythmogenic and should be used cautiously, if at all, in *acute* CHF. Check ECG, serum potassium, BUN, and creatinine before loading with digoxin. After digoxin loading, it can be difficult to distinguish ischemic changes on ECG from digoxin effect. Be aware of other medications that the patient takes that might affect digoxin levels such as amiodarone, flecainide, quinidine, and verapamil. Decrease digoxin dose if the patient has renal disease. The aim is to achieve serum levels of 1.0 to 1.5 ng/mL.

h. **Nitric oxide synthetase inhibitors (L-NAME)** significantly improve survival in those with cardiogenic shock in small trials. This is not yet standard of care or widely available (Cotter et al, 2003).

4. **Surgery** might be indicated under rare conditions such as valvular heart disease or rupture of ventricular septum after an MI. In severe LV failure, an intra-aortic balloon pump might be beneficial as a temporizing measure.

IV. **Outpatient Treatment of CHF Secondary to Systolic Dysfunction.**

A. **Nonpharmacologic therapy.** Avoid excessive physical stress (but encourage exercise), reduce dietary salt, consider compressive stockings if needed to reduce risk of DVT (consider SQ heparin for inpatients), and weight loss if obese. Work on walking and endurance training.

B. **Drugs to avoid in CHF** include NSAIDS (including COX-2 inhibitors), metformin, cilostazol, sildenafil and other medications of this class, glitazones (class III and IV failure), many antiarrhythmics, calcium channel blockers with negative inotropic effects (e.g., diltiazem, verapamil), and many others.

C. **Drugs that have been shown to reduce mortality in CHF** include ACE inhibitors, β-blockers (e.g., metoprolol), spironolactone/eplerenone, and the combination of hydralazine plus isosorbide dinitrate.

D. **Pharmacologic and other therapy:** Consider checking a BNP after each intervention to see if your intervention is effective.

1. **Diuretics.** Loop diuretics are usually recommended (e.g., furosemide). Some patients develop resistance to loop diuretics after chronic use. A single dose of metolazone (5-20 mg qd) often results in significant diuresis in such patients. Monitor K^+ and Mg^{2+} levels in patients with heart failure who are receiving diuretics. Supplementation should be provided if necessary, because hypokalemia and hypomagnesemia are risk factors for the development of arrhythmias.

2. **Spironolactone at low dose (25-50 mg qd)** reduces mortality in patients with class III and IV heart failure. A more expensive alternative is **eplerenone,** which **has many more drug interactions** but causes less impotence and gynecomastia. Monitor closely for hyperkalemia and avoid in patients with a serum creatinine >2.5 (>2.0 for women) or preexisting hyperkalemia.

3. **β-Blocker** use in patients with CHF caused by systolic dysfunction is now the standard of care. The initiation and titration of these medications should be undertaken with care. These drugs should only be started in the stable patient; they can cause acute decompensation. Recommended agents include carvedilol and metoprolol (specifically Toprol-XL). Metoprolol is as effective and is much less expensive.

4. **ACE inhibitors** function primarily as afterload reducers and have been shown to reduce morbidity (CHF progression, MI, need for hospitalization) and mortality. ACE inhibitors also improve hemodynamics and increase exercise tolerance in heart failure. Begin therapy at low doses and titrate gradually. Observe the patient for hypotension, angioedema, or persistent cough. Monitor electrolytes and renal function because ACE inhibitors

can cause elevation of serum potassium and can cause a reversible decrease in renal function in some patients. Patients at high risk for adverse effects from ACE inhibitors include those with connective tissue diseases, preexisting renal insufficiency, and bilateral renal artery stenosis. **Contraindications to their use** include a history of hypersensitivity to ACE inhibitors, serum K$^+$ >5.5 mEq/L (consider evaluation for hypoaldosteronism or Addison's disease), or a previous episode of angioedema during their use. Relative contraindications include renal failure and hypotension. However, ACE inhibitors actually protect renal function in those with chronic renal failure (see Chapter 8 for details).

5. **Angiotensin-receptor blockers** function by afterload reduction. Consider stopping an ACE inhibitor if creatinine rises more than 30% over baseline. The limitations of ACE inhibitors (cough, angioedema) are not prevalent with these agents; however, their effects on renal function are still under investigation. **They should not supplant ACE inhibitors** but can be substituted for them for patients who are intolerant of ACE inhibitors. The combination of an ACE inhibitor and an ARB is no more efficacious than an ACE inhibitor alone. ARBs may not improve rate of reinfarction.

6. **Hydralazine and isosorbide dinitrate** used together increases survival but should only be used in those unresponsive to ACE inhibitors or ARBs. ACE inhibitors increase survival in heart failure more than combination hydralazine and isosorbide therapy. This combination is especially useful in patients of African ancestry, who tend not to respond as well to ACE inhibitors.

7. **Digoxin** improves symptoms in severe heart failure and in cases where atrial fibrillation is a complication of CHF. However, digoxin has no effect on mortality because of a proarrhythmic effect and should be considered a measure for symptom control only. Rapid digitalization is not necessary in patients with chronic CHF. The half-life of digoxin is 1.5 to 2 days in patients with normal renal function. The usual starting dose is 0.25 mg/day. Decrease the dose in small or elderly patients and in those receiving other drugs (such as quinidine, amiodarone, and verapamil) that raise digoxin levels. Decrease the dose in patients with impaired renal function. Monitor levels, especially after dose adjustments or after changes in other medications that can affect digoxin levels (such as quinidine, verapamil, and oral azole antifungals). Avoid digoxin in patients with idiopathic hypertrophic subaortic stenosis (IHSS) and those with diastolic dysfunction. Watch potassium levels closely; hypokalemia renders the heart more sensitive to digoxin and will predispose to digoxin toxicity.

8. **Positive inotrope infusions** such as dobutamine or milrinone have no benefit and can be harmful when used as chronic intermittent therapy.

9. **Calcium channel blockers should generally be avoided in CHF,** especially verapamil and diltiazem, which are relatively potent negative inotropic agents, and nifedipine, which can increase mortality. In patients with

CHF and hypertension, amlodipine (a second-generation dihydropyridine calcium channel blocker with no negative inotropic effect) has been shown to be efficacious but is not first line.

10. **Antithrombotic therapy.** Patients with a previous history of embolism or A Fib are at high risk for thromboembolic complications and should be considered for warfarin therapy unless a contraindication exists. Titrate the dose to an INR of 2.0 to 3.0 (prothrombin time not more than 1.5 times normal) to prevent increased risk of bleeding complications. If warfarin cannot be used, consider aspirin for the antiplatelet effect (80-300 mg/d).

11. **Ventricular assist devices (VADs)** have been shown to improve morbidity and survival in selected patients waiting to undergo transplantation. The decision to implant such a device should be made only after careful evaluation by a surgeon trained in their insertion. Follow-up care involves close collaboration with the transplant facility. VADs are being studied as stand-alone therapy for patients not considered candidates for transplantation.

12. **Enhanced external counterpulsation** involves intermittent compression of the legs and can improve CHF. Although it is promising, there are still scant data supporting this modality.

13. **Biventricular pacing with cardiac resynchronization** improves symptoms in some patients.

14. **Implantable defibrillator.** Indications for an ICD in CHF (among others) include:

   a. Ischemic cardiomyopathy without revascularization procedure within 3 months *and* documented MI more than 30 days ago *and* LVEF <35% *and* NYHA class II or III disease.

   b. Nonischemic cardiomyopathy for more than 9 months, LVEF <35%, functional NYHA class II or III disease.

   c. LVEF <30% with ischemic or nonischemic cardiomyopathy and no CHF symptoms.

   d. Any cardiomyopathy with NYHA class III or IV disease if QRS >120 ms.

15. **Follow-up.** Periodic assay of BNP to monitor the effectiveness of interventions is suggested, although no firm guidelines exist.

V. **Obstructive Hypertrophic Cardiomyopathy.** This is also known as idiopathic hypertrophic subaortic stenosis. It most commonly occurs in young adults before the third decade.

A. **Etiology and examination.** Obstructive hypertrophic cardiomyopathy is caused by a thickened septum impinging on anterior mitral leaflet and creating a variable dynamic obstruction in the left ventricular outflow tract. It is an autosomal dominant mutation with 50% penetrance and equal male-to-female ratio. Signs are commonly dyspnea, angina, syncope, and fatigue. Examination is notable for a laterally displaced apical impulse, rapid rise and biphasic carotid pulse, variably split S_2

and loud S_4, and harsh crescendo–decrescendo murmur at the lower left sternal border and apex. The murmur classically increases and lengthens with Valsalva and decreases with handgrip and squatting.

B. Management and treatment are aimed at reducing ventricular rate and allowing increased ventricular volume and outflow tract dimensions. It is most commonly treated with β-blockers or calcium channel blockers; do not use digitalis preparations. Patients must avoid strenuous physical activity, especially competitive sports. Some recommend dual chamber pacing. **Surgical therapy may be helpful in selected cases:** left ventricular myomectomy or heart transplantation for cases with severe left ventricular failure.

VI. Diastolic Dysfunction, Diastolic Heart Failure, Heart Failure with Preserved Systolic Function.

A. General. *Diastolic dysfunction* refers to abnormal filling of the left ventricle. Heart failure with preserved systolic function is a poorly understood yet exceedingly common syndrome (30%-50% of all heart failure cases, especially in older hypertensive women) and probably has a multifactorial etiology. Reversible causes should be sought, such as renal artery stenosis and other causes of hypertension, paroxysmal A Fib, sleep apnea, anemia, aortic stenosis with preserved ejection fraction, hypertrophic cardiomyopathy, and coronary disease. Constrictive cardiomyopathy should always be considered if there is substantial fluid overload with normal ejection fraction, and the echocardiography lab should be alerted to investigate (e.g., discordant RV and LV filling patterns with respiration). If there is a history of pulmonary edema, consider exercise-induced mitral regurgitation.

B. Clinical. Diastolic dysfunction is usually indistinguishable from CHF secondary to systolic dysfunction. However, echocardiography can clarify the etiology, evaluate ejection fraction, estimate left atrial size (an excellent marker of diastolic dysfunction providing useful prognostic information), and hypertrophy of the ventricle wall. Tachycardia, hypertension, and A Fib are particularly poorly tolerated in these patients.

C. Treatment

1. There is no evidence-based treatment. It seems reasonable to treat symptoms (e.g., diuretics for volume overload) and to extrapolate treatment from randomized, controlled trials involving systolic heart failure and atherosclerotic disease. β-Blockers and ACE inhibitors might therefore be helpful. Control of blood pressure is likely to be important in the long term to halt progression of LV hypertrophy.

2. Diltiazem and verapamil can be of benefit by slowing heart rate and increasing left ventricular filling. There might be some additional benefit secondary to cardiac muscle relaxation.

3. Cardiac output is generally fixed, so anything that drops afterload can cause hypotension.

HYPERTENSION

I. Overview.

A. Hypertension is defined as a sustained systolic blood pressure (SBP) of ≥140 mm Hg *or* a sustained diastolic blood pressure (DBP) of ≥90 mm Hg. See **Box 3-7** for the JNC 7 classification of hypertension. Note that SBP is as important as (if not more important than) DBP.

1. **Goals for patients with no special risk factors** are SBP <140 mg Hg and DBP <90 mm Hg.
2. **Goals for diabetic patients and patients with early renal insufficiency (<1 g proteinuria)** are SBP 130 mm Hg and DBP 80 mm Hg.
3. **Goals for patients with renal insufficiency** (>1 g proteinuria in 24 h) are SBP 125 mm Hg and DBP 75 mm Hg.

B. Before diagnosing HTN, document an elevated BP on at least three occasions over a 2-week period. The patient should be free of stress at the time of the exam, including being free of pain and anxiety (e.g., white coat hypertension).

C. Use a cuff of the proper size (small size gives falsely elevated readings); the arm should be resting comfortably on an armrest. **If the results are still inconclusive, consider 24-hour ambulatory monitoring** (see later). Treatment of HTN can reduce many potential complications such as CHF, nephropathy, and cerebrovascular events.

D. White coat hypertension. Some patients become hypertensive in response to stress (such as seeing you!). They have intermediate outcomes when compared to "hypertensive" and normotensive patients. Many clinicians elect to treat these patients. Another option is 24-hour ambulatory monitoring (see later).

E. Ambulatory Blood Pressure Monitoring.

1. **Ambulatory BP monitoring** is indicated for patients who have suspected white coat hypertension, difficult to control hypertension, hypotensive symptoms on antihypertensives (e.g., near syncope), possible autonomic dysfunction, and inconsistent blood pressure readings (so HTN cannot be ruled in or out).
2. Positive 24-hour ambulatory monitor is considered an average blood pressure of >135/85 during the day *and* >125/75 at night. Another published criterion is a blood pressure of >140/90 more than 40% of the time.

BOX 3-7
JNC 7 CLASSIFICATION OF HYPERTENSION
<120/80: normal
120/80 to 139/89: Prehypertension
140/90 to 159/99: Stage 1 hypertension
>160/100: Stage II hypertension

3

CARDIOLOGY

II. Etiology.

A. Essential hypertension is the most common form in all age groups except children. The cause of essential HTN is not completely understood.

B. Secondary hypertension, the result a pathologic process, is present in 1% of those with mild HTN but in 10% to 45% of those with hard-to-control hypertension. Causes of secondary HTN include renal artery stenosis (or other cause of increased plasma renin), renal parenchymal disease (glomerulonephritis, diabetic nephropathy, polycystic disease, obstructive uropathy), drugs (oral contraceptives, steroids, OTC meds), increased levels of catecholamines (pheochromocytoma), glucocorticoids (Cushing's syndrome), or mineralocorticoids (hyperaldosteronism, which is manifested by hypokalemia, HTN, and possibly edema). Consider also thyroid disease and sleep apnea.

C. Whom to evaluate for secondary HTN

1. **Patients with difficult-to-control hypertension and those with laboratory or clinical evidence of a secondary cause** (e.g., increased creatinine, low potassium).

2. **Patients with hyperaldosteronism,** which is characterized by hypertension, hypokalemia (but not in all patients), and possibly edema. Check potassium when the patient has an unrestricted salt intake and is off diuretics, ACE inhibitors, and ARBs. Draw renin and aldosterone levels at 8:00 AM; aldosterone-to-renin ratio should be increased.

3. **Patients with renal artery stenosis.** After traditional angiography, MR angiography is the most sensitive test for renal artery stenosis, followed by captopril-enhanced Doppler ultrasound, followed by captopril renal scan (90%, 63%, and 33% respectively). **Treatment:** PTCA is only 30% effective in those with atherosclerotic disease, and outcomes are the same as compared to BP controlled with medication (although it might allow reduction of medications). PTCA is 60% effective in those with fibromuscular dysplasia. ACE inhibitors are okay to use but follow creatinine closely.

4. See appropriate sections elsewhere for evaluation and treatment of other secondary causes.

III. Evaluation.

A. The initial evaluation of the patient with newly detected mild to moderately elevated blood pressure (not yet defined as HTN) should include the following:

1. **Thorough history** regarding diabetes, HTN, and cardiovascular disease in the family; personal history of cardiovascular symptoms, drug and alcohol use, level of physical activity, and diet.

2. **Physical exam** including weight, fundoscopic exam for evidence of retinopathy, cardiac exam, auscultation of abdomen and neck for bruits, and palpation of kidneys.

3. **Laboratory evaluation** may be postponed until follow-up visits have established the diagnosis of HTN.

4. **Recommend** salt restriction, increased exercise, weight reduction if indicated, and follow-up exam in 2 to 4 weeks for BP recheck.

B. **Once the formal diagnosis of hypertension is made, the evaluation should consist of the following:**

1. Urinalysis and serum creatinine to evaluate for renal disease, CBC, ECG, cholesterol and triglycerides (as part of CAD risk factor assessment), electrolytes and uric acid as baseline for determining appropriate medications, and serum glucose to evaluate for diabetes.

2. Other tests may be suggested by physical exam or lab results that point to a possible cause of secondary HTN.

IV. **Treatment.**

A. **Education.** All patients with HTN should be counseled regarding the nature of the disorder and the importance of long-term compliance with particular treatment regimens. Home BP monitoring should be taught.

B. **Lifestyle interventions.** Exercise, salt restriction, and weight reduction are appropriate for many patients with HTN but may be of limited efficacy due to poor compliance. Smoking cessation should be encouraged. If the patient abuses alcohol or other substances, appropriate treatment should be encouraged and arranged. Increased intake of calcium and magnesium should be encouraged to help reduce blood pressure unless a contraindication is present.

C. **Medications.** Numerous medications are available for pharmacologic treatment of HTN. The widely varying side-effects, costs, and dosing schedules allow tailoring of the medications to the particular needs of each patient. **A diuretic such as hydrochlorothiazide should be the first drug for most patients unless there is another indication** (e.g., ACE in diabetic patients and those with renal disease, β-blocker in those with angina). **β-Blockers are a good second choice.** In the past, patients were placed on a maximum dose of a single agent before a second agent was added. The thinking has changed, and moderate doses of several agents can allow good BP control without significant dose-related side effects (e.g., hypokalemia, edema, impotence).

1. **Patients of African ancestry tend to respond better to diuretics and not as well to ACE inhibitors, ARBs, and β-blockers** (but this is a generalization; individualize therapy).

2. **Diuretics.** Thiazide diuretics are effective alone and are useful in offsetting the fluid retention caused by other agents. Loop diuretics are more effective in patients with impaired renal function. Examples of thiazides are hydrochlorothiazide and chlorothiazide. The dosing range of HCTZ is 6.25 to 50 mg PO daily, with little additional benefit above 25 mg per day. **Advantages:** safe, inexpensive. **Disadvantages:** possible hypokalemia, impaired glucose tolerance (usually not clinically significant), increased uric acid levels and risk of gout, and increased plasma lipids. Dyazide and Maxide are potassium-sparing combinations of HCTZ and triamterene. Long term, the potassium-sparing diuretics are less expensive because they do not require

3

CARDIOLOGY

potassium monitoring and replacement. Compared to thiazide diuretics alone, potassium-sparing combinations are associated with a lower risk of sudden cardiac death.

3. **β-Blockers** (e.g., nadolol, metoprolol, propranolol) reduce cardiac output (negative inotropic and chronotropic effects). They are also useful for treating angina and arrhythmias and as prophylaxis against migraines. They are generally considered most effective in the younger patient with a "hyperdynamic" cardiovascular system as evidenced by elevated resting pulse (high normal or tachycardic) and excessive response of BP to exercise. **Advantages:** many are relatively inexpensive and effective. **Disadvantages:** they can cause significant bradycardia or AV block, sedation, fatigue, bronchospasm in patients with asthma, erectile dysfunction, impaired glucose tolerance, and possibly elevated uric acid and plasma lipids (except those with intrinsic sympathomimetic activity). They should not be withdrawn abruptly, especially in patients with CAD, because rebound tachycardia and HTN can occur. Labetalol is a unique agent that provides both α-blockade and (predominantly) β-blockade. It tends to cause less bradycardia than other agents and has a direct peripheral vasodilating effect. It is not clear if atenolol reduces mortality. Consider using metoprolol.

4. **Central sympatholytics** include methyldopa, clonidine, guanabenz, and guanfacine. Sedation and fatigue can occur. A withdrawal syndrome can occur with abrupt cessation (especially with clonidine).

5. **α-Blockers** (prazosin and terazosin) are good choices in elderly men who have hypertension and benign prostatic hypertrophy. However, α-blockers are less effective at reducing mortality and cardiovascular events than other classes. Severe orthostatic hypotension can occur with the first dose. Fluid retention can occur. Sedation and headache are commonly seen early during treatment but tend to diminish with time. Avoid using Viagra, etc. with α-blockers. This may result in prolonged hypotension.

6. **Arterial vasodilators** include hydralazine and minoxidil. Both are potent vasodilators and can cause reflex tachycardia and fluid retention. They should be used only with a diuretic and sympathetic inhibitor (such as a β-blocker). They should not be used in patients with angina. Minoxidil is usually reserved for severe hypertension. A lupus-like syndrome has been seen with hydralazine.

7. **Calcium channel blockers** include verapamil, diltiazem, nicardipine, nifedipine, amlodipine, and others. Verapamil and diltiazem both slow AV nodal conduction. Both also have some negative inotropic effect (especially verapamil) and peripheral vasodilative effects. Calcium channel blockers generally do not adversely affect glucose tolerance or plasma lipids. They may be especially appropriate in the patient who needs both an antianginal and antihypertensive drug. Mild edema and constipation are frequent side effects of calcium channel blockers. Orthostatic hypotension and reflex tachycardia can occur, particularly with nifedipine. Short-acting nifedipine can increase cardiac mortality.

8. **ACE inhibitors** include captopril, enalapril, lisinopril, and others. All are effective for HTN and have been used in CHF. All can contribute to hyperkalemia and cause reversible decreased renal function. Consider lowering the dose or stopping the ACE inhibitor if the creatinine increases more than 30% above baseline. Side effects tend to be minimal, with no significant sedation, fatigue, or exercise intolerance in most patients. Occasional patients have trouble with persistent cough; aspirin 325 mg PO daily can decrease cough, as can indomethacin, oral iron supplements, or inhaled cromolyn. Switching to another ACE inhibitor does not improve the cough caused by these agents. Angioedema occurs in a small subset of patients taking ACE inhibitors and could be life threatening. Patients should be warned about this possibility. Patients at high risk for adverse renal effects include those with connective tissue disease, bilateral renal artery stenosis, or preexisting renal insufficiency. ACE inhibitors can have a favorable effect in preserving renal function or in slowing the progression of proteinuria in chronic renal failure. They also facilitate cardiac remodeling.

9. **Angiotensin II type 1 receptor blockers** include losartan, irbesartan, and valsartan. If ACE inhibitors are poorly tolerated, ARBs should be considered. These drugs antagonize the action of angiotensin II by displacing it from its receptor; this inhibits angiotensin II–induced vascular smooth muscle contraction, adrenal release of aldosterone, and presynaptic release of catecholamines, among other effects. They do not stimulate cough and are as effective as enalapril in controlling HTN. They do not adversely affect lipid parameters or glucose levels. Because of their uricosuric activity they reduce serum uric acid levels.

10. **Aldosterone blockers** include spironolactone and eplerenone. **Adding these drugs to a regimen often results in good BP control in cases of difficult-to-control HTN.** Start with 25 mg/day. Watch for hyperkalemia, especially if used with an ACE inhibitor or ARB. Eplerenone has more drug interactions and is expensive. Avoid if renal insufficiency is present.

D. **Follow-up.** Initially patients should be scheduled for frequent office visits until BP is adequately controlled and potential side effects are evaluated. Thereafter, visits may be scheduled every 3 to 6 months. Lab evaluation should include those indicated by the medications they are using (K^+, BUN, and Cr for ACEIs and ARBs; Na^+, K^+, and Cr for diuretics, etc.).

DYSLIPIDEMIAS

I. **Classification.**

A. Dyslipidemias may be grouped on the basis of serum lipid concentrations and electrophoretic patterns, by genotype, or by pathophysiologic features **(Table 3-4).** They may be classified as primary, which includes familial hyperlipidemia, or as secondary.

3

CARDIOLOGY

TABLE 3-4

CLASSIFICATION OF LIPOPROTEIN DISORDERS BY PHENOTYPES, GENOTYPES, AND CORRESPONDING CLINICAL MANIFESTATIONS

Phenotype	Plasma Lipid Levels		Lipoprotein in Excess	Genotype	Xanthomas	Other Clinical Manifestations
	Cholesterol	Triglyceride				
I	Normal or elevated	Elevated lipemia	Chylomicrons	Familial lipoprotein lipase deficiency, Apo C-II deficiency	Eruptive, tuberoeruptive	Recurrent abdominal pain, other gastrointestinal symptoms, hepatosplenomegaly
IIA	Normal	Elevated	LDL	FHC, familial combined hyperlipidemia—polygenic and sporadic hypercholesterolemia	Tendinous, xanthelasma, tuberous; planar (homozygous)	Premature CAD, arcus corneae, aortic stenosis (homozygous FHC), arthritis symptoms
IIB	Elevated	Elevated	LDL and VLDL	Familial combined hyperlipidemia, FHC		
III	Elevated	Elevated	VLDL and LDL	Familial dysbetalipoproteinemia	Planar (especially palmar), tuberous	Premature CAD and peripheral vascular disease, male > female, obesity, abnormal glucose tolerance, hyperuricemia, aggravated by hypothyroidism, good response to therapy

| IV | Normal or elevated | Elevated | VLDL | Familial hypertriglyceridemia, familial combined hyperlipidemia, sporadic hypertriglyceridemia | Usually none; rarely eruptive or tuberoeruptive | CAD and peripheral vascular disease, obesity, abnormal glucose tolerance, hyperuricemia, arthritic symptoms, gallbladder disease |
| V | Normal or elevated | Elevated | Chylomicrons and VLDL | Homozygous FHC | Eruptive, tuberoeruptive | Recurrent abdominal pain, other gastrointestinal symptoms, hepatosplenomegaly, peripheral paresthesia |

CAD, coronary artery disease; FHC, familial hypercholesterolemia; IDL, intermediate-density lipoprotein; LDL, low-density lipoprotein; VLDL, very-low-density lipoprotein.

CARDIOLOGY 3

BOX 3-8

RISK FACTORS WHEN CALCULATING LDL RISK CATEGORY

First-degree male relative with CAD at age < 55 or first-degree female relative with
  CAD at age < 65

Smoking

HDL < 40mg/dL

Hypertension

Age: men >45 years, women >55 years

Elevated LDL

B. **Secondary causes.**
1. **Exogenous:** alcohol, oral contraceptives, estrogens, androgens,
   corticosteroids, diuretics (thiazides), β-blockers, obesity, and high-
   cholesterol diet.
2. **Endocrine and metabolic:** diabetes, hypothyroidism, Cushing's disease,
   Addison's disease, hepatic disease, nephrotic syndrome.
3. **Miscellaneous:** pregnancy, pancreatitis, SLE.
II. **Evaluation and Initiation of Therapy.**
A. Step 1. **Obtain fasting lipid profile.**
B. Step 2. **Determine risk factors, including CAD equivalents (Box 3-8,
   Box 3-9). Ten-year cardiac risk** (see Fig. 3-1).
C. Step 3. **Determine patient's goal (Table 3-5) and initiate treatment.**
III. **Treatment of Elevated Cholesterol.**
A. **Initiate lifestyle changes** including exercise and diet modification.
1. Initiate TLC (therapeutic lifestyle change) diet. Modify total fat to less
   than 25% to 35% of calories, saturated fat to less than 7% of calories,
   cholesterol to less than 200 mg/day, carbohydrates to 50% to 60% of
   calories, polyunsaturated fat up to 10% of calories, monounsaturated
   fat up to 20% of calories.
2. Add 10 to 25 g soluble fiber and 2 g/d of plant sterols or stanols
   (found in some new margarines).
B. **Initiate drug therapy**
1. **HMG CoA reductase inhibitors** (statins: lovastatin, simvastatin,
   pravastatin, atorvastatin, others) inhibit HMG CoA reductase, which is
   the rate-limiting enzyme in the production of cholesterol by the liver.
   Statins are an excellent initial choice for many people because of

BOX 3-9

CHD EQUIVALENTS WHEN CALCULATING LDL RISK CATEGORY

Diabetes

Symptomatic carotid disease

Peripheral vascular disease

Abdominal aortic aneurysm.

TABLE 3-5

LDL CHOLESTEROL GOALS AND CUTPOINTS FOR THERAPEUTIC LIFESTYLE CHANGES AND DRUG THERAPY IN DIFFERENT RISK CATEGORIES

Risk Category	LDL Goal	LDL Level for Lifestyle Changes	LDL Level for Drug Therapy
CHD or CHD risk equivalents (10-y risk >20%)	<100 mg/dL	≥100 mg/dL	≥130 mg/dL (100-129 mg/dL: drug optional)* 10-y risk 10-20%: ≥130 mg/dL
2+ risk factors (10-y risk ≤20%)	<130 mg/dL	≥130 mg/dL	10-y risk <10%: ≥160 mg/dL
0-1 risk factor†	<160 mg/dL	≥160 mg/dL	≥190 mg/dL (160-189 mg/dL: LDL-lowering drug optional)

Note: In very high risk patients (CHD plus risk factors), an LDL goal of <70 mg/dL is recommended.
*Some authorities recommend use of LDL-lowering drugs in this category if an LDL cholesterol <100 mg/dL cannot be achieved by therapeutic lifestyle changes. Others prefer to use drugs that primarily modify triglycerides and HDL (e.g., nicotinic acid or fibrate). Clinical judgment may also call for deferring drug therapy in this category.
†Almost all people with no risk or one risk factor have a 10-year risk <10%; thus 10-year risk assessment in people with no risk or one risk factor is not necessary.
From National Cholesterol Education Program: Third Report of the Expert Panel on Detection, Evaluation, and Treatment of High Blood Cholesterol in Adults (Adult Treatment Panel III): ATP III at-a-Glance: Quick Desk Reference. Available online at http://www.nhlbi.nih.gov/guidelines/cholesterol/atglance.htm (accessed December 16, 2005).

established efficacy in preventing primary and secondary cardiovascular disease. These agents reduce total cholesterol, LDL, and triglycerides and can increase HDL. For example, atorvastatin can reduce cholesterol by up to 60% and triglycerides by up to 45% and can increase HDL by up to 12%. Side effects are rare and include elevated liver function test results, elevated muscle creatinine phosphokinase secondary to myopathy, and rarely rhabdomyolysis. Myopathy can occur in the absence of pain; peripheral neuropathy is a recently recognized side effect. Titrate doses at 4- to 6-week intervals until the desired LDL levels are achieved. Obtain liver enzymes at baseline, 12 weeks, and then every 6 months. Stop the statin if liver enzymes increase to three times baseline. Some guidelines no longer recommend monitoring LFTs but many consider it prudent.

2. **Bile acid sequestrants and resins (colestipol, cholestyramine, and colesevelam)** decrease total and LDL cholesterol by 20% to 40%. Constipation and GI upset are frequent side effects; they can be alleviated somewhat by increasing dietary fiber and adding psyllium laxatives. Resins can increase triglycerides and should be used with caution in patients with elevated triglycerides. They are often used with other agents such as niacin, a statin, or gemfibrozil. They can affect GI absorption of other drugs; other medications should be taken

1 to 2 hours before or 4 hours after a resin dose. Levels of concurrent medications (such as digoxin or PT/INR for patients receiving warfarin) should be monitored.

3. **Nicotinic acid (niacin)** decreases LDL and triglycerides and increases HDL. It also lowers blood levels of lipoprotein A. Common side effects include skin flushing, GI upset, and elevated liver enzymes, serum glucose, and uric acid. Rare side effects can include headaches, worsening of peptic ulcer disease, cardiac dysrhythmias, and elevations in serum muscle enzymes. Tolerance of minor side effects (flushing, nausea) can be improved by starting with low doses (100 mg bid or tid) and taking with meals. The maximum dose is 3 g daily. Taking 325 mg of aspirin 30 to 60 minutes before taking niacin decreases flushing. The sustained-release preparations of niacin are hepatotoxic and should not be used. Monitor liver enzymes every 6 to 12 weeks for a year and then every 6 months.

4. **Fibric acid derivatives (fibrates) (gemfibrozil, fenofibrate)** are used to decrease synthesis of VLDL and to lower fasting triglycerides. They can increase HDL and have a variable effect on LDL. GI side effects are common. Rare side effects include myalgias, increase in liver or muscle enzymes, headache, gallstones, arrhythmias, hypokalemia, anemia, and leukopenia. They can potentiate oral hypoglycemics and warfarin. Avoid clofibrate; it increases mortality. Use of these agents with statins has resulted in rhabdomyolysis.

5. **Probucol** was developed as an antioxidant; it decreases total, HDL, and LDL cholesterol. It is a common cause of QT prolongation on ECG and is no longer on the market in the United States because of the risk of sudden death.

6. **Fish oils and flax seed oil** (omega-3 fatty acids) decrease synthesis of VLDL and can decrease chylomicrons (and therefore TG). They can reduce risk of acute pancreatitis in patients with severe hypertriglyceridemia. Omega-3 fatty acids have proven benefit when eaten as fish. They are likely beneficial in capsule form.

7. **Ezetimibe (Zetia)** reduces cholesterol absorption and is approved as monotherapy or as an add-on to the statins. It is less effective than statins (13%-18% reduction in cholesterol vs. 40%-50%). It has few drug interactions and few side effects but is expensive.

8. **Psyllium (e.g., Metamucil)** contains soluble fiber; 7 grams of soluble fiber per day can reduce cholesterol and might decrease cardiovascular mortality.

IV. **Treatment of Elevated Triglycerides.** Primary goal is to lower LDL. If triglycerides are still elevated when LDL is within an acceptable range, initiate treatment for triglycerides.

1. **If triglycerides are 200 to 499 mg/dL** once the LDL goal is met, intensify LDL lowering or add nicotinic acid or a fibrate.

2. **If triglycerides are >500 mg/dL** once the LDL goal is met, lower triglycerides as a primary goal. Institute a very low fat diet (<15% of total

calories), increase physical activity, institute weight lowering, and initiate a fibrate or nicotinic acid. Once triglycerides are <500 mg/dL, proceed with more aggressive LDL lowering as for TG 200 to 499 mg/dL.

V. **Treatment of Low HDL.** Address HDL <40 mg/dL. Options are limited but include exercise, fish oil, flax seed oil, moderate alcohol intake, niacin, A-1 Milano phospholipid complex infusion (experimental), CEPT inhibitors (e.g., torcetrapib [experimental]).

SYNCOPE

I. **Definition.** Differentiate between near syncope and vertigo, because the differential diagnosis is different. See Chapter 9 for work-up and differential of vertigo.

A. **Syncope is a sudden, brief loss of consciousness and, strictly speaking, is related to abrupt cerebral hypoperfusion.** Only two CNS lesions can cause syncope: bilateral cortical dysfunction (e.g., from hypoperfusion) and reticular activating system injury.

B. **Near syncope** is a sense of impending LOC or weakness, occurs more frequently, and provides valuable diagnostic clues, because the patient usually has better recollection of the event.

C. **Frequency of causes**

1. Frequency ≥55%: vasovagal, vasodepressor, neurocardiogenic, cardioinhibitory (all of which mean the same thing)

2. Frequency 10%: cardiac, neurologic, undiagnosed causes

3. Frequency 5%: metabolic or drug-induced, "other"

II. **Causes.**

A. **Cardiac and circulatory**

1. **Cardioinhibitory (bradycardia, enhanced parasympathetics), neurocardiogenic (e.g., vasovagal), and vasodepressor (decreased systemic vascular resistance)** are the most common causes and tend to be familial. Cardioinhibitory syncope occurs when a susceptible person is confronted with a stressful situation or with prolonged standing, heat exposure, severe pain, etc. **Prodromal symptoms:** restlessness, pallor, weakness, sighing, yawning, diaphoresis, and nausea. These symptoms may be followed by light-headedness, blurred vision, collapse, and LOC as patients become bradycardic and lose autonomic tone. Occasionally, mild clonic seizures occur, but a seizure work-up is not indicated unless other signs point in this direction. Spells are brief, with prompt recovery on recumbency. These episodes may be recurrent.

2. **Orthostatic hypotension** is a fall in blood pressure upon assuming an upright position. It is seen in a variety of settings. **Orthostatic fall in BP or increase in pulse is neither sensitive nor specific for hypovolemia.**

a. Hypovolemia (hemorrhage, vomiting, diarrhea, diuretics).

b. Interference with normal reflexes (e.g., nitrates, vasodilators, β-blockers, calcium channel blockers, neuroleptics).

c. Autonomic failure, primary or secondary. Diabetes is the most common form of secondary autonomic neuropathy, whereas advanced age is a common cause of primary autonomic failure. Also consider Shy–Drager syndrome (autonomic failure with parkinsonian features, amyloid, paraneoplastic syndromes, collagen-vascular disorders, etc.)

d. Postprandial syncope in the elderly.

3. Outflow obstruction includes IHSS, aortic stenosis, mitral stenosis, pulmonic stenosis, atrial myxoma, pulmonary embolism, and subclavian steal syndrome. These patients might present with exertional syncope. Mechanical valve malfunction can also cause outflow obstruction.

4. Myocardial ischemia or infarction

5. Arrhythmias

a. Bradyarrhythmias: sick sinus syndrome, AV-node blocks, etc.

b. Tachyarrhythmias: PSVT, Wolf–Parkinson–White syndrome, ventricular tachycardia (including from prolonged QT interval, Brugada's syndrome), etc.

6. Carotid sinus hypersensitivity. Syncope can occur with shaving or wearing a tight collar. Rarely the carotid sinus is stimulated by tumor. Many consider this a subtype of cardioinhibitory syncope.

B. Metabolic. Episodes are usually amplified by exertion but can occur when patient is supine. The onset and resolution are usually prolonged.

1. Hypoxia, as with shunting in congenital heart disease.

2. Hyperventilation results in cerebral vasoconstriction with symptoms of breathlessness, anxiety, circumoral tingling, paresthesias of hands or feet, carpopedal spasm, and, occasionally, unilateral or bilateral chest pain. Patients can reproduce these spells by hyperventilating in a controlled environment.

3. Hypoglycemia

4. Alcohol intoxication or other drug

C. Neurologic. TIAs rarely, if ever, cause syncope. The reticular activating system must be involved in syncope. When this occurs, there are almost always other neurologic manifestations such as cranial nerve abnormalities.

1. Migraine is the second most common cause in adolescents. LOC is followed by headache.

2. Seizure is usually easily differentiated by aura, history of tonic–clonic movements, and postictal state.

3. Abrupt rise of intracranial pressure is seen with subarachnoid hemorrhage or obstructive colloid cyst of the third ventricle.

D. Reflex syncope results from impaired right-sided heart filling and global cerebral hypoperfusion. The patient is usually standing upright before an episode because gravitational pooling of blood plays a causal role. Potential etiologies include pulmonary embolism or infarction, pericardial tamponade, pulmonary hypertension, a pregnant uterus as it compresses the inferior vena cava, and coughing, which decreases preload by increasing intrathoracic pressure.

E. **Miscellaneous:** Cough, postmicturition, psychogenic, severe visceral or ligamentous pain, and subsequent to severe vertigo.

III. **Evaluation.** Not everyone needs every test. Use clinical judgment. EEG and CT generally have low yield unless the history supports the diagnosis of seizure, CNS bleed, etc.

A. **History is the most important part of the evaluation.** The patient and witnesses should be questioned about precipitating circumstances, prodromal symptoms, time course of onset and recovery, and medication history.

B. **Physical exam**

1. Blood pressure and pulse supine and standing (however, orthostatic vital signs are neither sensitive nor specific for hypovolemia).
2. Auscultation of subclavian and carotid arteries.
3. Cardiac exam with attention to murmurs and extra heart sounds. Provocative maneuvers (Valsalva) as indicated.
4. Careful neurologic exam.

C. **Laboratory studies** should be directed by history and physical exam and can include blood glucose, blood gases, electrolytes, and Hct.

D. **ECG/Holter ambulatory monitoring or event monitor.** Every patient deserves one ECG (even children) to rule out WPW, prolonged QT, and Brugada's syndrome. Event monitors that are worn for a month and activated when patient has a feeling of palpitations or near syncope are more cost-effective and sensitive than 24 to 48 hours of ambulatory monitoring, but only if the patient is going to be able to activate the monitor in the presyncopal period.

E. **Signal-averaged ECG** may be helpful in patients suspected of having ventricular arrhythmias.

F. **Echocardiography** is useful in evaluating valvular and myocardial disease.

G. **EEG.** Obtain if seizure disorder is suspected; however, it may be falsely negative in 50% of cases. Nasopharyngeal leads, sleep deprivation, and hyperventilation can all increase yield.

H. **Electrophysiologic** invasive cardiac studies may be indicated in patients with structural heart disease and unexplained syncope or with a history that suggests an arrhythmia.

I. **Tilt testing** is up to 80% sensitive for cardioinhibitory syncope but as low as 55% specific. Specificity is worse if pharmacologic stimulus is used (nitroglycerin, isoproterenol).

J. **GXT** is important and useful in patients with a history of exercise-related syncope. **Echocardiogram and ECG should be done first, however.**

IV. **Treatment** depends on cause.

A. **Vasovagal syncope** usually responds to avoiding stimuli that trigger syncope. If it is clinically severe, β-blockers, cardiac pacing, and SSRI antidepressants have all been used. However, the success rate is poor. The frequency of cough syncope might be reduced by antitussives.

3

CARDIOLOGY

B. **Medical.** See appropriate section based on diagnosis. Antiepileptics, antiarrhythmics, mineralocorticoids (for chronic orthostatic hypotension), support hose (to prevent blood pooling) or migraine prophylaxis are useful in selected cases. Midodrine, an α-antagonist, has been used successfully for orthostatic syncope but can cause recumbent hypertension.

C. **Surgical.** For critical aortic stenosis, carotid artery disease, etc.

PROPHYLAXIS AGAINST BACTERIAL ENDOCARDITIS

I. **General Comments.** Endocarditis can occur from transient bacteremia. Because a variety of health care procedures can result in bacteremia, prophylaxis against bacteria that can adhere to endocardium is recommended, particularly in patients at high risk for endocarditis. The frequency of bacteremia is highest subsequent to oral and dental procedures (because of the abundant oral flora), intermediate for genitourinary procedures, and lowest for diagnostic procedures of the gastrointestinal tract. It is important to give prophylactic antibiotics before a procedure because bacterial adhesion can occur within minutes after bacteremia develops.

II. **Endocarditis Prophylaxis Recommended.**

A. **Cardiac conditions**

1. Prosthetic cardiac valves (including bioprosthetic, homograft, and mechanical).

2. Previous episode of bacterial endocarditis.

3. Most congenital cardiac defects (especially cyanotic congenital heart disease, PDA, VSD, and surgically repaired intracardiac defects with residual hemodynamic abnormalities).

4. Valvular heart disease resulting from rheumatic or other disease (aortic regurgitation and stenosis, mitral regurgitation and stenosis).

5. Hypertrophic cardiomyopathy.

6. Mitral valve prolapse with regurgitation.

B. **Dental or surgical procedures**

1. Dental or surgical procedures that cause gingival or mucosal bleeding, including mechanical dental hygiene procedures.

2. Tonsillectomy or adenoidectomy.

3. Surgical procedures involving upper respiratory or gastrointestinal mucosa.

4. Rigid bronchoscopy.

5. Sclerotherapy of esophageal varices.

6. Esophageal dilation.

7. Transesophageal echocardiography.

8. Gallbladder surgery.

9. Urethral catheterization or urinary tract surgery if infection is present.

10. Prostate surgery.

11. I&D of infected tissue.

12. Vaginal hysterectomy.
13. Vaginal delivery in the presence of infection (e.g., chorioamnionitis).

III. Endocarditis Prophylaxis Not Recommended.

A. Cardiac conditions

1. Previous coronary artery bypass surgery.
2. Mitral valve prolapse without regurgitation. (If MVP is associated with thickening or redundancy of valve leaflets, patients can have increased risk of endocarditis, especially men >45 years of age).
3. Functional or innocuous heart murmurs.
4. Cardiac pacemakers and implantable defibrillators.
5. Isolated secundum atrial septal defect.
6. Six months or longer after surgical repair of PDA or VSD without residua.
7. Previous rheumatic heart disease or Kawasaki disease without valve dysfunction.

B. Dental or surgical procedures

1. Dental procedures not likely to cause gingival bleeding, such as fillings above the gum line or adjustment of orthodontic appliances.
2. Injection of intraoral anesthetics.
3. Shedding of primary teeth.
4. Insertion of tympanostomy tube.
5. Endotracheal intubation or flexible bronchoscopy with or without biopsy specimens.
6. Cardiac catheterization.
7. Endoscopy with or without biopsy.
8. Urethral catheterization, D&C, uncomplicated vaginal delivery, abortion, sterilization procedures, insertion or removal of an IUD, or laparoscopy *in absence of infection*.

IV. Standard Regimens.

A. Dental, oral, upper respiratory tract (total children's dose should not exceed adult dose).

1. **For adults:** amoxicillin 2.0 g (children, 50 mg/kg) PO 1 hour before procedure.
2. **In penicillin-allergic patients:** clindamycin 600 mg (children, 20 mg/kg) PO *or* cephalexin or cefadroxil 2.0 g (children, 50 mg/kg) PO *or* azithromycin or clarithromycin 500 mg (children, 15 mg/kg) PO 1 hour before procedure.
3. **In patients unable to take oral medications:** ampicillin 2.0 g (children 20 mg/kg) IV or IM 30 minutes before procedure *or* clindamycin 600 mg (children 20 mg/kg) IV 30 minutes before procedure.
4. **In penicillin-allergic high-risk patients:** vancomycin 1.0 g IV over 1 hour, starting 1 hour before surgery. A repeat dose is not necessary.

B. GI or GU procedures (total children's dose should not exceed adult dose).

1. **High risk:** ampicillin 2.0 g IV (children, 50 mg/kg) *plus* gentamicin 1.5 mg/kg IV (for adults and children, not to exceed 120 mg) 30 minutes before procedure, then amoxicillin 1.0 g (children, 25 mg/kg)

CARDIOLOGY **3**

PO 6 hours later *or* ampicillin 1.0 g (children, 25 mg/kg) IV 6 hours after first dose.

2. **High risk, penicillin allergic:** Vancomycin 1.0 g (children, 20 mg/kg) IV (over 1 h) starting 1 hour before procedure *plus* gentamicin 1.5 mg/kg IV (both adults and children, not to exceed 120 mg) 1 hour before procedure. Complete infusion 30 minutes before procedure.

3. **Moderate or low risk:** Amoxicillin 2.0 g (children, 50 mg/kg) PO 1 hour before procedure *or* ampicillin 2.0 g (children 50 mg/kg) IM or IV 30 minutes before procedure.

4. **Moderate or low risk, penicillin allergic:** Vancomycin 1.0 g (children, 20 mg/kg) over 1 hour. Complete infusion 30 minutes before procedure.

BIBLIOGRAPHY

Alboni P, Botto GL, Baldi N, et al: Outpatient treatment of recent-onset atrial fibrillation with the "pill-in-the-pocket" approach. *N Engl J Med* 351:2384-2391, 2004.

American College of Chest Physicians: Seventh ACCP Conference on Antithrombotic and Thrombolytic Therapy: Evidence-based guidelines. *Chest* 126(3 Suppl): 163S-696S [entire issue], 2004.

Antman EM, Anbe DT, Armstrong PW, et al: ACC/AHA guidelines for the management of Patients with ST-elevation myocardial infarction. *Circulation* 110:588-636, 2004.

Aurigemma GP, Gaasch WH. Clinical practice: Diastolic heart failure. *N Engl J Med* 351:1097-1105, 2004.

Bonow RO et al: ACC/AHA Guidelines for the management of patients with valvular heart disease: A report of the American College of Cardiology/American Heart Association Task Force on Practice Guidelines (Committee on Management of Patients with Valvular Heart Disease). *J Am Coll Cardiol* 32:1486-1588, 1998.

Braunwald E, Antman EM, Beasley JW, et al: ACC/AHA guideline update for the management of patients with unstable angina and non–ST segment elevation myocardial infarction. *Circulation* 106:1893-1900, 2002.

Chobanian AV, Bakris GL, Black HR, et al: The seventh report of the Joint National Committee on Prevention, Detection, Evaluaion and Treatment of High Blood Pressure. *JAMA* 289:2560-2572, 2003; erratum in *JAMA* 290:197, 2003.

Cotter G, Kaluski E,Milo O, et al: LINCS: L-NAME (a NO synthetase inhibitor) in the treatment of refractory cardiogenic shock: A prospective randomized study. *Eur Heart J* 24:1287-1295, 2003.

Freed LA, Levy D, Levine RA, et al: Prevalence and clinical outcome of mitral-valve prolapse. *N Engl J Med* 341:1-7, 1999.

Gregoratos G, Cheitlin MD, Conill A, et al: ACC/AHA guidelines for implantation of cardiac pacemakers and antiarrhythmia devices: A report of the American College of Cardiology/American Heart Association Task Force on Practice Guidelines (Committee on Pacemaker Implantation). *J Am Coll Cardiol* 31:1175-1209, 1998.

Heart Outcomes Prevention Evaluation Study Investigators: Effects of an angiotensin-converting-enzyme inhibitor, ramipril, on cardiovascular events in high-risk patients. *N Engl J Med* 342:145-153, 2000.

Heart Outcomes Prevention Evaluation Study Investigators: Vitamin E supplementation and cardiovascular events in high-risk patients, *N Engl J Med* 342:154-160, 2000.

Kinch JW, Ryan TJ: Right ventricular infarction. *N Engl J Med* 330:1211-1217, 1994.

Menon V, Harrington RA, Hochman JS, et al: Thrombolysis and adjunctive therapy in acute myocardial infarction. *Chest* 126(3 Suppl):549S-575S, 2004.

Naccarelli GV, Wolbrette DL, Dell'Orfano JT, et al: Amiodarone: What have we learned from clinical trials? *Clin Cardiol* 23:73-83, 2000.

Pitt B, Zannad F, Remme WJ, et al: The effect of spironolactone on morbidity and mortality in patients with severe heart failure. *N Engl J Med* 341:709-718, 1999.

Platelet Receptor Inhibition in Ischemic Syndrome Management in Patients Limited by Unstable Signs and Symptoms (PRISM) Study Investigators: A comparison of aspirin plus tirofiban with aspirin plus heparin for unstable angina. *N Engl J Med* 338:1498-1505, 1998.

Platelet Receptor Inhibition in Ischemic Syndrome Management in Patients Limited by Unstable Signs and Symptoms (PRISM-PLUS) Study Investigators: Inhibition of the platelet glycoprotein IIb/IIIa receptor with tirofiban in unstable angina and non-Q-wave myocardial infarction. *N Engl J Med* 338:1488-1497, 1998.

Roongsirtong C. Common causes of troponin elevation in the absence of myocardial infarction: Incidence and clinical significance. *Chest* 125:1877-1884, 2004.

Toole JF, Malinow MR, Chambless ME, et al: Lowering homocysteine in patients with ischemic stroke to prevent recurrent stroke, myocardial infarction, and death: The Vitamin Intervention for Stroke Prevention (VISP) randomized controlled trial. *JAMA* 291:565-575, 2004.

Wyse DG, Waldo AL, DiMarco JP, et al: A comparison of rate control and rhythm control in patients with atrial fibrillation. *N Engl J Med* 347:1825-1833, 2002.

Yamamoto K, Wilson DJ, Canzanello VJ, Redfield MM: Left ventricular diastolic dysfunction in patients with hypertension and preserved systolic function. *Mayo Clin Proc* 75:148-155, 2000.

3

CARDIOLOGY

Pulmonary Medicine

M. Brian Hartz, Devang R. Doshi, and Kevin C. Doerschug

DEEP VENOUS THROMBOSIS AND PULMONARY EMBOLISM

Deep Venous Thrombosis (DVT)

I. **Lower Extremity DVT.** Classically characterized by unilateral swelling and tenderness of the calf and thigh, which may be erythematous and warm. **However, the majority of lower extremity DVTs are in the calf and are clinically silent.**

II. **Upper Extremity DVT.** Occurs especially in patients with indwelling venous catheters in subclavian or internal jugular veins, but also in active individuals with repetitive upper arm motion or sports activities. Patients may present clinically up to several weeks out from the inciting factor.

III. **Superficial Thrombophlebitis.** Characterized by tenderness, erythema, and edema in the area of a superficial vein. **Superficial thrombophlebitis may propagate into the deep veins in up to 40% of cases;** in one study of 21 patients, 33% also had silent PE. Treat with NSAIDs and heat. **Follow superficial thrombophlebitis with Doppler US and anticoagulate if it propagates into the deep venous system.**

IV. **DVT in any location can migrate from the site of origin to the lungs, causing PE.** Calf DVTs embolize in 8% to 34% of cases. Overall, 52% to 67% of all lower extremity DVTs lead to PE.

V. **Risk Factors for DVT and PE.**

A. Pregnancy, smoking, recent surgery or trauma, immobilization, CHF, travel, and prior history of DVT or PE.

B. **Hypercoagulable states:** protein C or protein S deficiency, protein C activation resistance, antithrombin III deficiency, factor V Leiden mutation, prothrombin gene mutation, estrogen use, cancer, anticardiolipin antibodies, nephrotic syndrome, hyperhomocystinemia. **The timing of the evaluation for a hypercoagulable state is critical. Not all testing can be done in a patient with an active clot or in those who are anticoagulated.** Prothrombotic abnormalities do not increase the risk of recurrent DVT/PE beyond what can be predicted by clinical factors (cancer, use of OCPs, prior PE/DVT, etc.). Thus, evaluation of prothrombotic states is generally not very helpful clinically.

1. **The following can be tested for in the anticoagulated patient:** Protein C resistance (using newer tests), factor V Leiden (using PCR DNA analysis), prothrombin gene mutation (DNA PCR), anticardiolipin antibodies, and homocysteine levels.

2. **The following tests cannot be performed in the anticoagulated patient or in persons on estrogen:** Protein C level (patient must be off

warfarin for 10 days), protein S level (must be off warfarin for 10 days, has not been pregnant or received estrogen for 1-2 months), antithrombin III (must be off heparin and warfarin, and no pregnancy or estrogens for 1-2 months). In addition, liver disease, renal disease, surgery, and active thrombosis (e.g., PE or DVT) can all decrease antithrombin III levels, giving a false-positive result.

3. **Homocysteine levels** should be checked after a 12-hour fast.

VI. **Diagnosis of DVT.**

A. **Physical exam, including Homans' sign, does not reliably predict the presence or absence of DVT,** but can change pretest probability.

B. **Venous Doppler US.**

1. **One negative Doppler cannot rule out a DVT in high- or medium-risk patients** because of the lack of sensitivity of Doppler for calf DVTs. Must repeat in 1 week if following a patient not on anticoagulation.

2. **Venous Doppler:**

a. **Performs well (e.g., is sensitive and specific):**
   (1) In symptomatic patients (e.g., those with a swollen leg).
   (2) For clots above the knee (>95% sensitivity and specificity).

b. **Does not perform well (e.g., is not sensitive or specific):**
   (1) As a screening test in those without symptoms (e.g., postoperative patients or those with suspected PE but no swollen leg).
   (2) For clots below the knee (70% sensitivity).
   (3) **For pelvic vein DVT.**
   (4) In those with symmetrically swollen legs.

C. **Impedance plethysmography is not useful.**

D. **D-Dimer.** A negative high-sensitivity D-dimer (e.g., ELISA) in a low-risk patient is enough to rule out a DVT. See further discussion in the section on PE, later.

E. **Venography** is very rarely performed now, and can itself precipitate DVT.

VII. **DVT Prophylaxis in the Nonsurgical Patient (see Chapter 15 for prophylaxis regimens).**

A. **Patients admitted to medical floors, trauma service, or an ICU** should be assessed for risk and, if appropriate, treated with SQ heparin or enoxaparin and intermittent compression stockings. **Aspirin alone is ineffective for prophylaxis of the inpatient.**

B. **For airline travel,** avoid constrictive clothing and dehydration. Practice calf-stretching exercises during the flight; whether to pursue further prophylactic measures (graded compression stockings or single-dose LMWH) in high-risk patients should be decided on an individual basis. Again, aspirin is ineffective for this indication.

VIII. **Treatment of DVT.**

A. **Anticoagulation. See Chapter 6 for a complete discussion of anticoagulation, dosing, initiation of warfarin, etc.**

B. Consider outpatient treatment of stable, otherwise healthy low-risk patients.

C. **Drugs.** Weight-based unfractionated IV heparin or subcutaneous LMWH are the initial drugs of choice. **SQ LMWH is as effective as**

unfractionated heparin and may be safer, with a lower risk of
bleeding and thrombocytopenia. (See Chapter 6 for dosing.)

D. **If suspicion for DVT is high, but diagnostic tests are unavailable,** empiric anticoagulation with unfractionated heparin or LMWH is recommended until testing is completed.

E. **Duration of treatment.** Patients should be anticoagulated with warfarin after a DVT.

1. Low-dose warfarin (INR 1.5-1.9) is not beneficial over the long term and should not be used.

2. **For first DVT:**

a. **If due to an identifiable *and* transient or reversible cause,** 3 months.

b. **If there is no obvious predisposing condition,** then treat at least 6 to 12 months. **However, when warfarin is discontinued, patients return to their pretreatment risk of recurrent DVT/PE.**

c. **For recurrent DVT,** lifelong anticoagulation is indicated.

d. **Pregnancy.** Unfractionated IV heparin (adjusted-dose) or SQ LMWH heparin is used. Warfarin is contraindicated during pregnancy.

e. **For patients with active cancer,** current guidelines recommend use of LMWH for chronic anticoagulation rather than warfarin (class IA recommendation).

f. **Post-thrombotic syndrome** consists of chronic leg swelling secondary to venous obstruction or incompetence, leg pain, and ulcer formation. **Compression stockings can help prevent post-thrombotic syndrome and should be used in most patients after a first episode of DVT.**

Pulmonary Embolism (PE)

I. **Characterized by** hypoxia (80%), dyspnea/tachypnea (73%), pleuritic chest pain (66%), tachycardia (30%), cough (37%), and hemoptysis (13%). However, even patients with large clots may be asymptomatic.

II. **Testing for PE** (see **Box 4-1** and **Tables 4-1** and **4-2** for a summary of the approach to PE).

A. **Oxygen saturation and ABG may be normal in up to 15% of patients with a PE** and cannot be used to differentiate between those with or without PE, although they do change the pretest probability.

B. **Look for $\dot{V}/\dot{Q}$ mismatch by calculating the alveolar–arterial (A-a) gradient.** An elevated A-a gradient is present in 80% to 90% of those with PE. **The A-a gradient is normal in 10% to 20% of patients with PE.**

1. **A-a gradient** = Pa_{O_2} (alveolar) − Pa_{O_2} (arterial)

a. Pa_{O_2} (alveolar) = 150 − (Pa_{CO_2}) (1.2) assuming FiO_2 of 21% (room air)

b. Normal A-a gradient is 5 to 20 torr, but increases with age (normal = [age/4] + 4 torr).

2. **Other causes of a $\dot{V}/\dot{Q}$ mismatch (abnormal A-a gradient)** include resolving severe asthma, other causes of emboli (fat, air), sickle cell crisis, hepatopulmonary syndrome, pulmonary artery hypoplasia, lung

---

BOX 4-1

APPROACH TO THE PATIENT WITH SUSPECTED PULMONARY EMBOLISM

This approach will miss <5% of pulmonary emboli and has a specificity of >85%. There will still be some false positives. This approach requires a multirow detector CT and an ELISA D dimer. Single-row detector CT and non–ELISA D dimer do not have a negative predictive value adequate to rule out PE. If you have a single-row detector CT, CT can be used to *rule in* PE but not *rule out* PE! High-sensitivity ELISA D dimer can be used as the first step in low- and medium-probability patients but not in high-probability patients.*

STEPS IN EVALUATION

1. Perform Doppler ultrasound of legs. If Doppler is positive, anticoagulate; if negative, continue evaluation. Note that high-sensitivity ELISA D dimer can be used as the first step in the low-probability patient.
2. Determine clinical probability based on Wells criteria (see Table 4-1).
3. Perform further evaluation based on clinical probability.

LOW CLINICAL PROBABILITY (<10%)*

- Negative highly sensitive ELISA D dimer: PE ruled out.
- Normal V̇/Q̇ scan: PE ruled out.
- Low-probability V̇/Q̇ scan and normal leg Doppler: PE ruled out.*
- Positive CT scan: PE ruled in.
- Negative multirow detector CT scan: PE ruled out.

INTERMEDIATE CLINICAL PROBABILITY (35%)

- Normal V̇/Q̇ scan: PE ruled out. Note that this is *normal* V̇/Q̇, *not* low-probability V̇/Q̇.†
- Low-, intermediate-, or high-probability V̇/Q̇ scan: Proceed to angiography or CT plus leg Doppler.
- Negative multirow detector CT scan *and* negative lower-extremity Doppler: PE ruled out.
- Positive CT: PE ruled in.
- Negative ELISA D dimer: PE ruled out. *Note:* Many authors (including those of this chapter and book) do not consider a negative D dimer adequate to rule out PE in the intermediate-clinical-probability patient and would continue evaluation, including CT and leg Doppler.

HIGH CLINICAL PROBABILITY (70%)

- Normal V̇/Q̇ scan: PE ruled out. Note that this is *normal* V̇/Q̇, *not* low-probability V̇/Q̇.†
- High-probability V̇/Q̇ scan: PE ruled in.
- Low- or intermediate-probability V̇/Q̇ scan: Proceed to angiography or CT.‡
- Negative CT: Proceed to angiography.
- Positive CT: PE ruled in.

Evaluation modified from Fedullo PE, Tapson VE: *N Engl J Med* 349:1247-1256, 2003; and Roy PM, Colombet I, Durieux P, et al: *BMJ* 331:259, 2005.

*Intermediate- or high-probability V̇/Q̇ scans *are not helpful in the low-clinical-probability patient.* Low-clinical-probability patients with intermediate- or high-probability V̇/Q̇ scans need further testing (CT, angiogram, leg Doppler).

†Data suggest that this is a safe strategy (Fedullo and Tapson, 2005), but it is not universally accepted, and some would pursue additional testing (CT, angiography, leg Doppler) in these patients.

‡Low-probability or intermediate-probability V̇/Q̇ scan *is not helpful in the high-clinical-probability patient.* High-clinical-probability patients with a low- or intermediate-probability V̇/Q̇ scan need further testing (CT, angiography, leg Doppler) to rule in DVT/PE.

TABLE 4-1

WELLS' CRITERIA FOR PULMONARY EMBOLISM

Variable	Points
Signs and symptoms of DVT	3
Alternative diagnosis is less likely than PE (PE is the highest on the differential)	3
Heart rate >100 bpm	1.5
Immobilization or surgery within last 4 wk	1.5
History of DVT or PE in past	1.5
Hemoptysis	1
Cancer (currently under treatment, treated in past 6 mo, or in palliative care)	1

Clinical probability of PE: low, <2 points; intermediate, 2-6 points; high, >6 points.

vasculitis, post-radiation therapy, interstitial lung disease, atelectasis, pneumonia, and pulmonary edema (including ARDS).

C. **A CXR and ECG should be done** to rule out other causes of dyspnea and tachypnea, but they are not sensitive or specific for PE.

D. **Angiography is the gold standard,** but it is invasive and interpretation can be difficult if infrequently performed (up to an 8% miss rate).

E. **V̇/Q̇ scanning.** Must interpret with caution, and best done only in a situation where the CXR is near normal—pretest probability should be determined first (see Table 4-2).

F. **Spiral CT is up to 95% sensitive, but in some studies this value is as low as 60% for segmental PE.**

G. **Doppler US of the lower extremity is negative in 50% of patients with PE** but is helpful if positive.

H. **D-Dimer is helpful only if it is negative and clinical suspicion is low.** D-dimer is highly sensitive in some studies, but the technique of determining the D-dimer varies among labs. **You must know which technique your laboratory is using.** The sensitivity of latex agglutination is not sufficient to rule out PE (30% with PE have normal D-dimer). The whole-blood assay has an intermediate sensitivity (15% with PE have a normal D-dimer). ELISA has a 0.3% to 4% false-negative rate,

TABLE 4-2

INTERPRETATION OF THE V̇/Q̇ SCAN RESULTS IN LIGHT OF PRETEST CLINICAL PROBABILITY USING WELLS' CRITERIA*

V̇/Q̇ Scan Interpretation	Pretest Clinical Probability of Pulmonary Embolism (%)		
	High	Intermediate	Low
High	96	88	56
Intermediate	66	28	16
Low	40	16	4
Normal	0	6	2

*Wells' criteria are shown in Table 4-1.

From The PIOPED Investigators: Value of the ventilation/perfusion scan in acute pulmonary embolism: Results of the Prospective Investigation of Pulmonary Embolism Diagnosis (PIOPED). *JAMA* 263:2753-2759, 1990.

possibly as good as $\dot{V}/\dot{Q}$ scanning. **Most people with an elevated D-dimer do not have a PE. It is almost always elevated in many common conditions such as pregnancy, trauma, MI, postoperative state, heart failure, infection, and cancer.**

III. **Treatment of nonmassive PE is the same as for DVT.** The patient with a large PE may have right-sided heart failure and become relatively preload dependent, necessitating fluid resuscitation. **Mechanical ventilation or inotrope support can precipitate complete circulatory collapse but should be used as needed in the patient at risk of respiratory failure.**

A. **Anticoagulation.** Either unfractionated heparin or LMWH may be used for nonmassive PE. Because LMWH has a long half-life and is not easily reversed, consideration must be given to any potential for bleeding before choosing LMWH over unfractionated heparin; LMWH should be used with caution in those with renal failure. **See Chapter 6 for anticoagulation dosing and guidelines.**

B. **Thrombolytics may be beneficial** in cases of hypotension or circulatory collapse during PE; however, the data are mixed, with some trials showing increased mortality. There is ongoing controversy regarding whether they are helpful in patients with evidence of right heart strain who are not hypotensive.

C. **Vena caval filters.** If anticoagulation is contraindicated or ineffective, consider vena caval interruption with an IVC filter. **IVC filters are less effective than anticoagulation, and there is no 1-year difference in the PE rate in those with a vena caval filter and those without (clots form on the filter), even if used with concurrent anticoagulation. There is also an increased risk of DVT with IVC filters. IVC filters have not improved survival.**

PULMONARY FUNCTION TESTS

Figure 4-1 shows PFT results for normal lungs and in restrictive and obstructive lung disease.

I. **Spirometry** is most useful for diagnosing presence of obstructive lung disease **(Figure 4-2).**

A. **Forced vital capacity (FVC)** is the maximum volume of gas that can be exhaled forcefully after a maximum inspiration.

B. **Forced expiratory volume in 1 second (FEV$_1$)** is the volume of gas exhaled during the first second of an FVC maneuver. When <80%, and when the ratio of FEV$_1$/FVC is <0.7, it reveals obstructive physiology.

C. **Forced expiratory flow, midexpiratory phase (FEF$_{25-75\%}$),** measured in the middle one-half of forced expiration, represents flow through small airways. If <50% of that predicted, consider obstructive disease if the FEV$_1$/FVC ratio is also decreased despite a normal FEV$_1$.

D. **Lung volumes.**

1. **Total lung capacity (TLC):** The volume in lungs at maximum inspiration—a decreased TLC is the hallmark of a restrictive pattern.

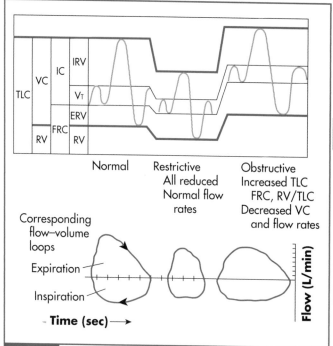

FIG. 4-1

Pulmonary function test results for normal lungs and in restrictive and obstructive lung disease.

2. **Residual volume (RV):** The volume left in the lungs after maximal expiration. Increased RV indicates air trapping.
3. **Tidal volume (V_T):** The volume of air inspired and expired during normal breathing.

II. **Diffusing Capacity.**

A. **Diffusing capacity of the lung for carbon monoxide (D_{LCO})** measures the diffusion of CO (which is used as a surrogate for oxygen) across the alveolar surface. D_{LCO} is affected by hemoglobin, so this should be measured simultaneously.

1. **D_{LCO} is decreased (defined as <80% of normal) by** interstitial thickening (fibrosis, sarcoid), decrease in alveolar surface area (emphysema, pneumonectomy, and pneumonia), inflammation (pneumonitis, bronchiolitis), carbon monoxide poisoning, or decrease in lung perfusion (pulmonary hypertension, anemia, PE).

2. **D_{LCO} is increased (defined as >140% of normal) by** significant pulmonary hemorrhage, obesity, polycythemia, large lung volumes, left-to-right shunt, and asthma.

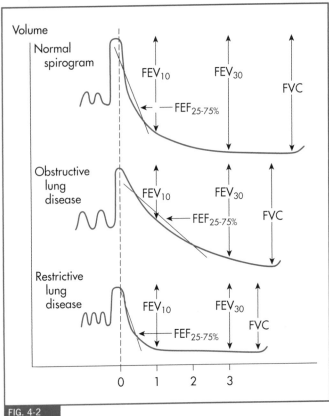

FIG. 4-2
Spirometry results for normal lungs and in restrictive and obstructive lung disease.

III. Interpreting Patterns of Abnormal PFTs.

A. **Obstructive disorders are defined by an FEV_1/FVC of <0.7.** Differential diagnosis includes emphysema, chronic bronchitis, and asthma. With bullous disease and air trapping, the TLC and RV will be increased, with a normal to decreased vital capacity (VC) and V_T.

B. **Restrictive disorders are suggested by a decrease in both FEV_1 and FVC, but with an FEV_1/FVC ratio of ≥ 0.7. However, restrictive disease is defined by a decrease in TLC.** Differential diagnosis includes interstitial lung disease, obesity, kyphoscoliosis, muscle weakness (such as with Guillain-Barré syndrome or myasthenia gravis), postsurgical state, paralysis, ascites, pleuritis, pleural effusions, pulmonary edema, pregnancy, peritonitis, chest/abdomen injuries.

IV. **Average Values.**
A. **Vital capacity** (predicted):
- Women = $(21.78 - [0.101 \times \text{age in y}]) \times$ height in cm
- Men = $(27.63 - [0.112 \times \text{age in y}]) \times$ height in cm
B. **Tidal volume:**
- Children: 7.5 mL/kg
- Adult women: 6.6 mL/kg
- Adult men: 7.8 mL/kg

POSITIVE-PRESSURE VENTILATION AND OXYGEN THERAPY

I. **General.** Respiratory failure is defined as the inability of the lungs to meet the metabolic demands of the body. This can involve failure of tissue oxygenation or failure of CO_2 homeostasis, or both. Acute respiratory failure should be suspected when a patient breathing room air has a Po_2 <60 torr or a Pco_2 >50 torr with a pH <7.3. **However, the decision to intubate is a clinical one and is not based on any absolute number.**

II. **Oxygen therapy.**
A. **Oxygen delivery systems:** see Table 4-3.
B. **Complications of oxygen therapy.**
1. **Pulmonary oxygen toxicity.** Mucosal drying, mucociliary dysfunction, atelectasis, interstitial and alveolar edema, and alveolar hemorrhage. Toxicity is especially problematic in those with a history of bleomycin use, even if the exposure was in the remote past.
2. **Decreased respiratory drive,** CO_2 retention (hypercapnia and acidosis), and respiratory failure in patients with chronic hypoxemia, who have a respiratory drive based on hypoxia (as in those with COPD). **However, oxygen should be given to maintain Po_2 >55 to 60 torr (88%-90% oxygen saturation); treat hypercapnia with ventilatory support as indicated.**
3. **Retrolental fibroplasia in neonates** of low birth weight or gestational age <34 weeks.
4. **Bronchopulmonary dysplasia** in infants who require mechanical ventilation after birth.
5. **Risk of fire and explosion.**

III. **Positive-Pressure Ventilation** can be achieved with either noninvasive, tight-fitting masks (continuous positive airway pressure [CPAP], bilevel positive airway pressure [BiPAP]) and high-pressure inspiratory gases, or the traditional mechanical ventilator with an endotracheal tube. Noninvasive ventilation can reduce the need for intubation and improve outcomes. Any invasive mode of ventilation increases the risk of a ventilator-associated pneumonia, which will prolong the patient's time on the ventilator and potentially lead to further complications. **Noninvasive positive-pressure ventilation (e.g., CPAP, BiPAP) is contraindicated in uncooperative or somnolent patients.**

4

PULMONARY MEDICINE

TABLE 4-3
OXYGEN DELIVERY SYSTEMS

Type	O_2 Flow (L/min)	Percentage O_2 Delivered	Comments
LOW-FLOW SYSTEMS			
Nasal cannula	0.25-8	22-45	Precise regulation of FIO_2 not possible Comfortable but limited to effective flow rate of <4 L/min Nasal mucosa drying is common
Simple mask	6-10	35-55	Offers little over nasal cannula Less comfortable, hot; skin irritation Not low enough FIO_2 for COPD O_2 rates must be at least 5 L/min to clear CO_2
Reservoir masks: nonrebreathing	12-15	90-95	High FIO_2 delivered; reservoir fills during expiration, which provides increased volume of O_2
Reservoir masks: partial rebreathing	8-12	50-80	Flow must be sufficient to keep reservoir bag from deflating upon inspiration
HIGH-FLOW SYSTEMS			
Venturi mask	4-12	21-100	Exact FIO_2 can be delivered Poor humidification Uncomfortable
Aerosol mask, face tent	0-12	30-100	Used to deliver precise FIO_2 or aerosol, or both Can provide controlled temperature of gas May need two or three setups to meet inspirational flows for $FIO_2 > 0.5$ Aerosol may induce bronchospasm, fluid overload, overmobilization of secretions, or contamination
Mask CPAP and BiPAP	0-12	≤100	Useful in COPD and CHF but not in asthma. May prevent intubation and decrease hospital stays.
T-tube	0-12	30-100	For spontaneous breathing through endotracheal tube Flow rates should be two or three times minute ventilation

A. Indications for positive pressure ventilation.

Note: *The decision to intubate a patient is a clinical decision and is not dependent on any particular laboratory parameter!*

1. **Hypercapnia.** Increased P_{CO_2} with inability to maintain adequate alveolar ventilation suggests respiratory failure. Some patients with chronic lung disease will tolerate an increased P_{CO_2}, remaining awake and comfortable; they tend to have a compensated respiratory acidosis with elevated serum bicarbonate, and usually maintain pH >7.3.

2. **Hypoxemia is indicated by a P_{AO_2} <40 to 60 torr on maximal fraction of inspired oxygen (F_{IO_2}). However, the decision to intubate or use noninvasive pressure support (CPAP, BiPAP) is a clinical one and is not based on a blood gas or any absolute criterion.**

3. **Other indications** include increasing obtundation, rapidly progressing respiratory disease, increased work of breathing or use of accessory muscles of respiration, acute hypercapnia with pH <7.2, or severe metabolic acidosis with inadequate ventilatory response.

B. Modes of positive-pressure ventilation.

1. Endotracheal tube–based mechanical ventilation.

a. **Volume-cycled ventilation. A tidal volume is set and the specified volume of gas is delivered.** Examples of volume-cycled ventilation include controlled mandatory ventilation (a fixed rate and volume are delivered), assist control (fixed minimum rate and volume are delivered, with the patient's respirations triggering additional breaths), and volume support. **In volume-cycled ventilation, the minute ventilation is guaranteed, but the airway pressures are variable, allowing for generation of high airway pressures and increased risk of barotrauma, such as pneumothorax.**

b. **Pressure-cycled ventilation. An inspiratory pressure is set, with the V_T dependent on pressure and patient compliance: V_T actually varies from breath to breath.** Examples include pressure-control and pressure-support ventilation. **The minute ventilation can change because delivery of a set volume is not guaranteed. Hence, gas exchange can vary, making hypercapnia or alkalosis possible. However, because inspiratory pressures are controlled, the risk of barotrauma is less.** Because ventilator-associated pneumothorax may be rapidly life threatening, pressure-cycled ventilation may be preferred in patients with variable compliance (pneumonia, ARDS).

2. **Noninvasive ventilation: CPAP or BiPAP, either continuously or intermittently.** The patient must be cooperative. CPAP or BiPAP may obviate the need for intubation and is associated with better outcomes. Settings for CPAP/BiPAP must be individualized. Start with 8 to 12 cm H_2O inspiratory pressure and 3 to 5 cm H_2O expiratory pressure. Gradually increase to 10 to 20 cm H_2O inspiratory pressure and up to

6 cm H_2O expiratory pressure for optimal results. **Patients must be closely observed for hemodynamic instability the first 8 hours after starting CPAP or BiPAP.**

3. **Ventilator management.**

a. **Oxygenation.** Generally, initiate mechanical ventilation with an FIO_2 of 100%, then taper 10% every 10 to 15 minutes to find the lowest FIO_2 necessary to maintain adequate oxygenation. **Initial V_T should be 8 to 10 mL/kg body weight.** Arterial oxygen content should be maintained at 60 torr or higher, or saturations at 90% or higher. An FIO_2 of >60% for over 24 hours has been associated with lung injury. **Positive end-expiratory pressure (PEEP) may be added to decrease the A-a gradient, allowing a lower FIO_2 while maintaining oxygenation (see later).** In patients with ARDS, some experts pursue a "lung protective" strategy using lower tidal volumes (6-8 mL/kg); see discussion of permissive hypercapnia, later.

b. **Ventilation.** Reflected by the PCO_2. Minute ventilation (minute ventilation = tidal volume × respiratory rate) is approximately 5 to 10 L/min or 100 mL/kg/min. Increases in minute ventilation will cause a decrease in PCO_2. Decreased minute ventilation (hypoventilation) will result in a rising PCO_2. Goal should be to maintain a normal pH.

c. **Permissive hypercapnia.** In certain situations (e.g., ARDS), low tidal volumes may lead to hypoventilation, and the PCO_2 will rise. When purposefully allowed to occur, this is called *permissive hypercapnia*, and can decrease injury (and mortality) from mechanical ventilation **as long as the patient maintains hemodynamic stability and good oxygenation.** There is no known safe upper limit for PCO_2 or lower limit for pH during permissive hypercapnia; closely watch both arterial pH and PCO_2 for signs of clinical deterioration.

d. **V_T.** Higher V_T may decrease venous return and may increase risk of barotrauma and lung injury.

e. **PEEP** may increase compliance of the lung and decrease the work of breathing by recruiting alveolar units, thus preventing atelectasis and decreasing shunting. It is usually begun at 3 to 5 cm H_2O and increased in small increments. **High levels of PEEP may result in decreased venous return and severe hemodynamic compromise.** Other negative consequences include overventilation, barotrauma, and elevated intracranial pressure. Cardiac output should be measured if there is an indication of problems because it may increase or decrease with increased PEEP.

f. **Peak airway pressure** reflects the pressure required to overcome airway resistance and is the peak pressure during the inspiratory cycle. If the level is >35 cm H_2O, consider obstruction in the endotracheal tube, bronchospasm, decreased lung compliance, or a pneumothorax from barotrauma.

g. **Sedation during mechanical ventilation is essential** and allows the patient to rest, decreases anxiety, and ensures better compliance with the ventilator. However, periodic interruption of sedation (e.g., early each morning) reduces the total number of days on a ventilator and in an ICU. **Initial therapy may include fentanyl, midazolam, diazepam, lorazepam, or propofol.** Propofol has the advantage of being very short acting and patients recover quickly once the infusion is stopped.

h. **Neuromuscular paralysis is occasionally needed but patients still need to be sedated and given analgesics.** Ventilator apnea alarm must be functional. For long- term paralysis, use nondepolarizing agents such as pancuronium, vecuronium, or cisatracurium. **Prolonged use of these agents, especially in continuous infusions and with concurrent corticosteroid use, is associated with prolonged (days to months) muscle weakness and ventilator dependence.** If repeated dosing or continuous drips are necessary, consider nerve stimulation testing to avoid overmedication. If a patient is seizing, paralysis should be continued only if continuous EEG monitoring is available. If necessary, a neostigmine-atropine combination can be used to reverse the nondepolarizing agents.

4. **Prevention of ventilator-associated complications.**

a. **Airway secretions have been shown to travel past inflated endotracheal tube cuffs. Continuous subglottic aspiration of secretions reduces the incidence of nosocomial pneumonia.** Frequent oral care and a semirecumbent position in bed will minimize the risk of ventilator-associated pneumonia.

b. **Stress ulcer prophylaxis.** Enteral feeding, H_2 blockers, and proton-pump inhibitors prevent upper GI tract stress ulcers in patients needing mechanical ventilation. However, H_2 blockers and proton-pump inhibitors may be associated with a higher risk of pneumonia because of bacterial overgrowth in the stomach.

c. **DVT prophylaxis.** See Chapter 15 for regimens.

d. **Occasional surveillance cultures** of tracheal aspirate may help tailor the treatment of pneumonia should it occur.

5. **Withdrawal of mechanical ventilation—guidelines for weaning from mechanical ventilation:**

a. **Ensure underlying process that led to need for ventilation has resolved and the patient is awake, alert, and off sedatives.**

b. **Ideal parameters.** Po_2 >60 torr with an Fio_2 <40%, Pco_2 and pH in acceptable range, PEEP <5 cm H_2O, minute ventilation <10 L/min. Although used in the past, maximal inspiratory pressure (> –20 cm H_2O) has been shown to be a poor predictor of successful weaning.

c. **Weaning from the ventilator:**
   - Place the patient in an upright position.
   - Have tube feeds turned off for several hours before extubation.
   - Explain the process to the patient and encourage cooperation.
   - Begin during the daytime; allow the patient to rest at night and between trials of weaning.
   - Causes of weaning failure include poor respiratory or cardiac function, underlying infection, high metabolic demands, poor nutrition and energy stores, and inadequate rest.

d. **Discontinue attempts at weaning if:**
  - pH <7.3, Pco_2 >50 torr, or Po_2 <60 torr.
  - The patient becomes anxious, fatigued, demonstrates increasing respiratory distress, or develops significant arrhythmias or hemodynamic deterioration.
e. **Methods of weaning from ventilator:**
  - **Pressure-support method.** Switch from an assisted mode of breathing to pressure support (see earlier), setting pressures to generate tidal volumes similar to the assisted volumes with a ventilation rate <20. Gradually decrease the inspiratory pressure until 8 to 10 cm H_2O above expiratory pressure. If patient can maintain adequate volumes with a ventilation rate of less than 20 for 30 to 60 minutes, consider extubation.
  - **T-piece method.** A T-piece trial involves having the patient breathe through the endotracheal tube for up to an hour without assistance from the ventilator. This will require increased work of breathing, and the patient may not tolerate it, as evidenced by increased respiratory rate or desaturation. However, if the patient does tolerate it, extubation is possible.

CHRONIC OBSTRUCTIVE PULMONARY DISEASE

I. **Definition.** A generalized increased resistance to airflow during expiration due to several different diseases, including chronic bronchitis, emphysema, chronic asthma, bronchiolitis, and bronchiectasis. Most patients have a combination of these entities, rather than pure emphysema or chronic bronchitis. COPD occurs in 10% to 15% of smokers. Asthma, bronchiectasis, and bronchiolitis are discussed separately elsewhere in this chapter.

II. **Chronic Bronchitis.** Characterized by chronic cough productive of mucus for at least 3 months in each of last 2 years with inflammatory changes in the bronchial mucosa. Results from prolonged exposure to pulmonary irritants, including cigarettes, allergens, pollutants, and recurrent infections.

III. **Emphysema.** Characterized by destruction of the lung parenchyma beyond the terminal bronchioles with coalescence of alveoli. **Divided into:**

A. **Centrilobular,** which is the result of smoking.

B. **Panlobular,** which is the result of α_1-antitrypsin deficiency. α_1-**Antitrypsin deficiency is the only form of COPD in which the underlying cause is treatable and the decline in pulmonary function can be slowed,** although the obstructive physiology does not resolve.

IV. **Diagnosis.** Diagnose with PFTs, including spirometry (before and after bronchodilators), lung volumes, and D_{LCO}.

A. **Spirometry shows obstructive airflow patterns** (reduced FEV_1 and reduced FEV_1/FVC), which generally are nonreversible. **However, there is usually some reversible component if more sensitive tests are done.**

Although degree of decrease in FEV_1 does not correlate with symptoms, it is a strong prognostic factor. When FEV_1 is <1 L, the 5-year survival rate is 50%.

B. Diffusion capacity is decreased as lung tissue is destroyed, as in emphysema. It may be low or normal in chronic bronchitis.

C. Lung volumes may show hyperinflation (increased TLC) and air trapping (increased RV).

D. CXR may be normal, or show evidence of bullous disease, hyperinflation, or increased interstitial markings from chronic airway inflammation

E. Blood gases can show hypoxia or compensated hypercapnia (normal pH) in late stages.

F. Laboratory data. See Chapter 2 for acute exacerbations.

1. **Hypercapnia with acidosis** is suggestive of acute decompensation.

2. **A high serum CO_2 level with a normal pH** is suggestive of a compensated chronic state.

3. **ECG may show multifocal atrial tachycardia,** which may be due to theophylline toxicity.

4. **Consider testing for α_1-antitrypsin deficiency** in relatively young patients with documented emphysema or obstructive physiology on PFTs and those with a positive family history of COPD.

G. Cor pulmonale can result from chronic hypoxemia. Hypoxemia causes pulmonary arterial constriction and, over time, can lead to right-sided heart failure. Patients then present with leg edema, JVD, and possibly a palpable liver with elevated liver enzymes. This may respond to long-term oxygen therapy, which will help reduce pulmonary hypertension.

H. Acute treatment of COPD (see Chapter 2 for details).

1. **Evaluate the patient for any underlying infection and begin appropriate antibiotics** (doxycycline and TMP-SMX are good choices. Fluoroquinolones show no additional benefit and are more expensive).

2. **Hospitalize if clinically indicated** (worsening tachypnea, falling Po_2, acidosis, increasing Pco_2).

3. **Provide supplemental oxygen if needed.**

4. **Corticosteroids** may be helpful in those who are hospitalized; maximal efficacy was seen during a 2-week course.

5. **Consider noninvasive ventilation early.**

6. **Beware if the patient seems too calm. It may indicate CO_2 retention with CO_2 narcosis.** This can occur as the result of giving high-flow oxygen to a patient with chronic COPD. However, do not withhold oxygen from a symptomatic, hypoxic patient even if it leads to the need for intubation.

I. Long-term management of COPD.

1. **Smoking cessation** is critical in the treatment of COPD!

2. **Pulmonary rehabilitation,** including conditioning and breathing techniques, improves exercise tolerance.

3. **Immunization.** All patients with COPD should have the pneumococcal vaccine at the time COPD is diagnosed as well as an annual flu shot.

4. **Low-flow oxygen** has been shown to be useful in reducing pulmonary arterial vasoconstriction, which, if uncontrolled, leads to cor pulmonale.

a. **Use continuous oxygen in those with either a Po_2 <55 torr, an O_2 saturation of <89%, or a Po_2 <59 torr with evidence of cor pulmonale (peripheral edema, hematocrit >55%, P pulmonale on ECG).**

b. **For borderline patients, testing oxygen saturation with exertion** may show a clear need for oxygen.

c. **Survival of hypoxemic patients is significantly enhanced with oxygen use 24 hours a day.** Patients should be encouraged to use oxygen at least 16 hours a day

d. **Oxygen saturation should be kept above 90% (Po_2 of 60-80 torr).** This usually can be accomplished with 2 L/min O_2 by nasal cannula, but titrate to patient's needs. Often, the patient with COPD does well with a saturation around 89% to 92%.

5. **Inhaled bronchodilators.** The effective use of these medications is predicated on instruction of the patient in their proper use. Many patients have difficulty properly using MDIs. A spacer can help, as can routine reeducation in inhaler technique.

a. **Anticholinergic agents (e.g., ipratropium) are the bronchodilators of choice in COPD.** Anticholinergics also decrease secretions, which can cause mucus plugging. The normal dose of ipratropium is 2 puffs every 6 hours. It is also available for nebulization. The equivalence of MDI versus nebulization is not as well studied as it is for β-agonists (see later). However, it is probably similar, and higher doses with an MDI may be helpful. Anticholinergics have an effect that is additive to the inhaled β-agonists. Tiotropium, an anticholinergic whose main benefit is that of once-daily dosing, is also available. It offers the potential for increased compliance and therefore increased efficacy, but at a greater expense than generic ipratropium. **However, if used properly, ipratropium and tiotropium are equivalent.** Combined β-agonist-anticholinergic inhalers are available.

b. **β-Adrenergic agonists** (e.g., albuterol, pirbuterol, and metaproterenol) can be used as needed for symptoms.

c. **One nebulizer of albuterol (2.5 mg) is equal to about 6 to 10 puffs from an MDI via spacer. Patients can use 4 to 10 puffs every 3 to 4 hours as needed, while watching for signs of toxicity.** Using it with a spacer increases efficacy and decreases side effects.

d. **A trial of inhaled albuterol is appropriate, even for those with no reversibility on spirometry.** They may have an improvement in symptoms. Many do have reversible disease that is not detectable on spirometry but can be detected on more sensitive tests.

e. **Long-acting β-agonists, such as salmeterol or formoterol, may be used to prevent nocturnal symptoms** and control symptoms during the day. However, these are not useful for control of acute bronchospasm. **Although the risk is not entirely clear, these agents likely should not** be used without a concomitant inhaled steroid because of a trend toward increased mortality.

f. **Not all patients with COPD need inhaled corticosteroids.** Inhaled corticosteroids have not been shown to slow the rate of decline in FEV_1 in patients with COPD, although they are recommended for patients with FEV1 <50% by one international consensus group. They may prevent exacerbations in patients with severe COPD, but overall it is difficult to say exactly which patients benefit from inhaled corticosteroids (although it is generally those with some reversible disease on PFTs).

g. **Oral steroids (e.g., prednisone) are a last resort** in a small subset of COPD patients. Their use should be limited to acute exacerbations of COPD.

h. **Leukotriene inhibitors (e.g., montelukast, zafirlukast) have no role in COPD.**

i. **Theophylline has an extremely limited role in COPD** because of its narrow therapeutic window and high potential for complications (arrhythmias, drug-drug interactions, and altered drug clearance).

j. **Long-term antibiotics are generally not helpful** but should be used to treat acute **purulent** exacerbations.

k. **Lung volume reduction surgery** is controversial, but referral may be appropriate for some patients (<75 years of age, no longer smoking, no cor pulmonale, and disease primarily affecting the upper lungs) with severe emphysema refractory to other therapy. Lung reduction increases mortality in other groups.

ASTHMA

I. Definition. Asthma is an inflammatory disease of the airways characterized by reversible airway obstruction.

II. Diagnosis.

A. History. Symptoms include wheezing, coughing at rest, shortness of breath, and nocturnal coughing with sleep disruption.

1. **Exacerbating factors** include viral URIs, sinusitis, reflux esophagitis, and aeroallergen exposure (including pollens, dust mites, cockroach and pet dander).

2. **Episodic bronchospasm may be secondary to exacerbating factors** such as exercise, cold air, exposure to tobacco smoke or chemical irritants (cleaners, perfume, potpourri, etc.).

a. **Exercise-induced asthma.** Pretreat patients with prn albuterol. Leukotriene inhibitors have been used but are more expensive and not as effective.

3. **Aspirin hypersensitivity.** Look for the triad of aspirin hypersensitivity, nasal polyps, and asthma. Aspirin use in this group of patients should strictly be avoided. **However, leukotriene inhibitors can be used to treat asthma exacerbation secondary to aspirin sensitivity.**

III. Physical Exam. The physical exam may be negative between exacerbations. Wheezing, prolonged expirations, depressed diaphragms (hyperinflation) on CXR, tachypnea, and retractions may be present especially with acute exacerbations. It is also important to evaluate for nasal polyps, GERD, rhinitis (hay fever), and sinusitis.

IV. Additional Tests.

A. Pulmonary function testing is the foundation of asthma diagnosis. Spirometry demonstrates evidence of airway **obstruction, which reverses by 12% or more** after inhaled β-agonist administration. Note that spirometry may be normal when the patient is asymptomatic or between exacerbations. Chronic asthma may lead to remodeling and irreversible airway obstruction.

B. Serial peak flow readings taken at home (e.g., before and after work/school) may show airflow variability. Use should be encouraged in patients with a poor perception of symptoms or unclear history of symptoms. **Peak flow measurements are effort dependent and overall do not improve treatment outcomes.**

C. Bronchoprovocation with methacholine or histamine may aid in establishing the diagnosis of asthma.

D. Skin testing for common aeroallergens may be indicated in patients with either a seasonal pattern or moderate to severe asthma. Immunotherapy may be of benefit in this group of patients.

E. Specific testing for sinusitis (rhinoscopy) or reflux (pH probe) to identify contributing factors may be indicated.

V. Disease Severity. Patients are classified by severity into two main classes, intermittent or persistent (Tables 4-4 and 4-5). Patients are further classified in persistent asthma according to severity of symptoms. **Patients in any category of asthma are at risk for severe, life-threatening exacerbations.**

VI. Viral Infections play a major role in acute exacerbations of asthma, especially in children. Common respiratory bacterial pathogens such as *Streptococcus pneumoniae* and *Haemophilus influenzae* do not trigger asthma exacerbations. **Consider starting steroids at the first sign of a URI in patients known to have exacerbations with URIs.**

VII. Management (see Tables 4-4 and 4-5).

A. Education. Increasing patient (family/caregiver) awareness of the disease, along with education (written and verbal), is the most important part of treating all patients with asthma. Demonstration and review of the technique of all devices used to treat asthma should be done at each visit.

B. Anti-inflammatory medications should be considered the mainstay of asthma therapy. Medications used for maintenance and rescue therapy are very different and should not be interchanged.

C. Written plan. All patients should have clear instructions with an outlined plan for dealing with acute symptoms and exacerbations (e.g., start oral steroids, increase β-agonist use, and what should prompt a call to their health care provider).

TABLE 4-4

GUIDELINES FOR ASTHMA IN PATIENTS OLDER THAN 5 YEARS

Classification	Definition	Treatment
Mild intermittent asthma	Symptoms occur ≤2 d/wk; nocturnal symptoms no more than twice a month; FEV_1 ≥80%, peak flow variability <20%	Inhaled bronchodilator use prn only. Daily anti-inflammatory medication is not recommended.
Mild persistent asthma	Symptoms occur more than twice a week but less than once a day; nocturnal symptoms more than twice a month; FEV_1 ≥80%; peak flow variability 20%-30%	Low-dose inhaled corticosteroids and prn use of short acting β-agonist.
Moderate persistent asthma	Symptoms occur daily; nocturnal symptoms >1 night/wk; FEV_1 >60% but <80%; peak flow variability >30%	Low- to medium-dose inhaled corticosteroids *plus* long-acting inhaled β-agonists.
Severe persistent asthma	Continual daytime symptoms; FEV_1 <60%; frequent nocturnal symptoms	High-dose inhaled corticosteroids *plus* long-acting β-agonists *plus* oral steroids if needed.

TABLE 4-5

GUIDELINES FOR ASTHMA IN CHILDREN YOUNGER THAN 5 YEARS

Classification	Definition	Treatment
Mild intermittent asthma	Symptoms occur ≤2 d/wk; nocturnal symptoms no more than twice a month; FEV_1 ≥80%; peak flow variability <20%	*Inhaled* prn β-agonist (e.g., albuterol)
Mild persistent asthma	Symptoms occur more than twice a week but less than once a day; nocturnal symptoms more than twice a month	Low-dose inhaled corticosteroid therapy *plus* inhaled bronchodilator prn only
Moderate persistent asthma	Symptoms occur daily; nocturnal symptoms more than 1 night a week	Low-dose inhaled corticosteroids *plus* long-acting inhaled β-agonists *or* medium-dose inhaled corticosteroids as monotherapy
Severe persistent asthma	Symptoms are continual; frequent nocturnal symptoms	High-dose inhaled corticosteroids *plus* long acting β-agonists *plus* oral steroids if needed

4

PULMONARY MEDICINE

D. Inhalers. All MDIs should be administered with the use of a spacer. In infants and children, spacers with masks should be encouraged to assist in delivery of all MDI medications. **Six to 10 puffs of an MDI equals one nebulizer treatment. If an MDI is used in adequate doses, there is no benefit to nebulizers.**

E. Nebulizers. The use of nebulizers is expensive, cumbersome, and time consuming. The use of MDIs with spacers (with masks in infants/toddlers) should be encouraged.

F. Monitoring. Monitoring of patients at each visit should include a history, including frequency of symptoms at rest, activity, and with sleep. Objective measurement should also be completed by measuring airflow obstruction by formal spirometry **(see Tables 22-9 and 22-10 for normal values).** Diary sheets may also be reviewed at each visit along with peak flow meter data where applicable. **The teaching about asthma that goes along with a peak flow meter is what gives the benefit.**

G. Indicators of control. Indicators of poor asthma control include nocturnal symptoms, urgent care or ED visits, and increased need for rescue inhaled β-agonists (daily use for a week or more than one canister per month).

VIII. Medications.

A. Quick relief (rescue) medications. See Chapter 2 for treatment of acute exacerbations.

1. **Short-acting β-agonists (inhaled albuterol, terbutaline, and pirbuterol).** All are available as MDIs, as well as nebulized solutions. Patients may safely use 6 to 8 puffs of an albuterol MDI every 2 to 4 hours. However, patients should be instructed to contact their health care practitioner if increasing doses are needed. Over-the-counter inhaled bronchodilators, such as metaproterenol or epinephrine, should be discouraged because of potential for excessive cardiac stimulation from nonselective adrenergic properties.

2. **Anticholinergics.** Ipratropium and tiotropium bromide produce bronchodilation by reducing vagal tone to the airways. This group of medications may be particularly helpful in conjunction with β-agonists in certain patients.

3. **Methylxanthines.** Theophylline and aminophylline are not recommended for use as rescue medications. They provide no additional benefit over inhaled β-agonists, and may cause significant adverse effects.

B. Maintenance medications.

1. **Anti-inflammatory drugs are the mainstay of asthma therapy.**

2. **Inhaled corticosteroids.** Indicated in all forms of persistent asthma. Several formulations are available (beclomethasone, budesonide, flunisolide, fluticasone, and triamcinolone) with varying potencies. However, effectiveness is equal in equipotent doses.

3. **Leukotriene Inhibitors (montelukast, zafirlukast).** The role of leukotriene inhibitors is not well defined and they are only marginally effective. *These medications are recommended as alternative agents only in persistent asthma.* In addition, they should be used as an

adjunct to inhaled corticosteroids (e.g., all patients on leukotriene inhibitors should also be on an inhaled steroid).

a. **Churg-Strauss syndrome, a necrotizing angitis, is a potential adverse effect associated with leukotriene inhibitor use.** It is seen in patients with preexisting asthma (especially if on systemic steroids) as well as those with allergies, sinus disease, or polyps. Features include peripheral eosinophilia, positive peripheral antineutrophil cytoplasmic antibody (p-ANCA), fever, and vasculitis of various organs, including skin (purpura and nodules), lungs, nerves, and kidneys. An abnormal CXR is seen in 25%, and mononeuritis multiplex is common. Treatment is with steroids and the prognosis is generally good if the diagnosis is made early.

3. **Cromolyn and nedocromil.** These drugs may be used as monotherapy only as **alternative agents** to low-dose inhaled corticosteroids in mild persistent asthma.

4. **Oral corticosteroids.** With adequate dosing of maintenance therapy using anti-inflammatory agents (primarily inhaled corticosteroids), chronic systemic steroids are rarely needed. If used for chronic asthma, attempt to decrease to a low dose or alternate-day dosing to limit side effects. The long-term goal should be to discontinue oral corticosteroids as maintenance therapy.

5. **Short-acting β-agonists. The** *scheduled* **use of short-acting bronchodilators is not recommended.** This leads to reduced receptor sensitivity. Control of symptoms actually is better achieved when β-agonists are used on a prn basis. Short-acting β-agonists (e.g., albuterol, terbutaline, and pirbuterol) should be used for coughing episodes, wheezing, symptom exacerbation, and before exercise. **There is no evidence suggesting a side effect advantage or better outcome with levalbuterol (Xopenex), which is the L-isomer of albuterol. It is more expensive and requires nebulization for administration.**

6. **Long-acting β-agonists.** Examples include salmeterol and formoterol (inhaled), extended-release albuterol (systemic). **These are not used as rescue medications but rather for long-term control. They should not be used as monotherapy** or as a replacement for inhaled corticosteroids, but may allow a reduction in the dose of inhaled steroid. They should always be used with an inhaled corticosteroid.

7. **Theophylline.** May add additional long-term control as an adjunct to inhaled corticosteroids only as an alternative agent in treating patients with mild to moderate persistent asthma. **There are considerable side effects with this class along with a low therapeutic window. If used, serum drug levels should be monitored regularly and maintained at 10 to 15 µg/mL.**

C. **Goals in managing persistent asthma. Patients should be maintained on the lowest dosage of drugs possible that is consistent with good asthma control.** Consider decreasing steroids to as low a dose as possible that will still maintain good asthma control. If adequate control is not obtained with maximal doses of inhaled steroids, use the lowest dose of leukotriene inhibitor or prednisone possible to maintain control.

BRONCHIECTASIS

I. Definition: Bronchiectasis is a chronic dilation and inflammation of medium-sized bronchi. Its hallmark is chronic and copious mucopurulent sputum, often containing *Pseudomonas*. Bronchiectasis can occur in anyone but is especially common in patients with cystic fibrosis (CF).

II. Predisposed to by recurrent pneumonias, granulomatous disease, carcinoma, or any process that can lead to a sequestered lobe.

III. CT scan shows enlarged peripheral airways with thickened walls.

IV. Treatment is based on prolonged courses of antibiotics targeted at organisms contained in sputum. Suppressive antibiotics on a monthly basis may be beneficial (e.g., doxycycline alternating with TMP-SMX or ciprofloxacin for 10 days per month). If only an isolated area is involved, it may be surgically resected. Mucolytics have variable results. Steroids are ineffective.

ALLERGIC BRONCHOPULMONARY ASPERGILLOSIS

I. Allergic Bronchopulmonary Aspergillosis (ABPA) is a condition that affects patients primarily with severe asthma and up to 10% of patients with CF. It occurs after exposure to spores of *Aspergillus fumigatus*, which worsens airway inflammation, leading to central bronchiectasis. **Prompt diagnosis and early intervention may prevent progression to severe bronchiectasis and pulmonary fibrosis.** Aspergillosis may erode into a pulmonary vessel, causing hemoptysis.

II. Symptoms include recurrent bronchial obstruction, fever, malaise, eosinophilia, hemoptysis, brownish mucus plugs. Wheezing may not be evident and there may be pulmonary consolidation.

III. Diagnostic Criteria.

A. Essential criteria:

1. Asthma or CF.
2. Central bronchiectasis.
3. Elevated serum total IgE.
4. Immediate skin test reactivity to *Aspergillus.*
5. Elevated serum-specific IgE or IgG to *Aspergillus fumigatus*.

B. Other common features not considered essential for diagnosis:

1. Positive sputum cultures for *A. fumigatus*.
2. Expectoration of brown sputum plugs containing *Aspergillus* hyphae.
3. Arthus late response after interdermal injection of *A. fumigatus*.
4. *A. fumigatus* precipitins detected in serum.
5. Peripheral eosinophilia.
6. Fleeting pulmonary infiltrates, often in the upper lobes.

IV. Treatment of ABPA.

A. Oral corticosteroids are the mainstay of therapy. Early and aggressive therapy may delay or prevent progression of ABPA to its advanced stages.

Therapy usually consists of daily use (prednisone 40 mg/day) for 2 weeks followed by alternate-day prednisone for 2 months.

B. Antifungal agents may be of some benefit in some patients; however, studies detailing dosing and length of treatment are lacking.

PNEUMONIA

I. **General.** An infection of the lower respiratory tract, including bacterial, viral, or fungal etiologies. Clinical manifestations include fevers, cough with or without sputum production, shortness of breath, and pleuritic chest pain.

II. **Physical Exam** *may* reveal crackles (rales) in the lungs with dullness to percussion and egophony. Infiltrates with or without pleural effusions may be seen on CXR. Patients may have few of these findings, particularly the very young and very old, or those with chronic illnesses. **In addition, these findings are nonspecific, and other diagnoses deserve consideration.**

III. **In children and the elderly, tachypnea is the most sensitive physical finding and warrants a CXR, even in the absence of rales.**

IV. **The Differential Diagnosis includes** heart failure, malignancy, pulmonary embolism, pulmonary vasculitis, eosinophilic pneumonia, and inflammatory lung diseases.

V. **Absence of an Infiltrate on CXR Does Not Rule Out Pneumonia!** An infiltrate may not appear on the initial CXR, but may develop as a patient is rehydrated.

VI. **Diagnosis.**

A. **Diagnosis is based on physical exam, CXR (PA and lateral), and clinical scenario** (see later for differential diagnosis of pulmonary infiltrates). However, the clinical exam for pneumonia is imprecise (even among pulmonologists), and a CXR should be done if there is any question. **The appearance on CXR (lobar vs. diffuse) does not relate to the causative organism and cannot be used to differentiate "typical" from "atypical" pneumonia.** The "atypicals" include *Mycoplasma pneumoniae, Chlamydia pneumoniae, Legionella pneumophila, Coxiella burnetii,* and viruses, especially influenza type A or B, among others.

B. **Blood gases and analysis of comorbidities and clinical judgment are helpful in making the decision whether to admit the patient.** The WBC count is less helpful because many patients may have pneumonia with a normal WBC count.

C. **For inpatients, most believe that attempts at defining the etiology are warranted, but a specific pathogen is identified in only 50% of patients even with extensive evaluation.** Treatment should not be delayed awaiting results. Blood cultures should be obtained and are frequently positive in pneumococcal pneumonia. **Gram stain of sputum analysis may be helpful, but be aware of significant**

PULMONARY MEDICINE

4

false-negative and false-positive results (especially for *Streptococcus pneumoniae*). Sputum cultures are rarely helpful. A diagnostic thoracentesis should be done if effusion is present. Testing for *Legionella* urinary antigen and other pathogen-specific tests should be considered. Cold agglutinins and *Mycoplasma* serology are rarely helpful.

D. **For outpatients, blood cultures and sputum cultures are a waste of resources and need not be done.**

E. **Immunosuppressed patients have a high incidence of opportunistic pathogens not covered by standard regimens,** and early chest CT and bronchoscopic lavage or biopsy should be considered.

VII. **Management.**

A. Clinical guidelines have been developed for determining which patients should be managed as inpatients, but clinical judgment is critical. **The decision to admit is not a commitment to long-term hospitalization, but it says you want to observe the patient for a time until it is clear that the patient will do well managed as an outpatient.**

B. **Empiric therapy is based on patient population and regional variances (Table 4-6).** Specific populations are discussed later. Starting antibiotics within 4 hours of arrival at the hospital has been shown to reduce mortality. **Antimicrobial therapy can be adjusted based on culture results when possible.**

C. **Bacterial pneumonia.** Treatment should continue for 7 to 10 days (depending on severity and clinical response); longer durations of treatment have not been shown necessary if the patient is not bacteremic. IV antibiotics may be switched to oral agents 24 to 48 hours after defervescence. *Mycoplasma* and *Chlamydia* pneumonias need to be treated 10 to 14 days.

VIII. **Course.** Patients may continue to be febrile 3 days into treatment, but up to 7 days for gram-negative infections and in patients with comorbid conditions. Therefore, treatment changes are not indicated as long as the patient is not worsening.

A. **The CXR appearance may lag behind clinical symptoms,** but a change in therapy is not indicated if the patient is stable. Rates of radiographic resolution will vary based on age and comorbidities; traditional thinking is that it should normalize within 6 weeks, but in the elderly it may take much longer. **Infiltrates not resolving in 12 to 14 weeks usually need further work-up (chest CT) because they sometimes represent noninfectious processes, such as malignancy.**

B. **Initiation of treatment for community-acquired pneumonia is empiric.** Once specific organism sensitivity is known, one may narrow the antibiotics.

IX. **Management of Patients Who Do Not Respond to Initial Therapy.**

A. **If the patient deteriorates, or infiltrates fail to resolve, consider further testing and change in treatment.**

TABLE 4-6
EMPIRIC TREATMENT OF PNEUMONIA BASED ON PATIENT POPULATION

Age	Organism	Primary* Regimen	Secondary Regimen	Comments
Neonates (birth to 1 mo)	Maternal vaginal flora: Escherichia coli, group B streptococci, S. aureus, Listeria monocytogenes	Ampicillin and gentamicin ± cefotaxime		Vancomycin if MRSA is possible, erythromycin if chlamydia is a concern.
1 mo to 3 mo†	Chlamydia trachomatis; Streptococcus and Staphylococcus spp	Erythromycin, clarithromycin		Generally afebrile with chlamydia; add cefotaxime if febrile
4 mo to 5 y	Viral,‡ pneumococcus, chlamydia	None or amoxicillin	If hospitalized: cefuroxime, cefotaxime	Authors prefer a macrolide to cover atypical organisms
Children older than 5 years	S. pneumoniae, Mycoplasma pneumoniae, Chlamydia	Amoxicillin or a macrolide (azithromycin, clarithromycin) or doxycycline if >10 years of age	If hospitalized: cefuroxime, ceftriaxone, or cefotaxime plus a macrolide	Authors prefer a macrolide Mycoplasma requires 2-3 wk of therapy
Adult outpatients with no comorbid factors	S. pneumoniae, Mycoplasma, Chlamydia spp	Azithromycin, clarithromycin, or doxycycline	Levofloxacin, gatifloxacin, moxifloxacin	Fluoroquinolones are second line
Adult outpatients with comorbid factors	S. pneumoniae (including drug resistant), gram-negative rods	β-Lactam plus extended-spectrum macrolide or doxycycline	Levofloxacin	Fluoroquinolones are overused and should be used only for appropriate indications

Continued

PULMONARY MEDICINE

4

TABLE 4-6

EMPIRIC TREATMENT OF PNEUMONIA BASED ON PATIENT POPULATION—cont'd

Age	Organism	Primary* Regimen	Secondary Regimen	Comments
Community acquired: Adult inpatients not requiring ICU	S. pneumoniae (including drug resistant), gram-negative rods	Third-generation cephalosporin *plus* a macrolide	Levofloxacin or other antipneumococcal fluoroquinolone	
Community acquired: Adult inpatients requiring ICU	S. pneumoniae, gram-negative rods, Legionella, Pseudomonas, Mycoplasma spp	Third-generation cephalosporin *plus* a macrolide		Consider adding vancomycin for MRSA
Hospital-acquired pneumonia	Pseudomonas and others Generally develops 2-5 days after admission	Antipseudomonal β-lactam (e.g., piperacillin, piperacillin/tazobactam) plus a fluoroquinolone or aminoglycoside		

*Add vancomycin to any regimen if MRSA is a concern.

†Chlamydia suggested by cough, infiltrate, conjunctivitis, absence of fever. Conjunctivitis may be absent.

‡Bordetella pertussis can cause whooping cough. If the diagnosis is considered, obtain a nasopharyngeal swab for PCR and treat with erythromycin (estolate preparation preferred) or clarithromycin for 14 days. Chemoprophylaxis is indicated for close contacts.

B. Consider unusual pathogens. Histoplasmosis in the Mississippi and Ohio River valleys, coccidioidomycosis in southwestern U.S., *Chlamydia psittaci* (psittacosis) with bird exposure, *Coxiella* with various farm animal exposures, TB.

C. Consider noninfectious diagnoses, such as the following:

1. Unifocal infiltrates: Pulmonary contusion, pulmonary embolism, bronchoalveolar cell and other lung carcinoma, pulmonary hemorrhage, lymphoma, radiation pneumonitis, lipoid pneumonia, and, rarely, lobe torsion or foreign body.

2. Multifocal infiltrates: Hypersensitivity pneumonitis, TB, fungal infections, bronchoalveolar cell and other lung carcinoma, Hodgkin's lymphoma, eosinophilic pneumonia, allergic granulomatosis and angiitis, collagen-vascular diseases, Wegener's granulomatosis, silicosis, black lung disease, amyloidosis, sarcoidosis, SARS, ARDS.

D. Reimage chest, particularly looking for effusions, abscess, and tumor causing a postobstructive pneumonia. Further testing with CT, bronchoscopy, or open lung biopsy may be useful.

X. Organism-Specific Notes.

A. *S. pneumoniae.* Penicillin-resistant *S. pneumoniae* (PRSP) is becoming more prevalent, but this depends on the region. With MIC >4 to penicillin, studies have shown using an antipneumococcal fluoroquinolone, vancomycin, or clindamycin may provide the best coverage until sensitivities return. With MIC <4, β-lactams (ceftriaxone) are appropriate. There are a few reports of levofloxacin-resistant pneumococci.

B. *H. influenzae.* Chronic colonizer in smokers. Most have β-lactamase, therefore β-lactamase inhibitors are needed, such as clavulanate or sulbactam. Also resistant to erythromycin, but clarithromycin and azithromycin give good coverage.

C. *Staphylococcus aureus.* Resistant to most β-lactams, except synthetics like methicillin and nafcillin, or those with β-lactamase inhibitors. Where methicillin-resistant *S. aureus* (MRSA) is prevalent, consider vancomycin.

D. *Legionella* is underdiagnosed. We recommend testing all inpatients in whom the etiology of community-acquired pneumonia is unclear. Legionella causes up to 6% of inpatient-treated pneumonia, with up to a 25% mortality rate.

XI. Other Pneumonia Syndromes.

A. Atypical organisms. *Mycoplasma pneumoniae, Chlamydia pneumoniae, Coxiella burnetii* (Q fever), *Chlamydia psittaci* (especially in bird owners), *Legionella pneumophila.* Viruses, such as influenza A and B, adenovirus, and RSV. *Pneumocystis carinii* pneumonia occurs in the immunocompromised, especially those with HIV infection **(Table 4-7).**

B. Aspiration pneumonia is common in elderly and sick patients, and is underdiagnosed; if likely, consider using measures to minimize aspiration (elevate head of bed, dietary measures) as well as broader-spectrum treatment to cover gram-negative organisms (see later).

PULMONARY MEDICINE

4

TABLE 4-7
COMMON ATYPICAL PNEUMONIAS*

Organism	Clinical Presentation	Diagnosis and Treatment
Chlamydia pneumoniae (TWAR)	Ten percent of all pneumonias in U.S. Hoarseness may be present, clinically similar to *Mycoplasma* pneumonia without neurologic and GI symptoms May also cause bronchitis and asthma	WBC usually normal, IgG antibody test available, self-limited but may use tetracyclines or macrolide
Fungal pneumonias (coccidioidomycosis, blastomycosis, histoplasmosis) Coccidioidomycosis may be associated with cavitary lesions, pulmonary hemorrhage, erythema nodosum	Occur in a geographic distribution: Coccidioidomycosis in southwest and California, blastomycosis in southeast/south central, histoplasmosis in east to midwest All cause an influenza-like illness with pneumonia	Coccidioidomycosis: spoors in sputum, skin test, IgG antibody; treat with fluconazole, itraconazole, or amphotericin B Blastomycosis: culture from sputum (4 wk!), KOH of sputum; treat with itraconazole, ketoconazole, amphotericin B Histoplasmosis: organism culture, skin test (not specific), identify polysaccharide in urine and blood (with disseminated disease); treat with itraconazole, but amphotericin B if moderately or severely ill
Hantavirus	Mice and rats are vectors, occurs throughout the U.S. (most common in southwest) Myalgias, fever, headache, abdominal pain, cough, rapid onset of respiratory failure, ARDS	Hemoconcentration, thrombocytopenia, hypoxia; IgM and IgG antibody tests available; ribavirin may be useful, contact the CDC
Legionnaires' disease (*Legionella pneumophila*)	One- to 2-day prodrome of headache, myalgias, then fever, chills, tachypnea, dry cough May become obtunded. Associated vomiting, diarrhea	WBC mildly elevated (8000-10,000), cold agglutinins negative, sputum immunofluorescent antibody available; look for Legionella antigen in urine (90% sensitive but only for one serotype); serum antibody titers available Treat with erythromycin (500 mg q6h), clarithromycin, or azithromycin

Pneumocystis *Mycoplasma pneumoniae*	See Chapter 11, HIV–AIDS Occurs in epidemics; associated pharyngitis, fever, headache Dry cough, may have clear exam but infiltrate on x-ray May have cold agglutinin–mediated hemolysis, meningeal signs, cranial nerve deficits, nausea, vomiting, diarrhea	See Chapter 11, HIV–AIDS WBC usually normal (<25% elevated 10,000-20,000) Cold agglutinin titer 1:128 (other pneumonias might have lower titers) IgG and IgM antibodies PCR testing available Treat with erythromycin, azithromycin, clarithromycin
Psittacosis (*Chlamydia psittaci*)	Especially in bird owners Headache, high fever, dry cough, myalgias, chest pain, perhaps vomiting and diarrhea Splenomegaly common and suggests the diagnosis; hepatomegaly, myocarditis possible	WBC usually normal but may be up or down; antibody titers diagnostic Treat with doxycycline 100 mg bid X-ray might not clear for 6 wk
Q fever (*Coxiella burnetii*)	Especially in dairy and slaughterhouse workers and those with livestock contact Fever, cough, headache, malaise, hepatitis, endocarditis	Antibody titers against "*Chlamydia burnetii*" diagnostic Treat with tetracycline 500 mg q6h
Tularemia (*Francisella tularensis*)	From rabbits (nonpulmonary variants as well) Tracheitis, pneumonia, cough, dyspnea, hemoptysis	Antibody titers and culture to diagnose Treat with streptomycin
Viral (influenza, parainfluenza, RSV, adenovirus)	Varies by virus	Generally normal WBC unless secondary infection

*See also Chapter 10, Infectious Diseases.

C. **Aspiration (chemical) pneumonitis. Sudden-onset fever, hypoxia, respiratory distress suggest aspiration pneumonitis (not pneumonia). This is sterile and occurs rapidly after aspiration. Most commonly this is gastric fluid, but may also occur with hydrocarbons, etc.**
1. **Predisposed by** CVA, NG tube, mental status changes, tube feedings.
2. **Requires** pH <2.5, 1 to 4 mL/kg aspirated.
3. **Mechanism** is chemical injury, surfactant/macrophage abnormalities.
4. **May progress to ARDS** and may see ARDS picture on radiograph.
5. **Does not require antibiotic treatment** but as a practical matter most patients are started on an antibiotic. If treating, cover anaerobes. Metronidazole **is not** adequate treatment. Consider clindamycin, cefoxitin, ticarcillin/clavulanate.

HYPERSENSITIVITY PNEUMONITIS

I. **Epidemiology.** Best known for affecting farmers, it can take many forms and affect people involved in other occupations and hobbies. This disease is difficult to diagnose.
II. **Etiology.** There are various etiologies **(Table 4-8)**. In farmers it is due to inhalation of *Actinomyces* spores found in moldy hay, moldy grain, and silage.
III. **Onset of Illness may range from weeks to years after first exposure** to an antigen.
IV. **Clinical Differentiation.** Not all exposed individuals will develop the disease. In contrast, toxic organic dust syndrome is a different entity that results from inhalation of endotoxin on the grain dust and affects all individuals exposed.
V. **Clinical Presentation.**
A. **Acute form.** Cough, dyspnea, chills, malaise and fever (flulike symptoms) occurring 4 to 8 hours after exposure to the antigen, as opposed to asthma, which tends to occur immediately. Wheezing is rare but there may be tachypnea and rales.

TABLE 4-8
COMMON CAUSES OF HYPERSENSITIVITY PNEUMONITIS

Source	Antigen	Disease Name
Hay, straw	Thermophilic bacteria	Farmer's lung
Heater water (e.g., humidifiers, including in the home)	Thermophilic bacteria	Humidifier lung
Sugar cane	Thermophilic bacteria	Bagassosis
Parrots, pigeons, ducks, chickens, etc.	Animal protein and excreta	Bird breeder's lung
Many other sources too numerous to list, including industrial solvents, rubber, cork, plastics	Various	Detergent worker's lung, chemical worker's lung, etc.

B. **Subacute form.** The subacute form constitutes the majority of cases. Patients note no flulike symptoms, but intermittent episodes of exertional dyspnea, fatigue, and cough after repeated low-dose exposure to the antigen. Physical exam and CXR may be negative, or there may be a reticulonodular infiltrate. Over time, subacute hypersensitivity pneumonitis may lead to chronic hypersensitivity pneumonitis.

C. **Chronic form** represents approximately 5% of cases and has a poor prognosis, usually leading to respiratory failure, cor pulmonale, and death. It has an insidious onset, with no episodes of acute systemic symptoms, but may present with cough, dyspnea on exertion, and fatigue with clubbing of fingers, etc. Will not have fever. Up to 50% will not have a clinically recognized primary illness. Exam reveals diffuse crackles; CXR shows alveolar or interstitial infiltrates in mid-upper lung fields. CXR does not improve after resolution of symptoms.

VI. **Testing.**

A. **Peripheral blood exhibits** lymphopenia, whereas bronchoalveolar lavage reveals lymphocytosis.

B. **CXR may reveal** a reticulonodular (interstitial) pattern, especially in lower lobes, or patchy alveolar infiltrate. This progresses to a ground-glass appearance.

C. **PFTs may show restriction.** Patients may be hypoxemic.

D. **Biopsy,** if done, shows interstitial inflammation with granuloma formation.

E. If exposure is not ongoing, the CXR, Po_2, and PFTs normalize after resolution of symptoms in 1 to 2 days.

VII. **Diagnostic Criteria. Determining the probability of hypersensitivity pneumonitis is complex but is determined by a combination of the following criteria:**

A. **Exposure to antigen,** including history of exposure, presence of antigen-specific antibodies in blood.

B. **Compatible CXR, clinical or physiologic findings.** Clinical/physiologic findings may include consistent time frame after exposure, hypoxia, dyspnea, fever.

C. **Bronchoalveolar lavage showing lymphocytes.**

D. **Positive inhalation challenge test.**

E. **Biopsy that is consistent.**

VIII. **Differential Diagnosis** includes asthma, atypical pneumonia, organic dust toxic syndrome, sarcoidosis, metal fume fever, and idiopathic interstitial pneumonia.

IX. **Treatment.**

A. **Generally supportive.** Remove patient from the exposure (use respirator, eliminate pets, wet down hay, etc., before resorting to moving). **Corticosteroids are indicated for acute severe systemic disease** but do not have an effect on long-term prognosis. Inhaled corticosteroids are ineffective.

B. Once fibrosis starts, it may be irreversible and progressive, even if antigen exposure is eliminated. Follow antibody levels as a measure of compliance with avoidance of etiologic agent.

VIRAL RESPIRATORY TRACT INFECTIONS

I. General. Approximately 80% of acute respiratory illnesses result from viral infections. These are usually self-limited infections caused by a large variety of viruses, including rhinovirus, adenovirus, echovirus, coxsackievirus, RSV, influenza and parainfluenza viruses. Occasionally, pneumonia may complicate these infections, either primary viral pneumonia or secondary bacterial pneumonia.

II. The Common Cold.

A. Causes. Rhinovirus, adenovirus, echovirus, coxsackievirus, RSV, and human metapneumovirus.

B. Clinical presentation. Symptoms include congestion, sneezing, clear to mucopurulent nasal discharge, dry or sore throat, low-grade fever, and cough.

C. Physical exam reveals erythematous nasal and oropharyngeal mucosa. Other signs may include conjunctival injection, clear fluid behind the tympanic membrane, clear to purulent rhinorrhea, and mild cervical lymphadenopathy. The chest exam is generally negative.

D. Management. The mainstay of treatment is symptom control, primarily rest, and hydration. Decongestants such as pseudoephedrine may be used for comfort. Acetaminophen or ibuprofen may be used for analgesia and fever.

1. **Antihistamines** have no proven benefit in controlling symptoms. **If they are used, use first-generation antihistamines with an anticholinergic effect. It is likely that anticholinergic effects are beneficial at reducing symptoms (e.g., nasal discharge).**

2. **Ipratropium bromide nasal spray.** The use of an anticholinergic nasal spray may help dry the nasal mucosa. Symptomatic relief may be achieved with 0.06% spray, 2 sprays in each nostril bid to tid.

3. **Zinc gluconate and echinacea.** Lozenges and echinacea likely have no effect on the course of the illness. The majority of studies are negative. Zinc nasal spray may cause loss of sense of smell.

4. **Education.** One of the most important things to encourage is frequent hand washing. This will prevent the spread of the illness to coworkers and family members. It is also important to discourage the use of antibiotics because they do not work in viral infections.

III. Influenza.

A. Overview. Influenza is a systemic illness resulting from infection with influenza viruses, which are orthomyxovirus, types A, B, and, rarely, C. These viruses can change their envelope proteins as their host population develops immunity, thereby maintaining the ability to cause recurrent infections. Influenza vaccinations for the predicted virulent strains are available in the fall months every year. They are generally effective in either preventing or decreasing the severity and duration of infection. The response to vaccine wanes with increasing age so that in the nursing home population, approximately 50% will mount a significant response.

B. Clinical presentation. There is usually an abrupt onset of high fever, chills, dry cough, headache, myalgia, and prostration. Physical examination is usually unremarkable with the exception of basilar rales in some patients. CXR is usually negative; however, perihilar prominence and increased markings may sometimes be present. Any evidence of an infiltrate is suggestive of a complicating pneumonia, either viral or bacterial. The diagnosis of influenza can be confirmed by either nasal swabs or viral cultures.

C. Management. The illness is usually self-limited, lasting 4 to 7 days in general. Rest, hydration, and acetaminophen or ibuprofen are recommended. Resistance patterns vary by year. Check with the CDC or local health authorities.

1. **Amantadine hydrochloride** 100 mg PO bid or **rimantadine** 100 mg PO bid **within 48 hours of symptom onset** can shorten the course of influenza type A. It may also be used for prophylaxis in compromised close contacts of infected individuals (also administer the vaccine if not already done). Rimantadine has a lower incidence of side effects. Reduce the dosage of both drugs in the elderly, for renal or liver impairment, and in the presence of a seizure disorder. These agents should be continued for 5 days or 24 to 48 hours after symptoms resolve.

2. **Neuraminidase inhibitors.** Zanamivir (Relenza) and oseltamivir (Tamiflu) cover both influenza types A and B. They are available for both treatment of acute symptoms or as prophylaxis (if started within 48 hours of symptom onset or exposure). **Both agents are fairly expensive and influenza type B is relatively uncommon in the U.S.** These agents may be used when contraindications are present for other agents or during outbreaks of influenza.

D. Complications of influenza. Myocarditis, myositis (including rhabdomyolysis), pericarditis, Reye's syndrome, and Guillain-Barré syndrome have all been reported as complications of influenza. In addition, secondary bacterial pneumonia can occur as well as respiratory failure and death.

E. Prevention. Immunization remains the primary method of prevention. The vaccine is recommended for anyone at an increased risk for complications of influenza: children aged 6 to 23 months, adults aged ≥65 years, pregnant women in their second or third trimester during influenza season, and persons aged ≥2 years with certain underlying chronic conditions. In addition, all health care workers and household contacts of patients at high risk should be vaccinated. The vaccine is contraindicated in patients with an egg allergy. The inactivated or killed vaccine is recommended for health care workers and household contacts of high-risk patients because of the risk of transmission

PULMONARY MEDICINE 4

of the virus from a live influenza nasal vaccine (FluMist) to immunocompromised hosts. Visit http://www.cdc.gov/flu/ for additional information.

IV. Bronchitis.

A. Characterized by cough with purulent sputum, rhonchi, and sometimes fever. Most cases are caused by viral infections, but also consider *H. influenza, S. pneumoniae,* and *Moraxella* as bacterial causes.

B. Treatment. There is no evidence that antibiotics are useful in nonsmokers with bronchitis. Cough suppression and inhaled β-agonists are generally the mainstay of treatment. Smoking cessation is highly encouraged in smokers and is the most beneficial long-term treatment.

1. Antibiotics. Erythromycin, doxycycline, and TMP-SMX are good antibiotic choices if antibiotics are indicated **(only in acute exacerbations of chronic bronchitis in smokers).**

2. Cough suppression. Albuterol 2 to 8 puffs with a spacer is most effective. Benzonatate 100 mg PO q6h will suppress cough; codeine (e.g., acetaminophen with codeine and various cough syrup preparations) is less effective.

CHRONIC COUGH

I. By Definition, symptoms should be present >8 weeks to diagnose chronic cough.

II. Most common causes in order of frequency: Postnasal drip/chronic sinusitis, asthma, including postviral reactive airways, GERD. Consider also medication (ACE inhibitors), CHF, pertussis, eosinophilic bronchitis (see eosinophils in sputum),and TB. **Pertussis in adults may present only with chronic cough and may be present despite childhood immunization, and represents 21% of those with chronic cough in one series (check acute and convalescent titers).**

III. History will often uncover the cause, especially history of smoking, smoke exposure, occupational exposure, foods, GERD, etc.

IV. CXR to rule out severe disease such as bronchogenic carcinoma, sarcoid, TB, bronchiectasis.

V. Nasopharyngeal PCR for pertussis.

VI. One Approach.

A. Treat with antihistamine or decongestant empirically. Consider course of antibiotics for sinusitis if appropriate.

B. If positive titer for pertussis, treat with erythromycin or other macrolide.

C. Give a therapeutic trial of an H_2 blocker or proton pump inhibitor for GERD.

D. Give a trial of a short acting β-agonist or steroids.

E. Bronchoprovocation testing for asthma may be considered in patients with an unclear history with incomplete response to β-agonists and corticosteroids.

F. Evaluate for habit cough. This is a diagnosis of exclusion. It is usually a reflex or habit type of cough or frequent throat clearing without a pathologic cause.

G. Persistent cough may require further evaluation, including sputum evaluation, barium swallow, 24-hour esophageal pH probe monitoring, esophagoscopy, high-resolution CT scan of the chest, and bronchoscopy.

H. This approach leads to successful treatment in 96% of cases (although there are recurrences).

EVALUATION OF CHRONIC COUGH IN CHILDREN

I. Causes of chronic cough in children can be differentiated according to age groups: infants, preschool, and school age/adolescence.

A. Infants. Consider congenital anomalies (tracheoesophageal fistula), primary ciliary dyskinesia, infections, including viral pathogens (RSV, CMV), chlamydia, pertussis, asthma, GERD, and CF.

B. Preschool age. Consider foreign body aspiration, infections (viral, mycoplasma, and bacterial), asthma, CF, GERD, and passive exposure to tobacco smoke.

C. School age/adolescence. Asthma and postnasal drip are the most common causes of cough in this age group. Other conditions to consider also include GERD, infections (mycoplasma), irritation due to smoking or pollution, and habit cough.

II. Diagnosis and evaluation in children.

A. Two warning signs for serious lung disease include neonatal onset and chronic purulent cough. Further studies should include evaluation for congenital anomalies, ciliary dyskinesia, α_1-antitrypsin deficiency, and CF.

OBSTRUCTIVE SLEEP APNEA

I. Affects 2% to 4% of the population. Anatomic closure of the airway occurs during sleep, but respiratory effort still occurs.

II. OSA predisposes to cardiovascular disease, hypertension, pulmonary hypertension (from chronic nocturnal hypoxia), MI, dysrhythmias, CVA, and MVA (sevenfold increase).

III. Clinical Picture.

A. Daytime sleepiness, snoring, headache, personality changes, intellectual deterioration, sexual dysfunction. Partners may note restless sleep, periods of apnea. Daytime sleepiness, mood instability, and nonrefreshing sleep are nonspecific and may occur with other sleep disorders, and depression.

B. Forty percent of women with sleep apnea have amenorrhea or dysmenorrhea that resolves with treatment.

C. Not all patients are obese. OSA occurs in those with a thin neck diameter as well.

IV. Diagnosis.
A. Polysomnography (sleep study) is the gold standard, but expensive.
1. Criteria for diagnosis of OSA include:
a. Cessation of airflow for 10 seconds with maintenance of respiratory effort.
b. Five or more episodes of apnea per hour.
c. Decrease in oxygen saturation of at least 4% during episodes.
B. Continuous nocturnal oxygen saturation measurement at home.
1. Using 10 desaturations per hour as the cutoff, it has 98% sensitivity but only 48% specificity, with a positive predictive value of 61% and a negative predictive value of 97% in those with a history suggestive of sleep apnea.
2. Not valid in those receiving oxygen therapy.
3. Home oximetry can be used to screen before ordering a sleep study because it has a high negative predictive value and is inexpensive.
V. Treatment.
A. Relieve nasal obstruction, including polyps, allergic causes, and structural abnormalities (e.g., septal deviation).
B. Weight loss.
C. Treat hypothyroidism if present.
D. Mask or nasal CPAP is the treatment of choice. Need to customize positive pressure to the patient during the sleep study. Only 46% will have adequate compliance.
E. Drugs have proven of little benefit. It is important to avoid medicines with sedating properties, as well as alcohol.
F. Surgical therapy, including tonsillectomy, uvulopalatopharyngoplasty (efficacy less than 50%, but there is a lack of good controlled studies). **Tracheostomy is the definitive treatment but should be saved as a last resort.**

SARCOIDOSIS

I. General. A diffuse, multisystem inflammatory process of unknown cause, characterized by the formation of noncaseating granulomas most commonly affecting the lungs and lymph nodes. Sarcoid strikes people of any age, but is most common among patients 20 to 40 years of age; African Americans are disproportionately affected.
II. Manifestations vary according to organ affected.
A. Pulmonary. Most commonly involved site. Signs/symptoms include hilar adenopathy, dyspnea, cough, pleural effusion, reduced D_{LCO}. **Ninety-five percent of patients will have some CXR abnormality.**
B. Systemic. Fever.
C. Skin. Erythema nodosum, other skin lesions.
D. Eye. Uveitis.
E. CNS. Seizure, meningitis, cranial nerve abnormalities.
F. Endocrine. Hypercalcemia, pituitary dysfunction.
G. Heart. Arrhythmias.

III. **Diagnosis.**
A. **Initial work-up.** In a patient with suspected sarcoidosis, a thorough evaluation, including neurologic exam, ECG, and ophthalmologic exam (even in patients without ocular or visual symptoms), is essential. PFTs, CXR, kidney and liver function tests, urinalysis, blood count, and calcium level should be obtained. Targeted investigations also should be performed to pursue specific organ-related symptoms.
B. **Biopsy.** Transbronchial biopsy or mediastinal lymph node aspiration may be diagnostic. Skin lesions also potentially a target.
C. **Serum ACE level.** Nonspecific and generally not helpful, although elevated in 75% of patients with sarcoid. ACE levels may be elevated in miliary TB, silicosis, asbestosis, and other conditions. Once diagnosis is made, one can follow ACE levels as measure of disease activity, although this usually is not needed.
IV. **Differential Diagnosis.** Must differentiate from fungal *(Histoplasma)* infection, TB, and lymphoma.
V. **Treatment.** Many people are asymptomatic, and can be observed without treatment. Monitoring for disease progression is recommended during the observation period.
A. **Corticosteroids. Reserved for the minority of patients with severe or progressive symptoms and cardiac, CNS, or other organ dysfunction, as well as for patients with eye involvement.** If used, doses, frequency, and duration of treatment should be minimized. **The use of steroids may actually prolong the course in patients with mild disease and increase the likelihood of relapse.**
B. **Steroid-sparing agents may be beneficial, but no evidence demonstrating their efficacy is available.**
C. Patients with severe disease are best managed in consultation with a pulmonologist.

HEMOPTYSIS

I. **Characterized** as scant (blood-tinged sputum), frank hemoptysis, or massive hemoptysis that interferes with respiration. Basing on volume of blood expectorated is a less useful classification because it depends on 24-hour observation and may not reflect the clinical urgency.
A. **Massive hemoptysis** is a potentially life-threatening problem. Most patients with massive hemoptysis should be observed in the hospital and have bronchoscopy urgently. Pulmonary consultation should be obtained early.
B. **Nonmassive hemoptysis.** Production of lesser amounts of blood, but still requiring a timely work-up.
II. **Sources.**
A. **Intrapulmonary.**
1. **Infectious:** Bronchitis, pneumonia, abscess, fungus.
2. **Structural:** AVM, foreign body, tumor.

PULMONARY MEDICINE

4

3. **Vascular:** Goodpasture's syndrome, Wegener's granulomatosis, Henoch-Schönlein purpura.

4. **Connective tissue disease:** RA, SLE, other vasculitides.

5. **Cardiac:** Severe mitral regurgitation can cause right upper lung infiltrate and hemoptysis.

6. **Pulmonary hemosiderosis:** Idiopathic diffuse alveolar hemorrhage—majority are young adults and children, with episodic hemoptysis, occasionally massive.

B. **Extrapulmonary (pseudohemoptysis).**

1. **GI tract:** Swallowed blood. Consider hemoptysis in patients who complain of hematemesis.

2. **Epistaxis:** Nasopharyngeal lesions.

3. **Bleeding diathesis** such as DIC.

4. **Drugs:** Cocaine, penicillamine, anticoagulants, etc.

III. **Evaluation.**

A. **Radiographs.** CXR should be done in all patients. CT can be used as a follow-up study in those with a high risk of disease.

B. **Blood work,** including coagulation tests.

C. **Bronchoscopy. Virtually all patients with massive hemoptysis need bronchoscopy** to identify the source and rule out airway lesions, such as tumor. **CT is generally more rewarding in the early stages of evaluation.**

IV. **Treatment.**

A. **Emergent. Death is usually from drowning.** Place patient with bleeding side down, consider mainstem intubation of good lung to protect that lung from fluid.

B. **Interventional bronchoscopy–based therapeutic measures** are sometimes possible. Modalities include cryotherapy, cautery/coagulation and endoscopically blocking the bleeding segment.

C. **Surgery** is occasionally helpful for bleeding lesions.

D. Embolization of bleeding source is possible by interventional radiology.

PLEURAL EFFUSION

I. **Definition.** An abnormal collection of fluid within the pleural space.

II. **Clinical Symptoms and Signs are nonspecific.** Dyspnea, orthopnea, and pleuritic pain are common. Physical exam reveals decreased breath sounds, dullness to percussion, and decreased tactile fremitus over the effusion.

III. **Diagnosis.**

A. **Radiographs. Lateral film is more sensitive** and can detect smaller amounts of fluid than a PA film. Blunting of a costophrenic angle on PA view suggests at least 500 mL of fluid. Decubitus films show layering of fluid, unless it is loculated. CT and US may help to clarify any uncertainties.

B. **Thoracentesis.** Defining whether the fluid is a transudate or exudate is the goal, and will help define the etiology of the effusion. **Send fluid for total protein, LDH, glucose, cell count and differential, Gram stain, and bacterial culture.** Pleural fluid pH should be determined on a blood gas machine. Other studies, such as cytology or AFB stain, may be needed depending on the clinical picture (suspicion of cancer or TB, respectively). **Compare lab results with those in Table 4-9 to differentiate a transudate from an exudate.**

IV. **Etiologies.**

A. **Exudate.** Due to an active process in the pleural space. Meets "Lights criteria" (see Table 4-9).

B. **Transudate.** Passive accumulation of fluid in the pleural space. The pleura is a bystander for some other systemic disease.

C. **Differential diagnosis** (see Table 4-9).

V. **Treatment.** Treat the underlying problem (e.g., diuresis for CHF, antibiotics for pneumonia). Draining a large effusion may relieve dyspnea. Caution is advised if doing large-volume thoracentesis: draining >1500 mL may lead to reexpansion pulmonary edema and clinical deterioration. Loculated effusions usually are not easily tapped, and sometimes require surgical drainage. Malignant pleural effusions will recur, sometimes rapidly, and may respond to pleurodesis.

4

PULMONARY MEDICINE

TABLE 4-9

DIFFERENTIAL DIAGNOSIS OF PLEURAL EFFUSION

Type of Effusion	Lab Criteria	Differential Diagnosis
Exudate	Lights criteria: Pleural fluid to serum total protein ratio >0.5 *or* Pleural fluid to serum LDH ratio >0.6 *or* Pleural fluid LDH >150 mg/dL or 2/3 the upper limit of the normal serum LDH	Parapneumonic effusion, malignancy, empyema, collagen vascular disease, TB, and other inflammatory diseases. An *empyema* is characterized by a pH <7.1 or positive Gram's stain. Empyemas usually require urgent chest tube or surgical drainage, and consultation is advised.
Transudate	Anything but above	Caused by transcapillary leak in patients with elevated hydrostatic pressure (LV dysfunction, renal failure, and portal hypertension), decreased oncotic pressure (nephrotic syndrome, liver failure), or thoracic duct obstruction. Also can see fluid migrate across the diaphragm in patients with ascites.

SARS (SEVERE ACUTE RESPIRATORY SYNDROME)

I. **Definition.** SARS is a newly identified atypical pneumonia, caused by a previously unrecognized coronavirus, thought to have originated in China in late 2002. In the spring of 2003, it infected more than 8000 people

II. **Symptoms are nonspecific** and include fever, headache, dyspnea, and dry cough that may rapidly progress to respiratory failure. **It is clear that there is a wide spectrum of severity, with some patients manifesting only URI symptoms.**

III. **Transmission** is by droplet spread and perhaps oral ingestion (water, sewage).

IV. **Incubation is 2 to 10 days.** Observe exposed patients in isolation for 10 days.

V. **Lab:** CXR shows bilateral infiltrates, lung consolidation, and an ARDS-like picture.

VI. **Treatment** is symptomatic. No antivirals have been shown to be effective.

VII. **Our knowledge of this disease is changing rapidly; check with your state health department, CDC (http://www.cdc.gov/ncidod/sars/index.htm), and WHO (http://www.who.int/csr/sars/en/) for updated information.**

WEGENER'S GRANULOMATOSIS

I. **General.** Wegener's granulomatosis is a systemic illness that primarily affects the nasal and sinus mucosa, the lung, and the kidney. Necrotizing granulomas are found in the perivascular areas. Usually occurs in middle-aged adults but may occur in younger patients (mean age, 40 years).

II. **Clinical Symptoms.**

A. **Pulmonary symptoms,** such as cough, recurrent pneumonia, hemoptysis.

B. **Renal symptoms,** including hematuria, pyuria, renal failure from glomerulonephritis.

C. **Recurrent sinusitis.**

D. **Systemic symptoms,** including fever, arthralgias, polyarthritis, weight loss.

III. **Diagnosis.**

A. **c-ANCA** (central antineutrophil cytoplasmic antibody) is 85% sensitive. However, it is not 100% specific because other vasculitides may also present with a positive c-ANCA.

B. **Multiple pulmonary nodules** (may be cavitary) or infiltrates on chest radiograph (90%).

C. **Biopsy specimen** that shows classic granulomas.

D. **Lab.** May have anemia, elevated ESR, leukocytosis, pyuria, and hematuria. Complement levels are normal, and the ANA is negative.

IV. Treatment and Course.

A. It is suggested that a consultation be obtained before you initiate the treatment of Wegener's granulomatosis. Wegener's has a 90% mortality rate within 1 to 2 years if not treated.

B. Steroids alone have been used for treatment but are not particularly effective.

C. Cyclophosphamide plus corticosteroids is the treatment of choice early in the disease before there is frank renal failure. **This should be initiated after consultation with rheumatology and immunology staff.**

BIBLIOGRAPHY

Bateman ED, Bantje TA, Joao Gomes M, et al: Combination therapy with single inhaler budesonide/formoterol compared with high dose of fluticasone propionate alone in patients with moderate persistent asthma. *Am J Respir Med* 2:275-281, 2003.

Centers for Disease Control and Prevention: Severe acute respiratory syndrome (SARS): Frequently asked questions. Available at http://www.cdc.gov/ncidod/sars/faq.htm#disease (accessed November 30, 2005).

de Jongste JC, Shields MD: Cough 2: Chronic cough in children. *Thorax* 58:998-1003, 2003.

Esteban A, Frutos F, Tobin MJ, et al: A comparison of four methods of weaning patients from mechanical ventilation. Spanish Lung Failure Collaboration Group [see comments]. *N Engl J Med* 332:345-350, 1995.

Fedullo PE, Tapson VE: Clinical practice: The evaluation of suspected pulmonary embolism. *N Engl J Med* 349:1247-1256, 2003.

Irwin RS, Madison JM: The diagnosis and treatment of cough. *N Engl J Med* 343:1715-1721, 2000.

Mandell LA, Bartlett JG, Dowell SF, et al: Update of practice guidelines for the management of community-acquired pneumonia in immunocompetent adults. *Clin Infect Dis* 37:1405-1433, 2003.

Mustafa S, Stein PD, Patel KC, et al: Upper extremity deep venous thrombosis. *Chest* 123:1953-1956, 2003.

National Heart, Lung, and Blood Institute: National Asthma Education and Prevention Program. Available at http://www.nhlbi.nih.gov/guidelines/asthma/index.htm (accessed November 30, 2005).

PIOPED Investigators: Value of the ventilation/perfusion scan in acute pulmonary embolism: Results of the Prospective Investigation of Pulmonary Embolism Diagnosis (PIOPED). *JAMA* 263:2753-2759, 1990.

Schuh S, Coates AL, Binnie R, et al: Efficacy of oral dexamethasone in outpatients with acute bronchiolitis. *J Pediatr* 140:27-32, 2002.

Spiro CE: Evaluating chronic cough: A systematic approach. *Clinician Rev* 13(10):52, 2003. Available at http://www.findarticles.com/p/articles/mi_m0BUY/is_10_13/ai_110401358 (accessed November 30, 2005).

Thorburn K, Kerr S, Taylor N, van Saene HK: RSV outbreak in a paediatric intensive care unit. *J Hosp Infect* 57:194-201, 2004.

Wainwright C, Altamirano L, Cheney M, et al: A multicenter, randomized, double-blind, controlled trial of nebulized epinephrine in infants with acute bronchiolitis. *N Engl J Med* 349:27-35, 2003.

Wark P: Pathogenesis of allergic bronchopulmonary aspergillosis and an evidence-based review of azoles in treatment. *Respir Med* 98:915-923, 2004.

Weinberger M: Clinical patterns and natural history of asthma. *J Pediatr* 142(2 Suppl): S15-S19; discussion S19-S20, 2003.

Weinberger M: Respiratory infections and asthma: Current treatment strategies. *Drug Discov Today* 9:831-837, 2004.

Weinberger M: Treatment strategies for viral respiratory infection–induced asthma. *J Pediatr* 142(2 Suppl):S34-S38; discussion S38-S39, 2003.

Wells PS, Anderson DR, Rodger M, et al: Evaluation of D-dimer in the diagnosis of suspected deep-vein thrombosis. *N Engl J Med* 349:1227-1235, 2003.

Williams JV, Harris PA, Tollefson SJ, et al: Human metapneumovirus and lower respiratory tract disease in otherwise healthy infants and children. *N Engl J Med* 350:443-450, 2004.

World Health Organization: Severe acute respiratory syndrome (SARS). Available at http://www.who.int/csr/sars/en/ (accessed November 30, 2005).

Gastroenterology

Rogelio G. Silva, Ali J. Husain, and Jatinder P.S. Ahluwalia

DYSPEPSIA AND GASTROESOPHAGEAL REFLUX

I. **Dyspepsia.**
A. **General.** Dyspepsia can include intermittent or persistent pain and discomfort in the upper abdomen or lower part of the chest, regurgitation, postprandial bloating or distention, heartburn, nausea, early satiety, and a feeling of postprandial fullness. These symptoms can also be present in patients with ulcer disease. **It is not possible to differentiate nonulcer dyspepsia from ulcer-related dyspepsia based on history and physical.**
B. **Etiology** is multi-factorial and can include food intolerance, motility problems (30%-80% have delayed gastric emptying), psychological overlay, and visceral hypersensitivity to distention.
C. **Differential includes** ulcer disease, gastritis, reflux esophagitis, and aerophagia (see later).
D. **Evaluation** can include an empiric trial of therapy, endoscopy, testing for food intolerance (e.g., elimination diet), ultrasound, CT scan, and gastric emptying studies.
E. **Treatment** for *H. pylori* in patients with dyspepsia and no ulcer is controversial and does not seem to yield any benefit. A trial of H_2 blockers, proton pump inhibitors, and/or a promotility agent (e.g., metoclopramide) is reasonable. Have patients slow their eating and chew well. However, treatment is often unsatisfactory.

II. **Gastroesophageal Reflux Disease.**
A. GERD is the reflux of gastric contents into the esophagus. It is subdivided into **nonerosive reflux disease** (no mucosal damage), **erosive esophagitis** (mucosal injury), and **Barrett's esophagus** (replacement of the normal squamous epithelium with columnar epithelium).
B. **Etiology.** incompetence of the lower esophageal sphincter and anatomic abnormality such as hiatal hernia. **Predisposing factors include** increased gastric volume (from meals, pyloric obstruction, or diabetic gastroparesis), increased abdominal pressure (obesity, pregnancy, ascites, or hiatal hernia), smoking, caffeine, alcohol, chocolate, and fatty meals.
C. **Clinical manifestations**
1. **Symptoms include** heartburn (or pyrosis), regurgitation, and dysphagia or odynophagia. **Dysphagia in the presence of chronic heartburn should raise concern for stricture or malignancy.**
2. **Extraesophageal manifestations of GERD** include asthma, laryngitis, hoarseness, chronic cough, and dental disease.
D. **Diagnostic evaluation**

1. **Testing should be reserved for patients with alarm symptoms (e.g., dysphagia, odynophagia, or weight loss),** those in whom the diagnosis is not clear, and those with chronic or refractory symptoms. **Symptomatic improvement after treatment is considered diagnostic of GERD in the appropriate clinical setting.**
2. **If the diagnosis of GERD is not clear or there are other symptoms, consider:**
a. **Esophagoscopy** with biopsy. **Normal mucosa on esophagoscopy does not rule out GERD.**
b. **Ambulatory 24-hour esophageal pH monitoring** for atypical or refractory symptoms and those considering antireflux surgery.
c. **Esophageal manometry** to measure LES pressure. This is only useful in those considering antireflux surgery.
d. **Double contrast barium swallow** to diagnose strictures noninvasively; sensitivity diminishes with mild disease.
E. **Complications of GERD** include aspiration pneumonia, acid laryngitis, asthma, pulmonary fibrosis, Barrett's esophagus, stricture formation, and adenocarcinoma.
F. **Treatment**
1. **Lifestyle modification:** smoking cessation, weight loss, and avoidance of tight-fitting clothing.
2. **Dietary modification:** restriction of fatty foods, citrus juices, chocolate, peppermint, excess alcohol, carbonated beverages, and red wine.
3. **Elevate the head of the bed** by 6 to 9 inches (using blocks under the legs at the head of the bed).
4. **Avoid the supine position** immediately after meals and **avoid meals before bedtime.**
5. **Drug therapy** consists of acid suppression. Consider endoscopy if the patient does not respond to maximal dose therapy or if symptoms recur after discontinuing therapy.
a. **Acid-suppressive therapy** (increases pneumonia risk: H_2 blockers 1:500, PPI 1:200)
   (1) **Histamine receptor antagonists (H_2 blockers:** Cimetidine, ranitidine, nizatidine, and famotidine) **are first-line therapy.** Titrate to effect.
   (2) **Proton pump inhibitors** are more expensive (except OTC omeprazole); **reserve for H_2 blocker failure** or proven esophagitis. Omeprazole 20 mg, lansoprazole 30 mg, rabeprazole 20 mg, and pantoprazole 40 mg given daily are effective in 85% to 90% of patients. For maximum benefit, administer 30 minutes before breakfast.
b. **Patients with breakthough pain on a PPI** can benefit from a bedtime dose of an H_2 blocker.
c. **Prokinetic agents** increase LES pressure and gastric emptying and improve peristalsis. **Metoclopramide (Reglan) 5 to 10 mg PO ½ h qac**

and qhs usually given in conjunction with H_2 blockers is effective in refractory cases; watch for extrapyramidal effects and fatigue. Cisapride causes cardiac arrhythmias and is off the market in the United States. Erythromycin can also cause QT prolongation.

6. **Surgical therapy or endoscopic therapy** are reserved for those who fail medical therapy. Fundoplication (open or laparoscopic) is the surgery of choice.

7. **GERD in pregnancy** is treated with lifestyle modification, antacid therapy, or sucralfate; these should be the first line of treatment. In refractory cases, H_2 blockers appear to be safe. PPIs are category B in pregnancy.

ESOPHAGEAL DISEASES

I. Presentation.

A. Dysphagia is the sensation of difficulty swallowing and feeling as though food is getting stuck in the esophagus. **The test of choice to evaluate dysphagia is a barium swallow study.** Dysphagia can be classified into one of two categories:

1. **Oropharyngeal dysphagia** (or transfer dysphagia): inability to initiate a swallow and often associated with cough and aspiration, choking, nasal regurgitation, or complaints of food sticking in the cervical esophagus. May be secondary to CVA or other neurologic disease.

2. **Esophageal dysphagia** is the sensation of difficulty passing the food bolus down the esophagus, typically described as food getting stuck behind the sternum.

B. Intolerance to different food consistencies helps narrow the differential diagnosis (Table 5-1).

C. Odynophagia is painful swallowing; it can manifest as retrosternal pain. **Odynophagia usually implies mucosal inflammation** (infectious esophagitis [candida, herpes, or CMV], pill-induced esophagitis, ulcerative esophagitis, and caustic or radiation injury).

TABLE 5-1
DIAGNOSIS OF DYSPHAGIA BASED ON SYMPTOMS

Diagnosis	Dysphagia to:	Constant or intermittent	Heartburn?	Progressive?
Malignancy or obstruction	Solids, then liquids	Constant	Yes	Yes
Esophageal ring	Solids	Intermittent	±	Possible
Motility disorder	Solids and liquids	Intermittent	Generally no	Generally no
Achalasia, scleroderma	Solids and liquids	Constant	Possible	Yes

GASTROENTEROLOGY 5

D. **Globus is the sensation of a lump or tightness in the throat that need not be associated with swallowing.** The sensation may be temporarily relieved with the ingestion of food or liquids and worsened with emotional stress or frequent dry swallowing. **Globus is commonly seen in patients with psychiatric illness (e.g., anxiety, depression, hypochondria) but is also related to GERD and upper esophageal sphincter dysfunction.**

E. **Noncardiac chest pain.** Esophageal disease can manifest as angina-like chest pain and may be relieved by NTG.

II. **Esophageal Foreign Bodies.**

A. **Esophageal foreign bodies may be due to** food bolus impaction (generally large bolus of meat, especially with strictures or dysmotility), accidental ingestion (children), or intentional ingestion (psychiatric patients, prisoners).

B. **Clinical manifestations include** pain, inability to swallow saliva (with complete obstruction), rarely esophageal perforation.

C. **Diagnostic evaluation.** History provides the diagnosis in most cases. **Chest and abdominal radiographs** can often identify ingested foreign bodies. **If esophageal perforation is suspected, consider a Gastrografin esophagram.** Barium should be avoided because it can affect visibility during upper endoscopy.

D. **Treatment (see Swallowed Foreign Bodies)**

III. **Food bolus impaction** should be cleared within 12 hours to prevent perforation and pulmonary aspiration.

A. **Glucagon 1 mg IV followed by a repeat 2-mg dose at 20 minutes** can relax the LES and allow spontaneous passage.

B. **Alternative therapies include** administration of a carbonated beverage (such as Pepsi), intravenous diazepam, oral nifedipine, or sublingual nitroglycerin. **Proteolytic enzymes (e.g., Adolf's meat tenderizer) have been associated with esophageal perforation and are *not* recommended.**

C. **Endoscopy is the treatment of choice if the above are not successful.**

IV. **Swallowed Foreign Bodies.**

A. **Coins**

1. Up to 35% may be asymptomatic.

2. Esophageal coins are generally visible as a disk on AP radiograph, whereas those in the trachea tend to be on edge.

3. **Endoscopy is the treatment of choice.** If the coin passes into the stomach, there is no need to proceed to endoscopy. Simply observe the patient and confirm passage by radiograph or observation of stool.

B. **Button batteries**

1. **This requires emergency management! Batteries can perforate the esophagus within 4 hours after ingestion.**

2. Urgent endoscopic removal is required if a button battery is lodged in the esophagus.

3. If it passes into the stomach, you may watch for 24 to 48 hours with repeat radiographs. If the battery has not passed into the intestinal tract or is larger than 20 mm, then endoscopic retrieval is necessary.
4. Call the National Button Battery Ingestion Hotline (202–625–3333) for questions.

C. Sharp or pointed objects

1. This is a medical emergency. Remove these endoscopically as soon as possible to prevent perforation. If the object has passed beyond the reach of an endoscope, serial daily radiographs should be performed to follow progress along the GI tract.
2. If there is no advancement in 3 consecutive days or symptoms occur, then surgical removal is warranted.

V. Achalasia.

A. General background. Achalasia is a motility disorder that affects men and women equally (generally 20-40 years old) secondary to the loss of innervation resulting in insufficient LES relaxation, aperistalsis of the esophageal body, and elevated LES pressures. Patients have increased risk of esophageal cancer (usually squamous cell).

B. Clinical manifestations

1. Dysphagia to solids and liquids, chest pain.
2. Regurgitation with nocturnal aspiration, difficulty belching, weight loss.

C. Diagnostic evaluation

1. **Barium swallow demonstrates narrowing of the distal esophagus (bird beaking), dilation of the proximal esophagus, an epiphrenic diverticulum, or a tortuous esophagus.** Esophageal dilation may be absent early on.
2. **Esophageal manometry** establishes the diagnosis, especially if the barium swallow is equivocal.
3. All patients must have upper endoscopy to rule out pseudoachalasia (caused by tumors of the GE junction and cardia).

D. Treatment. The goal of treatment is to relieve the pressure gradient and facilitate esophageal emptying. No therapy can restore motility.

1. **Drug therapy.** Efficacy is variable and tends to decrease with time.
   a. **Nitrates.** Isosorbide dinitrate 5 to 10 mg sublingually before meals; nitroglycerin 0.4 mg SL half an hour before meals and at bedtime.
   b. **Calcium channel blockers.** Nifedipine 10 to 30 mg PO half an hour before meals.
2. **Pneumatic dilation** is the most effective nonsurgical treatment; however, 30% require repeat dilations.
3. **Surgical myotomy.** Symptomatic improvement is seen in 80% to 100% of patients.
4. **Botulinum toxin injection.** Endoscopic injection of botulinum toxin type A into the LES is initially effective in 85% of patients, but symptoms recur in more than 50% of patients after 6 months.

VI. Diffuse Esophageal Spasm.

A. General background. Diffuse esophageal spasm is most commonly seen in patients older than 50 years and is characterized by large amplitude, long duration, repetitive contractions of the esophagus. The cause is unknown but it may be due to esophageal hypersensitivity.

B. Patients have recurrent chest pain (commonly indistinguishable from cardiac angina) and dysphagia. Dysphagia is associated with both liquids and solids and is intermittent and nonprogressive. Symptoms may be precipitated by stress or cold liquids.

C. Diagnostic evaluation. Esophageal manometry shows intermittent diffuse contractions mixed with periods of normal peristalsis. **Barium esophagram** findings are variable and may be normal.

D. Treatment

1. Treat GERD if present.

2. Smooth muscle relaxants: nitroglycerin 0.4 mg SL prn for pain; isosorbide dinitrate 10-30 mg PO bid; nifedipine 10-30 mg PO qid; diltiazem 90 mg PO qid.

3. Other potential therapies include trazodone, imipramine, botulinum injection, or pneumatic dilation.

VII. Scleroderma.

A. General background. Esophageal motility disorders are present in 80% of patients with scleroderma and are due to fibrosis of the esophageal smooth muscle.

B. Clinical manifestations. Dysphagia and acid reflux with or without esophagitis and an increased risk for Barrett's metaplasia, adenocarcinoma, and stricture formation.

C. Diagnostic evaluation. Barium swallow shows dilation of the lower esophagus and poor sphincter tone. Manometry reveals low pressures at the LES and low-amplitude ineffective distal motility.

D. Treatment is directed at controlling acid reflux and esophagitis (see discussion of GERD treatment).

VIII. Zenker's Diverticulum.

A. Zenker's diverticulum (pharyngoesophageal diverticulum) is an outpouching of mucosa in the posterior upper esophagus. It generally occurs after age 60 years, but some patients report years of symptoms.

B. Typical manifestations include regurgitation of undigested food when the patient bends over or lies down, transient dysphagia, pulmonary aspiration, gurgling in the throat, halitosis, or regurgitation of foul-smelling food into the mouth.

C. The diagnosis is confirmed by barium esophagram or endoscopy. The treatment of choice is surgical resection.

PEPTIC ULCER DISEASE

I. General. Predisposing factors for both duodenal and gastric ulcers include infection by *H. pylori*, use of alcohol, tobacco, aspirin, and/or

NSAIDS, and physiologic stress such as multiple trauma, sepsis, neurosurgical problems, gastrinoma, and other "ICU" stresses.

II. **Clinical Manifestations.**

A. **There is no symptom complex that can adequately differentiate among gastric ulcers, duodenal ulcers, and nonulcer dyspepsia.**

B. Food might exacerbate or relieve the pain of either type of peptic ulcer. The pain of gastritis is reliably worsened by food. The pain of either type of ulcer may be felt as a gnawing pain in the chest, back, mid abdomen, or either upper quadrant. Many ulcers are asymptomatic (especially those related to NSAIDS) and first manifest with a perforated viscus or GI bleed.

III. **Diagnostic Evaluation.**

A. **History and physical**

1. **The presence of alarm symptoms such as early satiety, dysphagia, or weight loss should be carefully investigated.** History of NSAID, aspirin, or anticoagulant use is critical.

2. **Examine the abdomen.** Evaluate for melena, hematochezia, or occult blood either in a passed stool or with a rectal exam.

B. **Lab testing.** Obtain a CBC and fecal occult blood test × 3 (if initially negative). Consider LFTs, amylase, and lipase to exclude pancreatic or biliary causes of epigastric pain in the proper clinical scenario.

C. **Gastrointestinal imaging. Patients older than 45 years who have new onset of dyspeptic/ulcer symptoms or with alarm symptoms suggesting malignancy (fever, weight loss, early satiety, occult GI bleeding, or vomiting) should be referred for endoscopy.** Others can be treated empirically but should undergo endoscopic evaluation if they have little or no response to therapy after 7 to 10 days or have persistent symptoms after 6 to 8 weeks. Alternative evaluation can include barium upper GI radiography, but endoscopy offers several advantages including direct visualization and the ability to obtain biopsies to diagnose *H. pylori* infection and exclude malignancy.

IV. *H. pylori* **Infection.**

A. *H. pylori* **(a urease-producing flagellated bacterium) infection plays an etiologic role in up to 95% of those with duodenal ulcers and more than 80% of those with gastric ulcer.** *H. pylori* infection is highly correlated with atrophic gastritis, intestinal metaplasia, gastric carcinoma, gastric non-Hodgkin's lymphoma, and mucosa-associated lymphoid tissue (MALT) lymphomas of the stomach. **Other potential causes of peptic ulcer disease include** NSAIDs, Zollinger-Ellison syndrome, infiltrative or granulomatous disorders, Crohn's disease, and other infections.

B. *H. pylori* **testing. A recommended approach includes noninvasive *H. pylori* testing (e.g., antibody testing) followed by antibiotic therapy if positive.** If the noninvasive *H. pylori* test is negative, then empiric antisecretory therapy with a PPI for 1 month can be instituted. **The rapid urease test (CLO test), stomach biopsy, urea breath test,** and stool antigen tests have decreased sensitivity (more false negatives) in patients who have recently been treated with antibiotics, bismuth, PPIs, or H_2 blockers. Discontinue antibiotics for 4 weeks prior to testing and other drugs 2 weeks prior to testing. Sensitivities given next assume therapy has been discontinued. Available *H. pylori* tests include:

1. **Invasive tests. Rapid urease test or CLO test.** The reported sensitivity is 80% to 90% and specificity is 95%. It requires gastric mucosal biopsy. **Alternatively, gastric biopsy for histology** offers direct visualization of the *H. pylori* organism with standard H&E stains or special stains for *H. pylori*. The reported sensitivity is 91%.

2. **Noninvasive tests**

a. **Qualitative serum *H. pylori* antibody test** has a sensitivity of 67% to 90% and specificity of 75% to 91%. The antibody test cannot be used for post-treatment follow-up or in patients with a history of prior *H. pylori* infection because the antibody titers persist (43% positive remain antibody positive at 1 year).

b. **Urea breath test (UBT)** requires ingestion of urea labeled with a carbon isotope (^{13}C or ^{14}C), and if *H. pylori* is present, the urea is split into CO_2 and ammonia. The labeled CO_2 then diffuses into the blood and is exhaled and measured. Sensitivity is 90% to 100%. The UBT can be used to confirm successful eradication of *H. pylori*.

c. **Stool antigen test** is available to diagnose *H. pylori* infection and for post-treatment follow-up. This test is accurate (sensitivity, 91%; specificity, 94%) and cost effective, and it can be used safely in children and pregnant women. It is available in an office-based kit providing results within 5 to 10 minutes.

V. **Treatment.**

A. **Treatment of *H. pylori*.** Treat all *H. pylori*-positive patients; treatment decreases ulcer recurrence and improves healing **(Table 5-2)**. All of the options have a greater than 90% eradication rate. Confirmation of

TABLE 5-2

TREATMENT FOR *H. PYLORI*

Regimen	Number of Days
Omeprazole 20 mg bid *plus* clarithromycin 500 mg bid *plus* amoxicillin 1 g bid (Prevpac)	14 days
Lansoprazole 30 mg bid *plus* clarithromycin 500 mg bid *plus* metronidazole 500 mg bid	14 days
Bismuth subsulfate 525 mg (2 tablets) bid *plus* metronidazole 500 mg PO tid *plus* tetracycline 500 mg qid *plus* lansoprazole 30 mg PO qd	14 days
Omeprazole 20 mg bid *plus* clarithromycin 500 mg bid *plus* metronidazole 500 mg bid	10 days
Helidac (bismuth subsalicylate, metronidazole, tetracycline) qid *plus* famotidine 40 mg qd	14 days

H. pylori eradication (urea breath testing or endoscopy with biopsy) is warranted in patients with complicated duodenal ulcers or gastric ulcers.

B. Antisecretory therapy

1. The H_2 blockers (cimetidine, ranitidine, famotidine, etc.) and PPIs (omeprazole, esomeprazole, lansoprazole, rabeprazole, pantoprazole, etc.) are all effective in treating peptic ulcers when given for 6 to 8 weeks. PPIs are generally considered first line-therapy due to increased efficacy and fewer drug interactions. Gastric ulcers can require longer duration of therapy (up to 12 weeks). **Using acid-control measures alone is not optimal treatment of *H. pylori*–infected patients.** Sucralfate is an alternative therapy for duodenal ulcers but it only works in the presence of acid (cannot be used with H_2 blockers or PPIs concurrently); compliance is difficult because of qid dosing.

2. **Lifestyle modification is also important.** The patient should be advised to avoid factors that predispose to ulceration, including alcohol, NSAIDS, aspirin, and tobacco.

C. Special considerations

1. **Duodenal ulcers**

a. **Recurrent ulcers**

   (1) Exclude persistent *H. pylori* infection or continued NSAID use.

   (2) Patients with recurrent duodenal ulcers should have an evaluation to exclude Zollinger–Ellison syndrome, including endoscopy and serum gastrin levels. **See Discussion of Zollinger-Ellison syndrome below.**

   (3) Surgical consultation may be warranted for vagotomy or antrectomy.

   (4) Carcinoma can manifest as a refractory ulcer.

   (5) Evaluate for CMV infection in immunosuppressed patients.

b. **Complications of duodenal ulcer disease include:**

   (1) **Bleeding** (see discussion of gastrointestinal bleeding).

   (2) **Perforation** usually occurs posteriorly and manifests as an acute abdomen with free air in the abdomen. Elderly patients taking NSAIDs are at increased risk of perforation.

   (3) **Gastric outlet obstruction** is a rare complication. Symptoms include early satiety, nausea, vomiting, and abdominal pain. Endoscopic evaluation with dilation or surgical consultation is necessary if conservative efforts are ineffective.

2. **Gastric ulcers require endoscopy at the end of therapy in order to exclude gastric carcinoma.** Resolution of symptoms and healing of the ulcer with treatment does not exclude carcinoma.

VI. Prevention of Recurrence (Table 5-3).

A. Continue maintenance therapy for 2 additional weeks after 6 to 8 weeks of treatment and consider long-term suppression in those at high risk for recurrence (smokers, alcoholics) and in those with long-term aspirin use, refractory ulcers, and complicated ulcers or in those at high risk for bleeding.

B. Treatment for *H. pylori* is effective in preventing recurrence.

GASTROENTEROLOGY 5

TABLE 5-3

PEPTIC ULCER DISEASE MAINTENANCE THERAPY

H$_2$-Receptor Antagonist	Maintenance Dose
Cimetidine	400 mg qhs
Ranitidine	150 mg qhs
Famotidine	20 mg qhs

Note: PPI maintenance therapy is indicated in patients who fail H$_2$-blocker therapy.

VII. NSAID-Induced Gastroduodenal Ulcers.

A. General. NSAIDs inhibit the production of protective mucus and bicarbonate. Risk factors for NSAID-induced PUD include age older than 60 years, NSAID use, and concomitant glucocorticoid or anticoagulant use. If the patient is *H. pylori* positive, treat before starting long-term NSAID therapy.

B. Clinically, many NSAID-related ulcers are painless. Dyspeptic symptoms do not correlate well with NSAID-induced ulcers; patients with symptoms often do not have ulcers and those without symptoms often do.

C. Treatment. Stop the offending drug and use acetaminophen for pain control. If that is not possible, consider one of the following strategies:

1. **Use an NSAID with lower GI toxicity such as ibuprofen.** COX-2 inhibitors are not recommended because of an increased risk of strokes and MIs and little if any GI benefit during long-term use. Low-dose aspirin (81 mg) negate any potential GI benefit of COX-2 inhibitors.

2. Consider adding misoprostol (200 μg bid) to the NSAID therapy, although this is poorly tolerated secondary to side effects (e.g., diarrhea, abdominal pain).

3. Start lansoprazole 30 mg daily, which is better tolerated and has fewer drug interactions.

VIII. Zollinger–Ellison Syndrome.

A. General background. ZES is caused by hypersecretion of gastrin from a gastrinoma and is responsible for 0.1% to 1% of all cases of peptic ulcer disease.

B. Diagnostic evaluation

1. **Measurement of serum gastrin level is the initial screening test.** Serum gastrin can be elevated both in acid hypersecretory states (e.g., ZES) and, ironically, in states of low acid secretion (e.g., PPI or H$_2$ blocker therapy, gastric atrophy, stomach surgery, and pernicious anemia with achlorhydria).

2. **A normal gastrin level reliably rules out ZES. If the serum gastrin level is elevated, the test should be repeated simultaneously with a gastric pH.** If the gastrin level remains high with gastric pH <2.5, the diagnosis of ZES is highly likely. In this scenario, refer to an appropriate specialist for definitive diagnosis and treatment.

3. **ZES is associated with hyperparathyroidism and pituitary dysfunction** (multiple endocrine neoplasia [MEN I]) at a rate of 20% to 25%. Appropriate tests to evaluate for the presence of MEN I include serum calcium and PTH levels, as well as tests for pituitary function.

ACUTE GASTROINTESTINAL BLEEDING

Note: *Stabilizing the bleeding patient is paramount. See discussion of shock in chapter 2 for guidelines.*

I. Types.
A. **Hematemesis** is vomiting of bright red blood or coffee grounds–like material. It usually implies bleeding proximal to the ligament of Treitz.
B. **Melena** is black, tarry stool secondary to GI bleeding with digestion of hemoglobin. It may occur in both upper and lower GI bleeding (particularly bleeding from the distal small bowel or right colon). **Dark stools can also occur after ingestion of iron, Pepto-Bismol, or licorice but the stool guaiac will be negative.**
C. **Hematochezia** is bright red blood per rectum that usually implies a lower GI source of blood loss and less commonly massive upper GI bleeding with rapid transit. **Red stools can be related to ingestion of red foods such as beets or Kool-Aid.**
II. Laboratory Evaluation.
A. If an acute abdomen is present, consider CXR and an upright abdominal film to exclude free intraperitoneal air.
B. **Laboratory studies should include** CBC, platelets, PT/PTT, electrolytes, and BUN/creatinine (upper GI bleeders often have elevated BUN due to increased uptake of nitrogen from digested blood). Type and crossmatch for at least 2 units of blood and more as needed.
C. **Angiography or ^{99}Tc-tagged RBC scanning can be useful to localize bleeding in the lower GI tract** and rarely from an upper GI source.
III. **Clinical Considerations and Differential Diagnosis in Upper GI Bleeding.** (Table 5-4).
A. Causes
1. **Peptic ulcer disease** may be asymptomatic until first bleed, especially in patients taking NSAIDS.
2. **In alcoholic patients or those with chronic liver disease** consider erosive gastritis or bleeding related to portal hypertension (gastropathy or varices).
3. **Mallory–Weiss tear** is a linear tear of the gastroesophageal mucosa that occurs after prolonged vomiting or retching and causes minor self-limited bleeding. Mediastinal air on CXR portends a poor course **(Boerhaave's tear with mediastinitis).**
4. **Boerhaave's tear occurs** when the esophagus ruptures into the mediastinum, often as a result of vomiting. Patients present with rapid onset of chest pain, odynophagia, tachypnea, tachycardia, fever, and possible shock. Chest radiograph shows free mediastinal air. Diagnosis is by Gastrografin swallow demonstrating esophageal leak.

5

GASTROENTEROLOGY

TABLE 5-4
ETIOLOGY OF GI BLEEDING

Category	Upper GI Bleed	Lower GI Bleed
Inflammatory	Peptic ulcer	Ulcerative colitis
	Esophagitis	Crohn's disease
	Gastritis	Diverticulitis
	Stress ulcer	Enterocolitis
		Radiation colitis
Mechanical	Mallory–Weiss tear	Anal fissure
	Hiatal hernia	Diverticulosis
		Intussusception
Vascular	Esophageal varices	Hemorrhoids
		AV malformations
		Angiodysplasia
		Aortoenteric fistula
Neoplastic	Carcinoma	Carcinoma, polyps
Systemic	Blood dyscrasias	Blood dyscrasias

Treatment includes NPO, continuous NG suction, antibiotics, and surgical repair. Antibiotics must include aerobic and anaerobic coverage (e.g., ceftriaxone plus clindamycin).

5. Aortoenteric fistula should be considered in patients with a prior history of abdominal aortic aneurysm repair.
6. **Dieulafoy's lesions** are abnormal submucosal arterioles commonly seen in older patients with a prior history of coronary artery disease, hypertension, and diabetes.

B. Evaluation

1. **NG tube placement with aspiration and lavage is indicated** both as a diagnostic tool and to improve visualization during endoscopy. However, **NG aspirate is only 43% sensitive for upper GI bleeding in those without hematemesis.** If the aspirate is bloody and fails to clear with *warm saline* lavage, consider urgent endoscopy. Remove the NG tube unless it is needed to prevent nausea and vomiting. **Ice saline lavage is not useful and can prolong bleeding. A properly placed NG tube does not induce variceal bleeding.**
2. **Endoscopy may be done acutely for upper GI bleeding** to help define and potentially treat the source of bleeding.
3. In patients with ulcer bleeding, evaluate for *H. pylori* infection and treat if positive (see discussion of peptic ulcer disease).

C. Treatment

1. **Most patients with an upper GI bleed should be hospitalized. The exception is Mallory–Weiss tears in a healthy patient with a stable hemoglobin and hematocrit.**
2. **High-dose IV PPIs (pantoprazole 80-mg bolus followed by 8 mg/h drip for 24 h) should be started in high-risk bleeding *ulcers*.** This decreases rebleeding from 22% to 6.7%. If no bleeding recurs after 24 hours, IV PPI can be switched to an oral form (e.g., lansoprazole).

3. **Erythromycin.** Consider giving IV erythromycin 3mg/kg over 20 to 30 minutes, 30 to 90 minutes before endoscopy to facilitate gastric emptying of blood and improve visualization during endoscopy (remember the risk of arrhythmias, however).

4. **If esophageal variceal bleeding is suspected:**

a. If bleeding has stopped, there is no need to completely normalize PT/INR.

b. **Start IV octreotide (a synthetic somatostatin analogue, 50-mg bolus followed by 50-mg/h drip × 5 days).** Octreotide in combination with endoscopic therapy is superior to endoscopic therapy alone in controlling acute variceal bleeding in patients with cirrhosis but does not improve mortality. **Octreotide in the absence of endoscopy is of limited benefit.**

c. **Transjugular intrahepatic portosystemic shunt (TIPS)** is safe and effective in treating variceal hemorrhage in patients with portal hypertension who fail endoscopic therapy.

d. **β-Blocker.** Once the patient is hemodynamically stable and before discontinuing octreotide, a noncardioselective β-blocker should be initiated to decrease portal pressures. Propranolol (10 mg bid) or nadolol (20 mg qd) can be titrated to achieve a 25% reduction in heart rate. In patients intolerant of β-blockers or those with bronchospasm, isosorbide mononitrate may be used.

e. **Balloon tamponade** with a 4 lumen Sengstaken–Blakemore (Minnesota) tube can be used as a temporizing measure to control variceal bleeding. **Its use is fraught with complications including esophageal perforation, aspiration pneumonia, and asphyxia.** The tube should be used for no more than 24 hours due to the risk of necrotic ulcers at compression sites.

f. Antibiotics should be administered prophylactically in variceal bleeders with ascites due to an increased risk of spontaneous bacterial peritonitis (see section on ascites and SBP).

g. Up to 50% of patients die with their first variceal bleed.

h. Although traditionally used, **vasopressin causes splanchnic ischemia and should be avoided.**

5. **Bleeding *gastric* varices** can be difficult to treat and rebleeding is common. Endoscopy is not thought to be effective. Current treatment recommendations are IV octreotide and balloon tamponade followed by TIPS or surgical shunting. The triad of isolated gastric varices, splenomegaly, and normal hepatic function should raise the suspicion for **splenic vein thrombosis.**

IV. **Clinical Considerations and Differential Diagnosis in Lower GI Bleeding** (see Table 5-4).

A. **Causes. Most causes of lower GI bleeding are initially self-limited.**

1. Diverticular bleeding is usually acute and painless.

2. Hemorrhoidal or anal fissure bleeding is usually minor.

3. Neoplasms can manifest with iron-deficiency anemia.

5

GASTROENTEROLOGY

4. Consider ischemic colitis, particularly in patients who have recently undergone abdominal vascular surgery or in patients with A Fib.
5. Consider infectious colitis (amebiasis, *Campylobacter*, shigella, *E. coli*, etc.) in recent travelers and campers and in case of unsanitary water intake.
6. Consider solitary rectal ulcer.
7. Consider internal hemorrhoids in young healthy patients with self-limited bleeding.
8. Patients with a significant bleed or comorbidities should be hospitalized.

B. **Evaluation of high risk, ongoing, bleeding**
1. **Perform NG lavage** to exclude the possibility of upper GI bleeding manifesting as hematochezia (remember that NG aspirate is only 43% sensitive in those without hematemesis).
2. **Colonoscopy.** If NG aspirate is negative, proceed with a colonoscopy when practical. Preparation with polyethylene glycol solution (1 gallon orally over 2 h) improves visualization and has not been shown to reactivate bleeding.
3. If bleeding persists, obtain a radionuclide bleeding study and/or angiography. **Coil placement via interventional radiology may be useful in stopping the bleeding.** Barium studies are *not* recommended due to the risk of perforation.
4. A surgical consultation should be obtained in case operative intervention is needed.

ACUTE DIARRHEA

I. **Definition.** Abnormally increased frequency (>3/d) **or** decreased consistency of stools compared to a patient's normal for less than 3 weeks.

II. **Classification of diarrhea can help establish the diagnosis.**

A. **Osmotic diarrhea is caused by ingestion of a poorly absorbed solute** (carbohydrate malabsorption): ingestion of mannitol, sorbitol, lactulose; disaccharidase deficiency (lactose intolerance, fructose intolerance); pancreatic insufficiency; small intestinal mucosal disease (celiac sprue); and excessive ingestion of osmotic laxatives and/or magnesium-containing antacids).

B. **Secretory diarrhea** is caused by increased small intestinal secretion or reduced absorption of fluid. This can result from bacterial enterotoxins (e.g., cholera toxin), infections in patients with AIDS (*Cryptosporidium* spp., *M. avium* complex); hormonal secretagogues, (e.g., vasoactive intestinal peptide [VIP] secreted by pancreatic tumors); carcinoid (5-HIAA excess); gastrin hypersecretion (e.g., Zollinger–Ellison syndrome); or nonosmotic (irritant) laxatives. Clinical manifestation is large-volume, watery stools without blood or leukocytes.

C. **Exudative (inflammatory) diarrhea** can be caused by inflammatory bowel disease and eosinophilic gastroenteritis, radiation enterocolitis, infection with invasive organisms, cytotoxins, ischemia, or vasculitis.

Intestinal mucosa is inflamed, causing mucus, blood, and pus to leak into the lumen.

D. Motility disturbance. Normal stool output is 250 g/day. Diarrhea due to dysmotility is characterized by small, frequent and formed stools associated with urgency. Causes include hyperthyroidism, anorectal disease, proctitis, intraperitoneal blood, fecal impaction, and irritable bowel syndrome.

III. Causes.

A. Infectious. Contaminated food is the most frequent source of organisms causing diarrhea (contaminated water is less common in the United States). **Table 5-5** contains details of common causes of food poisoning.

1. **Bacteria:** *Campylobacter jejuni*, enterotoxigenic *Escherichia coli*, *Salmonella*, shigella, *Clostridium difficile, Yersinia enterocolitica, Vibrio cholerae, Aeromonas, Plesiomonas shigelloides*, and noncholera vibrios.

2. **Viruses:** Rotavirus, Norwalk agent, enterovirus, and hepatitis-associated virus.

3. **Fungi:** *Candida, Actinomyces, Histoplasma*.

4. **Parasites:** *Giardia lamblia* (fairly ubiquitous), *Entamoeba histolytica* and *Cryptosporidium, Strongyloides*.

B. Toxins

1. **Bacterial toxins:** Staphylococcus (food poisoning), *Clostridium perfringens, C. botulinum, C. difficile, Bacillus cereus*, shigella spp, and certain strains of *E. coli* produce toxins.

2. **Chemical poisons:** Heavy metals and mushroom poisoning.

C. Dietary: Intake of nonabsorbable sugar substitutes (sorbitol), food intolerance or allergy, irritating foods, milk, and excessive caffeine.

D. Drugs: Laxatives, magnesium-containing antacids, colchicine, antibiotics, cholinergic agents, lactulose, and quinidine.

E. Visceral causes: Appendicitis, diverticulitis, GI hemorrhage, fecal impaction, ischemic colitis, and pseudomembranous colitis.

IV. Diagnosis.

A. Acute diarrhea is often self-limited, and the diagnosis can be made by history and physical examination.

B. If the patient develops systemic toxicity, severe pain, dehydration, or bloody stools, or if symptoms persist more than 24 hours without improvement, consider checking:

1. **CBC** with differential.

2. **Stool studies,** including culture (× 1), ova and parasites × 3, occult blood, and *Giardia* and *Cryptosporidium* antigens. **Stool for occult blood is only 36% sensitive and 86% specific in patients with culture-proven *Salmonella, Shigella,* and *Campylobacter*.** Stool for leukocytes is only 57% sensitive and 86% specific for infectious diarrhea. **Fecal testing for lactoferrin is more sensitive.**

3. *C. difficile* toxin, particularly with recent antibiotic use, operation, or other intervention. Refer to *C. difficile* section for details.

TABLE 5-5
SOME COMMON FOOD POISONINGS

Poisoning	Foods	Food Taste	Symptoms	Onset	Lasts	Heat Stability, Other Toxin Characteristics	Treatment
Bacillus cereus	Fried rice, other cooled rice or vegetables	Normal	Vomiting	½-3 h	10 h	Heat stable	Supportive
			Diarrheal form	6-10 h	20-36 h	Heat labile	Supportive
Ciguatera poisoning	Red snapper, amberjack, grouper, warm water fish	Normal	GI symptoms (75%) followed by perioral numbness, diffuse dysesthesias, hot/cold reversal on face (pathognomonic), cranial nerve palsies, hallucinations, unusual sensory symptoms (e.g., feel teeth are loose), cardiac abnormalities, hypotension	Minutes to 30 h (most common 1-6 h)	Up to months or years	Heat stable; calcium channel blocker	Gastric decontamination, supportive; calcium gluconate and atropine as needed
Clostridium perfringens	Meats ubiquitously infected	Normal	Watery diarrhea, nausea, cramps; vomiting rare	6 to 12 h (but up to 24 h)	24 h	Ingest live organisms; usually meats cooked and improperly cooled	Supportive (IV fluids, etc.)

Salmonella	Eggs, poultry	Normal	Diarrhea with blood, cramps; occasional sepsis	8-48 h	2-5 d	Heat labile, but organisms occasionally survive cooking	Supportive; if severe, levofloxacin or IV ceftriaxone
Scombroid poisoning	Dark-meat fish (tuna, mackerel, swordfish, mahi mahi, etc.) including canned	Peppery, metallic	Skin flushing, wheezing, diarrhea, headache, urticaria	20-30 min	3 h to days	Heat stable; histamine like	Like anaphylaxis (see Chapter 2)
Shigella	Poor hygiene, person to person	N/A	Nausea, vomiting, diarrhea with progression to invasive diarrhea (heme-positive stool); neurologic symptoms including seizures in young patients	36-72 h	3 d to 2 wk	Shiga toxin inhibits water resorption.	Supportive, fluoroquinolones
Staphylococcal	Any protein-rich food	Normal	Cramps, vomiting, mild diarrhea, occasional fever	1-2 h	5-8 h (occasionally days)	Heat stable, CNS toxin	Supportive

GASTROENTEROLOGY 5

4. **Serum electrolytes** are useful if history suggests voluminous diarrhea with possible secondary hypomagnesemia, hypokalemia, and contraction alkalosis.

5. **Sigmoidoscopy** with biopsy is particularly indicated in patients with bloody diarrhea. It can also be useful in diagnosing inflammatory bowel disease, shigellosis, *C. difficile* toxin (in colonic aspirate in cases when stool is negative), and amebic dysentery. It is particularly useful in immunocompromised patients to determine etiologies such as GVHD, CMV colitis, and protozoal diseases (e.g., cryptosporidium, microsporidia).

6. **Abdominal radiographs, flat and upright,** should be taken if you suspect obstruction or perforation. Significant enteritis may be associated with air-fluid levels. **In general, abdominal radiographs are not useful in the patient with diarrhea.**

V. **Treatment.**

A. **Volume repletion** (see also Chapter 12)

1. **Oral** (clear liquids, sodium- and glucose-containing oral rehydration solutions). See Chapter 12 for instructions on making a rehydration solution at home.

2. **Intravenous** normal saline or lactated Ringer's if the patient has intractable vomiting.

B. **Absorbents** (Kaopectate, aluminum hydroxide) **do not alter the course of the disease or reduce fluid loss,** but they allow the patient more control over the timing of defecation. Medications should be taken at least ½ hour before or 2 hours after absorbents are used.

C. **Antisecretory agents** such as bismuth subsalicylate (Pepto-Bismol). Usual dose is 30 mL every 30 minutes up to 8 doses.

D. **Antiperistaltics,** such as anticholinergics and opiate derivatives. **Do not use in patients with fever, systemic toxicity, or bloody diarrhea.** Discontinue if there is no improvement or if patient's condition deteriorates. However, antiperistaltics are otherwise safe in the adult patient with diarrhea. **Antiperistaltics have been safely used in children, but this is not the standard of care and they should be used only after careful consideration.**

1. **Diphenoxylate with atropine (Lomotil)** is available in tablets (2.5 mg of diphenoxylate) and liquid (2.5 mg of diphenoxylate per 5 mL). The initial dose for adults is two tablets qid (20 mg/day). For children the dose is 0.1 mg/kg per dose qid. The dose is tapered as diarrhea improves. It is not indicated for diarrhea caused by pseudomembranous colitis or enterotoxin-producing or invasive bacteria. **Lomotil should not be used in ulcerative colitis or in children younger than 2 years. Lomotil is quite toxic and has a low therapeutic range in children.**

2. **Loperamide (Imodium)** is available over the counter in 2-mg capsules and liquid (1 mg/5 mL). It increases intestinal absorption of electrolytes and water and decreases intestinal motility and secretion. The dose in adults is 4 mg initially, followed by 2 mg after each diarrhea stool, not

to exceed 16 mg in a 24-hour period. In children, the dose is based on age: 2 to 5 year olds take 1 mg tid, 6 to 8 year olds 2 mg bid, and 9 to 12 year olds 2 mg tid on the first day of treatment. Thereafter, 0.1 mg/kg is administered after each diarrheal stool, not to exceed the total daily dose recommended for the first day of therapy. Loperamide is safe and decreases the number of unformed stools and the duration of diarrhea in patients with *Shigella*-induced dysentery who are treated with ciprofloxacin.

E. Antibiotics are not necessary for most episodes of diarrhea. Once cultures are done, empiric treatment with an agent that covers *Shigella* and *Campylobacter* is reasonable **in those with severe diarrhea, systemic signs or heme-positive diarrhea.** A 3-day course of a fluoroquinolone (ciprofloxacin 500 mg PO bid or norfloxacin 400 mg PO bid) is the first-line therapy. TMP–SMX (Bactrim DS 1 tab PO qd) is an alternative therapy, but resistant organisms are common. If the diarrhea is caused by seafood ingestion, infection with either *V. cholerae* or *Vibrio parahaemolyticus* is possible and can be treated with either a fluoroquinolone or with doxycycline 100 mg PO bid. **It is not clear if antibiotics can increase the risk of hemolytic-uremic syndrome in those infected with *E. coli* O157:H7.** Also see Traveler's Diarrhea.

CHRONIC DIARRHEA

I. **Definition.** Chronic diarrhea is defined as loose stools with or without increased stool frequency persisting for more than 4 weeks.

II. **Etiology** (see Acute Diarrhea earlier for additional discussion).

A. **Infection.** See previous section. Also consider Whipple's disease, which is caused by *Tropheryma whippelii* and is associated with nondeforming arthritis, abdominal pain, fever, weight loss, lymphadenopathy, and occasionally CNS symptoms.

B. **Inflammation:** Ulcerative colitis, Crohn's disease, ischemic colitis, diverticulitis, AIDS-related chronic diarrhea, **collagenous colitis (very common in middle-aged and elderly women),** and lymphocytic colitis.

C. **Drugs:** Laxatives, antibiotics, NSAIDs, magnesium-containing antacids, and alcohol.

D. **Malabsorption:** Short-bowel syndrome, celiac sprue (gluten-sensitive enteropathy), carbohydrate malabsorption, pancreatic insufficiency, and small bowel bacterial overgrowth.

E. **Endocrine:** Hyperthyroidism, diabetes, adrenal insufficiency, hypoparathyroidism, Zollinger–Ellison syndrome, VIPoma, carcinoid tumor, pheochromocytoma, ganglioneuroma, villous adenoma, medullary thyroid carcinoma, or systemic mastocytosis.

F. **Motility disorders:** Irritable bowel syndrome and dumping syndrome.

G. **Infiltrative disorders:** Amyloidosis, diffuse intestinal lymphoma, and scleroderma.

H. **Other disorders:** Fecal incontinence, food allergy, radiation enteritis or colitis. **Chronic watery diarrhea without abdominal pain cannot be**

GASTROENTEROLOGY 5

considered a variant of irritable bowel syndrome and warrants a thorough work-up.

III. Evaluation.

A. A useful strategy for evaluation of chronic diarrhea is to categorize the diarrhea as secretory or osmotic. Calculate the fecal osmotic gap:

$$\text{Fecal osmotic gap} = 290 - [2 \times (\text{fecal Na}^+ + \text{fecal K}^+)]$$

1. **Secretory** diarrhea is defined by a fecal osmotic gap <50 mOsm/kg.
2. **Osmotic** diarrhea is defined by a fecal osmotic gap >125 mOsm/kg.

B. **History**

1. Inquire about diet history (e.g., caffeine, wheat products, lactose), medications, relationship to meals and character of stools, fecal incontinence.
2. How long have symptoms been present? Long symptom duration (>1 y), lack of significant weight loss (<5 kg), absence of nocturnal diarrhea, and straining with defecation have a 70% specificity for functional problems.

C. **Physical examination.** Look for abdominal tenderness, distention, organomegaly, anal fistulas, rectal mass, and hyperactive bowel sounds.

D. **Laboratory analyses. Not every patient needs every test. Use clinical judgment.**

1. **CBC with differential.** Anemia suggests chronic blood loss, infection, malabsorption, or neoplasm. Eosinophilia may be secondary to parasitic disease or allergic reaction. Megaloblastic anemia can result from vitamin B_{12} or folate malabsorption.
2. **Stool exam** for occult blood, leukocytes, and ova and parasites. **Stool lactoferrin is highly sensitive and specific for detection of neutrophils** (e.g., with infectious diarrhea and pseudomembranous colitis). A stool specimen should be sent for culture and sensitivity; **one culture is sufficient. Stool antigen test (sensitivity 92%, specificity 98%) is available for *Giardia* and *Cryptosporidium* and is more sensitive than O&P. Generally three separate stool samples are sent for ova and parasites to increase diagnostic yield.**
3. **Serum electrolytes,** magnesium, iron, creatinine, albumin, cholesterol; calcium and phosphate to evaluate for vitamin D malabsorption and parathyroid disease (also alkaline phosphatase); fasting or random glucose to screen for diabetes. Carotene levels may be low because of fat malabsorption. PT/PTT may be abnormal because of decreased vitamin K absorption. Check TSH to rule out thyroid disease.
4. **ESR and C-reactive protein,** if elevated, could indicate chronic inflammation.
5. **Special tests**
   a. **A 72-hour fecal fat quantitation** could be useful if steatorrhea (fat malabsorption) is suspected. The interpretation of Sudan stain of a

random stool sample is fraught with difficulties because the amount of fat ingested is variable.

b. **D-Xylose absorption** is decreased in disorders of the proximal small intestine.

c. **A stool pH < 5.3 is diagnostic of a carbohydrate intolerance.** Breath hydrogen test can suggest lactase deficiency or fructose malabsorption. You can also check for reducing substances in stool or try a therapeutic lactose-free diet.

d. **Small intestinal biopsy** is useful for Whipple's disease, celiac sprue, GVHD, regional enteritis, giardiasis, and other parasitic infestations.

e. **Celiac disease.** See later.

f. **Small bowel aspirate culture for bacterial overgrowth.**

g. **Stool test for phenolphthalein (test for factitious laxative abuse). Note that phenolphthalein is no longer available in the United States.** Bring stool pH to 8.0. If the specimen turns maroon, this indicates the presence of phenolphthalein, an ingredient in over-the-counter laxative products. Urine tests are available to detect aloes, senna alkaloids, and bisacodyl.

h. **Endoscopy.** Sigmoidoscopy or colonoscopy, especially if Crohn's disease, neoplasm, or AIDs-associated diarrhea are suspected.

i. **Radiographic studies.** Barium studies of the upper GI tract, small intestine, and colon are useful if inflammatory bowel disease or GI tract tumors are suspected.

IV. Treatment.

A. **Treatment should be directed at the underlying cause of the chronic diarrhea,** not control of diarrhea alone.

B. **Occasionally, when a definitive diagnosis cannot be made, empirically try:**

1. **Diet restriction:** restricting lactose, gluten, or long-chain fatty acids in the diet. Restrictions should be done systematically so that if symptoms improve, the restricted factor can be identified and removed permanently from the diet. Lactase replacements (such as Lactaid caplets) are available OTC for patients intolerant to lactose.

2. **Pancreatic enzyme supplementation** (Creon [pancrelipase] capsules) for suspected pancreatic exocrine deficiency (such as cystic fibrosis or chronic pancreatitis).

3. **Increase dietary or supplemental fiber.**

4. **Cholestyramine** tends to have a constipating effect mostly due to binding bile salts, especially in patients who have <100 cm of ileum resected.

5. **Antimicrobials** (such as metronidazole or ciprofloxacin)

6. **Judicious use of antidiarrheal medication** may be appropriate for symptomatic relief in some patients. Opiates should generally be avoided in the treatment of chronic diarrhea. See acute diarrhea section for dosages and cautions.

GASTROENTEROLOGY   5

CLOSTRIDIUM DIFFICILE INFECTION

I. **General.**
A. *Clostridium difficile* is a gram-positive, anaerobic, spore-forming bacterium associated with antecedent antibiotic therapy responsible for antibiotic-associated diarrhea and colitis.
B. The infection clinically ranges from asymptomatic carrier states (two thirds of infected hospitalized patients) to severe pseudomembranous colitis. More virulent, deadly, strains are emerging, especially after treatment with fluoroquinolones.
C. *C. difficile* colitis must be considered in patients presenting with presumed flares of inflammatory bowel disease.

II. **Etiology.**
A. *C. difficile* colitis can be caused by almost any antibiotic, including cephalosporins and penicillins.
B. Symptoms can develop within a few days or even 6 to 10 weeks after antibiotic therapy. Risk depends on the number of antibiotics and duration.

III. **Clinical Manifestations.** Any of these manifestations may be absent, and pseudomembranous colitis should be considered in any patient with otherwise unexplainable diarrhea.
A. **Symptoms include profuse watery diarrhea** that may be foul smelling, abdominal pain, cramping, tenderness, and low-grade fever.
B. **Stools may be guaiac positive** and occasionally grossly bloody.
C. **White blood cell count is 12,000 to 20,000.**
D. **In severe cases, toxic megacolon, colonic perforation, and peritonitis can develop.** Other complications include electrolyte abnormalities, hypovolemic shock, anasarca caused by hypoalbuminemia, sepsis, and hemorrhage.

IV. **Diagnosis.**
A. **Because *C. difficile* may be a normal bowel organism (especially in children), simply culturing the organism does not mean that diarrhea is caused by *C. difficile.*** Tests generally detect "Toxin A." ELISA assays have 70% to 90% sensitivity and 99% specificity.
B. **If there is a high suspicion and the initial *C. difficile* toxin test is negative, sending an additional two specimens will increase the yield. In rare cases, a false-negative ELISA will be obtained if there is a toxin A mutation.** These cases can be detected by performing toxin B assays, cytotoxicity assays, or flexible sigmoidoscopy with diagnostic histopathology noted on colon biopsy

V. **Treatment.**
A. Mild symptoms sometimes resolve spontaneously once the causative antibiotic is withdrawn. Contact precautions to prevent transmission.
B. More severe cases warrant therapy with oral antibiotic therapy. Metronidazole (500 mg PO qid) for 10 to14 days is an effective initial therapy. Oral vancomycin (125 mg PO qid) for 10 to 14 days

can be used in patients not responding to metronidazole or for critically ill patients. Relapsing patients (25%) can be treated with another course of the aforementioned antibiotics.

VI. Lactobacillus. There is some evidence to suggest that using live lactobacillus helps to prevent antibiotic-related diarrhea and can prevent recurrences of *C. difficile* diarrhea in those who are predisposed.

TRAVELER'S DIARRHEA

I. Definition and Clinical Features.

A. Traveler's diarrhea is loose stools with or without increased frequency acquired when traveling from an industrialized country to a developing country or starting up to 7 to 10 days after return to a developed area.

B. Classically, most people have 3 to 5 loose stools per day and the illness generally lasts for 3 to 5 days in untreated persons. Fever, bloody stools, or both can be found in 2% to 10%. Other associated symptoms include nausea, vomiting, and abdominal pain or cramps. Although the diarrhea is mostly benign and self-limited, significant volume loss may cause dehydration.

II. Etiology.

A. Bacterial pathogens are responsible for 90% of cases and include enterotoxigenic *E. coli* (predominant cause), *Campylobacter jejuni*, *Aeromonas*, *Shigella*, *Salmonella*, and noncholera vibrios.

B. Viral pathogens account for approximately 10% of the cases, and rotaviruses are the most common.

C. *Giardia*, *Cryptosporidium*, and *Cyclospora* organisms are rare causes of traveler's diarrhea.

III. Prophylaxis and Prevention.

A. Educate travelers prior to departure about water purification, food and drink selection (local ice contaminates beverages; foods washed with unsterilized water could be contaminated).

B. Prophylactic antibiotic use is not recommended for routine travelers because of the risk of adverse effects from the drugs and the development of resistant gut flora. **Routine prophylaxis is recommended for high-risk persons including travelers with inflammatory bowel disease, HIV, hypochlorhydria, and genetic immunodeficiency syndromes, as well as those with significant chronic medical conditions such as severe heart disease or organ transplantation for whom the development of diarrhea could be especially detrimental.** Ciprofloxacin 500 mg PO daily or norfloxacin 400 mg PO daily are the drugs of choice for prophylaxis. These agents afford >94% protection.

C. Prophylactic use of bismuth subsalicylate (Pepto-Bismol) 524 mg PO qid with meals and qhs provides protection rates of up to 65% against traveler's diarrhea. Attapulgite (Kaopectate) 1200-3000 mg per dose with a maximum of 8 doses is suggested to bind bacteria and toxins and absorb excess fluid.

5

GASTROENTEROLOGY

IV. Treatment.

A. For mild cases of nonbloody traveler's diarrhea, increased oral fluid and salt intake may be sufficient.

B. Adding loperamide is safe for nonbloody traveler's diarrhea without fever.

C. **Although routine prophylaxis with antibiotics is discouraged, sending the traveler with a prescription to take at the onset of acute diarrhea is reasonable.** Doxycycline 100 mg PO qd (resistant strains common), TMP–SMX 160 mg/800 mg (1 double-strength tablet) PO qd (resistant strains common except in Mexico), norfloxacin 400 mg PO qd, or ciprofloxacin 500 mg PO qd may be used for 3 days. **However, fluoroquinolones should not be prescribed to children or pregnant women.** No significant resistance to the fluoroquinolones has yet been reported in high-risk areas. These medications should be continued for 1 or 2 days after the patient returns home. A course of metronidazole to cover for *Giardia* organisms may also be sent with the patient. Rifaximin (Xiraxan 200 mg PO tid) is a new (but expensive), nonabsorbed, gut-selective oral antibiotic. A dose of 200 mg tid for 3 days has been shown to reduce duration of symptoms in patients with traveler's diarrhea.

GIARDIASIS

I. General.

A. Giardiasis is caused by the flagellated protozoan parasite *Giardia intestinalis* (aka *G. lamblia*), which is transmitted through water (wells on farms, streams, or lakes), person-to-person transmission or by food. The disease varies from asymptomatic colonization (15%) to explosive diarrhea (25% to 50%) with weight loss and malabsorption.

B. **Approximately 50% of those ingesting the parasite will not become colonized or develop diarrhea.**

II. Groups at increased risk include travelers to developing countries, campers, children in daycare and their families, homosexual men, and immunocompromised persons (especially with AIDS).

III. Clinical Presentation.

A. Incubation is 7 to 10 days.

B. Diarrhea (may initially be watery), weight loss, and abdominal cramping are the most common symptoms. Nausea, vomiting, increased flatulence, and chronic malabsorptive diarrhea may occur. The infection may also be asymptomatic.

IV. Diagnosis.

A. Detect *Giardia* antigen in the stool by immunofluorescence (most common) or ELISA. It is 85% to 98% sensitive and 95% specific.

B. *Giardia* can also be diagnosed by duodenal biopsy (90% sensitivity) or checking stool for O&P (50%-70% sensitivity with one and 90% sensitivity with three stool specimens). PCR stool assays are experimental.

V. Treatment.

A. Mainstay of treatment is metronidazole 250 mg PO tid for 5 days, which is effective in about 90% of the cases. Higher dose of 750 mg PO tid for 5 days is indicated for treatment failures. Quinacrine 100 mg PO tid after meals for 5 days is an alternative but is no longer available in the United States. Nitazoxanide is a recently approved agent that is administered at a dose of 100-500 mg PO bid for 3 days with an efficacy of 81% to 85%. **Albendazole is useful for metronidazole-resistant strains** and in travelers with additional helminthic infections; 400 mg PO qd × 5 days has a 95% cure rate.

B. Because giardiasis causes shortening and disruption of microvilli with deficiencies in epithelial brush border enzymes (e.g. lactase), it is best to avoid dairy products until eradication of the parasite.

VI. Prevention.

A. Boiling or heating water to >70°C for 10 minutes eliminates *Giardia* cysts. Iodine-based water treatments are more efficacious than chlorine-based treatments, but iodine disinfection must be conducted for at least 8 hours. Water filtration devices also remove *Giardia* cysts.

B. Strict hand washing and personal hygiene are useful in preventing person-to-person spread. There are no vaccines for giardiasis.

INFLAMMATORY BOWEL DISEASE

I. Crohn's Disease (Regional Enteritis, Granulomatous Colitis).

A. Definition and general information: Crohn's is an idiopathic inflammatory disorder that can involve any portion of the GI tract and can produce extraintestinal manifestations. It most commonly involves the ileum and colon. Both small intestine and colon are involved in approximately half of the patients. It is more common in teenagers and young adults, although any age group can be affected.

B. Clinical presentation includes chronic or nocturnal diarrhea, abdominal pain especially in the right lower quadrant, anorexia, weight loss, fever, fatigue, recurrent oral aphthous ulcers, and bowel obstruction. Recurrent perianal fissures, fistulous tracts, strictures, and abscess formation are not uncommon. Extraintestinal manifestations involve the skin, eyes, and joints. **Acute presentation of ileitis can be confused with appendicitis.** Patients with colon involvement present with rectal bleeding and perianal complications. Gastric and duodenal involvement manifests with epigastric pain, nausea, vomiting, or gastric outlet obstruction. Disease involving the small bowel can result in partial or complete small bowel obstruction, bacterial overgrowth, or protein-losing enteropathy causing cachexia and growth retardation. Mineral and vitamin malabsorption causes anemia (iron deficiency, anemia of chronic disease, or B_{12} deficiency), osteopenia, cholelithiasis, or nephrolithiasis (oxalate stones).

C. Diagnosis and evaluation
1. **Endoscopy with biopsies** is the gold standard.
2. **X-ray contrast studies** (small-bowel follow through more so than air-contrast barium enema) are useful if they reveal areas of small bowel stricturing, fistulas, or mucosal abnormalities. Small bowel enteroclysis is more sensitive to evaluate jejunal or ileal involvement. **Contrast studies should be avoided in patients with severe disease to prevent inducing toxic megacolon and in patients with possible bowel obstruction.**
3. **Video capsule endoscopy** is assuming a greater role for detecting ulcerations beyond the reach of endoscopes.
4. **CT** is helpful in evaluating for abscesses. CT is less costly, faster, more readily available, and as sensitive as MRI for detecting abdominal abscesses.
5. **Laboratory studies.** Patients can have anemia or elevated ESR or CRP.
6. **Serological evaluation.** Antisaccharomyces cerevisiae (ASCA) positivity is seen in 60% of patients with Crohn's disease, 5% of patients with ulcerative colitis, and less than 5% of patients without inflammatory bowel disease. High expression of ASCA is associated with worse prognosis: younger age of symptom onset, fibro-stenosing course, and increased risk for multiple surgeries.

D. Complications
1. **Dehydration** and malnutrition from diarrhea and malabsorption. Fat-soluble vitamins and vitamin B_{12} tend to be particularly affected.
2. **Strictures** and bowel obstruction.
3. **Bowel perforation** and abscess formation with **chronic fistula formation** (enterocutaneous, enterovaginal, enterovesicular, enteroenteric).
4. **Metabolic bone disease** due to chronic steroid use or calcium or vitamin D malabsorption.
5. **Renal disease including urolithiasis** (due to steatorrhea promoting excess colonic absorption of oxalate-causing hyperoxaluria).
6. **Colon cancer** (two times the rate of age-matched controls). Small bowel cancer risk is 17-fold higher, but the absolute risk remains low because of the rarity of these types of tumors.
7. **Toxic megacolon** (more common with ulcerative colitis).
8. **Approximately twofold increase in incidence of lymphoma (increased further to approximately sixfold with infliximab infusions).**
E. Other extraintestinal manifestations include arthritis, erythema nodosum, pyoderma gangrenosum, episcleritis or keratoconjunctivitis, and sclerosing cholangitis.
F. Severity of disease
1. **Mild or moderate disease.** Ambulatory patients who can tolerate oral alimentation and who have no manifestations of dehydration, toxicity (high fevers, rigors, prostration), abdominal tenderness, painful mass, obstruction, or >10% weight loss.

2. **Severe disease.** Hospitalized patients or those who are unable to tolerate oral alimentation or who show signs of dehydration, toxicity, abdominal tenderness, painful mass, obstruction, or >10% weight loss.

3. **Remission.** Patients who are asymptomatic or without inflammatory sequelae, including patients who have responded to acute medical intervention or have undergone surgical resection without gross evidence of residual disease. **Patients requiring steroids to maintain well-being are considered to be steroid-dependent and not in remission.**

4. **Flares can be caused by** recent antibiotic use, infection (especially *C. difficile*), physiological or psychological stress, NSAID use, or medical noncompliance.

G. **Table 5-6 lists drug therapy.**

1. **Acute treatment (see Table 5-6 for details). Steroids are the mainstay of acute treatment.** Switch to oral when possible and taper rapidly. **Aminosalicylates and sulfasalazine** can be used to acutely to treat disease and continued long term. **Antibiotics may be useful in the short term. Biologic therapy** (infliximab [Remicade]) should only be used if the patient is failing other therapy. **Parenteral nutrition is critical in the severely ill patient (e.g., those admitted).** Resume feedings once symptoms have subsided.

2. **Long-term management and maintenance of remission (see Table 5-6 for details):** Steroids (taper rapidly); 5-ASA chosen by site of disease needing therapy; azathioprine (Imuran) or 6-mercaptopurine (6-MP) are effective steroid-sparing agents. Antibiotics and infliximab are not particularly useful long term.

a. Antidiarrheal agents, including loperamide or Lomotil (atropine sulfate-diphenoxylate HCl) can be helpful.

b. **Other agents.** Multiple therapies are being evaluated. These include agents directed against TNF (thalidomide) and leukocyte adhesion molecules (natalizumab). Modulation of the cytokine response (helminths) is also being explored. Humanized monoclonal antibody to TNF (adalimumab, Humira) has just become available.

3. **Surgical intervention** is not curative for Crohn's disease but is vital in the management of several complications including: abscess, strictures with obstruction, fistulas, and focal activity that prevents tapering of steroids.

II. **Ulcerative Colitis.**

A. **Definition.** Ulcerative colitis is an idiopathic inflammatory disorder that involves colonic mucosa and submucosa in a continuous pattern and can extend from the rectum to the cecum. Unlike Crohn's disease, there are no skip lesions, transmural inflammation, fistulas, or small bowel involvement.

B. **Clinical presentation** consists of diarrhea (often bloody), passage of blood and mucus per rectum, abdominal pain, fever, tenesmus, and toxic megacolon. **Although extent of disease might not correlate with**

5

GASTROENTEROLOGY

TABLE 5-6

TREATMENT FOR INFLAMMATORY BOWEL DISEASE

Drug	Dose	Indication	Delivery	Useful in	Comments
STEROIDS					
Prednisone or other systemic steroid	Prednisone 20-60 mg; methylprednisolone 60 mg IV. Higher doses have been used IV.	I, M	Systemic	UC, Crohn's disease	Response within 7-10 d Taper rapidly to lowest effective dose
Budesonide	9 mg/day dose	I, M	Right colon, terminal ilium	UC, Crohn's	Fewer side effects than other steroids; not absorbed.
Hydrocortisone enema	100 mg	M	Distal colon	UC, Crohn's	
5-ASA DRUGS*					
Sulfasalazine (sulfa moiety plus ASA)	Start at 500 mg bid, increase to 3-6 g/d divided qid Supplement with folate	I, M	Colon, less effective for ileitis	UC, Crohn's	Sulfa moiety responsible for most side effects: rash, headache, fever, male infertility (reversible)
Mesalamine (Pentasa)	Max: 4.8 g/d divided qid	I, M	Duodenum to anus	UC, Crohn's	
Mesalamine (Asacol)	Max: 3.2 g/d	I, M	Terminal ilium	Crohn's	
Mesalamine enema, suppositories, 5-ASA suppositories		I, M	Left colon, rectal disease	UC but also rectal/left colon Crohn's	Can be used in addition to oral therapy with good results.

Drug	Dose	I/M	Location	Disease	Comments
Balsalazide	6.75 g/d divided tid	M	Left colon	UC	Safety and efficacy not established longer than 8-12 wk Expensive
Olsalazine	500 mg bid but up to 1g bid	M	Colon	UC	Can cause diarrhea; less systemic absorption than mesalamine
ANTIBIOTICS					
Metronidazole	10-20 mg/kg/d divided qid	I	Systemic	UC, Crohn's	No studies of efficacy to maintain remission; peripheral neuropathy with metronidazole
Ciprofloxacin	500 mg bid	I	Systemic	UC, Crohn's	
BIOLOGIC THERAPY					
Infliximab	5-10 mg/kg week 0, 2, and 8 M: q6-8 weeks	I, M	Systemic	UC, Crohn's	Monoclonal antibody to TNF-α. Only 10% efficacy at 1 y. **Increases lymphoma risk.**
Other Agents					
Azathioprine (Imuran)	2 mg/kg/d	M	Systemic	UC, Crohn's	Bone marrow suppression, pancreatitis (2%-3%), Check CBC q1-2 mo. Can take 3 mo for max effect. Steroid sparing.
6-mercaptopurine†	1.5-2 mg/kg/d	M	Systemic	UC, Crohn's	
Methotrexate†	25 mg IM q wk × 16 wk followed by 15 mg q wk. Supplement with folate.	M	Systemic	Crohn's	Immunosuppression, liver toxicity

I, induction; M, maintenance.

*Induction dose should be continued as the maintenance dose. Try to taper drugs over time.

†If patients require steroids while on azathioprine or 6-MP, start infliximab or methotrexate. Patients should take vitamin D and calcium.

severity of disease and vice versa, presentation of ulcerative colitis can be divided into:

1. **Mild** disease limited to the rectum and rectosigmoid colon and manifesting with intermittent blood and mucus per rectum, mild crampy abdominal pain, and fewer than four loose stools per day.

2. **Moderate** disease extending to the splenic flexure and up to 10 loose bloody stools daily associated with mild anemia and low-grade fevers.

3. **Severe** disease usually involving the entire colon and fever, poor nutrition with weight loss, more than 10 loose stools daily, and anemia requiring transfusion.

C. Diagnosis

1. **Endoscopy (colonoscopy or sigmoidoscopy) and biopsy is the gold standard.**

2. **Contrast studies showing superficial ulcerations are supportive findings but not diagnostic.** As with Crohn's disease, contrast studies are contraindicated in those with acute disease because barium can induce a toxic megacolon.

3. **pANCA** is positive in 65% of ulcerative colitis patients, 15% of Crohn's disease patients, and less than 5% of patients without IBD.

D. Complications include anemia, dehydration, and osteoporosis. The risk of colon cancer is threefold to 10-fold higher than in the general population. Screening for dysplasia is recommended for patients with more than 10 years of disease. **Patients with ulcerative colitis are also at increased risk for primary sclerosing cholangitis,** even if they have had a colectomy.

E. Extracolonic manifestations are the same as those found in Crohn's disease except for renal disease, which is exclusively found in those with Crohn's disease.

F. Treatment is dictated by disease severity and the extent of colonic involvement. **Aminosalicylates are the mainstay of therapy** for induction of remission in mild to moderately active ulcerative colitis as well as to prevent relapses in quiescent disease. Parenteral nutrition is critical in the ill patient.

1. **Mild disease** (see Table 5-6): **5-ASA suppositories** (1000 mg; Canasa) bid, **5-ASA (Rowasa) or steroid foam** (e.g., Cortifoam; 100 mg hydrocortisone) enemas.

2. **Moderate disease:** Enemas plus oral 5-ASA agents if disease is still active (sulfasalazine or other formulation depending on site needing treatment).

a. Combined oral 5-ASA therapy with steroid or 5-ASA enemas is more effective in inducing remission in left-sided ulcerative colitis when compared with either therapy alone.

b. **Corticosteroids are indicated in patients not responding to 5-ASA therapy.** Prednisone can be started at a dose of 20-40 mg orally qd and taper as clinically tolerated.

c. **In patients who do not tolerate steroid tapering or in those who have disease refractory to 6 months of steroid therapy, azathioprine should be tried.**

3. **Severe or fulminant disease.** These patients usually need to be hospitalized, made NPO, and given parenteral nutrition and IV fluid and medications.

a. **Steroids are the cornerstone of treatment for severe disease activity** and in those who fail initial therapy with aminosalicylates (see Table 5-6).

b. **Broad-spectrum antibiotics** should be given to patients with fulminant ulcerative colitis that manifests with fever, leukocytosis with bandemia, and peritoneal signs or megacolon.

c. **Toxic-appearing patients with megacolon not responding to high-dose IV steroids within 72 hours may be spared surgery with IV cyclosporine** given at doses of 2 mg/kg per day as a continuous infusion for approximately 7 days used in conjunction with steroids in up to 40% of cases. **The 2 mg/kg dose is as effective as the 4 mg/kg dose with less nephrotoxicity.**

d. **Infliximab has been used successfully in severe refractory ulcerative colitis, but its efficacy has not been established by large randomized, controlled trials.**

e. It is prudent to consult general surgery in these cases.

4. **Surgical management** is indicated for uncontrolled hemorrhage, toxic colitis, perforation, and toxic megacolon. Total proctocolectomy is curative for ulcerative colitis.

5. **Maintenance therapy.** 5-ASA compounds or 6-MP/azathioprine are necessary to maintain remission in ulcerative colitis.

CELIAC DISEASE

I. **General.** Celiac disease (gluten-sensitive enteropathy) is a chronic disorder of the small intestine resulting in malabsorption. It occurs in whites worldwide. Its prevalence is between 1:100 and 1:200 in Northern Europe and the United States.

II. **Etiology.** Celiac disease is a cellular allergy to proteins in wheat, rye, and barley. Celiac disease requires HLA types HLA-DQ2 or HLA-DQ8.

III. **Clinical Manifestations.**

A. **Celiac disease can have both gastrointestinal and extraintestinal manifestations.**

1. **Children** usually present prior to 24 months (after introduction of cereal in the diet). Common signs and symptoms in children include failure to thrive, vomiting, diarrhea, poor school performance, and abdominal distention. Laboratory abnormalities include iron or folate deficiency anemia and abnormal transaminases.

2. **Adults** commonly present with iron-deficiency anemia, diarrhea, steatorrhea, flatulence, and weakness. The severity of symptoms depends upon the amount and the specific location of small

5

GASTROENTEROLOGY

intestine involved. Other laboratory abnormalities include macrocytic anemia (due to folate deficiency), coagulopathy (vitamin K deficiency), and vitamin D deficiency resulting in osteopenia.

B. Conditions associated with celiac disease include dermatitis herpetiformis, IgA deficiency, T1DM, autoimmune thyroid disease, Sjögren's syndrome, rheumatoid arthritis, Down's syndrome, hepatitis, infertility, neuropathy, anemia, and osteopenia.

IV. Diagnostic Evaluation.

A. Draw serum markers (see later). If these are negative and the patient is high risk (e.g., classic symptoms otherwise unexplained), proceed to endoscopic biopsy. Patients with low probability of celiac sprue can be excluded adequately with serologic markers alone.

B. Serologic tests include IgA antiendomysial and IgA tissue transglutaminase antibodies, which are found in up to 95% of patients with gluten sensitivity. Other tests include the IgA and IgG antigliadin antibodies, which are sensitive but far less specific.

C. Duodenal biopsy is the most sensitive means of making the diagnosis.

D. To make the diagnosis unequivocally, the patient's symptoms must be relieved with an adequate trial (a few weeks) of a gluten-free diet, with improvement in the intestinal biopsy or decreasing serum titers of antiendomysial antibodies.

V. Treatment.

A. A gluten-free diet is expensive and a major lifestyle modification. It should only be recommended when the diagnosis has been confirmed. There is no role for an empiric trial of gluten withdrawal.

B. Dietitian consultation or intensive instruction is recommended. The diet is based on avoiding all foods containing rye, barley, oat, or wheat gluten. **For the first 3 to 6 months, patients should avoid dairy products due to secondary lactase deficiency.** The patient must be encouraged to compulsively read food labels. Corn, rice, and soybean flours are safe. If there is an incomplete response, the diet must be reviewed and other potential sources of gluten removed. Symptomatic improvement is present at 2 weeks in the majority of patients, and the diet needs to be maintained lifelong. Patients commonly require vitamin and iron supplementation, including calcium and vitamin C. **Note that many medications include gluten in the binder, and this can vary from lot to lot of the same medication.**

VI. Complications. Patients with celiac sprue are at increased risk for both intestinal and extraintestinal T-cell lymphomas, esophageal squamous cell carcinomas, and small intestinal adenocarcinomas.

BELCHING, BLOATING AND GASSINESS

I. General.

A. Belching, bloating, and gassiness occur as a result of an imbalance in the production, transit, or expulsion of gas from the GI tract.

Although usually benign, gassiness can be a manifestation of a significant disorder (e.g., peptic ulcer disease, bowel obstruction, parasitic infections, malabsorption).

B. Fructose intolerance is an increasingly recognized problem from the growing use of sweeteners containing corn syrup.

II. Differential Diagnosis.

A. Recurrent belching, or eructation, may be caused by GERD or **excessive swallowing of air (aerophagia).**

B. Excessive production of gas can result from bacterial overgrowth, bacterial fermentation of indigestible food such as certain beans and legumes, or malabsorption of commonly consumed carbohydrates such as lactose, sorbitol or fructose.

C. Visceral hypersensitivity. Clinically, patients have bloating and abdominal discomfort from bowel distention that does not produce symptoms in normal subjects.

D. Consider **peptic ulcer disease and *H. pylori* gastritis.**

E. Consider gastroparesis, especially in diabetic patients.

III. Clinical Evaluation.

A. Differentiate emergent and serious from nonserious disorders, especially in cases involving abdominal distention of sudden onset. Nausea, vomiting, diarrhea, hematochezia, unintentional weight loss, or nocturnal symptoms suggests the possibility of an organic etiology.

B. In cases of chronic symptoms, the possibility of carbohydrate intolerance should be considered and a detailed diet history elicited (e.g., fructose, sorbitol). Surgical bowel resection, giardiasis, small bowel bacterial overgrowth, celiac disease, and Crohn's disease can all contribute to carbohydrate malabsorption.

C. Consider constipation or pseudo-obstruction, especially in the elderly.

D. Abdominal gassiness and bloating occurs in 10% to 20% of patients following Nissen fundoplication for surgical treatment of GERD.

IV. Physical Examination.

A. Rule out obstruction and infection by radiograph and appropriate cultures.

B. Physical examination should include a rectal examination, which, in conjunction with the abdominal flat plate, can suggest constipation or stool impaction. Stool should be checked for occult blood, especially in patients older than 50 years.

C. In those suspected of having an infection, stool should be sent for routine cultures and O&P, including *Cryptosporidium*, *Giardia*, and *E. histolytica*.

D. Rule out celiac disease, Crohn's disease, and gastritis or peptic ulcer disease in appropriate patients. (See section on these conditions earlier.)

E. Breath hydrogen test. Give test dose of lactulose, glucose or, if these tests are negative, fructose (found in soft drinks, fruit juices, and corn products). This testing has a 90% sensitivity for bacterial overgrowth syndromes. **May be false positive in lactase deficiency.**

F. **D-Xylose test** also has a 90% sensitivity for bacterial overgrowth but is more difficult to perform.

G. **For gastroparesis,** consider a gastric emptying study using radiopaque contrast material.

V. Treatment.

A. Treat underlying disease as appropriate.

B. **Withdraw offending sugars** (lactose, fructose). See later for a discussion of lactose intolerance. Withdrawal of fructose results in improvement in 70% of those who are fructose sensitive. Avoid carbonated beverages.

C. **Withdraw NSAIDS, narcotics, and other temporally related drugs** (e.g., anticholinergics).

D. **Treat *H. pylori* infection if present.**

E. **Small bowel bacterial overgrowth should be treated** with a 14- to 21-day course of amoxicillin/clavulanate, cephalexin, or TMP–SMX plus metronidazole 250 mg PO tid or norfloxacin. Some patients require up to 1 or 2 months of treatment, and symptoms can recur. For these patients, treatment for the first 7 to 10 days of the month is appropriate.

F. **Legumes.** In patients particularly sensitive to intake of legumes, use of α-D-galactosidase enzyme-containing products such as Beano may be beneficial.

G. **Aerophagia.** Patients should chew thoroughly, avoid gulping foods and liquids, and avoid carbonated beverages, chewing gum, and smoking. **Self-induced belching to relieve abdominal pressure is actually counterproductive in these patients and leads to additional air swallowing, causing a vicious cycle.**

H. If the work-up is negative, abdominal bloating and gassiness could be related to a functional disorder or irritable bowel syndrome. See section on irritable bowel.

LACTOSE INTOLERANCE

I. **General.** Lactose intolerance is caused by a deficiency of the enzyme lactase, a disaccharidase that hydrolyzes lactose into glucose and galactose. Lactase deficiency is the most prevalent genetic deficiency worldwide, commonly affecting persons from Asia and the Mediterranean, African Americans, Native Americans, and Mexicans.

II. **Types of Lactase Deficiency.**

A. **Late-onset or acquired.** Adult lactase deficiency is inherited as an autosomal recessive trait. Onset is most common in adolescence and early adulthood. Symptom severity depends on residual intestinal lactase activity and the size of the lactose load.

B. **Secondary.** Temporary lactase deficiency produced by acute infectious gastroenteritis or mucosal damage from NSAIDs, chronic alcohol use, or medications. Chronic small intestinal disorders (celiac sprue, cystic fibrosis, Whipple's disease, regional enteritis, HIV-induced enteropathy) may also cause a lactase deficiency.

C. **Congenital** (alactasia). This condition is extremely rare and is the result of complete absence of lactase expression because of a genetic defect.

III. **Clinical Presentation.**

A. Symptoms include abdominal distention and pain, gaseous bloating, borborygmi, flatulence, and diarrhea resulting from increased distention and decreased transit time of lactose in the small bowel and production of small chain fatty acids and gases in the colon.

B. Patients who are "lactose intolerant" by their own report rarely have symptoms if they limit themselves to about 250 mL of milk per day.

IV. **Diagnostic Evaluation.**

A. **Trial of lactose-free diet** involves withdrawal of lactose from diet for 2 weeks. Improvement in symptoms strongly implicates lactose intolerance.

B. **Breath hydrogen test** is the most practical and noninvasive test. However, false positives may occur in patients with bacterial overgrowth.

C. Small-bowel biopsy for lactase enzyme in intestinal brush border can be helpful, but it is not done routinely.

D. **Stool pH <5.3 is diagnostic of carbohydrate intolerance.**

V. **Management.**

A. **Diet measures.** Study ingredient labels on foods and decrease or avoid products that contain milk, lactose, and dry milk solids. Use lactose-reduced milks or milk supplemented with exogenous lactase.

B. **Lactase supplements** (Lactaid, Lactrase, Dairy Ease) may be taken 30 minutes before consuming a lactose-containing product. Two capsules provide enough lactase to hydrolyze the lactose in an 8-oz glass of whole milk.

C. Consumption of yogurt containing live bacterial cultures can result in release of bioactive bacterial lactase into the gut.

IRRITABLE BOWEL SYNDROME

I. **General.** IBS is the most commonly diagnosed gastrointestinal disorder; prevalence in North America is approximately 10% to 15%.

II. **Etiology.** IBS is a functional disorder characterized by abdominal pain or discomfort and altered defecation. The pathophysiology of IBS involves several factors: abnormal gut motility, increased visceral sensitivity, and dysregulation of the brain–gut axis, with increased stress reactivity and altered pain perception.

III. **Clinically,** patients often have a change in stool frequency or form and abdominal pain relieved with defecation. The diagnosis is confirmed by identifying the common symptoms of IBS **(Box 5-1)** and excluding other conditions with similar presentations.

IV. **Diagnostic Evaluation. Exclude organic disease. Blood in stools, nocturnal diarrhea, weight loss, etc., require further evaluation.** If appropriate, consider laboratory evaluation:

A. Stool examination for ova, parasites, occult blood, and laxatives (for diarrhea).

GASTROENTEROLOGY 5

> **BOX 5-1**
>
> **ROME II DIAGNOSTIC CRITERIA FOR IRRITABLE BOWEL SYNDROME**
>
> At least 3 months of continuous or recurrent symptoms of abdominal pain within a 12-month period; pain is:
> - Relieved by defecation *or*
> - Associated with a change in stool consistency *or*
> - Associated with a change in stool frequency
>
> Supporting (but not necessary) symptoms for the diagnosis of irritable bowel syndrome include:
> - Altered stool frequency (>3 times per day or <3 times per week)
> - Altered stool form
> - Altered stool passage (straining, urgency, incomplete evacuation)
> - Passage of mucus
> - Abdominal bloating

Note: The diagnosis of a functional bowel disorder always presumes the absence of a structural or biochemical explanation for the symptoms. Diarrhea should not be bloody unless accompanied by an anorectal lesion such as hemorrhoids or a fissure. Physical examination should be normal and systemic symptoms or weight loss absent.

B. Plain abdominal film, colonic transit study, anorectal manometry (for constipation).

C. CBC, ESR, and serum chemistries.

D. Upper GI series, flexible sigmoidoscopy, or colonoscopy with biopsies.

V. Treatment.

A. Nonpharmacologic therapies

1. **Stress reduction,** reassurance, patient education, and diet or lifestyle modification when needed.

2. **Fiber supplementation (25 g/day)** is effective in patients with constipation-predominant symptoms but not always for pain or diarrhea.

3. **Psychotherapy** may be effective.

B. Pharmacologic therapies. Drug therapy should be directed at several factors including abdominal pain, disturbance in defecation, and psychological features.

1. **For constipation:**

a. **Fiber supplementation** with psyllium, methylcellulose, or polycarbophil.

b. Consider magnesium salts or polyethylene glycol–based laxatives.

c. Stimulant cathartics such as bisacodyl and senna should be *avoided*.

2. **For diarrhea:**

a. **Diphenoxylate-atropine (Lomotil) or loperamide** (Imodium) inhibit peristalsis and fluid secretion. Benefits are moderate at best. Loperamide is preferred because it does not have an anticholinergic component and does not induce euphoria.

b. **Cholestyramine** may be added for refractory diarrhea.

3. **Antispasmodics** (NNT is 12 to benefit one patient), including anticholinergics, calcium channel blockers, and opiate antagonists.

Consider these for the treatment of abdominal pain, particularly when it is precipitated by meals. Side effects commonly limit their use. Commonly prescribed antispasmodics include dicyclomine (10-20 mg qid), hyoscyamine (0.125-0.25 mg qid), belladonna (0.3-1.2 mg qid), clidinium bromide (2.5-5.0 mg qid), and glycopyrrolate (1-2 mg tid).

4. **Tricyclic antidepressants** in patients with moderate to severe diarrhea-predominant symptoms and abdominal pain. Consider nortriptyline (less anticholinergic), amitriptyline, desipramine, clomipramine, and doxepin. Start at a low dose of 10 to 25 mg qhs and gradually increase to 100 mg. Efficacy is limited.

5. **Serotonin 3–receptor antagonists** reduce the rate of colonic transit, reduce gastrocolic reflex, and increase colonic compliance. Alosetron (Lotronex) 1 mg PO bid is effective in women with diarrhea-predominant IBS but is now available for compassionate use only. **Ischemic colitis has been reported rarely with this medication; thus its use is limited to exceptional cases under strict supervision.**

6. **Serotonin 4–receptor agonists.** Tegaserod (Zelnorm) at a dose of 6 mg PO bid for 12 weeks has been approved as a prokinetic agent in women with constipation-predominant IBS. Reserve it for women who fail laxative or fiber therapy.

DIVERTICULAR DISEASE

I. **Diverticulosis.**

A. **Definitions**

1. **Diverticulum** (plural, diverticula) is an outpouching of the bowel wall usually 0.1 to 1 cm in diameter. They occur mostly in the sigmoid and descending colon. Common colonic diverticula are pseudodiverticula, which are herniations of mucosa and submucosa but not muscularis at sites of penetration of nutrient arteries.

2. **Diverticulosis** is the presence of multiple diverticula, not necessarily a pathologic condition. Up to half of the population older than 50 years of age has it.

3. **Diverticulitis** is inflammation and infection in one or more diverticula.

B. **Clinically, diverticulosis is mostly (80% to 85%) asymptomatic.** Some have mild intermittent left lower quadrant abdominal pain, bloating, and constipation or diarrhea.

C. **Diagnostic evaluation. Studies are not indicated if symptoms are mild and the patient is otherwise healthy,** but they are indicated if symptoms are more severe or if the patient has occult blood in stool, weight loss, or other concerning symptoms. **Consider CBC, UA, and flexible sigmoidoscopy and barium enema or colonoscopy.**

D. **Treatment** includes high-fiber diet; antispasmodics such as dicyclomine can help with cramping. Avoid cathartic laxatives.

II. Diverticulitis (also see Chapter 15 for diagnosis of abdominal pain).

A. General. Microperforation of diverticulum leads to peridiverticulitis. Free perforation is rare, but localized abscess, sinus tracts, or fistulas into the bladder, vagina, etc. may occur. Most cases occur in the sigmoid colon, and the incidence increases with age.

B. Clinical manifestations

1. Diverticulitis can manifest with acute abdominal pain, chills, fever, and tachycardia but more often develops over hours to days with left lower quadrant pain, anorexia, fever, nausea, and vomiting.

2. **Pneumaturia** may be present if there is erosion into the bladder.

C. Diagnostic evaluation

1. **Differential includes** appendicitis, inflammatory bowel disease, ischemic colitis, colon cancer, other causes of bowel obstruction, and urologic or gynecologic disorders. See Chapter 15 for a more complete discussion.

2. **Physical exam** may reveal abdominal tenderness to palpation with possible rebound tenderness or guarding. A palpable mass may be present, representing an abscess or inflammatory phlegmon. Bowel sounds may be active if there is partial obstruction and hypoactive or absent if peritonitis has developed.

3. **Diagnostic studies** include a CBC with differential, UA, abdominal plain films (flat and upright), and CXR to evaluate for ileus, obstruction, and free air.

4. **CT scan is the diagnostic imaging procedure of choice,** although ultrasound has been used. CT scan can reveal the diverticulum or indirect signs of pericolonic inflammation such as fat stranding, thickening of the colonic wall, microperforations, and abscesses.

5. **Sigmoidoscopy is generally deferred** until after the patient has been treated and the acute symptoms are resolved. Likewise, **barium enema should be delayed** because of the risk of perforation and free barium in the peritoneal cavity. **Colonoscopy is contraindicated** in acute diverticulitis.

D. Treatment

1. **Uncomplicated diverticulitis**

a. **Outpatient management is feasible if the patient is reliable, tolerates oral intake, and has mild symptoms.** Lack of improvement after 2 to 3 days of therapy warrant hospitalization.

b. **Antimicrobials.** Treat for 7 to 10 days with one of these options: ciprofloxacin 500 mg PO bid (or equivalent quinolone) plus metronidazole 500 mg PO tid; TMP–SMX DS PO bid plus metronidazole 500 mg PO TID; amoxicillin–clavulanate 875/125 mg PO bid. For patients with significant comorbidities, the following antibiotics may be used in addition to those listed above: quinolone (ciprofloxacin 400 mg IV bid) plus metronidazole (500 mg IV tid); third-generation cephalosporin (ceftriaxone 1 g IV q12h) plus metronidazole (500 mg IV tid). Alternatives include ampicillin–sulbactam (Unasyn), ticarcillin–clavulanate (Timentin), or piperacillin–tazobactam (Zosyn). **Oral fluoroquinolones have the same** bioavailability as IV and are preferred in patients with a functioning bowel.

c. **Diet restrictions. Outpatients** should be kept on clear liquids for 2 to 3 days and advanced slowly as tolerated. **Inpatients** should be kept NPO with IV hydration or on clear liquids if tolerated. **Nasogastric** tube placement may be necessary if severe vomiting is present.

2. **Complicated diverticulitis**

a. **Diffuse peritonitis requires broad-spectrum IV antibiotics (see earlier), aggressive fluid resuscitation, and emergency exploratory laparotomy.**

b. **Resection with primary anastomosis is possible** if bowel preparation is complete; otherwise colostomy would be necessary.

c. **Perforation is rare.** If present, it usually requires emergent laparotomy.

d. **Abscesses should be drained percutaneously** under ultrasound or CT guidance. If this fails, surgical intervention is indicated.

e. **Fistulae are normally treated with bowel rest, antibiotics, and subsequent surgical repair.**

3. **Recommendations after treatment of acute diverticulitis.**

a. Patients should undergo a colonic evaluation to exclude other colonic pathology 2 to 6 weeks after recovery with a colonoscopy or flexible sigmoidoscopy plus barium enema.

b. Patients should follow a high-fiber diet.

c. One third of patients develop recurrent crampy abdominal pain without diverticulitis and one third develop recurrent diverticulitis.

4. **Indications for elective surgery** include recurrence with two or more attacks of diverticulitis or complications of diverticulitis. Immunosuppressed patients and patients younger than age 40 are generally referred for surgical resection after the first episode of diverticulitis.

CONSTIPATION AND FECAL INCONTINENCE

See Chapter 12 for pediatric considerations.

I. **Constipation.**

A. **General. Constipation is a symptom (not a disease). Constipation is defined as** two or more of the following for at least 12 weeks: excessive straining, passage of hard or lumpy stools, feeling of incomplete evacuation, sensation of anorectal blockage or obstruction, or manual maneuvers (digital evacuation, support of the pelvic floor) to facilitate defecation in greater than 25% of bowel movements; *or* fewer than 3 bowel movements per week. Additionally, there should be no loose stools and there are insufficient criteria for irritable bowel syndrome

B. **Constipation is generally considered a disorder of colorectal motility that can be subdivided into slow-transit constipation** (characterized by slower than normal movement of contents from the proximal colon to the rectum), **pelvic floor dysfunction** (normal colonic transit but inability to move stool from rectum), and **combination syndrome** (slow colonic transit and pelvic floor dysfunction).

GASTROENTEROLOGY 5

C. Etiology

1. **Drugs:** Aluminum-containing antacids, calcium, iron, opiates, antihypertensives (calcium channel blockers, clonidine, methyldopa), anticholinergic agents (antidepressants, neuroleptics, antihistamines), some antiparkinsonian drugs, antispasmodics, estrogen and progestins, among many others.
2. **Diet:** Inadequate fluid and fiber intake.
3. **Lack of exercise.**
4. **Metabolic/endocrine:** Hypercalcemia, hypokalemia, hypothyroidism, diabetes mellitus, Addison's disease, Cushing's syndrome, and other electrolyte abnormalities.
5. **Neurogenic:** Multiple sclerosis, parkinsonism, spinal cord disease, autonomic neuropathy, Chagas' disease, Hirschsprung's disease.
6. **Colon disease:** Tumors, diverticular disease, diverticulitis, irritable bowel syndrome, inflammatory strictures, abnormal colonic or anal musculature junction.
7. **Others:** Anal fissures (pain), hemorrhoids, ulcerative colitis (proctitis), rectal neoplasms, dementia.

D. Diagnostic evaluation

1. **History.** Ask about stool frequency and consistency; straining; sensation of incomplete evacuation; need for manual disimpaction; perineal/vaginal, abdominal, or pelvic pressure maneuvers; diet history; drug history; history of obstetric surgery, back injury, neurologic problems, and sexual abuse. Digital disimpaction or perineal pressure raise a concern for pelvic floor dysfunction.
2. **Physical exam.** The examiner might note palpable colonic loops in the left lower quadrant of the abdomen due to the presence of stool. Perianal inspection can reveal fissures or hemorrhoids. Rectal examination should include evaluation of anal sphincter tone both at rest and with a squeeze. Bearing down should cause relaxation of the anal sphincter along with perineal descent; absence of either component suggests obstructive defecation. The anal reflex can be tested by light touch with a cotton swab around the perianal area.
3. **Diagnostic studies.** Consider CBC, serum electrolytes including calcium, glucose, thyroid stimulating hormone, and stool for occult blood.
4. **Structural evaluation of the colon** is indicated to screen for colorectal cancer or colitis either by colonoscopy or flexible sigmoidoscopy plus barium enema, particularly if the patient is older than 50 years or has had a recent change in bowel habits.
5. **Infants and young adults usually need minimal work-up.** Exceptions include suspected Hirschsprung's disease or chronic refractory constipation. See Chapter 12.
6. **In older adults, the extent of the evaluation depends on the nature and duration of symptoms.** Presence of iron deficiency anemia, with or without blood in the stool (occult or frank), warrants a work-up for colon cancer in older adults with constipation.

7. **Exclusion of secondary causes listed above suggests idiopathic constipation, a colorectal motility disorder.** Consider a trial of treatment. If ineffective, evaluate colonic transit time radiographically with markers. The presence of 5 or more markers 120 hours after ingestion suggests slow colonic transit. In obstructive defecation, patients usually have more markers in the rectosigmoid colon.

8. After evaluation, in most patients the diagnosis should be one of the following entities: **IBS** (if pain and the other features of IBS are present), **slow-transit constipation, rectal outlet obstruction** (abnormal physical exam and anorectal manometry), combination of slow-transit constipation and rectal outlet obstruction, organic constipation (mechanical obstruction or drug side effect), or constipation secondary to systemic disease.

E. Treatment

1. **Patient education.** Avoid irritant and combination laxatives. Allow adequate time and a relaxed environment. Increase ambulation/exercise.

2. **Fluid and fiber.** If no pathology is uncovered by diagnostic tests indicated above, a trial of a high-fiber/high-water diet with or without fiber supplementation can be instituted. Tell patients that bloating and flatulence can occur initially with fiber (maybe less with methylcellulose) and that improvement takes a few days.

3. **If there is no significant improvement with fiber supplementation, then start an inexpensive saline laxative** such as milk of magnesia 15 to 30 mL PO qd or bid. Titrate to obtain soft but not loose stools. Other saline laxatives or hyperosmotic preparation options include magnesium citrate (half or full bottle PO 17.7 g/300 mL) or sorbitol (70%).

4. Stimulants such as bisacodyl (Dulcolax 10 mg PO qd), senna (2 to 4 tabs PO qd to bid) or more expensive osmotic laxatives such as lactulose (15 to 30 mL PO qd to bid) or polyethylene glycol (Miralax 17 g PO qd) should be reserved for patients failing the above-mentioned therapy.

5. **Local agents (enemas, suppositories).** Common enema solutions include water, saline, mineral oil, phosphate, and soap-suds enemas. Bisacodyl and glycerin suppositories work as local rectal stimulation.

6. Patients with obstructive defecation should be referred for further evaluation and bowel retraining.

7. Surgical treatment may be required in certain circumstances (Hirschsprung's disease, idiopathic megacolon, and pseudoobstruction).

8. Psychosocial issues concerning defecation (embarrassment, aversion, anxiety, and depression) may also have to be explored in some patients.

II. Fecal Impaction.

A. General: Fecal impaction is a firm, immobile mass of stool, most often in the rectum but also possible in the sigmoid or descending colon. It is most common in elderly, bed-bound, or inactive patients. See the constipation section for differential diagnosis.

B. Clinically, patients may have fever, symptoms of acute abdomen, or mental status changes (patients with dementia). Impaction can manifest with involuntary leakage of stool around the impaction, which may be mistaken for diarrhea (overflow diarrhea).

C. Treatment involves softening of stool with glycerin or bisacodyl suppositories and enemas (see earlier). Manual disimpaction may be necessary.

III. Fecal Incontinence.

A. General. Fecal incontinence is defined as the involuntary passage or the inability to control anal discharge of fecal material. Prevalence is high in institutionalized and geriatric patients. It may be classified as passive incontinence (involuntary passage of stool without awareness), urge incontinence (discharge of fecal matter despite active attempts to retain it), or fecal seepage (leakage of stool following otherwise normal evacuation).

B. Etiology

1. If normal pelvic floor

a. Fecal impaction, especially in the elderly.

b. Carcinoma of the anal canal or lower rectum.

c. Spinal cord injuries and other neurologic conditions (e.g., cauda equina, diabetes, frontal lobe lesions, MS).

d. Rectal prolapse.

e. Aging with decreased anal canal pressures and rectal compliance.

f. Other conditions that cause diarrhea can predispose to fecal incontinence.

2. If abnormal pelvic floor

a. Damage to the anal sphincter related to operative or obstetric injury, especially forceps deliveries.

b. Pudendal nerve injury associated with childbirth or stretch injury due to prolonged straining during defecation.

c. Anorectal surgery including hemorrhoidectomy and fissure repair.

C. History includes inquiring about onset of incontinence, precipitating event(s), frequency and severity of incontinence, and detailed obstetric history. Also ask about other conditions that may be associated with fecal incontinence (e.g., diabetes mellitus, neurologic disorders, pelvic irradiation, urinary incontinence).

D. Physical examination

1. Perineal inspection for soiling, chemical dermatitis, a gaping anus (indicative of loss of sphincter function), fistula, or rectal prolapse.

2. Assess perianal sensation and check the anocutaneous reflex by stroking the skin in all quadrants around the anus. Absence of this reflex indicates pudendal neuropathy.

3. Evaluate the length of the anal sphincter and its tone at rest and with a squeeze.

4. Ask the patient to strain (may reveal rectal prolapse or excessive perineal descent).

5. Perform a bimanual exam, including rectovaginal sweep, in females.

E. Diagnostic procedures. If diarrhea is present, consider flexible sigmoidoscopy plus barium enema or colonoscopy (see diagnostic evaluation of chronic diarrhea). Consider anorectal manometry, anal ultrasound, or electrophysiologic testing in appropriate patients. If rectal prolapse is suspected but not found on exam, refer for defecography.

F. Treat the underlying cause, if identified. Mild incontinence might respond to bulking agents, high-fiber diet, or antidiarrheals such as loperamide and Lomotil. Consider **bowel retraining (biofeedback therapy)** for elderly patients with fecal impaction and patients with mild pudendal neuropathy, weak anal sphincter, or impaired rectal sensation. Weak or damaged anal sphincter in a patient with an intact pudendal nerve could benefit from surgical repair of the sphincter. Patients with rectal prolapse should also be referred for surgical evaluation.

ANORECTAL DISEASES

I. Hemorrhoids.

A. General. Hemorrhoids are cushions of vascular tissue located within the anal canal. They are *not* varices and not related to portal hypertension. Factors associated with the development of hemorrhoids include increased abdominal pressure secondary to straining during bowel movements, heavy lifting, childbirth, and benign prostatic hypertrophy.

B. Etiology

1. **Internal hemorrhoids** are derived from the internal hemorrhoidal plexus above the dentate line and are covered by rectal mucosa. Chronic straining during defecation is thought to dilate these vascular cushions, which may eventually prolapse. Internal hemorrhoids are classified on the basis of the degree of prolapse:

a. **First-degree hemorrhoids:** No prolapse.

b. **Second-degree hemorrhoids:** Prolapses, but reduce spontaneously.

c. **Third-degree hemorrhoids:** Require manual reduction.

d. **Fourth-degree hemorrhoids:** Permanently prolapsed, will not reduce.

2. **External hemorrhoids** are derived from the external hemorrhoidal plexus below the dentate line and are covered by stratified squamous epithelium.

C. Diagnostic evaluation. Digital rectal examination followed by anoscopy is recommended for all patients with presumed hemorrhoidal disease or bleeding. During examination, the patient should be asked to strain to evaluate the degree of prolapse. Patients older than 50 years and with anemia or a family history of colon cancer should also undergo a colonoscopy.

D. Clinical manifestations

1. **Painless** bright-red bleeding per rectum associated with bowel movements is the most common sign of internal hemorrhoids. Pain suggests another condition such as thrombosed external hemorrhoid or fissure.

2. **External hemorrhoids** can manifest with a bulging associated with discomfort, irritation, or pruritus in the anal area or with severe pain in

5

GASTROENTEROLOGY

the case of acute thrombosis. Minor rectal bleeding may be seen during defecation or after cleansing.

E. Treatment

1. Internal hemorrhoids

a. **First- and second-degree internal hemorrhoids usually respond to high-fiber diet or bulking agents such as psyllium or methylcellulose.**

b. **Rubber-band ligation is the treatment of choice for first-, second-, and third-degree hemorrhoids not responding to conservative measures,** and this therapy is associated with fewer complications and less pain as compared to surgical hemorrhoidectomy.

c. **Infrared photocoagulation** is reserved for first- and second-degree hemorrhoids that fail conservative measures. There is a higher likelihood of requiring further intervention, but fewer adverse effects are seen as compared to rubber-band ligation.

d. **Injection sclerotherapy** is usually reserved for first- and second-degree internal hemorrhoids with persistent bleeding.

e. **Surgical hemorrhoidectomy** is usually reserved for third- and fourth-degree hemorrhoids. Long-term complications include anal stenosis (approximately 10%) or rarely incontinence.

2. External hemorrhoids

a. Conservative management of uncomplicated cases includes increased dietary fiber, stool bulking agents, warm sitz baths twice daily (reduces anal pressure), stool softeners, and avoidance of straining during bowel movements. Irritation may be treated with medicated suppositories or creams such as Anusol HC (contains hydrocortisone) to help decrease inflammation. Limit steroid-containing medications to less than 1 to 2 weeks of continuous use to avoid atrophy of anal tissues.

b. **Surgical therapy** should be limited to patients with acute thrombosis. Complete excision of the thrombosed vein is indicated.

II. Anal Fissures.

A. General. Anal fissure is a superficial tear in the distal lining of the anal canal, most often posteriorly in the midline, usually due to anal trauma associated with passage of hard stool. Increased anal sphincter pressure or local ischemia can also play a role. In cases of multiple fissures or lesions located outside of midline, consider inflammatory bowel disease, leukemia, syphilis, and TB.

B. Clinically, usually acute onset of sharp anal pain is brought on by a bowel movement. Pain lasts for several minutes to hours. A small amount of bleeding may be seen, and pruritus may be present. With digital rectal examination, a small split or tear in the anoderm near the anal verge can be identified. Skin tags or indurated edges may be seen with chronic fissures.

C. Treatment includes bulk laxatives, stool softeners, and sitz baths, with a 90% success rate. There is no proven benefit of topical ointments, suppositories, or local anesthetic injections. Most fissures usually heal in 2 to 4 weeks. If the fissure is present after 6 to

8 weeks of therapy, it is considered chronic and requires further therapy. **Pharmacotherapy aimed at reducing sphincter tone. Topical nitroglycerin ointment** 0.2% (1 inch 2% NTG paste mixed with 9 inches of petroleum jelly) applied bid for 8 weeks is successful in 60% to 80%.**Other treatments include topical or oral nifedipine, topical diltiazem** 2% gel bid, **and topical bethanechol** 0.1% gel applied tid. **Local injections of botulinum toxin** to relax the internal sphincter muscle results in healing in up to 96% of patients. **Surgical lateral internal sphincterotomy is the definitive therapy.**

III. **Anorectal Abscess.**

A. **General.** Obstruction of anal glands leads to infection and subsequent abscess formation. Associated conditions include Crohn's disease, HIV, carcinoma, TB, radiation, trauma, and foreign bodies, although the majority have no predisposing condition. Locations include perianal (40% to 50%), ischiorectal (20% to 30%), intersphincteric (20% to 25%), and supralevator (5% to 7%).

B. **Clinical manifestations.** Pain, erythema, swelling, and occasionally fever are common complaints with superficial abscesses. Deeper abscesses can manifest with systemic symptoms such as fever, malaise, and elevated WBC. Examination reveals an exquisitely tender and erythematous mass with or without cellulitis.

C. **Diagnostic evaluation.** Careful physical examination, including rectal examination, is usually sufficient to make the diagnosis. Imaging modalities (CT, MRI, or endorectal ultrasound) are occasionally needed, particularly in supralevator abscesses. Imaging offers the advantage of assessing associated conditions such as Crohn's disease, pelvic inflammatory disease, or diverticulitis.

D. **Treatment includes urgent incision, and drainage is critical to successful treatment. This is generally done in the OR.** Delay in drainage could result in further tissue destruction and severe necrotizing soft-tissue infection. **Antibiotic therapy** is important in patients with surrounding cellulitis and in immunocompromised or diabetic hosts. Broad-spectrum antibiotics with aerobic and anaerobic coverage are preferred (e.g., amoxicillin–clavulanate, second- or third-generation cephalosporins plus metronidazole). Patients should be warned that fistulas develop in approximately 25% of cases, usually occurring several weeks after the abscess is drained.

DIFFERENTIAL DIAGNOSIS OF ELEVATED LIVER ENZYMES

I. **General Principles.**

A. **Boxes 5-2, 5-3, and 5-4** list the differential diagnosis and evaluation of elevated liver enzymes.

B. Even mild elevation of liver enzymes can indicate potentially significant liver disease. Liver test elevations do not always correlate with extent of hepatocellular damage.

BOX 5-2

DIFFERENTIAL DIAGNOSIS OF ELEVATED TRANSAMINASES

Elevated ALT and AST can be caused by the following:

Viral agents: Hepatitis (A, B, C, D, E), CMV, Epstein–Barr, and other viruses

Drugs and chemicals: Acetaminophen overdose, the "glitizones", HMG-CoA reductase inhibitors, INH, griseofulvin, anticonvulsants, NSAIDs, chemicals (carbon tetrachloride, etc.), alcohol, and other hepatotoxins

Primary liver diseases: Primary sclerosing cholangitis, primary biliary cirrhosis (positive antimitochondrial antibody)

Metabolic diseases: Gilbert's disease (mild elevation in unconjugated bilirubin, especially with dehydration), Wilson's disease (decreased ceruloplasmin), hemochromatosis (see Chapter 6), α_1-antitrypsin deficiency, and cystic fibrosis

Mechanical difficulties: Ductal obstruction secondary to common duct stone or carcinoma (especially pancreatic, hepatoma, metastatic), Budd–Chiari syndrome (thrombosis of the hepatic vein)

Cholestasis from central venous nutrition, pregnancy, or ceftriaxone therapy

Infiltrative processes: Fatty liver (suspect in patients with diabetes, hypothyroidism, and obesity; determine fatty infiltration by US), amyloid, granulomatous hepatitis, liver abscess (including amebic or echinococcal; diagnosis by US or CT; may be accompanied by eosinophilia), AIDS-related lymphoma, or other neoplasm.

Other: CHF, celiac sprue, muscle diseases (e.g., polymyositis)

C. A complete history including new prescription or over-the-counter medications, drug overdoses, use of illicit drugs, and exposure to chemicals is of utmost importance.

D. Duration of liver test abnormalities, shaking chills, and signs and symptoms of chronic liver disease (see later) are helpful in narrowing the differential diagnosis.

II. Abnormal Liver Tests.

A. Mild elevations of transaminases (<2-3 times normal) are seen in patients with fatty liver, nonalcoholic steatohepatitis (NAFLD), and chronic viral hepatitis.

B. Moderate elevations of transaminases (3-20 times normal) are typical of acute or chronic hepatitis, including alcoholic hepatitis.

BOX 5-3

CAUSES OF ELEVATED ALKALINE PHOSPHATASE

Pregnancy

Type O or B blood after a fatty meal.

Liver: cholestasis, partial obstruction of the biliary ducts, primary sclerosing cholangitis, adult bile ductopenia, primary biliary cirrhosis, sarcoidosis, and other granulomatous diseases.

Bone diseases: Paget's disease, metastatic disease, etc.

Work-up: Includes imaging of the liver (e.g., ultrasound).

BOX 5-4

EVALUATION OF ELEVATED LIVER ENZYMES

First step is to repeat the test. If normal, no further work-up is necessary.

ELEVATED ALT/AST

- Look for toxin exposure (alcohol, medications, illicit drugs, herbs, chemicals, natural toxins)
- Hepatitis A, B, and C serology
- ANA and anti–smooth muscle antibody (sensitivity 28%-40%; autoimmune hepatitis); elevated serum γ globulins and IgG (1.5-3 × normal in autoimmune hepatitis)
- UC-ANCA (P-ANCA; characterize PSC but is also seen in autoimmune hepatitis)
- Antimitochondrial antibody (primary biliary cirrhosis)
- Serum Fe^{2+}, TIBC, and transferrin saturation (hemochromatosis)
- Serum α_1-antitrypsin level
- Serum ceruloplasmin (Wilson's disease), especially if age <40 y
- Antiendomysial IgA or tissue transglutaminase IgA (gluten-sensitive sprue)
- Ultrasound or CT imaging (ultrasound first)

ELEVATED ALKALINE PHOSPHATASE

- Check GGT
- If GGT is elevated, obtain an ultrasound or CT imaging (ultrasound first)
- Check antimitochondrial antibody
- If bile ducts are dilated, consult a gastroenterologist for an ERCP

C. High transaminase elevation occurs in acute viral hepatitis, drug reaction, other toxin-related injury (e.g., acetaminophen toxicity), and ischemic injury related to shock.

D. AST/ALT ratio of 2:1 is characteristic of alcoholic liver disease.

E. ALT and AST can rise in common duct obstruction (e.g., from cholelithiasis) and may be the first to rise in the case of a bile duct obstruction.

F. Coagulation factors reflect liver synthetic function. Less than 20% factor V activity, a non–vitamin K–dependent factor, is a poor prognostic factor in fulminant hepatic failure and indicates a need for liver transplant.

G. Prothrombin time may be prolonged in cholestatic liver disease due to vitamin K deficiency; try to correct with vitamin K 10 mg SC/IV qd × 3 days.

III. GGT and Alkaline Phosphatase.

A. GGT is too nonspecific to be helpful in the diagnosis of any specific liver disease. It is inducible by drugs, alcohol, renal failure, pancreatic disease, etc.

B. If the alkaline phosphatase is elevated, a GGT and 5'-nucleotidase should be drawn or the alkaline phosphatase should be fractionated to determine if it is of bone or liver origin. However, fractionation of alkaline phosphatase is more expensive and not widely available, and serum

5'-nucleotidase determination is not done commonly. A normal GGT in the presence of an elevated alkaline phosphatase suggests a bone origin of alkaline phosphatase.

VIRAL HEPATITIS

Hepatitis B, C, and D can cause acute (<6 months' duration) or chronic (>6 months' duration) liver injury. Hepatitis A and E have only acute forms. Table 5-7 gives a summary.

I. Hepatitis A Virus.

A. General: HAV is an RNA virus affecting 1.4 million people worldwide annually. The overall prevalence of positive serology to HAV in the United States is greater than 30%. Transmission is primarily fecal–oral (contaminated food and water), particularly in areas of poor sanitation. It is rarely transmitted by parenteral exposure. It is often subclinical in children, but its onset is usually abrupt in adults, and it is usually an acute self-limited infection.

B. Risk factors include traveling to developing countries, having personal contact with an infected person, consuming raw or undercooked shellfish, having homosexual contact, spending time in daycare centers or institutions, using intravenous drugs, and receiving blood transfusions.

C. Clinical manifestations. The usual incubation period is approximately 30 days. **Symptoms include** fatigue, malaise, fever, nausea, vomiting, anorexia, and right upper quadrant pain. **Fulminant hepatic failure is rare but can occur** in patients with underlying liver disease (chronic hepatitis C). **Other manifestations include** dark urine, light-colored stool, jaundice, hepatomegaly, and pruritus. **Laboratory abnormalities** include marked elevation of bilirubin (commonly >10 mg/dL), serum transaminases (ALT>AST, usually >1000), and alkaline phosphatase. **Extrahepatic manifestations** include arthritis, vasculitis, thrombocytopenia, and anemia.

D. Diagnostic evaluation. Acute infection is confirmed with positive anti-HAV IgM. IgM titers remain positive for 4 to 6 months after exposure. After 6 months anti-HAV IgG titers increase and remain elevated for decades, signifying past exposure or immunity.

E. Prophylaxis. Anti-HAV IgG (gamma globulin) 0.02 mL/kg IM can be administered to close contacts or travelers to endemic areas ideally within 2 weeks of exposure. This provides passive immunity for up to 6 months. **Immunization** is effective if given IM at least 4 weeks before anticipated exposure, with a booster dose 6 months to 1 year later. **Both IgG prophylaxis and hepatitis A vaccination can be administered at the same time but at different sites.**

F. Treatment is supportive in most cases. Complete recovery usually occurs within a few months. Rare cases of fulminant hepatitis A (1%-5%) require ICU monitoring and liver transplantation and occur in those with preexisting liver disease.

TABLE 5-7

COMPARISONS OF TYPE A, TYPE B, AND TYPE C HEPATITIS

Feature	Hepatitis A	Hepatitis B	Hepatitis C
Incubation	15-45 d (mean, 30 d)	30-180 d (mean, 60-90 d)	15-160 d (mean, 50 d)
Onset	Acute	Often insidious	Insidious
Age preference	Children, young adults	Any age	Any age, but more common in adults
TRANSMISSION ROUTE			
Fecal–oral	+++	–	Unknown
Other nonpercutaneous routes	±	++	++
Percutaneous	±	+++	+++
OTHER CHARACTERISTICS			
Severity	Mild	Often severe	Variable
Prognosis	Generally good	Worse with age, debility	Moderate
Progression to chronicity	None	Occasional (5%-10%)	Frequent (65%-85%)
Prophylaxis	Immunoglobulin or hepatitis A vaccine	Standard IG (efficacy unknown), HBIG, hepatitis B vaccine	Not indicated at this time.
Carrier	None	0.1%-30%	Exists but prevalence unknown

II. Hepatitis B Virus.

A. General. HBV can cause both acute and chronic hepatitis. **It is the leading cause of liver-related death from cirrhosis and hepatocellular carcinoma worldwide.** HBV is transmitted by perinatal, sexual, or parenteral exposure. The perinatal transmission is particularly important in Southeast Asia and sub-Saharan Africa, where prevalence of asymptomatic infection is higher than 10%.

B. Risk factors include IV drug use, male homosexual activity, multiple sexual partners, needle-stick injuries in health care workers, chronic dialysis, and blood transfusion (risk is 1/63,000 in the United States).

C. Clinical manifestations. Rate of chronic infection varies with age. It is 90% in case of perinatal infection and 20% to 50% if contracted between 1 and 5 years of age. Less than 5% of adult patients develop chronic hepatitis B infection that can progress to cirrhosis and hepatocellular carcinoma.

1. **Acute hepatitis B** can manifest as a subclinical process, as icteric hepatitis (30%), or as fulminant hepatic failure.

a. **Incubation and prodrome** (malaise, anorexia, nausea, vomiting, fever, RUQ pain, and myalgia) **generally last** 1 to 4 months. This may be followed by an acute symptomatic phase (1-3 mo) that rarely progresses to a chronic infection.

b. **Laboratory abnormalities include** transaminases >1000 (ALT>AST). Bilirubin usually rises after transaminase elevation. ALT elevation for longer than 6 months suggests chronic infection.

2. **Chronic hepatitis B is divided into two types:** an asymptomatic carrier state and chronic active hepatitis leading to possible cirrhosis or hepatocellular carcinoma. The asymptomatic carrier state is defined by **a positive HBsAg for greater than 6 months after the acute infection. Chronic active hepatitis is defined by positive HBsAg along with (possibly intermittent) mild to moderate elevation of transaminases.** If HBeAg is present, the risk of rapid progression of liver disease is increased.

3. **Fulminant hepatic failure** occurs in 0.1% to 0.5% of patients with acute hepatitis B. Patients present with typical features of hepatic failure including encephalopathy and coagulopathy. Up to 12% to 20% of patients with chronic HBV progress to cirrhosis over a 5-year period.

4. **Hepatocellular carcinoma** is reported in 6% to 15% of patients with cirrhosis due to HBV. **Screening for hepatocellular carcinoma is controversial and not well proven, but it has become the standard among hepatologists.** Serial AFP (sensitivity 45%-65%, specificity 80%-94%) and RUQ ultrasound (sensitivity 71%, specificity 93%, positive predictive value 15%) every 6 months is recommended for hepatocellular carcinoma surveillance in cirrhotic patients.

5. **Extrahepatic manifestations of chronic hepatitis B** include polyarteritis nodosa, glomerular disease, serum sickness–like syndrome, mixed cryoglobulinemia, papular acrodermatitis, and aplastic anemia in 10% to 20% of patients.

D. Diagnostic evaluation

1. **HBsAg is found in acute illness and becomes positive 1 to 7 weeks before clinical disease.** It remains positive 1 to 6 weeks after clinical disease and in chronic carrier states. **Blood containing HBsAg is considered potentially infectious.** As noted earlier, HBsAg is a marker for chronic active hepatitis and the carrier state.

2. **Hepatitis B surface antibody (Anti-HBs) appears weeks to months after clinical illness. The presence of this antibody confers immunity** and indicates prior disease (if HBcAb⁺) or vaccination (if HBcAb⁻).

3. **Hepatitis B antibody against the core antigen (Anti-HBc IgM) appears during the acute phase of the illness** and its presence can be used to diagnose acute HBV infection, especially in the window period when both HBsAg and HbsAb may be undetectable. It may be present for several months to as long as 2 years. HBc IgG titers appear thereafter and denote prior infection. Consider testing for HBV DNA and repeating HBc IgM in patients with isolated HBc IgG to rule out acute or active infection.

4. **HBeAg is a marker for active viral replication and infectivity.** Loss of the HBeAg and development of anti-HBe antibodies is termed *HBeAg seroconversion* and is usually associated with improved prognosis and remission of liver inflammation. An exception to this is the "precore" mutation, which manifests with persistent hepatitis B viremia and loss of HBeAg.

5. **Measurement of HBV DNA confirms active infection and replication.** It is useful to determine the need for antiviral therapy and efficacy of treatment.

6. Liver biopsy is useful in patients with chronic HBV infection to determine the severity of liver injury, overall prognosis, and response to therapy.

E. Prophylaxis

1. **HBV vaccination** IM in the deltoid muscle is recommended for all infants and children as well as adolescents with any risk of exposure at 0, 1, and 6 months. Adults in high-risk groups for exposure should also be vaccinated. High-risk groups include:

a. Health care workers or workers in contact with blood products

b. Staff or persons in institutions for the developmentally disabled or inmates of long-term correctional facilities

c. Hemodialysis patients or recipients of clotting factor concentrates

d. Household contacts and sexual partners of known hepatitis B carriers

e. International travelers staying longer than 6 months in endemic areas

f. IV drug users

g. Sexually active men or women with multiple partners (>1 in 6 months)

2. **Hepatitis B immune globulin (0.05-0.07 mL/kg) should be given soon (preferably within 48 hours) after a sexual or needle-stick exposure along with concurrent vaccination.** It is also recommended for liver transplant recipients with HBV infection and infants born to mothers who test positive for HBsAg, within 12 hours of birth with concurrent vaccination. See Chapter 24 for pediatric immunization schedule.

F. Treatment

1. **Treatment of acute hepatitis B** generally involves supportive measures only. In patients with fulminant hepatitis, ICU monitoring and early liver transplantation may be required. Instruct patients on barrier protection during intercourse. Contacts should be notified. Test for other viral infections, such as HIV and HCV.

2. **Treatment of chronic hepatitis B** includes interferon, lamivudine, and adefovir. **Candidates for therapy include those with established chronic infection (HBsAg+) with elevated viral DNA levels ($>10^5$ copies/mL) and active liver disease (elevated ALT [2× normal] and chronic hepatitis on biopsy).** Consider liver transplantation in decompensated cirrhotic patients with chronic HBV.

III. Hepatitis C Virus.

A. General. There are six known genotypes that vary in their geographic distribution as well as in their response to therapy. In the United States, up to 70% of infected persons have genotype 1, and 14% have genotype 2. HCV accounts for 70% of all cases of chronic hepatitis. It is the leading cause of liver transplantation and is detectable in 1.8% of the general population in the United States. It can be found in one third of all HIV-infected patients. The virus has an extremely high mutation rate and is thus not easily neutralized by the body's immune response.

B. Risk factors. Hepatitis C is transmitted parenterally. Risk factors include IV drug use, history of blood transfusion prior to 1991, hemodialysis, tattooing, body piercing, alcohol abuse, cocaine use, high-risk sexual behavior, health care work, and organ transplantation from HCV-positive donors. The risk of HCV infection through blood transfusion currently is 1:103,000. Perinatal transmission rate is 1 to 5%. Risk of sexual transmission is low.

C. Clinical manifestations

1. **Acute HCV infection is usually asymptomatic,** but 20% of patients develop jaundice. Typically, transaminases are elevated in the several hundred to one thousand range with variable hyperbilirubinemia, but these parameters are usually not as severe as in acute HBV. The abnormalities can last 2 to 12 weeks. **Some patients (20%-25%) clear the virus, but the majority go on to develop chronic HCV.** Fulminant hepatitis with HCV is exceedingly rare.

2. **Chronic hepatitis C** is usually asymptomatic and patients are found incidentally to have elevations of transaminases (2-8 times normal) or through blood donation screening. Vague symptoms of fatigue, malaise, anorexia, arthralgias, right upper quadrant pain, or weight loss are seen in 20%. ALT is more than two times normal in 25%.

a. **Cirrhosis develops in up to 25% of patients with long-term chronic HCV.**

b. **Risk factors for disease progression include** age at infection older than 40 years, duration of infection, post-transfusion acquisition, greater than 50 g of daily alcohol consumption, degree of damage on biopsy, male gender, coinfection with hepatitis B or HIV, and elevated ALT.

c. **HCV infection is a risk factor for developing hepatocellular carcinoma (5%).** Risk increases significantly with cirrhosis.

d. **Extrahepatic manifestations include** mixed cryoglobulinemia, glomerulonephritis, porphyria cutanea tarda, thyroid disease, Sjögren's syndrome, and lichen planus.

D. Diagnostic evaluation

1. **Serologic tests measuring HCV antibody** are more than 92% sensitive for the new-generation assays. False-positive tests can occur in low-risk patients and false negatives in immunocompromised patients. **A positive HCV antibody test requires further testing to distinguish among current infection, prior infection with clearance, or false-positive test.**

2. **HCV RIBA (recombinant immunoblot assay) is specific for hepatitis C.**

   a. A positive HCV antibody, negative viral RNA, and positive RIBA suggests prior exposure with viral clearance.

   b. A positive HCV antibody, negative viral RNA, and negative RIBA suggests a false-positive test.

3. **HCV viral RNA can be measured** to detect minute quantities of viral RNA in the blood as early as 1 to 2 weeks after infection. The best test to assure clearance of the virus is the qualitative HCV RNA test.

4. Determination of the HCV viral genotype is important to determine the duration and likelihood of response to therapy. Genotypes 2 and 3 have an 82% response rate compared to 42% for genotype 1.

E. Treatment

1. The aim is to eradicate the virus and halt progression of liver disease and its complications. **African Americans are less likely to respond to treatment for an as yet unknown reason.**

2. Sustained virologic response is defined as clearance of the virus by qualitative PCR 6 months after completion of therapy. It is usually associated with improvement in biochemical markers and liver histology.

3. **Treatment regimens and duration of therapy for *acute* hepatitis C are still controversial.** The current consensus is to begin treatment 3 months after initial infection if viremia persists. Treatment with IFN-α monotherapy has a reported rate of viral clearance of up to 98%. The use of pegylated interferon in this setting remains investigational but is probably as effective as standard interferon.

4. **Treatment for *chronic* HCV is indicated in patients with serum HCV RNA, abnormal ALT, compensated liver disease, ability to comply with treatment, 6 months' abstinence from drugs and alcohol, and liver biopsy indicating moderate inflammation or portal fibrosis.** Patients must not have ongoing depression or suicidal ideation.

5. **Treatment is controversial in those with a normal ALT.** Treatment choices in those with a normal ALT should be individualized based on risk, etc. Patients with a *low* risk of going on to cirrhosis include those infected before age 35, female patients, and those with no alcohol use

and no or minimal fibrosis on biopsy. The decision to treat must also take into account the genotype; **those with genotypes 2 and 3 are more likely to respond to treatment.**

6. **Current treatment regimens for chronic hepatitis include** a combination of weekly pegylated IFN-α injections plus ribavirin (IFN-α-2b 1.5 μg/kg SQ weekly and oral ribavirin 800 mg daily *or* IFN-α-2a 180 μg SQ weekly plus ribavirin 1000-1200 mg orally based on weight) for 24 weeks for genotypes 2 and 3 or 48 weeks for genotypes 1, 4, 5, and 6. The sustained virologic response rate is approximately 54% to 56% for combination therapy.

7. **Therapy should be monitored by a clinician experienced in HCV treatment if possible.** Prior to initiating therapy, a baseline liver profile, biochemistry profile, CBC, TSH, HCV RNA titer, and genotype should be obtained. Liver biopsy prior to therapy is recommended to stage disease. If the patient has clinical depression, a formal psychiatric evaluation or treatment for depression should be instituted prior to initiating therapy.

8. **Therapy can have multiple side effects** including flulike symptoms, anorexia, malaise, fatigue, myalgias, fever, myelosuppression, hair loss, thyroid dysfunction, and depression.

9. **Ribavirin is a teratogen and abortifacient and can cause a dose-related hemolytic anemia** (requiring the monitoring of hemoglobin throughout therapy). Other potential adverse effects include cough, dyspnea, rash, pruritus, and hyperuricemia among others. Female patients are required to use two forms of birth control for 6 months after completing therapy.

10. Therapies under investigation include immune modulators such as histamine dihydrochloride, thymosin, IL-10, and derivatives of current therapies including albuferon or ribavirin derivatives.

IV. **Hepatitis D Virus.**

A. **General.** The hepatitis D virus requires coinfection with hepatitis B. It can occur as a "superinfection" in the presence of chronic HBV infection or as a "coinfection" with HBV. Initially it was seen most often in IV drug users in North America, but this has decreased dramatically due to increased HBV vaccination, better hygiene, and control of risk factors. It is still seen in India, Africa, and the Mediterranean basin.

B. **Diagnosis** is made with detection of the HDV RNA in serum. An alternative is detection of HDV antigen (HDAg) in liver tissue.

C. **Clinical course** is identical to that of HBV, because it requires HBV coinfection to be active, but with increased likelihood for worsening of manifestations of HBV infection including fulminant hepatitis. The risk of hepatocellular carcinoma is similar for cirrhotic patients with hepatitis B alone. See the HBV section (earlier) for treatment.

V. Hepatitis E Virus.

A. General. HEV is transmitted by the fecal–oral route (particularly through contaminated water). Most cases occur in developing countries, so consider in travelers returning from abroad.

B. Clinical manifestations, diagnosis, and treatment. HEV usually causes a self-limited hepatitis. Signs and symptoms are similar to those of other acute viral hepatitides and usually last 1 to 4 weeks. Diagnosis is made by measuring anti-HEV antibodies (IgM appears first and can last 4 to 5 months; IgG can last 1 to 4.5 years); viral RNA can also be measured in the stool or serum. Treatment is supportive.

ALCOHOLIC LIVER DISEASE, LIVER FAILURE, AND CHRONIC LIVER DISEASE

I. Alcoholic Liver Disease.

A. General background

1. Alcoholic liver disease is caused by chronic alcohol consumption on average exceeding 80 g/day (equivalent to six 12-oz cans of beer, 1 liter of wine, or 5-6 liquor drinks) for men and 60 g/day for women.

2. Alcoholic liver disease is the second most prevalent form of liver disease in developed countries (after nonalcoholic fatty liver disease). Risk factors include female sex, obesity, and concomitant HCV infection.

3. **Three histologic forms of ALD are recognized:** hepatic steatosis (fatty liver), alcoholic hepatitis, and alcoholic cirrhosis. Among heavy, chronic alcohol users, 90% to 100% develop fatty liver but only 10% to 35% develop alcoholic hepatitis and 8% to 20% develop cirrhosis. **Patients with cirrhosis and superimposed alcoholic hepatitis have a 4-year mortality exceeding 60%.**

4. There is increased prevalence of HCV in patients with alcoholic liver disease.

B. Clinical presentation

1. Presenting features range from nonspecific signs and symptoms to frank liver failure. Also see discussion of chronic liver disease (later) for signs and symptoms. None of these signs and symptoms are pathognomonic for alcoholic liver disease.

2. Epigastric or right-sided abdominal pain, progressive jaundice, increasing abdominal girth, or lower extremity swelling might be the reasons compelling the patient to seek medical attention. Anorexia, nausea and vomiting, fever, tachycardia, and tender hepatomegaly in the absence of an infection could be due to alcoholic hepatitis.

3. Progressive jaundice, palmar erythema, Dupuytren's contractures, cutaneous telangiectasias, feminization (gynecomastia and testicular atrophy) and complications of portal hypertension (see later) are signs of chronic liver disease.

4. Alteration in mental status may be noted due to **hepatic encephalopathy** (see later) and/or alcohol intoxication or withdrawal.

5. Parotid gland hypertrophy may be present due to recurrent emesis.

C. Diagnosis and laboratory evaluation. A thorough history of alcohol use, complete liver panel, biochemical profile, CBC, and PT with INR should be obtained on all patients. The CAGE questionnaire (see Chapter 18) can be used to screen for alcohol dependency. Two positive responses on the CAGE questionnaire has >70% sensitivity and >90% specificity for alcohol dependency.

1. **AST/ALT ratio** is typically between 2:1 and 8:1, and both measures are usually <300 IU/L. Unless associated with acetaminophen toxicity, transaminase values higher than seven times the upper limit of normal should make one question the diagnosis of alcoholic liver disease.

2. **Elevated GGT and MCV.**

3. **Leukocytosis** (with neutrophilia) in the absence of an infection may be present due to alcoholic hepatitis.

4. **Coagulopathy** persisting despite replacement of vitamin K indicates decreased hepatic synthetic function.

D. Prognosis. Patients with alcoholic hepatitis and discriminant function (DF) >32 have a poor prognosis with a predicted mortality of approximately 50% in 1 month.

$$DF = 4.6 \, (PT_{patient} - PT_{normal}) + \text{total bilirubin (mg/dL)}$$

E. Liver biopsy may be necessary if the diagnosis is unclear or if there are atypical features. It aids in selecting patients being considered for steroid therapy, because **up to 28% of patients with a clinical picture of alcoholic hepatitis do not have histologic features consistent with alcoholic hepatitis on the biopsy.**

F. Treatment

1. **General principles. Alcohol abstinence** and supportive care are key to the successful treatment of ALD. Ensure good nutrition; protein intake should be at least 60 g/d. **Give thiamine 100 mg/d** to prevent Wernicke–Korsakoff's syndrome, orally or IV, and folate 1 mg daily. Treat alcohol withdrawal.

2. **Alcoholic hepatitis. Pentoxifylline** (inhibitor of TNF synthesis) 400 mg PO tid improves survival and decreases risk of hepatorenal syndrome. If an infectious process has been ruled out, patients with severe alcoholic hepatitis (hepatic encephalopathy or DF >32) might benefit from corticosteroids. Consider **prednizone or prednisolone 40 mg PO daily** for 4 weeks followed by tapering over several weeks.

3. **Chronic alcoholic liver disease.** Liver enzyme abnormalities persisting for 6 months after the cessation of alcohol intake should prompt further workup (up to liver biopsy). Consider **alternative medicines.** Milk thistle (silymarin) and S-adenosylmethionine (SAM-e) at 1200 g/d PO for 2 years was found to decrease mortality and need for liver transplantation (16% vs. 30% for placebo). **Liver transplantation** may be considered for patients who have been abstinent for more than 6 months. Survival after orthotopic liver transplant for ALD is similar to

that for end-stage liver disease from other causes. Recidivism is 11% to 50%.

II. Acute Liver Failure: Fulminant Hepatic Failure.

A. Definition. Acute liver failure is acute liver injury with synthetic dysfunction (coagulopathy) and encephalopathy in a person who previously had a healthy liver or well-compensated liver disease. Development of encephalopathy within 2 weeks (in patients with underlying liver disease) or 8 weeks (in patients with previously healthy livers) from the onset of symptoms such as jaundice defines FHF. *Subfulminant* liver failure is defined as development of encephalopathy between 2 and 6 months.

B. Etiology. Toxin-induced and viral hepatitis are the most common causes. Acetaminophen toxicity is the most common cause in the United States. Other less common causes include Wilson's disease, autoimmune hepatitis, fatty liver of pregnancy, and Reye's syndrome. **Box 5-5** lists common etiologies.

C. Clinically, one of the earliest signs is a change in personality including uncooperative and violent behavior. **Jaundice does not correlate with neuropsychiatric changes.** Fetor hepaticus, flapping tremor, and hyperreflexia may be present. Coagulopathy can cause spontaneous bleeding from mucosal surfaces. In later stages, decerebrate rigidity with spasticity can be noted. **In contrast to chronic liver disease, the liver is nonnodular, and splenomegaly and vascular telangiectasias are not present.** Cerebral edema is common in FHF but not in subfulminant cases. Renal failure and features of portal hypertension are more frequent in subfulminant failure. **Remember that fulminant hepatic failure can be superimposed on chronic liver disease. Table 5-8** shows the classification based on Child–Pugh score.

D. Evaluation

1. Obtain routine biochemical profile and complete liver panel. Serum albumin is usually normal initially. Expect hyponatremia and hypokalemia, especially in the later stages.
2. **Hypoglycemia is found in a large percentage of patients with FHF.** Lactic acidosis develops in approximately half the patients with grade 3 coma.
3. Coagulopathy develops due to decreased hepatic synthesis of coagulation factors. Monitor neurologic status and PT and INR (good prognostic indicator).
4. Cerebral edema can lead to respiratory depression and respiratory acidosis.

BOX 5-5
ABCD OF ACUTE LIVER FAILURE
A: Acetaminophen (20%), hepatitis A (7%), autoimmune hepatitis
B: Hepatitis B (10%)
C: Cryptogenic (15%)
D: Drugs (besides acetaminophen, 12%), hepatitis D

CHILD–PUGH CLASSIFICATION OF CIRRHOSIS

Feature	Points		
	1	2	3
Ascites	None	Slight	Moderate
Bilirubin (mg/dL)	<2	2-3	>3
Albumin (g/dL)	>3.5	2.8-3.5	<2.8
Encephalopathy	None	Grade I-II	Grade III-IV
INR	<1.7	1.8-2.3	>2.3

Class A: 5-6 points
Class B: 7-9 points
Class C: 10-15 points

E. Treatment

1. Consult with a hepatologist for consideration for liver transplantation. **Transfer the patient to a center that can do an orthotopic liver transplant; this is the only proven treatment for fulminant liver failure.**
2. Treat acetaminophen toxicity if present (see Chapter 2).
3. Correct hypoglycemia and electrolyte abnormalities. If the patient is to be moved to another medical center, start the patient on 20% glucose infusion during transport.
4. Coagulopathy is managed by parenteral vitamin K 5-10 mg SQ qd for 3 days and by transfusion of fresh frozen plasma.
5. Treat hepatic encephalopathy (described later).
6. Aggressively evaluate for infections.
7. Hypothermia to 34°C with cooling blankets improves mortality.

F. Prognosis. The decision to transplant depends on the probability of spontaneous liver recovery. The three most useful factors in determining need for referral to a transplant center are **degree of encephalopathy** (grade I or II, approximately 70% recover; grade IV, <20% recover), **age** (between 10 and 40 years have better prognosis), and **cause of liver failure.**

III. End-Stage Liver Disease.

A. General. Liver cirrhosis is a late-stage, diffuse process characterized by the formation of islands of regenerated liver surrounded by dense fibrosis (abnormal nodules) that occurs after a protracted insult such as alcohol, chronic active hepatitis, etc. Patients with cirrhosis may be classified based on the Child–Pugh classification (see Table 5-8). Those who are at least Child-Pugh B may be considered for orthotopic liver transplantation.

B. Symptoms and signs include weight loss, malnutrition, fatigue, easy bruising, jaundice and pruritus, edema, ascites, and encephalopathy with asterixis. Most complications of cirrhosis occur as a result of portal hypertension (edema, ascites, esophageal varices and bleeding, portal hypertensive gastropathy, and splenomegaly) or decreased synthetic function (coagulopathy, jaundice, encephalopathy, malnutrition) of the liver. **Cirrhotic patients are functionally immunosuppressed and therefore are more prone to infections.** GI bleeding is a common cause of hepatic encephalopathy (see later).

C. Diagnostic evaluation

1. **Laboratory evaluation can show normal liver enzymes in ESLD because of the small amount of residual hepatic tissue.**

2. Patients usually have low serum albumin, anemia, thrombocytopenia, and possibly elevated blood ammonia. Electrolyte abnormalities include hyponatremia, hypokalemia, and free water overload. There may also be concomitant acidosis or alkalosis.

2. **Histologic evaluation of liver biopsy is the gold standard for diagnosing cirrhosis. Ultrasound with Doppler evaluation of portal veins is a sensitive means of detecting cirrhosis.** Some acute inflammatory processes such as autoimmune hepatitis or alcoholic hepatitis can create findings typical of portal hypertension. Once the inflammation subsides, these findings can disappear.

D. Management of complications

1. **Varices**

a. **A nonselective β-blocker, such as propanolol or nadolol, reduces the risk of initial bleeding from esophageal varices.** Propanolol can be started at a dose of 10 mg bid and titrated (to 60 mg qd) to effect a 25% reduction in the baseline heart rate. Nonselective β-blockers are also the treatment of choice for bleeding from portal hypertensive gastropathy. **Isosorbide can have an additive effect to the β-blocker.**

b. **Endoscopic band ligation of esophageal varices is more effective than propanolol for the primary prevention of variceal bleeding.** Endoscopic ligation can be repeated every 4 to 6 weeks until the esophageal varices have all been obliterated.

2. Management of other complications of chronic liver disease (e.g., hepatic encephalopathy, ascites, coagulopathy, spontaneous bacterial peritonitis, hepatorenal syndrome) is as described under individual sections.

E. Liver transplantation has become a widely accepted therapy for ESLD. There are minimum listing criteria to allow a patient with ESLD to begin the process of evaluation for transplant, including Child-Pugh score higher than 7 (class B and C), documented spontaneous bacterial peritonitis, less than 10% predicted chance for survival without transplantation, and higher than grade 2 hepatic encephalopathy in acute liver failure.

IV. Nonalcoholic Fatty Liver Disease.

A. General background

1. Nonalcoholic fatty liver disease (NAFLD) is the most common cause of abnormal liver tests in the United States.

2. Often it is discovered incidentally when elevated liver tests or hepatomegaly are noted during evaluation of an unrelated medical problem.

5

GASTROENTEROLOGY

3. **NAFLD encompasses a spectrum of diseases ranging from fatty liver (steatosis) to nonalcoholic steatohepatitis (NASH) to cirrhosis.**
4. It is characterized by predominantly macrovesicular hepatic steatosis occurring in persons with no history of excessive alcohol consumption.
5. It is a common disorder; 10% to 24% of the population have some degree of NAFLD and 2% to 5% have NASH (fatty liver with inflammatory changes). Its prevalence increases to 50% to 75% in obese persons and 100% in severely obese persons with diabetes.
6. **Associated conditions include:**
a. **Metabolic syndrome.** NAFLD is considered the liver component of the metabolic syndrome. Hence, it is associated with obesity, diabetes, insulin resistance, and dyslipidemia.
b. **Other conditions associated with NAFLD include** rapid weight loss, TPN, prolonged starvation, inborn errors of metabolism (Wilson's disease, hypoproteinemia, abetalipoproteinemia, tyrosinemia), postsurgery (obesity surgery, small bowel bypass such as jejunoileal bypass), and drugs or toxins (e.g., amiodarone, corticosteroids, perhexiline maleate, estrogens, and tamoxifen).
7. Steatosis accelerates the development of fibrosis in patients with chronic hepatitis C.
B. **Clinical manifestations**
1. **The majority (48%-100%) of patients with NAFLD are asymptomatic.** Uncommon symptoms include vague RUQ pain, fatigue, and malaise.
2. Physical findings include hepatomegaly that is present in up to 75% of patients. Other less common findings include splenomegaly, spider angiomata, palmar erythema, and ascites.
3. **Laboratory abnormalities include:**
a. Two- to fourfold elevation of AST and ALT (AST/ALT ratio <1). The AST/ALT ratio increases as fibrosis advances.
b. Elevated alkaline phosphatase (one third of patients) and elevated ferritin level (nearly one half of patients), with normal bilirubin and albumin.
c. Low titer ANA (<1:320) is less common.
C. **Diagnostic evaluation**
1. Most patients undergo evaluation for abnormal liver tests, hepatomegaly, or both. The key to evaluating the patient with NAFLD is a complete history and physical examination, including risk factors for liver disease, followed by diagnostic studies to exclude other causes of hepatic disorders.
2. **Detailed history of alcohol consumption is important.** Absence of significant alcohol use is generally defined as intake of less than 20 to 40 grams of alcohol per day.
3. **Laboratory tests** should include a complete hepatic panel, CBC, and PT/INR; HCV antibody and HBsAg; iron studies; ceruloplasmin (in patients <40 y); $\alpha 1$ antitrypsin level; and ANA and antimitochondrial (AMA) antibodies.

4. **Imaging studies**
a. Liver ultrasound can reveal increased echogenicity of hepatic parenchyma, suggesting fatty infiltration. It has a sensitivity of about 89% and a specificity of 93% in detecting steatosis.
b. CT imaging can also reveal hepatic fat seen as a low-density parenchyma (93% sensitivity). It is mostly diffuse but can be focal, raising a question of a malignant liver mass. In such cases, an MRI can distinguish space-occupying lesion from fatty infiltration (characterized by isolated areas of fat infiltration) or focal fatty sparing (characterized by isolated areas of normal liver).
c. Imaging studies cannot definitively establish the diagnosis of NASH, and they do not predict the severity of disease.
5. Liver biopsy is the ultimate test to establish the diagnosis, severity, and prognosis. However, routine use of liver biopsy in patients with presumed NAFLD is controversial.

D. Treatment
1. There is no single effective therapy available for NASH at this time.
2. In patients with diabetes and hyperlipidemia, control of blood glucose and hyperlipidemia is recommended.
3. Gradual weight loss of 10% or more has been shown to improve liver enzyme abnormalities and steatosis on liver ultrasound, especially in obese adults and children. There is some evidence that weight loss can improve histologic features on liver biopsy. Very rapid weight loss should be avoided because it can worsen portal inflammation and fibrosis.
4. Vitamin E at a dose of 400 to 1200 IU has been shown to normalize liver transaminases in obese pediatric patients with NAFLD, and there is some evidence to suggest histologic improvement in inflammation and fibrosis.
5. Other agents studied with evidence of aminotransferase or histologic improvements include medications that improve insulin sensitivity such as metformin, rosiglitazone, and pioglitazone, agents with antioxidant properties such as *N*-acetylcysteine, and HMG-CoA reductase inhibitor. However, these agents remain poorly studied.
6. Patients not showing improvement in liver tests after control of diabetes and hyperlipidemia and after gradual weight loss of 10% or more of initial body weight should be referred to a gastroenterologist or hepatologist.

ASCITES

I. **General Background.** Ascites is a pathologic accumulation of serous fluid within the abdomen and it is the most common major complication of cirrhosis. It is associated with high morbidity and mortality (mortality 30% over 1 year and 60% to 80% in 5 years). An abrupt development of ascites after many years in a patient with stable cirrhosis should suggest the possibility of hepatocellular carcinoma.

II. Etiology.

A. Cirrhosis is the underlying cause in about 80% to 85% of patients with ascites. Up to 50% of cirrhotic patients develop ascites over 10 years.

B. Other causes include heart failure, abdominal carcinomatosis, tuberculosis, fulminant liver failure, pancreatic disease, pelvic inflammatory disease, connective tissue diseases, and hypoproteinemia.

C. Unlike non–alcohol-related causes of liver disease, ascites in alcoholic liver disease may be reversible with salt restriction and abstinence from alcohol.

III. Clinical and Radiologic Findings.

A. Presence of dullness to percussion of the flanks helps differentiate ascites from other causes of increased abdominal fullness and distention. The dullness should shift upon rotating the patient in the right or left lateral positions. Shifting dullness indicates the presence of at least 1.5 liters of ascitic fluid.

B. A plain abdominal x-ray might show the ground glass appearance with centrally located bowel loops, but it is not necessary or recommended in assessment or treatment of ascites.

C. Ultrasonography may be necessary to determine the presence or absence of ascites. Doppler studies of the portal system are helpful in cases in which Budd–Chiari syndrome or a vena caval web are suspected.

D. CXR and an echocardiogram are helpful in assessing patients suspected to have ascites of cardiac origin.

IV. Diagnostic Work-up and Evaluation.

A. **A diagnostic paracentesis should be performed routinely in all patients with new-onset ascites and in all patients admitted to the hospital with ascites to rule out spontaneous bacterial peritonitis** (see later). A 22-gauge needle can be inserted in a Z-track fashion (to minimize leakage of fluid after paracentesis) in midline between the umbilicus and the pubis symphysis in order to avoid collateral vessels. In the presence of a midline scar, a position about 1.5 in (4 cm) above and medial to the anterior superior iliac spine can be used safely.

B. **Ascitic fluid is mostly straw colored or yellow tinged.** Cloudiness or opacified appearance is due to the presence of neutrophils. Milky-appearing ascites is known as chylous ascites; it is due to the presence of triglycerides. Nontraumatic bloody ascites should raise the suspicion for tuberculosis and malignancy. A tea-colored fluid is occasionally seen in pancreatic ascites.

C. **Initial ascitic fluid analysis should include** cell count with WBC differential (mandatory), albumin, total protein, and culture (inoculation into blood culture bottles at bedside increases the yield). Cytology and smear and culture for mycobacteria should be considered in cases in which there is high suspicion of peritoneal carcinomatosis and TB, respectively. Glucose, amylase, and Gram stain are of little or no value except in cases of suspected gut perforation.

D. **Patients undergoing outpatient therapeutic paracentesis need testing for ascitic fluid cell count and differential only.**
1. Patients with PMN >250/mL are assumed to be infected and need to be treated. In cases of bloody taps, only 1 PMN per 250 red cells can be attributed to contamination of the ascitic fluid with blood.
2. In ascites due to tuberculous peritonitis and peritoneal carcinomatosis, **lymphocytes predominate.**
3. **A serum–ascites albumin gradient >1.1 g/dL indicates portal hypertension with greater than 90% reliability.**

$$SAAG = [albumin]_{serum} - [albumin]_{ascites}$$

V. **Other Causes of Ascites.**
A. **High SAAG (>1.1 g/dL)**
1. Cardiac ascites is due to congestion of hepatic sinusoids and has high total protein.
2. Nephrogenous ascites occurs in patients on hemodialysis with volume overload and tends to have high total protein as well.
3. Massive liver metastases can result in portal venous inflow obstruction, and tumor emboli in portal vein radicals cause portal hypertension. Ascitic fluid total protein is <2.5 mg/dL in two thirds of the cases of liver metastases. Budd–Chiari syndrome also needs to be considered.
4. In myxedema, ascites forms due to congestive heart failure and has high protein (>2.5 mg/dL).
B. **Low SAAG (<1.1 g/dL)**
1. Tuberculous peritonitis is most often found in Asians and immigrants from Central America.
2. Peritoneal carcinomatosis accounts for about half of all cases of ascites due to a malignancy. Cytology is positive in 97% to 100% of the cases.
3. Pancreatic ascites accounts for 1% of ascites. Patients often have underlying liver disease due to alcohol abuse. The fluid has high amylase and the total protein of the ascites is usually high also.
4. Biliary ascites is due to leakage of bile into the peritoneum. It is dark brown and has a bilirubin value >6 mg/dL and an ascitic fluid–to–serum bilirubin ratio of >1.
5. Ascites with low SAAG may be seen in patients with connective tissue diseases due to serositis in the absence of portal hypertension.
6. Nephrotic syndrome is a cause of ascites with low protein.
7. Ascites in a febrile, sexually active young woman should raise a suspicion for chlamydia peritonitis. This ascites has high protein and elevated WBC.
VI. **Treatment of Ascites and Other Considerations.** Successful treatment of ascites depends on the accurate diagnosis of the cause of ascites.
A. **Discontinue any prostaglandin inhibitors or other drugs that reduce GFR** (e.g., NSAIDS).
B. **Sodium restriction is key** to the success of treatment of ascites. Patient should be instructed to follow a 2 g/day sodium diet. Fluid restriction is not necessary in the absence of hyponatremia.

5

GASTROENTEROLOGY

C. Avoidance of salt substitutes that contain KCI and potassium-enriched foods should be emphasized, especially if the patient is also on a potassium-sparing diuretic to prevent hyperkalemia.

D. If salt restriction alone is not effective, initiate oral diuretics, which are the mainstay of treatment of ascites. A combination of spironolactone and furosemide is usually successful in causing natriuresis without precipitating hyper- or hypokalemia. The usual beginning doses are spironolactone 100 mg qd and furosemide 40 mg qd.

E. Random (spot) urinary sodium and urinary potassium can be checked and the doses of diuretic adjusted to effect Na^+/K^+ ratio >1. (Increase in furosemide dose causes increased urinary Na^+ and K^+ loss, and increase in spironolactone dose causes increased K^+ retention.)

F. The doses of spironolactone and furosemide can be titrated to a maximum of 400 mg qd and 160 mg qd, respectively, using the 100 mg–to–40 mg ratio to help maintain normokalemia. The goal of diuretic therapy should be to effect no more than 1 to 2 lb (0.5 to 1 kg) weight loss daily.

G. Body weight, serum electrolytes, BUN, and creatinine need to be followed closely.

H. Diuretic therapy should be stopped if encephalopathy, hyponatremia (Na <120 mmol/L despite fluid restriction), or renal insufficiency (creatinine >2 mg/dL) develop. Overaggressive diuresis can also lead to hepatorenal syndrome, a nonreversible condition resulting in progressive renal failure due to renal hypoperfusion in patients with advanced liver disease. Avoid diuresis of greater than 1 L per day.

I. Large-volume paracentesis (LVP) can be performed in patients with tense ascites affecting satiety and respiration. No albumin replacement is recommended for removal of less than 5 L of ascitic fluid. Intravenous albumin (6-8 g/L of ascitic fluid removed) is recommended for large-volume paracentesis in order to decrease risk of circulatory compromise and reaccumulation of ascites.

J. Refractory or diuretic-resistant ascites, defined as minimal to no weight loss despite maximal diuretic therapy or development of complications of diuretics, occurs in 5% to 10% of cirrhotic patients with ascites.

1. It can be managed by repeated LVP, peritoneovenous shunt, or TIPS placement.

2. TIPS is superior to repeated LVP in controlling the recurrence of ascites, but it has not been shown definitively to improve survival.

3. Patients with TIPS must be monitored for shunt malfunction and increased incidence of hepatic encephalopathy. Shunt stenosis occurs in upwards of 50% of the patients after 6 to 12 months.

4. A sudden worsening of refractory ascites or an improvement in hepatic encephalopathy without any interval change in medical regimen or salt restriction suggests shunt stenosis and requires shunt evaluation with duplex Doppler studies and shunt revision. Shunt stenosis may be minimized with use of new polytetrafluoroethylene-coated stents.

5. TIPS is contraindicated in patients with advanced liver failure, especially in the presence of renal failure.

6. While orthotopic liver transplantation should be considered initially after the onset of ascites, eligible patients who are diuretic resistant need to be prioritized for transplantation because 50% die in 6 months.

K. Prevention of spontaneous bacterial peritonitis. Patients with ascitic fluid total protein concentration <1.0 g/dL and gastrointestinal hemorrhage are at high risk for development of spontaneous bacterial peritonitis. There is good evidence that Bactrim (1 DS tablet daily 5 days a week) is effective in preventing spontaneous bacterial peritonitis and decreasing mortality. Norfloxacin 400 mg qd has been used but there is rapid development of resistant organisms. Ciprofloxacin 750 mg once a week or levofloxacin 250 mg daily are being used increasingly. Also see treatment for spontaneous bacterial peritonitis later.

HEPATIC HYDROTHORAX

I. Definition and General Information. Hepatic hydrothorax is the presence of a large pleural effusion in a patient with cirrhosis and portal hypertension in the absence of coexistent cardiopulmonary disease. It is seen in up to 9% of cirrhotic patients presenting with ascites, is often right-sided ($\sim$ 85%), and is often massive.

II. Etiology. Hepatic hydrothorax is thought to be due to defect(s) in the tendinous portion of the right (or left) hemidiaphragm. The pleural fluid tends to recur and is usually transudative. Because negative intrathoracic pressure favors unidirectional fluid transfer across the diaphragmatic defect, hepatic hydrothorax can occur in the absence of ascites, thus confusing the clinician and leading to an extensive diagnostic evaluation.

III. Clinical Presentation and Diagnosis.

A. Hepatic hydrothorax should be suspected in every cirrhotic patient presenting with a unilateral pleural effusion.

B. Because negative intrathoracic pressure favors unidirectional flow, it can occasionally be found in the absence of ascites.

C. Depending on its size, the patient can experience shortness of breath, cough, hypoxemia, and chest discomfort.

D. A thoracentesis is not always necessary to establish the diagnosis in asymptomatic cirrhotic patients with ascites, but it should be performed in those presenting with left-sided hydrothorax, fever, pleuritic chest pain, shortness of breath, or lack of ascites to exclude other diagnoses including spontaneous bacterial empyema.

E. Diagnosis is confirmed by obtaining a nuclear study that establishes the presence of a peritoneo–pleural communication. The study involves the instillation of ^{99m}Tc–sulfur colloid into the peritoneum and documenting the uptake and accumulation of the radiotracer in the pleural space.

5

GASTROENTEROLOGY

IV. Treatment.

A. Hepatic hydrothorax is treated like ascites (see earlier).

B. A large-volume thoracentesis may be performed to relieve shortness of breath due to a large effusion.

C. Chest tube placement is relatively contraindicated in hepatic hydrothorax due to the potential for life-threatening depletion of fluid and electrolytes as the leak continues.

D. In cases not responding to usual therapy, video-assisted thoracoscopy to repair diaphragmatic defect(s) combined with pleurodesis, or TIPS can be used.

SPONTANEOUS BACTERIAL PERITONITIS

I. General Information.

A. Spontaneous bacterial peritonitis is a common (10%-30%) complication in patients with cirrhosis and ascites and occurs mostly in the setting of low ascitic fluid total protein level (<1 g/dL).

B. Pathogenesis involves bacterial translocation from the gut to the systemic circulation and then to ascitic fluid with decreased antibacterial activity in a host with depressed reticuloendothelial phagocytic activity.

C. *E. coli*, *Klebseilla pneumoniae*, and *Pneumococcus* are the three most common isolates.

D. Renal failure occurs in approximately one third of the patients despite treatment of the infection.

II. Presentation and Diagnosis.

A. Abdominal pain and fever are the most characteristic symptoms, but hepatic encephalopathy, gastrointestinal bleeding, vomiting, diarrhea, shock, or hypothermia may be the presenting symptom(s) in a large number of patients.

B. It can also be totally **asymptomatic.** Therefore, one must have a low threshold for performing a paracentesis to obtain ascitic fluid for analysis.

C. Spontaneous bacterial peritonitis is diagnosed when there is a positive ascitic fluid culture or when the ascitic fluid PMN count is >250 cells/mm^3 in the absence of an identifiable intraabdominal source of infection.

D. Ascitic fluid culture must be placed directly into blood culture preferably at bedside to increase the sensitivity of culture.

E. Secondary peritonitis due to perforated viscus usually results in a PMN count in the thousands, multiple organisms on gram stain and culture, and at least two of the following: total protein >1 g/dL, LDH higher than the upper limit of normal for serum, and glucose <50 mg/dL.

III. Treatment.

A. Empiric antibiotic treatment should begin immediately if ascitic fluid PMN count is >250 cells/mm^3 or if spontaneous bacterial peritonitis is suspected to prevent deterioration of the patient. One should *not* wait for ascitic fluid culture results before beginning treatment.

B. A broad-spectrum therapy is recommended in suspected ascitic fluid infection until culture results and susceptibility are available. Cefotaxime 2 g IV q8h or a comparable third-generation cephalosporin is the treatment of choice. Aztreonam and vancomycin can be used in penicillin-allergic patients as guided by ascitic fluid cultures. Five days of treatment is recommended. A repeat paracentesis can be performed 48 hours after starting appropriate therapy if there is lack of clinical improvement.

C. IV albumin at a dose of 1.5 g/kg body weight on day 1 and 1 g/kg on day 3 is recommended to reduce the incidence of renal impairment and death in comparison to treatment with antibiotics alone. Subsequently, these patients should receive prophylaxis (norfloxacin 400 mg qd, levofloxacin 250 mg qd, ciprofloxacin 750 mg every week, or Bactrim DS 1 tablet qd × 5 days/week).

HEPATIC ENCEPHALOPATHY

I. General.

A. Hepatic encephalopathy is a reversible syndrome with global CNS depression that occurs as a result of hepatocellular failure. It is associated with increased portosystemic shunting of nitrogenous compounds derived from the gut.

B. Ammonia is thought to play an important role in the pathogenesis of hepatic encephalopathy, but plasma levels correlate poorly with the severity.

II. Etiology. Exacerbations of encephalopathy in cirrhotic patients may be precipitated by hypovolemia, GI hemorrhage, infection (SBP, UTI, or pneumonia), hypokalemia, metabolic alkalosis (systemically hypovolemic or hyperventilating), electrolyte disturbances (hyponatremia, hypokalemia), constipation, noncompliance with lactulose use, or sedative use.

III. Clinical Manifestations and Evaluation.

A. Table 5-9 lists symptoms and staging.

B. Subclinical hepatic encephalopathy can be detected by number connection tests (*Trails A or B test*) and asterixis.

C. Rule out other causes of encephalopathy and attempt to identify any precipitating factor(s). Absence of any precipitating factors of hepatic encephalopathy indicates worsening liver function.

D. Check ammonia level, electrolytes, glucose, BUN, creatinine, CBC, PT, and INR. Aggressively hunt for underlying infections by performing blood cultures, urinalysis, urine culture, diagnostic paracentesis, and CXR. Many cirrhotic patients do not mount a fever when infected.

E. Corroborate history with family and friends about medical compliance, bowel habits, and the potential use of alcohol, illicit drugs, benzodiazepines, and narcotics. If INR is >5 and the patient has localizing symptoms, obtain head CT to rule out intracranial hemorrhage.

TABLE 5-9
HEPATIC ENCEPHALOPATHY GRADING SYSTEM

Grade	Mental Status	Asterixis
I	Abnormal sleep pattern; euphoria/depression; mild confusion, asterixis	±
II	Lethargy, moderate confusion	+
III	Stuporous, marked confusion	+
IV	Coma	−

IV. **Treatment.**

A. **Correct hypovolemia,** treat any exacerbating cause that is identified, and initiate ammonia-lowering therapy.

B. **Lower the production and absorption of ammonia. Give lactulose,** a nonabsorbable disaccharide, in doses of 20 to 40 g (30-60 mL) daily. Titrate up to 20 to 40 g tid to qid to affect 2 or 3 semiformed bowel movements per day. If lactulose cannot be administered orally or by NG tube, it may be given as a 300-mL (200-g) retention enema. Lactitol is as effective as lactulose but has fewer side effects. **Other laxatives do not reduce ammonia and are not effective in this situation. There is contradictory evidence about the effectiveness of lactulose and lactitol.** There is no benefit on mortality.

C. **Correct hypokalemia (hypokalemia increases ammonia production by the kidney).**

D. **Antibiotics and sodium benzoate. In patients with inadequate response to lactulose alone,** sodium benzoate 2 to 8 g/day and/or neomycin 4 to 6 g/day PO can be added in divided doses, although long-term use of the latter drug is associated with ototoxicity and nephrotoxicity. Rifaximin 400 mg PO q8h has been shown to be as effective as lactitol for hepatic encephalopathy.

E. **Benzodiazepines and opiates should be avoided.** Use haloperidol intravenously at doses of 0.5 to 1.0 mg to treat agitation. Flumazenil is associated with limited success and is *not* recommended as a routine therapy in patients with hepatic encephalopathy.

F. **Do not restrict protein in cirrhotic patients unless they do not respond to all other treatment** modalities. In these rare cases, dietary protein may be restricted to 0.8 to 1 g/kg per day.

G. In the acute situation or in severely constipated patients, tap water enemas should be given to evacuate the bowels.

ACUTE PANCREATITIS

I. **Etiology.**

A. **Cholelithiasis,** including microlithiasis, is the most common cause in the United States, Western Europe, and in Asia (45% of cases).

B. **Chronic alcohol ingestion** is the second leading cause (35% of cases). It is unclear if acute alcoholic pancreatitis ever arises in the absence of chronic glandular damage.

C. **"Traumatic"** causes include postoperative stress, ERCP, direct trauma, manometry of the sphincter of Oddi, endoscopic sphincterotomy, and perforation of a duodenal ulcer.

D. **Metabolic insults include hypertriglyceridemia** (>1000 mg/dL), hypercalcemia (e.g., hyperparathyroidism), and renal failure.

E. **Drugs** include DDI, DDC, azathioprine, mercaptopurine, valproic acid, acetaminophen, and others.

F. **Infectious** causes include viruses (mumps, rubella, cytomegalovirus, adenovirus, HIV, coxsackievirus B), bacteria (mycoplasma, *Campylobacter*, legionella, *Mycobacterium tuberculosis*, *M. avium* complex), and parasites (ascariasis, clonorchiasis).

G. **Connective tissue disorders** (SLE, polyarteritis nodosa, sarcoidosis) and idiopathic causes.

II. **Pathophysiology.**

A. Acute pancreatitis is an acute inflammatory process with possible involvement of peripancreatic tissues and distant organ systems.

B. In mild disease there is interstitial edema. In severe disease there are areas of necrosis and hemorrhage in the gland, and a systemic inflammatory response syndrome (SIRS) may develop.

III. **Clinical Presentation.**

A. Abdominal pain in midepigastric region radiating to the left upper quadrant or back. **Always include acute pancreatitis in the differential diagnosis of acute abdomen.**

B. Symptoms and signs include nausea and vomiting, low-grade fever, ileus, and in severe disease signs of shock and multiorgan failure (ARDS, acute renal failure secondary to ATN), DIC, and pancreatic hemorrhage with CNS hypoperfusion, with confusion and lethargy in severe cases.

C. Other signs include pleural effusions, pneumonia, and atelectasis; pancreatic fluid collections, pseudocysts, and abscesses; and signs of retroperitoneal bleeding (Cullen's and Grey Turner's sign, but seen rarely).

IV. **Diagnostic Evaluation.**

A. **Amylase and lipase levels should be determined** (although whether both are necessary is a topic of heated debate). Amylase is elevated in 80% of those with pancreatitis and is more sensitive early in the course. Lipase is more sensitive if symptoms have been present for more than 24 hours. Lipase is more specific than amylase. Both the amylase and lipase may be normal in a patient with CT-proven pancreatitis. False-positive elevated amylase is seen with renal failure, alcoholic liver disease, GYN disease, other GI disease, bulimia, salivary gland disease, etc. False-negative amylase is seen with elevated triglycerides and others. False-positive lipase is seen with renal failure, cholecystitis, fat injury, multiple drugs (including furosemide), and HIV.

B. **Ultrasound or CT of the pancreas** might show pancreatic glandular edema, peripancreatic fat stranding, or pancreatic/peripancreatic fluid collections. Ultrasound of the gallbladder may show a common bile duct stone in gallstone pancreatitis.

C. **X-ray may reveal a sentinel loop,** a localized ileus in the midepigastric region. Pleural effusions (especially right sided) might also be present.

D. **Labs.** Order CBC, electrolytes, liver profile, calcium, magnesium, and PT/PTT. **Hypocalcemia can occur due to saponification of fat with resultant binding of calcium to fatty acid chains.** Leukocytosis is common. Amino-transaminases and bilirubin may be elevated from biliary obstruction in gallstone pancreatitis. Liver profile abnormalities are more sensitive (but less specific) for early common bile duct obstruction in acute biliary pancreatitis.

E. **Urinary trypsinogen activation peptide (TAP)** is a promising new test that can predict severity of acute pancreatitis 24 hours after onset. It is not yet available universally.

V. Prognosis.

A. **Ranson's criteria** were initially devised based on alcoholic pancreatitis but are applicable to all acute pancreatides. Assessment by these criteria takes 48 hours. Presence of fewer than three findings is associated with a <5% mortality risk, whereas the presence of 3 or 4 signs on admission is associated with a mortality of 15% to 20%.

1. On admission:
   a. Age >55 years.
   b. WBC >16,000.
   c. Blood glucose >200 mg/dL.
   d. LDH >350 IU/L.
   e. AST >250 IU/L.
2. At 48 hours:
   a. Fall in Hct >10% (third spacing and possible hemorrhage).
   b. Rise in BUN >5 mg/ dL.
   c. Serum calcium <8 mg/ dL.
   d. Arterial Po_2 <60 mm Hg.
   e. Base deficit >4 mEq/L.
   f. Estimated fluid third spacing of >6 L.

B. **The Apache II score is a better predictor of outcome than are Ranson's criteria and have the benefit of being able to be done on admission whereas Ranson's criteria cannot be fully scored until 48 hours after admission.**

VI. Acute Management. Treat the underlying cause and provide supportive care.

A. **Treat shock** (see Chapter 2). Invasive hemodynamic monitoring may be required. The patient might need up to 6 to 8 L of intravenous fluid per day.

B. Prevent or correct hypocalcemia, hypomagnesemia, and hypokalemia.

C. Suppress gastric acid with proton pump inhibitors (benefit is questionable).

D. **An NG tube helps relieve nausea.** However, NG tubes have not been shown to reduce the duration of hospitalization, nor do they decrease pain intensity associated with pancreatitis.

E. **Nutrition is critical to recovery.** While the patient is ill, avoid stimulation of the exocrine pancreas. **Classically, TPN was encouraged; however, this method increases the risk of sepsis and metabolic perturbations.** Placement of enteral feeding tube beyond the ligament of Treitz (nasojejunal tube or percutaneous jejunostomy) prevents pancreatic stimulation, maintains mucosal integrity, and decreases absorption of endotoxins and cytokines from the GI tract. This can be done even in moderate to severe cases.

F. **In mild/moderate cases, oral refeeding may be restarted in a few days** when the patient is pain free. Start with a low-fat, low-calorie diet and advance as tolerated.

G. **Antibiotics** are indicated if there is associated ascending cholangitis. **However, routine antibiotics are not helpful for mild or moderate acute pancreatitis.** The data in severe pancreatitis is contradictory, with the largest study to date suggesting no benefit. However, it is not unreasonable to treat **acute pancreatitis complicated by necrosis (>30% of the pancreas) with prophylactic, broad-spectrum antibiotics (e.g., imipenem).** Surgical consultation should be obtained for possible drainage of necrotic tissue.

H. **Pain control. Morphine or fentanyl are the preferred agents.** There is no evidence that meperidine is superior, and meperidine has active metabolites that can cause seizures and agitation.

I. **Octreotide has not been shown to be useful in treating pancreatitis.**

J. **Early ERCP to clear the** biliary tract has been shown to reduce morbidity and mortality in gallstone pancreatitis.

VII. **Long-Term Sequelae.**

A. **Chronic pancreatitis** is characterized by chronic and progressive loss of pancreatic parenchyma through repeated bouts of acute pancreatitis.

B. **Pseudocysts** are peripancreatic fluid collections that develop a wall of unepithelialized granulation tissue. Pseudocysts complicate less than 5% of acute pancreatitis cases. They take 4 to 6 weeks to mature. Treatment (percutaneous needle, endoscopic drainage, or surgical resection) is indicated if they are enlarging and/or symptomatic or persist for longer than 6 weeks. Although a threshold of >6 cm has been used in the past, it is not a strict guideline for intervention. If asymptomatic, they should generally be managed expectantly, because many resolve spontaneously.

C. **Pleural fistulas and pancreatic ascites** result from pancreatic fluid entering the pleural space or abdomen, respectively. Treatment includes octreotide, ERCP (with pancreatic duct stenting), or surgery.

D. **Splenic vein thrombus** may occur due to inflammation adjacent to the splenic vein. It can manifest with UGI bleeding. Patients usually have normal liver function and isolated gastric varices. Diagnosis can be made noninvasively by Doppler ultrasonography.

E. **Pancreatic insufficiency and glucose intolerance** only develop after loss of 90% of pancreatic function. These can be treated with diet modification (restricted fat diet or diabetic diet) or medications. In patients whose steatorrhea cannot be controlled with diet, consider oral lipase supplementation (e.g., Viokase, Creon) and fat-soluble vitamin (A, D, K, E) supplements.

BIBLIOGRAPHY

Angeloni S, Nicolini G, Merli M, et al: Validation of automated blood cell counter for the determination of polymorphonuclear cell count in the ascitic fluid of cirrhotic patients with or without spontaneous bacterial peritonitis. *Am J Gastroenterol* 98:1844-1848, 2003.

Angulo P, Lindor KD: Non-alcoholic fatty liver disease. *J Gastroenterol Hepatol* 17 Suppl:S186-S190, 2002.

Arteel G, Marsano L, Mendez C, et al: Advances in alcoholic liver disease. *Baillieres Best Pract Res Clin Gastroenterol* 17:625-647, 2003.

Avery ME, Snyder JD: Oral therapy for acute diarrhea: The underused simple solution. *N Engl J Med* 323:891-894, 1990.

Banerjee S, Lamont JT: Treatment of gastrointestinal infections. *Gastroenterology* 118:S48-S67, 2000.

Barkun A, Bardou M, Marshall JK: Consensus recommendations for managing patients with nonvariceal upper gastrointestinal bleeding. *Ann Intern Med* 139:843-857, 2003.

Bhattacharya A, Mittal BR, Biswas T, et al: Radioisotope scintigraphy in the diagnosis of hepatic hydrothorax. *J Gastroenterol Hepatol* 16:317-321, 2001.

Boyer TD: Transjugular intrahepatic portosystemic shunt: Current status. *Gastroenterology* 124:1700-1710, 2003.

Butterworth RF: Hepatic encephalopathy. *Alcohol Res Health* 27:240-246, 2003.

Cardenas A, Kelleher T, Chopra S: Review article: Hepatic hydrothorax. *Aliment Pharmacol Ther* 20:271-279, 2004.

Castellote J, Lopez C, Gornals J, et al: Rapid diagnosis of spontaneous bacterial peritonitis by use of reagent strips. *Hepatology* 37:893-896, 2003.

Chey WD: *Helicobacter pylori. Curr Treat Options Gastroenterol* 2:171-182, 1999.

Corley DA, Cello JP, Adkisson W, et al: Octreotide for acute esophageal variceal bleeding: A meta-analysis. *Gastroenterology* 120:946-954, 2001.

Czaja AJ, Freese DK: Diagnosis and treatment of autoimmune hepatitis. *Hepatology* 36:479-497, 2002.

DeVault KR, Castell DO: Updated guidelines for the diagnosis and treatment of gastroesophageal reflux disease. *Am J Gastroenterol* 100:190-200, 2005.

Egan LJ, Sandborn WJ: Drug therapy of inflammatory bowel disease. *Drugs Today (Barc.)* 34:431-446, 1998.

Eisen GM, Baron TH, Dominitz JA, et al: Guideline for the management of ingested foreign bodies. *Gastrointest Endosc* 55:802-806, 2002.

Elta GH: Urgent colonoscopy for acute lower-GI bleeding. *Gastrointest Endosc* 59:402-408, 2004.

Farrell RJ, Kelly CP: Current concepts—Celiac sprue. *N Engl J Med* 346:180-188, 2002.

Feagan BG: Maintenance therapy for inflammatory bowel disease. *Am J Gastroenterol* 98:S6-S17, 2003.

Feldman M, Friedman LS, Sleisenger MH: *Sleisenger and Fordtran's Gastrointestinal and Liver Disease*, 7th ed. Philadelphia, WB Saunders, 2002.

Fine KD, Schiller LR: AGA technical review on the evaluation and management of chronic diarrhea. *Gastroenterology* 116:1464-1486, 1999.

Flamm SL: Chronic hepatitis C virus infection. *JAMA* 289:2413-2417, 2003.

Friedman S: General principles of medical therapy of inflammatory bowel disease. *Gastroenterol Clin North Am* 33:191-208, viii, 2004.

Fung SK, Lok AS: Treatment of chronic hepatitis B: Who to treat, what to use, and for how long?. *Clin Gastroenterol Hepatol* 2:839-848, 2004.

Garcia-Tsao G: Current management of the complications of cirrhosis and portal hypertension: Variceal hemorrhage, ascites, and spontaneous bacterial peritonitis. *Gastroenterology* 120:726-748, 2001.

Gines P, Uriz J, Calahorra B, et al: Transjugular intrahepatic portosystemic shunting versus paracentesis plus albumin for refractory ascites in cirrhosis. *Gastroenterology* 123:1839-1847, 2002.

Gines P, Cardenas A, Arroyo V, Rodes J: Management of cirrhosis and ascites. *N Engl J Med* 350:1646-1654, 2004.

Hanauer SB, Feagan BG, Lichtenstein GR, et al: Maintenance infliximab for Crohn's disease: The ACCENT I randomised trial. *Lancet* 359:1541-1549, 2002.

Hanauer SB, Present DH: The state of the art in the management of inflammatory bowel disease. *Rev Gastroenterol Disord* 3:81-92, 2003.

Howden CW, Hunt RH: Guidelines for the management of *Helicobacter pylori* infection. Ad Hoc Committee on Practice Parameters of the American College of Gastroenterology. *Am J Gastroenterol* 93:2330-2338, 1998.

Jamal MM, Morgan TR: Liver disease in alcohol and hepatitis C. *Ballieres Best Pract Res Clin Gastroenterol* 17:649-662, 2003.

Kaviani MJ, Hashemi MR, Kazemifar AR, et al: Effect of oral omeprazole in reducing re-bleeding in bleeding peptic ulcers: A prospective, double-blind, randomized, clinical trial. *Aliment Pharmacol Ther* 17:211-216, 2003.

Lau JY, Sung JJ, Lee KK, et al: Effect of intravenous omeprazole on recurrent bleeding after endoscopic treatment of bleeding peptic ulcers. *N Engl J Med* 343:310-316, 2000.

Lau JY, Sung JJ: Management options for patients with ulcer hemorrhage. *Ann Intern Med* 140:845-846, 2004.

Lembo A, Camilleri M: Current concepts: Chronic constipation. *N Engl J Med* 349:1360-1368, 2003.

Levitsky J, Mailliard ME: Diagnosis and therapy of alcoholic liver disease. *Semin Liver Dis* 24:233-247, 2004.

Lichtenstein GR, Wu G: *Small And Large Intestine*. Requisites in Gastroenterology Series, vol 2. Philadelphia, Mosby, 2003.

Lin M, Triadafilopoulos G: Belching: Dyspepsia or gastroesophageal reflux disease? *Am J Gastroenter* 98:2139-2145, 2003.

Mas A, Rodes J, Sunyer L, et al: Comparison of rifaximin and lactitol in the treatment of acute hepatic encephalopathy: Results of a randomized, double-blind, double-dummy, controlled clinical trial. *J Hepatol* 38:51-58, 2003.

Mertz HR: Drug therapy: Irritable bowel syndrome. *N Eng J Med* 349:2136-2146, 2003.

Mitchell RM, Byrne MF, Baillie J: Pancreatitis. *Lancet* 361:1447-1455, 2003.

Morgan TR, Mandayam S, Jamal MM: Alcohol and hepatocellular carcinoma. *Gastroenterology* 127:S87-S96, 2004.

O'Grady JG, Alexander GJ, Hayllar KM, Williams R: Early indicators of prognosis in fulminant hepatic failure. *Gastroenterology* 97:439-445, 1989.

Olden KW: Diagnosis of irritable bowel syndrome. *Gastroenterology* 122:1701-1714, 2002.

Pratt DS, Kaplan MM: Evaluation of abnormal liver-enzyme results in asymptomatic patients. *N Engl J Med* 342:1266-1271, 2000.

5

GASTROENTEROLOGY

Rao SS: Constipation: Evaluation and treatment. *Gastroenterol Clin North Am* 32:659-683, 2003.

Rao SSC: Belching, bloating, and flatulence. How to help patients who have troublesome abdominal gas. *Postgrad Med* 101:263-269, 275-278, 1997.

Reddy KR, Long W: *Hepatobiliary And Pancreatic Disease*. Requisites in Gastroenterology Series, vol 3, Philadelphia, Mosby, 2003.

Reid BM, Sanyal AJ: Evaluation and management of non-alcoholic steatohepatitis. *Eur J Gastroenterol Hepatol* 16:1117-1122, 2004.

Rockey DC: Occult gastrointestinal bleeding. *N Engl J Med* 341:38-46, 1999.

Runyon BA, Greenblatt M, Ming RH: Hepatic hydrothorax is a relative contraindication to chest tube insertion. *Am J Gastroenterol* 81:566-567, 1986.

Runyon BA: Management of adult patients with ascites due to cirrhosis. *Hepatology* 39:841-856, 2004.

Schiller LR: Chronic diarrhea. *Gastroenterology* 127:287-293, 2004.

Sharma P, McQuaid K, Dent J, et al: A critical review of the diagnosis and management of Barrett's esophagus: The AGA Chicago Workshop. *Gastroenterology* 127:310-330, 2004.

Sifrim D, Castell D, Dent J. Kahrilas PJ: Gastro-oesophageal reflux monitoring: review and consensus report on detection and definitions of acid, non-acid, and gas reflux. *Gut* 53:1024-1031, 2004.

Singh N, Gayowski T, Yu VL, Wagener MM: Trimethoprim–sulfamethoxazole for the prevention of spontaneous bacterial peritonitis in cirrhosis: A randomized trial. *Ann Intern Med* 122:595-598, 1995.

Skoog SM, Bharucha AE: Dietary fructose and gastrointestinal symptoms: A review. *Am J Gastroenterol* 99:2046-2050, 2004.

Soriano G, Guarner C, Tomas A, et al: Norfloxacin prevents bacterial infection in cirrhotics with gastrointestinal hemorrhage. *Gastroenterology* 103:1267-1272, 1992.

Sort P, Navasa M, Arroyo V, et al: Effect of intravenous albumin on renal impairment and mortality in patients with cirrhosis and spontaneous bacterial peritonitis. *N Engl J Med* 341:403-409, 1999.

Spechler SJ: American Gastroenterological Association medical position statement on treatment of patients with dysphagia caused by benign disorders of the distal esophagus. *Gastroenterology* 117:229-233, 1999.

Steffen R, Sack DA, Riopel L, et al: Therapy of travelers' diarrhea with rifaximin on various continents. *Am J Gastroenterol* 98:1073-1078, 2003.

Stollman NH, Raskin JB: Diagnosis and management of diverticular disease of the colon in adults. Ad Hoc Practice Parameters Committee of the American College of Gastroenterology.[see comment]. *Am J Gastroenterol* 94(11):3110-21, 1999.

Strader DB, Wright T, Thomas DL, Seeff LB: Diagnosis, management, and treatment of hepatitis C. *Hepatology* 39:1147-1171, 2004.

Tack J, Bisschops R, Sarnelli G: Pathophysiology and treatment of functional dyspepsia. *Gastroenterology* 127:1239-1255, 2004.

Talley NJ, Silverstein MD, Agreus L, et al: AGA technical review: Evaluation of dyspepsia. American Gastroenterological Association. *Gastroenterology* 114:582-595, 1998.

Thielman NM, Guerrant RL: Acute infectious diarrhea. *N Eng J Med* 350:38-47, 2004.

Tome S, Lucey MR: Review article: Current management of alcoholic liver disease. *Aliment Pharmacol Ther* 19:707-714, 2004.

Tuteja AK, Rao SSC: Review article: Recent trends in diagnosis and treatment of fecal incontinence. *Aliment Pharmacol Ther* 19:829-840, 2004.

Uemura N, Okamoto S, Yamamoto S, et al: *Helicobacter pylori* infection and the development of gastric cancer. *N Engl J Med* 345:784-789, 2001.

Vaira D, Vakil N, Menegatti M, et al: The stool antigen test for detection of *Helicobacter pylori* after eradication therapy. *Ann Intern Med* 136:280-286, 2002.

Yassin SF, Young-Fadok TM, Zein NN, Pardi DS: *Clostridium difficile*–associated diarrhea and colitis. *Mayo Clin Proc* 76:725-730, 2001.

Zuccaro G, Jr.: Management of the adult patient with acute lower gastrointestinal bleeding. American College of Gastroenterology. Practice Parameters Committee. *Am J Gastroenterol* 93:1202-1208, 1998.

Hematologic, Metabolic, and Electrolyte Disorders

Deborah Wilbur and James Bonucchi

BLEEDING AND CLOTTING DISORDERS

I. **Presentation.**

A. **You can often determine type of bleeding disorder by history and physical.** Get family and personal history of bleeding (joints, GI bleeding, etc.). Has excess bleeding been present from birth or is it acquired? Remember that many drugs can contribute to bleeding, including β-lactam antibiotics, warfarin, calcium channel blockers, SSRIs, heparin, NSAIDs, and ASA among many others.

B. **Not all bleeding is from a hematologic abnormality.** Consider capillary fragility (Cushing's syndrome, Marfan's syndrome, senile purpura). Petechiae can be secondary to coughing, sneezing, Valsalva maneuver, blood pressure measurement, vasculitis (palpable purpura), scurvy (vitamin C deficiency), or exogenous steroids. Telangiectasias could suggest Osler–Weber–Rendu syndrome.

II. **Differentiation of Platelet versus Coagulation Defect.**

A. **Platelet defects.** Patients generally have immediate onset of bleeding after trauma. Bleeding is predominantly in skin, mucous membranes, nose, GI tract, and urinary tract. Bleeding may be observed as petechiae or ecchymoses. Must differentiate from vasculitic palpable purpura.

B. **Coagulation system defects.** Delayed, "deep" bleeding (in the joint spaces, muscles, and retroperitoneal spaces) is common. These are observed on exam as hematomas and hemarthroses.

III. **Physical Exam.** For acute bleeding, assess volume status and correct shock if present (see Chapter 2). Do a rectal exam for evidence of GI bleeding and examine oropharynx for evidence of bleeding. Look for hepatosplenomegaly (evidence of platelet destruction, extramedullary hematopoiesis).

IV. **Tests of Coagulation.**

A. **PT/INR (to assess extrinsic system)** is elevated in DIC, warfarin use, chronic liver disease, vitamin K deficiency, fat malabsorption, factor deficiencies (vitamin K dependent), etc.

B. **PTT (to assess intrinsic system)** is elevated in factor deficiencies (such as hemophilia), factor inhibitors, antiphospholipid antibodies (mix patient's serum with equal amount of normal serum; if PTT corrects, PTT elevation is caused by deficiency and not by a circulating anticoagulant, which will prevent coagulation even with adequate clotting factors present), heparin, and other drugs such as antipsychotics. **PTT is the best screening test for coagulation defects and rises when**

coagulation factors fall to less than 30% to 40% of normal plasma level. Patients with an elevated PTT can paradoxically have increased thrombotic events depending on cause (e.g., antiphospholipid antibody syndrome).

C. Platelet count. If less than 50,000, surgical bleeding can result. If less than 10,000 to 20,000, incidence of spontaneous bleeding is increased. **LP is safe at a platelet count greater than 50,000.**

D. Bleeding time is the traditional screening test of platelet function, but it is **poorly reproducible and has poor specificity and should not be used.**

E. Platelet function analysis is an in vitro test to evaluate platelet function. The most popular such test is the PFA-100. It is more reproducible than bleeding time and has largely replaced bleeding time.

F. Fibrin degradation products (or fibrin split products) provides a measure of fibrin destruction. It is elevated in DIC and can also be elevated in other states such as trauma, inflammatory diseases, and dysfibrinogenemias.

G. D dimer is a byproduct of clot breakdown. It is a sensitive measure of endogenous fibrinolysis (and therefore coagulation). An elevated D dimer is present in many patients (especially with cancer, trauma) so it is sensitive for active clotting but not specific for abnormal intravascular clotting (e.g., DVT, PE). See Chapter 4 for further details.

H. Assays for specific factors, such as V, VIII, X, can be performed.

V. Abnormal Bleeding Caused by Inherited Platelet Disorders.

A. Von Willebrand's disease

1. **Von Willebrand's disease is the most common hereditary coagulation disorder.** There are several variants, most of which are autosomal dominant. Abnormal synthesis of vWF causes decreased platelet adhesion and decreased serum levels of factor VIII (because vWF is the carrier for factor VIII). Type I is characterized by a quantitative deficiency in vWF, type II by a qualitatively abnormal vWF, and type III by severe quantitative deficiency in vWF.

2. **Testing. You might need to test a single patient several times because the level of vWF is variable within a patient.** Testing should include vWF antigen, vWF activity (also called *ristocetin cofactor activity*), and factor VIII activity.

3. **Treatment involves normalizing factor VIII and vWF activity. Mild bleeding in type I patients can be treated with desmopressin** (see the discussion of hemophilia for dose). **More significant bleeding in type I patients or bleeding in type II or III patients requires infusions of a factor VIII product that also contains vWF, such as Humate-P** (see the discussion of hemophilia for calculations). Another alternative is cryoprecipitate (1000-1250 U of factor VIII:C, generally about 10 bags). However, this carries the risk of virus transmission. Adjunctive antifibrinolytic therapy with aminocaproic acid or tranexamic acid is particularly useful for mucosal bleeding. **If none of these modalities works, consider platelet transfusion.** Finally, oral contraceptives are

often prescribed for control of menorrhagia in von Willebrand patients. For further information, see Manucci, 2004.

B. **Other inherited disorders of platelet function include adhesion defects** (e.g., Bernard-Soulier syndrome), decreased platelet aggregation, and secretion defects as in gray platelet syndrome or in storage pool disease. These disorders are exceedingly rare and can be treated with platelet transfusions.

VI. **Bleeding Caused by Acquired Disorders of Platelet Function.**

A. **Drugs:** NSAIDS, ticlopidine, clopidogrel, GPIIb/IIIa receptor antagonists, β-lactams, plasma expanders, calcium channel blockers, SSRIs, and quinidine are just some of the drugs that can impair platelet function.

B. **Uremia**

C. **Cardiopulmonary bypass surgery**

D. **Hematologic conditions,** such as paraproteinemias, myelodysplastic syndromes, and myeloproliferative disorders have been associated with qualitative platelet dysfunction. Treatment is directed at the underlying disorder.

VII. **Bleeding and Clotting Caused by Quantitative Platelet Disorders.**

A. **Thrombocytosis** occurs in myeloproliferative disease (including polycythemia vera, chronic idiopathic myelofibrosis, and essential thrombocythemia). **In these states, platelets are often poorly functioning, leading to a bleeding disorder,** although there may also be abnormal thrombosis. The platelets in patients who have a reactive thrombocytosis (e.g., cancer, inflammation, iron deficiency anemia) function well. Treatment of bleeding is by platelet transfusion to bring the pool of *normal* platelets to 50,000/mL. **For patients with thrombotic complications, aspirin 325 mg/day is indicated.** Definitive treatment of the underlying condition is critical.

B. **Thrombocytopenia can be caused by decreased production, increased splenic sequestration, or increased platelet destruction.** Consider also HELLP syndrome, and gestational thrombocytopenia in pregnant women. Always check the peripheral smear to rule out platelet clumping or pseudothrombocytopenia as a source of low platelet value.

1. **Decreased production can be caused by**

a. **Marrow failure,** including infiltration secondary to malignancy or fibrosis, B_{12} and folate deficiency, or myelodysplastic syndromes. Diagnose by bone marrow biopsy.

b. **Multiple drugs,** including ethanol, heparin, estrogens, thiazides, and chemotherapeutic drugs.

c. **Infectious causes,** including sepsis, AIDS, EBV, ehrlichiosis, Colorado tick fever, Rocky Mountain spotted fever, babesiosis, malaria, multiple viral infections, etc.

2. **Increased sequestration in spleen** can be secondary to portal hypertension (for example, from cirrhosis).

HEMATOLOGIC, METABOLIC, AND ELECTROLYTE DISORDERS

6

3. **Increased platelet destruction can be caused by**
   a. **Immunologic destruction:** Bacterial or viral infections, drugs (sulfonamides, quinidine, INH, sedative–hypnotics, digoxin, heparin), idiopathic thrombocytopenic purpura (ITP).
   b. **Nonimmunologic destruction:** Vasculitis, DIC, thrombotic thrombocytopenic purpura (TTP), hemolytic uremic syndrome (HUS), and prosthetic heart valves.
4. **ITP is an immunologic destruction of platelets (by antiplatelet antibodies).**
   a. **It is often preceded by URI or other viral infection,** particularly in children. It is more common in women and in persons with HIV, mononucleosis (EBV), Graves' disease, and hyperthyroidism.
   b. **ITP manifests as petechiae and other bleeding such as CNS bleeding or bleeding gums.** Women can have increased uterine bleeding.
   c. **Diagnosis. The patients might have antiplatelet antibodies, but testing has not been shown to have predictive value and is not recommended.** Diagnosis usually can be made based on presentation alone, although bone marrow biopsy is recommended in patients older than 60 years. Bone marrow should show normal or increased megakaryocytes.
   d. **Treatment**
      (1) **You may choose to follow and not treat if there is no bleeding.** In children, 70% recover in 4 to 6 weeks.
      (2) **Platelet transfusions are not helpful,** and infused platelets will be destroyed along with the patient's platelets. You might want to use platelet transfusions to try to stop acute bleeding, though.
      (3) **Steroids.** For bleeding or platelet count less than 20,000, treat with prednisone 1 to 2 mg/kg per day until there is a response, and then taper. Another option is high-dose steroids (methylprednisolone 1 g/d × 3-4 d) followed by oral steroids. It can take 2 to 3 weeks to see a response.
      (4) **Intravenous IgG** concentrates can increase platelet count (1 to 2 g/kg IV × 2 d). Rho(D) immune globulin (WinRho-SD) is indicated as IV therapy for ITP in nonsplenectomized patients who are Rh positive. The dose is 250 IU/kg given either at one time or as split doses and must be reduced for those with anemia. See package information for details.
      (5) **Splenectomy** is an option for patients who are bleeding and are not responding to other measures. Other options include rituximab, danazol, vincristine/vinblastine, cyclophosphamide, and azathioprine. Full treatment guidelines are available at http://www.hematology.org/policy/guidelines/idiopathic.cfm.
C. **Heparin-induced thrombocytopenia and thrombosis syndrome (HITTS)** is an antibody-mediated adverse effect of heparin associated with both venous and arterial thromboses. You also might see skin necrosis.

1. **Caveat:** Of patients receiving heparin, 10% to 20% have a nonimmune mediated drop in platelets 1 to 4 days after starting heparin. Typically, platelets reach a nadir of 100,000 and then return to normal. This rapid drop in platelets is not associated with thrombosis and does not require any therapy. **You must ensure that the patient has not had any heparin in the previous 100 days; if so, consider HITTS (see below).**

2. **Clinical presentation of HITTS typically involves a platelet count fall of 50% or greater with or without a** *thrombotic* **event occurring 4 to 14 days after initiating heparin.** HITTS can occur sooner if the patient has received heparin on a separate occasion within the past 100 days. HITTS occurs in 1% to 2% of those getting unfractionated heparin.

3. **Diagnosis.** Various tests exist, including heparin-induced platelet aggregation assays (80% sensitive, 90% specific) and ^{14}C serotonin release assay (100% sensitive, 97% specific).

4. **Further studies.** Approximately half of patients have thromboses at the time of diagnosis and up to a quarter more will develop thromboses. Therefore, it is reasonable to perform Doppler studies on all four limbs at the time of diagnosis and to have low threshold for repeating such studies.

5. **Therapy.** Immediately stop all heparin, including IV line flushes. Begin a nonheparin anticoagulant, such as lepirudin, argatroban, or danaparoid. Once platelet count has recovered, you may add warfarin at low maintenance doses. You must continue the nonheparin anticoagulant until platelet count is stable and INR has been therapeutic for at least 2 days. **Patients have increased risk of thrombosis for up to 1 month following antibody-mediated, heparin-induced decline in platelets.**

6. **Prevention.** LMWH, which is less frequently associated with HIT than unfractionated heparin, is recommended for postoperative orthopedic surgery patients (Warkentin and Greinacher, 2004).

VIII. **Bleeding Caused by Defects of the Intrinsic Pathway.**
   A. **Products available for factor replacement**

1. **Fresh frozen plasma** contains all the coagulation factors in nearly normal concentrations. This is useful for patients with liver disease who have multiple factor deficiencies. FFP contains about 200 to 250 U of each factor (about 1 U/mL of factor VIII).

2. **Cryoprecipitate** contains factor VIII, factor XIII, vWF, and fibrinogen. It contains about 100 IU of factor VIII per bag.

3. **Factor VIII concentrates** contain a high concentration of factor VIII and a variable amount of vWF (Humate-P or Koate-HS have adequate amounts). Ultrapure monoclonal preparations are available (Monarc-M and Hemofil-M). They are much more expensive but carry lower risk of viral contamination.

4. **Genetically engineered factor VIII** (Kogenate FS or Helixate FS) carries no risk of disease transmission but **does not contain vWF.**

5. **Prothrombin complex concentration** contains 500 to 1000 IU of prothrombin factor X and factor IX.

6. **Recombinant factor VIIa** is used in bleeding patients with hemophilia and inhibitors to factors VIII or IX.

B. Hemophilias. If possible, patients with bleeding disorders should be treated at a hemophilia treatment center (HTC). Patients treated at an HTC have been shown to live longer and have fewer hospitalizations for bleeding complications.

1. **Hemophilia A is a deficiency of factor VIII.** It is X-linked recessive, but **about 30% of cases are due to new mutations.** Diagnose by factor VIII assay. PT and thrombin clot time are normal. PTT generally is elevated. **Treatment of factor VIII deficiency** is as follows:

a. Minor cuts and abrasions, superficial ecchymosis, and nontraumatic hematuria might require no therapy. CNS trauma requires prophylactic therapy.

b. **Uncomplicated hemarthrosis, noncritical hematomas, and traumatic hematuria** are treated with factor VIII to achieve a factor VIII level of 30% to 40% for at least 72 hours.

c. **Life-threatening hemorrhage and hematomas** in critical locations require factor VIII to achieve a factor VIII level of 80% to 100% for 10 days.

d. **In mild hemophilia, desmopressin 0.3 mg/kg in 50 mL NS IV** over 15 to 30 minutes will transiently increase factor VIII and vWF enough for minor surgery. Levels will return to baseline value with a half-life of 8 to 10 hours. ε-Aminocaproic acid 75 mg/kg PO q6h (4 g q6h in adults) should be used to prevent fibrinolysis. An alternative is tranexamic acid 25 mg/kg tid (1.5 g PO tid in adults).

e. **To calculate the factor VIII dose needed,** first determine the required activity; 1 U/mL = 100% activity; 0.5 U/mL = 50% activity; etc.

Units of factor VIII needed =
  Wt in kg × 0.5 × ([Required activity %] − [Pt's current activity %])

For example, if a 25-kg patient has 10% activity and you want to raise it to 50% activity for an uncomplicated hemarthrosis:

Units of factor VIII needed = 25 kg × 0.5 × (50% − 10%) = 500 units

f. **Consider using ε-aminocaproic acid or tranexamic acid after factor is infused** (see discussion of mild hemophilia for dose).

2. **Hemophilia B is a deficiency of factor IX** (Christmas disease). It is X-linked recessive. Diagnose by factor IX assay. **Treatment of factor IX deficiency by monoclonal or recombinant factor IX product is preferred.**

3. **Factor XI deficiency** is an autosomal recessive disease occurring primarily in Ashkenazi Jews. Bleeding is minor, but when it occurs it is treated with FFP infusion.

IX. Bleeding Caused by Defects of the Extrinsic and Common Pathway.

A. Hepatocellular insufficiency. Patients have decreased production of vitamin K–dependent factors II, VII, IX, and X as well as Factor V, which is produced by the liver but is not vitamin K dependent.

B. Vitamin K deficiency

1. **Cholestasis and other GI disease can cause impaired absorption** of lipid-soluble vitamin K.

2. **Poor dietary intake of vitamin K** causes deficiency.

3. **Broad-spectrum antibiotics.** Gut bacteria produce vitamin K. Loss of these bacteria from antibiotics can lead to vitamin K deficiency.

C. Coumarin anticoagulants

D. Treatment

1. **Vitamin K deficiency**

a. **Mild vitamin K deficiencies can be treated with vitamin K 2.5 to 10 mg PO or SQ daily for 1 to 3 days.** Administration of vitamin K can make it difficult to achieve anticoagulation with warfarin for several days.

b. **For severe hemorrhage,** infuse FFP 15 mL/kg IV and then 5 to 8 mL/kg IV q8-12h.

2. **Liver disease**

a. Fresh frozen plasma.

b. Vitamin K 10 mg PO or SQ for 1 to 3 days.

c. In a patient with fulminant liver failure and severe bleeding not controlled by these treatments, consider recombinant factor VIIa to control bleeding. It is extraordinarily expensive and therefore not indicated if liver recovery or transplant is not expected.

3. **Warfarin overdose**

a. **Do not just treat the INR; you also must assess bleeding risk. If INR is <5 and the patient has a low risk of bleeding, observation and withholding of warfarin for one or two doses is adequate.** Expect a response in 24 to 48 hours. Alternatively, for an INR <9, give vitamin K 1 to 5 mg PO; for INR >9, give vitamin K 5 to 10 mg PO.

b. **For active bleeding,** administer vitamin K 10 mg IV. Also administer FFP or prothrombin complex. With a life-threatening bleed, consider infusing recombinant factor VIIa instead of prothrombin complex.

X. Bleeding Caused by Vascular Defects.

A. TTP–HUS in adults (TTP and HUS have a similar presentation and treatment in adults and thus are discussed together).

1. **Criteria for diagnosis** include thrombocytopenia, microangiopathic hemolytic anemia (schistocytes, helmet cells on smear) with elevated LDH (secondary to the hemolysis), fever, renal failure, and mental status changes or fluctuating focal neurologic deficits. **However, microangiopathic hemolytic anemia in the presence of an otherwise unexplainable thrombocytopenia is considered sufficient to initiate treatment.**

2. **Etiology.** TTP–HUS is often idiopathic. Familial variants exist. It is associated with several drugs, including tacrolimus, cyclosporine, ticlopidine, clopidogrel, quinine, and chemotherapeutic agents. It has been associated with HIV and *Escherichia coli* O157:H7 as well as other subtypes. It can occur in the postpartum period.

3. **Diagnose by clinical presentation**
4. **Outcome.** Mortality is now 5%, much better than in the past. There is a 40% 10-year recurrence rate if the patient survives the initial insult.
5. **Therapy. The most effective therapy is daily plasma exchange** until platelets and LDH normalize. Other modalities have been tried, including high-dose steroids (prednisone 200 mg/d). Plasma exchange has largely replaced other modalities of treatment (including steroids) and is more effective.
6. Transfusions are not recommended.
B. **Hemolytic uremic syndrome in children is distinct from that in adults and is treated differently.**
1. **HUS manifests with** thrombocytopenia, fever, microangiopathic hemolytic anemia, hypertension, and acute renal failure with anuria. It is one of the more common causes of renal failure in children younger than 4 years.
2. **Typical presentation.** Following an episode of bloody diarrhea, the patient develops acute renal failure, microangiopathic hemolytic anemia, and decreased platelets with or without CNS abnormalities.
3. **Etiology.** HUS is induced by a diarrheal illness caused by *E. coli* O157:H7, which produces Shiga toxin (also known as verocytotoxin) but also could be caused by *Shigella, Staphylococcus*, or other *E. coli* subtypes. *E. coli* O157:H7 has been found in pond water, apple cider, and uncooked or undercooked hamburger. Daycare is also a risk. The patient might not have a diarrheal prodrome. **Data suggest that treatment of *E. coli* O157:H7 with antibiotics increases the rate of HUS.**
4. **Therapy** consists of supportive care with early initiation of dialysis.
C. **Henoch–Schönlein purpura** is a generally self-limited vasculitis.
1. It can follow URI or streptococcal infection. Peak incidence is ages 4 to 11 years.
2. Patient presents with purpura, arthralgias, colicky abdominal pain, vomiting, diarrhea, and hematuria (from nephritis).
3. Aspirin and corticosteroids have been used for joint pain and GI symptoms, respectively. Corticosteroids do not change the course of the associated renal disease but may be given (prednisone 1 mg/kg/d or 60 mg in adults).
XI. **Disseminated Intravascular Coagulation.** DIC is uncontrolled activation of clotting factors and fibrinolytic enzymes; it consumes clotting factors and platelets.
A. **DIC occurs as a result of**
1. **Complications of obstetrics,** including abruptio placentae, retained products of conception, amniotic fluid embolism, and eclampsia.
2. **Infection,** especially gram negative with endotoxin release.
3. **Malignancy,** especially adenocarcinoma of pancreas and prostate, acute promyelocytic leukemia.
4. **Other:** Head trauma, heat stroke, venomous snake bites, etc.

B. **To distinguish between liver failure and DIC,** check factor V and factor VIII levels. Both are low in DIC, but only factor V is low in liver failure.

C. **Complications vary in acute versus subacute DIC.**

1. **Subacute DIC** has thromboembolic events including DVT, heart valve thrombosis, stroke, extremity infarction, etc.

2. **Acute DIC** has serious bleeding complications with depletion of clotting factors.

D. **Diagnosis is made on elevated PT/INR or elevated PTT, thrombocytopenia, reduced level of fibrinogen, elevated D dimer, and elevated fibrin degradation products (fibrin split products).** There is also evidence of microangiopathic hemolysis on peripheral smear.

E. **Treatment.** Correct the problems that led to DIC in the first place.

1. **If there are no complications of DIC (no bleeding or thrombosis), there is no need to institute replacement therapy.**

2. **For bleeding complications, you can infuse platelets to replace platelets and cryoprecipitate or FFP to replace clotting factors.** Maintain fibrinogen level at >100 mg/dL and other factors above 50% activity if possible.

3. **If patient has primarily thrombotic complications, you may use heparin 300 to 500 U/h (about 5-10 U/kg/h)** without a bolus but only if it can correct the underlying process. **However, no controlled trials demonstrate benefits from heparin.**

4. **ε-Aminocaproic acid and tranexamic acid, which prevent fibrinolysis, are not recommended** because they can increase thrombotic complications.

XII. **Bleeding Caused by Heparin.**

Treatment is protamine sulfate, which forms an inactive complex with heparin. Use 1 mg of protamine zinc to neutralize about 100 units of heparin. Calculate dose and administer over 10 minutes. Do not exceed 50 mg. Heparin half-life is 30 to 180 minutes; therefore, dose of protamine needed will decrease rapidly with time. Administer slowly to prevent hypotension. Protamine is an anticoagulant when not complexed with heparin. Therefore, follow dosing guidelines carefully.

MANAGEMENT OF ANTICOAGULATION

I. **Heparin** binds to antithrombin III, accelerating its activity.

A. **Initiating heparin (IV, unfractionated).** *Note that doses are different depending on the reason for treatment!* Therapeutic levels are reached much more quickly with weight-based dosing. **Check PT/INR/PTT in 6 hours.** Adjust dose as per protocol in **Table 6-1.** These are guidelines. Use clinical judgment!

6

HEMATOLOGIC, METABOLIC, AND ELECTROLYTE DISORDERS

TABLE 6-1
DOSING OF IV HEPARIN BASED ON BODY WEIGHT*

aPTT (sec)[†]	Dose Change (IU/kg/h)[‡]	Additional Action	Next aPTT (h)[§]
<35 (<1.2 × mean normal)	+4	Rebolus with 80 IU/kg	6
35-45 (1.2-1.5 × mean normal)	+2	Rebolus with 40 IU/kg	6
46-70 (1.5-2.3 × mean normal)	0	0	6[§]
71-90 (2.3-3.0 × mean normal)	−2	0	6
>90 (>3 × mean normal)	−3	Stop infusion 1 h	6

*Initial dosing; loading 80 IU/kg; maintenance infusion:18 IU/kg/h (check aPTT in 6 h).
[†]The therapeutic range in seconds should correspond to a plasma heparin level of 0.2-0.4 IU/mL by protamine sulfate or 0.3-0.6 IU/mL by amidolytic assay. When aPTT is checked at 6 h or longer, steady-state kinetics can be assumed.
[‡]Heparin 25,000 IU in 250 mL D_5W. Infuse at rate dictated by body weight through an infusion apparatus calibrated for low flow rates.
[§]During the first 24 h, repeat aPTT q6h. Thereafter, monitor APTT once every morning unless it is outside the therapeutic range.
From Hirsh J, Raschke R: *Chest* 126(3 Suppl):188S-203S, 2004.

1. **Thromboembolic disease.** Weight-based dosing (bolus of 80 U/kg and start a drip at 18 U/kg/h) is preferred over the traditional regimen (bolus of 5000 U and start a drip at 1000 U/h) **(Table 6-2).** Note that this dosing generally overshoots the PTT but improves outcomes overall.

2. **Acute coronary syndrome**

   a. Bolus of 60 to 70 U/kg (maximum 5000 units), then drip at 12 to 15 U/kg per hour (maximum 1000 U/h). Goal is aPTT of 1.5 to 2 times normal (50-75 sec).

   b. **If patient is receiving tPA or other thrombolytic,** bolus of 60 U/kg (max 4000 units) and drip at 15 U/kg/h (max 1000 U/h). Goal is aPTT of 1.5 to 2 times normal (50-75 sec).

3. See section XI for management of bleeding caused by heparin.

B. **LMW heparin.** Three different products have been approved. For enoxaparin, full-dose anticoagulation requires 1 mg/kg SQ bid. No need to follow PT/INR/PTT. Risk of heparin-induced thrombocytopenia is much less with LMWH (<1%).

1. **Special circumstances**

   a. **Unfractionated heparin is preferable in patients with a creatinine clearance of 25 to 30 mL/min or less who need full anticoagulation.** For DVT prophylaxis, LMWH can be used in patients with renal disease.

   b. No dose adjustment is required for obesity unless weight is greater than **150 kg** (see monitoring below).

2. **Monitoring**

   a. **Routine monitoring of LMWH is not recommended.**

   b. **Monitoring may be useful in the following situations:** critical ICU patients in whom LMWHs have variable effects, markedly obese patients (weight >150 kg), children, patients with creatinine clearance <30 mL/min (unfractionated heparin is recommended if CrCl < 30 mL/min).

TABLE 6-2

RECOMMENDED THERAPEUTIC RANGE FOR ORAL ANTICOAGULANT THERAPY

Indication	INR
Prophylaxis of venous thrombosis (high-risk surgery)	Optimal INR 2.0-3.0
Treatment of venous thrombosis	
Treatment of pulmonary embolism	
Atrial fibrillation	
Tissue heart valves	INR 2.0-3.0 for 3 mo, then low-dose daily aspirin.
DVT **while on warfarin** with INR 2.0-3.0	No good studies. Several strategies can be tried: increase INR to 3.5, add aspirin, or change to SQ LMW heparin. Vena caval filters can be used but are of questionable efficacy and are likely counterproductive.
Symptomatic anticardiolipin antibody syndrome (if no history of DVT, no need to anticoagulate).	For first thrombotic event, initial INR goal should be 2-3. If subsequent event while on warfarin, goal is 2.5-3.5.
Tilting disk valves and bileaflet valves in mitral position	2.5-3.5
Caged ball valves and caged disk valves	2.5-3.5 and ASA
Bileaflet mechanical valve in aortic position	2.0-3.0

Modified from Salem DM et al: *Chest* 126(3 Suppl):457S-482S, 2004.

c. **To monitor, check anti–factor Xa activity 4 hours after a dose is given.** It should be at steady state at this point. For those being treated bid, maintain 0.6 to 1.0 IU/mL of anti-Xa activity. The appropriate level for daily dosing is less well established.

3. **For bleeding complications,** give protamine 1 mg per 100 anti-Xa units administered if the last dose of LMWH was within 8 hours (for example enoxaparin contains anti-Xa 100 U/mg). A second dose of 0.5 mg per 100 anti-Xa units can be given if bleeding continues. Dosing has not been established for longer than 8 hours after administration of LMWH, but it seems reasonable to start with 0.5 mg per 100 anti-Xa units and repeat if needed. Anti-Xa is not as effective as when used with unfractionated heparin.

C. **Caveats**

1. **Unfractionated and LMW heparin can cause thrombocytopenia.** Due to risk of HITTS, monitor platelets at least every 2 days during the first 2 weeks of therapy. See section VII C for management of HITTS.

2. **Heparin should be given for at least 5 days and continued for 2 days after the INR is therapeutic.**

3. **A hypercoagulable state will exist when heparin is stopped if the duration of heparin administration has been at least 72 hours** from relative antithrombin III deficiency.

II. **Warfarin.**

A. **To initiate warfarin (Coumadin etc.) (see Table 6-2 for INR goals for various conditions.)**

B. **Warfarin should be started at the same time as heparin.** Remember that heparin should be continued for at least 2 days after a therapeutic INR is obtained.

C. **Start warfarin at 5 to 10 mg qhs in most patients.** A starting dose no higher than 5 mg is recommended for elderly patients. The INR will change 24 to 48 hours after a dose of warfarin. Therefore wait at least 48 hours to see how a change affects the INR before making any additional changes to the warfarin dose.

D. **Hereditary resistance to warfarin occurs,** which might require doses that are larger than the usual dose to achieve a therapeutic INR. **However, noncompliance is by far the most common cause of a subtherapeutic INR.** Other patients are highly sensitive to warfarin and need only low doses of the drug to achieve a therapeutic INR.

E. **Monitor INR daily until level is therapeutic and has been therapeutic with a stable INR for 2 days;** then monitor 2 to 3 times weekly for 1 to 2 weeks and then every 4 weeks.

III. **Newer Anticoagulants.**

A. **Direct thrombin inhibitors** include lepirudin and argatroban, which are approved for the treatment of HITTS, as well as bivalirudin, which is approved for unstable angina patients undergoing PTCA.

B. **Factor X inhibitors** include fondaparinux, which has been approved for postoperative DVT prophylaxis in patients undergoing orthopedic procedures at a dose of 2.5 mg SQ daily. Factor X inhibitors are approved for use, along with warfarin, in patients with symptomatic acute PE or DVT. Dosing is weight based.

IV. **Risk of Embolic Event in the Absence of Anticoagulation (Table 6-3).**

V. **Management of Anticoagulation for Surgical Procedures (Box 6-1).**

VI. **Vena-caval Filters.** Vena-caval filters can be used in the short term. Over a 1-year period **there is no benefit in reduced pulmonary embolism and no reduced death, and there is actually an increased risk of DVT even when used with anticoagulation.**

ANEMIA

I. **Definition.**

A. Anemia is defined as a low Hct and Hb. Normal Hct is 36% to 48%, and normal Hb is 12 to 16 g/dL.

TABLE 6-3
ANNUALIZED RISK OF THROMBOTIC COMPLICATIONS IN THE ABSENCE OF ANTICOAGULANT THERAPY FOR SELECTED CONDITIONS

Condition	Annualized Thrombosis Risk, %
Lone atrial fibrillation	1
Average risk atrial fibrillation	5
Biologic heart valve (e.g. porcine), > 3 months	0.5-3.3%
Thromboembolic event, single, > 3 months	8%
High-risk atrial fibrillation with stroke, embolism in last 12 months	12
Dual-leaflet (St. Jude) aortic valve prosthesis	10–12
Recurrent thromboembolic events	15%
Biologic heart valve (e.g. porcine), first 3 months	6% over first 3 months (high risk)
Single-leaflet (Bjork-Shiley) aortic valve prosthesis	23
Dual-leaflet (St. Jude) mitral valve prosthesis	22
Thromboembolic event, < 3 months	1% per day over first 1 month. Still high risk up to 3 months, though
Multiple St. Jude prostheses	91

Thromboembolic event = DVT, PE

B. **Changes in intravascular volume can be reflected in the hematocrit.** Fluid overload leads to hemodilution and a lower Hct, whereas volume contraction can yield a spuriously elevated Hct even in the face of anemia. **Fluids and blood products equilibrate in the circulation within 15 to 30 minutes so there is no need to wait hours to recheck a Hb/Hct after blood administration.**

II. **Signs and Symptoms of Anemia.** (Signs and symptoms are neither sensitive nor specific.)
A. **Symptoms** include dyspnea on exertion, palpitations, angina pectoris, light-headedness, syncope, anorexia, and tinnitus.
B. **Signs** include pallor of mucous membranes and skin, mild tachycardia, peripheral edema, and systolic ejection murmurs from increased flow.
C. **Anemia may be asymptomatic if it is long-standing.** Patients can adapt to a gradual change in Hb and Hct.

III. **History.** Obtain history, including presence of jaundice or gallstones (hemolysis), history of blood loss, alcohol abuse, presence of pica, diarrhea, other chronic illnesses, drugs.

IV. **Laboratory Evaluation. All anemic patients should have the following labs:**
A. **CBC with differential,** peripheral smear.
B. **Mean corpuscular volume.** In hemolysis, elevated MCV reflects reticulocytosis.
C. **Serum ferritin** (estimate of Fe stores)
D. **TIBC** (mmol/L) = transferrin (mg/L) × 0.025. Transferrin saturation = serum iron/TIBC (normal is >16).

BOX 6-1

RECOMMENDATIONS FOR MANAGING ANTICOAGULATION THERAPY
IN PATIENTS REQUIRING INVASIVE PROCEDURES (SEE TABLE 6-3 FOR RISK)

LOW RISK OF THROMBOEMBOLISM (< 8%)

Stop warfarin therapy approximately 4 d before surgery. Allow the INR to return to near normal. Briefly use postoperative prophylaxis (if the intervention itself creates a higher risk of thrombosis) with a low dose of UFH (5000 units SC) or a prophylactic dose of LMWH and simultaneously begin warfarin therapy. Alternatively, a low dose of UFH or a prophylactic dose of LMWH can also be used preoperatively.

INTERMEDIATE RISK OF THROMBOEMBOLISM ≈ 9-12%

Stop warfarin approximately 4 d before surgery. Allow the INR to fall. Cover the patient beginning 2 d preoperatively with a low dose of UFH (5000 units SC) or a prophylactic dose of LMWH and then commence therapy with low-dose UFH (or LMWH) and warfarin postoperatively. Some authors recommend a higher dose of UFH or a full dose of LMWH in this setting.

HIGH RISK OF THROMBOEMBOLISM (> 12%)

Stop warfarin approximately 4 d before surgery. Allow the INR to return to normal. Begin therapy with a full dose of UFH or a full dose of LMWH as the INR falls (approximately 2 d preoperatively). UFH can be given as an SC injection before the patient is admitted. It can then be given as a continuous IV infusion after hospital admission in preparation for surgery and discontinued approximately 5 h before surgery with the expectation that the anticoagulant effect will have worn off at the time of surgery. It is also possible to continue with SC UFH or LMWH and to stop therapy 12-24 h before surgery with the expectation that the anticoagulant effect will be very low or have worn off at the time of surgery.

LOW RISK OF BLEEDING

Continue warfarin therapy at a lower dose and operate at an INR of 1.3-1.5, an intensity that has been shown to be safe in randomized trials of gynecologic and orthopedic surgical patients. The dose of warfarin can be lowered 4 or 5 d before surgery. Warfarin therapy can then be restarted postoperatively and supplemented with a low dose of UFH (5000 units SC) or a prophylactic dose of LMWH if necessary.

Adapted from Ansell J, Hirsh J, Poller L, et al: *Chest* 126(3 Suppl):204S-233S, 2004.

E. Reticulocyte count

1. **The reticulocyte count is expressed as a percentage of total cells counted and must be corrected to a total number of reticulocytes per microliter.** This is done by multiplying the RBC count by the percentage of reticulocytes. Normal is 50 to 100,000 reticulocytes/μL.
2. **Reticulocyte counts that are normal or low (in the face of anemia) suggest inability of the bone marrow to respond to anemia (marrow failure).**
3. **Increased reticulocyte counts indicate acute blood loss or hemolysis with a marrow that is able to respond.**
4. If reticulocyte count is low or normal, reflecting the inability of the marrow to respond to anemia ("marrow failure"), the MCV is helpful in

diagnosing anemia. The MCV is either normocytic at 80 to 100 fL, microcytic at <80 fL, or macrocytic at >100 fL.

F. **Consider serum haptoglobin and serum free hemoglobin** to evaluate for hemolysis.

G. **Consider serum transferrin receptor and transferrin receptor complex,** which **accurately reflect bone stores of iron and can substitute for a bone marrow evaluation of iron stores** in many cases. These are not needed in all cases but serum transferrin receptor and receptor complex are elevated in iron-deficiency anemia and can be used to tell if those with anemia of chronic disease have coexistent iron-deficiency anemia. **Be careful. Serum transferrin receptor and receptor complex will also be elevated in hemolysis because of increased demand for iron.** Thus it should only be used when trying to diagnose iron deficiency in those with coexistent anemia of chronic disease.

V. **Differential Diagnosis of anemia** is given in **Box 6-2** and **Table 6-4.**

VI. **Microcytosis and Unresponsive Marrow.** Low or normal reticulocyte count and anemia.

A. See Box 6-2 for differential diagnosis.

B. **Iron deficiency is the most common cause of microcytosis with a low reticulocyte count. Iron deficiency is occasionally normocytic.**

1. **Exam.** Skin and conjunctivae may show pallor; nails may be dry and brittle, with ridges; cardiovascular exam may reveal tachycardia and flow murmur. Stomatitis or glossitis may be present. However, physical signs and symptoms are not sensitive enough to rule in or out the diagnosis of anemia.

2. **Lab tests**

a. **CBC shows microcytic, hypochromic cells;** platelet count may be elevated.

b. **Low serum ferritin is the best overall test for outpatients but is not useful in many hospitalized patients or those with chronic illness.** Serum ferritin is an acute phase reactant and is elevated by fever, cancer, and other inflammatory processes. Thus, patients can be iron deficient but have a normal or elevated ferritin.

c. **In patients who are hospitalized or chronically ill, serum transferrin receptor and transferrin receptor complex are better tests for iron deficiency.** These levels are elevated in iron deficiency anemia (see earlier for a discussion of serum transferrin receptors and transferrin receptor complex) but are normal in isolated anemia of chronic disease.

d. **Increased TIBC with transferrin saturation <15% and low serum iron.**

e. **Bone marrow biopsy** specimen shows decreased iron stores.

f. Must differentiate from the thalassemias and anemia of chronic disease. Red cell distribution width (RDW) is increased in iron-deficiency anemia but usually normal in thalassemias.

g. **Other work-up.** All adults with iron-deficiency anemia should be evaluated for upper and lower GI bleeding.

3. **Treatment.** Identify and stop any source of blood loss. Give ferrous sulfate 325 mg PO tid. Enteric-coated and timed-release products are

BOX 6-2

DIFFERENTIAL DIAGNOSIS OF ANEMIA BASED ON CELL SIZE AND MARROW RESPONSE (RETICULOCYTE COUNT)

MICROCYTOSIS (MCV <70) WITH UNRESPONSIVE MARROW (LOW OR NORMAL RETICULOCYTE COUNT)

Iron deficiency anemia

Blood loss (GI, menses), etc.

Lead

Insufficient intake

Anemia of chronic disease (microcytic 30% of cases)

Thalassemias

Sideroblastic anemia

Increased iron need (infancy, pregnancy, etc.)

Decreased absorption of iron (gastrectomy, achlorhydria, chronic diarrhea)

NORMOCYTOSIS WITH UNRESPONSIVE MARROW (LOW OR NORMAL RETICULOCYTE COUNT)

Iron deficiency anemia (rarely)

Anemia of chronic disease

Primary marrow disorders

Aplastic anemia

Toxin-induced anemia (some)

Infectious anemia (e.g., HIV)

Graft versus host disease

MACROCYTOSIS WITH UNRESPONSIVE MARROW (LOW OR NORMAL RETICULOCYTE COUNT)

Vitamin B_{12} and folate deficiency

Some drugs

Arsenic

Alcohol (occasionally)

Hypothyroidism

Primary marrow disorders (e.g., myelodysplastic disorders)

Liver disease

ANEMIA WITH RESPONSIVE MARROW (RETICULOCYTOSIS)

Hemolytic anemia including microangiopathic

HUS–TTP

Warm and cold antibody induced

Valve prosthesis

Eclampsia/HELLP

Malignant hypertension

Red blood cell defects (e.g., spherocytosis, paroxysmal nocturnal hemoglobinuria)

Recent hemorrhage

TABLE 6-4
DIAGNOSIS OF ANEMIA BASED ON LABORATORY RESULTS

Anemia	MCV	Reticulocyte count	Ferritin	Iron	TIBC	Serum transferrin receptor/receptor complex	Comments
Iron deficiency anemia	Low	Low	Low	Low	High	High	Ferritin may be falsely high from inflammation, chronic illness
Anemia of chronic disease	Low or normal	Low	High or normal	Low	Low	Normal (unless coexistent iron deficiency)	
Hemolytic anemia	High or normal	High				High because of increased iron demand	Elevated LDH, bilirubin possible; low haptoglobin
B_{12}/folate deficiency	High	Low					Low B_{12} or folate; may have markedly elevated LDH
Sideroblastic anemia	Most decreased; variants with increased or normal MCVS exist.	Low or normal	High	High	Normal		
Thalassemia	Low	Low	Normal	Normal	Normal	High because of increased iron demand	These patients can develop iron overload with repeated transfusions

HEMATOLOGIC, METABOLIC, AND ELECTROLYTE DISORDERS **6**

poorly absorbed. Iron is better absorbed if administered between meals on an empty stomach but causes less GI upset if taken with meals. Vitamin C increases absorption. Calcium and magnesium can impair iron absorption. Iron can impair thyroxin absorption. Treat for 6 months to replace body stores. Iron is toxic and should be kept away from children. **If marrow does not respond to iron (the patient does not develop a higher reticulocyte count), consider an alternate diagnosis** such as thalassemia or another superimposed cause of anemia such as inflammation, vitamin B_{12} or folate deficiency, continued bleeding, etc.

C. **Anemia of chronic disease** is microcytic in 30% of cases. See VII B later in this section for details.

D. **Thalassemias.** Hemoglobin is made up of paired α and β chains. Thalassemia is caused by a defect in the synthesis of either α or β chains. **Normally there are four genes to produce α chains but only two to produce β chains.**

1. **α-Thalassemia** is caused by decreased synthesis of Hb α subchain.

a. **α-Thalassemia minima.** One of the four genes is deleted but there are no hematologic abnormalities.

b. **α-Thalassemia trait.** Two of four genes are deleted. RBCs are microcytic and hypochromic, and there is no significant anemia.

c. **Hemoglobin H disease.** Hb is composed of four **β chains** because three of four **α genes** are deleted. Moderate anemia results, and Hb carries oxygen poorly.

2. **β-Thalassemia minor** is caused by decreased synthesis of β chains. One of two genes is not present (heterozygous). There is mild anemia with pronounced microcytosis and possibly an increased RBC count.

a. **Diagnosis.** Hb electrophoresis shows increased HbA2, usually >4%, and possibly an increase of hemoglobin F.

b. **Treatment.** None. Genetic counseling is necessary.

3. **β-Thalassemia major.** Both genes for β-chain synthesis are defective or missing.

a. **Presentation.** Manifestations develop during first year of life as fetal hemoglobin levels decrease. Patients usually present with severe anemia (Hct <20%). There is pronounced wasting, jaundice, hepatosplenomegaly, slow growth and development, and delayed onset of secondary sex features. The patient has skeletal abnormalities secondary to bone marrow expansion.

b. **Diagnosis.** Hb electrophoresis shows large amounts of HbF, variable amounts of HbA, and increased HbA2.

c. **Treatment** includes transfusion, splenectomy, deferoxamine (to prevent iron overload from transfusions), and folic acid supplementation. Watch for development of hemochromatosis. Cord blood stem cell transplantation and compatible relative bone marrow transplantation have been used with success.

d. **Prognosis.** Many patients die before puberty secondary to hemochromatosis.

E. Sideroblastic anemia. Amorphous iron is deposited in RBC mitochondria, which may form a ring around the RBC nucleus during development (therefore ringed sideroblasts).

1. **Cause** is ineffective erythropoiesis.

a. **Hereditary.** Multiple forms; most are X-linked recessive.

b. **Acquired.** Drugs and toxins (alcohol, lead, INH, chloramphenicol), neoplasia and inflammation, malnutrition, copper deficiency, zinc excess, idiopathic. Sideroblastic anemia can also represent a myelodysplastic syndrome.

2. **Lab tests.** CBC might show normochromic or hypochromic cells; anisocytosis and poikilocytosis are pronounced; possibly normocytic or microcytic cells. Sideroblasts may or may not be present. Iron studies show increased serum iron, increased ferritin, increased transferrin saturation, decreased TIBC. LDH may be elevated.

3. **Presentation.** Patients can present with anemia or hemochromatosis.

4. **Treatment**

a. Withdraw offending agent, especially alcohol.

b. Pyridoxine 200 mg daily for 2 to 3 months with or without folate. One third of hereditary cases will respond.

c. **Depending on anemia and iron stores, phlebotomy or deferoxamine,** 40 mg/kg per day SQ by infusion pump over 12 hours for 5 days per week might be necessary.

d. **Splenectomy is contraindicated in hereditary forms.** There is a high rate of fatal thromboembolic events with splenectomy.

VII. **Normocytosis and Unresponsive Marrow.** Low or normal reticulocyte count and anemia.

A. **Iron deficiency.** Generally there is microcytosis, but normocytosis is possible (see earlier).

B. **Anemia of chronic disease** is probably the most common anemia except for blood loss–related iron-deficiency anemia.

1. **Causes** include chronic infections (subacute bacterial endocarditis, osteomyelitis, AIDS), chronic inflammatory disorders (RA, SLE, sarcoidosis, renal failure), neoplasms, hypothyroidism, liver disease, alcoholism, CHF, and diabetes. Some authors do not classify the anemias associated with kidney, liver, and endocrinologic diseases into this category.

2. **Multifactorial causes** include unresponsive bone marrow, inability to mobilize iron stores, slightly decreased RBC life span.

3. **Lab tests.** Hemoglobin is generally 9 to 11 mg/dL. Cells may be normocytic or microcytic. **Serum ferritin is usually increased but may be normal. Serum transferrin, TIBC, and serum iron are decreased. Transferrin saturation is decreased.** Erythropoietin levels will be low compared with similarly anemic patients with iron-deficiency anemia (but higher than those in normal persons). Bone marrow shows adequate iron stores.

4. **Treatment.** Treat underlying disease. Transfuse only as needed for symptoms. Erythropoietin along with supplemental iron is the

treatment of choice. Start with 40,000 units SQ weekly and increase to 60,000 units SQ weekly if no response in 4 weeks. If no response by 12 weeks, the patient is not going to respond, and erythropoietin should be discontinued. Reduce dose when Hct reaches 36% and hold dose if Hct reaches 40%.

C. Primary marrow disorders

1. **Primary marrow disorders include** congenital aplastic anemia, acquired aplastic anemia, and marrow depression from drugs and toxins (antineoplastic agents, immunosuppressive drugs, ionizing radiation, benzene, chloramphenicol, antithyroid agents, oral hypoglycemics, TMP–SMX, ticlopidine), and from infections (hepatitis, mononucleosis, GVHD, lupus, HIV).

2. **Clinical manifestations** include weakness and fatigue from anemia, bleeding from thrombocytopenia, and infection from leukopenia.

3. **Diagnosis requires bone marrow biopsy.** Hematology consultation is advised for therapy.

VIII. Macrocytosis with Unresponsive Marrow. Low or normal reticulocyte count and anemia.

A. Causes

1. **Vitamin B_{12} deficiency** from malabsorption from pernicious anemia, gastrectomy, Crohn's disease, celiac sprue. Strict vegetarians are at high risk; not a problem in lacto–ovo vegetarians. In the elderly, achlorhydria and lack of intrinsic factor can decrease vitamin B_{12} absorption.

2. **Folic acid deficiency** is usually caused by poor intake in alcoholics and indigent persons or by increased demand in pregnancy.

3. **Drugs** including methotrexate, trimethoprim, pentamidine, AZT, hydroxyurea, alkylating agents, and chloramphenicol.

4. **Alcohol** also causes macrocytosis independent of nutritional effects.

5. **Endocrine causes** including hypothyroidism.

B. Clinical presentation

1. **Vitamin B_{12} deficiency**

a. **Symptoms include** gastrointestinal symptoms (glossitis, taste bud atrophy, anorexia, weight loss, diarrhea). Neurologic symptoms include numbness, paresthesias, weakness, ataxia, sphincter dysfunction, positive Babinski sign (dorsiflexed big toe).

b. **Signs include those of anemia** (pallor, tachycardia, etc.) and neurologic signs of hyperreflexia or hyporeflexia, positive Romberg sign, impaired positional and vibratory sensation, depressed mentation, hallucinations, and personality changes. Neurologic disease can occur with normal hematocrit.

c. **Laboratory:** Low B_{12} level. High methylmalonate level which should drop with treatment.

d. **Some suggest periodic screening of patients older than 55 years, because symptoms of deficiency can exist before hematologic changes occur.** If 258 pmol/L is used as cutoff, 40.5% of the elderly may be deficient.

e. **Patients with pernicious anemia have a higher rate of esophageal, stomach, and colorectal tumors and hypothyroidism. Be particularly vigilant in screening these patients.**

2. **Folate deficiency.** Signs and symptoms are the same as in vitamin B_{12} deficiency, except that the patient is more likely to be malnourished; neurologic abnormalities are generally absent.

C. **Diagnosis.** Elevated MCV, low reticulocyte count. However, many have normal indices because of coexistent thalassemia or iron deficiency, etc. Patients have low vitamin B_{12} or low RBC folate levels, respectively. **RBC folate is preferred because serum folate level varies with meals and is an unreliable indicator of basal state. With borderline values, consider checking homocysteine and methylmalonic acid levels.** Both are elevated in B_{12} deficiency; only homocysteine is elevated in folate deficiency. Thrombocytopenia (50%) and leukopenia are late findings. Smear shows anisocytosis, poikilocytosis, basophilic stippling, and hypersegmentation of neutrophils.

D. **Therapy**

1. **Vitamin B_{12} deficiency.** Cyanocobalamin 1 mg IM daily for 7 days, then 1 mg IM weekly for 4 weeks, then 1 mg IM every month for life. Oral replacement in compliant patients works just as well, even in the presence of pernicious anemia. Use 1 to 2 mg PO qd.

2. **Folate deficiency.** Folic acid 1 mg PO qd is sufficient.

3. **Blood transfusions are usually not required.** Empiric therapy before a diagnosis is established can be dangerous. A patient deficient in vitamin B_{12} might have a hematologic response to folic acid but an exacerbation of neurologic symptoms.

IX. **Anemia with Increased Red Blood Cell Production.**

A. **Usually acute anemias are primarily associated with blood loss or hemolysis.** They can be caused by prolonged running or marching, as well as microangiopathic changes as with HUS–TTP or artificial valves.

B. **Hemolytic anemia**

1. **Presentation.** Patients usually have classic signs and symptoms of anemia (see section II A). Hemolytic crisis, which is rare, manifests with fever, chills, tachycardia, tachypnea, backache, and hemoglobinuria. This can progress to renal failure from hemoglobinuria. In addition to the causes discussed later, consider malaria, ehrlichiosis, etc. Patients with chronic hemolysis (e.g., sickle cell patients) can develop cholelithiasis secondary to pigment stones.

2. **Lab tests**

a. **Often normochromic–normocytic** but may be macrocytic.

b. **Generally elevated indirect bilirubin with normal direct bilirubin.** Haptoglobin is decreased; serum LDH is increased; hemosiderinuria and hemoglobinuria may be present. Serum free hemoglobin may be increased.

c. **Coombs' tests.** Direct Coombs' test measures antibody that is attached to RBCs (antibody directly on RBC). Indirect Coombs' test measures circulating anti-RBC antibodies in serum. Example: In Rh disease,

HEMATOLOGIC, METABOLIC, AND ELECTROLYTE DISORDERS

6

mother has positive indirect Coombs' test (circulating anti-D antibody). Rh-positive child has positive direct Coombs' test because mother's antibodies are coating cells (tested after birth).

3. **Hemolytic anemia secondary to acquired hemolytic disorders**

a. **Warm antibody–induced hemolytic anemia.** Antibodies are most active at temperature of 37° C. About 70% of those with antibody-related hemolytic disease have warm antibodies.

   (1) **May be primary (60%) or secondary (40%)** to underlying disease affecting the immune system (e.g., CLL, non-Hodgkin's lymphoma, SLE, myeloma, HIV). Commonly occurs with drugs (penicillin, α-methyldopa, INH, sulfonamides).

   (2) **Direct Coombs' test is usually positive,** and generally there is an IgG antibody.

   (3) **Anemia is often severe,** with Hb of 7.0 or less; can be fatal.

   (4) Patient can have enlarged spleen and liver, jaundice.

   (5) **No therapy is required if disease is mild.** With significant hemolysis, prednisone 1 to 1.5 mg/kg per day, transfusions, splenectomy (50%-75% respond; might relapse), and cytotoxic agents (cyclophosphamide 50-150 mg/d or azathioprine 50-200 mg/d) have been used with some success. Hematology consultation is recommended. Also need folic acid 1 mg/d.

b. **Cold-antibody–induced hemolytic anemia** represents about 15% of those with antibody-related hemolysis. Agglutination of cells is followed by hemolysis.

   (1) **These IgM antibodies agglutinate RBCs, generally at temperature of 4° to 35° C** but occasionally up to 37° C. Seen with *Mycoplasma pneumoniae*, infectious mononucleosis, lymphoid neoplasms (e.g., CLL, Waldenstrom's macroglobulinemia), etc. Most patients are older than 60 years.

   (2) **Diagnose by RBC agglutination on smear, absurdly elevated MCV (secondary to clumping);** blood bank will detect cold agglutinin.

   (3) **May note cold-related symptoms,** such as acrocyanosis, that improve on warming.

   (4) **Treatment.** Maintain patient in warm environment. Chlorambucil 4 to 6 mg/d is the most common agent used if antibody is due to a neoplastic process. Consider plasma exchange in seriously ill patients. Splenectomy and steroids are generally not helpful, but an occasional patient responds to prednisone 100 mg/d if there are low titers of cold agglutinins. If related to infectious process, anemia generally resolves spontaneously in weeks.

c. **Trauma in the circulation**

   (1) **Abnormalities of the vessel wall** are seen in malignant hypertension, eclampsia, TTP, valve prostheses, and microvascular thrombi.

   (2) **Diagnosis.** Fragmented and nucleated RBCs. See appropriate section on underlying disease.

   (3) **Therapy** is directed toward the underlying illness.

d. **Red blood cell defects.** Hereditary spherocytosis (incidence is about 220 persons per million in the general population; it is inherited, but one third of cases are de novo), hereditary elliptocytosis, hereditary stomatocytosis can cause a hemolytic anemia. May develop aplastic crisis secondary to parvovirus B19. Splenectomy generally prevents hemolysis.

e. **Paroxysmal nocturnal hemoglobinuria.** Onset is in adulthood, hemoglobinuria after sleep, venous thrombosis and embolism, evidence of chronic hemolysis. Diagnose with flow cytometry demonstrating absent CD 55 and CD 59. Average life span after diagnosis is 10 years.

SICKLE CELL ANEMIA

I. **Incidence.** About 0.3% of African Americans are homozygous (have sickle cell disease); 13% of African Americans are heterozygous (carriers; have sickle cell trait).

II. **Genetics.** Autosomal recessive. Abnormal hemoglobin S, leading to sickling of RBCs.

III. **Clinical.**

A. **Anemia** (see III A and III B in anemia section above for clinical symptoms).

B. **Sickle crisis** incidence is 60% per year. Sickle crisis is defined as sickling of cells causing vasoocclusive disease with bone, lung, and renal infarctions. It is often precipitated by exposure to cold and, importantly, infection. The most common sites of pain are lumbar spine, abdomen, femur, knees, sternum, ribs, shoulder, and elbows. Joint involvement may be symmetric. It may be associated with abdominal distention or ileus. Patients can have fever and pulmonary infarctions (see discussion of acute chest syndrome later). It may be difficult to differentiate abdominal pain of a sickle crisis from the pain of a surgical acute abdomen. Patients can develop priapism, skin ulcers, and retinal vessel obstruction.

C. **Fever** results from infections, especially pneumonia and especially in children. If temperature is >38° C (101° F), start broad-spectrum antibiotics (e.g., ceftriaxone) while searching for a cause of infection; patients are de facto splenectomized secondary to repeated infarction. You need to treat fever aggressively because encapsulated organisms such as pneumococci and *Haemophilus influenzae* cause high mortality.

D. **Bilirubin is increased secondary to increased RBC destruction.** Cholelithiasis is common (75%).

E. **Acute chest syndrome** occurs in 40% of patients with sickle cell anemia.

1. **It is characterized by** pleuritic chest pain, fever, hypoxia, cough, dyspnea, rales, and rhonchi (any combination). Usually there is a rapid decrease in Hb, with increased platelets and WBCs.

2. It is a major source of mortality in those with sickle cell disease (15% of deaths in adults). There may be a delayed development of infiltrates on CXR. It is difficult to differentiate from pneumonia.

F. **Acute splenic sequestration syndrome,** which causes hemoglobin to drop 3 to 6 g/dL, occurs in children younger than 3 years (requires mostly intact spleen). Spleen is palpable, and patients get rapidly shocky and require blood transfusions acutely. Mortality is 15% and recurrence is 50%. Splenectomy should be considered to prevent recurrence.

G. **Aplastic anemia** occurs in response to parvovirus B19 and others.

H. **Sickle trait.** Patients have hematuria and sloughing of papilla, trouble concentrating urine.

IV. Diagnosis.

A. Microscopic examination of blood smear shows typical sickle-shaped RBCs. Most states perform universal neonatal screening for sickle cell disease.

B. Hemoglobin electrophoresis is performed on patients with positive screening tests to confirm the diagnosis.

V. Treatment.

A. Acute treatment of sickle pain crisis and acute chest syndrome

1. **Pain control** (such as IV morphine), administration of oxygen, hydration, transfusion for evidence of cardiopulmonary failure, or Hb < 5 gm/dL.

2. **If fever is >38° C (101° F), start antibiotics** (e.g., ceftriaxone) while looking for source of infection.

3. **Treatment of acute chest syndrome.** Admission for hydration, oxygen, pain control, antibiotics, and simple blood transfusion or possibly exchange transfusion if seriously ill.

B. Chronic and prophylactic treatment

1. **Infection prophylaxis** including pneumococcal, meningococcal, and *H. influenzae* vaccines during childhood. Start prophylactic penicillin 125 mg PO bid at 2 months of age and increase to 250 mg PO bid starting at 3 years of age. **Can stop this prophylaxis at age 5 but only if the child has not had a severe pneumococcal infection.** However, any fever should be aggressively treated with antibiotics (e.g., ceftriaxone) regardless of whether the patient is taking penicillin or not.

2. **Folic acid,** 1 mg/d.

3. **Hydroxyurea** has been shown to increase fetal hemoglobin and decrease frequency of sickle cell crises. Long-term effects (e.g., malignancy induction) are unknown. Start at 500 mg/d in adults, 10 to 15 mg/kg per day in children (>2 years). Increase to 1000 to 2000 mg/day (20 to 30 mg/kg per day). Keep track of blood counts, etc.

4. **Indications for transfusions.** Any child with a stroke should have prophylactic transfusions. Exchange transfusions to keep HbS under 30% will prevent recurrent strokes. Allow HbS to increase to 50% at age 4 years. Even though it is not yet standard of care, prophylactic transfusions for those with abnormal intracranial blood flow by Doppler

will prevent strokes and should be considered (see Adams et al, 1998, for protocol). Patients age 2 through 16 years should be screened twice yearly by Doppler.

5. **Surgery.** Transfuse to Hct of 30% before surgery (as effective as getting HbS to below 30% and has fewer complications).
6. **Bone marrow transplantation** has been used with success in some cases.

G6PD DEFICIENCY

I. **Incidence.** G6PD deficiency is an X-linked disorder that is expressed in 10% of African American men and fewer African American women. It also occurs in persons of Mediterranean ancestry. There are several hundred known variants.
II. **Clinically.** The deficiency causes a variable degree of hemolysis in RBCs after exposure to substances or situations that cause oxidative stress.
A. **Drugs.** Sulfonamides, nitrofurantoin, salicylates, vitamin C, quinine, quinidine, and dapsone.
B. **Foods.** Fava beans cause particularly severe hemolysis (generally only in those with the Mediterranean variant).
C. **Infections.** Fever, viral illnesses, and bacterial infections.
D. **DKA and renal failure.**
III. **Diagnosis. Check G6PD levels when reticulocyte count is normal.** If levels are checked after acute hemolysis, the cells surviving in the circulation and the young reticulocytes might have a normal G6PD level.
IV. **Treatment.**
A. Because only old RBCs are vulnerable, generally less than 25% of the RBC mass is affected.
B. Patients can develop renal failure secondary to hemolysis. Maintain hydration and withdraw offending agents.
C. Educate the patient about risks of oxidative medications and fava beans.

HEMOCHROMATOSIS

I. **Hereditary Hemochromatosis.**
A. **General.** Hemochromatosis is an inherited disorder that results from excessive iron absorption from food. It is fairly common in European populations and is 10% heterozygous and 0.5% homozygous. It generally manifests in those 40 to 60 years of age. Men are more commonly symptomatic than women.
B. **Clinically** the patient can have evidence of liver failure (cirrhosis), pancreatic failure (diabetes, specifically "bronze diabetes"), arthritis, congestive heart failure, hypothyroidism, impotence (secondary to hypogonadism), CNS symptoms, nonspecific RUQ abdominal pain, and excess skin pigmentation.

6

HEMATOLOGIC, METABOLIC, AND ELECTROLYTE DISORDERS

C. **Alcohol intake** can exacerbate the disease and hasten the onset of symptoms.

D. **Diagnosis.** Elevated serum iron, elevated fasting transferrin saturation (>45%), elevated fasting serum ferritin. If transferrin saturation and ferritin are elevated, blood should be obtained for genotyping for mutations in the *HFE* gene. Liver biopsy can document presence of cirrhosis and can exclude other hepatic pathology. In patients who are homozygous for the C282Y mutation, are younger than 40 years, have a ferritin <1000 ng/mL, and have normal transaminases, liver biopsy is not recommended. (Guidelines are available in Tavill, 2001.)

E. **Treatment** is based on phlebotomy. Remove 500 mL of blood every week until the patient is iron deficient. Afterwards, the patient will require less frequent phlebotomies to prevent iron reaccumulation. Patients should be instructed to avoid Vitamin C.

II. **Transfusion-Related Hemochromatosis.**

A. **General.** Transfusion-related hemochromatosis is related to iron overload from transfusions, especially in those with sickle cell disease, myelodysplastic syndromes, aplastic anemia, and thalassemia.

B. **Diagnosis** is by blood testing as in idiopathic hemochromatosis.

C. **Treatment** is deferoxamine, 1 to 4 g/d IV or SQ. Hematology consultation is suggested.

TRANSFUSION MEDICINE

I. **Available Products.**

A. **Packed red blood cells** are used to reverse hemodynamically significant anemia in patients without compatibility problems. Expect the Hb to increase by 1 g/dL per unit in the patient without active bleeding. Rate of transfusion depends on clinical setting (faster with acute blood loss; over 3 to 4 hours with CHF).

B. **Leukocyte-poor RBCs** are used to prevent immunization against donor WBCs in those with a history of febrile reaction to packed RBCs and in those requiring many transfusions. They are also used for potential transplant patients and patients at particular risk for CMV infections.

C. **Washed RBCs** are used in those with a history of anaphylactic or allergic reactions to transfusions (such as those with IgA deficiency).

D. **Irradiated RBCs** are used in those with immunodeficiency (but not HIV) to prevent transfusion-associated GVHD. Examples include those with bone marrow transplants and premature infants.

II. **Blood hemoglobin will stabilize 15 to 30 minutes after transfusion. It is not necessary to wait hours before checking Hb/Hct after transfusion.**

III. **Indications for transfusion** (based on NIH, American College of Physicians guidelines). Following the guidelines in **Table 6-5** will minimize number of transfusions and improve mortality rates when compared with a more liberal transfusion policy. However, use clinical judgment!

TABLE 6-5

INDICATIONS FOR TRANSFUSION

Indication	Transfuse to maintain:
Transfuse any symptomatic patient (e.g. tachycardia, hypotension, CHF, angina)	Until no longer symptomatic
Asymptomatic, presurgical, stable patient	Hb 7-8g/dL
Hemodynamically stable postsurgical stable patient	Hb 8 g/dL
Postsurgical patient at risk for ischemic disease (e.g. cardiac, bowel)	Hb 10 g/dL
Hemodynamically stable, nonpregnant, ICU patients >16 years old without ongoing blood loss	Transfuse at 7 g/dL to maintain Hb at 7-9 g/dL
Elderly patients following MI	Transfuse to maintain Hct of >33%

IV. **Diuretics (e.g., furosemide; dose determined by underlying function) might be necessary to maintain hemodynamic stability in those with CHF, etc.**

V. **Transfusion Reactions.**

A. **Hemolytic reactions** may be acute or delayed.

1. **Symptoms** include fever with or without chills, flank pain, pain in the extremity that is accepting the transfused blood, tachycardia, hypotension, DIC, renal failure, chest pain, wheezing, nausea, vomiting, dark urine.

2. **Actions.** If transfusion reaction is suspected, immediately discontinue transfusion and return transfused unit to blood bank along with a specimen of patient's blood.

3. **Treatment** includes fluids and mannitol (0.5 to 2.5 g/kg) to maintain urine output and prevent renal failure. Furosemide may also be useful. Dopamine may be needed for blood pressure support. Treat pain with narcotic analgesics, wheezing with albuterol, etc., as appropriate.

B. **Febrile reactions** complicate about 2% of transfusions.

1. **Symptoms** include fever with or without shaking chills, headache, and malaise. Symptoms generally occur within 5 hours of transfusion. Must differentiate from sepsis.

2. **Treatment.** Stop transfusion; use meperidine in 25-mg aliquots IV to control symptoms such as chills; acetaminophen for fever. You can try to pretreat with acetaminophen and ASA and meperidine to prevent febrile reactions. After a febrile transfusion reaction, consider use of leukocyte-poor cells in future transfusions.

C. **Allergic reactions**

1. **Allergic reactions complicate about 2% of transfusions, especially in those who are IgA deficient.** True anaphylaxis occurs is 1 in 20,000.

2. **Symptoms** include allergic manifestations such as pruritus, urticaria, bronchospasm with wheezing, possibly shock.

3. **See Chapter 2 for treatment of anaphylaxis.**

4. Use washed cells if the patient is reacting to plasma protein.

6

HEMATOLOGIC, METABOLIC, AND ELECTROLYTE DISORDERS

D. Graft-versus-host disease
1. **GVHD is rare.** Patients clinically have fever, diarrhea, rash, pancytopenia, and elevated liver enzymes.
2. **It is most common in those with lymphoma, bone marrow transplants, and hereditary immune deficiencies and in premature infants, but not in persons with AIDS.**
3. **Treatment.** Mortality rate is high (>90%). Treatment is not generally effective and requires consultation with hematology staff. Prevent mortality by using irradiated cell products in those at risk.
E. Transfusion-related acute lung injury
1. Pulmonary infiltrates and noncardiogenic CHF (ARDS) related to lung injury.
2. **Clinically** note fever, chills, cough, and hypoxia.
3. **Treatment** is symptomatic and includes respiratory support, including mechanical ventilation if required. Notify blood bank to ensure that the patient does not receive any further blood products from the donor of the blood product that precipitated the symptoms.
F. Posttransfusion purpura
1. **Immunologically mediated severe thrombocytopenia that develops approximately 5 to 10 days following transfusion of red cells or platelets.** It is more common in women.
2. **Treatment.** IVIG 1 g/kg IV daily for two days.
G. Infection rate for hepatitis B is 1:200,000; hepatitis C is 1:1,900,000; hepatitis A is too low to categorize; HIV is 1:2,000,000.

MONOCLONAL GAMMOPATHY OF UNDETERMINED SIGNIFICANCE

I. **Definition.** MGUS is defined by the presence of a serum monoclonal (M) protein of no more than 3 g/dL with no or only very small amounts of urinary M protein and no anemia, renal insufficiency, bony lytic lesions, or hypercalcemia. It is often found when a serum protein electrophoresis (SPEP) is ordered after a clinician has noted an elevated total protein.
II. **Incidence.** MGUS occurs in 1% to 2% of adults in the United States. Incidence increases with age. It is more common in males and African Americans.
III. **Prognosis. Most patients do not progress to a malignancy, but up to 30% develop myeloma, Waldenstrom's, amyloidosis, or another lymphoproliferative disorder.** Higher initial concentration of the M protein correlates with higher risk of progression to malignancy.
IV. **Evaluation and Follow-Up**
A. All patients need a careful history and physical. Also obtain a CBC, creatinine, calcium, serum immunofixation electrophoresis, 24-hour urine sample for urine protein electrophoresis and urine immunofixation electrophoresis, and quantitative IgA, IgM, and IgG levels.

B. **If the patient has accompanying hypercalcemia, renal failure, anemia, or bone lesions or any other history of or evidence for a B-cell proliferative disorder (e.g., lymphadenopathy, "B symptoms" [fever, night sweats, weight loss, pruritus, fatigue]), patient should be immediately referred to a hematologist for evaluation of multiple myeloma, Waldenstrom's, or other malignant process.** Similarly, a patient with a monoclonal protein level of 3 g/dL or greater should also be evaluated by a hematologist.

C. **If none of the above features is present and the M-protein is <2.0 g/dL,** repeat SPEP in 6 months, and annually thereafter if stable.

D. **If the patient is asymptomatic and M-protein is >2.0 g/dL, perform bone marrow aspiration and biopsy.** Also obtain a skeletal bone survey to look for lytic lesions. (*Note:* A bone survey involves plain films. This is different from a nuclear medicine bone scan.) If these studies are negative, repeat SPEP in 3 months × 3, and then annually if stable.

HYPERVISCOSITY SYNDROME

I. **Etiology.** Elevated serum protein levels associated with Waldenström's macroglobulinemia or multiple myeloma increase serum viscosity to such a degree that microcirculation is impaired. More common is hyperviscosity secondary to elevated hematocrit (generally >60% when patients are symptomatic).

II. **Clinical Presentation.**

A. **CNS symptoms** include headache, blurred vision, dizziness, hearing loss, mental status changes, and seizures. CVA may also occur.

B. **Cardiac manifestations** include congestive heart failure.

C. **Hematologic symptoms** include easy bruising and mucosal bleeding.

III. **Diagnosis.**

A. **For protein-related hyperviscosity,** measure serum viscosity. Values are reported as a ratio of the flow time of serum to flow time of saline through the viscometer. Normal values are 1.6 to 1.9. Rarely patients with viscosities of 2 to 4 are symptomatic, whereas symptoms become increasingly common as patients' serums reach viscosity of 5 to 8.

B. **For polycythemia-related hyperviscosity** there is no direct relationship between the hematocrit and symptoms. Diagnosis and treatment are based on clinical criteria.

IV. **Treatment.**

A. **For protein-related hyperviscosity** for patients with mental status changes, plasma exchange should be performed emergently. Plasma exchange will rapidly but only temporarily lower serum viscosity. Therefore, the underlying process (e.g., Waldenström's or multiple myeloma) should be treated as well to prevent recurrence once plasma exchange has been performed.

B. **For polycythemia-related hyperviscosity,** phlebotomize 500 mL of blood while simultaneously replacing the blood with saline.

Up to 1 to 1.5 liters of blood can be removed in 24 hours in an emergency. **Simply phlebotomizing patients will not be effective. Blood volume must be replaced with saline.** Aim for a Hct of 60% initially and 55% as a long-term goal.

HYPOGLYCEMIA

I. Definition. Plasma glucose <50 mg/dL.
II. Symptoms. Tremulousness, palpitations, sweating, hunger, impaired concentration, irritability, blurred vision, lethargy, seizure, or coma.
III. Categories.
A. Iatrogenic hypoglycemia is the most common cause. It is a complication of insulin or oral hypoglycemic therapy.
B. Postprandial hypoglycemia is often idiopathic but can be caused by early diabetes, alcohol, renal failure, complication of gastrectomy, salicylates, β-blockers, pentamidine, or ACE inhibitors.
1. Patients generally have symptoms as above.
2. Hypoglycemia occurs 2 to 4 hours postprandially, has sudden onset, and generally subsides in 15 to 20 minutes.
3. Thought to be caused by epinephrine release.
C. Fasting hypoglycemia
1. Symptoms are generally of neuroglycopenia, including headache, mental dullness, and fatigue. Symptoms may progress to confusion, blurred vision, loss of consciousness, and seizures (especially in children).
2. Etiology
a. Excess insulin or insulinoma.
b. Alcohol abuse and liver disease secondary to decreased gluconeogenesis.
c. Pituitary or adrenal insufficiency secondary to decreased counterregulatory hormones.
d. Fasting hypoglycemia is common in young children.
e. Renal insufficiency with decreased gluconeogenesis.
D. Other medications include INH, haloperidol, TCAs, organophosphates, salicylates, warfarin, and many others.
IV. Evaluation.
A. To evaluate for postprandial hypoglycemia, do a 5-hour GTT. Give 75 g glucose load orally and measure serum glucose every 30 minutes for 5 hours. Twenty-five percent of otherwise symptom-free patients will become symptomatic and have blood glucose <50mg/dL when given this challenge, so the presence of symptoms does not always mean the patient's baseline symptoms are due to hypoglycemia. Others will be asymptomatic but have a blood glucose <50 mg/dL.
1. Early diabetes. Normal or elevated fasting glucose during first 2 hours, but may have low plasma glucose levels at 3 to 4 hours.
2. Postgastrectomy. Rapid elevation of glucose within 1 hour, rapid decline and trough in 2 to 3 hours.

3. **Idiopathic hypoglycemia.** Normal plasma glucose levels at 1 to 2 hours, low glucose at 3 hours, and return to baseline within 5 hours.
4. **Idiopathic postprandial syndrome.** Postprandial hypoglycemic symptoms with a normal GTT.
B. **To evaluate for fasting hypoglycemia:**
1. **Screen by measuring plasma glucose after overnight fast.**
2. If fasting level is normal, consider 72-hour hospitalized fast.
3. Some premenopausal women normally have serum glucose <50 mg/dL after 72-hour fast.
C. **To evaluate for other causes of hypoglycemia:**
1. **Insulinoma.** Patients usually have hunger, weight gain, and hypoglycemic symptoms. Diagnosis is by demonstrating high serum insulin levels when patient is hypoglycemic. Most are from islet cell tumors. Consultation with an endocrinologist is important.
2. **Surreptitious insulin administration or oral hypoglycemic administration**
a. Usually a diabetic patient or person with medical background.
b. Needle marks from insulin administration may be evident.
c. Can measure oral agents and some synthetic insulins in the blood.
d. Measure insulin level and C-peptide level. C-peptide will be low in exogenous insulin administration.
e. Presence of anti-insulin antibodies supports the diagnosis of exogenous insulin administration (especially beef or pork).
3. **Alcohol abuse.** Patient should have other stigmata of alcohol disease. Hypoglycemia occurs because of limited liver gluconeogenesis secondary to depletion of NADH.
4. **Liver disease**
a. Patients usually have elevated liver enzymes and other signs of liver failure.
b. Any patient with liver disease and hypoglycemia should be evaluated for a hepatoma.
5. **Pituitary or adrenal insufficiency** (see adrenal section).
6. **Renal failure. The kidneys are responsible for about 50% of gluconeogenesis.** Thus patients with renal failure might not tolerate oral hypoglycemic agents or insulin as well as those with normal renal function.
V. **Treatment.**
A. **Acute management**
1. **Oral carbohydrate** if the patient is conscious. Can administer by NG tube as well.
2. **IV D$_{50}$,** 1 ampule or more. No predictable response to IV glucose in terms of mg/dL rise.
3. **If no IV access, glucagon** 1 mg IM (can cause nausea, vomiting, and aspiration if the patient is unable to protect the airway). **This will not work with alcohol-related hypoglycemia and in small children who have depleted stores of glycogen.**

HEMATOLOGIC, METABOLIC, AND ELECTROLYTE DISORDERS

6

4. Monitor glucose every 15 to 30 minutes.
5. If hypoglycemia is secondary to oral agents, the patient should be admitted because hypoglycemia can recur for up to 48 hours.

B. Prevention and long-term management

1. Adjust dose of insulin or hypoglycemic agent.
2. Diabetes education.
3. ADA diet with complex carbohydrates.
4. Propantheline 7.5 to 15 mg PO ½ hour before meals can delay gastric emptying in postgastrectomy patients, avoiding rapid peaks in serum blood glucose levels. Not approved for this use.

DIABETES

I. Overview.

A. Definition. Diabetes mellitus is a metabolic disorder that is caused by either decreased insulin production or insulin resistance leading to hyperglycemia.

B. Classification

1. **Type 1 diabetes** is a result of autoimmune destruction of the pancreatic islet cells, which results in severe insulin deficiency. T1DM usually occurs in childhood or early adult life and accounts for less than 10% of cases. T1DM often results in ketoacidosis.
2. **Type 1.5 diabetes (adult-onset T1DM)** is adult-onset diabetes that is initially (poorly) responsive to diet and oral hypoglycemic agents. Patients progress rapidly to insulin dependence. Patients tend to be thin rather than obese and have circulating anti–islet cell antibodies and anti–glutamic dehydrogenase antibodies (anti-GAD). Approximately 10% of patients with apparent T2DM have this type of diabetes. **Consider type 1.5 diabetes in adults with new-onset diabetes that is poorly controlled with diet and oral hypoglycemic agents.**
3. **Type 2 diabetes** is associated with obesity, insulin resistance, and relative insulin deficiency. About 80% of diabetes in the United States is T2DM. It usually occurs in adults older than 40 years; however, prevalence in teenagers is rising. It affects 8% of the U.S. population and 19% of those older than 65 years. Ketosis can occur in association with T2DM; however, it is not as common as in T1DM.
4. **Gestational DM** occurs in association with pregnancy but resolves after delivery. These women are at increased risk for developing T2DM later in life.
5. **Other types of diabetes** are associated with exocrine pancreas diseases, Cushing's syndrome, pheochromocytoma, drugs and chemicals (β-blockers, oral contraceptives), pancreatectomy, and genetic syndromes such as lipodystrophies, which are rare causes.

II. Glycemic Control.

A. Tight glycemic control is critical in T1DM and will reduce complications.

B. Evidence for the benefit of tight control is less compelling in T2DM (and most of the benefit is seen in patients taking metformin). Control of blood pressure and lipids is critical for all diabetic patients. Those with T2DM actually benefit more from meticulous attention to blood pressure and lipids than from oral hypoglycemic agents.

III. Presentation and Evaluation.

A. Symptoms are polyuria, polydipsia, and polyphagia. Other symptoms include weight loss, blurred vision (from osmotic changes in the vitreous), dehydration, infections, or recurrent vaginal candidiasis. Many cases are asymptomatic and are found on routine screening.

B. Screening

1. Test all patients at age 45, and repeat fasting blood glucose every 3 years.

2. Test sooner and more often if the patient has any of the following risk factors: obesity (BMI >27 kg/m^2), first-degree relative with DM, member of high-risk group (African American, Hispanic, Native American, or Asian), history of GDM or delivering a baby heavier than 4 kg (9 lb), hypertension, HDL <35 mg/dL or triglycerides >250 mg/dL, history of impaired fasting glucose, or impaired GTT on previous screening.

C. Testing for diabetes. The fasting blood sugar is the test of choice for diabetes. **The oral glucose tolerance test has fallen out of favor because of poor reproducibility.** The glucose tolerance test must be performed after a 10- to 16-hour fast and when the patient is not under any metabolic stress (e.g., fever). Plasma glucose is measured before the test and 2 hours after glucose administration. **Fasting blood glucose results are as follows: Normal <100 mg/dL. Impaired is 100-125 mg/dL** (1%-5% of these patients will develop DM each year). **Diabetes is ≥126 mg/dL.**

D. Diagnosis of diabetes can be made if any one of the following is present:

1. **Random plasma glucose >200 mg/dL and symptoms of diabetes.**

2. **Two fasting plasma glucose results >126 mg/dL.**

3. **Two-hour postprandial plasma glucose >200 mg/dL after a 75-g oral glucose load**

4. **Elevated HbA1c is suggestive but not diagnostic for diabetes.**

E. Caveats. Of those with a fasting plasma glucose of 110-126 mg/dL, only 0.02% have an elevated HbA1c, 80% have a normal HbA1c, and the rest have an HbA1c only slightly elevated. Of those with a fasting glucose of 126 mg/dL to 140 mg/dL, 61% have a normal HbA1c, 35% have a slightly elevated HbA1c, and only 3% have a high HbA1c. If the HbA1c, which is a reflection of blood glucose over the past several months, is 1 percentage point above the reference laboratory's upper range of normal, it has a specificity of 98% for diagnosis of DM.

IV. Differentiating T1DM and T2DM. It is usually possible to differentiate between T1DM and T2DM based on the clinical situation. On occasion, however, this may be difficult.

A. The diagnosis can be clarified by the use of the C-peptide, a product of the cleavage of proinsulin to insulin. This is present in those with T2DM and is low or absent in those with T1DM. If the C-peptide is borderline, checking it after a glucose load can help. In those with T2DM, it will increase significantly after glucose load; this response will be absent in those with T1DM.

B. Islet cell antibodies can also be measured; they are typically elevated in T1DM and not present in T2DM.

C. Anti-GAD antibodies are present in T1DM.

V. Honeymoon Period.

A. After the initial diagnosis, there often occurs a honeymoon period during which only small amounts of a hypoglycemic agent or insulin are needed.

B. Often, diabetes first manifests during a situation of metabolic stress (such as infection or pregnancy). With the return to baseline metabolic demands, the pancreatic reserve may be adequate to maintain a normal or near-normal blood glucose.

VI. Somogyi phenomenon refers to hyperglycemia that occurs as a counterregulatory response (increased gluconeogenesis and sympathetic outflow) to a period of drug-induced hypoglycemia. If controlling high blood glucose becomes a problem (especially AM glucose), consider checking for hypoglycemia in the time leading up to high readings.

VII. Treatment.

A. Goal of therapy is to normalize the HbA1C, eliminate symptoms, and prevent microvascular and macrovascular complications of diabetes.

B. Patient education plays a crucial role in management of DM. Patients must have an understanding of diet planning, exercise, home glucose-monitoring techniques and frequency, foot care, signs of infection, and symptoms and management of hypoglycemia. This should be reviewed with patients at the onset of diabetes and periodically, often in conjunction with a diabetes educator.

C. Diet. With the help of a registered dietitian, proper diet plans can be reviewed with patients. Alcohol should be kept to a minimum because it increases the risk of hypoglycemia. Macronutrients should be balanced as 60% to 65% carbohydrates (higher in complex carbohydrates than simple carbohydrates), 10% to 20% protein, and 25% to 30% fat.

1. **T1DM.** Rigid diet plans must be followed to avoid fluctuations in plasma glucose. There is increased flexibility with newer intensive therapy such as insulin pumps or four-shots-a-day regimens. If a meal is delayed, patients may need to ingest 10 grams of carbohydrates per 30 minutes to avoid hypoglycemia. Calorie intake can be estimated at 40 kcal/kg/day for an adult. Moderate exercise requires additional 10 grams of carbohydrates per hour. Vigorous exercise may require up to 20 to 30 additional grams per hour. Another option is decreasing insulin intake in the meal prior to exercise if exercise is planned.

2. **T2DM.** In obese patients, glucose intolerance can be at least improved, if not reversed, with moderate weight loss. Plasma glucose levels can decline to normal ranges with as little as 2.5 to 4.5 kg (5-10 lb) weight loss. This should be highly encouraged in all obese patients because it can delay the use of pharmacologic therapy. It can also help offset the weight gain many patients experience when they start oral or insulin therapy.

D. **Pharmacologic therapy. Hypoglycemia is the main side effect of pharmacologic therapy.** Symptoms include shakiness, tachycardia, weakness, sweating, hunger, and nightmares. If not treated promptly with glucose, symptoms can progress to stupor and coma. Over time, with the loss of autonomic responsiveness from autonomic neuropathy, patients might not have typical hypoglycemic symptoms (hypoglycemia unawareness).

1. **T1DM.** Studies suggest that intensive therapy with tight glycemic control decreases the risk of developing complications from diabetes. However, intensive therapy is complicated by more frequent hypoglycemic episodes. Insulin is the only currently available treatment for T1DM. Many forms of insulin are available including beef, pork, recombinant human insulin, and synthetic insulin. Beef and pork tend to be more immunogenic, with the development of anti-insulin antibodies.

a. **Initiating insulin.** Typically, a patient with T1DM requires 0.5 to 1.0 U/kg of insulin per day, divided into multiple doses. **Control is initially obtained with a sliding scale** of regular insulin. Measure serum glucose every 6 hours and give SQ regular insulin to cover sugars. Once the glucose is stabilized with q6h injections, a split-dosing regimen is introduced. Traditionally, NPH is given, with two thirds of the total insulin requirement given as an AM dose and one third given as a PM dose. Short-acting insulin (regular, lispro, or aspart) can be added to cover high sugars. Alternatively, a long-acting insulin (Ultralente or glargine) or an insulin pump can be used to deliver a basal rate of insulin that can be supplemented by shorter-acting insulin to achieve control.

b. **Goal of therapy is HbA1c <7.** Blood sugars are typically measured before meals. Insulin can be adjusted to cover meal carbohydrates as well as to correct for premeal plasma hyperglycemia.

c. **Types of insulin. *Note:* Only regular insulin should be given IV.**
   (1) **Insulin lispro and aspart** are short acting, with an onset of action of less than 30 minutes and a duration of less than 4 hours. The benefit of short-[acting insulin is that it can be tailored to cover the carbohydrate intake in each meal. It must be used with long-acting insulin to cover basal insulin needs. There is no advantage over traditional insulin regimens at reaching target HbA1c goals or preventing hypoglycemia. However, short-acting insulin increases flexibility with diet and lifestyles.
   (2) **Regular insulin** is short acting, with an onset of less than 30 minutes, peaks at 2 to 4 hours, and has a duration of 4 to 6 hours.

   (3) **NPH and Lente** are intermediate acting. Onset is 1 to 3 hours, peak is 6 to 12 hours, and duration is typically up to 18 hours.

   (4) **Ultralente** is long acting. Onset is 4 to 8 hours, peak is 14 to 24 hours, and duration is 28 to 36 hours.

   (5) **Insulin glargine (Lantus)** is ultralong-acting synthetic insulin that allows reliable once-a-day administration for basal insulin therapy. Onset of action is within 4 hours. Duration of action is longer than 24 hours without a peak activity. Glargine must be used with short-acting insulin to cover meal insulin needs. **It cannot be mixed in a syringe with other insulin preparations.**

   (6) Inhaled insulin (e.g., Exubara), is now available.

2. **T2DM**

a. **Initial therapy should be aimed at weight loss** because this can decrease plasma glucose levels and increase insulin sensitization in the patient. HbA1c can be decreased 0.5 to 2 percentage points with weight loss.

b. When diet is not sufficient, oral agents and/or insulin can be added to the regimen. **Oral agents (for T2DM only)** include the following:

   (1) **Metformin is generally the drug of choice for T2DM in patients for whom it is appropriate.** Of all of the hypoglycemic agents, it has been shown to improve outcomes. Another advantage is that metformin does not cause hypoglycemia.

     (a) Metformin can be used as monotherapy or in combination with sulfonylureas or insulin. **It is especially useful in overweight patients because it does not cause weight gain.** Metformin also improves plasma lipid and fibrinolytic profiles associated with T2DM. Initial dose is 500 mg PO qd until initial nausea and anorexia are tolerated and then advanced to 500 mg bid and then increased 500 mg/day weekly to a maximum dose of 2500 mg if needed to control sugars. Taking it with or after food can lessen the GI side effects.

     (b) **The main risk of metformin is the rare induction of lactic acidosis.** This risk is minimized if metformin is avoided in patients with renal disease (creatinine $\geq$1.4 mg/dL), any type of acidosis, liver disease, or severe hypoxia. Use in mild CHF is controversial.

     (c) **If possible, discontinue metformin for 48 hours prior to using intravenous contrast material and 48 hours after IV contrast material because contrast material can contribute to the development of lactic acidosis. There are also cases of lactic acidosis after the initiation of NSAIDs.** Expect a decrease of 1 to 2 percentage points in HbA1c levels.

   (2) **Sulfonylureas** stimulate pancreatic beta cells to secrete insulin. Glyburide 1.25 to 20 mg or glipizide 5 to 40 mg are good choices for an oral hypoglycemic. There is little evidence that glipizide doses higher than 20 mg/day are helpful and they can actually result in decreased beta cell function. Glyburide is more likely to result in

glycemic control when used once a day than glipizide is. Glyburide should be used in a twice-daily dosing if 20 mg/day total is required. Newer agents, such as glipizide GITS and glimepiride, have persistent hypoglycemic effect with once-daily dosing. Expect a decrease in HbA1c levels by 1 to 2 percentage points.

- (a) **Effectiveness typically declines annually,** up to 10%, as beta cell dysfunction progresses.
- (b) **Sulfonylureas are contraindicated in T1DM,** pregnancy (although currently under investigation), severe renal and liver diseases, and lactation. They should be avoided in children.
- (c) **Complications include** hypoglycemia, disulfiram-like effect, flushing, headache, tachycardia, nausea and vomiting, severe hyponatremia, and fluid retention (especially in the elderly).
- (d) **Drug interactions include** propranolol and clonidine (can mask the signs and symptoms of hypoglycemia); thiazide diuretics, chlorthalidone, furosemide, ethacrynic acid, and phenytoin (may have antagonistic effects on sulfonylureas); β-blockers, ACE inhibitors, salicylates, sulfonamides, phenylbutazone, methyldopa, clofibrate, warfarin, MAO inhibitors, and chloramphenicol (hypoglycemic effects of the sulfonylureas can be potentiated by these drugs).
- (e) **Sulfonylureas may increase mortality despite glycemic control.**

(3) **α-Glucosidase inhibitors.** Acarbose and miglitol are oral agents that decrease absorption of carbohydrates from the GI tract. The main side effects include asymptomatic elevation of liver enzymes, flatulence, and diarrhea. These drugs are generally less effective than other classes, can decrease HbA1c levels by 0.5 to 1 percentage point, and may be used in combination with other agents.

(4) **Thiazolidinediones** such as rosiglitazone (Avandia) and pioglitazone (Actos) increase the body's sensitivity to endogenous insulin. They can be used as monotherapy or in combination with metformin or insulin for T2DM; combination therapy leads to decrease in HbA1c of 0.6 to 1.3 percentage points. Side effects include anemia, edema, and elevated LFT. Use with caution in CHF. Pioglitazone has the benefit of lowering triglycerides and increasing HDL. Troglitazone is no longer on the market in the United States because of significant liver toxicity.

(5) **Meglitinides. Nateglinide** (Starlix) and **repaglinide** (NovoNorm, Prandin) are short acting and expensive and must be used before each meal. Mechanism of action is similar to sulfonylureas'. They may be used as monotherapy or in combination with metformin or glitazones **(but not sulfonylureas).** Side effects include hypoglycemia. They should be avoided in liver disease. They are useful in patients with erratic eating schedules.

(6) **Insulin.** In T2DM, insulin is usually added to oral agent(s) when glycemic control is suboptimal. Adding a daily injection of an

intermediate-acting insulin such as NPH or long-acting insulin such as insulin glargine can improve HbA1c. Starting doses typically are 5 to 10 units. This can be increased as needed every 5 to 7 days until adequate control is achieved. Giving NPH at bedtime can result in better glycemic control (there is significant gluconeogenesis at night). See above for further insulin regimen details. **Insulin may increase macrovascular complications in T2DM.**

(7) **Glitizars (e.g., Muraglitazar).** These new drugs improve glucose control and lipid profile. They are expensive, however, and can increase edema and CHF more than the glitazones.

(8) **Incretin mimetics (e.g. exenatide) are expensive. They can be added to sulfonylureas or metformin to improve control. Injectable.** Pramlintide can also be used in T1DM.

VIII. Complications. There is a relationship between level of hyperglycemia and modification of risk factors, on the one hand, and death from CAD and all causes, on the other. Intensive glycemic control has been shown to delay the development and progression of diabetic retinopathy, nephropathy, and neuropathy in T1DM. However, the benefit of treatment is less compelling in T2DM. Routine screening studies are listed in **Table 6-6.**

A. Goals are as follows:

1. **Glycemic control.** Target HbA1c is <7. This correlates to a fasting plasma glucose of 90 to 130 mg/dL. Postprandial glucose goal is <180. Incidence of hypoglycemia can increase with intensive therapy, however.

2. **Blood pressure.** JNC 7 recommends target blood pressure of 125/75 mm Hg or less. This can prevent more complications than glycemic control in T2DM.

3. **Lipids**

a. **LDL.** Without CAD, target LDL is 100 mg/dL or less. With CAD, target LDL is less than 70 mg/dL. Therapy should be initiated with LDL greater than 70 mg/dL (see Grundy et al, 2004).

b. **HDL** >45 mg/dL

c. **Triglycerides** <200 mg/dL

B. Specific complications

1. **Diabetic nephropathy** is the most common cause of end-stage renal disease in the United States. Risk factors associated with the development of diabetic nephropathy include hypertension, albuminuria or proteinuria, poor glycemic control, smoking, high-protein diets, and hyperlipidemia, although the last two are somewhat controversial in the literature.

a. There is clear evidence to indicate that the use of ACE inhibitors in diabetics who have microalbuminuria can delay the development of renal failure; this is true even in the absence of hypertension. Angiotensin receptor blockers (ARBs) and non–dihydropyridine

TABLE 6-6

SUMMARY OF ROUTINE DIABETIC FOLLOW-UP

Follow-up	T1DM	T2DM
Eye exam by ophthalmologist	5 years after diagnosis and then every year	At time of diagnosis and every year thereafter
HbA1c	Every 3 months	Every 3 months
Blood pressure	Every visit	Every visit
Foot check	Every visit (use 10-g monofilament nylon)	Every visit (use 10-g monofilament nylon)
Urine microalbumin	Every 6 months to 1 year after 12 years of age	Every 6 months to 1 year
Lipid panel	Every 12 months	Every 12 months
Diabetic education	Annually	Annually

calcium channel blockers (verapamil, diltiazem) are (likely less effective) alternatives. ARBs likely do not reduce cardiovascular events. Accordingly, all diabetic patients older than 12 years should be screened for microalbuminuria at least yearly.

b. **There are three ways to reliably measure microalbumin:** measurement of the albumin-to-creatinine ratio in a random, spot collection (the best method), a 24-hour urine collection (can also measure creatinine clearance), or a timed collection (e.g., a 4-h collection). **Dipsticks are also available to check for microalbumin. However, routine UA dipsticks are not sensitive enough and should not be used.** A positive test is considered >30 mg in 24 hours of albumin or >20 μg/min of albumin.

2. **Coronary artery disease.** The leading cause of death in DM patients is MI. Thirty percent of myocardial infarctions in diabetic patients are "silent" (i.e., painless). Therefore, the possibility of an MI must be considered whenever a diabetic patient presents with CHF, dyspnea, diabetic ketoacidosis, or other secondary event.

3. **Peripheral vascular disease.** The most important risk is smoking. Other risk factors (in addition to DM) include HTN and elevated LDL and triglyceride levels. This disease results in ischemia with ulceration, polymicrobial infection, and gangrene of the lower extremities.

4. **Diabetic neuropathy**

a. **Polyneuropathy** is the most common type of neuropathy and results in distal pain, numbness, hyperesthesia, variable weakness, and possibly muscle wasting. Conditions such as vitamin B_{12} deficiency, uremia, and alcohol abuse should be excluded. Polyneuropathy has been shown to be associated with poor glycemic control. Screening is done using a 10-g monofilament nylon to the feet. Therapy includes tight glucose control, pain management, low-dose tricyclic antidepressants, carbamazepine, gabapentin, nasal calcitonin, oral anesthetics (mexiletine, tocainide) and topical capsaicin cream.

b. **Mononeuropathy** can result in sudden motor or sensory deficit or pain. It is most commonly associated with the femoral, sciatic, and peroneal nerves. Cranial nerves may be involved. Usually resolves in a few months.

c. **Autonomic neuropathy** may affect the cardiovascular reflexes, gastrointestinal function (diabetic gastroparesis, gastric atony), and genitourinary function. Symptoms can include syncope, resting tachycardia, nausea, vomiting, impotence, neurogenic bladder, diarrhea, and urinary or fecal incontinence. Orthostatic hypotension can be treated with compression hose, fludrocortisone 0.1- 0.3 mg/d or with NaCl 1 to 4 g PO qid (may cause fluid overload). Midodrine has also been approved for orthostatic hypotension and fluoxetine (Prozac) and venlafaxine (Effexor) may also be used; care must be taken to avoid recumbent hypertension. Gastroparesis may be treated with metoclopramide 10 mg $1/2$ hour ac and hs. Erythromycin and cisapride (no longer on the market in the United States) have also been used to promote gastric emptying but have more drug interactions.

d. **Diabetic amyopathy** is a rare complication of DM, with proximal muscle weakness and pain, most commonly involving the pelvic girdle. Onset may be rapid, and the patient may have a low-grade fever and an elevated ESR. Prognosis for improvement is good over months. **Diabetic patients may also suffer spontaneous muscle infarctions that can be seen on MRI.**

e. **Neuropathic arthropathy** (Charcot's joints) are degenerative changes of the joints of the feet and ankles that occasionally progress to complete joint destruction. This process is often painless and secondary to recurrent trauma, which may have gone unnoticed by the patient.

5. **Diabetic foot disease.** Diabetic foot ulcers, a result of neuropathy, arthropathy, trauma, and peripheral vascular disease, affects 15% of patients with diabetes. Eighty-five percent of amputations to the lower limbs in diabetic patients are preceded by foot ulcerations. **Patients must be educated to inspect feet daily to evaluate for the early signs of ulcer formation.** Proper-fitting shoes are essential. Ulcers can become infected, most typically with *Staphylococcus, Streptococcus*, gram-negative organisms, or anaerobic bacteria. If ulcers are infected, outpatient therapy can include ciprofloxacin, cefalexin, clindamycin, or amoxicillin–clavulanic acid. More serious infections require intravenous antibiotics such as imipenem–cilastatin, ampicillin–sulbactam, piperacillin–tazobactam, and broad-spectrum cephalosporins. Vancomycin should be used if MRSA is suspected. Aggressive therapy includes dressing changes and debridement. Investigation for osteomyelitis with surgical debridement may be necessary. Amputation may be necessary. Tight glycemic control promotes wound healing.

6. **Diabetic retinopathy** is one of the leading causes of blindness in the United States. Earliest clinical findings are microaneurysms and intraretinal dot hemorrhages. These are present in almost all patients with T1DM after 20 years and 80% of patients with T2DM after the same duration of disease. Changes progress to increased intraretinal hemorrhages and cotton wool spots, signs of ischemic disease. This is followed by proliferative diabetic retinopathy with the formation

of new vessels. As neovascularization occurs, vitreous hemorrhages and retinal detachment can result. Therefore, an annual exam with an ophthalmologist is essential for all T1DM patients older than 12 years and all T2DM patients of any age. Glucose and blood pressure control can prevent or delay diabetic retinopathy. There are many experimental drugs on the horizon for treatment and prevention of diabetic retinopathy.

IX. Diabetic Ketoacidosis.

A. Overview. With severe insulin deficiency, a ketotic state develops from the breakdown of free fatty acids. This leads to increased acetoacetic acid and β-hydroxybutyric acid levels, resulting in acidosis. It occurs typically in T1DM but can occur rarely in T2DM. Thirty percent of patients with T1DM present with DKA as their initial presentation, and there is a 1% to 3% mortality rate with each episode.

B. Causes. DKA often results from infection, poor compliance with insulin, trauma, myocardial infarction, pregnancy, or dehydration.

C. Evaluation

1. **Symptoms:** mental status changes, rapid breathing with Kussmaul respiration (compensation for acidosis), acetone (fruity) odor on breath, nausea, vomiting, dehydration, and history of DM (except initial presentation). **Often patients present with abdominal pain and vomiting.**

2. **Hyperglycemia** can be detected rapidly with a blood glucose monitor. Urine dipsticks are 99% sensitive for serum ketones. Plasma glucose is typically >250 mg/dL; arterial pH is <7.35 or serum bicarbonate <15 mEq/L with serum or urine ketosis. **Twenty percent of patients with DKA have "euglycemic" DKA with a glucose of less than 300 mg/dL.**

3. **Additional laboratory evaluation** should include serum glucose determined by the laboratory, serum ketones, electrolytes (in particular, potassium), anion gap, BUN, creatinine, and serum osmolarity. **Evaluation for infection is a must with a CXR, blood cultures, and urinalysis with microscopy and culture.** Be mindful of hypokalemia and hypomagnesemia during therapy. Glucose should be monitored hourly during treatment and electrolytes every 1 to 2 hours initially. An ABG adds nothing to the treatment of DKA and is optional as long as the serum bicarbonate can be followed.

D. Treatment

1. **Acute management in adults**

a. **Supportive therapy** includes ABCs, airway management, and treatment of shock.

b. **Fluid.** Patient can have up to a 3- to 6-liter deficit. Isotonic saline should be used initially. 1 liter should be rapidly infused, followed by 1 L/h until volume depletion is corrected (slower if the patient has a history of heart failure). If the patient is initially hypernatremic, this can worsen with treatment, and rapid conversion to ½ NS once the patient is hemodynamically stable is recommended. The next goal is to correct free water deficit using 0.45% saline infusion. Finally, maintenance fluids (0.9%-0.45% saline) should be continued for 12 to 24 hours until the patient is euvolemic and glucose is stable.

c. **Insulin.** Intravenous insulin therapy is indicated; 5 to 10 units of regular insulin can be given IV followed by a drip of 0.1 U/kg per hour (5-10 u/h). **Ideal rate of fall of serum glucose is 50 to 75 mg/dL per hour,** no more than 100 mg/dL per hour, to prevent osmotic encephalopathy. If the glucose fails to fall by at least 10%, insulin infusion should be increased each hour until response occurs. Once the serum glucose reaches 250 mg/dL, IV glucose should be administered as $D_{10}W$ to maintain serum glucose concentrations. Insulin infusion should be adjusted if needed to maintain glucose level at goal, but it should not be stopped. **It is preferable to give $D_{10}W$ with the infusion than it is to stop the insulin, because insulin is still required to clear the acidosis and ketotic state!**

d. **Potassium.** Patients typically require 10 to 20 mEq/h of potassium during therapy unless initial K^+ is >6 mEq/dL or the patient is oliguric or has renal failure. **Table 6-7** gives guidelines.

e. **Bicarbonate.** Routine use of HCO_3^- is discouraged at any pH. HCO_3^- causes rapid K^+ and osmolarity shifts and does not improve outcomes. **In fact, HCO_3^- can cause a prolonged ketosis (it is also associated with the development of cerebral edema in children).** Consider the use of HCO_3^- if the pH is <7.0 (although this is still discouraged). HCO_3^- may be administered with one of the initial liters of fluid by mixing two ampules of HCO_3^- (88 mEq) in a liter of 0.45% saline, which is substituted for one of the liters of normal saline.

f. **Phosphate supplementation is generally discouraged because the PO_4^{3-} will usually return to normal when the metabolic state normalizes. PO_4^{3-} generally does more harm than good.** Potassium phosphate (4 mEq K^+/93 mg P) may be added to maintenance fluids if necessary. Do not exceed total dose of 20 mEq K^+, and great caution is required in renal insufficiency.

g. **Magnesium** should be replaced. Give $MgSO_4$ 2.5 g in 50 mL NS over the first hour. Serum Mg^{2+} does not reflect total body stores, and patients with prolonged diuresis secondary to hyperglycemia are likely hypomagnesemic. Use caution in patients with renal failure.

TABLE 6-7

POTASSIUM REPLACEMENT IN ACIDOTIC ADULTS

Serum K^+ (mEq/dL)	mEq/h KCl in NS
<3	40
3-4	30
4-5	20
5-6	10
>6	0

These are rough guidelines only. Use clinical judgment!

h. **Diet.** Oral intake may resume as mental status, nausea, and vomiting allow. Full diet is usually withheld until ketosis resolves.

i. **Termination of therapy.** IV insulin should be continued as described above and for 1 hour after administration of the usual insulin dose (typically given prior to first full meal).

2. **Acute management in children.** Avoid too-rapid glucose lowering or overcorrection to prevent CNS injury. Assume 10% to 15% (100-150 mg/kg) fluid deficit. **Although it has been traditional to avoid fluids in pediatric DKA because of worries of cerebral edema, this has been disproved. The only predictors of cerebral edema are the use of bicarbonate and the severity of the DKA.**

a. **Fluids.** In the first hour, give 20 mL/kg boluses of 0.9% saline until the patient is out of shock. For hours 2 through 8 give 50% of total deficit (include the amount given in the first hour when calculating the additional need). Change to D_5 0.45% saline when glucose is <250 mg/dL. For hours 9 through 24, continue to replace fluid deficit using ¼ to ½ normal saline plus maintenance fluids as described in the pediatric section.

b. **Insulin** can be given as a bolus of 0.1 U/kg followed by a 0.1 U/kg per hour drip. Correct other abnormalities as indicated above.

HYPERGLYCEMIC–HYPEROSMOLAR NONKETOTIC STATE

I. **Overview.** Severe hyperglycemia can lead to mental status changes and volume depletion with absence of serum ketones. It occurs primarily in T2DM.

II. **Causes.** Severe hyperglycemia leads to osmotic diuresis and secondary volume depletion. This causes elevation of plasma osmolarity and hypernatremia with little or no ketosis.

III. **Evaluation.**

A. **Symptoms** include mental status changes, volume depletion, obtundation, coma, or shock.

B. **Laboratory studies** include serum glucose, ketones, osmolarity, electrolytes, BUN, creatinine, and arterial blood gases. ECG should also be obtained. Treatment should not be delayed pending results.

IV. **Treatment.**

A. **Acute management**

1. **Supportive measures.** Provide adequate airway and ventilation, treatment of shock.

2. **Fluid.** Patient may have a deficit up to 8 to 10 liters. Initial therapy should be with NS at 1L/h until intravascular volume is restored. If hypernatremia is present, fluid may be switched to 0.45% saline. Caution must be exercised in the setting of renal impairment, CHF, or possible MI.

3. **Insulin.** Treatment is initiated with 5 to 10 units of regular IV bolus for serum glucose >600 mg/dL, and insulin drip is begun as above under DKA.

6

HEMATOLOGIC, METABOLIC, AND ELECTROLYTE DISORDERS

B. Additional management

1. **Monitor** glucose and electrolytes initially every hour. Urine output should be monitored continuously (via Foley catheter). ABGs should be followed if bicarbonate is given. Serum osmolarity should be checked every 2 to 3 hours initially to aid in fluid therapy.

2. **Fluid.** After intravascular volume is restored, therapy should be guided by electrolyte determinations. Generally 0.45% saline will be appropriate. If significant hypernatremia is present, see the discussion of hypernatremia. Fluid should be administered at 150 mL/h, adjusted according to vitals and urine output.

3. **Electrolytes.** Potassium depletion can occur, and supplementation should be provided if levels approach low normal; give 10mEq/h of KCl initially, then adjust accordingly.

4. **Insulin.** After initial bolus, constant infusion of regular insulin should be started at 5 to 10 U/h. Gradual decline in blood glucose (around 75 mg/dL/h) is the desired goal. Glucose should be added to the maintenance fluids when blood glucose drops to the 200 to 300 mg/dL range.

5. Patient should be evaluated for possible precipitating causes, including infection, MI, and stroke.

THYROID DISORDERS

Hyperthyroidism

I. **Definition.** Hyperthyroidism is defined as high levels of circulating thyroid hormone.

II. **Symptoms.**

A. Patients can have nervousness, heat intolerance, palpitations, tachycardia, weight loss, weakness, dyspnea on exertion (also CHF), emotional lability, poor concentration, itching and burning of eyes, fullness in the throat, diarrhea, and dysmenorrhea or amenorrhea.

B. Diarrhea is a bad sign and can herald the onset of thyroid storm.

C. Geriatric patients may show withdrawal or depression (apathetic hyperthyroidism).

III. **Laboratory Evaluation of Hyperthyroidism.**

A. **Ultrasensitive thyroid stimulating hormone** is the best method for diagnosing hyperthyroidism. TSH is decreased in response to increased circulating thyroid hormone in 98% of cases.

B. **Free T_4,** a measure of the active thyroid hormone, is unaffected by changes in the thyroxine-binding globulin (TBG). Free T_4 is elevated in most cases of hyperthyroidism.

C. **Total T_4** measurement is affected by increases in TBG. Therefore elevated total T_4 is not sensitive or specific. Total T_4 is elevated in states that increase the TBG, including pregnancy, estrogen therapy and oral contraceptives, infectious hepatitis, cirrhosis, breast carcinoma, hypothyroidism, and acute intermittent porphyria.

D. **Free T_4 index** corrects the total T_4 for the serum TBG to allow one to estimate the free T_4.

E. **Free T_4/T_3 RIA.** About 5% of hyperthyroid patients have a normal T_4 level but an elevated T_3 level, indicating an isolated T_3 hyperthyroidism. If the patient is clinically hyperthyroid but the free T_4 is normal, checking a T_3 RIA is prudent.

F. **Antithyroid antibodies**

1. **Anti-TSH receptor antibodies are relatively specific for Graves' disease** but are found in 10% to 20% of patients with autoimmune thyroiditis. Levels should decrease with antithyroid treatment. If levels persist after treatment, hyperthyroidism is likely to recur when antithyroid treatment is discontinued.

2. **Anti-thyroglobulin (anti-TG) and anti–thyroid peroxidase (anti-TPO, formerly known as antimicrosomal antibody)** may be elevated in chronic autoimmune thyroiditis (Hashimoto's thyroiditis) but also in lower levels with Graves' disease.

IV. **Etiology.**

A. **Graves' disease** is the most common cause of hyperthyroidism in the third and fourth decades. It causes a diffuse, symmetrically enlarged thyroid gland with normal to slightly soft consistency and possibly pretibial myxedema. **About 80% to 95% of patients have anti-TSH receptor antibodies.** The classic infiltrative ophthalmopathy can occur with or without overt hyperthyroidism.

B. **Toxic multinodular goiter** results in an irregular, asymmetric, nodular thyroid gland. It usually develops insidiously in the sixth or seventh decade in a patient who has had a nontoxic nodular goiter for years. A thyroid scan can be useful in establishing the diagnosis.

C. **Solitary hyperfunctioning adenomas** usually occur during the fourth and fifth decades. The thyroid gland contains a smooth, well-defined, soft to firm nodule that shows intense radioactive uptake on scan with absence of uptake in the rest of the gland. Most patients with solitary adenomas do not become thyrotoxic. When they do, they are usually less toxic than those with Graves' disease, and they do not develop ophthalmopathy or pretibial myxedema.

D. **Autoimmune thyroiditis** involves a normal-sized or enlarged nontender thyroid gland. Thyroid antibodies, when present, are high in titer (see later for a discussion of thyroid antibodies). Uptake of ^{131}I is suppressed or zero. **About 80% to 100% will be anti-TG and/or anti-TSO positive.** This disorder improves spontaneously but often recurs. Autoimmune thyroiditis, painless thyroiditis, lymphocytic thyroiditis, and Hashimoto's thyroiditis are probably all the same disorder.

E. **Excess exogenous thyroid** can occur because of dosage errors or if large doses of thyroid hormones are taken to lose weight or increase energy. The thyroid gland is normal-sized or small, and ^{131}I uptake is suppressed.

F. Subacute thyroiditis and viral thyroiditis involve a tender, diffusely enlarged thyroid gland with a normal or elevated T_4, a depressed ^{131}I uptake, and an elevated ESR. It is probably of viral origin and can manifest as a sore throat.

G. Subclinical hyperthyroidism has suppressed TSH with normal free T_4 levels. The patient might or might not have symptoms. It can progress to Graves' disease, multinodular goiter, or hypothyroidism. In patients with multinodular goiter the progression rate to clinical hyperthyroidism is 5% per year (Toft, 2001).

H. Rare causes include radiation thyroiditis, amiodarone (can cause both hyper- and hypothyroidism), thyroid carcinoma, excessive TSH stimulation, excessive iodine intake, struma ovarii, and trophoblastic disease.

V. Treatment.

A. Graves' disease

1. **Propylthiouracil (PTU) 100 to 150 mg q8h, or methimazole 15 to 60 mg divided bid or tid** depending on severity of illness. Clinical improvement may be seen in 1 to 2 weeks, and the patient becomes euthyroid 2 to 3 months after beginning therapy. PTU achieves results faster because it prevents the peripheral conversion of T_4 to active T_3. After the euthyroid state is reached, the medication dose should be decreased by a third every few months if the patient remains euthyroid. A free T_4 level should be checked after 1 month of therapy and then every 2 to 3 months. These drugs are usually continued for 6 months to 1 year. Low-dose thyroxine may be needed during therapy. A significant number of patients experience permanent remission of hyperthyroidism after discontinuing these medications. **Side effects (which are more common with PTU) include rashes, agranulocytosis, thrombocytopenia, anemia, hepatitis, arthritis, and fever.** WBC count and liver enzymes should be obtained before drug therapy is started and rechecked after 1 month and 3 months of treatment; after that labs should be rechecked only if new symptoms arise. These drugs cause no permanent thyroid damage.

2. **Inorganic iodine** rapidly controls hyperthyroidism by inhibiting hormone synthesis and release from the gland. One drop of saturated potassium iodide solution in juice is taken daily. This should not be used as the sole form of therapy. It may be used for 7 to 10 days before surgery to decrease the vascularity of the thyroid gland. It should not be used for at least 3 days after ^{131}I therapy but thereafter may be used alone until the ^{131}I becomes effective.

3. **Levothyroxine.** Despite initially positive data, it is unlikely that routine use of levothyroxine during treatment reduces the recurrence of Graves' disease.

4. **Propranolol 80 to 200 mg/d divided q6h or atenolol 25 to 100 mg/day** divided bid reduces symptoms of tachycardia, palpitations, heat intolerance, and nervousness but does not normalize the metabolic rate.

It should not be used alone except in the case of transient hyperthyroidism secondary to autoimmune (viral) thyroiditis.

5. ^{131}I **5 to 15 mCi** in a single dose can render 90% of patients euthyroid within 3 to 6 months. This will not control symptoms; therefore, treatment should be preceded and followed by antithyroid therapy. Most patients eventually become hypothyroid. Pregnancy is an absolute contraindication to ^{131}I therapy.

6. **Surgery** is usually reserved for those who are unable to take antithyroid drugs. Complications include hypoparathyroidism and hypothyroidism.

7. **Ophthalmopathy.** Smoking can worsen ophthalmopathy. **Ophthalmopathy can also worsen (usually transiently) with radioactive iodine. This can be prevented by treatment with prednisone 0.5 mg/kg PO for 3 months starting 2 to 3 days after radioactive iodine.** However, this carries the risk of prednisone exposure. Symptomatic treatment for ophthalmopathy includes artificial tears or methylcellulose drops for the discomfort, patching or prisms for diplopia, and diuretics and raising the head of the bed for circumorbital edema.

B. **Toxic multinodular goiter is treated with ^{131}I or surgery.** Antithyroid drugs do not induce permanent remission and should be used only as interim therapy. Large multinodular goiters do not respond well to ^{131}I. Hypothyroidism is rare after ^{131}I therapy for toxic multinodular goiter because normal thyroid tissue is suppressed as a result of the disease and does not take up ^{131}I.

C. **Solitary hyperfunctioning adenomas are treated with ^{131}I or surgery;** antithyroid drugs are used only as interim therapy when needed. Hypothyroidism is rare after therapy.

D. **Autoimmune thyroiditis is transient and does not require definitive treatment except in patients with recurrent hyperthyroidism. Propranolol may be used alone if symptoms are mild.** Antithyroid drugs may be needed for a short time in some patients.

E. **Subacute thyroiditis and viral thyroiditis are generally self-limited but should be treated with aspirin 650 mg qid. In more severe cases, prednisone may be used** at 40 mg PO qd, tapering to 10 mg over 2 weeks, and then continued for 1 month after the patient becomes asymptomatic. A β-blocker (e.g. propranolol) can be used to control tachycardia, etc. Resolution of symptoms usually occurs in 1 to 6 months, but relapse is common. Hypothyroidism can occur but is rare.

Thyroid Storm

I. **Overview.** Thyroid storm is a severe, life-threatening form of hyperthyroidism that may be precipitated in a mildly hyperthyroid patient by increasing stress such as trauma or illness.

II. **Clinical.** Patients have signs and symptoms consistent with thyrotoxicosis (tachycardia, heat intolerance, weight loss), as well as fever, confusion, agitation, weakness, dyspnea, diarrhea, and shock.

HEMATOLOGIC, METABOLIC, AND ELECTROLYTE DISORDERS   6

III. Treatment. When thyroid storm is suspected, treatment should be instituted immediately. If defervescence does not occur within several hours, concurrent infection should be suspected. Other signs of hyperthyroidism can require several days of therapy before improvement is seen.

A. Propranolol 20 to 40 mg q4h to control tachycardia, tremor, etc. (can give 0.5 to 1.0 mg IV q5min to keep pulse at about 100; might need >15 mg IV).

B. Give PTU 250 mg PO or per NG q6h (alternative is methimazole 20-40 mg PO or per NG q6-8h). PTU is preferred in this situation and prevents conversion of T_4 to T_3.

C. SSKI 30 gtt PO 1 hour after giving PTU to prevent iodine from being used for additional thyroid hormone synthesis. Continue with 5 to 10 gtt qid. Alternative is 0.5 g sodium iodide (NaI) in 1 L NS over 12 hours.

D. Fluid and electrolytes should be replaced and fever controlled with acetaminophen and a cooling blanket.

E. Give steroids equivalent to about 300 mg of hydrocortisone per day (100 mg IV q8h). Dexamethasone has some theoretical advantage because it prevents conversion of T_4 to T_3 peripherally. (This is about 12 mg of dexamethasone divided tid.)

F. Avoid aspirin because it can increase circulating active T_3 and T_4 by reducing protein binding.

Hypothyroidism

I. Definition. Prevalence of hypothyroidism is 1% to 6%.

A. Primary hypothyroidism is a thyroid hormone deficiency resulting from thyroid gland dysfunction.

B. Secondary hypothyroidism results from TSH deficiency.

C. Tertiary hypothyroidism results from a deficiency in thyrotropin-releasing hormone (TRH).

II. Etiology.

A. Without thyroid enlargement. Most common cause is radioactive iodine therapy or thyroidectomy for hyperthyroidism. Second most common is idiopathic hypothyroidism. Less common are developmental defects and TSH or TRH deficiency. Amiodarone therapy can cause hypothyroidism in up to 20% of patients, as can lithium.

B. With thyroid enlargement. Most common cause is "burned out" Hashimoto's thyroiditis (autoimmune).

C. Miscellaneous causes. Drugs (e.g., lithium, amiodarone), iodine deficiency, and inherited defects in hormone synthesis are rare causes.

III. Evaluation.

A. Signs and symptoms. Fatigue, weakness, slow movement, cold intolerance, constipation, hair loss, menorrhagia, carpal tunnel syndrome, dry skin, edema of the face and extremities, memory impairment, hearing loss, hoarseness, and occasionally bradycardia and hypothermia. Sparse eyebrows with loss of the lateral half is a nonspecific sign. Pericardial effusion and ascites occasionally occur. A delay in the relaxation phase of the deep tendon reflexes, especially at the ankles, is a specific finding. Some patients have myalgias and arthralgias. Psychosis can develop with long-standing hypothyroidism and may be precipitated by thyroid hormone replacement. Infants can have hypotonia, umbilical hernia, delayed mental and physical development, and other signs and symptoms typical of adult patients. Mental retardation can result if hypothyroidism goes untreated in the first few years of life.

B. Laboratory findings. Primary hypothyroidism has elevated TSH and low free T_4. **Secondary hypothyroidism** (pituitary cause) has low TSH and low free T_4. The ^{131}I uptake is not helpful. Other laboratory abnormalities can include high AST, low sodium, low blood glucose, elevated CPK, elevated cholesterol and triglycerides, mild anemia, and elevated prolactin levels secondary to high TRH levels.

C. Treatment. Mainstay of therapy is levothyroxine. All preparations are considered equivalent; generics are just as good as the brand-name agent. **Because of variable dose in each lot, "natural" thyroid hormone is not recommended.** Average daily dose is 0.1 to 0.15 mg a day. Patients older than 40 years or with heart disease should be started with one fourth to one third the normal dose, with increases every 2 to 4 weeks until 0.1 mg is reached. The goal is to normalize TSH. Check TSH 2 to 3 months after changing the levothyroxine dose. Elective surgery should be postponed until euthyroid state is achieved with therapy. Increased sensitivity to narcotics and hypnotics is also common in the hypothyroid patient. **Some patients believe that they need doses of T_3 to feel euthyroid. This is not supported by the literature. Concurrent use of iron decreases thyroid absorption. Avoid oversuppression of the TSH; this can lead to osteoporosis.**

IV. Pregnancy and Hypothyroidism.

A. Recent data (Alexander, 2004) suggest that serum TSH levels should be checked as early as 5 weeks after conception in pregnant patients who have hypothyroidism. TSH levels should be monitored every 2 weeks until levels are stable, roughly at 20 weeks' gestation.

B. Thyroid replacement hormone doses should be adjusted to keep TSH within normal limits. Most women require increased doses of levothyroxine during pregnancy secondary to the increase in TBG caused by estrogen.

V. Subclinical Hypothyroidism. Slightly elevated TSH (<10) with normal free T_4 should be treated only if the patient is symptomatic, has a goiter, or has hypercholesterolemia. **In general, treating these asymptomatic patients can actually worsen quality of life.**

VI. Myxedema Coma.

A. Overview. *Myxedema coma* is the term used to describe patients who are in a coma or in shock with concurrent severe hypothyroidism causing bradycardia, hypothermia, hypoventilation, etc. The precipitating event is often another systemic illness. **Patients often have concurrent hypoglycemia and hyponatremia.**

B. Etiology. Severe hypothyroidism that is exacerbated by another illness such as infection, hypoglycemia, respiratory depressants, allergic reactions, hypothermia, or other metabolic stress. Cases have occurred in those on lithium or amiodarone.

C. Treatment

1. **Levothyroxine** 200 µg to 500 µg IV as a loading dose, then 50 µg/day and titrate dose until patient is euthyroid. **Some data suggest better outcomes with the use of the 500-µg dose, but use caution in those with underlying cardiac disease.** Also give T_3 5 to 20 µg PO or IV followed by 2.5 to 10 µg q8h until patient stabilizes.

2. **Hydrocortisone** 100 mg IV q8h should be given to prevent precipitation of adrenal crisis.

3. **Treat** other underlying illnesses as necessary. Mortality is 30% to 40% even with optimal care.

Thyroid Enlargement

I. **Goiter.** A goiter is a simple enlargement of the thyroid gland. It is more common in females; the highest incidence is in the second through sixth decades of life.

A. **Diffuse goiters are caused by** iodine deficiency or excess, congenital defects in thyroid hormone synthesis, and drugs (e.g., lithium carbonate).

B. **Most patients are asymptomatic.** It is unusual to have pain and rare to have hoarseness and tracheal obstruction. Thyroid function tests should be performed on all patients with goiter because it can be associated with hypothyroidism, euthyroidism, or hyperthyroidism.

II. **Multinodular goiter** is a multinodular enlargement of the thyroid gland. The most common cause is iodine deficiency.

A. **Clinical presentation**

1. **Symptoms** include thyromegaly, occasionally with rapid enlargement and tenderness secondary to hemorrhage into a cyst. Rarely, tracheal compression can occur, causing coughing or choking. Some patients may complain of a lump in the throat.

2. **Physical exam.** Many nodules of varying sizes are usually palpable. Occasionally it is difficult to distinguish from the typically lobular, irregular Hashimoto's gland.

3. **Thyroid function tests** are performed to rule out toxicity. A thyroid scan is useful only if the diagnosis of multinodular goiter is in doubt based on physical exam. A scan will show a patchy radioisotope distribution. **Malignancy is rare but should be considered if the gland is enlarging rapidly or hoarseness develops.**

B. **Treatment.** The main indications for treatment are compression of the trachea or esophagus and venous-outflow obstruction. For nontoxic multinodular goiter, the treatments include surgery, radioiodine, or thyroxine therapy. Oversuppression of the TSH can cause bone demineralization. For toxic multinodular goiter, options are antithyroid agent, surgery, radioiodine, and more recently percutaneous injection of ethanol. Levothyroxine suppression should not be given to patients with angina or other known heart disease unless the patient is hypothyroid. If thyroid enlargement persists despite adequate TSH suppression, a needle biopsy or subtotal thyroidectomy should be considered.

III. Solitary Nodules.
A. **Solitary nodules are usually benign. Suspect malignancy** in a patient with a history of radiation exposure, rapid enlargement, hoarseness or obstruction, and a solid nodule that is cold on scan.
B. **Diagnosis.** History and a thyroid scan should be done on every patient with a solitary nodule. Hot nodules that take up the radioisotope are generally benign, but **fine-needle aspiration of any solitary nodule is prudent.**
C. **Treatment** is indicated with signs of compression of trachea or esophagus, significant growth, and recurrence of a cystic nodule after aspiration. Treatment is similar to multinodular goiter: surgery, thyroxine, or radioiodine for nontoxic nodule; antithyroid agent, surgery, radioiodine for toxic nodule. Suppressive therapy with levothyroxine is usually not effective, however.

Other Thyroid Disorders

I. **Subacute thyroiditis** causes diffuse enlargement of the thyroid gland and may be associated with hyperthyroidism, hypothyroidism, or euthyroidism. See the section on hyperthyroidism for discussion of this entity.
II. **Euthyroid sick syndrome** involves decreased peripheral conversion of T_4 to active T_3. Labs show a decreased serum T_3, an increased reverse T_3, a decreased T_4, and a low or normal TSH. It is possible that these patients have a transient central hypothyroidism. However, this syndrome may be protective in the ill patient, and treatment with thyroid replacement does not improve outcomes. Treat the underlying illness.

ADRENAL DISEASE

I. **Adrenal Insufficiency.**
A. **Etiology**
1. **Primary adrenal insufficiency (Addison's disease)** is most commonly caused by autoimmune disease. This can be associated with other autoimmune endocrinopathies such as thyroid disease or diabetes. Other causes include hemorrhage into the adrenal glands especially during sepsis, metastatic disease, TB, histoplasmosis, amyloidosis, AIDS, and treatment with ketoconazole. Serum Na^+ <130 mEq/L and K^+ >5 mEq/L with metabolic acidosis suggests primary adrenal insufficiency.

6

HEMATOLOGIC, METABOLIC, AND ELECTROLYTE DISORDERS

2. **Secondary adrenal insufficiency** is caused by hypothalamus or pituitary destruction or suppression. It can occur from steroid administration that is abruptly discontinued. **With this form of adrenal disease, the renin–angiotensin–aldosterone system remains intact; therefore, the electrolyte abnormalities of Addison's disease are rarely observed.**

B. **Symptoms**

1. Weakness, fatigue, orthostatic hypotension, anorexia, nausea, vomiting, and weight loss.

2. Hyperpigmentation (especially in skin folds or creases) and freckling secondary to ACTH stimulation of melanocytes. This is not seen with secondary adrenal insufficiency where the ACTH is low.

3. Cold intolerance and hypometabolism.

4. Disease may be insidious and manifest with shock during acute illness or injury

C. **Diagnosis**

1. **Cosyntropin stimulation test:**

a. Draw baseline plasma cortisol level.

b. Give cosyntropin 250 µg (0.25 mg) IV before 9:00 AM.

c. Draw plasma cortisol levels 30 to 60 minutes later.

d. A level greater than 20 µg/dL after stimulation is normal. An 8 AM level of less than 5 µg/dL prior to stimulation is diagnostic for adrenal insufficiency; a level less than 10 µg/dL is suggestive. This test can be normal in the setting of recent-onset (1-2 weeks) *secondary* adrenal insufficiency.

e. If testing is normal but you still strongly suspect adrenal insufficiency, consider metyrapone test (next).

2. **Metyrapone test** is used to diagnose recent-onset secondary adrenal insufficiency. It should be performed in the hospital.

a. Draw baseline cortisol level.

b. Administer metyrapone 3 g orally at midnight.

c. Measure serum cortisol and deoxycortisol at 8:00 AM the next day. If the hypothalamic–pituitary–adrenal axis is intact, the plasma cortisol level should be less than 5 µg/dL and the 11-deoxycortisol level greater than 10 µg/dL.

4. Serum ACTH is elevated in primary adrenal insufficiency and low in secondary adrenal insufficiency.

D. **Treatment**

1. **Adrenal crisis**

a. Draw serum electrolytes, glucose, plasma cortisol, and ACTH if diagnosis is suspected but not known. Start therapy immediately without waiting on lab results.

b. **Infuse 1 to 2 L NS or D$_5$ NS rapidly.** Correct hypoglycemia, hyponatremia, hyperkalemia, and hypercalcemia.

c. **Hydrocortisone 100 mg IV stat, then q6h.** An alternative that does not interfere with cortisol testing is dexamethasone 4 mg or more IV q6h.

d. **Search for infection or other causes for precipitation of adrenal crisis.**

e. **Taper steroids over the next 2 to 3 days to maintenance dosing** (hydrocortisone succinate 150 mg IV on day 2, 75 mg IV on day 3).

2. **Maintenance therapy**

a. **Prednisone** 5 to 7.5 mg PO qhs *or* dexamethasone 0.5 mg PO qhs (0.25-0.75 mg) *plus* fludrocortisone 0.1 mg PO qd if a mineralocorticoid is needed. Bedtime dosing more closely mimics the diurnal variation in the ACTH (lowest in the morning).

b. **Add hydrocortisone 5 to 10 mg PO in midafternoon if needed for symptom control (weakness, fatigue).**

c. **Hydrocortisone as a maintenance agent is falling out of favor** with some endocrinologists, but you can use hydrocortisone 15 to 20 mg PO every morning and 5 to 10 mg PO in the midafternoon.

d. Women may need long-term androgen replacement.

3. **Management of adrenal disease during acute illness or surgery**

a. **For minor febrile illness or stress (physiologic),** increase steroid 2 to 3 times usual daily dose for 3 days. No need to increase fludrocortisone.

b. **For severe illness, vomiting, or trauma,** hydrocortisone or equivalent 100 mg IV q6-8h.

4. **Surgery**

a. **Minor procedures** may be performed under local anesthetic, normal daily dosing.

b. **Moderately stressful procedures** require a single dose of hydrocortisone 100 mg IV before the procedure.

c. **Major surgery** requires hydrocortisone 100 mg IV immediately before induction anesthesia and continue 100 mg IV q8h. Taper dose by half each day over 3 days, then resume maintenance dosing.

II. **Cushing's Syndrome (Glucocorticoid Excess).**

A. **Etiology.** Most commonly secondary to exogenous steroid administration. ACTH-secreting pituitary microadenoma (Cushing's disease), adrenal tumors, and ectopic ACTH-secreting tumors (small cell lung cancer) make up a minority of causes.

B. **Clinical findings.** Moon (rounded) facies, truncal obesity, buffalo hump, abdominal stria, poor wound healing, hirsutism, amenorrhea, hypertension, glucose intolerance, atrophic skin with "senile purpura," and psychiatric abnormalities.

C. **Diagnosis**

1. **Elevated AM fasting cortisol** of greater than 14.3 μg/dL with lack of diurnal variation (100% specific at this level but not 100% sensitive).

2. **Elevated 24-hour urine free cortisol** is sensitive for Cushing's syndrome (usually >150 mg/24 h in Cushing's). Urine 17-OHS is not helpful because of false positive results in obesity.

3. **Dexamethasone suppression test.** Administer dexamethasone 1 mg PO at midnight.

a. Measure 8 AM serum cortisol next day; normal is <2 μg/dL. However, 8% of those with Cushing's syndrome suppress to <2 μg/dL. **Therefore, the dexamethasone suppression test should not be the only test to rule out Cushing's in the patient with high clinical probability.**

b. **If above is equivocal, give dexamethasone 0.5 mg PO q6h for 48 hours.** Collect 24-hour urine during last 24 hours of test. Urine free

cortisol should be low. Alternatively, draw blood at hour 6 after the test ends and check serum levels of cortisol, dexamethasone, and ACTH.
c. You can also administer dexamethasone IV 1 mg/h for 7 hours by constant infusion. At the end of this time, a normal person should have reduced plasma cortisol by at least 7 mg/dL over baseline value.
d. Further diagnosis for cause and therapy should be performed in consultation with an endocrinologist.

METABOLIC ACIDOSIS

I. Definition.
A. Metabolic acidosis is a pH <7.4 and implies a loss of bicarbonate or accumulation of fixed acids.
B. Patients are divided into two groups based on the calculated anion gap $(Na^+ - [Cl^- + HCO_3^-])$. A normal anion gap is ≤12. The body will try to compensate for a metabolic acidosis with hyperventilation, which drops the Pco_2 and partially corrects the acidosis.
II. Urine Ion Gap.
A. Calculating the urine ion gap ($[Na^+ + K^+] - Cl^-$) can help determine if acidosis is related to kidney function. A normal urine anion gap $(-20$ to -50 mEq/L) implies normal renal NH_4^+ excretion and a nonrenal cause for the acidosis. An abnormal (e.g., elevated) positive gap denotes the opposite.
B. Caveat: Ion gap calculation is only valid in the absence of diuretics. Also, if the patient is volume depleted secondary to GI losses, urine ion gap could be falsely elevated.
III. Normal Anion Gap Acidosis.
A. GI bicarbonate (HCO_3^-) losses, including causes relating to diarrhea, ileostomy, and colostomy.
B. Renal tubular acidosis
1. **Distal (type I) RTA** is caused by a distal nephron acidification defect. The patient is hypokalemic and urine pH is >5.3. Causes include familial and idiopathic hypercalciuria, Sjögren's syndrome, rheumatoid arthritis, primary hyperparathyroidism, multiple myeloma, and severe dehydration as well as lithium, amphotericin B, and toluene. Distal RTA is occasionally seen in a hyperkalemic form with SLE, obstructive uropathy, or sickle cell uropathy. Treat with bicarbonate repletion at 1 to 2 mEq/kg/day with any acute K^+ deficit corrected and maintenance oral K^+ if needed.
2. **Proximal (type II) RTA** is caused by a defect in the ability of proximal tubules to recover bicarbonate. Acutely the urine pH is usually >5.5, but it decreases with falling serum bicarbonate levels, resulting in increased proximal reabsorption of bicarbonate; the final result is urine pH 5.5. Causes include autoimmune diseases (see type I RTA), multiple myeloma, heavy metals, acetazolamide, and outdated tetracycline. Treatment is to identify the primary cause and treat it. Bicarbonate at 5 to 15 mEq/kg

per day may be required and can result in severe hypokalemia. Consider use of thiazide diuretics to cause ECF volume contraction to promote HCO_3^- reabsorption proximally.

3. **Type IV RTA** is generally caused by moderate renal insufficiency with renal resistance to aldosterone (as in diabetes). Presentation is similar to that for hyporeninemic hypoaldosteronism. K^+ may be normal but generally is increased. Bicarbonate is typically >15 mEq/L. Urine pH, done under mineral oil at time of collection, is usually <5.5. Treat with K^+ restriction and consider use of loop diuretics such as furosemide (Lasix and others). Bicarbonate may be needed (see above for dosing). Fludrocortisone (Florinef) at 0.1 to 0.2 mg PO qd may be useful if primary adrenal insufficiency is the cause.

C. **Interstitial renal disease** is the same as type IV RTA; the kidney is insensitive to aldosterone, leading to a hypoaldosterone state and an elevated serum K^+.

D. **Ureterosigmoid loop**

E. **Ingestion** of acetazolamide, ammonium chloride, cholestyramine, calcium chloride, or magnesium chloride.

F. **Small bowel drainage** or fistula, biliary drainage or fistula, or pancreatic drainage or fistulas.

IV. **Increased Anion Gap Acidosis.**

A. **Ingestions** including methanol, ethanol, ethylene glycol (antifreeze), salicylates, paraldehyde, cyanide (including from nitroprusside). **You can measure for these substances directly, but the first step is to determine the osmolar gap:** measured osmolarity – calculated osmolarity.

$$\text{Calculated osmolarity} = (2 \times [Na^+]) + (glucose/18) + (BUN/2.8)$$

An osmolar gap indicates the presence of an unmeasured substance (e.g., ethanol, methanol, ethylene glycol, lactate) or ESRD without dialysis (GFR <10). Treatment depends on the underlying condition.

B. **Uremia** or renal failure.

C. **Lactic acidosis.**

D. **Alcoholic ketoacidosis or diabetic ketoacidosis.**

V. **Treatment.**

A. Acidosis usually resolves with aggressive IV hydration and correction of the underlying disease (e.g., DKA).

B. Consider sodium bicarbonate therapy if the patient has severe acidemia (blood pH <7.0, bicarbonate <8 mmol/L). **However, there is no evidence that bicarbonate changes outcomes, and it can be harmful.**

METABOLIC ALKALOSIS

I. **Definition.**

A. Metabolic alkalosis is defined as serum pH >7.40. It implies a loss of acid or gain of bicarbonate.

B. ECF volume contraction, hypokalemia, and increased mineralocorticoids or glucocorticoids all impair the normal kidney's ability to excrete excess HCO_3^- and can result in a metabolic alkalosis. Additionally, excess exogenous bicarbonate ingestion should be in the differential.

C. Metabolic alkalosis is separated into the two categories; chloride responsive and non–chloride responsive. The urine Cl⁻ level is measured to help differentiate the causes of metabolic alkalosis. A urine Cl⁻ of <25 mEq/L suggests normal renal function (in the absence of diuretics). ECF contraction secondary to overzealous diuretic use or other cause of dehydration is commonly termed *contraction alkalosis*.

II. Clinical findings include carpal–pedal spasms, tetany, neuromuscular irritability, hypotension, hypoventilation, impaired cognition, cardiac arrhythmias, and decreased levels of ionized Ca^{2+}.

III. Diagnosis.

A. Elevated serum HCO_3^- levels and alkalotic serum pH.

B. There may be a compensatory respiratory acidosis with a decrease in the respiratory rate.

C. The urine may be alkaline or paradoxically acidic, especially in the presence of K^+ wasting (hyperaldosteronism and diuretic use).

IV. Treatment.

A. Chloride-responsive alkalosis is the more commonly seen form, with urine Cl⁻ <10-25 mEq/L. It is usually secondary to contraction alkalosis caused by GI HCl losses (emesis, NG suctioning) or diuretic use. It is occasionally seen with villous adenomas or cystic fibrosis. Treat the underlying cause and correct concurrent hypokalemia (for IV KCl see following section on hypokalemia). Chloride may be administered as NaCl tablets or as NS if the patient is volume depleted. Use caution in those with CHF and those who are fluid overloaded. Consider acetazolamide if renal function is intact. Some physicians also recommend use of H_2-blockers to decrease gastric HCl losses.

B. Non–chloride-responsive alkalosis has urine Cl⁻ generally >25 mEq/L and even >45 mEq/L. It is seen in primary hyperaldosteronism, Cushing's syndrome, and renal artery stenosis. It is occasionally seen in patients who consume excessive amounts of licorice or secondary to severe hypokalemia (<2.0 mEq/L) or Bartter's syndrome (see hypokalemia discussion later). The primary treatment is to determine the underlying cause and to correct it. See hypokalemia discussion for treatment of low levels of potassium.

C. Other rare causes of alkalosis include massive citrated blood transfusions, hypercalcemia of malignancy, sarcoidosis, vitamin D toxicity, and high-dose penicillin–carbenicillin. Also consider milk-alkali syndrome.

D. If the metabolic alkalosis is severe (pH >7.55 or bicarbonate >45 mmol/L) with systemic effects, consider HCl acid therapy, which is typically done in an ICU setting.

POTASSIUM

I. **Total body K$^+$** is approximately 50 mEq/kg body weight; 98% is intracellular. A serum decrease of 1 mEq of K$^+$ corresponds to a 10% to 20% deficit in total body K$^+$.

II. **Serum K$^+$ concentration** is not always a reliable indicator of total body K$^+$. Distribution is affected by multiple factors (see hyperkalemia and hypokalemia sections). Total body K$^+$ is largely controlled by the kidney, with 90% of ingested K$^+$ excreted in the urine and 10% of the daily K$^+$ load excreted in the GI tract (in uremic patients this can increase to 33%). **Aldosterone promotes potassium excretion (and thereby can cause hypokalemia).** Normally there is no significant K$^+$ loss through the skin. However, with profuse sweating the K$^+$ loss through the skin can approach 24% of the daily K$^+$ load. From 5 to 15 mEq of K$^+$ is lost daily in the urine even with no K$^+$ intake.

Hypokalemia

I. **Hypokalemia is defined** as serum K$^+$ level <3.5 mEq/L (note that for K$^+$, Na$^+$, and Cl$^-$, mmol/L = mEq/L).

II. **Etiology**

A. **GI losses of K$+$** are seen in vomiting, NG suction, diarrhea, malabsorption syndrome, and laxative or enema abuse. Villous adenomas can excrete K$^+$ and are associated with a large amount of mucus in the stools. GI losses distal to the stomach result in a low urine K$^+$ concentration and metabolic acidosis secondary to high bicarbonate losses. GI losses from the stomach result in a high urine K$^+$ concentration (usually >40 mEq/L) and metabolic alkalosis secondary to high hydrochloride loss. Hydrogen ions are retained by the kidney in an attempt to maintain acid–base balance in exchange for potassium.

B. **Drug-induced hypokalemia** can be due to abnormal losses (diuretics such as thiazides, furosemide, ethacrynic acid; mineralocorticoid or glucocorticoid; penicillin and aminoglycosides). It can also be secondary to transcellular K$^+$ shift (epinephrine, decongestant, bronchodilators, tocolytics, theophylline, caffeine, insulin, and verapamil). Significant K$^+$ loss is more likely if the patient has edema (edematous states are associated with elevated aldosterone level, which stimulates K$^+$ excretion). Serum K$^+$ concentration should be measured before initiating a diuretic and 1 week after initiation or increase in dose of the diuretic.

C. **Other causes of hypokalemia**

1. **Insufficient dietary K$^+$ is an unusual cause** and is seen occasionally in alcoholics or cachectic patients.

2. **Excessive renal losses.** Hypokalemia occurs with a urine K$^+$ concentration of >20 mEq/L. **Causes** include hyperaldosteronism, Barter's syndrome (hypokalemia, normotension, no edema, sodium

wasting, and metabolic alkalosis), glucocorticoid excess, Mg^{2+} deficiency, osmotic diuresis, and some types of RTA (see earlier).

3. **Extracellular to intracellular shift.** Metabolic alkalosis shifts potassium intracellularly (in exchange for hydrogen), as do insulin and adrenergic excess (MI, inhaled β-agonists).

4. **Hyperaldosteronism.** Patients can have hypertension and edema when severe. To evaluate, stop all antihypertensives that can change the test (diuretics, ACE inhibitors, ARBs) and liberalize diet (must have normal Na^+ intake); get baseline serum aldosterone value, and then give fludrocortisone 0.2 mg PO tid for 3 days. Recheck serum aldosterone, which should be <3 ng/dL. See "Hypertension" in Chapter 3 as well. Other protocols are also used, such as spironolactone challenge.

5. **Rarely hypokalemic familial periodic paralysis.**

III. **Presentation.**

A. Patients are mostly asymptomatic. However, hypokalemia can cause weakness (especially of proximal muscles), perhaps areflexia, and decreased GI motility, resulting in ileus.

B. Hyperpolarization of the myocardium occurs with hypokalemia and can cause ventricular ectopy, reentry phenomena, and conduction abnormalities. The ECG usually shows flattened T and U waves and ST-segment depression. Hypokalemia also causes increased sensitivity of cardiac cells to digitalis preparations, which can result in toxicity at therapeutic plasma levels of digitalis.

IV. **Treatment** goal in all patients is 4.0 mEq/L.

A. **Magnesium. It is difficult or impossible to correct a K^+ deficit in the face of hypomagnesemia, a frequent occurrence with potassium-wasting diuretics.** A Mg^{2+} level should be checked if there is any difficulty increasing the serum potassium. Mg^{2+} should be replaced if the serum level is low. **Because serum Mg^{2+} levels do not reflect total body stores, empiric use of Mg^{2+} is indicated despite a normal serum Mg^{2+} if it is still difficult to increase the serum potassium (see section on hypomagnesemia).**

B. **Oral therapy. K^+ supplementation** (20 mEq KCl) should be given at the start of non–potassium-sparing diuretic therapy if indicated. **A rule of thumb that can be used is 10 mEq of KCl should raise serum K^+ levels by approximately 0.1 mEq/L.** Recheck K^+ concentration 2 to 4 weeks after starting supplementation. Check periodically thereafter. In hypokalemic–hypochloremic metabolic alkalosis, a chloride supplement should be given as well (KCl). Consider potassium-sparing diuretics, which might not require potassium supplementation. Renal failure and ACE inhibitors are relative (but not absolute) contraindications to potassium-sparing diuretics.

C. **IV therapy should be used for severe hypokalemia** and in patients unable to tolerate oral supplementation. If serum K^+ concentration is >2.4 mEq/L and there are no ECG changes, K^+ can be given at a rate up to 10 to 20 mEq/h, with maximum daily administration of 200 mEq.

Rapid treatment may be required if K⁺ concentration is <2 mEq/L with ECG changes; up to 40 mEq/h can be given if the patient is on a monitor and the K⁺ is given, diluted, through a peripheral line. Serum K⁺ concentrations should be measured every 4 to 6 hours with the patient under continuous ECG monitoring. Use a nondextrose solution to prevent insulin release, which causes potassium to shift intracellularly.

Hyperkalemia

I. **Hyperkalemia is defined** as serum K⁺ above laboratory normal (generally 5.0 mEq/L).

II. **Etiology.**

A. **Inadequate renal excretion** results from acute or chronic renal failure, potassium-sparing diuretics, ACE inhibitors, and ARBs,.

B. **Potassium load from massive cell death** is caused by crush injuries, major surgery, burns, acute arterial emboli, hemolysis, GI bleeding, or rhabdomyolysis. **Exogenous sources** such as ingestion of potassium supplements and salt substitutes, blood transfusions, IV potassium administration, and high-dose penicillin therapy must also be considered. Also consider water softeners as a potential source of exogenous potassium.

C. **Intracellular to extracellular shift** is caused by acidosis, digitalis toxicity, insulin deficiency, or rapid increase of blood osmolality.

D. **Adrenal insufficiency/hypoaldosteronism** (Addison's disease) (see section above).

E. **Pseudohyperkalemia** is secondary to hemolysis of blood sample or prolonged tourniquet time.

III. **Presentation.**

A. **The most important effect is a change in cardiac excitability.** ECG shows sequential changes with a rising serum potassium level. Initially, tall peaked T waves are seen (K⁺ >6.5 mEq/dL). This is followed by prolonged PR intervals, diminished P-wave amplitude, and widened QRS complexes (K⁺ 5.7-8 mEq/L). Eventually the QT interval prolongs and leads to a sine-wave pattern. Ventricular fibrillation and asystole are likely with K⁺ >10 mEq/L.

B. Other findings include paresthesias, weakness, areflexia, and ascending paralysis.

IV. **Treatment.** Continuous ECG monitoring is warranted if ECG changes are present or if serum potassium is >7 mEq/L.

A. **Calcium gluconate** may be administered IV as 10 mL of a 10% solution over 10 minutes to stabilize myocardium and cardiac conduction system (1 ampule). This can be repeated twice at 5-minute intervals if no response. Administration of calcium can cause digitalis toxicity in patients receiving digitalis therapy. **Calcium gluconate should not be used in the face of digitalis toxicity.**

6

HEMATOLOGIC, METABOLIC, AND ELECTROLYTE DISORDERS

B. **Sodium bicarbonate** alkalinizes the blood, causing a shift of potassium from the extracellular fluid to the intracellular space. This is given as 40 to 150 mEq of $NaHCO_3$ IV over 30 minutes or as an IV bolus in an emergency; it can worsen CHF because of sodium load. The effect is temporary but will work even when serum pH is normal.

C. **Insulin** causes a shift of K^+ from the extracellular fluid into cells; 5 to 10 U of regular insulin should be administered with 1 ampule of 50% glucose IV over 5 minutes. A response might not be seen for 50 to 60 minutes, and the effect usually lasts for several hours.

D. **Cation-exchange resins** such as sodium polystyrene sulfonate (e.g., Kayexalate) remove K^+ from the body by binding K^+ in the GI tract in exchange for another cation (Na^+ in the case of sodium polystyrene sulfonate and most other drugs in this class). These drugs may be given orally or rectally. The initial oral dose is 15 to 30 g of sodium polystyrene sulfonate mixed with 50 to 100 mL of 70% sorbitol to counteract its constipating effect. The dose may be repeated every 3 to 4 hours if needed. A retention enema is given as 50 g of sodium polystyrene sulfonate mixed with 200 mL of 20% sorbitol or $D_{20}W$ and may be repeated every 1 to 2 hours initially and then every 6 hours or as necessary. These agents cause a significant sodium load and can precipitate CHF.

E. **Dialysis** may be required in severe, refractory cases of hyperkalemia.

F. **Aerosolized β_2-agonists** drive K^+ intracellularly and are particularly useful in renal failure. You can use constant nebulization of albuterol.

G. **Potassium restriction** is indicated in the late stages of renal failure (GFR <15 mL/min).

H. **Adrenal insufficiency is treated acutely with hydrocortisone succinate.** See the discussion of adrenal insufficiency in this chapter.

SODIUM

Hyponatremia

I. **Hyponatremia** is defined as serum sodium below normal (generally 135 mEq/L). There are **four possible states; Box 6-3** gives an overview. Initial assessment is to measure urine osmolality and urine sodium. Then assess the patient's volume status based on clinical exam and lab data such as urine specific gravity and BUN/Cr. Hyponatremia is then classified as follows: artifactual or spurious, dilutional (hypervolemic with expansion of total body water), hypovolemic (sodium depletion in excess of water depletion), and euvolemic (sodium and water depletion in equal amounts).

II. **Types of Hyponatremia.**

A. **Artifactual or spurious are due to lab reporting error secondary to hyperglycemia or hyperlipidemia.**

BOX 6-3
DIFFERENTIAL DIAGNOSIS OF HYPONATREMIA BASED ON VOLUME STATUS AND URINE SODIUM
SPURIOUS (SODIUM DECREASED BECAUSE OF LABORATORY INTERACTION)*
Hyperglycemia
Hyperlipidemia
Hyperproteinemia (myeloma, macroglobulinemia, etc.)
Mannitol
Other osmotically active substances
HYPOVOLEMIA (DRY) AND URINE SODIUM >20 mEq/L (RENAL LOSS)
Diuretics
RTA, Metabolic acidosis
Osmotic Diuresis (e.g. mannitol, DM)
Mineralocorticoid deficiency
Hypoaldosteronism
Addison's disease
HYPOVOLEMIA (DRY) AND URINE SODIUM <10 mEq/L (EXTRARENAL LOSS)
Vomiting, diarrhea, NG suction
Third-spacing such as with burns, pancreatitis, surgery, etc.
Sweating
EUVOLEMIA (NO EDEMA) AND URINE SODIUM > 20 mEq/L
Glucocorticoid deficiency
Stress (physical, emotional)
Drugs
SIADH
Hypothyroidism
HYPERVOLEMIA (EDEMA) AND URINE SODIUM >20 mEq/L
Renal failure
HYPERVOLEMIA (EDEMA) AND URINE SODIUM <10 mEq/L
Other causes of fluid overload such as cirrhosis, CHF, nephrotic syndrome, etc.
SIADH (pt might not appear edematous)

*This occurs only if using flame photometer and *not if measured by ion-selective electrode.*

1. **Hyperglycemia.** Correct sodium for glucose. Each increase of blood glucose of 100 mg/dL decreases serum sodium by 1.7 to 2.4 mEq/L depending on how high the glucose is; 2.4 mEq/L is used as the correction factor when the glucose is >300 mEq/L. **No need to correct if ion-specific laboratory probe is used.**
2. **Hyperlipidemia.** Measured serum osmolality is normal and greater than the calculated osmolality:

$$Osm = (2 \times Na^+) + (Glucose/18) + (BUN/2.8)$$

B. **Dilutional or hypervolemic (SIADH is discussed separately later)**
1. **Etiology is defect in water excretion** including sodium-retaining (edematous) states, CHF, renal failure, nephrotic syndrome, cirrhosis, and ascites.

2. **Diagnosis of dilutional or hypervolemic hyponatremia** (to diagnose most causes of hypervolemic or dilutional hyponatremia [renal failure, CHF, hypothyroidism, and Addison's disease], see the section appropriate to the individual illness).

a. Clinical situation and underlying disease are key to determining the cause.

b. Urine sodium concentration is usually very low (<10 mEq/L). However, with acute and chronic renal failure, patients can have urine Na^+ and Cl^- concentrations >20 mEq/L.

c. Urine osmolality is elevated (only valid in absence of diuretics).

d. **Excessive water intake without sodium retention can cause hyponatremia in the presence of renal failure, hypothyroidism, or Addison's disease.**

C. **SIADH** is nonosmotically driven ADH secretion and may be euvolemic or hypervolemic.

1. **Etiology**

a. SIADH can be caused by CNS disorders including Guillain-Barré and subarachnoid hemorrhage, by acute intermittent porphyria, and by many drugs including MAO inhibitors, desmopressin, paregoric, oral hypoglycemic agents, opioids, barbiturates, vincristine, clofibrate, carbamazepine, and NSAIDs. SIADH is also seen with physical stress, including postoperatively. Postoperative hyponatremia is more common and more severe in menstruating females.

b. **Reset osmostat accounts for 20% to 30% of cases of apparent SIADH.** The Na^+ is generally 125 to 135 mEq/dL and stable despite treatment (alteration of fluids, solutes, etc.).

2. **Diagnosis.**

a. Patients with SIADH generally have a normal GFR and urine osmoles of >130 mOsm/kg. This is an inappropriately hypertonic urine with respect to serum Na^+. Urine osmolality should be <130 mOsm/kg if the patient is hyponatremic because the kidneys should be conserving sodium and getting rid of free water. In SIADH, urine osmoles are >130 mOsm/kg, indicating the kidneys cannot properly conserve sodium and excrete free water.

b. **ADH can be measured in the blood.** However, ADH excretion can be erratic and might not be elevated at all times in SIADH.

c. To differentiate SIADH from a reset osmostat (for example, when treatment for SIADH is not working): **Give a 10 to 15 mL/kg water bolus (oral or via D_5W IV).** Normal patients and those with a reset osmostat will excrete 80% within 4 hours. Those with SIADH will not respond and excretion will be impaired. **Patients with a reset osmostat will not respond to therapy for SIADH.** Therapy is unnecessary because the patient has achieved a new equilibrium. Try to correct underlying abnormalities, however.

3. **Treatment (try in the order listed)**
a. Restrict fluid to 1 L/d.
b. Give salt tablets or hypertonic saline with or without a loop diuretic to clear free water.
c. Demeclocycline 3.25 to 3.75 mg/kg q6h to antagonize the effect of ADH on the kidney might help. Doses up to 1200 mg/day (400 mg q6h) have been used. Use with caution in those with liver disease, CHF, or renal failure.
d. Give IV urea (30 g/d) to increase free fluid excretion. **Use only if first three fail and patient is symptomatic.**

C. **Hypovolemic**
1. **Causes** are combined water and sodium loss: GI loss such as vomiting, NG suction, diarrhea; third-space losses as with burns, surgery; excessive sweating, diuretics; renal and adrenal disease including uncontrolled diabetes mellitus, hypoaldosteronism, Addison's disease, recovery phase of renal disease.
2. **Diagnosis**
a. **If renal function is normal, the urine osmolality is high and the urine Na⁺ usually less than 10 to 15 mEq/L;** thus the kidney is responding appropriately by conserving Na⁺. The FE_{Na} is <1%. (See Chapter 24 for calculations.)
b. In those with kidney or adrenal disease, the urine Na⁺ is usually >20 mEq/L and is not helpful. (See section on renal failure.)
c. In the presence of metabolic alkalosis, urine Na⁺ may be high with a low urine chloride (<10 mEq/L).

D. **Euvolemic hyponatremia** is caused by SIADH; see earlier for diagnosis and treatment. It can also be caused by water intoxication but usually requires intake of >10 L/day. Other causes include hypothyroidism, stress, and adrenal insufficiency. With these latter three, the urine Na⁺ is >20 mEq/L. Fluid restriction is diagnostic (see diabetes insipidus discussion later for protocol).

III. **Clinical presentation of hyponatremia** depends on severity and time course of onset.

A. Rapidly developing hyponatremia is more symptomatic.

B. If plasma Na⁺ drops 10 mEq/L over several hours, patients can have nausea, vomiting, headache, and muscle cramps.

C. If plasma Na⁺ drops 10 mEq/L in an hour, patients can have severe headache, lethargy, seizures, disorientation, and coma.

1. Mortality is 50% if Na⁺ concentration falls rapidly to less than 113 mEq/L.

2. Serum electrolytes should be checked in any patient with a change in mental status.

D. Patient might have signs of the underlying illness (such as CHF, Addison's disease). If hyponatremia is secondary to fluid loss, patient might have signs of shock including hypotension and tachycardia.

HEMATOLOGIC, METABOLIC, AND ELECTROLYTE DISORDERS

6

IV. **Treatment.**
A. **Treat underlying condition** (CHF, Addison's disease, hypothyroidism, SIADH). See specific section on treatment of underlying disease.
B. **Stop any contributing drugs.**
C. **Correct a long-standing hyponatremia slowly and a rapidly developing hyponatremia more aggressively.** Do not overcorrect hyponatremia. Overcorrection can precipitate central pontine myelinolysis. Consider early therapy with IV NaCl. This is associated with better outcomes than fluid restriction.
1. **Do not raise serum Na+ more than 12 mEq/L in 24 hours in asymptomatic patients.** If the patient is symptomatic, increase serum Na+ by 1 to 1.5 mEq/L per hour until symptoms resolve.
2. **To calculate the amount of Na+ needed to raise the serum Na+ to 125 mEq/L:**

$$Na \ (mEq) = 125 \ mEq/L \times Actual \ serum \ Na^+ \ (mEq/L) \times TBW \ (L)$$

$$TBW = 0.6 \times Body \ weight \ (kg)$$

3. You may replace Na+ with 3% or 5% NaCl solution (provide 0.51 mEq/mL and 0.86 mEq/mL, respectively).
4. In those with ECF volume expansion, diuretics may be necessary.

Hypernatremia

I. **Hypernatremia** is defined as a serum sodium above normal (generally >145 mEq/L).
II. **Etiology.**
A. **Hypernatremia results if hypotonic fluid losses are not adequately replaced.**
1. If fluid losses are extrarenal (GI losses, perspiration, or hyperventilation), the urine osmolality will be greater than that of the serum, and urinary Na+ will be <20 mEq/L.
2. A urine osmolality less than or equal to that of the serum implies renal fluid losses (diuretic therapy, osmotic diuresis, diabetes insipidus, acute tubular necrosis, postobstructive uropathy, hypokalemic nephropathy, or hypercalcemic nephropathy).
B. **Hypernatremia can occur with hyperalimentation or other hypertonic fluid administration.**
III. **Signs and symptoms.** Muscle irritability, confusion, ataxia, tremulousness, seizures, and finally coma. Additional manifestations usually occur secondary to the underlying abnormality and volume status (tachycardia and orthostatic hypotension with volume depletion; edema with fluid excess).
IV. **Treatment.**
A. **Hypernatremia with volume depletion should be treated by administration of isotonic saline until hemodynamic stability is achieved.** You can then correct the remaining water deficit with D_5W or hypotonic saline.

B. Hypernatremia with volume excess is treated with diuresis or, if necessary, with dialysis. D_5W is then administered to replace the water deficit.

C. Body water deficit is estimated by:

$$Deficit = Desired\ TBW - Current\ TBW$$

$$Desired\ TBW = Measured\ serum\ Na \times (Current\ TBW/Normal\ serum\ Na)$$

$$Current\ TBW = 0.6 \times Current\ body\ weight$$

where TBW is measured in liters and body weight is measured in kilograms.

D. One half the calculated water deficit should be given in the first 24 hours, and the remaining deficit is corrected over 1 or 2 days to avoid cerebral edema secondary to abrupt change in serum sodium concentration.

E. Diabetes insipidus (serum sodium might be normal if patient has no access to free water) is caused by either renal resistance to ADH or decreased secretion of ADH, including granulomatous disease, CNS trauma or hypoxia, tumor, drugs (especially lithium carbonate), etc. Patient can have polyuria and polydipsia.

1. **Diagnosis.** An initial urine osmolality of <300 mOsm/kg indicates possibility of diabetes insipidus (though occasionally urine osmolality is 300-500 mOsm/kg). Patients with hypernatremia should have a maximally concentrated urine (800-1200 mOsm/kg). **Next step is water deprivation under direct observation** because of risk of hypovolemia for 6 to 12 hours. **Check urine and serum osmolality.** If patient can concentrate urine to normal with fluid deprivation (>800 mOsm/kg), the problem is not diabetes insipidus (consider water intoxication, etc.). **If patient is not able to concentrate urine, the problem is probably diabetes insipidus.** Confirm by administration of 10 to 20 mU of DDAVP by nasal spray or 5 units SQ. If urine concentrates by 50%, the diagnosis is central diabetes insipidus. If urine does not concentrate, consider nephrogenic diabetes insipidus (e.g., kidney unresponsive to ADH) or other diagnosis causing hypernatremia.

2. **Treatment.** DDAVP 10 to 25 mg intranasally bid to reduce polydipsia or polyuria.

CALCIUM

Hypercalcemia

I. Hypercalcemia is elevated serum Ca^{2+} of >10.5 mg/dL after correction for serum albumin:

$$Corrected\ calcium = Serum\ calcium +$$
$$(0.8 \times [Normal\ serum\ albumin - Patient's\ albumin])$$

Another option is to measure ionized calcium.

II. History. "Bones, stones, abdominal groans, and psychic overtones."

A. If hypercalcemia is mild, patient may be asymptomatic.
Hypercalcemia is often found on routine screening labs. Asymptomatic, incidental hypercalcemia secondary to hyperparathyroidism need not be treated.

B. Moderate elevations cause constipation, anorexia, nausea, vomiting, abdominal pain, and ileus.

C. More severe elevations (>12 mg/dL) cause emotional lability, confusion, delirium, psychosis, stupor, coma, weaknesses, and seizures. Nephrolithiasis or urolithiasis is common. Patient can have associated renal failure or QT shortening.

D. No symptom complex is sensitive enough to be diagnostic.

III. Etiology and pathophysiology. Overabsorption of calcium as with milk-alkali syndrome; too little calcium excretion as with thiazide use, or excess mobilization of bone as with hyperparathyroidism or metastatic cancer.

IV. Differential diagnosis. See specific topic for additional information.

A. Spurious. High-calcium meal before blood draw, long tourniquet application time; 53% are normocalcemic when calcium level is repeated.

B. Hyperparathyroidism. Patients generally have high calcium, low phosphate, and elevated serum parathyroid hormone.

C. Malignancy: Breast cancer (50% of cases with malignant causes), lung cancer, multiple myeloma, renal cancer, colon cancer, prostate cancer, ovarian cancer, and others.

D. Together, hyperparathyroidism and malignancy account for 80% to 90% of cases of hypercalcemia in adults.

E. Drugs and Foods: Lithium carbonate, vitamin D, vitamin A, thiazide diuretics, milk, as in milk-alkali syndrome.

F. Hyperthyroidism or hypothyroidism. See section above.

G. Immobilization and bed rest.

H. Addison's disease. See section above.

I. Cushing's disease. See section above.

J. Multiple endocrine neoplasia. MEN type I: tumors of parathyroid, pituitary, pancreas, and possibly Zollinger–Ellison syndrome; MEN type II: medullary thyroid carcinoma, hyperparathyroidism, pheochromocytoma.

K. Paget's disease of the bone (see Chapter 7).

V. Evaluation.

A. History and physical exam, including drug and vitamin history.

B. Repeat calcium level to rule out artifact. Get fasting AM calcium, electrolytes, BUN, creatinine, and alkaline phosphatase; look for evidence of renal failure, adrenal failure, and bone disease. Measure TSH to rule out hyperthyroidism or hypothyroidism. If repeat calcium level is elevated and no other abnormality is noted, continue work-up.

C. Check parathyroid hormone level, preferably using a two-site, double-antibody, immunoradiometric assay (immunoassay for intact parathyroid hormone). Also obtain a parathyroid hormone–related peptide (PTHrp), which can be elevated in hypercalcemia secondary to malignancy. Obtain a simultaneous calcium. If parathyroid hormone is high, the diagnosis is hyperparathyroidism. Consider surgical referral for parathyroidectomy. Normal or low parathyroid hormone suggests malignancy; continue work-up.

D. Search for malignancy, including breast exam, mammogram, chest radiograph, stool guaiac, PSA value, abdominal CT, bone scan, bone radiographs, etc., as dictated by patient age, history, and physical. Obtain serum and urine protein electrophoresis looking for myeloma if indicated (urine dipstick will not pick up Bence Jones proteins).

E. If this work-up is negative and patient has uveitis or erythema nodosum and has bilateral hilar adenopathy on CXR, sarcoid can be assumed. Serum ACE levels are unreliable (see sarcoid section, Chapter 4).

F. If work-up is negative and patient is asymptomatic, repeat calcium level and work-up in 6 months.

G. If work-up remains negative and calcium remains high, consider neck exploration for parathyroid adenoma.

VI. Laboratory Results.

A. High chloride and low phosphate levels suggest hyperparathyroidism.

B. Anemia, high sedimentation rate, abnormal serum globulins, low albumin level, and proteinuria suggest malignancy.

C. Elevated parathyroid hormone defines hyperparathyroidism.

D. Elevated BUN and creatinine levels suggest renal failure.

E. Elevated alkaline phosphatase levels suggest a bone process such as Paget's disease of the bone or metastatic breast or prostate cancer.

VII. Treatment. Address underlying disorder (see under specific diagnosis).

A. Acute treatment

1. **If patient is severely symptomatic or if serum Ca^{2+} is >15 mg/dL, reduce serum Ca^{2+} rapidly.**

2. **Promote diuresis and replace intravascular volume with normal saline.** If renal function is intact, give 1 to 2 L NS and furosemide 80 to 100 mg IV q2-12h for the first 24 hours. Adjust furosemide and saline rates to prevent fluid overload and intravascular depletion. Replace urine losses with NS and KCl to prevent hypokalemia. Avoid thiazide diuretics, which can cause calcium retention.

3. **If renal function is compromised and the patient is symptomatic, consider acute hemodialysis.**

4. **Calcitonin** 4 to 8 units SQ q6-12h is not very potent but is rapid acting. It will lower serum Ca^{2+} by 1 to 3 mg/dL. Use one or two

doses as emergency therapy while waiting for other modalities to work. Calcitonin is short acting. Side effects include abdominal cramping, nausea, flushing, and allergic reaction (to salmon calcitonin). Calcitonin nasal spray is now available for maintenance.

5. **Bisphosphonates** inhibit osteoclastic activity and are helpful in hyperparathyroidism and malignancy.
   (1) **Pamidronate** 60 to 90 mg IV over 4 to 24 hours is more potent than etidronate and achieves control in 70% to 100% of cases. It is effective within 2 days and reaches nadir at 7 days. Side effects are mild and include a transient increase in temperature ($<2°$ C), transient leukopenia, and a small decrease in serum phosphate. Pamidronate is generally preferred over etidronate and plicamycin.
   (2) **Disodium etidronate** 7.5 mg/kg IV daily over 4 hours for 3 to 7 days; can cause increase in serum creatinine and phosphate. Long-term administration can lead to osteomalacia. Calcium drops within 2 days and reaches nadir at 7 days. Disodium etidronate achieves control in 60% to 100%.

6. **Plicamycin (mithramycin)** 25 mg/kg IV in 500 mL D_5W over 3 to 6 hours is useful. May be repeated several times at 24- to 48-hour intervals. It is especially useful in hypercalcemia from malignancy. Side effects include nausea, local irritation, cellulitis if extravasation occurs, hepatic toxicity, nephrotoxicity, and thrombocytopenia. It is contraindicated in hepatic or renal dysfunction and in thrombocytopenia and other coagulopathies. Plicamycin works in 12 hours with peak at 72 hours. Use is becoming less common as bisphosphonates become more common. It is less well tolerated and less effective than pamidronate.

7. **Steroids.** Prednisone 60 mg/day PO or hydrocortisone succinate 200 to 300 mg IV. These are helpful for hypercalcemia from vitamin D intoxication, myeloma, and breast carcinoma.

8. **A very risky approach is to administer 1 L of disodium phosphate and monopotassium phosphate (0.5-1 g can be given over 24 h). This can cause soft-tissue calcification, renal failure, and death. This approach should be tried only if all other measures fail, hypercalcemia is life threatening, and hemodialysis is unavailable. A nephrology or endocrinology consultation is suggested before using this modality.**

B. **Chronic treatment.**

1. **Oral calcium binders** including phosphates (elemental phosphorus 1-3 g/d). Do not use in patients with renal failure. See Chapter 8, section on renal osteodystrophy for details.

2. **Oral etidronate** 1200 to 1600 mg/d. Can cause osteomalacia. Alendronate and risedronate may also be used but are not FDA approved for this indication.

3. **Pamidronate** may be repeated in initial dose (see earlier) weekly if needed. It does not cause osteomalacia.

Hypocalcemia

I. Hypocalcemia is defined as serum Ca^+ <8.8 mg/dL (usually <7 mg/dL when symptoms are present). Correct for serum albumin.

Corrected calcium = Measured serum calcium +
$$(0.8 \times [\text{normal serum albumin} - \text{Patient's albumin}]).$$

II. Causes include hypoparathyroidism, vitamin D deficiency or resistance, renal tubular acidosis and renal failure, magnesium depletion, acute pancreatitis, septic shock, and drugs (cisplatin, pentamidine, foscarnet, furosemide, ketoconazole). Hypocalcemia can also be spurious.

III. Clinical Symptoms.

A. Primarily neurologic

B. If hypocalcemia develops slowly, symptoms include confusion, encephalopathy, depression, and psychosis. Tetany, convulsions, laryngospasm, carpopedal spasm, and muscle aches may also be noted.

C. Look for Chvostek's sign (contraction of facial muscles elicited by light tapping of facial nerve).

D. Trousseau's sign. Carpopedal spasms elicited by application of tourniquet to extremity for 3 minutes. Avoid in those with vascular disease or coagulopathy.

IV. Treatment.

A. If tetany is present, administer 10 mL of 10% calcium gluconate over 15 to 30 minutes. The effect lasts only a few hours and repeat infusions might be required (calcium gluconate 60 mL in 500 mL D_5W at 0.5-2 mg/kg/h). Measure calcium every 2 hours.

B. Calcium can cause digoxin toxicity and can cause arrhythmias in those taking digitalis.

C. Correct any hypomagnesemia (see hypomagnesemia and hypokalemia discussion).

D. Administer oral calcium 1 to 7 g/d, divided, with meals.

E. If secondary to renal failure see renal osteodystrophy (Chapter 8).

F. If hypocalcemia is secondary to vitamin D deficiency, give vitamin D replacement, such as calcitriol (Rocaltrol), calcifediol (Calderol), etc.

G. If the patient is vitamin D resistant, treat with inorganic phosphate 1 to 3.5 g/d and calcitriol 0.25 to 1 mg/d.

MAGNESIUM

Hypermagnesemia

I. Hypermagnesemia is defined as serum Mg^{2+} >2.5 mg/dL. Distribution of Mg^{2+} is as follows: 50% of body stores is in bone, the remainder is mostly in muscle, <1% in ECF; 20% to 30% is protein bound and the remainder is free cation. Most is absorbed in small bowel and excreted by kidneys.

II. Causes.

A. Renal failure in patients administered magnesium-containing products (laxatives and antacids).

B. IV administration of Mg^{2+} (as in preeclampsia).

III. Clinical signs include impairment of neuromuscular transmission, which manifests as muscle weakness, respiratory depression, absence of deep tendon reflexes, widened QRS and prolonged PR interval, hypotension, heart block, and asystole.

IV. Treatment.

A. Administer 10 to 20 mL of 10% calcium gluconate IV over 10 minutes or 10% $CaCl_2$ 5 to 10 mg/kg IV to temporize. In patients without severe renal dysfunction, 20 mL of 10% calcium gluconate in a liter of NS can be given at 100 to 200 mL/h.

B. Administration of furosemide or ethacrynic acid can enhance excretion.

C. Hemodialysis is effective.

Hypomagnesemia

I. Hypomagnesemia is defined as serum $Mg^{2+} < 1.9$ mg/dL. However, serum levels do not reflect total body stores, and a patient (especially in CHF, using a diuretic, etc.) can be total body depleted and still have normal serum levels of Mg^{2+}.

II. Causes.

A. Hypomagnesemia is relatively common in stress situations such as myocardial infarction and shock.

B. Alcoholism and nutritional deficiency (chronic TPN).

C. Loss from diarrhea, diuretics (diuretics are a major cause of hypomagnesemia in those with CHF), and osmotic diuresis (diabetes).

D. Renal causes include hyperaldosteronism and hypoparathyroidism. Hypercalcemia causes increased renal Mg^{2+} excretion.

E. Amphotericin B and cyclosporin A.

III. Clinical signs and symptoms include anorexia, lethargy, vomiting, tetany, arrhythmias, seizures, and prolonged PR and QT intervals.

IV. Treatment.

A. In an emergency, give 2 to 4 g $MgSO_4$ in 50 mL D_5W over 5 to 15 minutes. Dose can be repeated to a total of 10 g over the next 6 hours. Continue replacement for 3 to 7 days with 48 mEq/L per 24 hours.

B. In a less severe situation, replace 0.03 to 0.06 g/kg per day in four to six doses until serum Mg^{2+} is normal.

C. Continue oral replacement therapy as long as precipitating factor is present (such as oral Mag-Ox one PO bid).

BIBLIOGRAPHY

Adams RJ, McKie VC, Hsu L, et al: Prevention of a first stroke by transfusions in children with sickle cell anemia and abnormal results on transcranial Doppler ultrasonography. *N Engl J Med* 339:5-11, 1998.

Adrogue HJ, Madias NE: Hypernatremia. *N Engl J Med* 342:1493-1499, 2000.

Adrogue HJ, Madias NE: Hyponatremia. *N Engl J Med* 342:1581-1589, 2000.

Adrogue HJ, Madias NE: Management of life-threatening acid-base disorders. First of two parts. *N Engl J Med* 338:26-34, 1998.

Adrogue HJ, Madias NE: Management of life-threatening acid-base disorders. Second of two parts. *N Engl J Med* 338:107-111, 1998.

Ahya SN (ed): *Manual of Medical therapeutics*, 30th ed, Philadelphia, Lippincott Williams & Wilkins, 2001.

Alexander EK, Marqusee E, Lawrence J, et al: Timing and magnitude of increases in levothyroxine requirements during pregnancy in women with hypothyroidism. *N Engl J Med* 351:241-249, 2004.

American Diabetes Association: Screening for type 2 diabetes. *Diabetes Care* 27: S11-S14, 2004.

Beers MH, Berkow R (eds): *The Merck Manual of Diagnosis and Therapy*, 17th ed. Rahway, NJ, 1Merck, 1999.

Boulton AJ, Kirsner RS, Vileikyte L: Clinical Practice. Neuropathic diabetic foot ulcers. *N Engl J Med* 351:48-55, 2004.

Cines D, Blanchette VS: Immune thrombocytopenic purpura. *N Engl J Med* 346: 995-1008, 2002.

Cooper DS: Subclinical hypothyroidism. *N Engl J Med* 345:260, 2001.

Diabetes Control and Complications Trial Research Group: The effect of intensive treatment of diabetes on the development and progression of long-term complications of diabetes mellitus. *N Engl J Med* 329(14):977, 1993.

Eisenbarth GS, Gottlieb PA: Autoimmune polyendocrine syndromes. *N Engl J Med* 350:2068-2079, 2004.

Elizalde JI, Clemente J, Marin JL, et al: Early changes in hemoglobin and hematocrit levels after packed red cell transfusion in patients with acute anemia. *Transfusion* 37(6):573-576, 1997.

Fajan SS, Bell GI, Polonsky KS: Molecular mechanism and clinical pathophysiology of mature onset diabetes of the young. *N Engl J Med* 345:971-980, 2001.

Frank RN: Diabetic Retinopathy. *N Engl J Med* 350:48, 2004.

Ganguly A: Primary aldosteronism *N Engl J Med* 339, 1828, 1998.

Gennari FJ: Hypokalemia, *N Engl J Med* 339:451-458, 1998.

Goodnough LT, Basch RG: Anemia, transfusion, and mortality. *N Engl J Med* 345: 1272-1274, 2001.

Grundy SM, Cleeman JI, Marz CN, et al: Implications of RECENT Clinical trials for the National Cholesterol Education Program Adult Treatment Panel III guidelines. *Circulation* 110:227-239, 2004.

Hebert PC, Wells G, Blajchman MA, et al: A multicenter, randomized, controlled clinical trial of transfusion requirements in critical care. *N Engl J Med* 340: 409-417, 1999.

Hermus AR, Huysmans DA: Treatment of benign nodular thyroid disease. *N Engl J Med* 338:1438-1447, 1998.

Joshi N, Caputo GM, Weitekamp MR, Karchmer AW: Infections in patients with diabetes mellitus, *N Engl J Med* 341:1906-1912, 1999.

Kasper DL, Braunwald E, Fauci A, et al (eds): *Harrison's Principles of Internal Medicine*, 16th ed. New York, McGraw-Hill, 2002.

6

HEMATOLOGIC, METABOLIC, AND ELECTROLYTE DISORDERS

Kitabchi AE, Wall BM: Management of diabetic ketoacidosis. *Am Fam Physician* 60:455-464, 1999.

Kjos SL, Buchanan TA: Gestational diabetes mellitus. *N Engl J Med* 341:1749-1756, 1999.

Klein J, Ojamaa K: Thyroid hormone and the cardiovascular system. *N Engl J Med* 344:501-509, 2001.

Kyle R: A long-term study of prognosis in monoclonal gammopathy of undetermined significance. *N Engl J Med* 346:564-569, 2002.

Greer JP, Foerster J, Lukens JN (eds): *Wintrobe's Clinical Hematology*. 11th ed. Philadelphia, Lippincott Williams & Wilkins, 2003.

Mannucci P: Treatment of von Willebrand's disease. *N Engl J Med* 351:683-694, 2004.

Mannucci PM, Tuddenham EG: The hemophilias—from royal genes to gene therapy. *N Engl J Med* 344:1773-1779, 2001.

Marx SJ: Hyperparathyroid and hypoparathyroid disorders. *N Engl J Med* 343:1863, 2000.

McCartney MM, Gilbert FJ, Murchison LE, et al: Metformin and contrast media: A dangerous combination? *Clin Radiol* 54:29-33, 1999.

Nathan DM: Initial management of glycemia in type 2 diabetes mellitus. *N Engl J Med* 347:1342, 2002.

Pearce EN, Farwell AP, Braverman LE: Thyroiditis. *N Engl J Med* 348:2646-2655, 2003.

Ritz E, Orth SR: Nephropathy in patients with type 2 diabetes mellitus. *N Engl J Med* 341:1127-1133, 1999.

Robertson RP: Islet transplantation as a treatment for diabetes. A work in progress, *N Engl J Med* 350:694, 2004.

Sanford JP: *Guide to Antimicrobial Therapy*. Dallas, Anti-Microbial Therapy, 2004.

Section on Hematology/Oncology, Committee on Genetics; American Academy of Pediatrics: Health supervision for children with sickle cell disease. *Pediatrics* 109:526-535, 2002.

Shumak KH, Rock GA, Nair RC: Late relapses in patients successfully treated for thrombotic thrombocytopenic purpura. Canadian Apheresis Group. *Ann Intern Med* 122:569, 1995.

Silverberg SJ, Shane E, Jacobs TP, et al: A 10-year prospective study of primary hyperparathyroidism with or without parathyroid surgery. *N Engl J Med* 341:1249-1255, 1999.

Steinberg MH: Drug therapy: Management of sickle cell disease. *N Engl J Med* 13:340, 1999.

Tavill AS, American Association for the Study of Liver Diseases, American College of Gastroenterology, American Gastroenterological Association: Diagnosis and management of hemochromatosis. *Hepatology* 33:1321-1328, 2001.

Toft AD: Subclinical hyperthyroidism. *N Engl J Med* 345:512, 2001.

U.K. Prospective Diabetes Study Group: UKPDS 28: A randomized trial of efficacy of early addition of metformin in sulfonylurea-treated type 2 diabetes. *Diabetes Care* 21:87-92, 1998.

Warkentin TE, Greinacher A: Heparin-induced thrombocytopenia: Recognition, treatment, and prevention: The Seventh ACCP Conference on Antithrombotic and Thormbolytic Therapy. *Chest* 126:311S-337S, 2004.

Yanovski SZ, Yanovski JA: Obesity. *N Engl J Med* 346:591-602, 2002.

Rheumatology

Jennifer L. Jones

GENERAL RHEUMATOLOGY

Laboratory data can be used to support the diagnosis of a rheumatologic syndrome (Tables 7-1 and 7-2). **However, rheumatologic diagnosis is primarily clinical, based on specific criteria outlined in the following sections.** Ordering "arthritis panels" is discouraged because the presence of an antibody in the absence of physical criteria is meaningless.

RHEUMATOID ARTHRITIS

I. **Overview.** RA is a chronic systemic inflammatory disease principally involving joints but also with extra-articular manifestations. It has a prevalence of 1% to 3% in the U.S. population, and females are affected 2 to 3 times more often than males. Life span is decreased on average by 7.5 years for men and 3.5 years for women. Incidence and severity increase with HLA-DR4 genotype. Disease onset is acute, subacute, or gradual; clinical course is self-limited or progressive.

II. **Diagnosis.**

A. To make a diagnosis of RA, at least four of the seven criteria of the American Rheumatology Association (ARA) must be present; the first four must be present for at least 6 weeks. **Be aware that a positive rheumatoid factor is only one criterion, and a positive rheumatoid factor need not be present for a diagnosis of RA to be made.** Additionally, there should not be evidence of other disease that could account for the symptoms, such as polyarteritis nodosa or lupus.

1. Morning stiffness in and around joints, lasting more than 1 hour.
2. Arthritis (must include soft tissue swelling or edema) of three or more joint areas simultaneously.
3. Arthritis of at least one of the following: wrist, metacarpophalangeal (MCP), or proximal interphalangeal (PIP) joint.
4. Symmetric arthritis involving the same joint areas bilaterally.
5. Rheumatoid nodules.
6. Positive serum rheumatoid factor.
7. Radiographic changes typical of RA on hand and wrist radiographs, including erosions or unequivocal bony decalcification in or adjacent to the involved joints.

B. **Most patients have an insidious onset; however, a third of patients experience rapid onset in days or weeks.** The disease may be rapidly progressive, causing joint destruction and other sequelae, or it can progress slowly; many have a fluctuating course of exacerbations and remissions. Symptoms remit in 70% of women during pregnancy.

TABLE 7-1
LABORATORY PROFILES OF RHEUMATOLOGIC DISEASES

Disease	Rheumatoid Factor	ANA	Denatured DNA	Anti-native DNA (anti ds-DNA)	Anti-Smith	Anti-Ro (SSA)	Anti-LA (SSB)	Anti-SCL70	Anti-centromere	Anti-Jo	ANCA	Ribosomal RNP	U1nRNP	Histone
RA*	+ (90%)	+ (40%)	− (20%)	− (<5%)	−	− (<5%)	−	−	−	−	−	−	−	− (15%)
SLE	− (20%)	+ (95%)	+ (75%)	+ (60%)	(15%)	(15%)	(15%)	−	−	−	−	− (10%) †	− (40%)	+ (70%)
Drug-induced SLE	−	+	+ (80%)	−	−	−	−	−	−	−	−	−	−	+ (90%)
SS	− (25%)	+ (90%)	−	−	−	−	−	(45%)	− (<1%)	−	−	−	−	−
SS-L	− (25%)	+ (90%)	−	−	−	−	−	− (10%)	+ (50%–80%)	−	−	−	−	−
PM/DM	− (30%)	+ (90%)	−	−	−	−	−	(10%)	−	(30%)	−	−	− (25%)	−
Wegener's	+ (50%)	− (15%)	−	−	−	−	−	−	−	−	+ (>90%)	−	−	−
MCTD	−	−	−	−	−	−	−	−	−	−	−	−	+ (100%)	−
Sjog	+ (75%)	+ (95%)	−	−	−	+ (65%)	+ (65%)	−	−	−	−	−	−	−

Note: Percentages in parentheses indicate the approximate positive percentage.

* Anticyclic citrullinated peptide (anti-CCP) is more specific than RF.

†But 85+ for SLE with cerebritis/psychosis.

+, positive in most cases; −, negative in most cases; MCTD, mixed connective tissue disorder; PM/DM, polymyositis/dermatomyositis; RA, rheumatoid arthritis; Sjog, Sjogren's syndrome; SLE, systemic lupus erythematosus; SS, scleroderma; SS-L, scleroderma, limited (aka CREST syndrome).

TABLE 7-2
PATTERN REPORTED BY LABORATORY FOR EACH TYPE OF ANTIBODY

ANTIBODY:	Anti-native DNA (anti-ds-DNA)	Anti-Smith	Anti-Ro (SSA)	Anti-LA (SSB)	Anti-SCL70	Anti-centromere	Anti-Jo	ANCA	Ribosomal RNP	U1nRNP	Histone
PATTERN:	Dif +/- Rim	Sp	Sp	Sp	Dif + Nuc	Cent	Cyto	P-ANCA: Perinuclear C-ANCA: Coarse	Nuc + Cyto	Sp	Dif

ANCA, antineutrophil cytoplasmic antibody; Cent, centromeric; Cyto, cytoplasmic; Dif, diffuse; ds, double stranded; Nuc, Nucleolar; Sp, speckled.

RHEUMATOLOGY

7

III. Clinical Features.

A. Articular manifestations

1. **Pathogenesis.** Synovium (synovial membrane) is the site of onset of inflammation; proliferation and hyperplasia of synovia occurs ("pannus" is the inflammatory synovium that contacts the cartilage). The pannus invades subchondral tissue and juxta-articular bone, resulting in erosions around the margins and joint destruction. You can see subchondral cysts, loss of cartilage, and bony erosion; thickened pannus may be palpated around joints, and a joint effusion may be present. There is also inflammatory destruction of soft tissues, resulting in laxity of ligaments and tendons.

2. **Sites.** The most commonly involved joints are MCP and PIP joints and wrists. Distribution is symmetric; small joints are predominantly involved, but elbows, shoulders, hips, knees, and ankles can also be involved.

3. **Specific joint involvement**

   a. **The hand is involved in 85% of patients.** You may notice fusiform swelling of fingers and MCP joints, ulnar deviation of fingers, and palmar subluxation of proximal area of phalanges. DIP and first CMC joints are usually spared (in contrast to osteoarthritis). Ulnar deviation at MCP joints often is associated with radial deviation at the wrist. Swan-neck and boutonnière deformities are also common. Patient may develop tendon rupture of fourth and fifth finger extensor tendons.

   b. **Cervical spine is commonly affected (40%).** Laxity of the transverse ligaments can lead to atlantoaxial subluxation or, less commonly, subluxation at lower levels, with possibility of resultant cord compression. Symptoms are those of a radiculopathy, including pain radiating up into the occiput, paresthesia, acute deterioration in hand function, sensory loss, abnormal gait, and urinary retention or incontinence.

   c. **Feet are also commonly involved,** including MTP, talonavicular, and ankle joints, in descending order of frequency. Severe disease can lead to pes planus, midfoot collapse, and hammertoe deformities.

B. Extraarticular complications

1. **Constitutional features** include fatigue, weight loss, muscle pain, excessive sweating, and low-grade fevers.

2. **Rheumatoid nodules** are characteristic of RA and seen in up to 25% to 50% of patients, especially those with more severe disease and high rheumatoid factor level. They occur in the lungs, heart, kidney, and dura mater, in addition to the extensor surface of the forearm, olecranon, Achilles tendons, ischial area, and other bony prominences. They are usually asymptomatic.

3. **Rheumatoid vasculitis.** Vasculitic lesions include rheumatoid nodules, small nail fold infarcts, and palpable purpura. It can also manifest by mononeuritis multiplex, organ ischemia, CNS infarctions, and MI.

4. **Ophthalmic.** Keratoconjunctivitis sicca is the most common eye complication and results in dry eyes with slight redness and normal vision. Episcleritis (usually asymptomatic), and scleritis (pain, photophobia; untreated may lead to vision loss) also occur.

5. **Respiratory.** Up to 40% have asymptomatic pleural disease, including pleural effusion and subpleural nodules. Patients can also develop symptomatic disease, including diffuse interstitial fibrosis with or without pneumonitis, bronchiectasis, bronchiolitis obliterans, or pulmonary hypertension. COPD is more common in RA patients than in the general public.

6. **Cardiac.** Symptomatic cardiac disease is not common, although asymptomatic cardiac involvement is common in seropositive patients. The most common type is acute pericarditis (unrelated to duration of arthritis), which can develop into tamponade. Rheumatoid nodules can involve valves, pericardium, and myocardium, leading to conduction defects or heart failure; coronary artery vasculitis can lead to MI.

7. **Neurologic.** Patient can have entrapment neuropathy secondary to tissue swelling (as in carpal tunnel). Mononeuritis multiplex can occur and is related to ischemic neuropathy from vasculitis.

C. Laboratory findings

1. **Anemia of chronic disease** (normochromic or hypochromic, normocytic) or thrombocytosis reflecting inflammation (see Chapter 6).

2. **Rheumatoid factor (RF) and anti-cyclic citrullinated peptide (anti-CCP).** RF occurs in 85% of patients but is not specific for the diagnosis of RA. RF is an immunoglobulin directed against IgG. Generally higher titers are found in those with more generalized disease and destructive arthritis. Extremely high titers are associated with the presence of rheumatoid nodules. **False positives occur with infection, TB, sarcoid, syphilis, various cancers, and lung and liver disease.** Anti-CCP antibodies have sensitivity similar to RF but are 90% to 96% specific for rheumatoid arthritis.

3. **Synovial fluid white blood cell count** is 5000 to 20,000/mm^3 with 50% to 70% neutrophils; cultures should be negative.

4. **Felty's syndrome** is a combination of (generally severe) seropositive RA, splenomegaly, and leukopenia (WBC <3500/mL, neutropenia). It is associated with serious infections, vasculitis (leg ulcers, mononeuritis), anemia, thrombocytopenia, and lymphadenopathy.

D. **Radiographic findings:** Characteristic changes in RA include periarticular osteopenia, symmetric narrowing of the joint space, and marginal bone erosions.

IV. **Treatment. Early and aggressive therapy with disease-modifying drugs at time of diagnosis is important.** Goal is to decrease joint destruction by controlling disease within 2 years of onset. More than 95% of seropositive patients respond to therapy, and 70% of patients have partial or complete remission.

7

RHEUMATOLOGY

A. **Education.** The basic treatment program consists of patient education and balancing rest, exercise, and medication. Physical and occupational therapy are important for preserving joint function.

B. **Analgesics and NSAIDs** provide symptomatic relief but **do nothing to suppress the rate of cartilage erosion or to alter the course of the disease.** Doses should be increased to the recommended maximum over 1 to 2 weeks; a medication should not be abandoned until the patient has been on a maximum dose for at least 2 weeks, because it can take this much time to reach maximal efficacy. In continued treatment failure, consider switching to another category of NSAID. Naproxen 500 mg PO bid and ibuprofen 600 mg PO tid are some of the least-expensive NSAIDs. Proton pump inhibitors taken with NSAIDs reduce incidence of gastric and duodenal ulcers.

C. **COX-2 inhibitors.** Celecoxib (Celebrex) and valdecoxib (Bextra) have no effect on disease progression, have the same efficacy as other NSAIDs, are likely to increase stroke and MI (valdecoxib), and have no GI advantage over ibuprofen in the long run (celecoxib). Up to 12% of patients on a COX-2 inhibitor develop ulcers, and these drugs are expensive. Both have renal side effects but no direct effects on platelets. *Note:* **Studies suggest that even one aspirin a day (e.g., for cardiac or stroke prophylaxis) negates any GI advantage of the COX-2 inhibitors.** The authors do not recommend the use of COX-2 inhibitors except in unusual circumstances.

D. **Disease-modifying antirheumatic drugs (DMARDs).** These drugs modify the fundamental pathologic process, limit bone loss, and should be started within 3 months of diagnosis. Aggressive treatment with a combination of DMARDs is the standard of care, although study data do not yet support one combination over another. Treatment must be individualized. Because of the spontaneous waxing and waning of RA, these drugs should be used for approximately 6 months before one decides on efficacy.

1. **Methotrexate is the most prescribed DMARD.** Use of methotrexate in combination with other drugs is increasing, and combination therapy of methotrexate, sulfasalazine, and hydroxychloroquine works better than either drug alone and better than sulfasalazine plus hydroxychloroquine. Methotrexate has also been used with cyclosporine. Dosing is 7.5 to 15 mg PO weekly. **Contraindications:** concomitant therapy with sulfonamide-containing antibiotics or HIV seropositivity. Alcohol consumption, gross obesity, and diabetes predispose to hepatic toxicity. Patient may have nausea, vomiting, and abdominal cramps. Serious side effects are bone marrow toxicity, alveolitis, and hepatic fibrosis. CBC every month and liver enzyme studies every 2 to 3 months are recommended. Persistent elevation of liver enzymes or significant hypoalbuminemia can indicate the need for a liver biopsy. Drug should be administered with folic acid, at least 5 mg/wk, which decreases side effects but not efficacy.

2. **Biologic response modifiers** modify the cytokines that mediate inflammation. These drugs are used as monotherapy or in combination with other agents and are commonly used in patients who have failed more inexpensive therapies. Combining them with another agent such as methotrexate seems to allow a sustained response and provide better control of disease progression than either drug alone. They are all given as injections and are quite expensive.

a. **TNF-α inhibitors** include infliximab (Remicade; approved in combination with methotrexate, not as monotherapy), etanercept (Enbrel), and adalimumab (Humira). TNF-α inhibitors are contraindicated in patients with ongoing infections or NYHA class III or IV heart failure and cannot be used with live virus vaccines.

b. **IL-1 inhibitor** is anakinra (Kineret) as mono- or combination therapy. May not be used in combination with TNF-α inhibitors due to increased risk of immunosuppression.

3. **Steroids.** Glucocorticoids have anti-inflammatory and immunosuppressive effects and modestly reduce joint erosion when used long term (e.g., prednisolone 7.5 mg qd for 2 years). **Because of their side-effect profile, they should mainly be used for treating acute flares or as bridging therapy until DMARDs become therapeutic.** Low-dose corticosteroids (<10 mg prednisone qd or equivalent) can be used in combination with other DMARDs. Keep steroid doses at the minimum effective dose because of osteopenia and other side effects such as insulin resistance, increased susceptibility to infection, ecchymoses, cataracts, and cushingoid appearance. Patients on chronic steroids should also take vitamin D, calcium, and possibly alendronate or risedronate (depending on degree of bone mineral loss).

4. **Leflunomide** is a pyrimidine synthesis inhibitor shown to reduce bone erosions. Efficacy is similar to methotrexate and sulfasalazine. It has a long half-life of 14 to 16 days. A loading dose of 100 mg qd for 3 days is suggested, followed by 20 mg/d. Leflunomide requires 4 to 6 weeks to reach a steady state. Monitor CBCc for bone marrow suppression and LFTs for hepatotoxicity.

5. **Antimalarials.** Hydroxychloroquine 400 to 600 mg PO daily for 4 to 6 weeks and then 200 to 400 mg daily. Baseline ophthalmologic examination with subsequent examinations every 6 months can allow one to detect early eye changes. Patient can have ciliary muscle dysfunction or corneal opacities. Having the patient view an Ansler grid daily will give an early warning of vision changes.

6. **Sulfasalazine** 500 mg PO qd, and then increase doses to a maximum of 3000 mg daily. Reduce to 500 mg qid for maintenance. Contraindications include sulfonamide allergy. Side effects include bone marrow toxicity, hepatitis, reversible oligospermia, yellow discoloration of urine and of soft contact lenses, nausea, headache, and abdominal discomfort. Monitoring CBCs and liver enzymes is recommended as well as semiannual visual field checks.

7

RHEUMATOLOGY

7. **Penicillamine.** Start with 125 to 250 mg PO qd 1 hour before or 2 hours after eating, and then increase the dose by 125 to 250 mg daily every 1 to 2 months to a maximum of 750 to 1000 mg daily. Metallic taste and nausea are common early problems that resolve with continued use. Skin rashes, bone marrow toxicity, and proteinuria may occur. Autoimmune syndromes, including myasthenia gravis, polymyositis, pemphigus, and Goodpasture's syndrome, have been reported to result from penicillamine. A monthly urinalysis and CBC count are recommended, and penicillamine should not be used in those with renal disease.

8. **Antibiotics.** Minocycline 100 mg PO bid has been shown to be effective for mild to moderate RA in a double-blind placebo-controlled trial. This is probably secondary to its anti-inflammatory effects.

9. **Azathioprine** 50 to 100 mg PO qd (1.0 to 1.5 mg/kg/d, which may be increased by 0.5 mg/kg/d weekly to 3 mg/kg/d after 3 months). Nausea is the main limiting factor. Azathioprine is more toxic than other disease-modifying drugs. Monthly CBC and quarterly LFTs are recommended. The concomitant use of allopurinol increases toxicity and should be avoided. Dosage should be reduced if renal impairment is present.

10. **Cyclophosphamide tends to be toxic,** and many patients have one or more side effects. These include nausea or vomiting (58%), alopecia (26%), dysuria (26%), hemorrhagic cystitis (14%), and herpes zoster (5%). Other adverse reactions included leukopenia, thrombocytopenia, and amenorrhea in premenopausal women.

11. **Cyclosporine** can be used for patients with severe, refractory disease. However, the potential for irreversible toxicity suggests limiting the drug to patients who are unresponsive to other therapy.

12. **Gold salts.** Oral gold tends to be less toxic than other medications but is less effective. Injectable gold is more toxic and no more effective than hydroxychloroquine and sulfasalazine. Parenteral form is gold sodium thiomalate and aurothioglucose, given IM as a single dose of 10 mg, followed by 25 mg 1 week later to test for sensitivity. Maintenance therapy is 25 to 50 mg weekly. If there is no improvement with a cumulative dose of 1 or 2 g or if toxicity develops, therapy should be discontinued. Oral therapy with Auranofin 3 to 6 mg PO qd commonly causes diarrhea. With either form, monthly urinalysis and CBC counts should be performed. Common side effects include pruritic skin rash, mouth ulcers, transient leukopenia, eosinophilia, and diarrhea (oral gold). Treatment can sometimes be temporarily halted and then restarted at lower doses, and side effects might not recur, but rash must be allowed to clear because it can lead to an exfoliative dermatitis. From 3% to 10% of patients develop transient proteinuria; this usually only requires cessation of treatment until the urine clears. Other less common

adverse effects include thrombocytopenia, pancytopenia, agranulocytosis, and aplastic anemia. These side effects usually respond to stopping drug; a gold-chelating agent (dimercaprol) can be used if response is not fast enough.

OSTEOARTHRITIS

I. **Overview.** OA is the most common joint disease worldwide. It is a condition of synovial joints characterized by focal cartilage loss and an accompanying reparative bone response. Typical radiographic features are joint space narrowing, osteophytes, and sclerosis. OA is strongly related to age. It is rare under 45 years of age without trauma, but at least half of those older than 65 years have radiographic evidence of OA.

II. **Types.**

A. **Primary OA** is a wear-and-tear phenomenon. Commonly affected joints include PIP and DIP joints, first CMC joint, knees, and hips. OA generally spares the shoulders and MCP joints. Increased body mass speeds the rate of OA development in weight-bearing joints.

B. **Secondary OA** can involve joints that are generally not involved with primary OA, including MCP joints, shoulder, or isolated large joints. It may be related to chondrocalcinosis or another secondary cause (see later).

1. **Traumatic arthritis** secondary to slipped capital femoral epiphysis, congenital hip dislocation, destruction secondary to septic joint, hemophilia, or other injury.

2. **Paget's disease** is a defect of bone resorption and redeposition in older persons. Radiograph shows typical scalloped pattern of bone deposition, and 85% have an elevated alkaline phosphatase with a normal GGT and serum 5'-nucleotidase. The serum 5'-nucleotidase has fewer false positives and is the preferred test to rule out a hepatic cause of alkaline phosphatase elevation. An alternative is to fractionate the alkaline phosphatase into bone and hepatic subtypes. Patients can have associated deafness, cardiac abnormalities, etc. Urine hydroxyproline does not accurately reflect disease activity. However, *N*-telopeptides and pyridinoline crosslink assays can be used to follow disease course. Risedronate or alendronate may be used for treatment.

3. **Alkaptonuria with ochronosis** is a rare disorder of tyrosine metabolism causing pigmentation and eventual breakdown of cartilage.

4. **Hemochromatosis.** About 50% of patients show chronic progressive arthritis, affecting predominantly MCP and wrist joints, as well as large joints, including shoulders, hips, and knees. Treatment for arthritis is symptomatic; see Chapter 6 for treatment of the underlying disease.

5. **Wilson's disease.** About 50% of adults with Wilson's disease have arthropathy, characterized by mild OA of the wrists, MCP joints, knees, and spine.

7

RHEUMATOLOGY

6. **Neuroarthropathy (Charcot's joint)** is a severe destructive arthropathy caused by impaired joint sensation. Diabetes mellitus, tabes dorsalis, and syringomyelia are common causes. The foot is involved most commonly.

III. **Clinical Features.**

A. **Pain after joint use progressing to pain with minimal movement, at rest, and at night.** As opposed to RA, there is generally no early morning stiffness (or <30 min of stiffness) or gelling.

B. **Pain and crepitus on passive movement** and joint enlargement are often noted.

C. **Some patients develop genu valgus or varus deformity at knee** if there is a disproportionate loss of cartilage on one side.

D. Pseudolaxity of collateral ligaments develops with degeneration of cartilage.

IV. **Radiographic Features.** Characteristic progressive changes include joint-space narrowing (may be asymmetrical), subchondral osteosclerosis, marginal osteophyte formation, and subchondral cysts. Spondylolisthesis (subluxation of one vertebra on another with lateral spondylosis) can occur.

V. **Laboratory.** None.

VI. **Treatment.**

A. **Goal of treatment** is to relieve pain, preserve joint motion and function, and prevent further injury and wear of cartilage.

B. **Biomechanical factors** including weight loss, use of canes or crutches, correction of postural abnormalities, and proper shoe support are helpful corrective measures. Regular exercise improves biomechanics.

C. **Pain control**

1. **Analgesics,** such as acetaminophen 1 g PO qid in scheduled doses, are important. **OA is not an inflammatory disorder, and acetaminophen is equal or superior to NSAIDs in efficacy and is without NSAID side effects.**

2. **NSAIDs** are helpful in those who have failed acetaminophen. However, they have many side effects and can hasten joint destruction. When an NSAID is being chosen, the patient's coexisting illnesses and the cost should be a consideration. Two weeks at maximum dose is needed before one decides that a particular drug is a therapeutic failure. Naproxen 500 mg PO bid or ibuprofen 600 mg PO qid are relatively inexpensive and well tolerated. COX-2 inhibitors are expensive and not recommended (see earlier discussion under RA).

3. **Corticosteroids.** Oral or parenteral corticosteroid therapy is not indicated. Intra-articular injection of steroid can be helpful in acute flares.

4. **Surgery.** Joint arthroplasty can relieve pain, stabilize joints, and improve function. Total joint arthroplasty is successful for the knee and hip. Arthroscopic "washing" of a joint is of no benefit.

5. **Sodium hyaluronate (Synvisc/Hyalgan)** can be injected directly into the joint and may provide up to 6 months of pain relief; the patient might need several injections before effect is noted. **It is expensive and data of efficacy are questionable. It seems to have at best a modest benefit.**

6. **Alternative therapies.** Chondroitin sulfate (400 mg tid) has been shown to decrease pain, has fewer GI side effects as compared with NSAIDs, and can have a longer duration of action. Glucosamine (500 mg tid) may be superior to placebo in controlling OA pain and might help repair cartilage; studies have given mixed results. S-adenosylmethionine (SAMe) assists in proteoglycan production. Several studies suggest that it may be as effective as NSAIDs for controlling OA pain but with decreased GI side effects. Capsaicin cream causes release of substance P from nerve fibers, modulating pain, and may be effective topically.

CRYSTAL-INDUCED SYNOVITIS

RHEUMATOLOGY 7

I. **Primary Gouty Arthritis.**

A. **Overview:** Primary gouty arthritis is an illness secondary to a chronic increase in serum uric acid. Deposition of uric acid crystals occurs throughout the body and results in multiple acute episodes of inflammatory arthritis; chronic, low-grade inflammation of joints; accumulation of articular, osseous, soft tissue, and cartilaginous crystalline deposits (tophi); renal injury (gouty nephropathy); and uric acid kidney stones.

B. **Acute gouty arthritis**

1. **Clinical features.** Onset is usually acute with (generally) nocturnal onset of monoarticular pain; rarely more than one joint is involved acutely. Involved joints are red, swollen, warm, and exquisitely tender. Fever and leukocytosis may occur. The big toe (first MTP joint) is the classic site of gout (also called podagra). Other sites, such as foot, knee, hand, or shoulder, may also be involved. Acute attack lasts 3 to 10 days without treatment. It may be difficult to differentiate from a septic joint, so joint aspiration for synovial fluid examination is critical, especially with the first attack.

2. **Precipitating events** include trauma, surgery, major medical illness (myocardial infarction, cerebrovascular accident, pulmonary embolus), fasting, alcohol ingestion, infection, and medications (thiazide and loop diuretics, niacin, low-dose salicylates). Overeating and emotional stress can also trigger attacks.

3. **Differential diagnosis** includes septic arthritis, other arthritis including pseudogout, and RA.

4. **Diagnosis.** Definite diagnosis can be made by demonstration of the presence of needle-shaped monosodium urate (MSU) crystals within synovial leukocytes or in material derived from tophi under polarizing or regular microscopy.

a. **Joint aspiration.** Synovial fluid typically reveals 2000 to 100,000 cells/mm^3, predominantly PMNs. **Urate crystals are needle shaped and negatively birefringent but can also be easily seen using a regular light microscope. Crystals can be recovered from joints during asymptomatic periods.** Fluid should be sent for Gram stain and culture to rule out infection.

b. **Serum uric acid levels** are generally not helpful in acute attacks and may be normal. However, when levels are chronically >10 mg/dL, the chance of having an acute attack is higher than 90%.

5. **Treatment. Do not administer allopurinol or probenecid until acute attack completely subsides; these can prolong the attack.**

a. **Pain management.** Oral narcotics (e.g., hydrocodone [Lortab]) can be used for pain management in addition to other medications.

b. **NSAIDs.** No studies support one NSAID over another for acute gouty attack. Indomethicin has historically been used; others include ibuprofen, nabumetone, and naproxen. **Avoid aspirin because it can have a paradoxical effect on serum urate.**

c. **Corticosteroids.** Methylprednisolone 10 to 40 mg intra-articular injection is effective for monoarticular presentation. Alternatively you may use methylprednisolone 125 mg IV or IM or **oral prednisone 60 mg** followed by prednisone 40 to 60 mg/d PO with or without colchicine 0.5 mg PO once or twice per day until symptoms resolve. No steroid taper is needed if the course is going to be limited to 7 days.

d. **Colchicine.**

(1) Colchicine should be reserved for cases in which the diagnosis of gout is not confirmed and a response may have diagnostic value, and for cases in which NSAIDs and steroids are contraindicated or have failed. However, colchicine also works for calcium pyrophosphate disease.

(2) Administer 1.2 mg PO initially, followed by 0.6 mg q2h up to 6 times on first day. On the second day, give 0.6 mg q6h and then q12h until side effects occur. Side effects include abdominal cramps, diarrhea, nausea, and vomiting. If diarrhea develops, discontinue the drug.

(3) The dose should be reduced in older patients and in patients with renal or hepatic disease.

(4) **Intercritical period** is the period between acute attacks; see section on treatment of hyperuricemia (later). The goal is to prevent recurrent attacks of acute gout. Oral colchicine 0.6 to 1.2 mg qd is the most effective dosing. **Side effects are uncommon at this dose, and the drug may be discontinued after the serum urate level becomes normal** and stable for 2 to 3 months. A low dose of NSAIDs (indomethacin 25 mg PO bid) is effective, but the incidence of side effects is higher than that of colchicine.

C. Chronic gout

1. **Clinical features** include chronic polyarticular changes as the result of persistent hyperuricemia without intercritical period. Tophi may develop in the helix of the ear, the ulnar aspects of the forearm, olecranon, prepatellar bursae, Achilles tendons, and hands. Extra-articular locations for tophi formation include myocardium, pericardium, aortic valves, and extradural spinal regions. Elderly patients often present with tophi.

2. **Clinical picture.** Gout can mimic rheumatoid arthritis, although it is generally less symmetric.

3. **Characteristic radiographic appearance** is bony erosion with an overhanging margin in the involved joint.

4. **Treatment of hyperuricemia.** Treatment depends on cause: increased uric acid production (about 10%) versus decreased excretion (about 90%). To differentiate, obtain a 24-hour urine specimen for uric acid or obtain spot urine for calculation of urate-to-creatinine ratio adjusted for GFR. If excretion is >800 mg/d, patient is an overproducer of uric acid. **Because allopurinol works for both types of gout, a 24-hour urine is often not done.** Asymptomatic hyperuricemia should not be treated. Treatment should be undertaken only after the second attack of gout or in the presence of a history of uric acid stones. The goal is to reduce serum uric acid level below its saturation point in extracellular fluid (6.4 mg/dL). Chronic hyperuricemia in the elderly is often due to diuretic use.

a. **Uricosurics** are drugs that increase the excretion of uric acid. They are used for patients who under-excrete uric acid.

   (1) Probenecid blocks tubular resorption of filtered uric acid. Initial dose is 250 mg PO bid and gradually increased by 500 mg every 4 weeks until the daily maximum dose of 2000 mg is achieved. The goal is to decrease serum uric acid levels to 5 to 6 mg/dL. It is recommended for patients younger than 60 years and those with normal renal function, uric acid excretion of less than 800 to 1000 mg/d, no history of kidney stones, and those not taking a medication that inhibits uric acid secretion. Advise the patient to increase fluid intake and consider alkalinization of the urine to a pH of 6.5 or more with sodium bicarbonate, 2 to 6 g/d, or acetazolamide (Diamox) 250 mg/d PO. Aspirin blocks probenecid's effect. Continue colchicine for prophylaxis as above.

   (2) Sulfinpyrazone (Anturane) 50 to 100 mg PO bid initial dose. The dose may be gradually increased by 100 mg every week until the maximum dose of 800 mg/day is attained. This is especially useful for patients who must take aspirin. Sulfinpyrazone is contraindicated in patients with a history of kidney stones.

b. **Allopurinol (Zyloprim)** is the only drug that decreases uric acid production; it can precipitate gouty attack at initiation of therapy (use concurrent colchicine until uric acid levels stabilize). It may be used to treat either overproducers or underexcreters. Starting dose is 100 mg PO qd. Usual dose is 200 to 300 mg/d, and maximum is 800 mg/d. Indications include a history of kidney stones, presence of tophi, renal insufficiency (GFR <60 mL/min), inability to lower the serum urate level below 7 mg/dL with other agents, urinary urate excretion higher than 800 to 1000 mg/d, allergy to uricosurics, and hyperuricemia caused by hypoxanthine-guanine phosphoribosyltransferase deficiency. Side effects are rare but can be serious. These include drug fever, rash (including Stevens–Johnson syndrome), bone marrow suppression, vasculitis, and hepatitis.

c. **Other measures.** A low purine diet is hard to adhere to but may have some mild benefit. Decreased alcohol consumption (beer in particular), weight loss if obese, and discontinuation of diuretics can help prevent further attacks.

II. Calcium Pyrophosphate Deposition Disease.

A. Overview. Calcium pyrophosphate deposition disease is a degenerative joint disease characterized by the accumulation of calcium pyrophosphate crystals in articular cartilage and periarticular tissues. It may be idiopathic or associated with a variety of metabolic and familial diseases such as hyperparathyroidism, hypothyroidism, hemochromatosis, and Wilson's disease.

B. Three distinct presentations of calcium pyrophosphate disease occur.

1. **Pseudogout** is an acute inflammatory attack that involves one or more joints and can last for several days. Attacks can be very similar to gout, though usually not so severe. The knees are involved in about half of patients, but any joint can be affected. Patients may have less-severe attacks between acute flares. Crystal deposition can occur in tendons, ligaments, and synovia, as well as in cartilage. Surgery or illness can predispose to attacks.

2. **Pseudo-osteoarthritis** is a chronic calcium pyrophosphate disease that can appear similar to osteoarthritis, with progressive degeneration of multiple joints. Knees are most commonly affected, followed by wrists, MCP joints, hips, shoulders, and elbows. Involvement may be symmetric.

3. **Pseudorheumatoid arthritis.** In 5%, calcium pyrophosphate disease causes symptoms similar to rheumatoid arthritis, including morning stiffness, fatigue, synovial membrane thickening, and elevated ESR. About 10% of patients with calcium pyrophosphate dihydrate (CPPD) have a positive rheumatoid factor.

C. Diagnosis

1. **Laboratory.** Joint should be tapped and will reveal CPPD crystals. **Crystals are rhomboid shaped, often intracellular, and positively birefringent, or blue when parallel to the axis of a polarizing microscope compensator. However, crystals can also easily be seen under a light microscope.** Evaluation should include serum calcium, magnesium, phosphorus, alkaline phosphatase, ferritin, serum iron and iron-binding capacity, glucose, T_4, TSH, and uric acid.

2. **Radiographic findings.** Typical findings are punctate and linear densities in articular hyaline or fibrocartilaginous tissues. Characteristic sites include articular cartilage of knee, acetabular labrum, symphysis pubis, articular disk of wrist, and anulus fibrosus of intervertebral disks. Radiologic screen for CPPD disease should include AP view of both knees, AP view of pelvis including hips and symphysis pubis, and PA view of both hands.

D. **Treatment of pseudogout**
1. **NSAIDS are effective.** No one drug is superior. NSAIDs may be used in a manner similar to that in acute episodes of gouty arthritis.
2. **Colchicine.** See section on gout for dosing. Oral form is less predictable than when used with gout but has been proved to reduce the number and duration of attacks (with 1.2 mg daily).
3. **Corticosteroid injections** are often combined with aspiration for large joints.

SPONDYLOARTHROPATHIES

I. **General.** The spondyloarthropathies are characterized by involvement of spine and entheses (insertions of tendons and ligaments) and are associated with HLA-B27. The target organs are not only joints but also the axial skeleton, enthesis, eye, gut, urogenital tract, skin, and sometimes the heart. The prevalence of this entity in the general population is estimated at 1%, equal to the prevalence of rheumatoid arthritis. Diseases included within this classification are ankylosing spondylitis, reactive arthritis (Reiter's disease), undifferentiated spondyloarthropathies, some forms of psoriatic arthritis, juvenile chronic arthritis, acute anterior uveitis, and arthritis associated with inflammatory bowel diseases such as Crohn's disease and ulcerative colitis.

II. **Ankylosing Spondylitis (Marie-Strumpell Disease).**
A. **General.** Ankylosing spondylitis is a disease primarily affecting the sacroiliac joints with varying involvement of the spine and less so the appendicular skeleton.

B. **Clinical presentation**
1. Onset is usually insidious, generally between 10 and 40 years of age. Patients generally have back pain that is worse after rest and improves with exercise. Patients may notice morning back stiffness that improves during the day; the pain may be so severe at night that it keeps the patient awake or prompts the patient to get up and become mobile to reduce the symptoms. By definition, the back is always involved. However, peripheral joints are involved in up to 25% of cases. Proximal large joints, such as hips, knees, shoulders, and ankles, are preferentially affected. TMJ involvement is common. Involvement is usually asymmetric but not always. Patients may have mild systemic manifestations such as fever, malaise, or anorexia.

7

RHEUMATOLOGY

2. **Enthesopathy.** Involvement of the sites of insertion of ligaments and tendons (entheses) is manifested clinically as Achilles tendinitis, plantar fasciitis, and costochondritis.
3. **Extraarticular manifestations** include uveitis in 25%; cardiac involvement in 10%, especially aortic insufficiency, cardiomegaly, conduction defects, and heart block; and renal and neurologic complications. Pulmonary involvement consists principally of upper lobe fibrocystic changes and chest wall restriction but can include *Aspergillus* infection in the pulmonary cavities.
4. **Late complications** secondary to bone involvement can include cord compression caused by spinal fractures, cauda equina syndrome (neurogenic bladder, fecal incontinence, leg pain and weakness), and severe chest wall restriction.

C. **Diagnosis**
1. **Physical examination**
   a. **Flexion test** (Schober test). Mark two points on the back, at the lumbosacral junction and 10 cm above, with patient standing erect. Have the patient bend forward and measure the distance between the two points. The normal spine should have an increase of more than 5 cm. Less than 5 cm is suggestive of decreased spinal mobility.
   b. **Chest expansion.** Normally, chest circumference increases by 5 cm with full inspiration. This is decreased in those with ankylosing spondylitis.
2. **Radiographic findings** include sacroiliitis with sclerosis and fusion of the sacroiliac joints. Patient may have an asymmetric erosive arthropathy. Spine involvement may be manifested by squaring of superior and inferior margins of vertebral body, syndesmophytes, and "bamboo spine."
3. **Lab tests.** The sedimentation rate is elevated in 75% of patients, as is the CRP. However, this does not always correlate with the activity of the disease. Immunofluorescence shows IgM deposition in the superficial vessels of the skin. HLA-B27 is present not only in 95% of whites with ankylosing spondylitis but also 6% to 8% of normal population. HLA-B27 should not be obtained as a screening test; the diagnosis is made on clinical and radiographic findings.

D. **Treatment**
1. **NSAIDs.** Indomethacin is the drug of choice, with a starting dose of 25 mg PO tid; may be increased to 50 mg tid. Side effects include nausea, gastric discomfort and diarrhea, headache, and vertigo; depression is common in the elderly. Other NSAIDs, such as naproxen and sulindac, are also effective. NSAIDs relieve pain but do not alter disease course.
2. **Aspirin** for unknown reasons is generally not effective.
3. **Sulfasalazine** 2 to 3 g PO qd may be helpful, especially for peripheral joint disease; it does not decrease axial skeleton inflammation. The effect starts within the first 2 to 3 months, and the drug continues to

be effective. The effect seems to be best in patients with high peak of disease activity and in early disease. In very chronic cases, the response has not been different from the placebo. Monitoring includes CBC and liver enzymes every 2 weeks during the first 3 months.

4. **Methotrexate and cyclophosphamide** have been used in recalcitrant cases.

5. **TNF-α inhibitors** are not FDA approved for this indication. A few studies have shown etanercept and infliximab to be effective in decreasing both axial and peripheral skeletal disease activity as well as significantly decreasing symptoms. Side effects include bone marrow suppression, serious infections, and local site reactions.

6. **Bisphosphonates.** A study of pamidronate IV showed decrease in pain and morning stiffness; results were not significant until 6 months of therapy. Further studies with oral agents are needed.

7. **Education** to maintain good posture, stop smoking, and avoid pillows at night and encouraging sleep in the prone position is important.

8. **Physical therapy exercises** (especially swimming) and attention to posture are critical. Range-of-motion exercises, especially extension of the back, are important to maintain flexibility.

9. **Genetic counseling should be recommended.** Offspring of those with the disease have a 10% to 20% risk of having disease.

III. **Reactive Arthritis (including Reiter's syndrome).**

A. **Clinical features**

1. **Overview.** Reactive arthritis is a seronegative arthropathy that preferentially involves the lower extremities; if urethritis or conjunctivitis are also present, it is termed *Reiter's syndrome*. Reactive arthritis is the most common type of polyarthritis in young men. It can manifest with insidious joint pain or acutely with fever (as high as 39°C), swollen, hot joints, severe weight loss, and diffuse polyarticular involvement. When synovitis is limited to a few joints, low-grade fever or no fever at all is the rule. **For diagnosis of reactive arthritis, onset must be temporally related to urethritis, diarrhea, or other infection with organisms such as *Yersinia, Salmonella, Shigella, Campylobacter*, or *Chlamydia*. However, initial infection may be asymptomatic.** The triad of arthritis, conjunctivitis, and urethritis should suggest a diagnosis of Reiter's syndrome. However, the manifestation of these symptoms can be separated by months. Up to 20% develop chronic disease. Relapses begin 3 to 4 years after the first episode and can consist of recurrence of peripheral arthritis or enthesopathic pain of pelviaxial symptoms or of iritis or other extraarticular symptoms. These symptoms can be isolated or associated. Radiographic changes may now be observed.

2. **Other associated findings** include skin disorders (balanitis, oral ulcerations, or keratoderma blennorrhagicum), conjunctivitis, and urethritis. In chronic disease, heart block or aortic regurgitation may occur. Diarrhea can precede the development of Reiter's syndrome.

RHEUMATOLOGY   7

There is an association of Reiter's disease with HIV infection, and arthritis may be present before symptoms or signs related to the HIV infection appear.

3. **Lab tests.** There is no definitive laboratory test to diagnose reactive arthritis. Findings can include an elevated ESR/CRP and anemia of chronic disease; 80% of patients are HLA-B27 positive. Stool cultures and urethral cultures should be done, although causative organism is rarely recovered. Offer HIV testing in the appropriate population.

B. **Treatment**

1. **NSAIDs.** Indomethacin 25 mg PO qid (can be increased to 50 mg PO qid) as well as others.

2. **Antibiotics.** Treatment of the underlying bacterial infection may hasten resolution but studies do not routinely support this. A 3-month course of tetracycline has been shown to hasten resolution of symptoms in those with disease related to *Chlamydia* organisms.

3. **Immunosuppressive drugs,** such as methotrexate or azathioprine, may be effective.

4. **Steroids.** Patients with large-joint involvement may benefit from intra-articular corticosteroid injection.

IV. **Arthritis Associated with Inflammatory Bowel Disease (Enteropathic Arthritis).** There are two types of arthritis associated with ulcerative colitis, Crohn's disease, and other GI problems: a nondestructive oligoarthritis of peripheral joints and ankylosing spondylitis. Arthritis affects 11% to 20% of patients with IBD.

V. **Psoriatic Arthritis.**

A. **Clinical features.** Psoriatic arthritis occurs in up to 7% of patients with psoriasis and is strongly associated with nail pitting. Most patients (95%) have involvement of multiple small joints of the hands and feet. Others have solely spine involvement or, more commonly (35%-50%), a combination of spine involvement and peripheral joint involvement. There is a high prevalence (10%-30%) of atlantoaxial subluxation in severe, chronic disease. The inflamed joints in patients with psoriatic arthritis often have a purplish discoloration, which is not commonly seen in other forms of arthritis.

B. **Treatment.** Mild forms can be successfully treated with NSAIDs, exercise, physical therapy, and education; control of psoriasis is important. Intra-articular steroid injections may be used when limited joints are involved. For progressive and severe disease, DMARDs should be initiated. Methotrexate, sulfasalazine, and cyclosporine are commonly used because there are some trial data to support their efficacy. Other DMARDs such as gold salts, antimalarials, and leflunomide are less studied and have shown only limited benefit. TNF-α inhibitors are also being used and appear quite effective in treating psoriatic arthritis, although there are few studies to date.

SEPTIC ARTHRITIS

I. **Overview.**

A. Any infectious agent can cause arthritis, but bacterial arthritis is the most rapidly destructive form. The major responsible organisms are *Neisseria gonorrhoeae* and *Staphylococcus aureus*. *Streptococcus* species (including those causing pneumococcal infections), *Enterobacter*, *H. influenzae*, and other gram-negative species are much less common. Brucellosis is rarely found as a joint pathogen in those who work with cattle.

B. **Source of infection**

1. **Hematogenous spread** secondary to a puncture wound, a skin infection, or an adjacent osteomyelitis. Rarely, septic arthritis is secondary to intra-articular injection or joint aspiration (incidence ranges from 1:500 to 1:5000).

2. **IV drug use** can cause infections in unusual joints such as the sternoclavicular or sacroiliac joints. Infections in IV drug users are often secondary to unusual organisms such as *Pseudomonas*, *Serratia*, and MRSA.

3. **Underlying illness.** Steroid use, RA, and joint prostheses also predispose to the development of septic arthritis. Patients with underlying illness such as lupus, RA, renal failure, and diabetes may have gram-negative organisms.

II. **Gonococcal Arthritis.**

A. **Clinical features.** Patients can have an acute arthritis involving one or more joints, usually the knees, ankles, or wrists, with the knee being the most commonly involved. Two thirds of patients have a dermatitis with one or multiple, usually asymptomatic, lesions that progress from macular to papular and finally vesicular or pustular. Any new acute inflammatory monoarthritis in a sexually active person should be considered related to gonococcal infection until proved otherwise. Fever may be present, and genitourinary symptoms occur in 25%. Physical exam reveals an acute arthritis, synovitis, or tenosynovitis, or all three. In gonococcal infection the arthritis should subside dramatically within 3 days and completely within 10 days after the start of antibiotics.

B. **Laboratory features (Table 7-3)**

1. **The synovial fluid WBC count averages more than 60,000/mL, but low WBC counts have been reported.** Gram stain is positive in less than 25%, and only 25% to 50% of synovial fluid cultures are positive in gonococcal arthritis.

2. Obtain blood cultures (<10% will grow organism) and cultures of the throat, joint, anorectum, blood, and genitourinary tract.

III. **Nongonococcal Bacterial Arthritis.**

A. **Clinical features** are acute onset of arthritis with a hot, swollen joint or joints. Generally one or two joints are involved. The knee is most

TABLE 7-3
SYNOVIAL FLUID ANALYSIS

Classification	Condition	Color	Clarity	Viscosity	WBC/µL	% NTP	Crystals	Glucose (% Serum)	Complement	Culture/ Smear
Normal	Normal	Yellow	Translucent	High	<200	<25	0	Same	Normal	0
Group 1 (noninflammatory)	Osteoarthritis	Yellow	Transparent	High	<2000	<25	0	Same	Normal	0
	Trauma	Pink or red	Transparent	High	<2000	<25	0	Same	Normal	0
Group 2 (inflammatory)	SLE	Yellow	Translucent	Slightly decreased	0-9000	<25	0	Same	Normal	0
	Acute rheumatic fever	Yellow	Translucent	Slightly decreased	0-60,000	25-50	0	Same	Normal	0
	Pseudogout	Yellow or white	Translucent or opaque	Low	50-75,000	90	+	Same	Normal	0
	Gout	Yellow or white	Translucent or opaque	Low	100-160,000	90	+	Same	Normal	0
	Rheumatoid arthritis	Yellow or purulent	Translucent or opaque	Low	3000-50,000	50-75	0	75-100	Normal or low	0
	Tuberculosis	Purulent	Opaque	Low	2500-100,000	50	0	50-75	Normal or low	+
Group 3 (purulent)	Bacterial arthritis	Purulent	Opaque	Low	50,000-300,000	>90	0	<50	Normal or low	+*

NTP, neutrophils; SLE, systemic lupus erythematosus; WBC, white blood cells.
*Often negative in gonococcal arthritis.
From Paget S et al: *Rheumatology and Outpatient Orthopedics.* Philadelphia, Lippincott-Raven, 1993.

commonly affected in adults, whereas the hip and knee are the most commonly involved joints in children. Fever is common but may be low grade; chills are less common.

B. Diagnosis

1. **Obtaining a synovial fluid sample is critical.** The definitive test is joint aspiration with fluid sent for Gram staining (75% positive for gram-positive cocci), culture (90% will grow causative organism), synovial fluid leukocyte count and differential (>50,000 cells/mL in 70% of patients, with >80% neutrophils), and synovial fluid glucose (decreased). **As with gonococcal arthritis, the synovial fluid leukocyte count might not be in the range classically considered to be positive.**

2. **Blood cultures should be done.** They are positive in 50% of patients with nongonococcal bacterial arthritis.

3. **An elevated WBC count** with a left shift and an elevated ESR often occur but are nonspecific.

4. **Radiographic examination** should include plain films obtained for baseline view and to look for osteomyelitis. Usually no initial changes are visible except effusions and perhaps juxta-articular osteopenia. The changes of osteomyelitis take 10 to 20 days to appear on plain films. Radionuclide imaging, gallium scanning, and CT or MRI can be helpful, particularly with suspected hip or axial joint infections. Ultrasonography may be used to establish the presence of effusion in the hip joint and aid with aspiration.

5. **Surgical exploration** may be necessary to obtain fluid from joints such as the sternoclavicular or sacroiliac.

6. **Diagnostic considerations.** Differential includes occult celiac disease, sarcoid arthritis, Lyme disease, parvovirus arthropathies, Hepatitis B or C, Behçet's syndrome (recurrent oral or genital ulcers [>97%], uveitis [50%], meningoencephalitis, arthritis [40%-50%]), and HIV-associated arthritis.

IV. Treatment.

A. Antibiotic therapy

1. **Gonococcal arthritis.** Ceftriaxone 1 g IV qd or cefotaxime 2 g IV q8h, for at least 3 days, followed by cefuroxime axetil 500 mg PO bid. For penicillin-allergic patients, an alternative is spectinomycin 2 g IM q12h.

2. **Nongonococcal arthritis**

a. **In adults,** make the initial choice based on gram-stain results and clinical likelihood. Essentially all antibiotics reach high levels of activity within an inflamed joint after oral or parenteral administration. Consider a penicillinase-resistant penicillin (such as methicillin or nafcillin) or vancomycin plus an aminoglycoside or aztreonam. Imipenem has been proposed for single-agent therapy.

b. **In neonates,** give methicillin, nafcillin, or vancomycin plus a third-generation cephalosporin.

c. **In infants and young children,** give methicillin, nafcillin, or vancomycin plus cefuroxime.

d. **For prosthetic joint infections,** give vancomycin plus aztreonam.

B. **Drainage**

1. **Needle drainage** is as good as open drainage in most situations but is not adequate for hip infections, especially in children. **Aspirate with a large-bore needle daily while effusions are accumulating rapidly.** You can irrigate with sterile saline; antibiotic irrigation can cause synovitis.

2. **Open drainage** is the method of choice for hip infections.

3. **Arthroscopy.** Early arthroscopy has been reported to be helpful, especially in knees and shoulders, for better visualization and irrigation.

C. **Immobilize the joint** in the functional position during the acute phase of infection and follow with early mobilization and muscle-strengthening exercises.

D. **Reassess therapy** if synovial fluid cultures are not negative within 72 hours (tap and reculture) or if synovial fluid leukocyte count is not substantially lower after 7 days.

E. **Prognosis**

1. Up to 10% mortality rate.

2. Only 60% recover completely; many are left with a joint problem, especially if they are symptomatic for more than 7 days before therapy. *Staphylococcus aureus* and gram-negative bacilli tend to be more destructive. *Neisseria gonorrhoeae* and pneumococci are rarely destructive.

3. Sterile synovitis can develop after treatment but is usually self-limited and responds to NSAIDs.

RHEUMATIC FEVER AND RHEUMATIC CARDITIS

I. **Etiology and Present Significance.**

A. Acute rheumatic fever and rheumatic carditis represent the clinical sequelae of infection with group A streptococci.

B. Peak age of incidence is 5 to 15 years. Primary and recurrent illness occurs in adulthood as well. The incidence has decreased markedly, but it is still a common problem in developing countries and is increasing again in developed nations.

C. Among patients with rheumatic heart disease, the incidence of valvular disease is: mitral valve 85%, aortic valve 44%, and tricuspid valve 10% to 16%.

D. In developed countries, patients with rheumatic fever might not meet the Jones criteria for diagnosis **(Box 7-1).**

II. **Clinical Features.**

A. From 40% to 60% of patients develop carditis during the initial episode of acute rheumatic fever. Manifestations include cardiomegaly, heart murmur (mitral regurgitation, aortic regurgitation), friction rub secondary to pericarditis, and congestive heart failure.

BOX 7-1

JONES CRITERIA FOR RHEUMATIC FEVER

The revised Jones criteria recognize both major and minor manifestations of the disease. The development of two major criteria or one major and two minor criteria suggests a high probability of rheumatic fever.

MAJOR CRITERIA

Polyarthritis: Any degree of arthritis. Generally migratory and in large joints. Resolves in about 1 month.

Carditis.

Sydenham's chorea ("St. Vitus' Dance")

Erythema marginatum

Subcutaneous (Aschoff) nodules (painless subcutaneous nodules over bony surfaces)

MINOR CRITERIA

Arthralgia

Fever

Elevations in acute phase reactants (ESR, CRP)

Prolonged PR interval on EKG

Evidence of recent group A strep infection by positive rapid strep test, positive throat culture, or rising streptococcal antibody titer

---

B. All patients suspected of having acute rheumatic fever should be evaluated by echocardiography. Arthritis may be very short-lived and migratory; the clinician must have a high suspicion for acute rheumatic fever.

III. Treatment and Prophylaxis.

A. Antibiotics (e.g., benzathine penicillin G) are given to eradicate tonsillar and pharyngeal group A streptococci. Aspirin is used to treat the acute polyarthritis. Corticosteroids (e.g., prednisone) are used to treat carditis and are administered for 3 to 6 weeks.

B. Secondary prevention consists of chronic administration of antibiotics to patients who have already sustained significant damage from rheumatic carditis. Monthly IM injection of 1.2 million units of penicillin G benzathine appears to provide optimal prophylaxis. Prophylaxis in these patients should be lifelong, although some authors argue that prophylaxis may be discontinued 5 years after the last acute attack or after full-time education is completed and the patient has fewer exposures to streptococcus.

FIBROMYALGIA SYNDROME

I. Clinical Features.

A. Fibromyalgia is characterized by diffuse aches, stiffness, and fatigue coupled with multiple symmetric tender spots in specific areas **(Fig. 7-1).** More than 75% of patients are women, and the peak incidence is

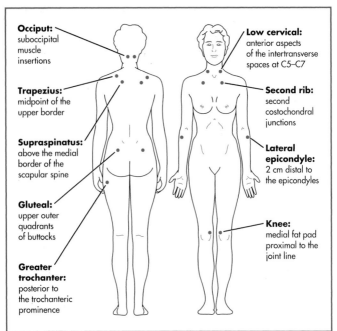

Occiput:
suboccipital muscle insertions

Trapezius:
midpoint of the upper border

Supraspinatus:
above the medial border of the scapular spine

Gluteal:
upper outer quadrants of buttocks

Greater trochanter:
posterior to the trochanteric prominence

Low cervical:
anterior aspects of the intertransverse spaces at C5–C7

Second rib:
second costochondral junctions

Lateral epicondyle:
2 cm distal to the epicondyles

Knee:
medial fat pad proximal to the joint line

FIG. 7-1

Location of specific tender points in fibromyalgia. *(From Schumacher HR Jr, Klippel JH, Koopman WJ [eds]: Primer on the Rheumatic Diseases, 11th ed. Atlanta, Arthritis Foundation, 1997.)*

20 to 60 years of age. There is often discordance between symptoms and objective findings. The cause may actually be related to a sleep disturbance but is not well understood.

B. **Pain** is often aggravated by stress, cold, and activity. Patients often complain of subjective swelling of hands and feet, as well as paresthesia and dysesthesia of hands and feet.

C. **Fatigability** is often extreme, occurring after minimal exertion.

D. **Sleep disturbance.** Patients complain of nonrestorative sleep, and waking unrefreshed. Research has shown alpha wave intrusion into non-REM delta wave sleep 70% greater than controls and decreased amount of stage III and IV sleep. Patients can have depression, irritability, and mood instability.

E. **Headache** is common, as are **diffuse abdominal pain** and alternating diarrhea or constipation.

F. **Miscellaneous** symptoms include paresthesias, numbness, decreased mentation, and feeling of swollen hands and feet.

G. **Associated syndromes** include irritable bowel syndrome (35% to 65%), reflex sympathetic syndrome (1% to 10%), female urethral syndrome (urethral spasm with dysuria and urgency, 12%), and migraine headaches.

II. **Diagnosis.**

A. **Fibromyalgia is a diagnosis of exclusion** (normal CBC, ESR, thyroid functions, rheumatoid factor, electrolytes, creatinine, calcium, phosphorus, UA). Patients must meet the American College of Rheumatology (ACR) criteria: widespread pain of at least 3 months' duration in combination with at least 11 of 18 specified tender points; pain on both sides of the body, both above and below the waist, and pain in the axial skeleton. Diagnosis may need to be established over time.

B. The World Health Organization views the ACR criteria as primarily for research purposes and determines that a patient has fibromyalgia based on the history and the finding of a nonspecific number of tender points.

III. **Treatment.**

A. **Treatment is aimed at controlling symptoms, improving function, and restoring adequate sleep.** Exercise programs and self-help strategies are the mainstay of treatment.

B. Treatment includes reassurance, education, graded aerobic exercise, massage, cognitive therapy, and increased flexibility. Patients may be assured that fibromyalgia is generally a self-limited illness that typically resolves within 2 to 3 years. **Low-dose amitriptyline (Elavil), 10 to 75 mg PO qhs, or other tricyclic such as doxepin or nortriptyline taken before bedtime are the drugs of choice.** Add an SSRI in the morning if needed for depression or anxiety. Duloxetine (and likely venlafaxine) might have some moderate benefit. Benzodiazepines should be avoided. NSAIDs and acetaminophen have spotty efficacy but are worth a try. Acupuncture may be a useful adjunct to improve pain. Vitamin D supplementation may be helpful in some patients. Narcotics are generally not effective.

CHRONIC FATIGUE SYNDROME

I. **Clinical Picture.**

A. The condition is characterized by 6 months of severe disabling fatigue and a combination of symptoms described in **Box 7-2.**

B. The patient is classified as having idiopathic chronic fatigue if diagnosis is suggested but inclusion criteria are not met.

II. **Laboratory Evaluation.** CBC with differential, ESR/CRP, ALT, protein, albumin, globulin, alkaline phosphatase, calcium, phosphorus, glucose, BUN, electrolytes, creatinine, TSH, urinalysis, and laboratory tests based on specific findings to exclude other diagnoses.

III. **Treatment.** There are no established treatment guidelines. Exercise and cognitive behavior programs have shown promise. Self-help and support groups may also be beneficial.

RHEUMATOLOGY 7

BOX 7-2

CRITERIA FOR CHRONIC FATIGUE SYNDROME

Chronic fatigue is defined as self-reported persistent or relapsing fatigue lasting 6 or more consecutive months, with four or more inclusion criteria concurrently present for at least 6 months.

INCLUSION CRITERIA

Impaired memory or concentration

Sore throat

Tender cervical or axillary adenopathy

Muscle pain

Multijoint pain

New headaches

Unrefreshing sleep

Postexertion malaise

EXCLUSION CRITERIA

Active medical conditions that can explain fatigue (e.g., hypothyroidism)

Previously diagnosed condition whose resolution is not documented (e.g., hepatitis C)

Numerous psychiatric conditions (e.g., major depressive disorder, schizophrenia, dementia, anorexia)

Current alcohol or substance abuse or within last 2 years

Unexplained physical, laboratory, or radiographic finding suggesting cause of fatigue

---

POLYMYALGIA RHEUMATICA AND GIANT CELL ARTERITIS

I. **General.** Polymyalgia rheumatica (PMR) and giant cell arteritis form a spectrum of disease and affect patients of older than 50 years; up to 15% of patients with PMR have giant cell arteritis and 40% of patients with active giant cell arteritis have symptoms of PMR.

II. **Polymyalgia Rheumatica.**

A. **Clinical features**

1. Pain and stiffness in the neck, shoulder, and pelvic girdle. Symptoms are bilateral and symmetric and more prolonged in the morning. May have diffuse aching.

2. Systemic features may be present such as low-grade fever, fatigue, and weight loss.

3. ESR and C-reactive protein are elevated, with ESR elevation of 50 to 100 mm common. However, 15% of those with PMR may have a normal sedimentation rate and C-reactive protein. **CRP is no more sensitive for PMR than is the ESR.**

B. **Diagnosis**

1. Rule out other causes such as claudication, disk disease, hypothyroidism, and myositis. In PMR, thyroid functions are normal, CPK and aldolase are not elevated, ANA should be "normal" for age, and rheumatoid factor usually is negative. Patients can have normocytic, normochromic anemia.

2. Giant cell arteritis should be excluded.

C. Treatment includes prednisone: initial dose of 10 to 20 mg PO qd for 1 month and then reduce by 2.5 mg every 2 to 4 weeks until the lowest dose is reached that controls symptoms. Most patients require treatment for 3 to 4 years, but withdrawal after 2 years is worth attempting. Low-dose treatment should not be used in patients with symptoms suggestive of temporal arteritis.

III. Giant Cell Arteritis (Temporal Arteritis).

A. Clinical features. Giant cell arteritis predominantly affects persons older than 50 years with early symptoms of headache, fever, fatigue, and perhaps upper-limb girdle pain. Patients may have associated ocular symptoms including partial vision loss and field cuts, diplopia, ptosis, and blindness. Tongue or jaw claudication can occur.

B. Laboratory abnormalities include greatly elevated ESR, but 10% have normal ESR and CRP; moderate normochromic anemia, and thrombocytosis may be present.

C. Diagnosis. Temporal artery biopsy is most useful within 24 hours of starting treatment; however, steroids have little effect on the sensitivity of the biopsy, and treatment should not be delayed. A positive result helps to prevent later doubt about the diagnosis. Sensitivity of a biopsy is determined by length of artery taken and thinness of sections on microscopy. If biopsy is negative but there is high clinical suspicion for temporal arteritis with large vessel involvement, imaging such as MRA can aid in diagnosis.

D. Treatment is prednisone: initial dose of 20 to 40 mg PO qd for 8 weeks. Patients with ocular symptoms may need up to 80 mg PO qd. Reduce the dose by 5 mg every 3 to 4 weeks until it is 10 mg qd and then taper slowly, based on symptoms and ESR. Treatment should last 24 to 30 months, at which time a trial off of steroids may be tried.

RAYNAUD'S PHENOMENON

I. Overview.

A. Episodic, biphasic or triphasic color change: white (ischemia), then often blue (stasis), then red (reactive hyperemia), of fingers or toes in response to cold or emotion.

B. More than 90% of patients with Raynaud's phenomenon are female.

II. Types.

A. Raynaud's disease (primary Raynaud's phenomenon). The cause is unknown, and the symptoms are usually stable. Phenomenon is thought to represent an exaggeration of normal physiologic response to cold in approximately 80% of cases.

B. Secondary Raynaud's phenomenon. Predisposing factors include atherosclerosis, arteritis, cancer, collagen vascular disease, thoracic outlet syndrome, embolic occlusions, occupational disease (working

7

RHEUMATOLOGY

outdoors, using vibrating tools), and certain drugs (β-adrenergic blockers, nicotine, ergotamine).

III. Diagnosis.

A. Diagnosis is made on clinical grounds.

B. The UK Scleroderma Study Group diagnostic terms for diagnosis of Raynaud's phenomenon:

1. Definite Raynaud's phenomenon consists of repeated episodes of biphasic color changes.

2. Possible Raynaud's phenomenon consists of uniphasic color changes, plus numbness or paresthesia.

3. No Raynaud's phenomenon is marked by no color changes on cold exposure.

IV. Treatment.

A. Treat the underlying condition.

B. Simple conservative measures include dressing warmly, relaxation and behavior modification (e.g., cold avoidance and stress management), and cessation of cigarette smoking.

C. Medications may be helpful; most studied are the calcium channel blockers.

1. Calcium channel blockers: nifedipine extended release 30 mg PO daily, amlodipine 5 to 20 mg PO daily, felodipine 2.5 to 10mg PO bid.

2. ACEIs and ARBs: captopril 6.25 mg PO daily (may increase to 25 mg daily); losartan 25 to 100 mg daily.

3. Transdermal nitroglycerin: $1/4$ to $1/2$ inch of 2% ointment topically daily.

4. Viagra, 200 mg bid, may be effective in refractory cases.

LUPUS

Systemic Lupus Erythematosus

I. Overview.

A. SLE is a systemic illness characterized by chronic inflammation; clinical manifestations are varied.

B. Genetic, environmental, and hormonal factors play a role in its etiology.

C. The incidence is 2.9 to 4 per 100,000 persons per year in the United States. SLE is more common in African Americans and some Asian populations. It most commonly has its onset between 15 and 40 years of age and has an 8:1 female-to-male ratio.

II. Diagnosis.

A. SLE diagnosis requires the presence of 4 of 11 signs:

1. Malar rash (fixed, raised, or flat); nasolabial folds are typically spared.

2. Discoid rash (raised erythematous patches with overlying scale).

3. Photosensitivity (by history or observation).

4. Oral ulcers (oral or nasopharyngeal, usually painless).

5. Arthritis (in two or more peripheral joints with tenderness, swelling, or effusion).
6. Serositis (pleuritis or pericarditis).
7. Renal disorder (proteinuria >0.5 g/d, >3+ proteinuria) or Red cell casts.
8. Neurologic disorder (seizures or psychosis in the absence of other causes).
9. Hematologic disorder (hemolytic anemia, leukopenia <4000/mm, lymphopenia <1500/mm, or thrombocytopenia all in the absence of offending drugs and on two occasions).
10. Immunologic disorder (positive lupus anticoagulant, abnormal titer of anti–double-stranded DNA antigen, positive anti-Smith antigen, abnormal IgG or IgM anticardiolipin antibodies, or false-positive VDRL test for 6 months with a negative confirmatory TPI or FTA).
11. Positive results of fluorescent antinuclear antibody.
B. **Keep in mind that a positive ANA is neither required for a diagnosis of lupus nor sufficient in itself to make a diagnosis of lupus.** Initial workup for suspected lupus should include CBC, chemistry panel, ANA, ESR or CRP, CK, UA, ECG, and CXR.

III. **Clinical Features.**
A. **Symmetric arthritis and arthralgias that are nondeforming and nonerosive.** SLE can be confused with RA early in the course. Patients can have long-term deformity secondary to contractures. Tenosynovitis occurs in up to 10%, sometimes in absence of arthropathy. Ulnar deviation at MCP joints can be confused for RA.
B. **Mucocutaneous manifestations**
1. **Acute cutaneous lupus.** Characteristic butterfly malar rash, often accompanied by a more widespread morbilliform eruption. Rash flares with exacerbation of systemic disease or from sun exposure.
2. **Discoid lupus.** Erythematous raised patches with keratotic scaling, mostly on scalp, face, or neck. Alopecia and scarring are common (especially older lesions). Many patients with discoid lupus have no other systemic involvement.
3. **Subacute cutaneous lupus.** Skin lesions are symmetric, superficial, nonscarring, often annular, occurring on shoulders, upper arms, chest, back, and neck. More than half of patients have diffuse nonscarring alopecia, and 20% have discoid lesions. Photosensitivity is prominent, but the incidence of nephritis is low.
4. **Mucosal manifestations** include recurrent oral and vaginal ulcers.
C. **Cardiac involvement**
1. **Pericarditis** can occur in up to 30% and may be asymptomatic. It is often accompanied by pleural effusions and is rarely complicated by tamponade or restrictive pericarditis.
2. **Myocarditis** can occur in up to 25% and is often associated with pericarditis. It is suggested by tachycardia, ST–T wave changes, and cardiomegaly. CK-MB can be elevated and can result in CHF or arrhythmias.

RHEUMATOLOGY 7

3. **Endocarditis** is typically asymptomatic without murmur or hemodynamic dysfunction. Mitral and aortic are the most commonly involved valves, and damage can be severe. Emboli are relatively rare.

4. **Myocardial infarction** is usually considered secondary to accelerated atherosclerosis from long-term steroid use. Risk of coronary artery disease is significantly increased in SLE.

D. Renal involvement affects 50% of patients, with any pathologic form of glomerulonephritis. Clinical presentations include hematuria, proteinuria, hypertension, and uremia. Only 0.5% go on to end-stage renal disease. However, lupus nephritis is a poor prognostic marker, with a survival rate of 85% at 5 years and 65% at 10 years.

E. Pulmonary involvement. Lung or pleura involved in 40% to 50%, with pleuritis or pleural effusion most common. May also develop acute pneumonitis. Myopathy may affect the diaphragm.

F. Central nervous system is often involved, with highly varied presentation; depression is common. Headaches, strokes, TIAs, and memory loss or encephalopathy can occur. Seizures, chorea, and frank psychosis also occur.

G. Gastrointestinal system is less commonly involved but includes hepatitis, peritonitis, pancreatitis, protein-losing enteropathy, or esophageal dysmotility. Liver involvement is not uncommon, but jaundice is rare.

H. Raynaud's phenomenon is present in about half of patients at presentation.

I. Vascular. Terminal arterioles may be involved in vasculitis, manifesting as purpura, petechiae, ulcers, and livedo reticularis.

J. Reticuloendothelial system. Lymphadenopathy is common. Urinary and pulmonary infections are common.

IV. Laboratory Findings.

A. ANA is found in 95% of those with SLE, but it is also found in other connective tissue disorders, so the specificity is low. The most common pattern is homogeneous and diffuse. **Anti–double-stranded DNA and anti-Smith antigens are found *only* in SLE,** whereas other antibodies such as anti–single-stranded DNA may also be present in other illnesses. Other antibodies such as anti-Ro and anti-La may also be present, suggesting Sjögren's syndrome. Those who are ANA positive with inflammatory arthritis or Raynaud's but who do not meet criteria for SLE are classified as having undifferentiated connective tissue disorder (UCTD). Of these, one third progress to SLE, one third maintain UCTD, and one third remit.

B. Hematologic abnormalities. A normochromic, normocytic anemia is seen in up to 40% of patients. Evidence of hemolytic anemia may be present, including decreased haptoglobin (see Chapter 6). Thrombocytopenia is found in up to 25% of patients. The ESR may be elevated but does not correlate with disease activity.

C. **Lupus anticoagulant.** SLE is characterized by circulating anticoagulant with an elevated PTT or with circulating antiphospholipid (50% of those with lupus) or anticardiolipin antibodies (see later). It is associated with venous or arterial thrombosis (see later).

D. **Patients with SLE can have a false-positive VDRL test.** However, FTA will be negative.

E. **Hypocomplementemia** (C3, C4) may be present and correlates with disease activity.

V. **Treatment.** Generally a rheumatologist should participate, although these patients can be followed by a primary care physician. Treatment should be individualized according to the activity of the disease and organs involved. Avoid sulfa antibiotics and be aware of oral contraceptives, both of which can induce flares.

A. **Preventive care**

1. **Regular monitoring.** Patients should be seen every 3 to 6 months even if they are doing well.

2. **Energy conservation.** Fatigue is a common complaint.

3. **Photoprotection** includes sunscreen and avoidance of excess sun.

4. **Infection control** includes pneumococcal vaccine and yearly influenza vaccine. Consider antibiotic prophylaxis for procedures.

5. **Contraception.** Avoid pregnancy at time of increased disease activity or while using immunosuppressive therapy. Women with anti-Ro in particular run a risk of antibodies crossing the placenta and inducing neonatal lupus, congenital heart block, and miscarriage. Estrogen containing contraceptives seem safe in stable patients with inactive disease.

6. **Symptomatic.** Heat to affected joints, conditioning exercises, weight loss if necessary, and relaxation techniques.

B. **Medication**

1. **NSAIDs** are useful for symptomatic relief of joint pain and the pain associated with pleurisy and pericarditis, as well as treatment of systemic symptoms such as fever and fatigue. May combine with a low-dose steroid to minimize side effects of higher doses of both. Watch for adverse renal effects, especially in those who already have lupus nephritis.

2. **Antimalarial drugs (chloroquine, hydroxychloroquine).** Hydroxychloroquine is the most commonly used. They are effective for cutaneous, musculoskeletal, and mild systemic symptoms. Mechanism of action is unknown. Begin 400 mg PO daily for 4 weeks and then taper to maintenance dose. Relapse is frequent with discontinuation of drug. See section on RA for side effects and monitoring.

3. **Steroids.** Topical preparations are effective for cutaneous manifestations. If fluorinated, limit exposure to 2 weeks. Low-dose oral prednisone (10 mg/day) can be used for minor disease activity. Dose should be once daily in morning to reduce effect on pituitary–adrenal axis and high dose limited to 4 to 6 weeks if possible. Maintenance should be the lowest possible dose, using alternate-day therapy

7

RHEUMATOLOGY

if possible. NSAIDs are used to try to lower steroid dose or for symptomatic treatment on the off day of alternate-day therapy. Prednisone at 1 mg/kg per day may be used for severe flares of joint symptoms, CNS symptoms, and nephritis. IV therapy with methylprednisolone may be needed in particularly severe disease. Consider alendronate, vitamin D, calcium, and low-cholesterol diet as prophylactic measures if oral steroids are required chronically.

4. **Immunosuppressive drugs (azathioprine, cyclophosphamide)** can be used for severe flare and renal or CNS involvement. These are generally reserved for patients who failed conventional therapy.

5. **Anticoagulation.** Persons with antiphospholipid syndrome should be treated with warfarin and low-dose aspirin but only if they have had symptomatic disease (e.g., thrombosis).

Drug-Induced Lupus

I. **Clinical Features.** Drug-induced lupus is a lupus-like syndrome characterized by arthralgias, myalgias, fever, and serositis (pleurisy and pericarditis). CNS and renal disease are rare.

II. **Laboratory Tests.** Lab tests reveal cytopenias and ANA in a diffuse-homogeneous pattern. Anti-dsDNA antibodies typically are not present. Antihistone antibodies are present in more than 90% of cases but are not specific for drug-induced lupus.

III. **Causative Agents.** Hydralazine and procainamide have been strongly implicated in drug-induced lupus. Other drugs include phenytoin, primidone, isoniazid, chlorpromazine, quinidine, penicillamine, minocycline, propylthiouracil, methylthiouracil, and methyldopa.

IV. **Treatment.** Symptoms usually resolve when the offending drug is withdrawn. Antinuclear antibodies can persist for months.

ANTIPHOSPHOLIPID SYNDROME

I. **General.**

A. Antiphospholipid syndrome is a disorder characterized by recurrent venous or arterial thrombosis, recurrent fetal loss, and thrombocytopenia associated with the presence of one or more of lupus anticoagulant, anticardiolipin antibody, or anti-β2-glycoprotein I antibodies. It can occur as a manifestation of lupus or as an isolated, discrete syndrome.

B. The female-to-male ratio is 2:1.

C. *Anticardiolipin* and *antiphospholipid* are essentially interchangeable terms. Depending on the assay used to detect them, they cross-react. Several subtypes that do not cross-react have been identified but are currently of little clinical significance.

II. **Clinical Features.**

A. **Pregnancy loss.** Obstetric complications include recurrent fetal loss (often but not always in the late second or third trimester), severe preeclampsia, uteroplacental insufficiency, premature delivery, chorea gravidarum, and intrauterine growth retardation. Patients can also have "postpartum syndrome," which is manifested by pleuropericarditis and fever.

B. **Thrombosis.** All venous and arterial systems can be involved. The most common site for venous thrombosis is in the lower extremities. Patients can have recurrent DVT or PE. The most common arterial complications are embolic cerebrovascular accidents and TIAs.

C. **Other features** include endocardial valvular vegetations, livedo reticularis, migraine headache, thrombocytopenia, and Coombs'-positive hemolytic anemia.

III. **Diagnosis.**

A. **Criteria for the presence of lupus anticoagulant (LA)** include prolonged PTT not corrected by addition of normal plasma but corrected by freeze-thawed platelets or phospholipids.

B. Anticardiolipin antibody (aCL) and anti-β2-glycoprotein I (aβ2g) antibodies are measured by immunoassays.

C. **Clinical diagnosis can be made** if the patient has experienced unexplained thromboembolism, thrombocytopenia, or recurrent fetal loss in conjunction with persistently elevated titers of aCL or LA.

IV. **Management.**

A. **There is no evidence that prophylactic anticoagulant therapy is helpful in patients who have been and are asymptomatic.**

B. **Thrombotic events.** Chronic anticoagulation with warfarin (goal INR 2-3) and antiplatelet drugs may be used; ASA alone is ineffective. Heparin is substituted for warfarin during pregnancy. Intravenous immunoglobulin during pregnancy in women with APS who have failed aspirin and subcutaneous heparin is controversial because studies have not shown consistent benefit. **Because patients can have an elevated PTT and occasionally PT, follow anticoagulation by measuring percent factor 2 activity.**

C. **Catastrophic antiphospholipid syndrome** involves acute onset of simultaneous occlusion of multiple vessels. Triggers include infection, surgery, and oral contraceptives. Treatment is based only on case reports and includes anticoagulants, steroids, IVIG, plasmapheresis, and fibrinolytics.

SYSTEMIC SCLEROSIS AND SCLERODERMA

I. **General.** Scleroderma is a diverse group of conditions that have in common fibrosis of skin and other tissues, including the microvascular system, visceral organs, and immunologic system. Pathogenesis is unclear but involves abnormalities of fibroblasts and cells of the

7

RHEUMATOLOGY

endoreticular system. Genetic and environmental factors are thought to contribute.

II. Clinical Features.

A. Skin. Bilateral symmetric swelling of the fingers ("sausage digits") and hands is often an early manifestation. Edema is replaced by induration in a few weeks to several months, resulting in thickened, hard skin. Skin thickness spreads rapidly and within months can affect the forearms, upper arms, face, and finally the trunk.

B. Raynaud's phenomenon occurs in almost all patients.

C. Joints are affected by nondeforming symmetric polyarthritis similar to rheumatoid arthritis.

D. Lungs. Diffuse interstitial fibrosis occurs in 70% of patients and treatment is difficult.

E. Heart. Cardiac abnormalities, such as conduction defects and supraventricular arrhythmias, are seen in up to 70%.

F. Gastrointestinal system is the most common internal organ system involved. Esophageal dysfunction is the most common gastrointestinal abnormality but patients can have malabsorption and other problems.

G. Kidney. Renal involvement often results in fulminant hypertension, renal failure, and death.

III. Treatment. No curative therapy is available.

A. Treatment of localized scleroderma. Options include topical corticosteroids, calcitriol 0.50 to 0.75 μg daily, and UVA therapy.

B. Antifibrotic medications. Penicillamine 125 mg PO qod can decrease skin thickness, delay internal organ involvement, and prolong life expectancy. Minocycline 50 mg PO, colchicine 0.6 mg bid, and IFN-α or IFN-γ have each been investigated in small studies and shown to have some benefit.

C. Other treatments are directed against symptoms including Raynaud's, hypertension, and gastroesophageal reflux; digital sympathectomy is indicated for a critically ischemic finger.

BIBLIOGRAPHY

Afari N, Buchwald D: Chronic fatigue syndrome: A review. *Am J Psychiatry* 160(2):221-236, 2003.

Amor B: Spondyloarthropathies, Reiter's syndrome. *Rheum Dis Clin North Am* 24(4):677, 1998.

Anandarajah AP, Ritchlin CT: Treatment update on spondyloarthropathy, *Postgrad Med* 116(5):31-40, 2004.

Breedveld FC: Osteoarthritis—The impact of a serious disease. *Rheumatology* 43(Suppl 1):4-8, 2004.

Brennan P, Silman A, Black C, et al: Validity and reliability of three methods used in the diagnosis of Raynaud's phenomenon. The UK Scleroderma Study Group. *Br J Rheumatol* 32:357, 1993.

Bruce I, Gladman DD: Psoriatic arthritis. Recognition and management. *BioDrugs* 9:27, 1998.

Cassetta M, Gorevic PD: Crystal arthritis. Gout and pseudogout in the geriatric patient. *Geriatrics* 59(9):25-30, 2004.

Cohen S: Risedronate therapy prevents corticosteroid-induced bone loss. *Arthritis Rheum* 42(11):2309, 1999.

Dall'Era M, Davis JC: Systemic lupus erythematosus. How to manage, when to refer. *Postgrad Med* 114(5):31-37, 40, 2003.

Deal CL, Moskowitz RW: Nutraceuticals as therapeutical agents in osteoarthritis. The role of glucosamine, chondroitin sulfate, and collagen hydrolysate. *Rheum Dis Clin North Am* 25(2):379, 1999.

Duhaut P, Berruyer M, Pinede L, et al: Anticardiolipin antibodies and giant cell arteritis: A prospective, multicenter case-control study. *Arthritis Rheum* 41: 701, 1998.

Ferrieri P: Proceedings of the Jones Criteria Workshop. *Circulation* 106(19): 2521-2523, 2002.

Fraenkel L: Different factors influencing the expression of Raynaud's phenomenon in men and women. *Arthritis Rheum* 42(2):306, 1999.

Gill JM, Quisel AM, Rocca PV, Walters DV: Diagnosis of systemic lupus erythematosus. *Am Fam Physician* 68(11):2179-2186, 2003.

Gladman DD: Psoriatic arthritis. *Rheum Dis Clin North Am* 24(4):829, 1998.

Goldenberg DL: Septic arthritis. *Lancet* 351(9097):197-202, 1998.

Issa SN, Ruderman EM: Damage control in rheumatoid arthritis. *Postgrad Med* 116(5):14-24, 2004.

Jimenez SA, Derk CT: Following the molecular pathways toward an understanding of the pathogenesis of systemic sclerosis. *Ann Intern Med* 140(1):37-50, 2004.

Jones G, Halbert J, Crotty M, et al: The effect of treatment on radiological progression in rheumatoid arthritis: A systematic review of randomized placebo-controlled trials. *Rheumatology* 42(1):6-13, 2003.

Laufer S: Osteoarthritis therapy—Are there still unmet needs? *Rheumatology* 43 Suppl 1:i9-15, 2004.

Leirisalo-Repo M: Prognosis, course of disease, and treatment of the spondyloarthropathies. *Rheum Dis Clin North Am* 24(4):737, 1998.

Levine JS, Branch DW, Rauch J: The antiphospholipid syndrome. *N Engl J Med* 346(10):752-763, 2002.

Littlejohn GO: Balanced treatments for fibromyalgia. *Arthritis Rheum* 50(9):2725-2729, 2004.

Maksymowych WP: Update in spondylarthropathy. *Arthritis Rheum* 51(1):143-146, 2004.

Millea PJ, Holloway RL: Treating fibromyalgia. *Am Fam Physician* 62(7):1575-1582, 87, 2000.

Morehead K, Sack KE: Osteoarthritis. What therapies for this disease of many causes? *Postgrad Med* 114(5):11-7, 2003.

Morelli V, Naquin C, Weaver V: Alternative therapies for traditional disease states: osteoarthritis. *Am Fam Physician* 67(2):339-344, 2003.

Olivieri I, van Tubergen A, Salvarani C, van der Linden S: Seronegative spondyloarthritides, *Best Pract Research Clin Rheum* 16(5):72372-9, 2002.

Pipitone N, Kingsley GH, Manzo A, et al: Current concepts and new developments in the treatment of psoriatic arthritis. *Rheumatology* 42(10):1138-1148, 2003.

Rott KT, Agudelo CA: Gout. *JAMA* 289(21):2857-2860, 2003.

Sapadin AN, Fleischmajer R: Treatment of scleroderma. *Arch Dermatol* 138(1): 99-105, 2002.

7

RHEUMATOLOGY

Sieper J, Rudwaleit M, Braun J, van der Heijde D: Diagnosing reactive arthritis: Role of clinical setting in the value of serologic and microbiologic assays. *Arthritis Rheum* 46(2):319-327, 2002.

Siva C, Velazquez C, Mody A, Brasington R: Diagnosing acute monoarthritis in adults: A practical approach for the family physician. *Am Fam Physician* 68(1): 83-90, 2003.

Toivanen A: Managing reactive arthritis. *Rheumatology* 39(2):117-119, 2000.

Weyand CM, Goronzy JJ: Giant-cell arteritis and polymyalgia rheumatica. *Ann Intern Med* 139(6):505-515, 2003.

Wigley FM: Clinical practice. Raynaud's phenomenon. *N Engl J Med* 347(13): 1001-1008, 2002.

Williams EA, Fye KH: Rheumatoid arthritis. Targeted interventions can minimize joint destruction. *Postgrad Med* 114(5):19-28, 2003.

Williamson L, Bowness P, Mowat A, Ostman-Smith I: Lesson of the week: Difficulties in diagnosing acute rheumatic fever-arthritis may be short lived and carditis silent. *BMJ* 320(7231):362-365, 2000.

Nephrology and Urology

Mark A. Graber and Jennifer L. Jones

URINARY TRACT INFECTIONS: WOMEN

I. **Acute Cystitis.**

A. **Signs and symptoms.** Dysuria, frequency, urgency, nocturia, enuresis, incontinence, urethral pain, suprapubic pain, low back pain, hematuria. Fever is unusual. The onset may follow intercourse ("honeymoon cystitis"). Up to 30% of patients with symptoms of cystitis may have a smoldering pyelonephritis (especially if symptoms have been present >1 week).

B. **Differential diagnosis of urinary symptoms.** Urinary frequency and urgency can be caused by UTI, diuretic use, caffeine, tea, drugs (e.g., theophylline), interstitial cystitis, vaginitis, pregnancy, pelvic mass, PID, BPH (in the man), as well as other causes.

1. **Uncomplicated UTI is defined as** no structural or metabolic abnormalities.

2. **Complicated UTI is defined as** structural, functional or metabolic abnormalities (e.g., polycystic, solitary, or transplanted kidney; diabetes; renal insufficiency; indwelling catheter; neurogenic bladder) or certain patient characteristics (e.g., elderly, pregnant, male, child, history of recurrent UTI).

C. **Causes of UTI.** Colonization by fecal flora, usually *Escherichia coli* (75% to 95%) or *Staphylococcus saprophyticus*. Complicated infection has more diverse causative organisms, including *Klebsiella, Enterobacter, Proteus, Serratia, Pseudomonas*, group B streptococci, or *Candida* species.

D. **Laboratory findings.**

1. **Urinalysis** (UA; from clean catch midstream).

a. **Positive leukocyte esterase, nitrite, hematuria or pyuria. Thirty percent of UA results are false negative, so patients may have bacterial cystitis and a negative UA.**

2. **Microscopy.**

a. **Bacteriuria.** Classically more than five organisms/HPF by microscopy or 10^5 organisms/mL on culture has been considered as a UTI. However, 10^2 organisms/mL is a better definition and correlates better with symptoms.

3. **C&S.** Not needed in uncomplicated UTI. Cultures should be done for recurrent UTIs, pyelonephritis, and complicated UTI, and in pregnant patients.

E. **Treatment.**

1. **Deciding whom to treat.** Presence of classic symptoms in a patient who has had a previous documented UTI is about 70% predictive of a UTI, so one can consider treatment even in the absence of positive urine findings. Presence of multiple classic symptoms (dysuria, frequency,

hematuria) increases likelihood of UTI to as great as 90%, so may treat without UA. However, also consider other causes as listed previously under signs and symptoms, especially vaginitis.

2. **Antibiotics** can be used in a 3-day regimen for young, sexually active women (preferred over single dose; decreases relapse rate without increasing side effects), or a standard oral regimen lasting 7 to 10 days. A 7- to 10-day course of antibiotics should be used for complicated UTIs and patients with symptoms for more than 1 week who have a higher risk for pyelonephritis.

3. All of the following drugs can be used in a 3-day or 7- to 10-day course. Failure of a short course of antibiotics generally indicates an upper tract infection and requires 10 to 14 days of antibiotics. **Failure of a 14-day course suggests a deep-seated kidney infection and may require 4 to 6 weeks of antibiotics.** Culture should be done in treatment failures to check for resistance patterns.

   a. **TMP–SMX DS** 1 tablet PO bid. If community *E. coli* resistance is <20%, this is the preferred treatment because it is inexpensive and has a cure rate superior to cephalosporins and amoxicillin. However, in some locations, up to 30% of *E. coli* may be resistant.

   b. **Fluoroquinolone.** Ciprofloxacin 250 to 500 mg PO bid; levofloxacin 250 to 500 mg PO qd. Resistance is low; drug is typically reserved for resistant organisms.

   c. **Oral cephalosporin.** Cephalexin 250 to 500 mg qid. Not as effective as TMP–SMX.

   d. **Nitrofurantoin** 50 to 100 mg PO qid with meals and at bedtime. Absorption is increased when taken with food. Has not been shown to be effective for pyelonephritis, but use may become more prevalent in simple cystitis because of resistance to TMP–SMX.

   e. **Other antibiotics.** Doxycycline 100 mg PO bid × 7 d; amoxicillin/clavulanic acid; amoxicillin alone has a lower cure rate than other drugs because of high resistance rates.

4. **Changing antibiotics. If a C&S is done and the organism is resistant to the drug prescribed, a change in antibiotics is indicated only if the patient is still symptomatic.** Many drugs reach such high levels in the urine that standard sensitivity testing may not reflect in vivo activity.

5. **Other measures.**

   a. **Consider a bladder anesthetic, such as phenazopyridine hydrochloride (Pyridium) 200 mg tid for 2 days, to relieve symptoms promptly.** Inform the patient that this will produce an orange tinge in tears and urine. Warn the patient not to wear contact lenses because they may become discolored.

   b. Instruct patient to increase fluid intake. See later for other measures.

II. **Chronic Cystitis.** Up to 20% of young women with acute cystitis develop recurrent UTIs. During these recurrences, the causative organism should be identified by urine cultures to differentiate between relapse and recurrence. Multiple infections caused by the same organism are by definition complicated UTIs.

A. Symptoms. Similar to simple cystitis but variable in severity.

B. Laboratory findings. UA shows a significant bacteriuria and may have any degree of pyuria. Urine culture will be positive, with *E. coli* most common. Pyuria without bacteriuria should be suggestive of *Mycobacterium tuberculosis* or *Chlamydia* infection.

C. Radiographs. Excretory and retrograde urograms and voiding cystograms may demonstrate associated conditions: obstructive uropathy, vesicoureteral reflux, atrophic pyelonephritis, and vesicoenteric or vesicovaginal fistulas.

D. Treatment. Treat based on susceptibility testing but empirically as per cystitis (see earlier) until sensitivities known.

E. Prevention. Women who have more than three UTI recurrences documented by urine cultures within 1 year can be managed using the following:

1. **Acute self-treatment** with a 3-day course of standard therapy.

2. **Postcoital prophylaxis** with TMP–SMX DS, 1 tablet after coitus; single-dose fluoroquinolone may be used as second-line treatment depending on resistance patterns in the community. Patients should void immediately after intercourse, although the benefit is questionable.

3. **Continuous daily prophylaxis** with either TMP–SMX, one single-strength tablet qd; nitrofurantoin 50 to 100 mg/day; or a fluoroquinolone (e.g., levofloxacin 250 mg qd).

F. Other preventive measures.

1. Cranberry, in juice or tablet form, has been proven to reduce pyuria and bacteriuria by preventing *E. coli* adherence to cells. Increasing fluids in general may be helpful as well.

2. The use of a diaphragm for birth control may exacerbate recurrent UTIs secondary to incomplete voiding. The use of nonoxynol-9 is associated with an increased incidence of bacteriuria.

3. Vaginal estrogen cream (0.5-2 g intravaginally qd) may be useful in post menopause, but evidence is limited. Oral estrogen does not work.

4. Women should be instructed to wipe from front to back after a bowel movement to avoid bringing infective organisms toward the urethra.

5. There is no evidence that avoiding baths reduces the incidence of cystitis. However, irritating soaps should be eliminated.

III. Interstitial Cystitis.

A. Signs and symptoms. Frequency, urgency, and, rarely, urge incontinence with periurethral and suprapubic pain on bladder filling that is improved by voiding. Terminal hematuria may be present.

B. Etiology. Unclear; may involve altered glycosaminoglycan (GAG) layer, or autoimmune or allergic processes. Often exacerbated by ingestion of certain foods, cigarette smoking.

8

NEPHROLOGY AND UROLOGY

C. **Treatment.** Refer to a urologist for cystoscopy and possible biopsy. Unable to diagnose without cystoscopy under anesthesia.

1. **Dietary modification.** Eliminate alcohol, carbonated beverages, caffeine, spicy foods, tyramine-containing foods, acidic foods.

2. **Behavior modification.** Eliminate cigarette smoking. Institute bladder training to increase time between voids. Pelvic floor exercises may benefit some.

3. **Oral medications.** Pyridium; pentosan polysulfate (Elmiron) 100 mg tid × 3 mo may replace GAG layer, improve symptoms. **However, pentosan takes at least 3 to 6 months and as much as 1 to 2 years to become effective and is expensive.** It is also an anticoagulant and can cause bleeding. Hydroxyzine (10-75 mg qhs) is thought to stabilize mast cells, but is limited by side effect of drowsiness. Amitriptyline (10-75 mg qhs) is thought to decrease symptoms secondary to anticholinergic effects.

4. **Intravesical therapies.** May be used in various combinations. Hydrodistention under anesthesia; dimethyl sulfoxide (DMSO) instillations q1-2 wk; BCG as an immunomodulator, instilled q1wk × 6-8 wk; hyaluronic acid to replace GAG, instilled q1wk × 4-6 wk; heparin.

IV. **Radiation Cystitis.** Symptoms may develop months after cessation of treatment, with history based on exposure to radiation. Urine may or may not be sterile.

V. **Noninfectious Hemorrhagic Cystitis.** Noninfectious hemorrhagic cystitis can occur after radiation therapy or treatment with cyclophosphamide. There is often serious vesical hemorrhage. Urgent consultation with a urologist should be sought.

VI. **Urethritis.**

A. Patient may have UTI symptoms, pyuria, but negative cultures.

B. **Causes.** Infections with a low colony count, *Chlamydia, Neisseria gonorrhoeae, Trichomonas*, or vaginitis.

C. **Treatment.** Treat as chlamydia and gonorrhea **(Table 8-1).**

VII. **Asymptomatic Bacteriuria.**

A. Diagnosis requires >10^5 CFU/mL of urine of the same organism in two clean-catch specimens or >100 organisms in a single catheterized specimen. Prevalence is as high as 5% in women.

B. Must be distinguished from contamination from vaginal or urethral organisms attributable to poor technique in specimen collection. Treat based on C&S, not empirically.

C. **The only patients who should be treated for asymptomatic bacteriuria include those who** are pregnant, have had a recent urologic procedure, have recently had the removal of an indwelling catheter, have diabetes mellitus, or are children. Asymptomatic bacteriuria is not an indication for treatment with antibiotics in men, the elderly, or most women because treatment does not affect the outcome in these patients.

TABLE 8-1

TREATMENT OF SEXUALLY TRANSMITTED DISEASES

Type and Location	Drug of Choice	Alternatives
CHLAMYDIA TRACHOMATIS DISEASES		
Urethritis, proctitis, cervicitis, nongonococcal urethritis (treat also for gonorrhea)	Doxycycline 100 mg PO bid × 7 days* Azithromycin 1 g as single dose*	Erythromycin base 500 mg PO qid × 7 days (preferred in pregnancy), or Ofloxacin 300 mg bid × 7 days. Levofloxacin 500 mg daily ×7 days.
Persistent urethritis	Metronidazole 2 g PO in a single dose, *plus* Erythromycin base 500 mg PO qid × 7 days, or Erythromycin ethylsuccinate 800 mg PO qid × 7 days.	
Lymphogranuloma venereum	Doxycycline 100 mg PO bid × 21 days.	Erythromycin 500 mg PO qid × 21 days.
NEISSERIA GONORRHOEAE: GONORRHEA		
Urethritis, proctitis, pharyngitis (treat also for chlamydia)	Cefixime 400 mg PO in a single dose, or Ceftriaxone 125 mg IM in a single dose, or †Ciprofloxacin 500 mg PO in a single dose, or †Ofloxacin 400 mg PO in a single dose, or †Levofloxacin 500 mg PO in a single dose, *plus*	Spectinomycin 2 g IM once or Ceftizoxime 500 mg IM once or Cefoxitin 2 g IM plus probenecid 1 g PO once or Gatifloxacin 400 mg PO once or Norfloxacin 800 mg PO once or

Continued

TABLE 8-1
TREATMENT OF SEXUALLY TRANSMITTED DISEASES—cont'd

Type and Location	Drug of Choice	Alternatives
	Azithromycin 1 g PO in a single dose,	
	or	
	Doxycycline 100 mg PO bid × 7 days.	Lomefloxacin 400 mg PO once.
Disseminated	Initial until 24 h asymptomatic:	Initial alternative:
	Ceftriaxone 1 g IV or IM q24h	Cefotaxime 1 g IV q8h,
	or	or
	Ceftizoxime 1 mg IV q8h.	Ceftizoxime 1 g IV q8h,
	Follow with (for a total of 7-10 d):	or
	Cefixime 400 mg PO bid,	For persons allergic to β-lactam drugs:
	or	Ciprofloxacin 500 mg IV q12h,
	Ciprofloxacin 500 mg PO bid,	or
	or	Ofloxacin 400 mg IV q12h,
	Ofloxacin 400 mg PO bid,	or
	or	Spectinomycin 2 g IM q12h; follow with
	Levofloxacin 500 mg PO qd.	regimen to left.
PELVIC INFLAMMATORY DISEASE		
Initial treatment	Cefotetan 2 g IV q12h,	Ofloxacin 400 mg IV q12h,
	or	plus
	Cefoxitin 2 g IV q6h,	Metronidazole 500 mg IV q8h.
	plus	or
	Doxycycline 100 mg IV or PO q12h.	Ampicillin/sulbactam 3 g IV q6h,
	or	plus
	Clindamycin 900 mg IV q8h,	Doxycycline 100 mg IV or PO q12h.
	plus	or

Follow up with	Gentamicin 2 mg/kg IV (loading dose) followed by 1.5 mg/kg IV q8h or 4.5 mg/kg qd.	Ciprofloxacin 200 mg IV q12h, *plus* Doxycycline 100 mg IV or PO q12h, *plus* Metronidazole 500 mg IV q8h.
	Ofloxacin 400 mg PO bid × 14 days, *or*	Ceftriaxone 250 mg IM once, *or*
	Levofloxacin 500 mg PO qd, *plus*	Cefoxitin 2 g IM plus Probenecid 1 g PO in a single dose concurrently once, *or*
	Metronidazole 500 mg PO bid × 14 days.	Other parenteral third-generation cephalosporin (e.g., ceftizoxime or cefotaxime), *plus*
		Doxycycline 100 mg PO bid × 14 days. (Include this regimen with one of the above regimens.)

EPIDIDYMO-ORCHITIS

| If likely an STD | Ceftriaxone 250 mg IM in a single dose, *plus* Doxycycline 100 mg PO bid × 10 days *or* Ofloxacin 300 mg PO bid × 10 days | |
| If likely enteric organism | Ciprofloxacin ER 500 mg PO qd × 10-14 days *or* Ciprofloxacin 400 mg IV bid × 10-14 days *or* Levofloxacin 750 mg IV or PO qd × 10-14 days. | Ampicillin/sulbactam or third-generation cephalosporin |

Continued

NEPHROLOGY AND UROLOGY 8

TABLE 8-1

TREATMENT OF SEXUALLY TRANSMITTED DISEASES—cont'd

Type and Location	Drug of Choice	Alternatives
TRICHOMONAS VAGINALIS		
Trichomonas urethritis or vaginitis	Metronidazole 2 g PO in single dose or 500 mg bid × 7 days. CDC recommends the single 2-g dose in pregnancy (after first trimester).	No effective alternatives.
GRANULOMA INGUINALE		
Granuloma inguinale (_Calymmatobacterium granulomatis_)	TMP–SMX one double-strength tablet PO bid for a minimum of 3 wk, _or_ Doxycycline 100 mg PO bid for a minimum of 3 wk. Therapy should be continued until all lesions have healed completely.	Ciprofloxacin 750 mg PO bid for a minimum of 3 wk, _or_ Erythromycin base 500 mg PO qid for a minimum of 3 wk. _or_ Azithromycin 1 g PO weekly for minimum of 3 wk.
CHANCROID		
Chancroid (_Haemophilus ducreyi_)	Ceftriaxone 250 mg IM once _or_ Azithromycin 1 g PO once.	Ciprofloxacin 500 mg PO bid × 3 days, _or_ Erythromycin base 500 mg PO qid × 7 days.
SYPHILIS		
Primary and secondary	Benzathine penicillin G 2.4 million U IM in a single dose.	Doxycycline 100 mg PO bid × 2 wk, _or_ Tetracycline 500 mg PO qid × 2 wk.

Latent	Early latent syphilis: Benzathine penicillin G 2.4 million U IM in a single dose.	Doxycycline 100 mg PO bid§ × 28 days
		or
	Late latent syphilis or latent syphilis of unknown duration:	Tetracycline 500 mg PO qid × 28 days.
	Benzathine penicillin G 7.2 million U total, administered as three doses of 2.4 million U IM each at 1-wk intervals.	
Tertiary	Benzathine penicillin G 7.2 million U total, administered as three doses of 2.4 million U IM at 1-wk intervals.	As for latent syphilis.

HERPES SIMPLEX

Initial episode†	Acyclovir 400 mg PO tid × 7-10 days	Valacyclovir 1000 mg PO bid × 10 days
	or	
	Famciclovir 250 mg PO tid × 7-10 days	
Chronic suppression	Acyclovir 400 mg PO bid,	
	or	
	Famciclovir 250 mg PO bid,	
	or	
	Valacyclovir 500 mg PO qd,‖	
	or	
	Valacyclovir 1 g PO qd.	
Recurrent	Acyclovir 400 mg PO tid × 5 days,	Valacyclovir 500 mg PO bid × 5 days
	or	
	Acyclovir 200 mg PO five times a day × 5 days,	
	or	

Continued

NEPHROLOGY AND UROLOGY   8

TABLE 8-1

TABLE 8-1
TREATMENT OF SEXUALLY TRANSMITTED DISEASES—cont'd

Type and Location	Drug of Choice	Alternatives
	Acyclovir 800 mg PO bid × 2 days,	
	or	
	Famciclovir 125 mg PO bid × 5 days,	
	or	
	Valacyclovir 500 mg PO bid × 3 days.	
Disseminated herpes	Acyclovir 5-10 mg/kg body weight IV q8h × 5-7 days or until clinical resolution is attained.	

From Centers for Disease Control and Prevention: Sexually transmitted diseases treatment guidelines—2002. *MMWR Recomm Rep* 51(RR-6):1-78, 2002. Available online at http://www.cdc.gov/mmwr/preview/mmwrhtml/rr5106a1.htm.

Note: If treating for either *N. gonorrhoeae* or *C. trachomatis*, treat for both organisms, because patients commonly have concurrent infections. Always treat sexual partners as well!

*Doxycycline is as efficacious as azithromycin for chlamydia even if the patient does not take all of the doses. Bacteriologic cure rates are 95% for both drugs (and doxycycline is less expensive).

†See notes in text about resistance patterns.

‡May continue for > 10 days if lesions do not resolve.

§For pregnancy, desensitize to penicillin and treat with penicillin.

‖Less efficacious than other regimens.

URINARY TRACT INFECTIONS: CHILDREN

I. **Clinical Presentation.** Differs from adults in that symptoms may include only fever, new incontinence in a previously toilet-trained youngster, abdominal pain, diarrhea, vomiting, or lethargy. UTI is a common cause of fever in the neonatal period. Uncircumcised boys <8 weeks of age are more prone to UTIs than are girls or circumcised boys of same age.

II. **Diagnostic Criteria.** Same as for cystitis in women, earlier. **However, fever may cause pyuria; therefore, culture is always indicated.** Quick catheterization should be done unless the child can give a clean-catch urine; "bag" urines generally yield poor specimens for culture because of contamination. Most common organism in uncomplicated infection is Enterobacteriaceae.

III. **Management.** All children with UTIs need a repeat culture 1 to 2 weeks after completing treatment. All children <3 months of age should be admitted for IV antibiotics, as should children who look ill. An older child with simple, uncomplicated UTI can be treated as an outpatient. A 10- to 14-day course of antibiotics is generally prescribed for UTI in children because of studies showing lower reinfection rates and fewer treatment failures with longer treatment duration.

A. **IV regimens** include ceftriaxone 50 to 100 mg/kg q24h; gentamicin 3 mg/kg per dose q24h for age <1 mo, 2.5 mg/kg per dose q12h if >1 mo of age **(adjust dose of gentamicin based on peak and trough levels);** cefotaxime 150 mg/kg per day divided tid. Ampicillin 100 mg/kg per day divided q6h can be added to gentamicin for better enterococcal coverage, but is often inadequate on its own because of resistance.

B. **PO regimens** include TMP–SMX, 8 to 10 mg TMP, 30 to 60 mg SMX per kilogram per day divided bid; cefixime 8 mg/kg per day qd; or cephalexin 25 to 50 mg/kg per day divided tid-qid, nitrofurantoin 5 to 7 mg/kg per day divided qid. Amoxicillin/clavulanate can also be used.

IV. **Evaluation.** Radiologic evaluation for anatomic abnormality (IVP, US, voiding cystourethrogram [VCUG]) can be considered for all girls <5 years of age, all boys regardless of age, children with evidence of pyelonephritis, and any girl >5 years of age with recurrent UTIs, as well as in those who are not responding as expected to antibiotics. The evidence for these recommendations is only fair, and is increasingly controversial given that the result often does not change management. Some authors would not work up first cystitis in a girl but would defer work-up until a second infection.

NEPHROLOGY AND UROLOGY

8

URINARY TRACT INFECTIONS: MEN

I. Overview.

A. Cause. Ascending infection from the urethra is the most common; reflux of infected urine into prostatic ducts and then into the posterior urethra is likely an important cause of prostatitis. Hematogenous, lymphatic spread, or extension from adjacent organs is also possible.

B. Pathogens. *E. coli* (80% to 91%), *Proteus, Enterobacter, Pseudomonas, Serratia, Streptococcus faecalis*, and *Staphylococcus* species are the most common.

C. Localization of infection. Divided urine collection may help localize the infection: urethra is represented by first voided 10 mL, bladder by midstream collection, and prostate by the last 10 mL of voided urine. Prostatic massage before the last voided 10 mL will increase the yield.

II. Urethritis.

A. Presentation. Generally complain of a urethral discharge most noticeable in AM (watery to purulent), with or without urethral burning or itching, and burning on urination. May not note discharge but may have spotting in underwear.

B. Cause. *N. gonorrhoeae* and *Chlamydia trachomatis* (causes 80% of nongonococcal [GC] disease) are most common, followed by *Ureaplasma urealyticum, Mycoplasma* spp., *Trichomonas vaginalis, Candida*, and herpesviruses.

C. History. Ask about first onset of symptoms, recent sexual contacts, prior history of STDs.

D. Work-up. Examination should be performed at least 1 hour after the last void. Notice character of discharge: watery and thin are suggestive of *Chlamydia*, whereas a purulent-looking discharge is suggestive of gonorrhea. Obtain a specimen by inserting a calcium alginate (Kalginate) swab 2 to 3 cm within the urethra (a drop of the discharge is not acceptable because *Chlamydia* organisms are intracellular and urethral cellular material is required for culture).

E. Laboratory findings. Gram stain of urethral discharge should show more than five WBCs/HPF. Demonstration of intracellular gram-negative diplococci within PMNs is strong evidence of gonorrhea. Absence of gram-negative cocci is strong evidence of non-GC urethritis (e.g., *Chlamydia*). However, Gram stain is only 95% sensitive for GC. Culture on modified Thayer-Martin medium for gonorrhea (<100% sensitive) and send for immunofluorescent testing and PCR, or culture for *Chlamydia*.

F. Treatment (see Table 8-1). Be sure to treat for both *Chlamydia* and *N. gonorrhoeae,* and treat partner(s).

III. Bacterial Cystitis.

A. Signs and symptoms. Similar to those in women. Also examine urethra for discharge (urethritis), prostate, and epididymis for tenderness to rule out other disorders.

B. **Laboratory findings.** UA shows pyuria, bacteriuria, no casts, occasionally gross or microscopic hematuria. **C&S should be done in men with history consistent with UTI.**

C. **Treatment.** Treat 10 to 14 days and then obtain follow-up culture. Antibiotic choices are similar to those for female UTI. After successful treatment (urine is sterile), consider IVP or cystoscopy to rule out structural obstruction to outflow.

IV. **Infections of the Prostate Gland.** Up to 95% of prostate complaints in men are related to nonbacterial prostatitis or prostatodynia. If symptoms are not relieved after a course of antibiotics, consider nonbacterial cause. The NIH classification system is commonly used to categorize symptoms/findings.

A. **NIH category I: Acute bacterial prostatitis.**

1. **Signs and symptoms.** Acute febrile illness, chills, malaise, lower back pain, perineal pain, urinary urgency or frequency, nocturia, or dysuria. Varying degrees of urinary retention, tenesmus, or pain with bowel movement. The prostate is very tender, boggy, and warm to touch. (Do not massage because of risk of bacteremia.)

2. **Laboratory findings.** Leukocytosis with left shift, bacteriuria, hematuria, and pyuria. C&S is required.

3. **Therapy.**

a. Hospitalization for IV antibiotics if sepsis is suspected. Start gentamycin or tobramycin and ampicillin pending culture results. An alternative is ofloxacin 400 mg PO then 300 mg PO bid.

b. If hospitalization is not necessary (no fever; patient not toxic), prescribe TMP–SMX DS bid, ciprofloxacin 500 bid, or ofloxacin 300 mg bid. In young, sexually active men, treat for gonorrhea and *Chlamydia* infections for 14 days as well. In general, the fluoroquinolones penetrate the prostate better and are preferred for this indication.

c. **Continuing oral antibiotics for a total of 1 month to 6 weeks after an episode of acute prostatitis may reduce recurrence and reduce transformation into chronic prostatitis.**

d. Avoid urethral catheterization unless patient unable to void spontaneously.

e. After completion of successful therapy, the patient should be followed for at least 4 months with periodic examinations and cultures of prostatic fluids to ensure cure.

B. **NIH category II: Chronic bacterial prostatitis.**

1. **Signs and symptoms.** Low back and perineal discomfort; voiding symptoms similar to those of acute bacterial prostatitis but with a more insidious onset. No systemic signs; rarely, painful ejaculation. Prostate may feel normal, boggy, or focally indurated. Chronic prostatitis is the most common cause of recurrent UTIs in men.

2. **Laboratory tests.** UA and cultures should be done; **must identify causative organism to be NIH category II.** Prostatic secretions reveal inflammatory cells, with macrophages containing oval fat bodies.

NEPHROLOGY AND UROLOGY

8

UA will show WBCs and bacteriuria if secondary cystitis is present. Causative agents are usually *E. coli, Klebsiella, Proteus*, or *Pseudomonas*. But many cases of chronic prostatitis are not bacterial (see later).

3. **Treatment.** Ciprofloxacin 500 mg PO or norfloxacin 400 mg PO bid × 6-12 wk. Levofloxacin 500 mg PO qd is another option. This yields about an 80% cure rate. TMP–SMX DS bid × 3 mo cures about one third of cases and improves symptoms in about three fourths. Failure of therapy may indicate the need for IV antibiotics or the presence of infected prostatic calculi. Chronic suppression with TMP–SMX or a quinolone at bedtime may be helpful.

C. **NIH category III: Chronic prostatitis/chronic pelvic pain syndrome (CP/CPPS).**

1. **Etiology.** Most cases will fall in this category; it is also the most difficult to treat. This is a diagnosis of exclusion of unknown etiology. Most likely multifactorial, with theories of causation including hormonal component, autoimmune role, defective androgen receptor, imbalance of inflammatory over anti-inflammatory cytokines, role of stress.

2. **Signs and symptoms.** Same as for chronic bacterial prostatitis.

3. **Laboratory findings.** Prostatic secretions reveal inflammatory cells but no bacteria. No causative organism is ever identified.

4. **Therapy.**

a. A clinical trial of antibiotic therapy directed to aforementioned organisms is recommended: doxycycline 100 mg bid, or ofloxacin 300 mg bid should be tried for at least 4 weeks. **Because CP/CPPS usually does not respond to antibiotics, their continued empiric use is not justified beyond an initial 4-week course.**

b. Symptomatic flare-ups often respond to anti-inflammatory agents, such as ibuprofen 400 to 600 mg PO q4-6h.

c. α-Adrenergic receptor blocking agent may help: prazosin 2 to 4 mg PO bid, or terazosin 5 to 10 mg PO bid. However, most data are negative.

d. Other measures: pelvic floor training, biofeedback, hot sitz baths, reassurance. The recurrent symptoms can often cause significant emotional stress, anxiety, and depression, resulting in significant morbidity.

D. **NIH category IV: Asymptomatic inflammatory prostatitis. Diagnosis:** Inflammatory cells are found in prostatic secretions incidentally; patient is asymptomatic. Chronic inflammation of prostate may lead to elevation of PSA, but this has not been shown to be associated with prostate cancer.

V. **Epididymitis.**

A. **Causes.**

1. Sexually transmitted form is associated with urethritis and commonly caused by *Chlamydia* or *N. gonorrhoeae*, or both.

2. Nonsexually transmitted form is associated with UTI or prostatitis; in older men, commonly caused by *Enterobacter, Klebsiella*, or *Pseudomonas* organisms.

3. Causes such as trauma, tuberculosis, urine reflux, or as a complication of transurethral prostatectomy (TURP) or systemic infection are less common.

B. Signs and symptoms. Epididymitis is painful, and swelling and tenderness may extend to groin, lower abdomen, or flank. Fever, urethral discharge, and reactive hydrocele may occur but are not common.

C. Laboratory findings. WBC count may be normal or elevated with left shift. UA may show pyuria or bacteriuria. C&S is indicated.

D. Differential diagnosis. Mumps orchitis, tumor, testicular abscess, torsion, hernia, and trauma must be considered.

E. Therapy.

1. **General measures.** Bed rest, scrotal elevation and support ("jock strap"), analgesics, and spermatic cord block with lidocaine may be used.

2. **Antibiotics** (see Table 8-1).

3. **NSAIDs.** Effective for inflammatory component.

UPPER URINARY TRACT INFECTIONS: ALL PATIENTS

I. **Acute Pyelonephritis.**

A. Definition. Infection of the parenchyma and pelvis of the kidney, which may affect one or occasionally both kidneys.

B. Causes. Aerobic gram-negative bacterium, most commonly *E. coli*. All organisms causing acute cystitis can cause acute pyelonephritis. *Proteus* species are especially important because they produce urease, which causes alkaline urine and favors formation of struvite and apatite stones. Staphylococci may infect by hematogenous route and cause renal abscesses.

C. Clinical findings. Abrupt onset of shaking chills and fever >38.5° C, flank pain, malaise, and urinary frequency and burning. Often have nausea, vomiting, and diarrhea as well. Generally have costovertebral angle tenderness. **May be septic. Children may complain of abdominal pain.**

D. Laboratory findings. Leukocytosis with left shift. UA will show pyuria, possibly WBC casts, hematuria, and mild proteinuria. C&S of urine is mandatory; some also obtain blood cultures, but the efficacy is questionable because the organism will be recovered in the urine. With the exception of WBC casts, bacteremia, and flank pain, none of the physical or lab findings is specific for pyelonephritis, so be sure to rule out other causes of fever, back pain, and so on. BUN and creatinine usually remain normal in uncomplicated pyelonephritis.

E. Treatment.

1. **Who to hospitalize. Hospitalize if** the patient is a child, is an infant, has a high fever, is dehydrated, appears acutely ill, or is septic. Data indicate that healthy-looking pregnant patients may be treated as outpatients. Treat hospitalized patients empirically with IV

8

NEPHROLOGY AND UROLOGY

third-generation cephalosporin with or without gentamicin,
IV or PO fluoroquinolone (PO fluoroquinolones attain the same serum
levels as IV), gentamicin and ampicillin, ampicillin-sulbactam, or
ticarcillin/clavulanic acid pending C&S results. Avoid gentamicin and
fluoroquinolones in pregnant patients. Treat IV for about 48 to 72 hours
or more according to clinical response. Continue oral antibiotics for
2 weeks in an uncomplicated case but up to 6 weeks for recurrent or
complicated disease. Medication should be given for pain, fever,
and nausea. Ensure adequate hydration and maintenance of good urine
output with either IV or PO fluids. See also discussion of septic shock in
Chapter 10.

2. **If the patient is not acutely ill,** treat as outpatient for 10 to 14 days
if a simple pyelonephritis but up to 6 weeks if recurrent pyelonephritis.
Treat based on C&S, but empiric treatment options include TMP–SMX,
fluoroquinolone (e.g., ciprofloxacin 500 mg PO bid, levofloxacin
500 mg PO qd), amoxicillin/clavulanic acid, or a cephalosporin.
Fluoroquinolones achieve the same levels in the blood PO and IV,
making these a good choice. Another good option is to give 1 g of
ceftriaxone IV or IM at the time of diagnosis and then follow up the
patient the next day. If required, an additional dose of ceftriaxone
can be given at the follow-up exam if the patient warrants more
than PO antibiotics but does not require hospitalization. Ensure good
communication in case of worsening condition, and establish
follow-up care.

3. **If the patient is not improving** after 72 hours of appropriate
antimicrobial therapy, consider infected stones or obstruction and
treat early to avoid complications. If the patient is not responding to
antibiotics and the organism is known to be sensitive to the current
antibiotics, consider emphysematous pyelonephritis or abscess
formation. CT scan will identify these patients. In the small percentage
of patients who relapse after a 2-week course, a 6-week course is
usually curative.

4. **Follow-up study.** Consider IVP or VCUG after resolution of UTI in all
children and men or in women with frequent recurrences or unusual
symptoms. One to 2 weeks after therapy is completed, urine culture
should be obtained in pregnant patients, children, patients who remain
symptomatic, and those for whom suppression therapy is being
considered. Follow-up cultures are optional for others.

SEXUALLY TRANSMITTED DISEASES

General note on testing: Because chlamydia can be asymptomatic,
it is important to screen high-risk populations such as those younger than
20 years of age, those with more than one sexual partner, and so on.
There are now screening tests (PCR) that can be performed on the urine for

Chlamydia as well as *N. gonorrhoeae*, making a pelvic exam unnecessary. The sensitivity of GC culture is highly dependent on technique, 85% at best. Gram stain is 95% sensitive in men and 48% in women. DNA testing and fluorescent antibody testing are also available for GC.

I. Syphilis. Caused by the spirochete *Treponema pallidum*. Incidence is increasing, especially among African-American women. **See Chapter 11, HIV–AIDS, for unique considerations in the HIV-positive patient.**

A. Primary syphilis.

1. **Clinical presentation.** Characteristic sign is the chancre, a painless sore that usually develops 2 to 4 weeks after exposure. These are 1 to 2 cm in diameter, may be multiple, appear as shallow ulcerations with noninflamed margins, and occur most commonly on mucous membranes abraded during sexual contact. Chancres heal spontaneously and slowly without scarring in 2 to 12 weeks. Unilateral or bilateral inguinal lymphadenopathy may be present.

2. **Laboratory findings.** Dark-field exam of suspect lesions will reveal spirochetes. VDRL test or RPR test is initially positive in 50% of patients but may remain negative for up to 3 weeks after the appearance of the chancre. The VDRL is nonspecific and may be positive in other disease states (e.g., connective tissue disorders, sarcoid). FTA-ABS is the quickest, least expensive, and most specific and sensitive examination. After therapy, the VDRL and RPR may revert to negative (although 28% to 44% remain positive 36 months after treatment). The FTA will remain positive in the great majority (80%).

3. **Therapy** (see Table 8-1). Patients may experience fever, chills, arthralgias, myalgias, and nausea several hours after treatment (the Jarisch-Herxheimer reaction), usually subsiding within 24 hours.

B. Secondary syphilis.

1. **Clinical presentation.** Widespread, symmetric rash, often involving palms or soles (80%). Rash is usually erythematous but is otherwise variable in appearance (e.g., morbilliform, similar to pityriasis rosea) and normally occurs 4 to 10 weeks after chancre. Condylomata lata, oral or genital mucous patches (superficial mucosal erosions), systemic symptoms (50%), and symmetric adenopathy also occur. The lesions of secondary syphilis resolve with or without treatment in 2 to 10 weeks. Approximately 25% of untreated patients will have recurrence of symptoms within 4 years.

2. **Laboratory findings.** Dark-field exam of condylomata lata is often positive. VDRL test is highly reactive in 90% but should be confirmed with FTA-ABS.

3. **Therapy** (see Table 8-1).

C. Tertiary syphilis. Symptoms may occur 1 to 50 years after initial infection. May have gumma formation, tabes dorsalis (sensory loss in legs and bowel and bladder dysfunction, secondary to dorsal column changes), lymphocytic meningitis, aortic insufficiency, and dementia.

8

NEPHROLOGY AND UROLOGY

D. Therapy. Treat based on duration of infection. Repeat the VDRL test at 3, 6, and 12 months in all patients with syphilis. If the treatment is adequate, the VDRL test results should decline fourfold.

II. Gonorrhea. Caused by gram-negative diplococcus *N. gonorrhoeae*. (For discussion of gonococcal disease in the man, see previous section on urethritis.)

A. Signs and symptoms. The primary site of infection is the endocervix. Yellow-white discharge may be present, but the infection is frequently asymptomatic. Findings may include friable cervix, yellow-green cervical discharge, sterile pyuria, positive cultures, or other evidence of gonorrhea. Other infections include proctitis, pharyngitis, salpingitis, and disseminated disease (pustulovesicular lesions with arthralgias and arthritis).

B. Laboratory findings. Gram stain of a vaginal smear reveals gram-negative intracellular diplococci (only 30% to 70%). Culture on Thayer-Martin (chocolate agar) medium to grow *Neisseria* organisms.

C. Therapy (see Table 8-1). There is increasing resistance to fluoroquinolones; these drugs should be avoided if possible. Repeat cultures should be obtained 3 to 7 days after treatment to ensure adequate treatment. Sexual partner(s) should also be treated.

III. Chancroid. Caused by a gram-negative rod, *Haemophilus ducreyi*.

A. Signs and symptoms. A papule that becomes a pustule that subsequently ulcerates. In contrast to syphilis, the ulcers of chancroid are painful. Lesions are deep with flat, ragged, erythematous borders that may extend into subcutaneous tissue. Adenopathy is common; systemic signs of fever, headache, and malaise occur in 50%. Presence of ulcers increases risk of HIV transmission.

B. Laboratory findings. Smear reveals gram-negative rods in chains ("school of fish"). Culture on enriched chocolate agar with vancomycin may be positive; biopsy specimen is diagnostic. Swab from base of lesion may be sent for PCR testing.

C. Therapy (see Table 8-1).

IV. Lymphogranuloma Venereum. Caused by a highly virulent strain of *C. trachomatis*.

A. Signs and symptoms. A papule or pustule that appears 5 to 21 days after exposure and ulcerates. This lesion often goes unnoticed. Painful adenopathy (usually unilateral) occurs 1 to 2 weeks later. May form buboes, become fluctuant, or form chronic draining sinuses. Generally have fever, chills, or rash. Rectal strictures from anorectal node involvement can be seen.

B. Laboratory findings. Complement fixation titers should show a fourfold increase after 4 weeks. Culture of aspirate for *C. trachomatis* is diagnostic but is positive in only 20% to 30%.

C. Therapy (see Table 8-1). I&D of nodes is rarely indicated.

V. Herpes Simplex Genitalis. Classically caused by herpes simplex virus type II, but can also be type I.

A. **Signs and symptoms.** Often asymptomatic. Incubation is 2 to 10 days. Primary lesion is manifest by grouped painful vesicles on an erythematous base that ulcerate and heal without scarring. Fever and adenopathy are common. Secondary lesions are similar to primary lesions except that the duration and severity are less and accompanying fever and adenopathy are rare.

B. **Laboratory findings.** Tzanck smear of a base of a fresh vesicle (Giemsa stain) reveals multinucleated giant cells. Culture requires 48 to 72 hours; rapid antigen test is available. Type-specific serologic tests are available and recommended by CDC for herpesvirus, but may be negative during a primary outbreak.

C. **Therapy** (see Table 8-1).

VI. **Condyloma Acuminatum.** Caused by human papillomavirus, commonly types 6, 11.

A. **Signs and symptoms.** Soft, flesh-colored, verrucous lesions in genital area. Type 16, which is typically asymptomatic, is associated with an increased risk of cervical dysplasia and cancer.

B. **Laboratory findings.** Serologic studies may be necessary to rule out condyloma latum of secondary syphilis. Biopsy specimen (rarely necessary) is diagnostic.

C. **Therapy.**

1. **Podophyllin (10% to 25% in tincture of benzoin),** applied and then thoroughly washed off in 1 to 4 hours. Alternatively, home therapy with the preparation Podofilox 0.5% can be tried. Warts are treated bid × 3 d; an area of no more than 10 cm^2 should be treated. No further applications should be made for 4 days. This cycle can be repeated three times (a total of four cycles of 3 days of treatment over a 4-week period). Frequently causes local irritation, erythema, swelling and erosions. If a poor or no response is noted, another therapeutic modality should be tried.

2. **Trichloroacetic acid.** Can be applied cautiously to lesions. It is highly caustic and will injure normal skin; protect unaffected skin with petroleum jelly.

3. **Imiquimod 5% cream.** Acts as immunomodulator. Apply contents of one packet to affected areas overnight (6-10 hours) then wash off (no limit to surface area); use three times a week for up to 16 weeks. Even if lesions do not clear, most note a significant decrease in size of lesions. Side effects include moderate erythema at site of application. Imiquimod is 73% successful in women after 16 weeks of treatment. Its efficacy is only 30% to 40% in men. It is expensive.

4. **Intravaginal 5-fluorouracil.** Not FDA approved for this purpose. Use 5% 5-FU cream and apply one fourth of applicator qhs × 1 wk and then once weekly for 10 weeks. Alternatively, the cream can be used twice per week for 10 weeks. Many women will not tolerate these regimens because of erosion of vaginal mucosa.

NEPHROLOGY AND UROLOGY

8

5. **Alternative therapies.** Cryotherapy, electrosurgery, excision, laser vaporization, or intralesional interferon. Also consider combination therapy of destructive method followed by Imiquimod.
6. Condylomata tend to recur in 75% to 80%; counsel patient regarding this.

VII. Molluscum Contagiosum. Caused by a poxvirus.
  A. Signs and symptoms. Dome-shaped, raised papules, 2 to 6 mm with central umbilication.
  B. Laboratory findings. Incision of a papule reveals white, waxy core. Smear of contents reveals swollen epithelial cells. Biopsy specimen is diagnostic.
  C. Therapy. Curettage, cryosurgery, or electrodesiccation. Several medical therapies have been tried, although none is currently FDA approved. These include trichloroacetic acid, Podofilox, and Imiquimod. Several trials suggest that 1% or 5% Imiquimod cream applied tid for 5 days of each week × 4 wk is successful at eradicating lesions.

VIII. Candidiasis. Yeast infection caused by *Candida albicans*. See Chapter 13.
  IX. Trichomoniasis. Caused by protozoon *T. vaginalis*. See Table 8-1 and Chapter 13.
  X. Chlamydia. Caused by *C. trachomatis*. See Table 8-1 and Chapter 13.
  XI. Bacterial Vaginosis. May present as malodorous vaginal discharge. See Chapter 13 for details.

BENIGN PROSTATIC HYPERPLASIA

  I. Cause. Benign prostatic hyperplasia (BPH) rarely affects men younger than 40 years of age, but generally becomes symptomatic from 60 to 65 years of age. Prevalence increases with age to >50% in those over age 60.
  II. Clinical Presentation.
  A. Signs and symptoms do not directly correlate with prostate size. These include decreased force and caliber of urinary stream, hesitancy, urinary retention, postmicturition dribbling, double voiding (patient voids and is able to void again in 5 to 10 minutes), and overflow urinary incontinence (on straining or coughing). Irritative symptoms such as dysuria, frequency, nocturia, urgency, hematuria, and incontinence occur frequently. Flank pain during micturition, suprapubic pain, and azotemic symptoms occur less commonly.
  B. Exam. The bladder may be distended, and the prostate is enlarged, smooth, and symmetric. The prostate gland may be soft or firm and possibly nodular. However, the nodules lack the stony-hard consistency associated with carcinoma.
  C. Laboratory findings. UA may reveal signs of infection. If the obstruction has been severe enough to impair renal function, BUN and creatinine may be elevated. PSA may be elevated.

D. **Radiographic findings.** IVP may show upper tract or bladder changes secondary to obstruction (hydroureteronephrosis, bladder trabeculation and thickening, bladder diverticula or calculi). VCUG may be indicated. Postvoid catheterization will reveal residual urine. Order US with rectal probe and biopsies if indicated, to rule out carcinoma; perform cystoscopy if indicated.

E. **Uroflowmetry.** It is the most frequently used and most informative although nonspecific method of diagnosing bladder neck obstruction. Peak flow rate should be >15 mL/sec. Flow rate of <10 mL/sec usually indicates outlet obstruction.

F. **Postvoid residual urine.** It is a useful tool for follow-up and evaluation of response to therapy.

G. **Pressure flow studies.** These are indicated in patients with normal peak flow rates but with symptoms suggestive of infravesical obstruction and patients with symptoms suggestive of bladder voiding dysfunction.

H. **Treatment.** Men with mild symptoms may be managed by watchful waiting. Those with moderate symptoms may be managed by medical treatment. Those with severe symptoms are candidates for surgical treatment. An indwelling Foley catheter may help acute episodes but is only a temporary measure.

1. **Medical measures. Terazosin** 1 to 20 mg/d is often helpful in relieving symptoms. **Tamsulosin** 0.4 to 0.8 mg/d may be helpful, but it is more expensive. **Finasteride** (Proscar) 5 mg PO qd, a 5α-reductase inhibitor, blocks transformation of testosterone to 5α-dihydrotestosterone, causing atrophy of prostate tissue, but may take 6 to 12 months to have a clinical effect. Hypertrophy recurs on stopping drug. **Dutasteride** is an alternative 5α-reductase inhibitor. **Saw palmetto** is likely ineffective, although there is conflicting data.

2. **Surgical measures.** TURP is the gold standard surgical treatment, but it should not be performed in patients who want to remain fertile. There is a significant incidence of incontinence and impotence after TURP. Many other destructive methods are available, including microwave, laser, and needle ablation, but vary in efficacy, duration of benefit, safety, and cost.

3. **Antibiotics** should be used to control infection when indicated.

4. If exam reveals nodularity of the gland, referral to a urologist is indicated.

HEMATURIA

I. **Definition.** For purposes of initiating an evaluation of microscopic hematuria, the American Urological Association defines microscopic hematuria as ≥3 RBC/HPF on two of three properly collected urine specimens. Others will use a definition of >2 RBC/HPF. Incidence is 13% to 40%, depending on the population studied. Hematuria in the anticoagulated patient has the same significance as that in the otherwise normal patient and should not be ignored. **If dipstick is positive for blood but microscopic exam is negative for cells, consider hemoglobinuria or myoglobinuria.**

II. **Who to Evaluate. All patients with gross hematuria should have an evaluation.** If there is microscopic hematuria, consider evaluation in all individuals over 40 years of age **or with risk factors for malignancy (e.g., smoking; dye exposure; chemical, textile, leather, or rubber industry work; cyclophosphamide history; use of phenacetin-containing products).** Any patients with urine evidence of possible glomerular disease (e.g., RBC casts, proteinuria) or with an elevated creatinine should be evaluated for glomerular disease (see discussion of glomerular disease, later in this chapter). **All children with unexplained hematuria need a complete work-up, including radiologic examination.**

III. **Cause.** Divide into glomerular and extrarenal causes.

A. **Glomerular causes.** Glomerulonephritis, systemic vasculitis (e.g., Wegener's granulomatosis, SLE), malignant hypertension, IgA nephropathy, familial thin basement membrane disease, among other causes.

B. **Extraglomerular causes.** Possible causes include trauma, tumor (urologic cancer accounts for only 5% of hematuria), kidney stones, cystitis, prostatitis, pyelonephritis, urethral stricture, foreign body, bacterial endocarditis, crystalluria; traumatic exercise such as running may cause hematuria. Schistosomiasis and sickle cell disease should be considered in the proper population.

IV. **Evaluation** (for trauma-related hematuria, see Chapter 2).

A. **History and physical exam.** May provide evidence to indicate cause.

B. **Laboratory and radiologic investigation.**

1. Obtain repeat **UA with microscopy, renal function tests** (BUN, creatinine, urine creatinine/protein ratio). If renal insufficiency or proteinuria present, consider glomerulonephritis among others (tumor, etc.). Other indications of glomerular disease include RBC casts, small, dysmorphic RBCs or acanthocytes. Consider referral to nephrologist if a glomerular source of bleeding is suspected once appropriate testing is done (see section on work-up of glomerulonephritis, later).

2. **Further work-up.** Extent of work-up is controversial.

a. **Image upper urinary tract.** If no signs of glomerular source, image with IVP, US, or CT scan.

b. **Image lower tract.** If negative imaging of upper tract, consider urine cytology (first AM sample), although not very sensitive or specific. Refer to urology for cystoscopy those with positive cytology or risk factors for urologic malignancy (smoking; dye exposure; chemical, textile, leather, or rubber industry work; cyclophosphamide history; use of phenacetin-containing products).

V. Treatment. Address underlying cause.

UROLITHIASIS

I. **Overview.** Urolithiasis is a common cause of both hematuria and abdominal, flank, or groin pain, affecting about 4% to 5% of the population. Of these, 50% will have a second stone within 5 years and 60% within 9 years. Stones can be composed of calcium, oxalate, urate, cystine, xanthine, phosphate, or all of these.

II. **Clinical Presentation and Evaluation.**

A. **History.** Pain is usually of sudden onset, severe and colicky, not improved by position, radiating from the back, down flank, and into groin. Hematuria may be noted. Nausea and vomiting are common. Predisposing factors may be present: recent reduction in fluid intake, medications that predispose to hyperuricemia, history of gout, increased exercise with dehydration. Children <16 years of age make up 7% of those with stones and may present with only painless hematuria.

B. **Physical examination.** May reveal costovertebral angle tenderness. Tachycardia may be present, or the patient may have bradycardia from a vasovagal reaction. Vital signs are usually stable, and there should be no abdominal peritoneal signs.

C. **Laboratory findings.** UA will demonstrate gross or microscopic hematuria in 75% to 90% of patients with stones. In the other 10% to 25% the urine may be normal. **A negative UA does not rule out urolithiasis.** Urine culture should be obtained, and a fresh urine sample should be examined for crystals. WBC count may be increased on CBC secondary to pain and demargination. BUN and creatinine should be obtained.

D. **Differential diagnosis. Abdominal aortic aneurysm dissection and bowel ischemia can mimic urolithiasis and must be ruled out clinically or by radiographic study in the proper population before pain is assumed to be from urolithiasis.** Also consider other causes of abdominal pain (see Chapter 15).

E. **Imaging studies. Noncontrast spiral CT has replaced IVP as the study of choice for the diagnosis of urolithiasis.** The sensitivity of CT is 96% (or higher) versus 86% for IVP. In addition, it is faster and requires less radiation and no dye exposure. However, CT will not demonstrate indinavir stones. **Plain films of the abdomen are not sensitive and are a waste of money.**

III. **Initial Treatment.** Provide analgesia and adequate hydration, and obtain a urine specimen for analysis. Prescribe antibiotics as indicated for pyelonephritis or concurrent UTI.

A. **Ketorolac** 15 to 30 mg IV and narcotics (e.g., **morphine** 2-10 mg or more or fentanyl 25-100 μg IV) are usually required for analgesia.

8

NEPHROLOGY AND UROLOGY

NSAIDs (e.g., ketorolac) are as effective, if not more effective for renal colic than are narcotics. **However, they should be used as supplements to IV narcotics. There is no indication for IM medications in treating renal colic.**

B. **IV fluids** should be used to maintain hydration. **However, the use of large volumes of fluid, although traditional, may increase pain in the patient with an obstructed ureter.** It also does nothing to help a kidney stone pass.

C. **As a rough guideline, the majority of stones <4 mm will pass spontaneously within 48 hours,** but may take a month or more. However, those ≥6 mm will pass spontaneously only 10% of the time, and those 4 to 6 mm 50% of the time. If pain persists or the stone does not pass, consideration of nephrostomy stent placement and urologic intervention (e.g., basket removal of stone) is suggested. Renal injury from obstruction generally does not occur for at least 72 hours or more (some urologists will wait up to 2 weeks to clear a stone).

IV. **Discharge from the office or ED.** If the patient is discharged, he or she should be sent home with indomethacin suppositories or other NSAID (reduces need for narcotics, decreases return visits to ED) and oral narcotics (such as hydrocodone). All urine should be strained, and any stones found brought for analysis.

V. **Hospital Admission.** Hospital admission is required if parenteral analgesics are required, if persistent vomiting prevents adequate oral hydration, if pyelonephritis is suspected, or if patient has elevated BUN and creatinine, oliguria, or anuria because may need urgent decompression with ureteral stents or percutaneous nephrostomy.

VI. **Continuing Care.** All patients with kidney stones should increase their daily fluid intake regardless of the composition of the stones. Analysis of the stones may identify specific preventive measures. **There is good evidence that reducing the dietary intake of animal protein can reduce stone formation.** Drinking caffeinated beverages (coffee, tea) may also help.

A. **Uric acid stones** represent 10% of stones. May be managed medically because alkalinizing urine will dissolve stones (potassium citrate 20 mEq bid-tid to obtain urine pH 6.5-7). Should evaluate for hyperuricosuria. Allopurinol 200 to 300 mg/d inhibits uric acid synthesis and can reduce stone formation. Purines in the diet should be limited.

B. **Calcium oxalate stones** represent 75% of all stones. Hypercalciuria is often idiopathic, but it may occur in hyperparathyroidism, sarcoidosis, and type I renal tubular acidosis (have associated non-anion gap acidosis, alkaline urine pH). Reducing sodium intake in diet can reduce hypercalciuria and stone formation. **Despite common wisdom, it is clear that decreasing calcium intake may actually lead to additional stone formation.** Patients should be instructed to continue a normal calcium intake during meals. This will help bind oxalate and reduce the incidence of stone formation. Thiazide diuretics (25-100 mg/d) decrease calcium excretion and lead to a reduction in stone formation within 1 to 2 years. Potassium phosphate also reduces stone formation but is falling out of favor because of need for qid administration. Citric acid (Lemonade, orange juice) may also help.

C. **Magnesium ammonium phosphate stones (struvite stones)** represent 10% of all stones. They occur in the setting of high urinary pH seen in chronic urinary infections with urease-producing organisms. Antibiotics and acidification of the urine are indicated. Lithotripsy should be used to remove all visible stones from the urinary tract.

D. **Urolithiasis in pregnancy** may present in second or third trimester. Limit radiation exposure to fetus; preferred imaging is US. If conservative management is unsuccessful, use ureteral stent or nephrostomy tube because lithotripsy is contraindicated in pregnancy.

ACUTE SCROTAL PAIN AND SCROTAL MASSES

I. **Acute Scrotal Pain.** Must be assessed immediately to exclude testicular torsion.

A. **Evaluation.**

1. **History.** Inquire about trauma; nature, location, and duration of pain; associated symptoms; or recent infection of urethra, bladder, and prostate.

2. **Examination.** Localization of the painful structure is important for diagnosis. Assess for inguinal hernia, urethritis, or possible prostatitis.

3. **Lab tests.** Will be directed by the findings on history and physical. UA should be obtained to assess for hematuria or evidence of infection.

B. **Causes.**

1. **Trauma.** May be difficult to get accurate history if unusual sexual practices involved. US of scrotum and testicles can be useful in assessing trauma.

2. **Urolithiasis.** Indicated by hematuria. Often there is or has been associated flank pain. Examination reveals normal scrotal contents.

3. **Hernia.** Incarcerated hernia may present with only scrotal pain. Examination may reveal the presence of bowel sounds in the scrotum. Signs of intestinal obstruction may be present. US showing air/fluid levels, peristalsis is diagnostic.

4. **Epididymitis.** Often a history of prior urethral symptoms. Commonly occurs in sexually active men. Culture urethral discharge and urine. There is swelling and tenderness of the epididymis. The pain of epididymitis is often lessened by elevation of the scrotum. See Table 8-1 for treatment.

5. **Torsion of the testicle.** A urologic emergency, torsion present for longer than 4 to 6 hours will result in loss of the testicle. Generally present in young men after physical activity (although the link with activity has recently been questioned). Frequently complain of abdominal pain

and nausea and may not initially notice testicular pain. Exam may be remarkable for localized tenderness of the testicle, elevated testis, or an abnormal testicular lie. If torsion has been present for some time, epididymis will also be swollen and tender, complicating differentiation. Cremasteric reflex will generally be absent on the affected side. **But no combination of physical findings is sufficiently sensitive to rule out torsion. US may be useful but has an 11% false-negative rate. However, in no case should urgent consultation with a urologist be delayed if torsion is clinically suspected.** Manual detorsion may be attempted (if immediate surgical evaluation is not possible) by infiltrating the spermatic cord near the external ring with lidocaine or bupivacaine and counter-rotating the affected testicle. Viewed from below the patient's scrotum, the patient's right testicle would be detorsed by counterclockwise rotation; the patient's left by clockwise rotation (done in a manner similar to opening a book).

6. **Referred pain** such as from entrapment of a nerve during appendectomy.

II. Painless Scrotal Masses.

A. **Possible causes** include tumors of the testicle or spermatic cord, spermatoceles, hydroceles, varicoceles, hernias, or lipomas. Most are painless or associated with only mild pain. Acute, severe pain should prompt an evaluation as discussed previously. Occasionally tumors will cause acute pain, possibly from hemorrhage.

B. **Varicocele.** Common. Usual clinical presentation is adolescent or young adult with incidentally noted swelling in (usually) the left scrotum. Physical examination is generally diagnostic, with varicosities (typically described as a feeling of "a bag of worms") palpated above and separate from testicle. Varicosities enlarge with Valsalva maneuver.

1. **Treatment.** Firm scrotal support if symptomatic.

2. **Further evaluation or referral is indicated for the following:**

a. Large or bilateral varicocele in young adolescent. May result in inhibited growth of left or both testicles, possibly resulting in decreased function (testosterone production, spermatogenesis).

b. Male adult who is a member of an infertile couple.

c. New-onset varicocele in man older than 30 years (may indicate intra-abdominal process that is impeding blood return).

d. Right-sided varicocele without concomitant left-sided varicocele.

C. **Hydrocele.** Typically manifests as a gradually enlarging painless cystic structure. Can be transilluminated. Communicating hydroceles usually resolve before age 1 year. US may be advisable in older age group because a hydrocele can be secondary to tumor.

D. **Spermatocele.** Usually asymptomatic. Firm but somewhat compressible mass located superior to and separate from the testicle in the spermatic cord. US can aid in diagnosis. Requires no treatment for small spermatoceles. Larger ones may cause discomfort and may require exploration and surgical excision.

E. **Testicular tumor.** Generally occurs in a young adult. Usually painless. Firm, nontender mass will be found on the testicle. Cannot be transilluminated. US will confirm location of mass. Urologic consultation is required for evaluation.

URINARY INCONTINENCE

I. **General.** Defined as involuntary loss of urine.
II. **Causes.** Causes of transient incontinence include delirium, infection, atrophic vaginitis or urethritis, drugs, including sedatives, hypnotics, diuretics, opiates, calcium channel blockers, anticholinergics (antidepressants, antihistamines), decongestants, and others. Less common causes include depression, excess urine production (diabetes, diabetes insipidus), restricted mobility (i.e., patient cannot get to the bathroom), and stool impaction.
III. **Types of Incontinence and Their Specific Causes.**
A. **Urge incontinence.** "Overactive bladder." Involuntary loss of urine associated with a sudden urge and desire to void. Associated with detrusor overactivity. Causes include neurologic disorders (e.g., stroke, multiple sclerosis), UTIs, and uroepithelial cancer.
B. **Stress incontinence.** Involuntary loss of urine during coughing, sneezing, laughing, or other increases in intra-abdominal pressure. Most commonly seen in women after middle age (especially with repeated pregnancies and vaginal deliveries), stress incontinence is often a result of weakness of the pelvic floor and poor support of the vesicourethral sphincter unit. Another cause is intrinsic urethral sphincter weakness such as that from myelomeningocele, epispadias, prostatectomy, trauma, radiation, or sacral cord lesion.
C. **Overflow incontinence.** Involuntary loss of urine associated with overdistention of the bladder. May have frequent dribbling or present as urge or stress incontinence. May be attributable to underactive bladder, bladder outlet obstruction (e.g., tumor, prostatic hypertrophy), drugs (e.g., diuretics), fecal impaction, diabetic neuropathy, or vitamin B_{12} deficiency.
D. **Functional incontinence.** Immobility, cognitive deficits, paraplegia, or poor bladder compliance.
IV. **Evaluation.** Confirm urinary incontinence and identify factors that might contribute:
A. **History.** Include medications and provoking factors.
B. **Physical.** Include abdominal exam, pelvic exam, rectal exam, sensation in the rectal and perineal area, edema, drugs.
C. **Do stress testing.** Have patient cough or sneeze and observe for loss of urine.
D. **UA** and microscopic examination of urine. Urine culture, if warranted.
E. **Check postvoid residual.** This will be increased by outlet obstruction, neurogenic bladder, etc.
F. **Cystometry** with flow rates, etc., may be needed if cause clinically inapparent.

8

NEPHROLOGY AND UROLOGY

V. Treatment. Set goals and scoring system ahead of time. Most patients will respond to behavioral techniques. Most require structured input from nursing personnel.

A. Bladder training. Need education, scheduled voiding, and rewards. Must inhibit urinating until a set time, and this set amount of time should be progressively increased. Start at 2 to 3 hours and progress upward. Twelve percent may become entirely continent, and 75% may have a 50% reduction in incontinent episodes. Works best in urge incontinence but also may help stress incontinence.

B. Habit training. Teach patients to void when they normally would (e.g., morning, before bed, after meals).

C. Prompted and scheduled voiding. Especially good in cognitively impaired individuals. Reduced incontinent episodes by about 50%.

D. Pelvic floor exercises (Kegel exercises). Especially useful in stress incontinence; cure in 16%, and 54% improve.

E. Intermittent catheterization may also be used.

F. Drugs.

1. For urge incontinence, bladder spasms, detrusor instability. Oxybutynin (Ditropan, Ditropan XL), tolterodine (Detrol; low incidence of dry mouth). Tolterodine is expensive and no more efficacious than oxybutynin. New, longer-acting medications are available, including trospium chloride (Sanctura); however, they are more expensive. Second-line drugs include propantheline (may affect smooth muscle in the small bowel), flavoxate (Urispas), hyoscyamine sulfate (Levsin, Levsinex), and tricyclic antidepressants.

2. For stress incontinence. Use agents that increase bladder outlet resistance (e.g., pseudoephedrine). Duloxetine, a serotonin/norepinephrine reuptake inhibitor, is also being used, although not FDA approved.

3. For men. Treating obstructive prostatic symptoms may help (see section on BPH).

4. In women. Estrogen has been used both orally and intravaginally for incontinence, but studies do not show a benefit and this practice is discouraged.

5. Newer products include Introl bladder neck support prosthesis (similar to pessary and assists women with incontinence secondary to urethral hypermobility), Reliance urinary control insert, magnetic innervation technology, periurethral collagen injections.

G. Surgery. Multiple procedures available. Consider urology referral.

PENILE PROBLEMS

I. Priapism. Pathologic prolongation of a penile erection associated with pain. Fever and difficulty voiding can also be present. May result in impotence in 17% to 50% of cases; **early intervention is paramount.**

A. Causes. Idiopathic, sickle cell disease, trauma, neoplastic disease, drugs (heparin, phenothiazines, alcohol, hydralazine, intracavernous injection of cocaine, papaverine, prostaglandin E_1).

B. Treatment.

1. Medical. Terbutaline 0.25 to 0.5 mg SQ has been used with limited success. Phenylephrine 0.5 to 1 mg instilled into each corpus followed by irrigation is the treatment of choice. Generally, IV narcotics are required for pain control. However, medical measures should not delay surgical intervention.

2. Surgical. Administer IV narcotics and sedate the patient. Anesthetize the glans with lidocaine and perform aspiration of blood with an 18-gauge needle inserted through the glans into each corpora cavernosa. After aspiration of 30 to 90 mL of blood, irrigate with normal saline. May take multiple irrigations and aspirations to resolve. Therapy is surgical intervention if symptoms persist.

ERECTILE DYSFUNCTION

I. Evaluation.

A. History. Includes a detailed sexual history on changes of libido, problems with ejaculation or orgasm, and daily stresses. Risk factors: age over 60, type 2 diabetes, hypertension, hyperlipidemia, smoking, renal failure, hyperthyroidism, depression, sickle cell disease, alcohol abuse, medication use (common examples are thiazide diuretics, β-blockers, α-blockers, cimetidine, spironolactone, psychotropic medications such as SSRIs, marijuana, morphine, cocaine, and metoclopramide).

B. Complete physical examination. Includes exam of vascular and thyroid changes in secondary sex characteristics, perianal sensation, and sphincter tone. Some advise measuring penile blood pressure. Penile:brachial index <0.6 indicates significant vascular stenosis.

C. Laboratory. Often it is not necessary to find out the cause before starting the treatment. Baseline labs, CBC, testosterone, prolactin, glucose, liver function test, fasting lipid profile, and PSA if patient is older than 40. Androgen levels should be checked (serum free testosterone). If androgens are low, FSH, LH, and prolactin levels should be checked. Do Doppler studies to assess blood flow.

D. Many are psychogenic (50%). The ability to have an erection with masturbation or REM sleep generally indicates a psychogenic disorder.

II. Treatment.

A. Treat the cause. Better management of diabetes, remove offending drugs, better control of hypertension and hyperlipidemia. Testosterone injection or transdermal testosterone for hypogonadism. Sexual counseling may be useful.

B. Pharmacologic treatment and devices. More than 90% of patients respond to the following interventions regardless of etiology.

8

NEPHROLOGY AND UROLOGY

1. **External vacuum device.** Highly effective and acceptable. Side effects include cool penile skin temperature, discomfort, bruising, and impaired ejaculation.
2. **Intracavernosal therapy.** Alprostadil is the only agent approved for this purpose. Dose has to be adjusted in office. Side effects include priapism. Only 30% of individuals respond, and it can be used only three times per week. Constriction band has to be used concomitantly in veno-occlusive deficits.
3. **Intraurethral suppository of prostaglandin** (alprostadil). Effective in two thirds of patients. Side effects include penile pain, hypotension. Cost is also a factor.
4. **Type V phosphodiesterase enzyme inhibitors.** Act to increase nitrous oxide in corpus cavernosum, causing increased smooth muscle relaxation and increased blood flow, leading to an erection. Side effects include headache, flushing, dyspepsia, rhinitis, and visual disturbances. **Contraindicated in patients on nitrates and α-blockers because they potentiate the hypotensive effect.**
   a. **Sildenafil** (Viagra), 25 to 100 mg has been effective. Taken orally 1 hour before anticipated sexual activity and is effective for about 4 hours; absorption decreased by high-fat meal. Response rates range from 43% to 68%.
   b. **Vardenafil** (Levitra), 5 to 20 mg per dose. Onset of action around 20 minutes, lasting 4 hours. Contraindicated for use in patients on nitrates or α-blockers.
   c. **Tadalafil** (Cialis), 5 to 20 mg per dose. Onset of action at 30 minutes, lasting 36 hours. Absorption not affected by food.
5. **Apomorphine** (Uprima, Apokyn) is FDA approved for male impotence. Vomiting and nausea are major side effects.
6. **Surgical implants.** Popular in 1970s and 1980s. Patients with cavernous veno-occlusive disease are not good candidates for this operation.

RENAL FAILURE

I. **Acute Renal Failure.** Sudden loss of renal function as evidenced by oliguria or anuria, increase in BUN or serum creatinine.
A. **Prerenal cause.** Diminished renal perfusion because of volume depletion, inadequate cardiac output, or volume redistribution ("third spacing" from cirrhosis, burns, nephrotic syndrome, etc.). Kidney retains sodium and fluid in attempt to increase circulating volume (and therefore renal perfusion). BUN-to-creatinine ratio generally >20:1. About 75% of cases of acute renal failure are secondary to diminished renal perfusion (prerenal causes) or acute tubular necrosis (ATN).
B. **Renal causes.** Glomerular (rapidly progressive glomerulonephritis), vascular (renal artery or vein thrombosis, vasculitis), interstitial nephritis, or tubulointerstitial (ATN most common; see later).

C. Postrenal causes. Obstruction of the urinary tract from prostate disease or retroperitoneal disease.

II. Diagnosis. May have urine output <400 mL/24 h, elevated BUN and creatinine, or decreased creatinine clearance. A progressive daily increase in serum creatinine is diagnostic of acute renal failure.

A. Estimated creatinine clearance = [(140 − age [y]) × (body weight [kg])] ÷ (72 × serum creatinine [mg/dL]). For women, multiply this figure by 0.85.

B. May not reflect early renal damage because of compensatory hypertrophy of remaining glomeruli.

C. Normal for healthy adult is 94 to 140 mL/min for men and 72 to 110 mL/min for women.

III. Differentiating the Causes of Renal Failure (Table 8-2).

A. Formulas. These formulas apply best when there is oliguria (<500 mL/day). Factors such as diuretic use or coexisting liver disease with ascites may invalidate the results.

1. **U/P** = Urine osmolality to plasma osmolality ratio.

2. **FE_{Na}** = Fractional excretion of Na = (urine sodium/plasma sodium)/(urine creatinine/plasma creatinine) × 100.

B. UA in renal failure (Table 8-3). Also, if prerenal cause, generally normal UA with only hyaline casts. If ATN, may have smoky urine with dark granular casts (however, 20% may be normal). In glomerulonephritis, hematuria and proteinuria will be present.

IV. Acute Tubular Necrosis.

A. Definition. Acute renal failure resulting from renal ischemia or toxic insult. Renal function generally returns to adequate level if patient survives. Sepsis is a major cause of death in ATN.

B. Course. May progress from oliguric renal failure (urine output <400 mL/day) to nonoliguric renal failure, which may be manifested by massive urine output. The duration of renal failure is generally

TABLE 8-2

DIFFERENTIATING CAUSES OF RENAL FAILURE

Type of Failure	BUN/Cr	Urine Sodium (mEq/L)	Fractional Excretion of Sodium	Urine Osmolality (mosm/kg)	Urine Findings
Prerenal	>20	<20	<1	>500	Hyaline casts
Renal azotemia	<20	>20	>1-2	<350	Granular casts, renal tubular cells.
Postrenal	>20:1	Variable	>1	<400	Normal RBC, WBC, crystals
Glomerulonephritis	>20:1	<20	<1	>500	Nephritic urine (see Table 8-4), RBC casts

---

TABLE 8-3

CASTS IN RENAL FAILURE

Cast Type	Disease
Fat droplets, fatty casts	Nephrotic syndrome, polycystic kidney disease, fat embolism (see Chapter 15, General Surgery)
Hyaline casts	Normal finding
RBC casts	Glomerulonephritis, vasculitis
Renal tubular casts	Acute tubular necrosis
Waxy casts	End-stage renal disease
WBC casts	Interstitial nephritis, some glomerular disease, occasionally pyelonephritis

---

1 day to 6 weeks (average, 10-14 days). **Oliguric renal failure generally indicates greater renal damage and may be associated with worse outcomes. However, using diuretics to convert oliguric to nonoliguric renal failure is of no benefit and may increase mortality.**

C. **Laboratory findings.** Progressive hyponatremia, hyperkalemia, azotemia (creatinine increase by 0.5-2.5 mg/dL per day) and acidosis.

D. **Causes of ATN.**

1. **Ischemic and hypoperfusion injury.** Shock, sepsis, hypoxia, hypotension, cardiac arrest, or surgery.

2. **Toxic sources.** Radiologic contrast media, heavy metals, aminoglycosides, myoglobinuria from burns, trauma, polymyositis, cisplatin, IV acyclovir, and many other drugs.

E. **Evaluation.** Diagnosis often apparent because of clinical history. Rule out obstructive process (US of kidneys and ureters helpful). UA may reveal renal epithelial cells or renal-tubular cell casts, or may be negative. See Table 8-2 for differentiation from other causes.

F. **Treatment.** Maintain fluid balance and blood pressure. Dopamine, mannitol, and diuretics have not been shown to have any renal-sparing effect. **In fact, trying to change oliguric to nonoliguric renal failure may increase mortality.** See treatment of acute renal failure, later, for details.

V. **Prerenal Azotemia.** (See Table 8-2.)

A. **Cause and diagnosis.** Commonly caused by dehydration (often attributable to excessive diuretic therapy). May be secondary to decreased renal perfusion as with cardiac dysfunction or liver failure. **Labs reveal evidence** of decreased renal function with BUN elevated out of proportion to serum creatinine, often greater than 20:1.

B. **Treatment.**

1. **Adequate intravascular volume** will prevent progression to oliguric or anuric failure if it is secondary to inadequate volume. There is no evidence that albumin is superior to crystalloids in restoring plasma volume.

2. **Treat cardiac failure** as per CHF in Chapter 3. In those with CHF, consider also prerenal azotemia secondary to excessive diuretic use, ACE inhibitor–induced renal failure, and use of NSAIDs.

3. **If prerenal azotemia is secondary to liver failure,** outcome is poor unless patient is transplantation candidate.

VI. **Postrenal Azotemia.** Usually caused in men by bladder outlet obstruction and is rapidly treatable with a Foley catheter. Other causes include pelvic tumors and surgical injury. (See Table 8-2.)

VII. **Glomerulonephritis.**

A. **Causes include** poststreptococcal glomerulonephritis, hemolytic uremic syndrome, Henoch-Schönlein purpura, collagen vascular diseases, and others.

B. **Clinical presentation.** Sudden or gradual onset of renal failure, hematuria, RBC casts, proteinuria, azotemia, and edema.

C. **Diagnosis.** See section on nephrotic syndrome and nephritis, later.

VIII. **Interstitial Nephritis.**

A. **Causes include** drugs (70% of cases) such as methicillin, NSAIDs, rifampin, ASA, allopurinol, fluoroquinolones, some ACE inhibitors, morphine, sulfonamides, many others. Infections (15% of cases) including *Legionella, Streptococcus*, etc. Sarcoid (1% of cases), miscellaneous. **If coexistent uveitis, consider tubulointerstitial nephritis/uveitis syndrome (a detailed discussion is beyond the scope of this manual).**

B. **Onset.** From first day of drug exposure (rifampin) to months after drug started (NSAIDs). Generally in the range of 2 to 5 days if prior exposure to drug and 10 to 14 days if no prior exposure.

C. **Clinical presentation.** Fever (30%), rash (15%), acute rise in plasma creatinine, eosinophilia (peripheral, 25%) and eosinophils in urine, WBC casts. **If secondary to NSAIDs, may have absence of fever, rash, eosinophilia.** Biopsy will give the definitive diagnosis.

D. **Treatment.** Withdraw offending agent, consider steroids.

IX. **Treatment of Acute Renal Failure.**

A. **Careful monitoring of fluid and electrolyte status.** Fluids should be restricted to replacement of losses (urine output, other losses [GI], and approximately 500 mL/d for insensible loss). Dietary intake of potassium and phosphates should be severely restricted. Hyperphosphatemia may be prevented by use of oral calcium carbonate or calcium acetate antacids to absorb dietary phosphates and maintain PO_4 <5.5 mg/dL. A more expensive option is sevelamer (another oral phosphate binder). Calcium should be monitored because it tends to fall if phosphorus rises. Hyperkalemia should be treated as noted in Chapter 6. Fluid overload may require dialysis or diuretics, such as furosemide 20 mg IV or more. Adding a thiazide diuretic (e.g., metolazone, hydrochlorothiazide) may improve the diuresis. Dopamine can be used for pressure support but "renal dose" dopamine does not increase GFR significantly.

B. **Monitor acidosis.** Mild to moderate metabolic acidosis should be anticipated and may be well tolerated. Severe acidosis may require oral bicarbonate solution, which contains significant quantities of sodium and may increase edema.

8

NEPHROLOGY AND UROLOGY

C. Monitor carefully for signs of infection (a common cause of death during acute renal failure).

D. Dialysis is indicated for uremic pericarditis, severe hyperkalemia or other unmanageable electrolyte abnormality, severe acidosis, significant fluid overload, and other uremic symptoms (especially neurologic). Hemodialysis has been shown to improve survival in acute renal failure.

CHRONIC RENAL FAILURE

I. Definition. Clinical syndrome of chronic compromise of renal function, which can be categorized into three major groups:

A. Inadequate renal reserve, characterized by inability to compensate for extreme water or solute loading or deprivation.

B. Renal insufficiency, characterized by elevated BUN and greatly diminished capacity for dealing with water solute fluctuations, but otherwise can maintain homeostasis.

C. Renal failure, characterized by progressive increase in BUN to the point of causing uremia, fluid, and electrolyte imbalance (GFR <6 mg/min per square meter).

II. Causes. Common causes include diabetes, hypertension, glomerulonephritis, polycystic kidney disease, obstructive uropathy, and amyloidosis. See section on nephritis and nephrotic syndrome, later, for differential diagnosis. Unfortunately, deterioration may continue even after initial insult resolves, perhaps because of a change in intrarenal hemodynamics.

III. Clinical Manifestation. Early manifestations may include only nocturia because of inability to concentrate urine (therefore mobilizing fluid at nighttime when recumbent). Fatigue, altered mental status, peripheral neuropathy, anorexia, nausea and vomiting, and pruritus may indicate uremia. Hypertension is common. Fluid and electrolyte imbalances result in varying signs and symptoms. Loss of erythropoietin and vitamin D function results in anemia and osteodystrophy. Patients may remain asymptomatic until GFR is <10% of normal. Bleeding occurs secondary to platelet dysfunction.

IV. Laboratory Diagnosis. Generally reflected in an elevated BUN and creatinine. A 24-hour urine study shows a decreased creatinine clearance. Acidosis is usually present, as is a normochromic-normocytic anemia (anemia of chronic disease; see Chapter 6). Hyperkalemia and hyponatremia are often present.

V. Prevention. ACE inhibitors have been shown to decrease progression to renal failure in both diabetic and nondiabetic patients and may be beneficial even when started when the Cr = 5.0 mg/L. Protein restriction may reduce progression of chronic renal disease, although the data are conflicting. It seems reasonable to limit patients with early renal insufficiency to 0.8 g/kg per day of high-biologic-value protein, those with GFR below 55 mL/min to 0.7 to 0.8 g/kg per day, and those with GFR <25 mL/min to 0.6 g/kg per day.

Angiotensin receptor blockers (ARBs) and nondihydropyridine calcium channel blockers (verapamil, diltiazem) can be used as second-line therapy. **ARBs are not as effective as ACE inhibitors in reducing proteinuria and do not reduce cardiac events.** BP should be controlled to below 130/80 mm Hg.

VI. Treatment.

A. **Sodium and fluid hemostasis.** Generally not a problem until late in the disease. The kidney maintains ability to regulate sodium until extremely late in course. Use diuretics (e.g., furosemide) to remove excess free water.

B. **Potassium.** May require potassium restriction to 2 g/d (<50 mEq) late in the course of renal failure. May develop aldosterone resistance (and therefore hyperkalemia) requiring more aggressive therapy such as fludrocortisone and potassium-binding resins. See Chapter 6 for details.

C. **Acidosis.** Can be treated with PO sodium bicarbonate (1.2-2.4 g/d) if symptomatic (lethargy, fatigue, tachypnea) or if serum bicarbonate levels <17 mEq/L. This will give a sodium load; therefore, be careful in setting of CHF, fluid retention, and similar conditions.

D. **Dietary restrictions.** Required to maintain appropriate fluid and electrolyte balance. Protein restriction as in Prevention section, earlier.

E. **Phosphate and calcium ions.** Phosphate intake should be limited, and hyperphosphatemia should be treated with phosphate binders such as PO calcium acetate, calcium carbonate, or sevelamer (expensive) to prevent the development of renal osteodystrophy (elevated parathyroid hormone levels and calcium mobilization leading to bone cysts and weakness). Start supplements of vitamin D (calcitriol 0.25-1 µg/d is generally a good choice) and calcium supplementation. If the patient becomes hypercalcemic and the phosphate is still not controlled, lower the dose of calcium and vitamin D and consider the use of lanthanum carbonate (Fosrenal; an expensive oral phosphate binder used primarily in patients on dialysis) or cinacalcet (Sensipar; expensive). Cinacalcet binds to the calcium receptors on the parathyroid, inhibiting parathyroid hormone release. Avoid magnesium- and aluminum-containing preparations because of possible toxicity.

F. **Anemia.** Generally attributable to decreased erythropoietin production in kidney. Rule out other causes such as slow GI bleed, etc. See Chapter 6 for details on treatment of anemia of chronic disease. Several factors, including adequate dialysis and control of hyperpara-thyroidism related to renal failure will improve the response to erythropoietin. Iron supplementation is also important.

G. **Bleeding.** Can be treated with DDAVP (to release von Willebrand's factor from platelets), FFP, or cryoprecipitate. Dialysis will also improve platelet function, but just transfusing platelets usually is not effective in those with adequate platelet counts. Transfused platelets will function poorly unless patient is on dialysis. See also Chapter 6.

H. Immunizations. Hepatitis B **(give double the usual dose and give additional dose at 6 months [four doses total, give boost if titer falls to less than 10 IU]).** Give also tetanus, pneumococcal, influenza, and varicella vaccines (in children and possibly adults).

I. Dialysis. Hemodialysis and chronic ambulatory peritoneal dialysis. **Absolutely indicated for** uremic pericarditis, progressive motor impairment, fluid overload not responsive to other interventions or producing CHF, severe acidosis, neurologic findings (e.g., confusion, ataxia, foot drop), bleeding diathesis, nausea/vomiting, creatinine >12 mg/dL, and hyperkalemia. **Relative indications** include depression, unresponsive anemia, anorexia. **Early consultation with nephrologist should be considered. But early dialysis may worsen outcomes secondary to infectious complications, etc.**

J. Transplantation. An alternative to dialysis. Decision to proceed with dialysis or transplantation requires the assistance of a nephrologist.

PROTEINURIA, NEPHROTIC SYNDROME, AND NEPHRITIC URINE

I. Nephrotic Urine Versus Nephritic Urine. The nephrotic urine contains a large amount of protein but does not contain elements indicating active inflammation such as WBCs and RBC casts. In contrast, the nephritic urine is suggestive of acute renal inflammation and will contain protein, casts (WBC, RBC), blood by dipstick, and WBCs. The differential diagnosis can be narrowed based on whether a nephritic or nephrotic urine is present.

II. Nephrotic Syndrome.

A. General. Nephrotic syndrome is not a disease but rather the renal manifestation of multiple underlying causes. The primary disease may be renal in origin, such as minimal-change disease, or may be a systemic illness with renal manifestations, such as diabetes mellitus with nephropathy. Nephrotic syndrome may be related to "burned out" glomerulonephritis, active "nil" disease, and other causes of nephritis. Once active renal disease (nephritis) is no longer ongoing, the patient may end up with nephrotic syndrome and a nephrotic urine.

B. Definition. Nephrotic syndrome manifests as proteinuria of >2 to 3 g/d, hypoalbuminemia, edema, and hyperlipidemia. Thrombotic events may also occur. Nephrotic syndrome may occur at any age, including in children (nil disease most common in children).

C. Presentation.

1. Anorexia, malaise, edema, anasarca, or pleural effusions.
2. Focal edema, especially ankles and genitalia.
3. May be hypertensive, especially in those with collagen vascular disease.
4. Thrombotic phenomena, including renal vein thrombosis. Mostly caused by decreased fibrinolytic activity.
5. Frothy urine (bubbles in the toilet) secondary to proteinuria, nocturia secondary to increased vascular volume at night from fluid mobilization.

D. Laboratory findings.

1. **Urine.** Pronounced proteinuria (excretion >2 g/d); urinary protein-to-creatinine ratio >2; casts: hyaline, granular, waxy, or epithelial; urine Na low (<10 mmol/L); urine K:Na ratio >1.

2. **Blood.**

a. Hypoalbuminemia.

b. Globulins, adrenocortical hormones, or thyroid hormones may be low.

c. BUN and creatinine are variable depending on progression of renal disease.

d. Aldosterone initially high (aldosterone causes K excretion, Na retention, and hypertension).

e. Lipemia, including elevated cholesterol and triglycerides. May have lipiduria.

f. Microcytic anemia from urinary loss of transferrin or poor erythropoietin production.

g. Coagulation disorders may be from loss of factor IX, factor XII, and thrombolytic factors (urokinase and antithrombin III) in the urine and increased serum levels of factor VIII, fibrinogen, and platelets.

E. Diagnosis.
Focused on determining underlying cause **(Table 8-4 and Box 8-1).** History and associated clinical findings go a long way in making the diagnosis. Family history is important because many causes may be familial.

F. Work-up.
Overlaps with that of glomerulonephritis (see later).

G. In children.
Orthostatic proteinuria, a benign condition, is frequently found in children. In orthostatic proteinuria, protein is found only in the urine after the child has been upright, so a first morning void should be free of protein (if the bladder was emptied just before bedtime). A 24-hour UA can be done in two containers—one that collects the first morning void and another that collects the urine while the patient is awake and upright. Diagnostic criteria include

TABLE 8-4

INCIDENCE OF DISEASES ASSOCIATED WITH THE NEPHROTIC SYNDROME OR NEPHRITIC URINE OR PROTEINURIA

	Approximate Incidence	
Disease	Children	Adults
Primary Renal Disease	90%	75%
Minimal-change disease	65%	15%
Focal glomerulosclerosis	10%	15%
Membranous glomerulonephritis	5%	30%
Membranoproliferative glomerulonephritis	10%	7%
Others: mesangial proliferative glomerulonephritis, IgA nephropathy, rapidly progressive glomerulonephritis	10%	3%
Secondary Disease	10%	25%

Adapted from Berkow R (ed): *The Merck Manual of Diagnosis and Therapy*, 17th ed. Rahway, NJ, Merck, 1992.

8

NEPHROLOGY AND UROLOGY

BOX 8-1

DISEASES ASSOCIATED WITH THE NEPHROTIC SYNDROME OR NEPHRITIC URINE OR PROTEINURIA

PRIMARY RENAL DISEASE

- Minimal-change disease
- Focal glomerulosclerosis
- Membranous glomerulonephritis
- Membranoproliferative glomerulonephritis
- Others: mesangial proliferative glomerulonephritis, IgA nephropathy, rapidly progressive glomerulonephritis

SECONDARY RENAL DISEASE

Metabolic
- Diabetes mellitus
- Amyloidosis

Immunogenic
- Systemic lupus erythematosus
- Henoch-Schönlein purpura
- Polyarteritis nodosa
- Sjögren's syndrome
- Sarcoidosis
- Serum sickness
- Erythema multiforme

Neoplastic
- Leukemias
- Lymphomas
- Hodgkin's lymphoma
- Multiple myeloma
- Carcinoma (bronchus, breast, colon, stomach, kidney)
- Melanoma

Nephrotoxic and drugs
- Gold salts
- Penicillamine
- NSAIDs
- Lithium carbonate
- Street heroin

Allergenic
- Insect stings
- Snake venoms
- Antitoxins
- Poison ivy
- Poison oak

Infective
- Bacterial: postinfective glomerulonephritis, vascular prosthetic nephritis, infective endocarditis, leprosy, syphilis
- Viral: hepatitis B and C, Epstein-Barr, herpes zoster, HIV

BOX 8-1

DISEASES ASSOCIATED WITH THE NEPHROTIC SYNDROME OR
NEPHRITIC URINE OR PROTEINURIA—cont'd

- Protozoal: malaria
- Helminthic: schistosomiasis, filariasis

Congenital Nephrotic Syndrome

- Finnish type

Heredofamilial

- Alport's syndrome
- Fabry's disease

Miscellaneous

- Toxemia of pregnancy
- Malignant hypertension

Adapted from Berkow R (ed): *The Merck Manual of Diagnosis and Therapy*, 17th ed. Rahway, NJ, Merck, 1992.

the following: no or little protein in the first morning void; not greater than a total of 1.5 g of protein in a 24-hour urine; and 80% to 100% of the protein in the specimen collected while the child is upright (fractionate collection into two 12-hour periods in separate containers). However, many physicians make the diagnosis with only the absence of protein in the urine from the morning void.

H. Prognosis and treatment. All patients with proteinuria should be considered for ACE inhibitor therapy. ACE inhibitors will slow the progression to renal failure even in the nondiabetic patient with proteinuria. If not tolerated, an ARB or nondihydropyridine calcium channel blockers (e.g., diltiazem, verapamil) may decrease the progression of proteinuria. These are both second-line therapies, however. Treat hyperlipidemia with HMG-CoA reductase inhibitors. Indomethacin or another NSAID may reduce proteinuria; it may take several weeks to see a response. Remember, however, that this decreases renal perfusion, increases creatinine, may increase edema, and is a two-edged sword. Treatment of specific syndromes (e.g., various types of glomerulonephritis) is beyond the scope of this manual and is frequently inadequate. The exception is minimal-change disease or nil disease. Minimal-change disease has the best prognosis, with 90% of children and 50% of adults responding to steroid therapy. A nephrology consult should be obtained.

GLOMERULONEPHRITIS AND NEPHRITIS

I. **General.** Discussion of specific entities is beyond the scope of this manual. However, diagnostic work-up should proceed as noted in the following.

II. **Diagnosis and Work-up for Nephrotic Syndrome, Nephritis, or Suspected Glomerulonephritis.** Use clinical judgment in ordering appropriate tests. This work-up may also be appropriate for those with nephrotic syndrome and proteinuria when looking for an underlying cause. Work-up may include the following:

A. Minimum: CXR, CBC, screening cancer tests (as appropriate for age and symptoms), pursue cancer diagnosis in appropriate clinical setting (e.g., weight loss, elderly, adenopathy, back pain), other routine chemical analyses.

B. Serum and urine protein electrophoresis and immunoelectrophoresis to detect Bence Jones protein and monoclonal gammopathy.

C. Check for diabetes mellitus, amyloid, and SLE.

D. Check for hepatitis B surface antigen (HepBsAg). This causes up to 22% of nephrotic syndrome, depending on the population. Also, check for hepatitis C and HIV.

E. Family history of renal failure or deafness (Alport's nephropathy).

F. Sexual history (syphilis, hepatitis B, or HIV).

G. Hemoptysis (Wegener's granulomatosis or Goodpasture's syndrome).

H. Paresthesias or neurologic deficits (Fabry's disease).

I. ANA or ANCA, or both (Wegener's granulomatosis, other vasculitides).

J. C3, C4 (low in endocarditis, poststreptococcal glomerulonephritis, SLE, membranoproliferative glomerulonephritis, or cryoglobulinemia).

K. ASO and other evidence of recent streptococcal infection (status poststreptococcal glomerulonephritis).

L. Anti-glomerular basement membrane antibodies: positive in Goodpasture's syndrome.

M. Cryoglobulins.

N. Evaluation for sarcoid (see Chapter 4).

O. Biopsy. Box 8-2 lists indications and contraindications.

BOX 8-2

INDICATIONS FOR AND CONTRAINDICATIONS TO RENAL BIOPSY

INDICATIONS

- Nephrotic syndrome of unknown etiology after work-up
- Hematuria from a glomerular source with hypertension or with a progressive rise in creatinine
- Nephritis without a systemic explanation after work-up
- Suspicion of Wegener's granulomatosis with no other tissue available for biopsy
- Acute or subacute renal failure not otherwise explained

CONTRAINDICATIONS

- Irreversible coagulopathy
- Uncontrolled, severe hypertension
- Multiple bilateral renal cysts
- Renal or perirenal infection
- Hydronephrosis
- Known tumor
- Irreversible disease (e.g., small, shrunken kidneys)
- Inability to get consent

BIBLIOGRAPHY

Bent S, Nallamothu BK, Simel DL, et al: Does this woman have an acute uncomplicated urinary tract infection? *JAMA* 287:2701-2710, 2002.

Burnett AL: Pathophysiology of priapism: Dysregulatory erection physiology thesis. *J Urol* 170:26-34, 2003.

Cantarovich F, Rangoonwala B, Lorenz H, et al: High-dose furosemide for established ARF: A prospective, randomized, double-blind, placebo-controlled, multicenter trial. *Am J Kidney Dis* 44:402-409, 2004.

Centers for Disease Control and Prevention: Sexually transmitted diseases treatment guidelines—2002. *MMWR Recomm Rep* 51(RR-6):1-78, 2002.

Cohen RA, Brown RS: Clinical practice: Microscopic hematuria. *N Engl J Med* 348:2330-2338, 2003.

Dinsmore W, Evans C: ABC of sexual health: Erectile dysfunction. *BMJ* 318:387, 1999.

Elmer GW, Surawicz CM, McFarland LV: Biotherapeutic agents: A neglected modality for the treatment and prevention of selected intestinal and vaginal infections. *JAMA* 275:870-876, 1996.

Galejs LE: Diagnosis and treatment of the acute scrotum. *Am Fam Physician* 59: 817-824, 1999.

Gerstenbluth RE, Resnick MI: Medical management of calcium oxalate urolithiasis. *Med Clin North Am* 88:431-442, 2004.

Gilbert DN, Moellering RC, Eliopoulos GM, Sande MA: *The Sanford Guide to Antimicrobial Therapy*, 34th ed. Hyde Park, NY, Antimicrobial Therapy, 2004.

Golden MR, Marra CM, Holmes KK: Update on syphilis: Resurgence of an old problem. *JAMA* 290:1510-1514, 2003.

Gordon AE, Shaughnessy AF: Saw palmetto for prostate disorders. *Am Fam Physician* 67:1281-1283, 2003.

Gunter J: Genital and perianal warts: New treatment opportunities for human papillomavirus infection. *Am J Obstet Gynecol* 189(3 Suppl):S3-S11, 2003.

Hoberman A, Charron M, Hickey RW, et al: Image studies after a first febrile urinary tract infection in young children. *N Engl J Med* 348:195-202, 2003.

Holroyd-Leduc JM, Straus SE: Management of urinary incontinence in women: Scientific review. *JAMA* 291:986-995, 2004.

Hooton TM, Scholes D, Stapleton AE, et al: A prospective study of asymptomatic bacteriuria in sexually active young women. *N Engl J Med* 343:992-997, 2000.

Hua VN, Schaeffer AJ: Acute and chronic prostatitis. *Med Clin North Am* 88: 483-494, 2004.

Jepson RG, Mihaljevic L: Cranberries for preventing urinary tract infections. *Cochrane Database Syst Rev* (2):CD001321, 2004.

Johnson TM, Ouslander JG: Urinary incontinence in the older man. *Med Clin North Am* 83:1247-1266, 1999.

Keren R, Chan E: A meta-analysis of randomized, controlled trials comparing short- and long-course antibiotic therapy for urinary tract infections in children. *Pediatrics* 109:E70-0, 2002.

Kloner RA: Cardiovascular risk and sildenafil. *Am J Cardiol* 86:57F-61F, 2000.

Kuritzky L, Ahmed O, Kosch S: Management of impotence in primary care. *Comp Ther* 24:137, 1998.

Loughlin KR, Ker LA: The current management of urolithiasis during pregnancy. *Urol Clin North Am* 29:701-704, 2002.

Lukban JC, Whitmore KE, Sant GR: Current management of interstitial cystitis. *Urol Clin North Am* 29:649-660, 2002.

8

NEPHROLOGY AND UROLOGY

Malonza IM, Tyndall MW, Ndinya-Achola JO, et al: A randomized, double-blind, placebo-controlled trial of single-dose ciprofloxacin versus erythromycin for the treatment of chancroid in Nairobi, Kenya. *J Infect Dis* 180:1886-1893, 1999.

Mazzulli T: Resistance trends in urinary tract pathogens and impact on management. *J Urol* 168(4 Pt 2):1720-1722, 2002.

Mehta RL, Pascual MT, Soroko S, et al: Diuretics, mortality, and nonrecovery of renal function in acute renal failure. *JAMA* 288:2547-2553, 2002.

Miller KE, Ruiz DE, Graves JC: Update on the prevention and treatment of sexually transmitted diseases. *Am Fam Physician* 67:1915-1922, 2003.

Pontari MA, Ruggieri MR: Mechanisms in prostatitis/chronic pelvic pain syndrome. *J Urol* 172:839-845, 2004.

Richens J: Main presentations of sexually transmitted infections in men. *BMJ* 328: 1251-1253, 2004.

Ronald A: The etiology of urinary tract infection: Traditional and emerging pathogens. *Am J Med* 113(Suppl 1A):14S-19S, 2002.

Rubenstein RA, Dogra VS, Seftel AD, Resnick MI: Benign intrascrotal lesions. *J Urol* 171:1765-1772, 2004.

Seftel AD, Mohammed MA, Althof SE: Erectile dysfunction: Etiology, evaluation, and treatment options. *Med Clin North Am* 88:387-416, xi, 2004.

Sharlip ID: Evaluation and nonsurgical management of erectile dysfunction. *Urol Clin North Am* 25:647, 1998.

Teichman JM: Clinical practice: Acute renal colic from ureteral calculus. *N Engl J Med* 350:684-693, 2004.

Thorpe A, Neal D: Benign prostatic hyperplasia. *Lancet* 361:1359-1367, 2003.

Tyring SK: Molluscum contagiosum: The importance of early diagnosis and treatment. *Am J Obstet Gynecol* 189(3 Suppl):S12-S6, 2003.

Wing DA, Hendershott DM, Debuque L, Millar LK: Outpatient treatment of acute pyelonephritis in pregnancy after 24 weeks. *Obstet Gynecol* 94:683-688, 1999.

Workowski KA, Levine WC, Wasserheit JN: U.S. Centers for Disease Control and Prevention guidelines for the treatment of sexually transmitted diseases: An opportunity to unify clinical and public health practice. *Ann Intern Med* 137: 255-262, 2002.

Ziada A, Rosenblum M, Crawford ED: Benign prostatic hyperplasia: An overview. *Urology* 53(3 Suppl 3a):1-6, 1999.

Neurology

Deepak Madhavan and Coleman O. Martin

HEADACHE

I. **Overview.** Headaches are a common problem. Although most headaches are benign, it is the responsibility of the health care provider to rule out dangerous causes of pain. Proper classification of a particular headache syndrome allows specific treatment.

II. **Approach to the Headache Patient.**

A. **History contributes most to the diagnostic process.** Pertinent points include when the headaches first started, rapidity of onset, time to maximal pain, headache duration, frequency, location, quality, triggers (such as chocolate or red wine), aura, associated symptoms, and response to previous medications.

B. **Physical exam.** Mental status should be normal during a benign headache. Delirium raises the specter of CNS infection, hemorrhage, or vasculitis (e.g., lupus). Check cranial nerves, with special attention to visual fields, extraocular movements, corneal reflexes, gag reflexes, and fundi. Screen for abnormalities of strength, coordination, reflexes, and gait. Palpate the temples (for temporal arteritis, TMJ syndrome, and muscle-tension headache) and occipital region (for occipital neuralgia), apply pressure over the sinuses, and visualize the tympanic membranes.

C. **Neuroimaging**

1. **Whom to image.** It is not necessary for every patient with a headache to have an imaging study. However, those with a headache pattern suggestive of an intracranial lesion (e.g., SAH, abscess, tumor), those with the "worst headache of their life," and those with any focal signs or symptoms or persistent nonmigraine headache should be imaged. The yield in those with a migraine type of headache is 0.4%. **Remember, however, that only 30% of those with an SAH will have an initially focal neurologic exam.**

2. **CT** is sensitive for hemorrhagic strokes and subarachnoid hemorrhages.

3. **MRI** is the test of choice to rule out brain tumors. Consider an MRI when patients have focal neurologic signs or a daily headache for more than 1 month. **MRI is more sensitive for intracranial blood than is CT.**

D. **Laboratory studies are generally unnecessary.** In the proper clinical setting consider sedimentation rate for temporal arteritis; LP should be performed when subarachnoid hemorrhage is the possible diagnosis and CT is negative or when CNS infection or pseudotumor cerebri is suspected.

E. **Remember simple causes such as sinusitis, toothache, and TMJ syndrome.**

III. **Characteristics.** It is sometimes difficult to classify a headache into any one type based on the definitions below. The headache characteristics defined by the Headache Classification Committee of the International Headache Society are meant as guidelines to the diagnosis rather than absolute diagnostic criteria. **Table 9-1** compares common headache characteristics.

Primary Headaches

I. Migraine. Migraine headache is a common problem in the United States, affecting nearly 18% of women and 6% of men.

A. Onset is gradual, escalating to maximum intensity over 1 to 2 hours. Headache may last from a few hours to 3 days. Frequency of attacks varies widely. Status migrainosis indicates a continuous migraine headache lasting more than 3 days. Because of the unilateral nature, occipital neuralgia (see later) is often mistaken for a migraine headache.

B. Migraine without aura (common migraine) accounts for 80% of migraine headaches **(Box 9-1).**

C. Migraine with aura (classical migraine) accounts for 20% of migraine headaches **(Box 9-2).**

D. Treatment

1. Abortive therapies are most effective when taken during the aura phase or early in the headache. **With the exception of antihistamines and antiemetics, all abortive therapies can lead to rebound headaches.** Ergotamine derivatives, triptans, and isometheptene combinations are contraindicated in coronary disease, peripheral vascular disease, uncontrolled hypertension, and migraines with other neurologic signs such as alteration of consciousness, weakness, and diplopia.

a. **Narcotics are for occasional use only and should not be considered first-line treatment in the migraineur. These should be prescribed with caution due to the risk of dependency and rebound headache.**

b. **NSAIDs are effective for many patients** with migraines. Ibuprofen (400-800 mg) and aspirin (650-975 mg) have the advantage of rapid onset. Naproxen (500 mg) has a longer duration and when taken twice daily for 2 weeks can terminate status migrainosus. OTC preparations with caffeine are also effective. **Metoclopramide 10 mg PO enhances the efficacy of oral medication** by promoting gastric emptying and decreasing vomiting. Consider **dexamethasone** 4 mg IM or a short course of **prednisone** (40-60 mg PO qd), combined with analgesics, if migraine continues for longer than 24 hours and is unresponsive to standard therapy.

c. **Antiemetics** combat nausea, provide adequate analgesia for many patients, and do not lead to analgesic rebound headaches. IV preparations are more effective than rectal, which are more effective than oral. **Note that prochlorperazine and haloperidol may themselves abort a migraine headache.** Dosing is as follows: prochlorperazine (Compazine) 10 mg PO/IV or 25 mg PR; haloperidol (Haldol) 2.5 to 5 mg IV; droperidol 1.25 to 2.5 mg IV/IM (may use up to 5 mg. *Note:* has a black box warning in the United States); promethazine

TABLE 9-1
CHARACTERISTICS OF HEADACHES

Headache	Patient Population	Family History	Aura	Quality	Location	Duration	Associated Symptoms
Chronic paroxysmal hemicrania	Mean age of onset: 33 y F:M = 2:1	Absent	No	Severe, sharp, boring, throbbing	Unilateral, orbital, supraorbital, or temporal pain, always on the same side	1-40 attacks a day lasting 2-25 min. No periods of remission	Conjunctival injection, ptosis, lacrimation, rhinorrhea. Relieved w/ Indocin
Cluster	Age 20-40 y M:F = 9:1	Occasionally positive	Uncommon (6%)	Severe, boring, tearing, like a "hot poker in the eye"	Unilateral especially orbit	15-120 min	Ipsilateral tearing, Horner's syndrome, nasal stuffiness, hemifacial sweating
Migraine with aura	Age 20-40 y M:F = 1:3	Occasionally positive	Yes	Throbbing	Unilateral	3-12 h	Visual prodrome, nausea, vomiting, photophobia, phonophobia

(Continued)

TABLE 9-1
CHARACTERISTICS OF HEADACHES—cont'd

Headache	Patient Population	Family History	Aura	Quality	Location	Duration	Associated Symptoms
Migraine without aura	Onset age 6-25 y F:M = 3:1, but 1:1 at extremes of age	Positive	No	Begins as dull, penetrating; progresses to moderate or severe throbbing	Unilateral or bilateral	6-48 h	Nausea, vomiting, photophobia, phonophobia
Subarachnoid hemorrhage				Throbbing, severe	Variable	Variable	Can have focal neurologic symptoms or decreased level of consciousness, but may be alert with nonfocal exam
Tension-type	Any age, either sex		No	Dull, squeezing, nonthrobbing; not exacerbated by routine activity	Diffuse bilateral	30 min to 7 d	Depression

---

BOX 9-1

CRITERIA FOR MIGRAINE WITHOUT AURA

Must have at least five attacks meeting the following criteria:

- Headache attacks last 4-72 h
- Headache has at least two of the following:
  - Unilateral location
  - Pulsating quality
  - Moderate or severe intensity (inhibits daily activity)
  - Aggravation by routine physical activity

During the headache, at least one of the following:

- Nausea and/or vomiting
- Photophobia and phonophobia
- No organic etiology found by history, physical exam, or neurologic exam

---

(Phenergan) 25 mg PO/IM/PR (can be used in combination with hydroxyzine 25 mg PO/IM/PR).

d. **Isometheptene combinations** are well tolerated. Midrin (isometheptene, dichloralphenazone, acetaminophen 65/100/325 mg) 2 tablets at onset followed by 1 tablet per hour until relief. Max 5 tabs per 12-hour period.

e. **Ergotamine derivatives**
   (1) **Ergotamine/caffeine** (Cafergot, Wigraine) 1 mg ergot and 100 mg caffeine, 2 tabs at onset and 1 q30min up to 6 in 24 hours.
   (2) **Dihydroergotamine** (DHE-45, Migranal) **is highly effective. It is advisable to premedicate with metoclopramide, haloperidol, or prochlorperazine before administering** to prevent nausea. May not be used within 24 hours of a triptan medication. Injectable: 1 mg IV/IM/SC. May repeat in 1 hour if necessary for max dose of 2 mg per 24 hours. Intranasal: 1 spray in each nostril, repeat after 15 minutes. Max dose 6 sprays in 24 hours or 8 sprays in 1 week.

BOX 9-2

CRITERIA FOR MIGRAINE WITH AURA

Must have at least two attacks fulfilling the following criteria, at least three of which are present:

One or more fully reversible aura symptoms indicating focal cerebral cortical and/or brainstem dysfunction

At least one aura symptom develops gradually over >4 min

No aura symptom lasts >60 min (duration proportionally increases if >1 aura symptom present)

Headache follows the aura within 60 min (but headache may begin before or with the aura). Headache usually lasts 4-72 h but may have only the aura

No organic etiology found by history, physical exam, or neurologic exam

---

Note: Common aura types include scintillating scotomata, multiple small dots, homonymous visual disturbance, hemisensory disturbance, difficulty communicating, and occasionally vertigo.

   f. **Triptans** may not be used within 24 hours of an ergot derivative. Primary drawback is cost ($15/dose). Lack of effectiveness of one triptan is generally not predictive of efficacy of other triptans.

     (1) **Sumatriptan** (Imitrex). Efficacy: SQ > intranasal > oral. Efficacy is 80% SQ and 50% PO in properly selected patients. However, because it is short acting, up to 50% require rescue medication. SQ: 6 mg at onset, may repeat once after 1 hour to a max dose of 12 mg/24 h. Intranasal: 20 mg at onset, may repeat once after 2 hours to a max dose of 40 mg/24 h. PO: 25 mg at onset; if no response, additional 25 to 100 mg q2h to a max dose of 300 mg/24 h.

     (2) **Naratriptan** (Amerge) 2.5 mg PO. May repeat after 4 hours. Max dose 5 mg/24 h.

     (3) **Rizatriptan** (Maxalt, Maxalt MLT) 5 to 10 mg PO. May repeat at 2 and 4 hours if needed. MLT form is placed on tongue for oral absorption (superior with prominent nausea). Use 5 mg dose only for patients also taking propranolol. Max dose 30 mg/24 h or 15 mg/24 h in patients taking propranolol.

     (4) **Zolmitriptan** (Zomig) 1.25 to 2.5 mg PO. May repeat after 2 hours. Max dose 10 mg/24 h.

     (5) **Eletriptan** (Relpax) 20 mg to 40 mg PO. May repeat after 2 hours. Max dose is 80 mg/24 h.

     (6) **Valproic acid IV** (500 mg over 15-30 min) has been used to abort migraines with success but is second line and less successful than other treatments at preventing the need for rescue medications.

  2. Prophylactic therapies are appropriate when headaches occur more than twice a month or they lead to significant loss of productivity or quality of life. Consider other medical problems when choosing a prophylactic (e.g., use a β-blocker if patient is also hypertensive or a tricyclic if patient is also depressed.)

  a. **β-Blockers.** Options include propranolol (Inderal) 30 to 80 mg bid or sustained-release 60 to 160 mg qd; atenolol (Tenormin) 50 to 100 mg qd; nadolol (Corgard) 40 to 120 mg qd; sustained-release metoprolol 50 to 200 mg qd. If one β-blocker fails after an adequate trial (6-8 wk), consider switching to an alternative β-blocker.

  b. **Calcium channel blockers** are less effective for migraine than β-blockers but have fewer side effects. Verapamil sustained release (Isoptin SR, Calan SR) 180 to 480 mg qd. Trial should be 2 months. Other calcium channel blockers are less effective.

  c. **Tricyclic antidepressants.** Start at low dose and titrate to efficacy over a few months; this is a good choice because it will also help tension-type headaches and sleep. Side effects include sedation, dry mouth, urinary retention, and other anticholinergic side effects. Contraindicated in cardiac arrhythmias, prolonged QT, etc. Options include amitriptyline (Elavil) 10 to 200 mg qhs; nortriptyline (Pamelor) 10 to 200 mg qhs; doxepin (Sinequan) 10 to 200 mg qhs; desipramine (Norpramine) 10 to 200 mg qhs.

d. **SSRI antidepressants are less effective** but well tolerated. Options include paroxetine (Paxil) 20 to 60 mg q AM; fluoxetine (Prozac) 20 to 80 mg q AM.

e. **Anticonvulsants**

(1) **Valproic acid** (Depakote, Depakene) 250 mg bid to 500 mg tid. Effective and FDA approved for migraine prophylaxis. Adjust dose by blood level if control is difficult or sedation is problematic. Possible side effects include increased appetite, weight gain, sedation, transient alopecia, and hepatotoxicity. Check AST at onset, 1 month, 3 months, and then every 6 months.

(2) **Gabapentin** (Neurontin) 300 mg bid to 800 mg tid is **less effective** but well tolerated. No monitoring required.

(3) **Topiramate** (Topamax) 25 mg bid to 100 mg bid. Effective for prophylactic headache prevention with mood-stabilizing effects. Also has side effect of weight loss, so could be considered in overweight patients. Other main side effects include prominent sedation in a few patients, paresthesias of the fingers and toes, and a 1% risk of kidney stones. Can also cause acute angle closure glaucoma.

f. **Antihistamines** can be effective and with the exception of mild sedation are well tolerated. Cyproheptadine (Periactin) 4 mg bid; may increase to maximum dose of 8 mg tid.

g. **Alternative medicines. Riboflavin** (vitamin B_2) 400 mg qd, **feverfew**, and **magnesium** are effective at reducing migraine frequency.

h. **ACE inhibitors and ARBs** have been shown to reduce the frequency of migraine headaches.

3. **Nonpharmacologic therapies**

a. **Diet:** Avoid monosodium glutamate, nitrates, and alcohol. Spread out caffeine evenly. Keeping a log can identify foods that trigger headaches.

b. **Lifestyle changes:** Regular eating, sleeping, and exercise.

c. **Behavioral therapies:** Biofeedback, stress management, and self-help groups.

II. **Tension-type headaches are the most common type of headache (Box 9-3).** They can be episodic or chronic. Although they affect quality of life, these headaches are rarely debilitating. Nearly everyone experiences tension headaches from time to time. Tension-type headaches are separated into two subtypes based on frequency.

BOX 9-3

CRITERIA FOR TENSION-TYPE HEADACHE

Headache with at least two of the following:

Pressing/tightening quality

Mild or moderate intensity

Bilateral location

No aggravation by routine physical activity

No organic etiology found by history or by physical or neurologic exam

---

NEUROLOGY 9

A. Episodic type

1. Headache lasts 30 minutes to 7 days.
2. Patient has no nausea or vomiting with headache.
3. Photophobia and phonophobia are absent, or one but not the other is present.
4. Patient has at least 10 previous headaches as above, with number of headache days less than 180 per year and less than 15 per month.

B. Chronic type

1. Headache averages 15 days per month (180 days per year), for at least 6 months.
2. Patient has no vomiting.
3. Patient has no more than one of the following: nausea, photophobia, or phonophobia.

C. Treatment

1. **Abortive therapy.** Simple analgesics, NSAIDs, antiemetics (chlorpromazine, haloperidol), and dihydroergotamine as per migraine section. **Overuse can lead to analgesic rebound headaches.** Encourage nonpharmacologic therapies such as heat, stretching, relaxation therapy, etc.
2. **Prophylactic therapy.** TCAs, β-blockers, or calcium channel blockers as per migraine section.

III. Cluster headaches (episodic or chronic). Cluster headaches **(Box 9-4)** are uncommon, occurring in 0.1% to 0.4% of the general population. They are named by their curious periodicity, typically occurring up to several times a day for weeks or months, then spontaneously remitting. Additionally, their unique head pain profile and autonomic features set

---

BOX 9-4

CRITERIA FOR CLUSTER HEADACHE

Severe unilateral orbital, supraorbital, and/or temporal pain peaking in 10-15 min and lasting 30-45 min (occasionally up to 180 min). Pain rapidly resolves. Cluster headaches have a propensity to occur at night and can lead to sleep deprivation. Cycles generally last for a few weeks or months but can last more than a year.

- Headache is associated with at least one of the following on the pain side:
  - Conjunctival injection
  - Rhinorrhea
  - Lacrimation
  - Miosis
  - Nasal congestion
  - Ptosis
  - Forehead and facial sweating
  - Eyelid edema
- Additionally
  - Frequency of attacks ranges from 1 to 8 daily
  - There have been at least five episodes of headache

them apart from other headache syndromes. Headaches are so severe that patients may threaten suicide. Indeed, suicide rates in this population are increased.

A. Abortive therapies. Usefulness is limited by the high frequency and short duration of the headaches.

1. **Oxygen** 8 L/min by face mask relieves headache in 60% to 70% of patients. Effect occurs in approximately 5 minutes.

2. **Sumatriptan** (Imitrex) 6 mg SQ is rapidly effective and appears to be safe up to twice daily. Intranasal administration may also be effective. Because, by definition, cluster headaches are short lived, sumatriptan is an excellent choice for these patients.

3. **Lidocaine** 4% on a long cotton swab placed intranasally against the sphenopalatine ganglion is helpful for some patients.

B. Prophylactic therapies. Most patients with daily cluster headaches should also be treated with a prophylactic medication. This medication is continued for a few weeks beyond the termination of the headaches. For patients who relapse, chronic prophylactic therapy can be considered. If patients are unresponsive to standard therapy, consider the diagnosis of chronic paroxysmal hemicrania.

1. **Prednisone** 60 mg qd for 3 days followed by a taper to 0 mg over 15 days is a rapid and effective short-term treatment.

2. **Ergotamine** tartrate 1 mg bid. It is contraindicated in coronary disease, peripheral vascular disease, and uncontrolled hypertension.

3. **Lithium carbonate.** Start 300 mg bid and titrate to level of 0.4 to 0.8 mEq/L. It is more effective in chronic cluster headaches.

4. **Verapamil or valproic acid** as per migraine headache.

IV. Chronic paroxysmal hemicrania (Box 9-5) is a severe unilateral throbbing orbital, supraorbital, or temporal pain always on the same side, lasting 2 to 45 minutes. The average age of onset is 33 years, and female-to-male ratio is 2:1. No aura. **Therapy** is indomethacin, up to 150 mg/day. Response to indomethacin is one of the diagnostic criteria.

9

NEUROLOGY

BOX 9-5

CHRONIC PAROXYSMAL HEMICRANIA

Attack frequency is generally 1 to 40 per day. Periods of lower frequency can occur, but there is rarely a total remission.

- Headache is associated with at least one of the following on the pain side:
  - Conjunctival injection
  - Eyelid edema
  - Lacrimation
  - Nasal congestion
  - Ptosis
  - Rhinorrhea
- Absolute effectiveness of indomethacin (150 mg/day or less)
- No organic etiology found by history, physical, or neurologic exam

V. Analgesic rebound headache is produced by the overzealous use of analgesics. It often coexists with migraine or tension headaches that prompted the analgesia overuse.
A. Patient population. All patients who use analgesics two or more times per week in the symptomatic treatment of headache are at risk for this syndrome. It occurs most commonly when analgesics are used daily.
B. Causal medications. NSAIDs, acetaminophen, ergotamine derivatives, triptans, isometheptene combinations, and narcotics.
C. Pain characteristics are similar to tension headache pain.
D. Time course. Daily or near-daily headache that is dulled or relieved by analgesics only to return when the analgesic wears off.
E. Treatment. Most effective therapy is to stop analgesics. Hydroxyzine 25 to 50 mg q6h prn with or without promethazine 25 to 50 mg q6h prn may be used to dull the rebound headache. Warn patients that they will probably experience a constant headache for 1 to 2 weeks. Sometimes a long-acting NSAID (such as naproxen) can be scheduled daily for 2 weeks and then discontinued without recurrence of the headache. Consider use of a prophylactic headache medication targeted at the primary headache syndrome that precipitated the analgesic overuse. Prophylactic medication will not alleviate the rebound headache, however. It is imperative that the causative analgesic be discontinued.
VI. Occipital neuralgia is an occipital headache with a retro-orbital or frontal component. It occurs secondary to entrapment of the occipital nerve, especially after cervical strain or secondary to muscle tension. It is often misdiagnosed as migraine headache because of the hemicranial nature. Pain can be reproduced by pressure to occipital notch and is treated by NSAIDs and muscle relaxants, by tricyclic antidepressants, or by injection with bupivacaine and triamcinolone.

Secondary Headaches

Headache accompanied by systemic illness, neurologic deficits, or mental status changes are likely to be secondary to other cranial pathology. Patients with benign headache syndromes are equally at risk for secondary headaches, mandating that a patient with a new type of headache be reevaluated.
I. Idiopathic increased intracranial pressure (pseudotumor cerebri) occurs in 19 per 100,000 with a predilection for obese young women (can occur in others). **Pseudotumor cerebri as been associated with corticosteroid, vitamin A, tetracycline, and ibuprofen use.** It often manifests as chronic retrobulbar headache exacerbated by eye movements. Loss of peripheral vision, diplopia, meningeal signs, and paresthesias can occur. Exam may reveal papilledema and cranial nerve VI palsy. CSF is normal except for elevated opening pressure (250-450 mm H_2O). **Treatment** includes weight loss, serial LPs each removing 20 to 40 mL of CSF, diuretics (e.g., furosemide), acetazolamide 500 to 1000 mg qd (reduces CSF production as well as

being a diuretic), prednisone 40 to 60 mg qd, optic nerve fenestration, and rarely a shunt. Consider referral to neuro-ophthalmology.

II. **Brain Tumor. Headache is the most common isolated complaint, although only 50% of tumors cause headache.** A classic tumor headache (worse in morning, exacerbated by bending over, and associated with nausea and vomiting) only occurs in 17%. **Most have only symptoms of a typical tension-type headache.** Other neurologic signs or symptoms can help localize tumor but may be absent. Be aware of this in new-onset headaches in people older than age 50.

III. **Temporal (Giant Cell) Arteritis** should be considered in people older than age 55 (rare younger patients). Tenderness at the temples, jaw claudication, vision changes, and constitutional symptoms all suggest the diagnosis. Sedimentation rate is usually elevated but is normal in 15%. CRP may be elevated but has the same sensitivity as sedimentation rate. Refer to an ophthalmologist for a detailed retinal exam; a temporal artery biopsy is suggested. Blindness can rapidly occur if treatment is delayed. See Chapter 7 for further details.

IV. **Meningitis and Herpes Encephalitis.** See CNS infections section.

V. **Carbon Monoxide Poisoning.** See Chapter 2.

VI. **Subarachnoid Hemorrhage.** Patients generally have the acute onset of the "worst headache of their life." They can have nausea, vomiting, mental status changes, or loss of consciousness, which may be transient. **Most (59%) have a "warning leak" before the severe event and might have antecedent headaches for weeks.** Mortality rate is 60% for each bleed; therefore diagnosis of a warning leak can prevent death and morbidity.

A. **Patients might have mental status changes and meningeal signs but might not (39% are initially free of CNS symptoms and signs). Only 10% have an initially focal exam.**

B. Patients can have fever and leukocytosis from meningeal irritation.

C. **CT should be done on those with a sudden-onset severe headache and in those with a severe headache that is different from their usual headache.** In one study, 33% of those with new onset of severe headache and no CNS signs or symptoms and no other obvious cause of headache had SAH. CT scan finds only about 90% of SAH (98% in third-generation scanners). **If SAH is suspected in the context of a negative head CT, LP is necessary for definitive diagnosis.**

D. **Response to nonnarcotic and narcotic analgesia does not rule out SAH.**

VII. **Miscellaneous Headaches (Benign)** include postcoital headache, cold-induced headache (e.g., from ice cream), jolts and jabs (also known as ice-pick headache: stabbing, sharp, headache in temple or retro-orbital area lasting seconds occurring multiple times), and cough- or Valsalva-related headache (benign in 80% to 90%). Arnold–Chiari malformation can cause headache associated with Valsalva, cough, etc., and can be diagnosed by MRI. Arnold–Chiari malformation can lead to permanent disability.

DEMENTIA

See Chapter 21 for nursing home management of the dementia patient.

I. **Overview.** The perception of memory impairment is common among the elderly; approximately one quarter to one third of nondemented healthy elderly complain of memory difficulty. Cognitive performance is reduced somewhat with advancing age, and speed of processing is most affected. As a rule, accuracy of responses should not suffer significantly. Formal neuropsychological testing can be especially helpful both for patient reassurance and to establish a baseline for future testing.

A. **Definition** (DSM-IV diagnostic criteria). Acquired memory impairment plus at least one additional acquired cognitive deficit such as aphasia, apraxia (difficulty in carrying out motor activities despite intact motor function), agnosia (difficulty recognizing objects despite intact sensory function), or disturbance in executive function (as in organizing, planning). To be considered dementia, symptoms must represent a decline from the patient's prior baseline and must not be better accounted for by delirium or mental illness. **Table 9-2** differentiates delirium, dementia, and psychosis.

B. **Prevalence.** At age 65, 1% of the population has dementia. This percentage doubles with every 5 years of age. Fifty percent of persons living to their tenth decade have some degree of dementia.

C. **Potentially reversible causes.** Overall, 3% to 15% of dementia cases are reversible. Reversible causes include Wernicke's encephalopathy, vitamin B_{12} deficiency, subdural hematoma, normal-pressure hydrocephalus (see later), CNS infections (such as syphilis), depression (pseudodementia, see later), and resectable brain tumors. Subacute delirium (see later) is often mistaken for dementia and can arise from a variety of causes including but not limited to medication side effects, systemic infections, malignant hypertension, dehydration, uremia, liver failure, hypothyroidism, hyponatremia, hypercalcemia, and hypoglycemia.

D. **Irreversible causes** include Alzheimer's disease, vascular dementia, frontotemporal dementias (e.g., Pick's disease), dementia with Lewy bodies, Huntington's chorea, Creutzfeldt–Jakob disease, AIDS-related dementia, bovine spongiform encephalopathy, Parkinson's-related dementia, and heavy-metal poisoning (including lead, mercury, arsenic, manganese, and thallium).

II. **Diagnostic Evaluation.**

A. **History and physical** with a complete neurologic exam are essential. Babinski's sign, asymmetry of reflexes, and visual-field deficits suggest multi-infarct dementia or focal CNS abnormality rather than Alzheimer's disease.

B. **Mini-Mental State Examination** is a useful office screening tool for a quick assessment and serial exams. A score of 25 or less increases odds of dementia. **Dementia can still be present despite a "normal" MMSE score** (more likely in younger or well-educated patients). The MMSE is copyrighted but can be found on the World Wide Web.

TABLE 9-2
CLINICAL FEATURES OF DELIRIUM DEMENTIA AND ACUTE FUNCTIONAL PSYCHOSIS

Clinical Feature	Delirium	Dementia	Psychosis
Onset	Sudden	Insidious	Sudden
Course over 24 h	Fluctuating, with nocturnal exacerbation	Stable	Stable
Consciousness	Reduced	Clear	Clear
Attention	Globally disordered	Normal, except in severe cases	May be disordered
Cognition	Globally disordered	Globally impaired	May be selectively impaired
Hallucinations	Usually visual or visual and auditory	Usually absent	Predominately auditory
Delusions	Fleeting, poorly systematized	Usually absent	Sustained, systematized
Orientation	Usually impaired, at least to time	Often impaired	May be impaired
Psychomotor activity	Increased, reduced, or shifting unpredictably	Often normal	Varies from psychomotor retardation to severe hyperactivity, depending on the type of psychosis
Speech	Often incoherent, slow or rapid	Patient has difficulty finding words, perseveration	Normal, slow, or rapid
Involuntary movements	Often asterixis or coarse tremor	None	Usually absent
Physical illness or drug toxicity	One or both are present	Often absent	Usually absent

Adapted from Bross MH, Tatum NO: Am Fam Physician 50:1325-1332, 1994.

NEUROLOGY 9

C. **Initial lab tests** should include CBC, ESR, chemistry panel (with electrolytes, BUN, creatinine LFTs, calcium, glucose), thyroid function tests, RPR, vitamin B_{12}, and folate. A brain CT without contrast is the minimum neuroimaging required to screen for subdural hematoma, brain tumor, normal-pressure hydrocephalus, and multi-infarct dementia.

D. **Additional tests.** May be obtained if indicated by history, physical exam, or initial lab tests. These additional tests include UA, HIV, 24-hour urine heavy-metal screen, ECG, chest radiograph, EEG, MRI, blood gas, serum ammonia, lumbar puncture, and drug levels.

E. **Neuropsychological testing** is useful for assessing cases that are atypical such as onset at a young age (<60), rapidly progressing dementia, early loss of language, or possible psychiatric component. Testing allows the progression of the dementia to be accurately monitored and can help address important issues such as driving, cooking, independence, and financial independence management.

III. **General Management of Dementia.** See Chapter 21 for the general management of dementia (e.g., nursing home care).

IV. **Common Types of Dementia.**

A. **Alzheimer's dementia** is the most common dementing illness and represents up to 60% of dementia. Alzheimer's dementia is of enormous medical and social importance.

1. **Characteristics.** In addition to meeting the definition of a dementia, Alzheimer's dementia is typified by the following:

a. Onset is gradual, with relentless progression, and rarely begins before age 60.

b. Memory impairment is most severe for recent events.

c. Spatial disorientation is common early in the disease, and patients may become lost or disoriented when performing simple tasks (e.g., driving to the store).

d. Social graces are relatively preserved, but there may be incontinence of urine and stool.

e. Patients are often unaware of their deficits (anosognosia).

f. Psychiatric disturbances (hallucinations and delusions) can occur, typically later in the course. However, depression is common early in the course. Sundowning, nocturnal hallucinations, wandering, and confusion are common later in the course.

2. **Diagnosis.** It is vitally important to exclude other treatable causes of dementia. Brain CT may initially be normal; later, diffuse atrophy is evident. However, this is nonspecific, and the use of CT is mainly to rule out other problems (tumor, subdural, etc.). Brain MRI highlights more evidence of degeneration than CT does. Disturbances of gait, sudden onset of dementia, focal neurologic exam, or new onset of seizures should call the diagnosis into question.

3. **Treatment. Generally, the response to drugs is poor and all have very limited efficacy.** NNT is 12 for minimal benefit in one patient (Lanctot et al., 2003).

a. **Cholinesterase inhibitors. Donepezil** (Aricept) is indicated for treatment of mild to moderate Alzheimer's dementia. Initial dose is 5 mg PO qhs for 4 to 6 weeks. Then the dose may be increased to 10 mg PO qhs if needed. Side effects are common and include cholinergic manifestations such as salivation, nausea, seizures, etc. **Rivastigmine** (Exelon) initial dose is 1.5 mg bid and advance to 3 to 6 mg bid over 2 months. **Galantamine** (Reminyl) initial dose is 4 mg bid, can increase by 4 mg bid after a minimum 4 weeks for a maximum dose of 32 mg/day. Side effects are similar to donepezil's.

b. **Memantine** (Namenda) is indicated for the treatment of moderate to severe Alzheimer's dementia. Initial dose is 5mg PO daily, titratable to a max dose of 20 mg (10 mg bid). The most common side effects include dizziness (7%) and constipation (5%).

c. **Vitamin E,** 2000 IU PO qd; efficacy is limited. It does not reverse but might slow the progression of dementia. It may be used in conjunction with other Alzheimer's treatments. Vitamin E can cause increased risk of bleeding and is relatively contraindicated in those taking anticoagulants or who have a bleeding disorder.

B. Vascular dementia (formerly multi-infarct dementia) accounts for up to 20% of dementia in the elderly.

1. **Characteristics.** Onset often progresses in a stepwise deteriorating manner. Risk factors include male gender, smoking, history of TIAs, strokes, hypertension, coronary artery disease, and atrial fibrillation. Associated symptoms include disturbances of gait and early incontinence.

2. **Diagnosis** requires evidence of strokes, such as focal neurologic deficits and neuroimaging showing evidence of multiple hemispheric infarcts. Dementia should not be better accounted for by AD or other illness.

3. **Treatment.** Reduce modifiable risks for stroke. See section on stroke later.

C. Frontotemporal dementias are a heterologous group of neurodegenerative diseases including Pick's disease. They are important to differentiate from Alzheimer's dementia because of differences in management.

1. **Characteristics.** Onset is insidious and the course is slowly progressive. Psychiatric manifestations occur early and include social inappropriateness, disinhibition, delusions, ritualistic behavior, and mood disorders. **Language** changes include progressive reduction in speech with overuse of stock phrases and sometimes echolalia. **Patient loses personal awareness** and neglects hygiene and grooming. Spatial orientation and praxis are often preserved. Other signs include incontinence, late rigidity, akinesia, and tremor.

2. **Diagnosis.** MRI reveals relative atrophy of the frontal lobes and the anterior temporal lobes.

3. **Management.** Unfortunately, no specific medications have proved beneficial. Treatment is symptomatic, with behavior-modifying environment and medications (short-acting benzodiazepines, antipsychotics, and SSRIs).

9

NEUROLOGY

D. Dementia with Lewy bodies represents as much as 25% of dementia cases. It is an interesting **crossroads of dementia and parkinsonism.** The extrapyramidal symptoms tend to be mild with rigidity, bradykinesia, and frequent falls. Sometimes syncope occurs. Tremor is not prominent.

1. **Characteristics.** Fluctuations of attention and alertness, with patients having good and bad days. **Visual hallucinations** are often detailed and recurrent. Hallucinations in other modalities can also occur. **Memory disturbance** is typified by inefficient memory retrieval. With prompting, memory can be surprisingly intact. Visual spatial ability may be particularly impaired.

2. **Treatment**

a. *Avoid antipsychotics.* Patients with dementia with Lewy bodies are markedly sensitive to antipsychotics, which exacerbate their parkinsonism. New atypical antipsychotics may be of benefit but may still have extrapyramidal side effects.

b. **Donepezil** (Aricept) (NNT = 12) may be helpful for both the memory and psychiatric disturbances.

c. **Dopamine agonists** can improve parkinsonism. Monitor for worsening hallucinations.

E. Normal-pressure hydrocephalus

1. **Characterized by** triad of gradual onset of dementia, gait disturbance, and urinary incontinence. **However, this triad is not specific for normal-pressure hydrocephalus.**

2. **Diagnosis.** CT scan shows enlarged ventricles with preserved cortical ribbon. MRI reveals transependymal flow.

3. **Treatment.** Surgical ventriculoperitoneal CSF shunting can greatly improve symptoms or even be curative. However, treatment must be undertaken early in the disease to see improvement.

F. Pseudodementia is named for depression masquerading as dementia. Often patients indicate depression directly when asked. Other clues include patients having the ability to pinpoint the onset of symptoms and give detailed accounts of their impairments. Remote memory may be sketchy at interview, unlike other dementias where remote memory is relatively intact. Neuropsychological testing shows poor effort and improvement on coaxing. Treatment is directed at the underlying depression (see Chapter 18).

DELIRIUM

I. **Overview.**

A. Prevalence. Delirium affects 10% of all hospitalized patients, 20% of burn patients, 30% of ICU patients, and 30% of hospitalized AIDS patients.

B. Predisposing factors include extremes of age (young and elderly) and patients with a history of brain damage, dementia, or prior delirium.

C. Delirium is a medical emergency and requires a prompt, thorough evaluation.

II. Diagnosis by DSM-IV Criteria. The three following criteria must be met:

A. Disturbance of consciousness with reduced ability to focus, shift, or sustain attention.

B. A change in cognition (such as memory deficit, disorientation) or development of a perceptual disturbance not better accounted for by dementia.

C. Symptoms develop over a short period and tend to fluctuate during the day.

III. Common Causes of Delirium.

A. Organ failure: Renal (uremia), hepatic (hyperammonemia), pulmonary (hypoxia), cardiac (hypotension, low-perfusion states).

B. Nutritional: Vitamin B_{12}, folate, and thiamine deficiencies; hypoglycemia.

C. Endocrine: Hypothyroidism, hyperthyroidism, hypercorticism, hypopituitarism, and hyperparathyroidism.

D. Trauma or pain: Burns, fractures (especially of hips).

E. Infectious: Pneumonia, sepsis, cystitis, pyelonephritis.

F. Drugs: Many, including, but not limited to, anticonvulsants, antidepressants, antihypertensive drugs, antiparkinsonian drugs, corticosteroids, digitalis, antihistamines, narcotics, phenothiazines, drugs with anticholinergic side effects, H_2 blockers, and alcohol or sedative–hypnotic intoxication or withdrawal.

G. Electrolyte and acid–base disturbances. Hypernatremia, hyponatremia, hyperkalemia, hypokalemia, hypermagnesemia, hypomagnesemia, hypercalcemia, hypocalcemia, acidosis, alkalosis.

H. Urinary retention or fecal impaction.

I. Primary brain disorder.

1. **Structural:** Trauma, tumor, subdural hematoma, subarachnoid hemorrhage, stroke, concussion.

2. **Seizure:** Postictal state, nonconvulsive status epilepticus.

3. **Infection:** Meningitis, encephalitis.

J. Change in environment. Demented patients are susceptible to confusion and disorientation with changes in location and sleep as commonly occurs with travel.

IV. Diagnostic Evaluation.

A. Bystander effect. Most commonly the brain is an "innocent bystander" to a serious process elsewhere in the body. Work-up should proceed from immediately life-threatening conditions to more indolent medical and neurologic causes.

B. See Table 9-2 to differentiate delirium, dementia, and acute psychosis.

C. History. Ask family or nurse about patient's baseline level of function, any recent medication changes, systemic illnesses, or a history of mental illness.

D. Physical examination. Perform a thorough physical exam, paying attention to signs of the causes listed above. Assess for neck stiffness. If possible, perform MMSE. A score of less than 24 indicates significant cognitive disturbance. Neurologic exam should include a careful cranial nerve assessment and sensory, motor, and reflex screening to detect a brainstem or hemispheric process.

E. **Laboratory tests** include CBC, electrolytes, blood chemistry panel, UA, ECG, oxygen saturation, CXR, and abdominal film. If cause is not rapidly apparent, obtain ABG, cultures, and brain CT. Other labs as indicated by patient's history, exam, and clinical situation: cardiac isoenzymes, vitamin B_{12}, folate, cortisol, ammonia, ANA, RPR, TSH, toxicologic analysis, drug levels, MRI, lumbar puncture, EEG, and HIV serology.

V. **Management.**

A. **Treat** the underlying medical conditions promptly to decrease risk of death (10% to 65%) from the cause of delirium.

B. **Minimize any aggravating medications, optimize nutrition and hydration, and create a supportive environment.**

C. **Reassurance.** Family members provide reassurance. Procure familiar items from home to reorient patient.

D. **Sleep** should be regular and uninterrupted. Avoid naps during the day.

E. **Location.** Place patient near a nursing station for easier monitoring.

F. **Agitation.** Treatment of associated agitation is difficult because sedatives prolong the delirium and cloud the diagnostic process. If absolutely necessary, treat with haloperidol (Haldol), initial dose 0.5 to 1 mg IM or IV. Orally, try haloperidol or one of the new atypical antipsychotics such as olanzapine (Zyprexa) (again, the new antipsychotics do not have any fewer adverse reactions in these patients). If antipsychotics are not effective, consider adjunctive lorazepam (Ativan) 0.5 to 1.0 mg IM or IV. Soft restraints may be necessary for safety.

G. **Bed rails are not protective and increase the number and severity of falls.**

SEIZURES

I. **Overview.**

A. **Epidemiology.** Prevalence of epilepsy in the United States is 0.5% to 1%. Approximately 2% to 5% of children have febrile seizures, with an approximate age range of 3 months to 5 years.

B. **Definition.** *Epilepsy* refers to recurrent seizures that reflect aberrant electrical activity of cerebral cortical neurons. *Convulsion* applies to a seizure in which motor manifestations predominate. **_Note:_ A single seizure is not sufficient to warrant a diagnosis of epilepsy.**

II. **Classification.**

A. **Primary generalized seizures** are bilateral and symmetric without focal onset and are usually idiopathic.

1. **Absence (petit mal).** Brief (2-10 sec) lapse of consciousness. Onset is 4 to 12 years of age, and frequency of attacks decreases in adolescence. No aura or postictal period. Manifested by staring, eye blinking, lip smacking. EEG characteristically shows a diffuse 3-Hz spike-and-wave pattern. Tends to remit in late adolescence or early adulthood.

2. **Myoclonic.** Quick paroxysmal contractions of part of a muscle, whole muscle, or groups of muscles. Can occur as single jerk or intermittently in the same or different part of the body. *Note:* Not all myoclonus is epileptic. Other causes include infection, anoxia, and metabolic disturbances.

3. **Clonic, tonic, and tonic–clonic (grand mal),** with or without aura. The patient abruptly loses consciousness and has a tonic, clonic, or tonic–clonic convulsion, followed by postictal confusion.

4. **Infantile spasms with hypsarrhythmic EEG (high amplitude, markedly disorganized).** These begin in the first year of life and manifest as a series of myoclonic spasms (also known as salaam seizures). These are generally from underlying brain or neurologic disease and mandate a complete evaluation.

B. **Partial (focal) seizures**

1. **Simple.** Consciousness is not impaired. Subjectively, patients are likely to experience déjà vu and sensory, motor, or autonomic symptoms. For example, patients might note vague abdominal or thoracic sensations. With motor involvement, patients are likely to exhibit hemifacial or hemibody twitching.

2. **Complex.** Consciousness is impaired. Patient can have automatic behavior such as lip smacking, fumbling with clothes, or even walking. Patients are amnestic for part or all of the episode.

III. **Causes.** Seizures result from electrical irritability of gray matter through many possible mechanisms, including CNS infection, inborn errors of metabolism, congenital malformations, acquired metabolic disorders (hypoglycemia, uremia, hepatic encephalopathy, disturbances of Na^+, Cl^-, Mg^{2+}, Ca^{2+}, pH), structural lesions (stroke, trauma, subarachnoid hemorrhage, subdural hematoma, tumors), gliosis from old brain injuries, new medications or medication withdrawal, drug or alcohol use or withdrawal, and familial epilepsy. Common causes of epilepsy based on age are shown in **Table 9-3**.

IV. **Diagnosis.**

A. **History.** Ask direct questions to accurately characterize the beginning, middle, and end of the spell. Collateral information from witnesses is essential. Ask about prior seizures, medications, fever, headache,

9

NEUROLOGY

TABLE 9-3

CAUSES OF EPILEPSY BY AGE GROUP

Age of Onset	Probable Cause
Infancy and childhood	Congenital malformation, inborn errors of metabolism, idiopathic, birth trauma
Adolescence	Idiopathic, trauma
Early adulthood	Idiopathic, trauma, tumor, alcohol or other hypnotic drug withdrawal
Middle age	Trauma, tumor, vascular disease, alcohol or other drug withdrawal
Late life	Vascular disease, tumor, degenerative disease

circumstances precipitating events, history of drug abuse, ingestions, and trauma.

B. Physical examination. Assess neurologic (responsiveness, fontanels, pupils, fundi, cranial nerves, and sensory, motor, and reflex asymmetry), cardiovascular (BP, perfusion), and pulmonary (cyanosis, irregular breathing) systems. Check for breath odor (fruity indicates DKA, fetor hepaticus), rash, signs and symptoms of infection (sepsis, meningitis), signs of trauma, and cirrhosis.

C. Laboratory tests. Electrolytes, Ca^{2+}, Mg^{2+}, glucose, BUN, CBC, anticonvulsant levels (if applicable), toxicology screen, sepsis work-up including LP if indicated. Consider LFTs, Pb^{2+}, ammonia, CT scan.

D. EEG supports diagnosis of seizures. In patients with a generalized epilepsy syndrome or those with an irritative electrical focus, distinctive EEG patterns can be detected. **A normal EEG does not preclude seizure activity. A single 30-minute interictal EEG recording has a sensitivity of approximately 60% for finding epileptiform activity. This increases to 90% after the third interictal study.** Therefore, if the diagnosis of epilepsy is strongly considered, it may be worthwhile to do a prolonged (2-3 hours) interictal EEG or to proceed to video EEG.

E. Video EEG monitoring is helpful in patients with frequent spells to differentiate epileptic seizures from other types of spells (see below).

F. MRI is sensitive for structural brain lesions, including tumors, strokes, and hippocampal sclerosis.

V. Differential Diagnosis.

A. Syncope. Global brain hypoperfusion secondary to decreased cardiac output or vasodilation. Convulsions are common if a syncopal patient is not immediately moved to a supine position. Patients often report that syncopal spells are preceded by light-headedness, and postevent confusion is minimal. These patients do not need an EEG or seizure work-up if there is simple syncope followed by brief tonic–clonic movements (but they should be evaluated for syncope). See Chapter 2 for details.

B. Pseudoseizures are often a manifestation of psychological illness. Pseudoseizures are usually poorly stereotyped, varying in form and duration. Most epileptic seizures last less than 3 minutes, but pseudoseizures may have a much longer duration. They are much more likely to occur during times of stress and do not typically occur while alone or during dangerous activities such as cooking or drinking. Without capturing a spell on EEG, it can be difficult to differentiate pseudoseizures from epileptic seizures. Comparing a prolactin level drawn within 15 minutes of a spell to another drawn 24 hours later can be informative. Epileptic seizures are usually accompanied by a significant rise in prolactin level over that of the normal circadian variation. However, a normal prolactin is not helpful because not all seizures are associated with a rise in prolactin level.

C. **Transient ischemic attacks,** like seizures, are usually of relatively short duration, although TIAs are characterized by *loss* of neurologic function and only rarely cause motor activity.

D. **Migraine aura** is also a cause of transient neurologic dysfunction, but these spells do not manifest as motor activity. They can cause alteration in sensation, dexterity, balance, vision, and alertness (see discussion of migraine headache earlier this chapter).

E. **Breath-holding spells** are seen in infants and small children. During crying, the infant voluntarily holds breath during expiration, becomes cyanotic, loses consciousness, and may have a few convulsive limb movements. Breath-holding spells are distinguished from seizures by occurring only during emotional outbursts and by the cyanosis preceding (not following) the convulsive movements. They resolve with maturity (usually by 5 years of age).

VI. **Treatment (Table 9-4).**

A. **Principles.** If a patient has a single seizure, there is a 30% to 60% chance that patient will have a recurrent event. The risk of a recurrent seizure is lower if it was due to a provoking factor (e.g., acute illness, binge drinking, sleep deprivation) and is higher if no provoking factor is present. **Optimally use single-drug therapy because polypharmacy impairs drug effectiveness and side effects accumulate.** In a study of monotherapy, 47% of patients with newly diagnosed epilepsy were controlled with the first drug tried, another 13% with the second drug tried, and another 1% with the third drug tried. In patients failing monotherapy, only 3% of cases were controlled with dual antiepileptic drug (AED) therapy and none with triple therapy.

Most AEDs have side effects, including sedation, mood changes, and dizziness. Some can cause anemias, and baseline, 3-month, and yearly LFTs and CBCs may be necessary (see Table 9-4). Anticonvulsant levels are useful for monitoring compliance and adjusting dosages when seizures are uncontrolled or side effects occur. Many anticonvulsants are notoriously nonlinear in their pharmacokinetics, making it useful to recheck anticonvulsant levels after a dosage adjustment or changing some other drug with a known anticonvulsant interaction. Otherwise, checking levels when the patient is doing well (controlled seizures, no side effects) is unnecessary.

Note: Most of the first-generation AEDs (phenytoin, phenobarbital, carbamazepine, primidone) induce liver enzymes. This can lead to a variety of interactions, such as disrupting INR in anticoagulated patients and decreasing the effectiveness of oral contraceptives. This second interaction, combined with the potential teratogenic effects of AEDs, necessitates folate and prenatal vitamin supplementation in female patients of childbearing age. The liver involvement of these AEDs can also lead to progressive bone thinning, so calcium and vitamin D supplementation is also recommended in patients are taking first-generation AEDs. Valproic acid can also have bone-thinning effects. This should be discussed with the patient.

TABLE 9-4
COMMON ANTIEPILEPTIC DRUGS

Drug	Principal Therapeutic Indications	Monitoring	Effective Levels (mg/L)
Carbamazepine (Tegretol)	Complex partial seizures, secondarily generalized partial seizures	LFTs, CBC	4-12
Clonazepam (Klonopin)	Myoclonic seizures	None	N/A
Ethosuximide (Zarontin)	Absence seizures only	CBC	40-100
Gabapentin (Neurontin)	Adjunct therapy in partial seizures age >12 y	None	N/A
Lamotrigine (Lamictal)	Monotherapy in partial-onset seizures	If rash occurs, discontinue drug immediately (risk of Stevens-Johnson syndrome); rash can be prevented by a slow titration	N/A
Levetiracetam (Keppra)	Adjunctive therapy for partial-onset seizures in adults	None	N/A
Oxcarbazepine (Trileptal)	Monotherapy of partial-onset seizures in adults and children	None	N/A
Phenobarbital (Luminal)	Generalized tonic–clonic, status epilepticus, simple and complex partial seizures	LFTs, CBC	10-30
Phenytoin (Dilantin)	Simple and complex partial seizures, status epilepticus	LFTs	10-20
Primidone (Mysoline)	Generalized tonic–clonic, simple and complex partial seizures	LFTs, CBC	5-15
Tiagabine (Gabatril)	Adjunctive therapy in partial onset seizures, age >12 y	None	N/A
Topiramate (Topamax)	Monotherapy in partial-onset seizures, generalized seizures, absence seizures age >3y	None	N/A
Valproic acid (Depakene)	Generalized tonic–clonic, absence, complex partial seizures	LFTs	50-100
Zonisamide (Zonegran)	Adjunctive therapy in partial-onset seizures in adults	None	N/A

B. Surgical treatment is becoming increasingly useful in modern epilepsy management.

1. **Temporal lobectomy** is the most effective method for patients with focal-onset intractable epilepsy. Consider a patient to be a candidate for surgery if seizures are socially disabling and refractory to maximum doses of standard medications. Moreover, certain epilepsy syndromes (mesial temporal lobe epilepsy and discrete neocortical lesion) have a poor prognosis with purely medical treatment but respond well to surgical treatment, with an 80% to 90% seizure-free outcome in suitable patients.

2. **Vagus nerve stimulator** is an implanted device that intermittently stimulates the left vagus nerve. It is well-tolerated, effective adjuvant therapy for refractory partial-onset seizures. Its efficacy is comparable to adding an AED. Its main effect is that of palliation; it is not intended as a cure.

C. Treatment of status epilepticus. Status epilepticus is defined as a seizure (convulsive or otherwise) persisting more than 30 minutes or when a patient fails to return to normal consciousness between seizures. A seizure lasting more than 5 minutes increases the risk of status epilepticus. Because permanent brain damage starts in as little as 30 minutes, a rapid systematic approach is necessary. See Chapter 2 for treatment.

PARKINSON'S DISEASE

I. **Overview.** Parkinson's disease is a slowly progressive movement disorder of unknown etiology that primarily affects the pigmented dopamine-containing neurons of the pars compacta of the substantia nigra. It usually occurs late in adult life but occasionally as early as the fourth decade. Family history is present in 5% to 10% of cases. Epidemiologic studies have identified the following risk factors: living in rural areas or near wood pulp mills, exposure to agrochemicals, and consumption of well water.

II. **Diagnosis.**

A. Diagnosis is made clinically. Onset is usually insidious and asymmetric.

B. Cardinal symptoms are gross resting tremor (often pill rolling) of the hands and sometimes feet, bradykinesia, rigidity (described as lead pipe with cogwheeling), and postural instability (e.g., unable to maintain balance when pulled from behind). The parkinsonian gait is classically festinating (rapid small steps); turning requires several steps, and propulsion, retropulsion, and falling are common. Other features include masked facies, decreased blinking, stooped posture, and salivation.

C. The risk of dementia is six times that in the normal population. A favorable response to levodopa helps confirm the diagnosis. **If symptoms fail to respond after 4 to 8 weeks of levodopa therapy, the diagnosis of Parkinson's is doubtful.**

III. Differential Diagnosis.

A. Essential tremor is a symmetric, fine, rapid, action tremor intensified by a sustained posture such as holding the hands extended at arm's length. It is relieved by alcohol and is usually familial; a head and voice tremor may be prominent. Exam is otherwise normal without other signs of PD. Treatments include propranolol 20 to 60 mg tid, primidone (Mysoline) 50 mg qhs increased slowly to 250 mg tid, topiramate 400 mg/day, or implanted brain stimulator. **Benzodiazepines are generally only modestly, if at all, effective.**

B. Parkinsonism from drugs such as antipsychotics, metoclopramide (Reglan), lithium, methanol, thyroid disease, or carbon monoxide poisoning is usually apparent from the history.

C. "Parkinsonism-plus" syndromes is a catch term for several degenerative disorders that have some of the above features of Parkinson's disease but have other accompanying neurologic signs. These include Shy–Drager syndrome (severe dysautonomia), progressive supranuclear palsy (marked axial rigidity, loss of postural reflexes, vertical gaze paresis with accompanying downgaze abnormalities), striatonigral degeneration (pyramidal involvement, including hyperreflexia and Babinski's sign), diffuse Lewy body disease (early dementia and hallucinations), corticobasal ganglionic degeneration (apraxia, alien limb, and sensory disturbances), multiple system atrophy (a combination of features from the above syndromes plus possibly ataxia and dyssynergia). Levodopa treatment is classically not effective, but a trial may be warranted, because some parkinsonian features might show improvement.

D. Normal-pressure hydrocephalus is characterized by triad of incontinence, dementia, and apraxic gait ("Le marche de petit pas," or magnetic gait). Patients are unable to fully lift their feet off the ground while walking and often trip and fall. Tremor and rigidity are absent (see earlier for details).

E. Miscellaneous causes of parkinsonian-like features include Wilson's disease, prion diseases, HIV, West Nile virus, and tumor or structural lesions.

IV. Treatment.

A. Nonpharmacologic strategies

1. **Support.** Caregivers often suffer from stress, sleep deprivation, depression, and financial hardship. It is important to discuss these issues openly and be prepared to make referrals to social workers and counselors who specialize in chronic illnesses.

2. **Nutrition.** Parkinson's patients often suffer from malnutrition. Establishing good eating habits early in the disease course with ample fiber and calcium is important. Dietary restriction of protein is useful only for patients taking levodopa who experience motor fluctuations (see later).

3. **Exercise.** Although exercise does not alter disease progression, it slows the development of comorbid deterioration.

B. Pharmacologic therapy. Medications should be initiated when patients experience functional impairment such as difficulty with activities of daily living, danger of falling, or losing employment. Which medication to start is controversial and depends on such factors as the severity of disease, age, cognitive status, projected life span, and risk of developing complications of levodopa therapy. Medications should be chosen based on the potency needed and a patient's predicted sensitivity to side effects. Similarly, drugs must be slowly withdrawn. Precipitously stopping dopaminergic drugs can lead to neuroleptic malignant syndrome.

1. **Levodopa (Sinemet)** is the most effective antiparkinson drug. Sinemet is a combination of carbidopa, which minimizes the gastrointestinal side effects, and levodopa, the neurologically active drug. Initially start with Sinemet 25/100 (carbidopa/levodopa) 1/2 tablet qd advancing over a few weeks to a clinically effective dose, typically 1 tablet tid or qid. Alternatively, Sinemet CR (controlled release) offers several advantages: convenient dosing, fewer motor fluctuations, and potentially fewer dyskinesias. Start 50/200 (carbidopa/levodopa) 1/2 tablet qd, advancing slowly to 1 tablet bid. Bioavailability of Sinemet CR is 30% less than immediate-release Sinemet, and switching between drugs might require a dosage adjustment. Patients who fail to respond to high-dose levodopa (1000 mg/day) might not have Parkinson's and are unlikely to respond to other dopaminergic drugs. Recent concerns have centered around the dopaminergic function of levodopa actually contributing to oxidative neurodegeneration, although this is controversial. This combined with the possibility of the development of dyskinesias has prompted most clinicians to use dopamine agonists in the treatment of mild to moderate disease, or with young patients (70 or younger).
   Levodopa has several side effects:
a. **Nausea and vomiting** usually occur from insufficient carbidopa, particularly when taking small doses of Sinemet. Adding more carbidopa (available directly from Dupont Pharmaceuticals at no charge) or increasing the total dose of Sinemet can treat GI symptoms. Antiemetics such as promethazine (Phenergan) can be useful. Avoid phenothiazines (e.g., prochlorperazine [Compazine] and metoclopramide [Reglan]).
b. **Orthostatic hypotension** is common late in the disease. It may also respond to additional carbidopa. If orthostatic hypotension is present early in the disease course, the patient may have multiple-system atrophy (Shy–Drager syndrome; see earlier).
c. **Motor fluctuations** are problematic later in the disease course. First, patients develop **"wearing off"** of the benefits of levodopa before their next dose; later they can develop "on/off phenomena" (unpredictable freezing up). Some patients respond to changing to Sinemet CR or adding a catechol *O*-methyltransferase (COMT) inhibitor that decreases the destruction of dopamine peripherally (see later).

9

NEUROLOGY

d. **Dyskinesias** develop in 50% to 90% of patients who take levodopa for 5 to 10 years. Dyskenesias typically occur at peak dose and are involuntary choreiform movements involving the neck or proximal arms or legs. Dyskinesias may respond to lowering the dose or switching to Sinemet CR.

e. **Psychosis.** Visual hallucinations and delusions are common in the elderly taking dopaminergic drugs. Try to taper off any unnecessary drugs, and consider lowering the levodopa dose. Avoid the standard neuroleptics because they worsen Parkinson's disease. Olanzapine (Zyprexa) 1 to 15 mg qhs, risperidone (Risperdal) 1 to 8 mg qhs, and quetiapine (Seroquel) 25 mg bid can all be effective. Clozapine (Clozaril) 12.5 mg qhs increased to 25 to 75 mg qhs can have remarkable effects but requires weekly CBCs.

2. **Selegiline** (Eldepryl) is a selective MAO-B inhibitor. It has mild dopaminergic effects and possible neuroprotective effects, making it a good choice for early, mild disease. Taking with an SSRI or tricyclic antidepressant can cause a hypertensive crisis, so selegiline must be stopped 2 weeks before starting these drugs. Other side effects include dry mouth, dizziness, syncope, and confusion (especially in the elderly).

3. **Dopamine agonists** work by directly stimulating dopamine receptors. They have a longer duration of action than immediate-release levodopa and offer several therapeutic advantages in the right patient: They may be neuroprotective for dopaminergic neurons for a variety of theoretic reasons; earlier in the disease course, they allow symptomatic relief while sparing the patient the dyskinesia risks of levodopa; later in the disease course, agonists can be added to levodopa to minimize "off time." In advanced disease it may be necessary to add the agonist back to avoid levodopa dosages greater than 600 mg/day and reduce motor fluctuations (see later). Side effects of agonists are similar to those of levodopa: nausea, orthostatic hypotension, and hallucinations. Note that although agonists do not appear to cause dyskinesias in patients naive to levodopa, they can exacerbate them in patients already taking levodopa. Nonergot agonists have more specific binding at the dopamine receptors and are rapidly being embraced by neurologists for early and late Parkinson's therapy. Sleep attacks are a rare idiosyncratic reaction to these drugs.

a. **Ropinirol** (Requip). Start 0.25 mg tid, slowly taper to efficacy or a maximum of 8 mg tid.

b. **Pramipexole** (Mirapex). Start 0.125 mg tid, slowly taper to efficacy or a maximum of 1.5 mg tid.

4. **COMT inhibitors** can reduce "off time" in patients with advanced PD by prolonging the half-life of levodopa. Be prepared to reduce the dose of levodopa by 30% if the patient develops worsened dyskinesias.

a. **Entacapone** (Comtan) 200 mg must be taken with each dose of levodopa up to 1200 mg/day. A combined levodopa, carbidopa, entacapone formulation is now available. No monitoring is required.

b. **Tolcapone** (Tasmar) requires monitoring of liver enzymes weekly for the first 6 months of therapy, then every other week for the duration of therapy because of a small risk of hepatic necrosis. Dose at 200 mg tid. Diarrhea develops in 5% of patients taking tolcapone.

5. **Apomorphine** is a dopamine agonist that is used SQ for **rescue therapy** in patients with substantial motor off-periods. Apomorphine causes nausea and other unpleasant side effects and should be saved for rescue therapy.

6. **Anticholinergics** are useful for improving resting tremor in younger (<70 years) cognitively intact patients. Trihexyphenidyl (Artane) and benztropine (Cogentin) starting dose is 0.5 mg bid. Slowly titrate to efficacy or a maximum dose of 2 mg tid. Side effects are numerous, including urinary retention, confusion, exacerbation of closed-angle glaucoma, and memory and psychiatric disturbances.

7. **Amantadine** (Symmetrel) is an antiviral drug incidentally discovered to have antiparkinsonian benefits. It is sometimes used in early disease with transient benefit ranging from 2 months to 1 year. Late in the disease, amantadine can help reduce dyskinesias. Start 100 mg qod for 1 week and then increase slowly to 100 mg bid or tid. Side effects are similar to other dopamine agonists'. Livedo reticularis and ankle edema can also occur but rarely mandate stopping this drug. Avoid in the elderly because of CNS side effects, and discontinue by taper.

8. **Surgical therapy.** Pallidotomy can provide relief for refractory dyskinesias, and brain stimulators are effective for refractory tremor. Fetal tissue transplantation continues to be an area of research.

V. When to Refer. It is useful to refer the patient to a neurologist at the disease onset to assess for other causes of parkinsonism and confirm the diagnosis. Patients might also need periodic follow-up, especially if complications of therapy arise, especially motor fluctuations, dyskinesias, or freezing.

BENIGN NOCTURNAL LEG CRAMPS

I. Definition and Overview.

A. Definition. A benign muscle cramp is an involuntary, localized, visible, and usually painful skeletal muscle contraction (calf muscles most commonly affected). Cramps are believed to arise from irritability of the motor neuron. The source of the irritability is unknown. Cramps typically occur at night, are sporadic and random, and usually last seconds to minutes.

B. Lifetime incidence is 35% to 95%. It is most common in older adults.

C. Precipitating factors include muscle fatigue and passive plantar flexion.

II. Diagnosis.

A. Predisposing factors can include

1. **Lower motor neuron disease:** polyneuropathy, peripheral nerve injury, radiculopathy, amyotrophic lateral sclerosis (starts with weakness and fasciculations).

9

NEUROLOGY

2. **Altered fluid and electrolyte levels:** hypoglycemia, severe hyponatremia, hypocalcemia, respiratory alkalosis, hypermagnesemia, hypokalemia, hyperkalemia.
3. **Drugs:** nifedipine (Procardia), β-agonists (terbutaline sulfate), clofibrate (Atromid-S), penicillamine (Cuprimine).
4. **Miscellaneous:** alcohol ingestion, thyroid disease, tetany, heat cramps, hemodialysis, dystonias, peripheral vascular disease, and pregnancy.
B. **Physical examination** is generally unrevealing unless a cramp is observed. Look for evidence of peripheral vascular disease, polyneuropathy, nerve injury, muscle wasting, weakness, and fasciculations.

III. **Treatment.**
A. **Acute muscle cramp.** Stretching of the affected muscle (as in walking).
B. **Mechanical prevention.** Advise to stretch calf muscles intermittently throughout the day, use a footboard during sleep, and dangle feet over the edge of bed when lying supine.
C. **Pharmacologic prevention**
1. **Quinine.** The efficacy of quinine sulfate at low doses (such as 300 mg PO qhs) has been supported by several recent analyses. Its use is controversial because of potential side effects, including fatal thrombocytopenia, hypersensitivity reactions, and cardiac arrhythmias.
2. **Other reportedly helpful medications** include vitamin E (800 U/d), verapamil (Calan), carbamazepine (Tegretol), diphenhydramine (Benadryl), phenytoin (Dilantin), methocarbamol (Robaxin), and riboflavin. However, no randomized, controlled studies are found in the literature.

RESTLESS LEGS SYNDROME

I. **Overview.** Restless legs syndrome (RLS) is a common condition afflicting 5% to 15% of the population. It is characterized by dysesthesias and restlessness of the legs and can be associated with other medical conditions. RLS is treatable, although therapy must be individually tailored.
II. **Signs and Symptoms.**
A. **Unpleasant limb sensations.** Sensations are described as crawling, creeping, aching, jittery, or fidgety. Legs are much more commonly effected than the arms (hence the name).
B. **Sensations are precipitated by rest.**
C. **Compelling motor restlessness**. Movement of the limb may briefly relieve the sensation.
D. **Worse at night.** RLS sometimes occurs in the evening or while riding in a car.
E. **Periodic limb movements during sleep.** Patients with RLS often have semirhythmic flexion/extension movements of the foot that occur every 20 to 40 seconds during non-REM sleep.

III. Etiology.

A. The etiology of RLS is unknown; however, familial cases clearly exist. Although no causative link has been established, several medical conditions are known to occur in high frequency in patients with RLS. Symptoms may respond to treatment of the underlying conditions.

B. Among the potential causes are iron deficiency anemia, diabetes mellitus, uremia, pregnancy, rheumatoid arthritis, vitamin deficiencies (e.g., B_{12}, folate), peripheral nerve injury (e.g., polyneuropathy or radiculopathy), and Parkinson's disease.

C. Medications that may contribute to RLS symptomatology include lithium, β-blockers, tricyclic antidepressants, caffeine, alcohol, and histamine blockers. Neuroleptics deserve special mention because they can lead to akathisia, which resembles RLS.

IV. Diagnosis is by history. Consider other conditions that cause nocturnal limb discomfort: benign nocturnal leg cramps (see earlier), peripheral vascular disease, polyneuropathy, fibromyalgia, meralgia paresthetica (burning in the thigh or upper leg secondary to lateral cutaneous nerve entrapment), and drug-induced akathisia. Lab tests detect associated conditions and should include BUN, creatinine, glucose, ferritin, folate, and CBC. Consider ankle brachial indices, EMG, and a sleep study.

V. Treatment.

A. General measures. Limit smoking, alcohol, and caffeine. Discontinue aggravating medications.

B. Treatment of associated conditions can improve RLS.

C. Pharmacologic treatment options

1. **Pramipexole** (Mirapex) is currently first-line therapy due to favorable side-effect profile compared to levodopa. Dose is 0.125 mg q8h increasing to 0.25 mg q8h. Efficacy is supported by a placebo-controlled study. Higher doses may be used if necessary.

2. **Levodopa** (Sinemet) is a proven and effective treatment for RLS. Dose is 25/100 mg (carbidopa/levodopa) 1 hour before bed. If breakthrough symptoms develop in the middle of the night, switch to Sinemet CR 50/200 mg. Commonly, patients taking levodopa begin to develop RLS during the day. If this occurs, switch to a dopamine agonist.

4. **Ropinirole** (Requip). Starting dose 0.25 mg qhs. Increase dose by 2.5 mg/week up to 4 mg qhs. If symptoms are present during the day, ropinirole may be advanced to a maximum dose of 4 mg tid. Efficacy is supported by an open-label trial. Mean effective dose was 2.8 mg/day.

5. **Clonidine** (Catapres) 0.1 to 0.3 mg 1/2 hour before bed. Efficacy is supported by a placebo-controlled study. Higher doses may be used if necessary.

6. **Gabapentin** (Neurontin) 300 mg qhs. May increase to 800 qhs and give additional doses for daytime symptoms to a maximum dose of 800 mg qid. Open-label trials suggest less efficacy than dopamine agonists, but gabapentin is well tolerated and lacks drug interactions.

7. **Clonazepam** (Klonopin) 0.5 to 4.0 mg $1/2$ hour before bed is effective in some patients. It can contribute to nighttime falling and worsening of sleep apnea and is addictive.
8. **Baclofen** was shown in a single study to reduce force and amplitude of restless leg movements, although frequency was increased. The reported dose was 20 to 40mg qhs.

CNS INFECTION

I. **Overview.** Infections of the CNS are broadly classified as meningitis, encephalitis, and abscess. Patients can have more than one type simultaneously (e.g., meningoencephalitis). CNS infections can be difficult to diagnose, and sometimes the survival of the patient relies on a high index of suspicion by the health care provider.

II. **Meningitis.**

A. **Bacterial meningitis is a true medical emergency.** Despite our best care, the overall mortality rate is approximately 25%. The goal is to have IV antibiotics infusing within 30 minutes of presentation. If the LP is going to be delayed (e.g., for CT), administer antibiotics before CT and LP. It is far better for a patient to receive an unnecessary dose of antibiotics than to allow the infection to progress while awaiting test results.

1. **Organisms (Table 9-5).** Common organisms include *Streptococcus pneumoniae, Neisseria meningitidis, Streptococcus agalactiae, Listeria monocytogenes*, and *Haemophilus influenzae. S. agalactiae* primarily affects neonates. *L. monocytogenes* affects people at both extremes of age.

2. **Presentation.** At presentation, the classic triad of headache, fever, and stiff neck is present in only two thirds of cases. However, at least one part of the triad is reliably present. Symptoms generally develop in less than 2 days but in some cases progress over 7 to 10 days. Nausea, vomiting, and photophobia are common. Seizure, decreased mental status, or focal neurologic deficits may also occur.

3. **Examination** should include assessment for papilledema, middle ear and sinus infections, petechiae (common with *N. meningitidis*), nuchal rigidity, and Kernig's sign (knee cannot be extended beyond 135 degrees

TABLE 9-5

AGENTS CAUSING BACTERIAL MENINGITIS

Organism	% of Meningitis Cases	Gram Stain
Streptococcus pneumoniae	47%	Positive cocci
Neisseria meningitidis	25%	Negative cocci in pairs
Streptococcus agalactiae	12%	Positive cocci
Listeria monocytogenes	8%	Positive bacilli
Haemophilus influenzae	7%	Negative bacilli

with hip flexed at 90 degrees). Kernig's and Brudzinski's signs are present in only 9%.

4. **Laboratory exam.** Always draw blood for cultures. A spinal fluid exam should be performed as soon as possible. A brain CT before LP is not necessary if the patient is alert, has no papilledema, has no focal neurologic finding, is HIV negative, and probably does not have a subarachnoid hemorrhage. If neuroimaging is necessary, draw blood and begin antibiotics before the study. Spinal fluid should be sent for cell count, WBC differential, glucose, protein, culture, and Gram stain. Acid-fast bacilli stain and cryptococcal antigen may be obtained when indicated. If subarachnoid hemorrhage is also suspected, xanthochromia should be sought and cell counts should be sent on tubes 1 and 4. As soon as spinal fluid is obtained, start antibiotics. CSF results are listed in **(Table 9-6).** Latex agglutination studies (for *H. influenzae* type b, *S. pneumoniae, N. meningitidis, E. coli* K1, and the group B streptococci) have good specificity but limited sensitivity, so do not defer treatment based on a negative latex agglutination study.

5. **Treatment.** Treatment of bacterial meningitis generally must begin before the causative organism is identified. Generally, broad-spectrum therapy with vancomycin and ceftriaxone is initiated. Other factors affecting treatment are the patient's age and immunocompetency and the local prevalence of cephalosporin-resistant strains of *S. pneumoniae.* Often, a phone call to the hospital's infectious disease specialist is helpful.

a. **Antibiotics (Table 9-7).** As information about Gram stain, species identification, and resistance becomes available, the therapy should be narrowed.

b. **Steroids.** Unless there is a contraindication, most patients with meningitis should receive steroids. Outcomes are better in both children and adults who receive steroids regardless of whether the organism is *H. influenzae* or *S. pneumoniae.* Dose is 0.15 mg/kg IV q6h × 4 days

9

NEUROLOGY

TABLE 9-6
CEREBROSPINAL FLUID FINDINGS IN LUMBAR PUNCTURE

Condition	Protein (mg/dL)	Glucose (mg/dL)	WBC (number/mm³)
Normal	15-45	45-80	≤5 lymphocytes
Bacterial meningitis	100-500	0-40	50-10,000, chiefly neutrophils
Herpes encephalitis	15-150	Normal	50-200, chiefly lymphocytes (also ≤10000 RBCs)
Viral meningitis or encephalitis	20-200	Normal	10-500, chiefly lymphocytes; neutrophils may dominate in acute phase
Tuberculous meningitis	45-500	10-45	25-1000, chiefly lymphocytes
Cryptococcal meningitis	<500 in 90%	Moderately decreased in 55%	<800, chiefly lymphocytes

TABLE 9-7
EMPIRICAL TREATMENT OF BACTERIAL MENINGITIS

Clinical Setting	Antimicrobial Therapy
0-4 weeks of age	Ampicillin + cefotaxime; or ampicillin + aminoglycoside
4-12 weeks of age	Ampicillin + ceftriaxone
3 mo to 18 years of age	Ceftriaxone (+/– vancomycin) or ampicillin plus chloramphenicol
18 to 50 years of age	Ceftriaxone (+/– vancomycin)
>50 years of age	Ampicillin + ceftriaxone (+/– vancomycin)
Immunocompromised state	Vancomycin + ampicillin + ceftazidime
Basilar skull fracture	Ceftriaxone (+/– vancomycin)
Head trauma; post neurosurgery	Vancomycin + ceftazidime
Cerebrospinal fluid shunt	Vancomycin + ceftazidime
Gram stain (most likely agent)	
Positive cocci (*S. pneumoniae*)	Ceftriaxone (+/– vancomycin)
Positive bacilli (*L. monocytogenes*)	Ampicillin or penicillin G + aminoglycoside
Negative cocci (*N. meningitidis*)	Penicillin G
Negative bacilli (*H. influenzae*)	Ceftazidime

Note: Many authors recommend adding vancomycin to initial therapy given the prevalence of resistant *Pneumococcus*.

    in children, 10 mg IV q6h × 4 days in adults. The first dose of steroid should precede antibiotics by 15 to 20 minutes if possible, but don't delay antibiotics therapy in the sick patient!

c. **Prophylaxis.** Direct contacts of patients with *N. meningitidis* infection should receive rifampin 20 mg/kg not to exceed 600 mg bid for 2 days or ciprofloxacin 500 mg as a single dose or ceftriaxone 250 mg IM as a single dose. For those exposed to *H. influenzae* meningitis, use rifampin 20 mg/kg not to exceed 600 mg qd for 4 days.

B. **Viral meningitis** manifests similarly to bacterial meningitis, although its course is rarely aggressive and its presentation is more benign. Consciousness is usually only mildly impaired, if at all, and the fever is low grade. The diagnostic process and exam is similar to that for bacterial meningitis.

1. **Organisms.** The most common causes of viral meningitis are enteroviruses, herpes simplex virus, and HIV.

2. **Presentation.** In addition to fever, photophobia, headache, myalgias, and nausea, the diagnosis of viral meningitis may be suggested by associated signs, including genital lesions (herpes simplex type 2), diarrhea, or a maculopapular rash (enteroviruses).

3. **Diagnosis** is made by the history, exam, and spinal fluid results. Early in the course, the CSF may show a predominantly neutrophilic inflammatory response. This necessitates hospitalization and IV antibiotics until cultures return negative. Consider HIV testing.

4. **Treatment is symptomatic.** If genital lesions are also present or there is another reason to suspect herpes meningitis, consider acyclovir.

III. Encephalitis is characterized by prominent changes in mental status, headache, seizures, and sometimes focal neurologic deficits.

A. Bacterial encephalitis is rare and usually occurs in the setting of meningoencephalitis. Agents known to invade brain parenchyma include *Listeria monocytogenes, Rickettsia rickettsii* (Rocky Mountain spotted fever from ticks), leptospirosis (from animal urine), and the ameba *Naegleria fowleri* (from swimming). Treatment is directed at the causative agent.

B. Viral encephalitis

1. **Mosquito-borne** West Nile, St. Louis, eastern equine, and western equine viruses are all causes of encephalitides found in the United States. They are characterized by a decreased mental status, fever, seizures, and sometimes other focal neurologic deficits.

2. **West Nile virus (WNV) deserves special mention.** WNV, a mosquito-borne Flavivirus, arrived in the United States in 1999 and has since become endemic. Transmission by blood transfusion and organ donation has occurred. **West Nile should be strongly considered in patients with an unexplained fever, meningitis, or encephalitis presentation in the late summer or early fall.**

a. **Incubation** is 3 to 14 days. **Only 20% of infected patients develop symptoms and only half of these seek medical care.**

b. **Symptoms**

   (1) The majority of symptomatic patients develop a flulike syndrome with fever, malaise, myalgias, anorexia, nausea, vomiting, eye pain, and headache (from a mild viral meningitis). This syndrome lasts for 3 to 6 days before resolving. About 20% have a nonpruritic maculopapular rash of the chest, back, and arms.

   (2) **Severe neurologic illness develops in 1 in 150 infected persons,** including encephalitis, seizures, high fevers, paralysis, or a Guillain-Barré–like illness. **Box 9-6** lists neurologic manifestations of WNV. **Risk factors for neurologic disease include age older than 50 years, immunosuppression, and other debilitating illness.**

c. **Laboratory findings.** IgM in the CSF is present in 90% at 8 days, and eventually 95% of symptomatic persons have an IgM response

---

BOX 9-6

MANIFESTATIONS OF WEST NILE VIRUS

Headache, mental status changes

50% have severe weakness

10% have flaccid paralysis similar to Guillain-Barré (e.g., areflexia, dysesthesias)

Movement disorders: including myoclonus, intention tremor (not resting), and parkinsonism (bradykinesia, postural instability, cogwheeling)

Optic neuritis, radiculopathy, seizures, cranial nerve (e.g., facial weakness) findings, ataxia

Other involvement: myocarditis, pancreatitis, rhabdomyolysis, etc.

in the blood. These antibodies cross-react with St. Louis and Japanese encephalitis. CSF might show a lymphocytic pleocytosis, elevated protein, and normal glucose. Viral culture and PCR have low yields because viremia is short lived and is rare beyond day 1 of symptoms.

d. **Treatment.** As with the other mosquito-borne encephalitides, treatment is symptomatic and can require ICU support for ventilation.

e. **Outcomes.** Mortality is 1:1000 persons overall, and 5% to 14% of those with encephalitis succumb. More than 50% of survivors note residual symptoms such as fatigue, memory loss, gait disturbance, or weakness; 38% note depression. Only a third of those with encephalitis are able to return to their baseline activities.

3. **Herpes simplex** accounts for 10% of encephalitis cases; it is a devastating but treatable CNS infection.

a. **Presentation.** Acute onset of decreased mental status, headache, possibly seizures and disturbances of language, memory, or behavior.

b. **Diagnosis.** CSF usually shows a lymphocytic pleocytosis. Occasionally CSF WBC is normal. RBC is often dramatically elevated and misinterpreted as a traumatic tap. PCR of the CSF has replaced brain biopsy and is now the standard test for diagnosing HSV encephalitis. MRI shows inflammation of the temporal lobes and is the best means of early diagnosis. EEG may be helpful. CT with contrast is less sensitive than MRI but will be positive in most cases of HSV encephalitis.

c. **Treatment.** Begin acyclovir immediately in all patients with encephalitis until the diagnosis of HSV is either confirmed or excluded. Dose is 10 mg/kg IV q8h × 14 days. Monitor renal function during treatment.

IV. Brain Abscess. Most commonly, brain abscesses arise from traumatic or hematogenous spread of infection. They can also occur from contiguous spread of a suppurative process such as sinusitis or otitis media.

A. Presentation is variable and can include focal neurologic signs, seizures, headache, and indicators of systemic infection.

B. Diagnosis is made by neuroimaging with contrast. Needle aspiration confirms the diagnosis. Lumbar puncture is contraindicated and can lead to abscess rupture. The diagnosis of brain abscess mandates other studies seeking the etiology, which can include HIV serology, sinus studies, and transesophageal echocardiogram.

C. Treatment is directed by the clinical setting and includes IV antibiotics and sometimes neurosurgical evacuation.

CEREBROVASCULAR DISEASE

I. Overview. Cerebrovascular disease annually affects 500,000 Americans, killing 30% of those afflicted, making it the third most common cause of death. The surviving 70% of stroke patients often suffer significant disability, further underscoring the importance of proper medical treatment and prevention of cerebrovascular disease.

II. Classification.

A. **Transient ischemic attacks (TIAs)** are an interruption of perfusion in a vascular territory typically lasting between 2 and 20 minutes, causing focal neurologic deficits. **Risk of ischemic stroke is about 10% in the first week and 20% in the first month after a TIA. Thus prompt evaluation is required.** Patients who present within 48 hours of onset with TIA symptoms should be admitted to the hospital for evaluation.

B. **Ischemic stroke** accounts for 70% of strokes. It can be secondary to a large number of diseases resulting in thrombosis or embolic occlusion of a cerebral artery.

C. **Hemorrhagic stroke.** Fifteen percent to 20% of all strokes result from a breach in the vascular tree, allowing a hematoma to form in the brain tissue. Hemorrhagic transformation of an ischemic stroke can occur after large infarctions or with heparin or tPA therapy.

D. **Subarachnoid hemorrhage** typically results from aneurysmal bleeding in the subarachnoid space and results in the sudden onset of severe headache, **usually without focal neurologic deficits** such as paralysis. Nausea, vomiting, and alterations in consciousness are often prominent. SAH accounts for 5% to 10% of strokes, with a 40% overall mortality rate and a 60% mortality rate with recurrent bleeding. Approximately 40% of survivors are disabled. Early diagnosis is critical. See also section on headaches earlier in this chapter.

III. Presentation.

A. **TIAs and ischemic stroke.** All cerebrovascular events are characterized by sudden onset over seconds to minutes. TIAs and strokes are typified by neurologic function loss such as weakness, anesthesia, incoordination, loss of vision, aphasia, and dysarthria. Occasionally, headache or vertigo may occur.

B. **Hemorrhagic stroke** is also typified by loss of function, but headache, nausea, and vomiting are common. **Hemorrhagic stroke cannot be accurately differentiated from ischemic stroke without CT scanning.**

IV. Differential Diagnosis.

A. **TIAs.** Episodes without abrupt onset and termination are rarely TIAs. Other considerations include hypoglycemia, hypotension, delirium, postictal state, and migraine aura.

B. **Stroke.** Differential includes hypoglycemia, head trauma, subdural and epidural hematomas, MS, postictal state, delirium, tumor, brain abscess, and radiculopathy.

C. **SAH.** Main differential diagnosis is migraine headache and meningitis. In migraine there is usually a prior history. The consequences of missing SAH and CNS infection are so grave that the clinician should err on the side of performing a diagnostic work-up (including CT and lumbar puncture) in all questionable headaches.

V. Emergency Evaluation and Treatment.

A. **TIAs.** Patients with TIAs should generally be admitted for observation. Brain CT without contrast should be performed (see discussions of etiology and prevention later). Deficits lasting beyond 20 minutes are likely to progress to infarction and should be approached as strokes. **The efficacy of IV heparin in TIAs is unproven and use is contraindicated.**

B. **Ischemic stroke.** History, examination, and brain CT are essential components of the initial stroke evaluation. Patients being treated within 3 hours of symptom onset should be emergently considered for tPA. Organize the health care team early. A neurologist should be contacted when a possible tPA candidate arrives. A radiologist or neurologist should be available to read the CT because of limited sensitivity in detecting hemorrhages among physicians who do not routinely read these studies. A systematic approach is essential for a prompt, thorough evaluation. The tPA checklist is recommended **(Box 9-7)**. **Most studies of thrombolytics in stroke are negative, and tPA is not without**

BOX 9-7
STROKE CHECK LIST FOR tPA

- **Onset <3 h.** Time of onset must be definitively known. Strokes recognized upon waking are assumed to have occurred at onset of sleep.
- **Labs.** Several parameters must be normal prior to thrombolytic therapy. When patient arrives, send stat glucose, INR, aPTT, electrolytes, and CBC. Note that coagulation studies take a minimum of 30 min to complete.
- **Exam.** Initially should be brief and pertinent. NIH stroke scale (NIHSS) provides a quick reliable means of classifying a stroke's severity.* Also assess for meningeal signs, evidence of head trauma, fractures, and dislocations.
- **Head CT without contrast.** Allows the exclusion of hemorrhagic strokes and subdural and epidural hematomas.
- **ECG.** Assess for concurrent myocardial infarction.
- **Blood Pressure Control.** Use IV labetalol to reduce SBP to <185 and DBP to <110. Be judicious with blood pressure control. Suddenly lowering the blood pressure below 185/110 is risky and can be associated with stroke progression secondary to decreased perfusion. **This reflects requirements for tPA; see note below on lowering BP in ischemic stroke.**
- **Informed consent.** Often stroke patients are aphasic. Do not lose contact with the next-of-kin. Overall the risk of serious hemorrhagic transformation of ischemic stroke is approximately 1 in 16 patients.
- **Other exclusion criteria:** Glucose <50; platelet count <100,000; INR >1.4; aPTT >2 sec above upper limit; trauma, surgery, myocardial infarction, or GI bleed within 2 wk; head trauma or other stroke within 6 wk; suspicion of SAH; CT demonstrating acute stroke involving more than on third of a hemisphere; NIHSS <3 or >22.
- **tPA dose:** 0.9 mg/kg up to total of 80 mg. Give 10% IV bolus over 5 min followed by infusion of the remaining drug over 1 h.
- **If neurosurgical support is not available on site,** arrange for fastest possible travel to tertiary care facility immediately after tPA infusion is completed.

*Available at http://www.ninds.nih.gov/doctors/index.htm.

substantial risk; however, it has gained a wide acceptance as a
treatment. Be sure to get informed consent.

1. **Heparin.** Few therapies are more controversial in neurology than
   IV heparin in acute ischemic stroke. No definitive studies have shown a
   clear benefit to using IV heparin, and adverse effects such as hemorrhagic
   transformation of stroke are common. For this reason, the use of
   IV heparin in stroke is not recommended. It certainly should not be
   used with tPA. Subcutaneous heparin (5000 U SQ q12h) is clearly
   beneficial for the prevention of DVTs in patients with ischemic stroke.
2. **Intraarterial thrombolysis** is currently being used as therapy for ischemic
   strokes of the anterior circulation that manifest after 3 hours but before
   6 hours or with posterior circulation strokes (time window is variable).
3. **Aspirin** (325 mg) should be started in those with ischemic stroke within
   24 hours of the event. Ticlopidine is an alternative in those who are
   aspirin allergic.
4. **Blood pressure control in ischemic stroke.** Unless SBP is >220 mm
   Hg and DBP is >120 mm Hg or MAP >120 mm Hg, **treatment is not
   indicated.** Lowering blood pressure actually worsens outcomes.
   **Generally, withholding antihypertensives for 10 days after an
   ischemic stroke is prudent unless there is some other indication for
   lowering the BP such as CAD or aortic dissection.** Blood pressure
   does need to be lowered in the tPA candidate (see Box 9-1).

C. **Hemorrhagic stroke (intracerebral hemorrhage).** The diagnosis is
   confirmed by brain CT. If the hemorrhage exerts significant mass effect
   or extends into the ventricular system, or if there is a clotting deficiency,
   a neurosurgical consultation should be obtained. BP should be monitored
   closely and treated somewhat more aggressively than with ischemic
   stroke. **Treat BP if SBP is >140, MAP is >120, or DBP is >100.
   Perfusion pressure (relative to the intracranial pressure) should be
   maintained above 60 mm Hg. If the patient deteriorates, the blood
   pressure may be too low to maintain cerebral perfusion.** Maintain
   systolic pressure at > 90 mm Hg at all times. If the patient is taking
   warfarin, reverse anticoagulation with fresh frozen plasma. Avoid any
   anticoagulants. Factor VIIa 40 to 160 μg/kg can be given within 3 hours
   of onset of bleed but is expensive and does not substantially change
   outcomes (NNT = 60).

D. **SAH** is usually evident on CT as blood surrounding the midbrain. If CT
   is negative but there is a clinical suspicion, an LP is required to exclude
   SAH. If the diagnosis is confirmed, an emergent neurosurgical consultation
   is necessary. Pending this evaluation, BP should be lowered if
   SBP is >140, MAP is >120, or DBP is >100 using labetalol **in the alert
   patient. Neurologic symptoms could be due to decreased cerebral
   perfusion, and less aggressive BP management is then indicated. See
   section on headache for further details on diagnosis and evaluation of
   SAH.** Prophylactic measures to prevent seizures (e.g., IV phenytoin) are
   often recommended. This reduces seizure occurrence in the first week
   following the event (NNT = 10 to prevent one seizure) but has no effect

9

NEUROLOGY

on long-term outcome. Screening of asymptomatic relatives of patients with SAH for an aneurysm is not generally helpful because the rate of morbidity and mortality from surgical repair is the same as that of watchful waiting.

VI. Supportive Care of Stroke.

A. Blood pressure. See specific section (ischemic, SAH, intracerebral hemorrhage) for information on the role of BP control.

B. Free water should be limited to 1200 mL in the first 48 hours of stroke. If IV fluids are needed, use isotonic saline. Free water increases the risk of edema in the infarcted brain tissue.

C. Ancillary services. Physical therapy, speech pathology, occupational therapy, and a social worker should be involved early in care.

D. Prevention of complications. Frequent turning in bed may be necessary to prevent skin ulcers. A swallowing study should be done to evaluate for aspiration. A feeding tube may be necessary to safely deliver medications and nutrition. Compression stockings or subcutaneous heparin should be employed to prevent DVTs.

VII. Uncovering the Etiology. Determining the etiology of the stroke is helpful for guiding future stroke prevention. Studies are tailored to the case in question.

A. Chest x-ray assesses cardiac size and screens for pulmonary complications.

B. ECG is useful for diagnosing atrial fibrillation, atrial enlargement, and myocardial infarction. Telemetry may be necessary, especially among patients with hemorrhages, because there is a direct myocardial depressant effect from CNS illness that can cause CHF. Additionally, arrhythmias can occur.

C. Echocardiogram. Transesophageal echocardiogram is useful to exclude vegetations, shunts, and intracardiac thrombi. This should be performed on most patients without other clear etiology for ischemic stroke.

D. Carotid duplex should be performed in all patients with ischemic stroke who would potentially be candidates for carotid endarterectomy. Endovascular stenting of the carotid is an alternative in patients who are at high surgical or anesthesia risks.

E. Fasting lipid profile should be checked in all stroke patients 3 months after the event.

F. Coagulation studies should be undertaken in patients younger than 55 years without other clear risk factors for stroke. In the acute setting, draw activated protein C resistance, prothrombin gene rearrangement, and factor V Leiden. Draw protein C, protein S, and antithrombin III after 3 months, because these will be falsely depressed in the acute period.

G. MRI is helpful for diagnosing small strokes, tumors, and lesions in the posterior fossa.

H. Cerebral angiogram is reserved for subarachnoid hemorrhage, nonhypertensive cerebral hemorrhages, and cases of suspected vasculitis, and perhaps in young patients without other known etiology.

VIII. Preventing TIAs and Stroke. Aspirin and clopidogrel are equally effective at preventing stroke; there is no benefit to clopidogrel versus aspirin in preventing strokes.

A. Aspirin 81 or 325 mg is the primary first-line therapy for prevention of TIAs and non–cardioembolic ischemic strokes.

B. Clopidogrel (Plavix) 75 mg qd is suitable for patients who failed or are intolerant of aspirin. A 300-mg loading dose is required for immediate antiplatelet effect. A 75-mg/day dose regimen takes 3 or 4 days to become effective.

C. Aggrenox (aspirin 25 mg plus sustained-release dipyridamole 200 mg) bid is also suitable for patients who failed aspirin alone. The principal side effect is headache. Patients may require supplemental ASA. Dipyridamole is considered second line after ASA and clopidogrel.

D. Ticlopidine (Ticlid) is discouraged because of risk of thrombotic thrombocytopenic purpura (which is less common with clopidogrel).

E. Dual platelet inhibitor therapy (e.g., ASA plus clopidogrel). Data have shown that **dual therapy with ASA and clopidogrel does not confer any added protection against stroke compared with clopidogrel alone and increases the risk of GI bleeding.** Therefore, in the event of ASA failure, patients should stop taking aspirin before starting on clopidogrel.

F. ACE inhibitors. Independent of their effect on blood pressure, ACE inhibitors are emerging as an important class of drugs to lower the risk of stroke, possibly through a direct effect on the cerebral vasculature.

G. Warfarin anticoagulation should only be considered in patients with known cardioembolic sources.

H. Lipid-lowering drugs and diet modification should be aggressively pursued in stroke patients with elevated lipids (see Chapter 3).

I. Hypertension requires careful control in the outpatient setting to lower the risk of future strokes. Unless otherwise indicated, preferentially use an ACE inhibitor (see Chapter 3).

J. Carotid endarterectomy is appropriate for good surgical candidates with 50% stenosis in a symptomatic arterial distribution or 60% in an asymptomatic distribution, provided the surgeon has a documented track record of a less than 3% complication rate.

K. Tobacco consumption is a strong risk factor for stroke and **should be stopped.**

NEUROLOGY 9

NEUROPATHY

I. Overview. *Neuropathy* is an umbrella term for nonradicular diseases of the peripheral nerves. Neuropathy can be acute and life threatening as in Guillain-Barré syndrome or chronic as in diabetic neuropathy. Assessment of the patient seeks to define the time course of the disease, identify which nerves are involved, and, if possible, determine the underlying cause.

II. Classification.

A. Anatomic classification

1. **Mononeuropathy** is involvement of a single nerve (e.g., carpal tunnel syndrome, meralgia paresthetica).
2. **Polyneuropathy** is diffuse involvement of the peripheral nerves (e.g., diabetic neuropathy).
3. **Mononeuritis multiplex** is seemingly random involvement of multiple isolated nerves. It can occur in vasculitis, porphyria, diabetes, HIV, and others. **Patients with mononeuritis multiplex may present with a stocking-and-glove pattern of symptoms and might not have noticed their symptoms until this point.**

B. Cellular classification

1. **Axonal neuropathy** is loss of function from loss of nerve cells. It typically affects the longest nerves first; patients describe loss of sensation or paresthesias of the feet. Axonal neuropathy is usually symmetric, although it can be asymmetric early in the course. Weakness occurs late, tends to involve the most distal muscles, and tends to progress over weeks to months. Neuropathy preferentially affects the small nerve fibers first, resulting in painful paresthesias and burning sensations. Pain and temperature sensation may be lost. Small-fiber axonal neuropathy can also result in dysautonomia.
2. **Demyelinating neuropathy** is damage to the Schwann cells, leading to impairment of nerve conduction. It can manifest acutely by severe weakness (Guillain-Barré) or more progressively (chronic inflammatory demyelinating polyneuropathy [CIDP]). Weakness tends to involve both proximal and distal muscles and predominates over sensory loss. Pain is not as common as in axonal neuropathy, and sensory changes can be manifested by loss of vibration and position sense.

III. Localization.

A. Muscle. Proximal arm and leg weakness (difficulty getting out of the car, climbing stairs, taking objects out of overhead cupboards). Muscle weakness is usually symmetric, with spared sensation and reflexes.

B. Neuromuscular junction. Fatigability of muscles, with waxing and waning complaints of weakness. Weakness tends to be worse in the evenings and can be accompanied by diplopia and dysarthria. Repetitive strength testing tends to cause significant proximal muscle weakness.

C. Peripheral nerve. Weakness is usually more distal than peripheral and may be accompanied by fasciculations and atrophy. Sensory symptoms usually tend to be symmetric (stocking-and-glove) except in the case of mononeuropathy multiplex. Patients often complain of pins-and-needles sensation or distal burning. Patient usually presents with distal weakness that is asymmetric (think foot/wrist drop). Reflexes tend to be depressed.

D. Nerve root/plexus. Patients often present with symptoms of pain and asymmetric weakness, usually in the distribution of a myotome. Sensory changes in a dermatomal pattern are also usually present, sometimes described as an electric sensation shooting down the affected limb.

Can be confused with peripheral neuropathy due to asymmetry of symptoms. Atrophy and fasciculations can also be present.

E. Spinal cord. Hyperactive reflexes (reflexes can be absent early in the course), bandlike sensation at level of cord injury, sensory level at or above level of cord injury, Babinski's sign, urinary incontinence or retention, loss of rectal tone.

F. Brain. Hyperactive reflexes, higher order sensory loss (stereognosis, two-point discrimination), loss of higher cognitive functions.

IV. Diagnosis.

A. Careful history should elicit the onset and rate of progression of symptoms. Assess for other medical problems, medications, and toxic exposures (see below for details). Inquire about weakness and autonomic dysfunction (erectile dysfunction, bladder disturbances, and orthostasis). Ask what sensory modalities are involved. Have the patient draw a line on the skin to separate areas of normal and abnormal sensation.

B. Physical exam includes cranial nerves, proximal and distal strength, reflexes, gait, Romberg's sign and sensation to pin, monofilament nylon (described under diabetes in Chapter 5), 128-Hz vibration, and position.

C. Laboratory testing

1. **Tests for all patients with unexplained neuropathy** include CBC, glucose tolerance test, Vitamin B_{12}, rheumatoid factor, TSH, free T_4, sedimentation rate, CRP, ANA, and serum protein electrophoresis with immunofixation. If monoclonal gammopathy is present, obtain quantitative immunoglobulins, urine protein electrophoresis, and skeletal x-ray survey.

2. **Other tests to consider strongly** include HIV antibody, VDRL, Lyme titer, and lumbar puncture.

3. **Tests useful in the proper clinical setting** include folate, urine heavy-metal screen, ganglioside antibodies (GM1, anti-MAG, antisulfatide), and paraneoplastic antibodies (anti-Hu).

4. **Ganglioside antibodies** can be found in multifocal motor neuropathy (positive in 80%-90%). This is a demyelinating neuropathy that is characterized by slowly progressive, asymmetric weakness that generally begins in the hands and the distal musculature rather than the proximal musculature. There are generally no or few sensory findings, and ALS can be excluded from the differential by the absence of hyperreflexia and spasticity.

5. **Paraneoplastic syndromes** are associated with a neoplasm (especially ovarian, lung, breast) and include Eaton–Lambert syndrome, which is manifested by weakness that improves with muscle use. Patients can have anti–presynaptic calcium channel (anti-PCC) antibodies. Some paraneoplastic syndromes are sensory neuropathies associated with anti-Hu antibodies; others are related to CNS injury (especially cerebellar degeneration associated with anti-Yo, anti-Hu, and anti-Ri antibodies). Some paraneoplastic syndromes are indistinguishable from Guillain-Barré syndrome.

9

NEUROLOGY

D. Electromyography and nerve-conduction studies are helpful to confirm a clinical impression. They can often differentiate a radiculopathy from a neuropathy and can classify a primarily axonal from a primarily demyelinating process. Electromyographers function best when asked specific questions; for example, "Is this carpal tunnel syndrome, C6 radiculopathy, or asymmetric polyneuropathy?"

E. Nerve biopsy is undertaken only when etiology remains unknown after electrodiagnostic and other laboratory tests have been completed.

V. Common and Important Neuropathies.

A. Guillain-Barré syndrome can be immediately life threatening and deserves special attention.

1. **General.** GBS is an acute immune-mediated demyelinating polyneuropathy. It manifests with progressive, usually symmetric, weakness over a span of 2 days to 4 weeks. Weakness progresses from distal to proximal. Sensory disturbances are variable. Often a history of a recent respiratory or GI illness (especially *Campylobacter jejuni*) can be elicited. In addition to weakness, physical exam is remarkable for absent reflexes.

2. **Lab studies.** Electrodiagnostic studies confirm the clinical impression, although these may be normal in the acute setting. The first nerve conduction abnormalities are usually noted 4 to 5 days after the onset of the disease. LP, usually showing elevated CSF protein, provides additional evidence. Some patients may also be anti-GM1 positive (see above).

3. **Pulmonary.** Patients with GBS can undergo acute pulmonary decompensation, and overall 33% require ventilatory support. Even patients with mild symptoms should be admitted for a minimum of 24 hours. **Forced vital capacity or negative inspiratory force (NIF) should be assessed every 2 to 4 hours until patients prove pulmonary stability. Patients with an FVC <20 cc/kg or NIF less forceful than −30 should be transferred to the ICU.** Elective intubation should also be discussed at this point in case of further worsening. ABG and pulse oximetry are insensitive to impending decompensation.

4. **Treatment.** IVIG or plasma exchanges may shorten the course of GBS. IVIG is more convenient and less invasive, and is therefore the preferred treatment modality if patients have the cardiovascular and renal capacity to tolerate a large osmotic protein load. If the patient has a diagnosis of congestive heart failure or renal insufficiency, plasma exchange may be preferred. Plasma exchange following recent IVIG treatment is not recommended.

B. Diabetic neuropathy is the most common cause of diffuse polyneuropathy. It arises in half of all diabetics, and the neuropathy is primarily axonal. It can manifest in the form of mononeuropathy multiplex. Tight glucose control reduces the risk of developing neuropathy and can help halt progression. Some patients continue to progress despite tight control. Immunologic therapy is under investigation.

C. **Carpal tunnel syndrome.** See Chapter 16.

D. **Hereditary neuropathies.** Charcot–Marie–Tooth (CMT) encompasses a group of largely autosomal dominant neuropathies. Both axonal (CMT type 2) and demyelinating (CMT type 1 and CMT X-linked) forms exist. Onset often occurs during adulthood. Patients have a stocking-and-glove sensory loss and distal weakness. Slender hands and feet and high arches (pes cavus) typify the physical exam. In addition to electrodiagnostic tests, genetic testing is available. Treatment is symptomatic.

E. **Drug-induced neuropathies.** Nitrofurantoin, dapsone, metronidazole, isoniazid, disulfiram, amiodarone, vincristine, cisplatin, paclitaxel, phenytoin, chloramphenicol, hydralazine, and high-dose pyridoxine (vitamin B_6) can all lead to neuropathies.

F. **Environmental toxins.** Lead is the most common environmental toxin and is usually associated with gastric distress, anemia, and radial nerve symptoms (weakness of finger and wrist extension). Inquire about recent work in radiator shops, battery factories, etc. Remote exposure to lead is rarely responsible for a neuropathy. Diagnosis is confirmed by 24-hour urine heavy-metal testing.

G. **Malnutrition.** Vitamin B_{12} deficiency leads to dysfunction in several areas of the nervous system, including a predominantly axonal neuropathy, dementia, and spasticity. A macrocytic anemia may or may not be present. Serum B_{12} testing usually confirms the diagnosis. If results are low normal, consider a Schilling test. Deficiencies of vitamin B_6 (pyridoxine), vitamin E, niacin, and folate are rare causes of neuropathy.

H. **Alcoholic neuropathy.** Controversy exists as to whether isolated alcoholism is sufficient to lead to a neuropathy. Usually there is comorbid malnutrition, with concomitant B_{12} and folate deficiencies. Macrocytic anemia is common. The neuropathy is predominately axonal and characterized by distal weakness, stocking-and-glove sensory loss, and unsteady gait.

I. **Collagen vascular diseases** can lead to a vasculitic neuropathy. Nerves infarct, resulting in an axonal neuropathy. Mononeuritis multiplex may lead to a confluent stocking-and-glove neuropathy. Screen with an ESR, CRP, ANA, and rheumatoid factor. Consider a referral to a neuromuscular specialist for possible nerve biopsy.

J. **Infectious causes.** Lyme disease, HIV, syphilis, and leprosy can all lead to neuropathy. Consider testing in the appropriate setting.

K. **Chronic inflammatory demyelinating polyradiculoneuropathy (CIDP)** is a progressive neuropathy with prominent weakness of the proximal and distal musculature leading to difficulty rising from a chair and an unsteady gait. Diagnosis is made by electrodiagnostic studies and LP, which shows an elevated total protein and a normal cell count. CIDP can herald a plasma cell dyscrasia, and the workup should include a skeletal survey and both urine and serum protein electrophoresis with immunofixation. Consider a hematologic consultation. Treatment is with IVIG or prednisone.

9

NEUROLOGY

L. Other metabolic neuropathies include symptomatic thyroid disease, porphyria, and renal or hepatic failure.

VI. Treatment. Symptomatic treatment of neuropathy pain and paresthesias is directed at reducing the pain. Possible treatments include amitriptyline (Elavil) 10 to 75 mg hs, nortriptyline (Pamelor) 10 to 100 mg hs, gabapentin (Neurontin) 400 mg hs to 800 mg tid, and carbamazepine (Tegretol) 200 to 400 mg tid. Capsaicin cream has also been used with some success.

MULTIPLE SCLEROSIS

I. Overview. MS typically begins in early adulthood and is characterized by multiple areas of demyelination and sclerosis of the brain or spinal cord, or both. The cause is unknown and the familial incidence is low. Whites are more susceptible than blacks and Asians. Pregnancy decreases the risk of exacerbations, but exacerbations increase immediately postpartum. Infection or trauma can trigger exacerbations.

II. Clinical Manifestations.

A. MS is characterized by episodes of focal neurologic dysfunction separated in both space and time. Onset of symptoms is usually acute and worsens over a few days. Symptoms can last up to several weeks followed by either partial or full resolution. Later, other deficits appear that again show a waxing and waning course.

B. Common symptoms include weakness or numbness of a limb, monocular vision loss, diplopia, vertigo, facial weakness or numbness, sphincter disturbances, ataxia, and nystagmus. A history of symptoms aggravated by a hot bath is sometimes obtained.

C. MS is classically divided into two forms:

1. **Relapsing remitting MS.** Episodes fully resolve with good neurologic function between exacerbations. Accumulation of deficits is slow over decades, if at all.

2. **Chronic progressive MS.** Episodes fail to fully resolve, and deficits accumulate steadily. Relapsing remitting MS can convert to chronic progressive MS.

III. Laboratory Tests. About 90% of patients have abnormal findings in CSF that include a mild mononuclear pleocytosis, a modest increase in total protein, a greatly increased γ-globulin fraction, a high IgG index, presence of oligoclonal bands, and an increase in myelin basic protein. **MRI with gadolinium enhancement** is highly sensitive and differentiates old from new lesions. Visual evoked responses are abnormal in 80% of patients with definite MS.

IV. Differential Diagnosis. Behçet's disease, SLE, metastatic tumors, vascular malformations, Arnold–Chiari malformation, herniated intervertebral disk, spinocerebellar degeneration, CNS vasculitis, primary CNS lymphoma, Lyme disease, HIV encephalitis and progressive multifocal leukoencephalopathy, and multiple strokes.

V. Prognosis. One study showed that a 25-year mortality rate was about 26% compared with 14% in the general population. After 25 years, two thirds of the survivors were still ambulatory. **Of those who present with only optic neuritis, 60% will develop full-blown MS over the next 40 years.** Unfortunately, it is not possible to accurately predict which patients will progress.

VI. Treatment.

A. Acute exacerbations

1. **Triggers.** Urinary tract or other infections or excessive heat exposure can mimic MS exacerbation. Treating a UTI often leads to resolution of the neurologic symptoms without the use of steroids.

2. **Methylprednisolone** (Solu-Medrol) is often used to shorten the duration of acute exacerbations, although its utility in preventing long-term disability is unproven. A typical regimen is 250 mg IV qid for 3 days or 1000 mg IV qd for 3 days. Infusions are followed by a taper of prednisone 1 mg/kg per day for 11 days followed by a rapid taper of 5 days. Some centers are employing pulsed monthly steroids, presumably in an attempt to minimize potential inflammation that can lead to clinical relapses. However, there is no definitive trial that endorses this as an effective treatment.

B. Maintenance immunomodulatory

1. **IFN-β-1b** (Betaseron) 250 mg SQ qod has been shown to significantly reduce frequency of exacerbations and long-term disability in relapsing remitting MS.

2. **IFN-β-1a** (Avonex) 30 mg IM weekly has similar efficacy to IFN-β-1b but is administered weekly.

3. **IFN-β-1a** (Rebif) 44 μg SQ three times weekly was shown in a multicenter randomized, controlled trial to be more effective than Avonex in both primary and secondary endpoints after 24 and 48 weeks of treatment.

4. **Glatiramer acetate** (Copaxone) 20 mg SQ qd has a different mechanism of action but similar efficacy to the above agents.

5. **Methotrexate** 7.5 mg PO weekly may be effective in reducing the rate of progression in chronic progressive MS. Monitor CBC and AST monthly for the duration of therapy.

6. **Mitoxantrone** (Novantrone) is a potent immunosuppressive that has been used with success and is FDA-approved for this indication. However, there is a lifetime dosing cap due to its numerous side effects, including potential risk of cardiomyopathy.

7. **Mycophenolate mofetil** (Cellcept) is another strong immunosuppressive with many fewer adverse effects than either methotrexate or mitoxantrone. Used off-label for MS treatment, it is steadily becoming more popular in patients with refractory disease.

9

NEUROLOGY

VERTIGO AND DIZZINESS

I. **Overview.** Disturbances of balance are common. Frustrating the evaluation is the poor vocabulary patients may use to describe their symptoms. "Dizziness" is a general term indicating spatial disorientation and can be avoided by asking patients to describe their symptoms without using the word "dizzy." When dizziness is categorized as vertigo, presyncope, or dysequilibrium, the evaluation becomes much more straightforward.

II. **Classification with Signs and Symptoms.**

A. **Vertigo is defined as the hallucination of movement,** a sense that the environment is spinning, a sensation of feeling impelled forward, backward, or to either side. Others describe "tilting" of their environment or a "back-and-forth" feeling. The evaluation of vertigo centers around two questions: Is it a single episode or is it recurrent? Is it likely to be of central or peripheral origin?

1. **Single episode or recurrent.** Careful questioning is required to define the symptoms over time. In vertiginous patients, motion exacerbates the symptoms, making it difficult to differentiate discrete episodes of movement-induced vertigo from mild baseline vertigo with movement-induced exacerbations. The questions "When are the symptoms present?" and "When are the symptoms absent?" are equally important.

2. **Central or peripheral** (Table 9-8)

a. **Central causes arise from damage or dysfunction of the pons or cerebellum.** With the exception of TIAs they manifest as single (though often prolonged) episodes of vertigo. Other neurologic deficits such as dysarthria, numbness, weakness, or diplopia can accompany the vertigo.

TABLE 9-8

COMPARISON OF PERIPHERAL AND CENTRAL VERTIGO

Feature	Peripheral	Central
SIGNS AND SYMPTOMS		
Occurrence of vertigo	Episodic	May be constant
Vertigo severity	++	+
Exacerbated by motion	++	+
Nausea, vomiting	++	+
Hearing loss	Possible	Possible
Tinnitus	Possible	−
Central compensation	Good	Fair
Loss of consciousness	No	Possible
Other neurologic signs/symptoms	No	Possible (diplopia, dysarthria)
DIX–HALLPIKE TEST		
Nystagmus latency	10-30 sec	None
Nystagmus duration	Brief	Long
Nystagmus fatigue with multiple trials	Yes	No
Vertigo improves with multiple trials	Yes	No

Nystagmus may be prominent. Difficulty walking is usually more severe with central causes.

b. **Peripheral causes arise from damage or dysfunction of the labyrinth or VIII nerve.** Nausea and vomiting are typically more prominent with peripheral vertigo. Other symptoms referable to the ear, including hearing loss, pain, ear fullness, and tinnitus, are common. Episodes can be single or recurrent, depending on the etiology. Compensation is more rapid and complete with peripheral vertigo.

B. **Other types of dizziness that must be differentiated from true vertigo**

1. **Presyncope.** Vertigo is distinctly different from presyncope. Presyncope is a feeling of light-headedness or faintness. It is often associated with generalized weakness, visual blurring, a sense of impending blacking out, diaphoresis, SOB, or palpitations. Typically it is episodic and caused by a transient decrease in cerebral perfusion.

2. **Disequilibrium** is primarily experienced when standing or walking and is absent when lying or sitting. Crowds and difficult walkways (such as stairs, ramps, and escalators) exacerbate the patient's symptoms. There is no clear hallucination of movement but rather a vague feeling of being off balance. This often reflects a neurologic motor deficit such as from a CVA.

3. **Anxiety** is a major cause of "dizziness."

III. **Vertigo Syndromes.**

A. **Vertigo by time frame**

1. **Benign positional vertigo.** Each episode lasts seconds to minutes.

2. **Meniere's disease.** Each episode lasts at least 20 minutes and up to hours.

3. **Toxic damage to labyrinth** (e.g., salicylates, alcohol). Variable depending on etiology.

4. **Labyrinthitis** (e.g., viral). Each episode of vertigo lasts days.

B. **Causes of recurrent episodes of vertigo**

1. **Benign paroxysmal positional vertigo (BPPV)** is the most common cause of recurrent vertigo. Historical characteristics: change in head position precipitates brief episodes of vertigo; not associated with tinnitus; may be associated with nausea but rarely emesis. It follows a waxing and waning course over months to years, but most cases resolve with time. Most common age of onset is between 60 and 70 years. Women with BPPV outnumber men by 2:1. This condition is caused by calcium carbonate crystals displaced within the posterior semicircular canal. Confirm by the Dix–Hallpike test (patient rapidly lies down from sitting position, allowing the head to hang over the edge of the bed while simultaneously turning the head to the left or right) plus classic time course, presence only with motion, etc. **A positive test manifests as vertigo and the observation of rotatory nystagmus within 30 seconds of the maneuver, which resolves within minutes.** With the diagnosis confirmed, a positioning procedure can be performed that relocates the offending crystal (see Furman and Cass, 1999). Literature cites success

rates in excess of 85% for patients treated in this manner. For refractory cases, brief therapy with benzodiazepines (e.g., diazepam 2-5 mg tid or qid) or vestibular rehabilitation exercises may be of use. Meclizine (Antivert) is an alternative. Dimenhydrinate (Dramamine) may be superior to the benzodiazepines, at least acutely.

2. **Meniere's disease** is a syndrome with recurrent attacks of vertigo and tinnitus lasting at least 20 minutes and up to hours and with associated hearing loss (low frequencies are lost first; discrimination is maintained). Patients generally have a feeling of ear fullness that resolves after episodes of vertigo. **Brief, transient vertigo is not Meniere's disease.** Patients can have nausea, vomiting, and ataxia. Onset age is 30 to 60 years. Patients with newly suspected cases should be evaluated with MRI and audiometry. About 60% resolve spontaneously without treatment. Treatment includes bed rest, IV fluids (if unable to maintain hydration), antihistamines, and phenothiazines or diazepam (as above). Salt restriction and diuretics (such as hydrochlorothiazide or furosemide) may be helpful. Data are poor, but two thirds are reported to respond to either sodium restriction or diuretics. If symptoms are severe, surgical ablation may be performed (labyrinthectomy if hearing is already lost; vestibular nerve section if hearing is preserved). See BPPV above for symptom control.

3. **Migraine aura.** Vertigo can arise as an aura to migraine. Other symptoms include scintillating scotoma, homonymous hemianopsia, cortical blindness, diplopia, dysarthria, ataxia, and paresthesias. Patients are typically young women and adolescents. Symptoms last up to 30 minutes, and migraine headache occurs after the vertigo. Treatment of basilar migraines should avoid vasoconstrictors; otherwise standard abortive and prophylactic migraine medications are appropriate.

4. **Perilymph fistula occurs from a perilymph leak.** Vertigo is often precipitated by prolonged standing, change in head position, coughing, sneezing, swallowing, straining, barotrauma, air travel, or loud noises. There is often an antecedent history of head trauma that results in a small tear in the oval or round window leading to a perilymph leak. It tends to be better in the morning and worse after being upright for a time. It may be associated tinnitus and hearing loss. **Diagnosis:** Pneumatic otoscopy reproduces symptoms. The fistula often heals spontaneously. Surgical correction may be performed if symptoms are ongoing.

5. **Miscellaneous.** Consider also Arnold–Chiari syndrome, paraneoplastic syndromes with cerebellar degeneration (especially from gynecologic malignancy), CSF leak.

C. **Causes of a single acute episode of vertigo**

1. **Acute peripheral vestibulopathy (viral labyrinthitis)** is acute onset of severe vertigo, nausea, and vomiting that lasts days and slowly returns to normal. Hearing loss and tinnitus are not typical. Nystagmus may be present in the first 48 hours. Occurs in all ages. The cause is unclear

but might be viral (45% cluster around viral infections). Consider performing audiogram and brainstem auditory evoked potentials to screen for structural causes of the symptoms. MRI is necessary if screening test is abnormal or if the patient is older than 60 years and has history or risk factors for vascular disease. Treatment is bed rest, antiemetics, IV fluids, diazepam, and antihistamines per BPPV. Some have used short-course steroids with success (e.g., methylprednisolone 32 mg on day 1, 16 mg bid on days 2 to 4, taper to 4 mg on day 8).

2. **Vertebrobasilar stroke** is sudden vertigo, often with symptoms less severe than other syndromes. Nausea and vomiting may be seen. Hearing loss and tinnitus are not seen. Nystagmus is often prominent. Other neurologic deficits such as dysarthria, numbness, weakness, ataxia, and diplopia can accompany the vertigo. Weakness or numbness affecting one side of the face and the opposite side of the body may be seen. Often there is a history of risk factors for cerebrovascular disease. Any patient at risk for stroke should have posterior fossa imaging (MRI preferred; CT if MRI is unavailable). Consider neurology consultation for further workup.

3. **Cerebellar hemorrhage** produces acute onset of vertigo, headache, inability to walk, nausea, and vomiting. Physical signs include horizontal nystagmus, ipsilateral limb ataxia, and facial palsy. Any patient with acute-onset headache and vertigo should be considered for an emergent head CT. Patients with cerebellar hemorrhage can deteriorate rapidly. Neurosurgical consult for the question of posterior fossa decompression is recommended.

4. **Multiple sclerosis** causes vertigo that is less severe than in peripheral disorders. Nausea, vomiting, and ataxia may be seen. Hearing loss is rare. It is usually associated with other neurologic symptoms of demyelination in CNS and is most common in young women.

5. **Head trauma** can cause dizziness that is usually attributable to postconcussion syndrome (i.e., disequilibrium dizziness). Less common: BPPV, perilymph fistula, or basilar skull fracture.

6. **Toxic damage to labyrinth** can be caused by antibiotics (especially aminoglycosides), salicylates, ethanol, phenytoin, quinine, benzene, and arsenic.

7. **Acoustic neuroma** is a benign tumor arising from cranial nerve VIII. Patient may have tinnitus and hearing loss, but discrimination is lost long before hearing loss is complete. Patient may have associated facial palsy. Auditory brainstem evoked potentials and MRI with contrast are the most sensitive tests and MRI is now the standard of care.

IV. **Presyncope and syncope** are discussed in Chapter 3.

V. **Disequilibrium.**

A. **Processes that disturb equilibrium.** Disequilibrium typically arises from dysfunction of multiple sensory channels with or without impaired higher cortical processing or motor responsiveness.

9

NEUROLOGY

B. Abnormalities of sensory input can result from diseases that decrease or distort vision, impair the vestibular system, or interfere with proprioception. Cumulatively, these impairments result in disorientation while ambulating. This can result in falling, especially in dark environments. This problem is an especially common cause of falls in the elderly.

C. Abnormalities of central integration. Dementia, metabolic encephalopathy, and sedative medications can all contribute.

D. Abnormalities of motor response. Disturbance in pyramidal, extrapyramidal (such as Parkinson's disease), or cerebellar function (such as alcohol-related, degenerative, or neoplastic disease) can further impair ambulation.

E. Diagnostic evaluation of disequilibrium. Review medications. Ask about visual problems, hearing loss, sensory loss, paresthesias, and a

TABLE 9-9
PARTIAL DIFFERENTIAL DIAGNOSIS OF WEAKNESS

Illness	Autonomic Involvement	Sensory Changes	Fever	Fasciculations/ Muscle Cramps	Cranial Nerve Involvement
ALS	No	No	No	Prominent but disappear in advanced disease	Early
Botulism	Dry mouth	No	No	No	Yes, early
Cord compression or injury (e.g., epidural abscess, hematoma, tumor)	Possible	Yes	Possible with abscess	No	No
Diphtheria	No	Occasional	Yes	No	Pharyngeal followed by other cranial nerves; may resolve before generalized weakness

history of vertigo. Check for hyporeflexia or hyperreflexia, Romberg's sign, and signs of Parkinson's disease. If the patient has hearing loss, obtain audiometry or brainstem auditory evoked potentials. Consider MRI and neurologic consultation.

F. Therapy for disequilibrium. Discontinue aggravating medications. Correct metabolic derangements. If visual symptoms are present, refer patient to ophthalmologist. If there is bilateral hearing abnormality on audiometry or brain stem auditory evoked response, refer to ENT. Treat peripheral neuropathy or Parkinson's disease as discussed earlier. Patients may benefit from use of a light cane, a soft cervical collar, vestibular exercises, or environmental improvements (e.g., lights at night) to their home.

VI. Nonstroke Weakness. Table 9-9 lists the differential diagnosis of weakness not related to stroke.

9

NEUROLOGY

Reflexes	GI Symptoms	CSF	Pattern of Paralysis	Comments
Hyperreflexia	No	Normal	Intrinsics of hand first, then upper extremities, then bulbar	Life expectancy <3 y Muscle biopsy, EMG helpful; consider cervical cord compression
Not lost until complete paralysis of muscle group	Nausea, diarrhea, constipation in children (unless wound related)	Normal	Face and upper extremities first	Not all who eat same food will be symptomatic
Flaccidity and hyporeflexia early, spasticity and hyperreflexia late	No	No	Discrete cord level; if central cord, distal worse than proximal; arms worse than legs	Consider also trauma, cord infarction, hemorrhage. Start dexamethasone (10-20 mg) if likely from tumor. Neurosurgical consult recommended
Absent when patient has generalized weakness	No	Normal	Starts distally and progresses proximally (like Guillain-Barré) 10 d to 3 mo after sore throat	Pharyngitis prominent, may have cardiac involvement (heart block, myocarditis)

(Continued)

TABLE 9-9
PARTIAL DIFFERENTIAL DIAGNOSIS OF WEAKNESS—cont'd

Illness	Autonomic Involvement	Sensory Changes	Fever	Fasciculations/ Muscle Cramps	Cranial Nerve Involvement
Eaton-Lambert	No	No	No	No	Yes
Guillain-Barré	Possible	Yes	No	No	Rare; pupil reactivity maintained
Myasthenia gravis	No	No	No	No	Yes
Organophosphate poisoning (or pyridostigmine OD)	Prominent sweating, bradycardia, other cholinergic signs	No	No	Yes	Yes
Polymyositis/ dermatomyositis	No	No	No	No	Pharyngeal only; ocular usually intact
Subacute multifocal motor neuropathy	No	Occasionally	No	No	No
Tick paralysis	No	Paresthesias	No	No	No
West Nile virus	Generally no	Yes	Yes	No	Possible

ACh, acetylcholine; OD, overdose; PCC, presynaptic calcium-channel; WNV, West Nile virus.

Reflexes	GI Symptoms	CSF	Pattern of Paralysis	Comments
Present	No	Anti-PCC antibody	Strength may improve with repeated stimulation	A paraneoplastic syndrome especially with small cell carcinoma of the lung
Absent	No	Elevated CSF protein; possibly anti-GM1 antibody	Lower extremity involvement first proceeding cephalad	Antecedent URI or diarrhea (weeks), especially *Campylobacter*
Present until muscle strength is lost	No	Normal	Diplopia and facial muscle commonly first, then extremities. Fatigable muscle strength	EMG, anti-ACh receptor antibody positive (85%)
Present	Diarrhea, salivation			
Present	Absent	Normal	Proximal musculature primarily involved	Elevated CPK, muscle tenderness; biopsy helpful
Hyporeflexia	No	Paraproteins (IgG and IgM)	Hands and distal first	Positive ganglioside antibody in 80%-90% (anti-GM1, MAG, and sulfatide)
Early loss	No	Normal	Lower extremity then ascending	Tick should be present, especially on head
Diminished	Possible	Pleocytosis, positive IgM for WNV	Ascending	Occurs in two forms: Guillain-Barré form as well as poliomyelitis form

BIBLIOGRAPHY

de Gans J, van de Beek D, European Dexamethasone in Adulthood Bacterial Meningitis Study Investigators: Dexamethasone in adults with acute bacterial meningitis. *N Engl J Med* 347:1549-1556, 2002.

Diener HC, Bogousslavsky, J, Brass LM, et al: Aspirin and clopidogrel compared with clopidogrel alone after recent ischaemic stroke or transient ischaemic attack in high-risk patients (MATCH): Randomised, double-blind, placebo-controlled trial. *Lancet* 364:331-337, 2004.

Furman JM, Cass SP: Benign paroxysmal positional vertigo. *N Engl J Med* 341: 1590-1596, 1999.

Haskell SG, Fiebach NH: Clinical epidemiology of nocturnal leg cramps in male veterans. *Am J Med Sci* 313:210-214, 1997.

Headache Classification Committee of the International Headache Society: Classification and diagnostic criteria for headache disorders, cranial neuralgias and facial pain. *Cephalalgia* 8(Suppl 7):1-96, 1988.

Kaye JA: Diagnostic challenges in dementia. *Neurology* 51(Suppl 1):S45-S52, 1998.

Lanctot KL, Herrmann N, Yau KK, et al: Efficacy and safety of cholinesterase inhibitors in Alzheimer's disease: A meta-analysis. *CMAJ* 169:557-564, 2003.

Lauerma H, Markkula J: Treatment of restless legs syndrome with tramadol: An open study. *J Clin Psychiatry* 60:241-244, 1999.

Lowenstein DH, Alldredge BK: Status epilepticus. *N Engl J Med* 338:970-976, 1998.

Man-Son-Hing M, Wells G, Lau A: Quinine for nocturnal leg cramps: A meta-analysis including unpublished data. *J Gen Intern Med* 13:600-606, 1998.

Marks DR, Rappoport AM: Diagnosis of migraine. *Semin Neurol* 17:303-306, 1997.

Mellick GA, Mellick LB: Management of restless legs syndrome with gabapentin (Neurontin). *Sleep* 19:224-226, 1996.

Miller A, Bourdette D, Cohen JA, et al: Multiple sclerosis. *Continuum* 5:1-196, 1999.

Montplaisir J, Nicolas A, Denesle R, Gomez-Mancillla B: Restless legs syndrome improved by pramipexole: A double-blind randomized trial. *Neurology* 52: 938-943, 1999.

Ondo W: Ropinirole for restless legs syndrome. *Mov Disord* 14:138-140, 1999.

Panitch H, Goodin DS, Francis G, et al: Randomized, comparative study of interferon beta-1a treatment regimens in MS: The EVIDENCE Trial. *Neurology* 59:1496-506, 2002.

Pruitt AA: Infections of the nervous system. *Neurol Clin* 16:419-447, 1998.

Silber MH: Restless legs syndrome. *Mayo Clin Proc* 72:261-264, 1997.

Silberstein SD, Niknam R, Rozen TD, Young WB: Cluster headache with aura. *Neurology* 54:219-221, 2000.

Tunkel AR, Scheld WM: Acute meningitis. In Mandell GL, Bennett JE, Dolin R (eds): *Douglas and Bennett's Principles and Practice of Infectious Diseases,* 5th ed. Philadelphia, Churchill Livingstone, 2000.

Wetter TC, Stiasny K, Winkelmann J, et al: A randomized controlled study of pergolide in patients with restless legs syndrome. *Neurology* 52:944-950, 1999.

Young WB, Silberstein SD, Dayno JM: Migraine treatment. *Semin Neurol* 17: 325-333, 1997.

Younger DS, Rosoklija G, Hays AP: Diabetic peripheral neuropathy. *Semin Neurol* 18:95-104, 1998.

Yusuf S, Sleight P, Pogue, et al: Effects of an angiotensin-converting-enzyme inhibitor, ramipril, on cardiovascular events in high-risk patients. The Heart Outcome Prevention Evaluation Study Investigators. *N Engl J Med* 342:145-153, 2000.

Infectious Diseases

Wissam El Atrouni and Philip M. Polgreen

ANTIBIOTIC USE

Overuse of antibiotics has led to a problem with microbial resistance. Be judicious in your use of antibiotics. Reserve newer agents (linezolid and quinupristin-dalfopristin for gram-positive organisms) for cases in which they are the *only* alternative. Gram stain results are interpreted in **Table 10-1.**

PROPHYLAXIS FOR SPECIFIC EXPOSURES

I. *Neisseria meningitidis.* Vaccine available for acute outbreak; consult local public health organization. Rifampin 20 mg/kg per day PO (not >600 mg/dose) divided q12h × 2 days is indicated for all intimate contacts, including household members of patient. Other options for adults include ciprofloxacin 500 mg PO or ceftriaxone 250 mg IM. For children <15 years of age, ceftriaxone 125 mg IM can be used.
II. *Haemophilus influenzae.* Active immunization recommended, given as three-dose vaccination at 2, 4, and 6 months with a booster at 15 months. When there are other children in the home, rifampin 20 mg/kg per day as single oral dose for 4 days is recommended for all household contacts including adults.
III. *Pertussis.* For close contacts: erythromycin—children, 50 mg/kg per day divided qid × 14 days; adults 500 mg PO qid × 14 days. Alternative: clarithromycin 7.5 mg/kg bid × 14 days; TMP–SMX—adults, TMP–SMX DS × 14 days; children, TMP 8 mg/kg per day, SMX 40 mg/kg per day.
IV. **HIV.** See Chapter 11, HIV–AIDS.

PRINCIPLES OF CULTURING

I. **Blood Cultures. Volume of blood is the most important factor in determining the rate of positive cultures.** Anaerobic cultures are most likely to be useful in those with underlying immunosuppression (e.g., patients on steroids), those with a suspected abdominal source of infection, and those with suspected endocarditis.
A. **Adults. How much? How often?**
1. Before antibiotics, 20 to 40 mL from two separate sites to eliminate possibility of skin contamination. Cultures can be drawn at the same time; drawing from an IV site is acceptable for one set.
2. For fever of unknown origin (FUO), an additional set should be drawn on a different day. See section on FUO later in this chapter.
3. First two cultures will detect 92% to 99.3% of septicemias and 98% of cases of endocarditis; only 20% of patients hospitalized for pneumonia will have positive blood culture.

MICROBIOLOGIC CHARACTERISTICS OF BACTERIA BASED ON GRAM
STAINING

Organism	Aerobic or Anaerobic	Catalase	Coagulase
	Microbiologic Characteristics		
GRAM-POSITIVE COCCI			
Aerococcus	aerobic	−	
Enterococcus	aerobic	−	
Lactococcus	aerobic	−	
Streptococcus	aerobic	−	
Staphylococcus aureus	aerobic	+	+
Staphylococcus epidermidis	aerobic	+	−
Micrococcus	aerobic	+	−
Peptostreptococcus	anaerobic		

Organism	Aerobic or Anaerobic	Catalase	Morphology
	Microbiologic Characteristics		
GRAM-POSITIVE BACILLI			
Bacillus	aerobic	+	Spore forming
Nocardia	aerobic		Branching
Clostridium	anaerobic		Spore forming
Corynebacterium	aerobic	+	
Listeria	aerobic	+	
Lactobacillus	aerobic	−	
Actinomyces	some aerobic, some anaerobic	−	Spore forming
Eubacterium	anaerobic		Non–spore forming
Propionibacterium	anaerobic		Non–spore forming

Organism	Aerobic or Anaerobic	Oxidase	Miscellaneous
	Microbiologic Characteristics		
GRAM-NEGATIVE BACILLI			
Haemophilus	aerobic		
Actinobacillus		−	
Bacteroides fragilis	aerobic		Bile resistant
Campylobacter	aerobic		No growth on sheep blood agar
Legionella	aerobic		No growth on sheep blood agar
Enterobacter*	aerobic	−	No growth on sheep blood agar
Pseudomonas	aerobic	+	Not glucose fermenting
Gardnerella	aerobic	−	Glucose fermenting
Acinetobacter	aerobic	−	Not glucose fermenting
Pasteurella	aerobic	+	Glucose fermenting
Brucella	aerobic	+	Glucose fermenting
Campylobacter	aerobic	+	Not glucose fermenting

TABLE 10-1

MICROBIOLOGIC CHARACTERISTICS OF BACTERIA BASED ON GRAM
STAINING—cont'd

| | Microbiologic Characteristics | | |
Organism	Aerobic or Anaerobic	Oxidase	Miscellaneous
GRAM-NEGATIVE BACILLI—cont'd			
Helicobacter pylori	aerobic	+	Not glucose fermenting
Pseudomonas	aerobic	+	Not glucose fermenting
Vibrio	aerobic	+	Not glucose fermenting
Bordetella	aerobic	+	Urease producing
Bacteroides ureolyticus	anaerobic		Not bile resistant
Fusobacterium	anaerobic		Not bile resistant
GRAM-NEGATIVE COCCI			
Neisseria	aerobic	+	
Moraxella	aerobic		Not glucose fermenting
GRAM-NEGATIVE ACID-FAST BACTERIA†			
Mycobacterium tuberculosis	aerobic	+	
Mycobacterium marinum	aerobic	+	
GRAM-NEGATIVE WEAKLY ACID-FAST ORGANISMS			
Nocardia			

*Includes *Escherichia coli*, *Klebsiella*, *Proteus*, *Salmonella*, *Serratia*, *Shigella*, and *Yersinia*.
†*Cryptosporidium* is also a gram-negative acid-fast organism.
+, positive; −, negative.

4. If the patient has received antibiotics, blood should be drawn for a resin-containing medium in addition to the aerobic and anaerobic bottles (30 mL/site).
B. **Children. How much? How often?**
1. One to 5 mL is adequate to detect serious disease because pediatric patients generally have higher bacterial loads.
2. **Multiple sites are unnecessary and do not increase yield.**
C. **Interpreting results.** Coagulase-negative *Staphylococcus* (e.g., *S. epidermidis*), *Corynebacterium* species, and *Propionibacterium acnes* are likely contaminants unless multiple cultures are positive.

INFESTATIONS

I. **Parasitic Infestation by Pinworms.**
A. **Presentation.** *Enterobius vermicularis* is a small roundworm (nematode). Humans are the only known host. Males measure 2 to 5 mm and females measure 8 to 13 mm. Gravid females migrate from the cecum out the anus at night to lay 15,000 eggs on the perineum, causing pruritus, vulvitis, and restless sleep. May cause acute nocturnal vaginal pain in girls, and rarely weight loss, UTI, and appendicitis. Often whole families are affected. Eggs are transmitted by the fecal–oral route.

B. Examination. Sometimes worms can be seen in the perianal area about an hour after the child goes to sleep. The definitive diagnostic test is to stick cellophane tape onto the perianal area in the morning before bathing. The tape is then placed on a slide and examined under a microscope for the characteristic oval egg. Ask the patient to obtain specimens over 3 to 5 mornings and store them in the refrigerator before bringing them to the office. The cellophane tape test done over 3 days has a sensitivity of 90%.

C. Treatment. All members of the household should be treated simultaneously along with daily laundering of the affected child's underclothes and bedding. The following treatment is for adults and children older than 2 years.

1. **Mebendazole** (Vermox) 100 mg PO once. Repeat in 2 weeks. Contraindicated in pregnancy.

2. **Albendazole** (Albenza) 400 mg PO once. Repeat in 2 weeks. Teratogenic in pregnancy.

3. **Pyrantel pamoate** (Antiminth) 11 mg/kg (up to 1 g PO in one dose) **for all ages.** Repeat q2wk twice.

D. Prevention. Good hand washing, keep affected child's fingernails short, clean bedroom and bedding.

II. Scabies.

A. Presentation. Caused by an obligate human parasitic mite, *Sarcoptes scabiei*, that burrows in the skin. Most common in children, but found in all ages. Usually transmitted by person-to-person transmission, but may be picked up from bedding and clothes. The organism causes an intensely pruritic, papular eruption that is especially pruritic at night. Areas most affected are interdigital folds, flexor aspect of wrists and elbows, belt line, thighs, navel, penis, areola, abdomen, and intergluteal fold. The head and neck are typically spared in adults but can be involved in infants and children.

B. Examination. Look for pruritic papules, vesicles, and linear burrows. May also see excoriations, crusting, and secondary infections. A high percentage of children with scabies have persistent reddish-brown nodules, which can make diagnosis difficult. Confirm by scraping the leading edge of the lesion or under the fingernails with a scalpel blade; place on slide with mineral oil and look for mites, ova, or fecal pellets. In elderly patients, lesions can be bullous, and in the immunocompromised, itching may be absent.

C. Treatment.

1. **Permethrin** 5% (Elimite) is the preferred treatment. Apply from chin to toes; 8 to 14 hours later rinse off and repeat in 1 week if needed. May be used on infants >2 months of age, children, and pregnant women (category B). Safety during breast feeding is unknown.

2. **Lindane** (Kwell). Use with caution on patients <2 years of age. Apply from neck to toes. For children, leave on for 6 to 8 hours and then rinse off. If used on infants, rinse off after 6 hours. Repeat in 1 week. Use is

contraindicated in pregnancy. Side effects include possible neurotoxicity with seizures, especially in infants and children and in crusted scabies. **The FDA discourages the use of lindane.**

3. **Crotamiton** 10% (Eurax). Apply thin layer of medication. Reapply 24 hours later. Do not bathe between applications.

4. **Precipitated sulfur (5%-10%) in petroleum** applied to entire body for three consecutive nights is an alternative in those <2 months of age and in pregnancy. Bathe before each application and after last application.

5. **Ivermectin** 200 μg/kg PO once can be given in the treatment of scabies. Not for pregnant women and children <15 kg. Generally reserved for severe cases.

6. **Household members should be treated even if asymptomatic.** Bed linens, clothing, and towels used in the past 4 days should be washed in hot water (120°F) or stored in tightly sealed bags for 1 week. Treatment must be simultaneous for all. Trim fingernails and reapply scabicide to hands. Itching can last up to 4 weeks after treatment; **continued itching is not necessarily an indication for repeat treatment.** Can use oral antihistamines and topical steroids after primary treatment given.

III. **Pediculosis.** Two species of lice affect humans: *Pediculus humanus (capitis* and *corporis)* and *Phthirus pubis*. Sensitization to louse saliva and antigens results in clinical manifestations.

A. *Pediculus humanus capitis* **(head lice).** Seen primarily in preschoolers and early elementary school ages but occurs in all ages and socioeconomic groups. Spread by direct contact or fomites (e.g., helmets, combs). Signs and symptoms: pruritus; erythematous papules, excoriation, and pyoderma usually on occiput, postauricular region, and nape of the neck; lice and nits (eggs firmly attached to hair shaft about 1 cm from scalp). Combing with a lice comb then examining the teeth of the comb is better than direct exam. Differential diagnosis includes seborrhea, psoriasis, tinea capitis, and impetigo.

B. *Pediculus humanus corporis* **(body lice).** Live in clothing or bedding and not on humans. Seen primarily in lower socioeconomic groups and homeless persons. The louse bites at night and leaves pruritic vesicles or papules (especially in the axilla, groin, and trunk). Diagnosis is by examination of clothing seams to find nits or lice. Body lice transmit epidemic typhus *(Rickettsia prowazekii)* and trench fever *(Bartonella quintana)*.

C. *Phthirus pubis* **(pubic lice).** Transmitted by intimate contact. Diagnosis is by symptoms (pubic or anogenital pruritus) and by lice or nits found especially in the pubic hair, but also trunk, beard, eyelashes, or axilla. Often associated with additional STDs.

D. **Treatment for all forms of pediculosis involves a pediculicide.**

1. **Treat all sexual partners and household members simultaneously.**

2. Wash all bedding, clothes, towels, and hats in hot water and use a hot dryer.

INFECTIOUS DISEASES 10

3. If eyelashes or eyebrows are infested, avoid a pediculicide in those areas. Instead apply petrolatum five times per day until clear. Remove nits with forceps.
4. Pruritus may last for several weeks after successful treatment.
5. **For head or pubic lice: Permethrin (Nix) 1% cream rinse is drug of choice,** applied to scalp or affected area after shampooing, left on 10 minutes, then rinsed off. Re-examine in 1 week; retreat if nits still present. **Alternative:** 4% piperonyl butoxide, 0.33% pyrethrins (e.g., Rid, Pronto), 0.5% Malathion lotion (Ovide). Not for neonates and infants because of flammability; if ingested can cause respiratory depression. Must leave on for 8-12 hours. Lindane 1% shampoo (Kwell, Scabene) again can be neurotoxic in children and use is discouraged by the FDA. **Ivermectin** 200 µg/kg PO once and repeated in 7 to 10 days can be used as well.
6. **For body lice, use permethrin, or pyrethrin,** over whole body and wash 10 minutes later. Repeat in 7 to 10 days. May use ivermectin as above.

TUBERCULOSIS

I. **TB Screening.** Recent recommendations by the American Thoracic Society (ATS)/CDC are to target testing to persons at high risk for development of TB and progressing to active disease once infected. High-risk groups include the following:
A. **Close contacts** of those with known or suspected TB.
B. **Persons infected with HIV.**
C. **IV drug users** or users of other illicit drugs.
D. **Chronically ill patients with conditions or diseases that increase the risk of progressing from latent to active TB:** diabetes, high-dose steroid use, immunosuppressive therapy, end-stage renal disease, lymphoma, leukemia, head and neck or lung cancer, malnourishment, weight loss >10% below ideal weight, silicosis, gastrectomy, and jejunoileal bypass.
E. **Foreign-born persons** and those arriving within the last 5 years from countries that have had a high incidence of TB.
F. **Residents and employees of high-risk institutions:** correctional facilities, nursing homes, mental health institutions, and homeless shelters.
G. **Health care workers** serving high-risk patients.
H. **Medically underserved and low-income populations,** especially homeless persons.
I. **Infants, children, and adolescents exposed to high-risk adults.**
II. **Screening Methods.**
A. **Protein purified derivative (PPD).** Use 5 tuberculin units of PPD in 0.1 mL injected intradermally; read in 48 to 72 hours. In the elderly, if the PPD is initially negative, administer a second dose 1 week later to boost latent positive reactions. (This process identifies positive PPD that is the result of a distant exposure to TB, instead of a true, new conversion.)

In addition, persons who will undergo annual testing should have two-step testing as above the first time they are screened.

1. **False-positive results are caused by** nontuberculotic mycobacteria; BCG-induced reactivity (decreases with time, frequently gone after 1 year and is unlikely to persist for more than 10 years).

2. **False-negative results are caused by** impaired immunity. Mumps and *Candida* controls can be used to test for anergy, but their usefulness is controversial.

III. **Interpretation of PPD. The PPD should be interpreted in the same way in those who have received BCG and those who have not.**

A. **Measure induration** (the elevated and firm area), **not the area of erythema.**

B. **Induration ≥5 mm is considered positive among:**

1. People with recent close contact with patients with active TB.

2. HIV-positive people or those with HIV risk factors with an unknown HIV status.

3. People with CXR consistent with healed TB.

4. Immunosuppressed persons receiving the equivalent of >15 mg prednisone daily for at least 1 month.

C. **Induration ≥10 mm: 90% of reactors are infected with TB (true-positive PPD). An induration ≥10 mm is considered positive among:**

1. IV drug users known to be HIV seronegative.

2. Those with medical conditions with increased risk for progressing from latent to active TB (see ID, earlier).

3. Residents and employees of prisons, nursing homes, residential mental health facilities, or homeless shelters.

4. Foreign-born persons and those arrived from countries with high incidence of TB within last 5 years.

5. Medically underserved, low-income populations.

6. Children <4 years of age.

7. Recent converter or increase induration by at least 10 mm within 2 years.

8. Health care workers.

D. **Induration ≥15 mm is positive for patients with no risk factors (e.g., they meet none of the preceding criteria).**

IV. **Treatment of Latent Tuberculosis Infection (LTBI).** *Age is no longer a factor in deciding whether or not to treat LTBI.* All new converters should be treated.

A. **Approximately 5% of patients (without HIV) with a new PPD conversion will develop active TB within 2 years of conversion if untreated, and another 5% will develop active TB later in life. Treatment of LTBI reduces the risk of active TB by 65% to 75%. Active disease should be ruled out with a negative CXR and/or sputum for AFB before deciding to treat LTBI.**

B. Combination chemotherapy for presumptive TB should be initiated pending cultures if there is high clinical suspicion of **active** TB.

C. The risk of hepatitis due to isoniazid (INH) treatment is about 0.1%, and almost all cases occur within the first 3 months of treatment.

D. Adults: INH 300 mg PO qd × 9 mo (12 if HIV positive or if the CXR is consistent with previous TB infection). Add pyridoxine 25 to 50 mg PO qd to prevent development of peripheral neuropathy.

E. Children: INH 10 to 20 mg/kg per day PO qd × 9 mo (up to 300 mg/d total).

F. If multidrug-resistant TB is likely (Southeast Asia, Korea, Haiti, Philippines, New York, New Jersey, California, Florida), consider rifampin-based regimens. Rifampin 10 mg/kg (maximum 600 mg/d) for 4 months for an INH-resistant exposure is a good choice. Rifampin causes orange-colored body fluids and hepatitis.

G. Strongly consider therapy that is directly observed (INH 15 mg/kg twice per week).

H. Obtain baseline liver function enzymes and continue to monitor clinically for 9 months. Suggest checking LFTs every 2 weeks for the first month then every month for 3 months. If aminotransferase levels increase to greater than five times the normal range in asymptomatic persons, or above the normal range with symptoms of elevated bilirubin, discontinue INH or rifampin.

V. Active TB.

A. TB affects the lungs in the majority of patients. Extrapulmonary TB is more common in HIV-positive patients, and in women and children. However, TB can affect almost any body system, especially pleura, meninges, brain (tuberculoma), bone (thoracic spine, Pott's disease), joints, and GU system, and can be disseminated.

B. Diagnosis with acid-fast stain on sputum and cultures. Culture can take 6 weeks on solid media, but can grow in 7 to 21 days on liquid media. PCR (DNA probe) can help differentiate tuberculous from nontuberculous mycobacteria in HIV-positive patients. TB is difficult to grow from CSF and pericardial, pleural, or peritoneal fluid; therefore, biopsy may be needed.

C. Treatment consists of an initiation phase followed by a continuation phase. The initiation phase includes four drugs: INH, rifampin, pyrazinamide, and ethambutol daily for 2 months. Ethambutol may be discontinued if the susceptibility testing shows sensitivity to the first three drugs. Ethambutol also not recommended in children unless they have adult-type (upper lobe) disease or INH-resistant organism. An initiation phase without pyrazinamide is acceptable in pregnant women and those with severe liver disease or gout.

D. The continuation phase includes INH, rifampin for 4 or 7 months. Different dosing intervals are possible (daily, 5×/wk, 3×/wk, 2×/wk). High-risk patients should have a 7-month continuation phase (cavitary disease, positive smear or culture at the end of 2 months). Also severe forms (meningitis, bone, joints) benefit from prolonged continuation phase. **Steroids should be considered concomitantly for pleural disease, pericardial disease, CNS disease or meningitis. Note that**

antimicrobial treatment must be initiated before starting steroids. Regimens include prednisone 60 mg/d tapered over 6 weeks for adults and 2-4 mg/d for children tapered over 4 weeks.

E. **Rifampin interacts with several of the medications used to treat HIV** (i.e., protease inhibitors) and with other medications. Check for drug interactions. Rifabutin is an alternative for HIV-positive patients on HAART.

F. Every patient should have baseline AST, ALT, bilirubin, alkaline phosphatase, creatinine, platelets, visual acuity testing, and red-green color discrimination (when ethambutol is used). Obtain sputum for AFB and culture monthly until 2 consecutive months are negative. Suggest follow-up LFTs as described for treatment of LTBI.

G. **Contact the local health department for the identification of contacts.**

H. **Directly observed therapy is recommended for all patients.**

I. **Antituberculous drugs are generally considered safe in pregnancy** and breast-feeding. In the United States, pyrazinamide is not recommended in pregnancy.

VI. **Prevention of TB.** Isolation is indicated for any patient known or suspected to have TB. Isolation should consist of a single-patient room with negative-pressure ventilation. Persons entering the room should wear appropriate respiratory protection. **Note that isolation at home may be preferable for stable patients. It is likely that household members have already been exposed.**

IMMUNOSUPPRESSED HOST

I. **Factors that predispose patients to infection include** neutropenia, diabetes, alcoholism, AIDS, lymphomas, leukemia, malnutrition, cirrhosis, skin breakdown, therapy with steroids or cytotoxic drugs, solid organ and bone marrow transplants, complement deficiencies, splenectomy, renal failure, and the extremes of age.

II. **Elderly.** Acute confusion or change in mental status often indicates an infection in an elderly patient. The presentation may be otherwise nonspecific, lacking fever and localizing signs and symptoms. Sepsis should be strongly suspected in any elderly person with vomiting, mental status changes, or an elevated WBC and band count. Hospital admission and a septic work-up are advisable for such a patient.

III. **Infections in the immunosuppressed patient may not manifest with the usual signs or symptoms even with septicemia.** Specifically, the patient may not mount a fever or have lymphadenopathy or WBC response. Localizing symptoms may be absent. UTIs may exist in the absence of pyuria (especially in a neutropenic patient).

IV. **Neutropenic Fever is defined as** temperature at any time of 38.3°C (101°F), or 38.0°C (100.3°F) for more than 1 hour **and** an absolute neutrophil count <500 cells/mL, **or** <1000 cells/mL with a predicted decrease to <500 cells/mL. The risk for an infection in a neutropenic patient is greatest when the neutrophil count is <100 cells/mL.

10

INFECTIOUS DISEASES

The risk also increases with the duration of the patient's neutropenia. Start empiric antibiotics as soon as possible after culturing.

V. Work-up for all immunosuppressed patients should include UA, blood and urine cultures, CXR, and a biopsy or aspirate from each site that may be infected. A microbiologic diagnosis is usually not made initially; thus, initial therapy is usually empiric.

VI. Treatment should be directed against gram-negative bacilli. **Box 10-1** gives recommendations.

A. If patient becomes afebrile in 3 to 5 days, change treatment to reflect culture results *or* if cultures are negative and patient is low risk, change to amoxicillin/clavulanate plus ciprofloxacin (adults) or cefixime (children). Otherwise, continue IV antibiotics.

B. If patient is still febrile at 3 to 5 days, consider changing antibiotics if patient worsening; add vancomycin if not used already. **If febrile after 5 days and resolution of neutropenia is not imminent, start antifungal treatment (amphotericin B, liposomal formulations, voriconazole, or caspofungin).**

C. Continue the antimicrobial therapy until one of these conditions is met:

1. Neutropenia has resolved for 2 days *and* patient is afebrile for 2 days, *or*
2. Neutropenia has not resolved but patient is afebrile for 5 days and has no complaints, *or*
3. Absolute neutrophil count is >500 cells/mL for 5 days, patient is still febrile, and if no focus identified, can stop antibiotics.
4. **If none of these conditions is met, continue antibiotic therapy for 14 additional days and consider stopping at that time if no**

BOX 10-1
REGIMENS FOR NEUTROPENIC FEVER*
MONOTHERAPY
Ceftazidime, imipenem, meropenem, cefepime
MULTIDRUG THERAPY
Aminoglycoside plus antipseudomonal penicillin (ticarcillin, piperacillin), a cephalosporin (cefepime, ceftazidime), or a carbapenem
INDICATIONS FOR ADDITION OF VANCOMYCIN
Add vancomycin if
■ Patient has a peripherally inserted central catheter or central line that might be infected
■ Has known colonization with MRSA or resistant *Pneumococcus*
■ Has extensive mucositis
■ Is hypotensive or has cardiovascular compromise
■ Is failing current regimen

*For low-risk adult patients who do not appear ill, are expected to have neutropenia for a short duration, and have ready access to health care, PO ciprofloxacin and amoxicillin/clavulanate with close monitoring is an option.

disease is found. Observe closely because, by definition, if you reach this point in therapy the patient is still neutropenic and febrile.

VII. Both G-CSF and GM-CSF reduce the length of neutropenia, but have not improved survival rates.

VIII. **Antibiotic Prophylaxis is not recommended for afebrile neutropenic patients** except for bone marrow transplant recipients (who should receive antifungals), and patients at risk for *Pneumocystis* pneumonia (use TMP–SMX). This recommendation may change, however.

SEPSIS

I. **Definitions.**

A. **Bacteremia is defined** as the presence of bacteria in the blood stream as detected by blood cultures. Transient bacteremia occurs daily in healthy patients.

B. **Systemic inflammatory response syndrome (SIRS).** A response to inflammation or injury that can be infectious or noninfectious (e.g., pancreatitis), defined by having more than two of the following:

1. Temperature >38.3°C or <36°C.

2. Heart rate >90 beats/min.

3. Respiration rate >20 or $Paco_2$ <32 torr.

4. WBC >12,000/mm^3 or <4000/mm^3, or >10% bands.

C. **Sepsis.** SIRS is thought to be caused by an infectious process.

D. **Severe sepsis is associated with organ dysfunction (altered mental status, acute oliguria, lactic acidosis, elevated liver enzymes) despite adequate volume resuscitation.**

E. **Septic shock** is defined as sepsis with a systolic BP <90 mm Hg or drop of 40 mm Hg from baseline value in absence of other causes.

II. **Causes.**

A. **Gram-negative bacteria:** *Escherichia coli, Klebsiella pneumoniae, Pseudomonas aeruginosa, Proteus* spp., *Serratia* spp., *Neisseria meningitidis*.

B. **Gram-positive bacteria:** *Staphylococcus aureus,* coagulase-negative staphylococci, *Streptococcus pneumoniae, Streptococcus pyogenes,* enterococci.

C. **Other causes:** Opportunistic fungi (5%; mostly *Candida*), viruses, rickettsiae, and protozoa.

III. **Risk Factors** include hospitalization, illness, and invasive procedures.

A. **Risk for gram-negative septicemia increases with** diabetes, cirrhosis, alcoholism, lymphoproliferative diseases, burns, cancer, iatrogenic immunosuppression (e.g., chemotherapy, steroids), total parenteral nutrition, and urinary, biliary, or GI infections. In addition, neonates and the elderly with urinary dysfunction are at very high risk.

B. **Risk for gram-positive septicemia increases with** indwelling IV catheters, indwelling mechanical devices, IV drug use, and burns.

C. Risk for fungal septicemia increases with immunosuppression (e.g., neutropenic patients), patients with central venous catheters, and those talking prolonged courses of broad-spectrum antibiotics.

D. Splenectomized patients are at risk for infections from *S. pneumoniae, H. influenzae, N. meningitidis, Capnocytophaga* species (dog bites).

IV. Clinical Manifestations. Presentation may vary greatly between patients and is often subtle at the extremes of age. Early signs and symptoms include fever, chills, and tachypnea. Later, they include mental status changes, cold and clammy extremities, and oliguria.

V. Work-up.

A. History, physical exam, and chart review with special attention directed toward medications (especially antibiotics, immunosuppressive drugs), **recent surgeries or dental procedures, previous illnesses and surgeries (splenectomy), HIV risk factors, IV drug use.**

B. Diagnostic tests.

1. CBC with a differential.

a. Leukocytosis with left shift or leukopenia.

b. Toxic granulations, Döhle bodies, or intracytoplasmic vacuolization in PMNs.

c. Thrombocytopenia is suggestive of DIC, as are an increase in fibrin degradation products, a decrease in fibrinogen, and an increase in PT/INR (see Chapter 6).

d. RBC morphology is generally normal except with DIC; then microangiopathic hemolytic anemia with schistocytes is a possibility.

2. Blood cultures. Obtain at least two sets from two sites (blood cultures are often negative).

3. Culture all possible sources of infection: sputum, urine, skin lesions, CSF.

4. Urinalysis with microscopic exam. UTIs are a common cause of sepsis in the elderly.

5. General labs. Electrolytes, glucose, BUN/creatinine, LFTs, PT/PTT, CXR, ABG. Patients generally have a respiratory alkalosis followed by a metabolic (lactic) acidosis.

6. LP puncture if patient has a headache or meningeal signs.

7. Abdominal US or CT if the abdomen is possible source (e.g., bowel perforation, ischemic bowel, cholecystitis, diverticulitis).

VI. Common Primary Infections. Pneumonia, UTIs, wounds, cellulitis, abscesses, IV line infection, sinusitis, meningitis, endocarditis, biliary infections, appendicitis, peritonitis.

VII. Differential Diagnosis. Other causes of shock include myocardial infarction, pulmonary embolus, drug overdose (especially salicylates, which may mimic sepsis), bleeding, cardiac tamponade, rupture of aortic aneurysm, aortic dissection, and toxic shock syndrome.

VIII. Causes of fever in the ICU include infected catheters, sinusitis/otitis media, acalculous cholecystitis, drug fever, central fever, *Clostridium difficile* colitis, postcardiotomy syndrome (see Chapter 3, Cardiology), resistant organisms, and fungal infections.
IX. Treatment. Table 10-2 lists empiric antibiotics in sepsis. Goal directed therapy markedly decreases mortality (NNT=6).
A. Check serum lactate. If greater than 4, place a central line and put patient in ICU.
B. Respiratory and hemodynamic support. Keep oxygen saturation >92%. Consider ventilator support for progressive hypoxia or respiratory muscle failure.

TABLE 10-2

EMPIRIC ANTIBIOTICS IN SEPSIS

Likely Source of Sepsis	Likely Organisms	Antibiotics
Urosepsis	Gram-negative rods, enterococci	Third-generation cephalosporin (ceftriaxone, cefotaxime) ± an aminoglycoside
		Ticarcillin/clavulanic acid ± an aminoglycoside
		Piperacillin/tazobactam ± an aminoglycoside
		Imipenem or meropenem ± an aminoglycoside
Intra-abdominal infection	Polymicrobial, anaerobes	Ampicillin/sulbactam ± an aminoglycoside
		Cefoxitin ± an aminoglycoside
		Cefotetan ± an aminoglycoside
		Ticarcillin/clavulanic acid ± an aminoglycoside
		Piperacillin/tazobactam ± an aminoglycoside
		Imipenem or meropenem ± an aminoglycoside
Nosocomial pneumonia	Resistant gram-negative rods	Aminoglycoside (gentamicin or tobramycin) plus an antipseudomonal (ticarcillin, piperacillin, ceftazidime)
		If pathogens are resistant to aminoglycosides, third-generation cephalosporins, and aztreonam, then they might be susceptible to imipenem or meropenem
Neutropenia		Ceftazidime ± an aminoglycoside
		Imipenem or meropenem ± an aminoglycoside
		Cefepime ± an aminoglycoside
IV catheter	*Staphylococcus aureus*, *Staphylococcus epidermidis*, MRSA	Vancomycin
Unknown primary site		Third- or fourth-generation cephalosporin plus an aminoglycoside
		Ticarcillin/clavulanic acid plus an aminoglycoside
		Piperacillin/tazobactam plus an aminoglycoside
		Imipenem or meropenem plus an aminoglycoside

INFECTIOUS DISEASES

10

C. **Fluid management.** IV normal saline fluid boluses with the goal of a mean arterial BP >60 mm Hg. To avoid pulmonary edema, keep the CVP between 10 and 12 cm H_2O and the PCWP between 14 and 18 mm Hg. Colloid solutions have no proven benefits over crystalloid solutions. **Ensure adequate volume before considering pressors.**

1. **Adults:** 1 to 1.5 L in first 1 to 2 hours; probably will need more (4-6 L on average).

2. **Children:** 20 mL/kg over 2 to 5 minutes (neonates over 20 minutes) repeated twice in first hour if needed to maintain good perfusion.

3. **Continuing support.**

a. Transfuse as needed.

b. Try to keep urine output between 30 and 60 mL/h in adults and 0.5 to 1.5 mL/kg per hour in pediatric patients.

D. **If a patient has failed volume resuscitation with normal saline, start dopamine and titrate up to 20 µg/kg.** In dopamine-unresponsive patients, use norepinephrine infusion. Dobutamine may be added later to keep cardiac output >4 L/m^2. These drugs should be used in an ICU usually in conjunction with intra-arterial and pulmonary artery catheters. **However, pulmonary artery catheters are associated with increased mortality rates.** Early volume resuscitation and aggressive inotropic support, to normalize mixed venous O_2 saturation, lactate, base deficit, and pH, increase survival in severe sepsis and shock.

E. Monitor serum lactate and if increasing reassess fluid status, etc.

X. **Adrenal insufficiency should be considered in any patient with refractory hypotension who has taken steroids for longer than 2 weeks within the last year or is infected with either TB or *N. meningitidis.* Recent studies have shown that physiologic steroid supplementation (200-300 mg of hydrocortisone/day) for 5 to 7 days improved survival regardless of adrenal status.** Some would do a cosyntropin test and only treat non-responders.

XI. **Activated protein C** has been shown to be effective with an absolute mortality reduction of 6% (NNT = 17). It should be used only in patients with end-organ failure; APACHE score = 25 because of the increased risk of bleeding (see Bernard et al., 2001).

XII. **Intensive insulin therapy** to target glucose of 80 to 110 mg/dL lowers mortality rate in critically ill patients without a history of diabetes.

XIII. **Treat the infectious agent** (surgical drainage may be needed in some cases). Start antibiotics as soon as possible, preferably after cultures are obtained; tailor to most likely source until culture results are available.

FEVER OF UNKNOWN ORIGIN

I. **Definition.** FUO is an illness of longer than 3 weeks' duration with a fever ≥38.3°C for which a diagnosis has not been found after 1 week of inpatient or outpatient investigation.

II. **Evaluation.** The diagnosis is usually made clinically with supporting evidence found on lab and radiographic studies. There is no substitute for a good history and physical exam. Patients who do not have a diagnosis made after an intensive investigation often have the best outcomes, and fever will generally resolve in 4 to 5 weeks. The minimal work-up to qualify as FUO is listed in **Box 10-2.** (See IV below, however.)

III. **A comprehensive list of illnesses known to cause an FUO is given in Box 10-3.**

IV. **An evidence-based approach to the work-up of FUO** has been suggested in a review article by Mourad et al. (2003). Evidence suggests that the following have diagnostic value. **Combine clinical judgment with work-up below and work-up in Box 10-2.**

A. **Stop all nonessential drugs;** monitor for resolution of fever.

B. **Abdominal CT scan** helps identify two of main causes of FUO, intra-abdominal abscess and lymphoproliferative disorders.

C. **Technetium-based nuclear scan** may help locate infectious or inflammatory source; highly specific.

D. **Apply Duke criteria for infectious endocarditis (Box 10-4):** 99% specific in FUO, 82% sensitive for infective endocarditis.

E. **Doppler of lower extremities.** DVT accounts only for a small proportion (2%-6%) of FUO, but is safe and noninvasive.

F. **Temporal artery biopsy.** Giant cell arteritis may account for a large proportion of FUO in the elderly.

G. **Liver biopsy.** Its diagnostic yield of 14% to 17% was felt by authors to outweigh risk of biopsy.

BOX 10-2

MINIMUM WORK-UP FOR FUO

- Comprehensive history
- Repeated physical examination
- CBC, including differential and platelet count
- Routine blood chemistry, including LDH, bilirubin, and liver enzymes
- Urinalysis, including microscopic examination
- CXR
- ESR
- Antinuclear antibodies, rheumatoid factor
- Angiotensin-converting enzyme (although nonspecific for sarcoid)
- Routine blood cultures (×3) while not receiving antibiotics
- Cytomegalovirus IgM antibodies or virus detection in blood; heterophile antibody test in children and young adults
- Tuberculin skin test
- CT of abdomen or radionuclide scan
- HIV antibodies or virus detection assay
- Further evaluation of any abnormalities detected by above tests

From Arnow P, Flaherty J: Fever of unknown origin. *Lancet* 350:575-580, 1997. Used with permission.

INFECTIOUS DISEASES   10

BOX 10-3

COMPREHENSIVE LIST OF ILLNESSES KNOWN TO CAUSE FUO

INFECTION

- Intra-abdominal abscess (e.g., periappendiceal, diverticular, subphrenic); liver, splenic, pancreatic, perinephric, psoas, or placental abscess; appendicitis, cholecystitis, cholangitis, aortoenteric fistula, mesenteric lymphadenitis, tubo-ovarian abscess, endometritis
- Intracranial abscess, sinusitis, mastoiditis, otitis media, dental abscess
- Chronic pharyngitis, tracheobronchitis, lung abscess
- Septic jugular phlebitis, mycotic aneurysm, endocarditis, IV catheter infection, vascular graft infection
- Wound infection, osteomyelitis, infected joint prosthesis, pyelonephritis, prostatitis
- Tuberculosis, *Mycobacterium avium* complex, leprosy, Lyme disease, relapsing fever, *Borrelia recurrentis*, syphilis, Q fever, legionellosis, yersiniosis
- Salmonellosis (including typhoid fever), listeriosis, *Campylobacter*, brucellosis, tularemia, bartonellosis, ehrlichiosis, psittacosis, *Chlamydia pneumoniae*, murine typhus, scrub typhus
- Gonococcemia, meningococcemia
- Actinomycosis, nocardiosis, melioidosis, Whipple's disease *(Trophermyma whippleii)*, candidemia, cryptococcosis, histoplasmosis, coccidioidomycosis, blastomycosis, sporotrichosis, aspergillosis, mucormycosis, *Malassezia furfur*, *Pneumocystis carinii*
- Visceral leishmaniasis, malaria, babesiosis, toxoplasmosis, schistosomiasis, fascioliases, toxocariasis, amebiasis, infected hydatid cyst, trichinosis, trypanosomiasis
- Cytomegalovirus, HIV, herpes simplex, Epstein-Barré virus, parvovirus B19

NEOPLASIA

FUO has been reported in association with all common malignant diseases and with 46 malignancies altogether.

COLLAGEN VASCULAR DISEASE

- Adult Still's disease, SLE, cryoglobulinemia, Reiter's syndrome, rheumatic fever, giant cell arteritis/polymyalgia rheumatica, Wegener's granulomatosis, ankylosing spondylitis, Behçet's syndrome, polyarteritis nodosa
- Hypersensitivity vasculitis, urticarial vasculitis, Sjögren's syndrome, polymyositis, rheumatoid arthritis, erythema multiforme, erythema nodosum, relapsing polychondritis, mixed connective tissue disease, Takayasu's arteritis, Weber-Christian disease, Felty's syndrome, eosinophilic fasciitis

MISCELLANEOUS

- Hematoma, thrombosis, recurrent pulmonary embolism, aortic dissection, femoral aneurysm, post–myocardial infarction syndrome, atrial myxoma
- Drug fever, Sweet's syndrome, familial Mediterranean fever, familial hibernian fever, hyperimmunoglobulin D syndrome, Crohn's disease, ulcerative colitis, sarcoidosis, granulomatosis hepatitis
- Subacute thyroiditis, hyperthyroidism, adrenal insufficiency, primary hyperparathyroidism, hypothalamic hypopituitarism, autoimmune hemolytic anemia
- Gout, pseudogout

BOX 10-3

COMPREHENSIVE LIST OF ILLNESSES KNOWN TO CAUSE FUO—cont'd

- Cirrhosis, chronic active hepatitis, alcoholic hepatitis, shunt nephritis
- Malacoplakia, Kawasaki syndrome, Kikuchi's syndrome
- Mesenteric fibromatosis, inflammatory pseudotumor
- Castleman's disease, Vogt-Koyanagi-Harada syndrome, Gaucher's disease, Schnitzler's syndrome, FAPA syndrome (fever, aphthous stomatitis, pharyngitis, adenitis; found in children, recurs monthly, responds to steroids), Fabry's disease
- Cholesterol emboli, silicone embolization, Teflon embolization
- Lymph node infarction, sickle cell disease, vaso-occlusive crisis, anhidrotic ectodermal dysplasia, cyclic neutropenia, brewer's yeast ingestion, Hamman-Rich syndrome
- Milk protein allergy, hypersensitivity pneumonitis, extrinsic allergic alveolitis, metal fume fever, polymer fume fever, idiopathic hypereosinophilic syndrome
- Complex partial status epilepticus, cerebrovascular accident, brain tumor, encephalitis
- Anomalous thoracic duct, psychogenic fever, habitual hyperthermia, factitious illness

From Arnow P, Flaherty J: Fever of unknown origin. *Lancet* 350:575-580, 1997. Used with permission.

LYME DISEASE

I. **Epidemiology.**
A. **Worldwide distribution. Three foci in the United States:**
1. Northeast: Massachusetts to Maryland.
2. Upper Midwest, especially Wisconsin and Minnesota.
3. Coastal California and Oregon.
B. **Onset of illness is usually May to November,** peaking in June and July.
II. **Pathogenesis.**
A. **Cause.** *Borrelia burgdorferi sensu lato*, a spirochete group. Most common cause in the United States is *B. burgdorferi sensu stricto*.
B. **Transmission.** Bite from deer tick, *Ixodes scapularis* or *Ixodes pacificus*, during spring nymph stage.
C. **An infected tick that is attached for <24 hours is unlikely** to transmit infection, but almost 100% transmission occurs when >72 hours has elapsed.
III. **Clinical Characteristics.**
A. **Stage I (first weeks to months).**
1. **Erythema chronicum migrans.** Red macules with central clearing start 3 to 32 days after infection at the site of the bite and enlarge centrifugally to >5 cm. Erythema chronicum migrans is **seen in 60% to 70% of patients** with Lyme disease.
2. **Flulike illness.** Myalgia, arthralgia, fatigue, headache, neck pain and stiffness, fever, chills, and sore throat.

BOX 10-4

DUKE CRITERIA FOR DIAGNOSIS OF INFECTIVE ENDOCARDITIS

MAJOR CRITERIA

- Persistently positive blood culture
  - Two separate blood cultures >12 h apart
  - Three or more cultures drawn >1 h apart
  - Majority of cultures if four or more drawn
- Echocardiographic evidence of endocardial involvement:
  - Intracardiac mass on valve or supporting structure
  - Abscess
  - New partial dehiscence of prosthetic valve
  - New valvular regurgitation

MINOR CRITERIA

- Predisposing heart condition or IV drug abuse
- Fever ≥38.0°C
- Vascular findings
  - Arterial emboli
  - Septic pulmonary infarct
  - Mycotic aneurysm
  - Intracranial or conjunctival hemorrhage
  - Janeway lesions
- Immunologic findings
  - Glomerulonephritis
  - Osler's nodes
  - Roth's spots
  - Positive rheumatoid factor
- Positive blood culture but not meeting a major criterion
- Echocardiogram consistent with infective endocarditis but not meeting a major criterion

Note: Definitive diagnosis requires presence of 2 major, 1 major and 3 minor, or 5 minor criteria.

---

3. *Borrelia* **lymphocytoma: rarely seen in the United States.** Red, firm nodule on ear pinna in children, on nipple and areola in adults.
B. **Stage II (begins weeks to months after bite/rash).**
1. **Neurologic involvement** in 15%, including lymphocytic meningitis, encephalitis, chorea, unilateral or bilateral facial nerve palsy or any cranial nerve palsy, radiculoneuritis, mononeuritis multiplex, diffuse peripheral sensorimotor neuropathy.
2. **Cardiac involvement** in 5%, including fluctuating AV block (can be first, second, or third degree), myopericarditis with ST segment changes, arrhythmias, syncope, presyncope, or palpitations. Valvular involvement is rare.
C. **Stage III (weeks to years after tick bite).**
1. **Varies from migratory musculoskeletal pain to overt inflammatory arthritis.** Asymmetric oligoarticular intermittent pain and swelling,

usually of large joints (most commonly the knee). Other chronic neurologic syndromes can also occur. Another late manifestation is acrodermatitis chronica atrophicans (indurated and erythematous plaques on knees, elbows, hands, and feet that become atrophic), mostly in elderly women and rare in the United States.

IV. Diagnosis.

A. Usually based on clinical and epidemiologic evidence. Diagnosis requires a positive ELISA confirmed by Western blot. *A positive ELISA by itself is not specific enough, and false-positive results occur.*

1. **False-negative results occur in the first 3 to 4 weeks of illness** (no significant antibody response) and because of variable assay sensitivities between labs.

2. **False-positive results can occur with** *Treponema pallidum*, other treponemes, *E. coli*, JRA, SLE, mononucleosis, and bacterial endocarditis.

B. Differential diagnosis.

1. **Dermatologic manifestations can mimic** erythema multiforme, SLE, prodromal phase of hepatitis B, erythema marginatum, aseptic meningitis, infectious mononucleosis, and lymphoproliferative disorder.

2. **Rheumatologic manifestations can mimic** rheumatic fever, reactive arthritis, and JRA.

3. **Neurologic manifestations can mimic** Bell's palsy, multiple sclerosis, Guillain-Barré syndrome, and brain tumor.

V. Treatment.

A. Early disease. Doxycycline 100 mg PO bid × 14 to 21 days or amoxicillin 500 mg tid (if <9 years of age, 50 mg/kg per day divided tid) × 14 to 21 days or erythromycin 250 mg qid (if <9 years of age, 30 mg/kg per day divided tid) × 14 to 21 days.

1. **Jarisch-Herxheimer–like reaction** (fever, chills, rash, and lymphadenopathy within 6 hours of beginning treatment) is seen in 15%.

2. **Constitutional, fibromyalgia-like, symptoms may continue** for extended periods despite adequate treatment. **This is not related to ongoing infection and will not respond to antibiotics.** Look for depression, fibromyalgia, etc.

3. **Facial palsy alone (even bilateral) may be treated the same as early disease.**

B. Late disease.

1. **If no meningitis, doxycycline 100 mg PO bid × 21 days has an equivalent cure rate to ceftriaxone** 2 gm IV or IM daily × 14 days. Doxycycline has the advantage of being PO, less expensive, and less painful than ceftriaxone.

2. Lyme meningitis, serious carditis, or persistent arthritis. Treat with ceftriaxone 2 g IV qd (children, 75-100 mg/kg per day) or penicillin G 20 to 24 million U/d (children, 300,000 U/kg per day) IV divided q4h × 14 to 28 days.

VI. Prevention.
  A. Protective clothing: long sleeves, long pants tucked into socks, DEET-containing insect repellent, check for ticks bid when in endemic areas.
  B. Prophylaxis within 72 hours after a tick bite with doxycycline 200 mg PO once can prevent disease in 87% of cases **(NNT 83, NNH 10 [rash, anaphylaxis]). However, most studies show no benefit. Because only 1.2% of those in endemic areas who are bitten develop Lyme disease, observation and treatment of symptomatic patients is an option, especially given the NNT and NNH.**
  C. A vaccine was introduced in the United States in 1998; although proven effective in studies, it was removed from the market in 2002 for economic reasons.

EHRLICHIOSIS

  I. Epidemiology.
  A. Onset. April to September, peaking in June and July; two thirds are rural residents.
  B. Human monocytic ehrlichiosis (HME) is more common in southeast and south-central United States (Oklahoma, Georgia, Arkansas, Missouri, North Carolina).
  C. Human granulocytic ehrlichiosis (HGE) is more common in Minnesota, Wisconsin, New York, and Maryland.
  II. Pathogenesis.
  A. HME is caused by *Ehrlichia chaffeensis* transmitted by *Amblyomma americanum* (lone star tick).
  B. HGE is caused by *Anaplasma phagocytophilia* transmitted by *Ixodes scapularis* (deer tick), the same tick that transmits Lyme disease.
  III. Clinical Characteristics.
  A. Fever, diaphoresis, myalgias, arthralgias, malaise, headache, nausea, vomiting.
  B. About 15% have severe complications: renal failure, DIC, pulmonary hemorrhage, interstitial pneumonitis, bronchiolitis obliterans with organizing pneumonia (BOOP), seizures, and coma. HGE is usually milder than HME and mostly asymptomatic.
  C. Lab findings include leukopenia, anemia, thrombocytopenia, and elevations of AST, ALT, and LDH. May see morulae in circulating peripheral WBCs.
  IV. Diagnosis.
  A. Usually clinical, because therapy should be started before lab results are obtained.
  B. Can be confirmed by serum antibody acute and convalescent titers or PCR testing.

V. **Treatment.** Doxycycline 100 mg bid for adults (3 mg/kg per day divided bid for children) × 7 to 14 days.

VI. **Prevention.** When outdoors in tick-infested areas, wear light-colored clothing, use insect repellent, and check thoroughly for ticks afterward.

BABESIOSIS

I. **Epidemiology.**

A. **Most cases in New England, Wisconsin, and California.**

B. **Transmission by** *Ixodes scapularis*, the same vector as for Lyme disease.

C. Rodents act as reservoirs.

II. **Causes.** *Babesia microti* and *Babesia divergens*, which are intraerythrocytic protozoan parasites.

III. **Clinical Features.**

A. **Malaria-like illness, but unlike malaria, fevers are irregular.**

B. Fever, chills, drenching sweats, lethargy, malaise, myalgias, arthralgias, and darkened or red urine.

C. **The most severe cases occur in the splenectomized patients and the elderly.**

IV. **Laboratory Findings.** Elevated liver enzymes, leukopenia, and hemolytic anemia, as well as hemoglobinuria.

V. **Diagnosis.** Can find the intracellular organisms with Giemsa stain of a peripheral blood smear.

A. Multiple parasites per RBC, with pronounced pleomorphism. Often 4% to 7% RBCs infected (rarely up to 40%).

B. Serologic characteristics may also be diagnostic (ELISA, IFA).

C. PCR appears most specific.

VI. **Treatment.** The illness is generally self-limited except in the splenectomized and elderly. Treatment consists of atovaquone 750 mg PO bid and azithromycin 500 mg once then 250 mg qd × 7 days. Alternatively, clindamycin 600 mg PO tid plus quinine 650 mg PO tid × 7 days. Children: clindamycin 20 mg/kg per day, quinine 25 mg/kg per day.

LEPTOSPIROSIS

I. **Epidemiology.**

A. **Worldwide but higher incidence in the tropics;** many domestic and wild animal carriers.

B. **Transmission by** direct contact with animal tissue or urine or indirect through contaminated water, soil, or vegetation (usually through conjunctivae, broken skin).

C. **More common in teenagers and young adults;** July through October. Associated with slum living, water sports, and historically with occupational exposure such as farmers, veterinarians, and abattoir workers.

10

INFECTIOUS DISEASES

II. **Pathogenesis.**

A. **Caused by spirochetes,** *Leptospira interrogans sensu lato* and *Leptospira biflexa sensu lato* species.

III. **Clinical Characteristics.**

A. Fever, chills, headache, conjunctivitis, severe myalgias.

B. Anorexia, nausea, vomiting in 50%, diarrhea less common.

C. Typically a biphasic illness, with fevers, myalgias, headaches, and pyuria in the first phase. Fever recurs often with aseptic meningitis in the second phase, or with a fulminant disease (icterohemorrhagic form in 5%-10%)

D. Children tend to have acalculous cholecystitis, pancreatitis, abdominal causalgia, hypertension, and a rash with severe peripheral desquamation (life threatening).

IV. **Clinical Syndromes.**

A. **Weil's syndrome:** leptospirosis with jaundice, often with renal failure, thrombocytopenia, hemorrhages, anemia, altered mentation, or fever.

B. **Atypical pneumonia syndrome:** bilateral bronchopneumonia may progress to ARDS.

C. **Aseptic meningitis:** CSF with 10 to 1000/mm^3 WBCs, normal glucose, high protein.

D. **Cardiac involvement:** nonspecific ECG changes, first-degree AV block, acute pericarditis, and rarely arrhythmias, myocarditis, or CHF.

E. **Rhabdomyolysis is rare,** characterized by elevated CK in a setting of jaundice and elevated aminotransferases.

F. Conjunctivitis, conjunctival suffusions, and uveitis are well documented.

V. **Diagnosis.**

A. Blood or CSF culture positive for *Leptospira* first 10 days and from urine second or third week of illness (needs special medium).

B. Detection of antibodies by microscopic agglutination test in second week of illness, with fourfold rise in titers, or rapid genus-specific IgM detection assays can be positive in the first week.

C. PCR is both sensitive and specific.

VI. **Treatment is mostly supportive.**

A. IV penicillin 1.5 million U q6h × 7 d or ceftriaxone 1g IV qd × 7 d.

B. Jarisch-Herxheimer reaction seen in 15% to 80% after penicillin treatment.

C. Disease seems to worsen within hours of first penicillin dose. Body temperature rises, then falls, and hypertension is followed by hypotension.

D. Doxycycline 100 mg PO bid × 7 d if allergic to penicillin. Other options include amoxicillin 500 mg PO qid and ampicillin 500 to 750 mg q6h.

VII. **Prognosis.** Mortality rate 7%, primarily among those with icterohemorrhagic form.

ROCKY MOUNTAIN SPOTTED FEVER

I. **Epidemiology.**

A. **All states except Maine and Alaska;** more common in South Atlantic and Midwest states than in the Rocky Mountain states.

B. Peak incidence between April and October.

C. Most cases are in children 5 to 9 years of age.

II. **Etiology.** A tick-borne illness caused by *Rickettsia rickettsii*, an intracellular organism. The dog tick *(Dermacentor variabilis)* or wood tick *(Dermacentor andersoni)* has to be attached for at least 4 hours for transmission to occur; disease can also be transmitted when a tick is crushed during removal.

III. **Physical Findings.** After an incubation period of 7 days, there is **sudden onset of spiking fever, headache, confusion, myalgias, and weakness.** The disease may progress to obtundation with CSF pleocytosis on LP. Patients may also have nausea, vomiting, diarrhea, and hepatosplenomegaly.

A. **Rash** starting on extremities and spreading to trunk is a hallmark feature of this disease. Generally appears as erythematous macules on wrist and ankle within 24 hours, becomes petechial by day 4 if not treated. **However, 4% to 10% have no rash, and in others it may be evanescent. Rash can occur from 3 to 5 days after the fever develops.**

B. **Rarely, there may be pulmonary involvement or myocardial vasculitis** with nonspecific ST-T segment changes.

C. **Case fatality rate is as high as 25%.**

IV. **Laboratory Tests.**

A. Slightly decreased WBCs, **thrombocytopenia** (may develop DIC), anemia, elevated aminotransferases.

B. **Serologic testing should be used to confirm the diagnosis.** The Weil-Felix reaction is no longer used, and diagnostic titers may not be elevated until 10 to 14 days into the course. Therefore, **empiric treatment should be started based on clinical suspicion, given the high mortality rate of the disease.**

C. Immunohistologic examination of a cutaneous biopsy is relatively sensitive and highly specific (if available).

V. **Treatment.**

A. **In adults,** doxycycline 100 mg PO bid or tetracycline 500 mg PO qid.

B. **In children,** doxycycline 2.2 mg/kg PO bid is recommended as first-line therapy.

C. **Chloramphenicol** 50 to 75 mg/kg per day divided qid is another alternative but with more side effects (gray baby syndrome, aplastic anemia).

D. Treat both children and adults for at least 7 days or until afebrile for 2 to 5 days.

10

INFECTIOUS DISEASES

INFECTIVE ENDOCARDITIS

I. General. Infective endocarditis is an infection of the endothelial lining of the heart caused by direct invasion of organisms, usually on valvular surfaces. The disease occurs most commonly in patients with underlying structural heart disease. Infective endocarditis can be classified as either acute or subacute, or by certain etiologic factors such as prosthetic valves versus native valves.

II. Risk Factors.

A. Underlying heart disease. Rheumatic valvular damage, congenital heart disease, mitral valve prolapse (with mitral regurgitation or thickened mitral leaflets), prosthetic valves, hypertrophic cardiomyopathy, and previous bacterial endocarditis are predisposing factors for endocarditis. With more virulent organisms, such as *S. aureus*, previous valvular damage is present only in about 50% of the cases.

B. Events predisposing patients to bacteremia including IV drug use, IV catheters, dental and GU procedures, poor dental hygiene, hemodialysis, DM, and HIV.

C. Age >50 years increases risk.

III. Etiology of Bacterial Endocarditis.

A. Native valve endocarditis. *Streptococcus viridans, S. aureus*, enterococci, HACEK (*Haemophilus, Actinobacillus, Cardiobacterium, Eikenella*, and *Kingella*), gram-negative bacilli, fungi.

B. Prosthetic valve endocarditis. Coagulase-negative staphylococci, *S. aureus*, enterococci, gram-negative bacilli, fungi.

C. Endocarditis in IV drug users. *S. aureus*, streptococci, gram-negative bacillus, enterococci, fungi, polymicrobial.

D. Culture-negative (marantic) endocarditis is a nonbacterial thrombotic endocarditis that constitutes about 5% of cases of endocarditis.

E. Acute bacterial endocarditis. *S. aureus*, pneumococci, group A streptococci.

IV. Clinical Manifestations.

A. Acute bacterial endocarditis. Acute onset of fever, chills, arthralgias, and myalgias. **Patients appear systemically ill and often develop sepsis. CNS symptoms** occur in about 30% of patients from systemic emboli causing cerebral infarctions, brain abscesses, mycotic aneurysms, intracranial hemorrhages, and aseptic meningitis. **Septic emboli** to the kidneys, spleen, liver, coronary arteries, and mesenteric arteries can also occur. Cardiac valvular destruction can lead to rapid ventricular failure, and extension into the septum can cause heart block. Peripherally, **Janeway lesions** (nonblanching, nontender, erythematous macules that occur on palms and soles) occur, but other peripheral stigmata of subacute endocarditis are uncommon.

B. **Subacute bacterial endocarditis.** Fever and chills are almost always present, but the onset of the disease is insidious. **Symptoms can be present from weeks to months before they are brought to medical attention.** Patients complain of night sweats, weakness, fatigue, arthralgias, and myalgias, anorexia, malaise, weight loss. Complications included septic emboli, heart failure from valvular destruction, and heart block. Sepsis is less common than in acute bacterial endocarditis. On exam, heart murmurs are usually found. Physical exam findings also include **splinter hemorrhages, Roth's spots (edematous, exudative retinal lesions), Osler's nodes (painful, violaceous nodules in pulp of fingers and toes), and splenomegaly.**

V. **Diagnosis.** See Box 10-4 for Duke Criteria for diagnosis of infective endocarditis.

A. **Blood cultures should be obtained in any patient suspected of having endocarditis.** Blood cultures are positive in >90% of the cases but can be negative if the patient has recently been given antimicrobial therapy. The bacteremia is usually continuous. Three sets during a 1-hour period usually suffice. The cultures should be obtained before starting empiric antibiotic therapy if at all possible. In the acutely ill patient, cultures should be drawn (two or three sets) and empiric antibiotic treatment should be given without delay. Antimicrobial treatment can be refined when the culture results are available. In suspected cases with a subacute onset, the cultures can be obtained over a 24-hour period before starting antibiotic therapy. If the blood cultures remain negative over several days and endocarditis is still suspected, the lab should be notified to hold the blood cultures for 3 weeks to increase the chance of recovering fastidious organisms.

B. **Echocardiograph is not absolutely essential to make the diagnosis, and absence of vegetation on echocardiography does not rule out the diagnosis.** Transthoracic and transesophageal echocardiograms have a sensitivity of about 65% and 90%, respectively; both have very high specificity for vegetations (98%).

VI. **Treatment.**

A. **Empiric therapy awaiting culture results.**

1. **Native valve.**

a. **Acute presentation:** nafcillin 2 g IV q4h **plus** penicillin 20 million U/d as continuous drip **plus** gentamicin 1mg/kg IV q8h **(once-daily dosing not recommended),** *or* vancomycin 15/kg mg IV q12h plus gentamicin 1 mg/kg IV q8h (if penicillin allergy). Adjust gentamicin dose with peak/trough levels.

b. **Subacute presentation:** penicillin G 20 million U IV q24h (continuous infusion over 24 hours) **plus** gentamicin 1 mg/kg IV q8h *or* vancomycin 15 mg/kg IV qQ12h **plus** gentamicin 1 mg/kg IV q8h (if penicillin allergy).

2. **Prosthetic valve.** Vancomycin 15 mg/kg IV q12h plus gentamicin 1 mg/kg IV q8h plus rifampin 600 mg PO qd.
B. **Switch antibiotics based on culture and sensitivity.**
C. **Duration of therapy varies from 2 to 6 weeks depending on the organism** (see Mylonakis and Calderwood, 2001).
D. **Indications for surgery include** progressive CHF, multiple embolic events, fungal endocarditis, *Pseudomonas, Brucella,* or *Coxiella* endocarditis, persistent bacteremia, extension of infection into the conducting system (new heart block on ECG), relapse of infection, abscess on echocardiography, and sometimes large vegetations. Culture-negative endocarditis also occurs (see Brouqui and Raoult, 2001).

MALARIA

I. **General.** Malaria is a systemic illness manifested by recurrent fever and chills occurring within 8 weeks to several months after returning from areas of the world in which the disease is endemic.
II. **Epidemiology.** Endemic in most of the tropical and subtropical world, including South and Central America, the Caribbean, Africa, the Middle East, Southeast Asia, and Oceania.
III. **Pathogenesis.** Four species of intraerythrocytic parasites transmitted by the female *Anopheles* mosquito:
A. *Plasmodium falciparum* is the most common and most serious and is responsible for most deaths. No relapses.
B. *Plasmodium vivax,* second most common, relapses.
C. *Plasmodium ovale,* relapses.
D. *Plasmodium malariae,* no relapses.
IV. **Clinical Characteristics.**
A. **Recurrent fevers and chills:** Fever patterns are mostly erratic. *P. vivax* and *P. ovale* typically occur at 48-hour intervals, *P. malariae* at 72-hour intervals, *P. falciparum* at irregular intervals.
B. **Headaches, malaise, arthralgias, myalgias, cough, nausea, vomiting, and diarrhea are common.** Patients may be free of symptoms between episodes of fevers and chills. On exam, fever and splenomegaly are common, and sometimes jaundice, hepatomegaly, and abdominal tenderness.
C. **Severe cases of *P. falciparum* malaria can cause prostration,** mental status changes including seizures and coma, bleeding, jaundice, renal failure, hypoglycemia, pulmonary edema, and severe anemia with hemoglobinuria.
D. **Severity of disease is proportional to the degree of parasitemia, typically >5%.**
V. **Laboratory findings.** WBC counts are almost always within normal limits, thrombocytopenia in 70% and anemia in 25%,

aminotransferases are elevated in 25%, bilirubin in 33%, and LDH in 80% of patients.

VI. Diagnosis. A definitive diagnosis depends on the identification of the parasites in a peripheral blood smear, preferably stained with Giemsa. Obtain three smears over a 48-hour period. Rapid antigen detection tests are available for *P. falciparum* and *P. vivax*, with sensitivity of 90%. PCR is also highly sensitive (>90%) and almost 100% specific. Serology has no role in diagnosing acute malaria.

VII. Treatment. Treatment is dependent on the *Plasmodium* species, the area of acquisition (likelihood of drug resistance), and the severity of infection. If the type of *Plasmodium* cannot be identified it should be assumed that the patient has a drug-resistant *P. falciparum* infection until proven otherwise. For CDC malaria treatment information, see www.cdc.gov or call (770) 488-7788.

VIII. Prevention.

A. Avoid outdoor exposures between dusk and dawn in endemic areas.

B. Use insect repellent with DEET.

C. Dress to minimize exposure of skin.

D. Use mosquito nets sprayed with permethrin when possible.

E. Chemoprophylaxis depends on the likelihood of drug resistance in the geographic area visited; see www.cdc.gov or call (888) 232-3228.

BIOTERRORISM SUMMARY

Syndromes that can be caused by bioterrorism are shown in **Table 10-3**. Ways of recognizing and diagnosing illnesses that could be caused by bioterrorism are shown in **Table 10-4**. Treatment and prophylaxis for bioterrorism agents are shown in **Table 10-5**. Infection control precautions for bioterrorism agents are shown in **Table 10-6**. For more details, see http://www.bt.cdc.gov/Agent/agentlist.asp.

10

INFECTIOUS DISEASES

TABLE 10-3

SYNDROMES AND POSSIBLE BIOTERRORISM CAUSES: USE THIS TABLE TO DETERMINE THE POSSIBLE PRESENCE OF A BIOTERRORISM AGENT WHEN PRESENTED WITH AN UNEXPLAINED CLUSTER OF ILLNESSES

Syndrome	Bioterrorism Diseases			Naturally Occurring Diseases
	Category A	Category B	Category C	
Respiratory tract infection with fever	Inhalational anthrax, pneumonic plague, tularemia	Inhalational glanders, inhalational ricin, melioidosis, Q fever, typhus	Hantavirus (second stage), legionellosis, SARS	Diphtheria, *Escherichia coli*, histoplasmosis, influenza, malaria, measles, RSV
Gastroenteritis	Anthrax, Ebola, plague, Marburg, tularemia	Acute brucellosis, cholera, *Cryptosporidium, Giardia*, Q fever, paralytic shellfish toxins, ricin/abrin toxins	Hantavirus, norovirus, legionellosis	*Cestodes, Clostridium difficile, Helicobacter pylori*, hepatitis A, hepatitis E, leishmaniasis (visceral), Rocky Mountain spotted fever, typhoid fever
Rash with fever	Ebola, Marburg, pneumonic plague, smallpox	Glanders, typhus	Dengue fever, Lyme disease	Chickenpox, measles, monkeypox, mumps, Rocky Mountain spotted fever, rubella
Influenza-like illness	Anthrax, Ebola, plague, smallpox, tularemia	Brucellosis, glanders, Q fever, typhus	Hantavirus, legionellosis, Lyme disease, Nipah virus, SARS	Diphtheria, influenza, malaria, measles, mononucleosis, Rift Valley fever, RSV, yellow fever

Sepsis, nontraumatic shock	Ebola, Lassa fever, Marburg fever	*E. coli*	Hantavirus	CMV, *Enterococcus faecium*, histoplasmosis, listeriosis, *Staphylococcus epidermidis*, *Streptococcus pneumoniae*, TSS
Meningitis, encephalitis-like syndrome	Anthrax, Ebola, Lassa fever	Eastern equine encephalitis, Q fever, Venezuelan equine encephalitis	Japanese encephalitis, Lyme disease, Nipah virus, St. Louis encephalitis, West Nile virus	Chickenpox, dengue, Epstein-Barr virus, *Haemophilus influenzae*, influenza A, influenza B, malaria, measles, Rift Valley fever, Rocky Mountain spotted fever, viral meningitis
Botulism-like	Botulism			Diphtheria, listeriosis

Adapted with permission from Kristin Uhde, PhD, and the University of South Florida Center for Biological Defense.

TABLE 10-4
RECOGNIZING ILLNESSES POSSIBLY DUE TO BIOTERRORISM

Disease	Incubation Period	Early Symptoms	Clinical Syndrome	Diagnostic Samples	Diagnostic Tests
Anthrax, inhalational	1–7 d (possibly up to 60 d)	Nonspecific: fever, malaise, cough, dyspnea, headache, vomiting, abdominal and chest pain	Widened mediastinum, pleural effusion on CXR; rapid onset of severe respiratory distress, respiratory failure, shock	Blood, semen, CSF, pleural or ascitic fluids	Gram stain or Wright stain, blood culture Specialized labs: IHC, serology, DFA, PCR
Anthrax, cutaneous	1–12 d	Painless or pruritic papule	Papule evolves into a vesicular or ulcerative lesion, then forms a black eschar after 3–7 d	Swab of lesion, skin biopsy, blood	Gram stain, culture of lesion; blood culture Specialized labs: PCR, serology
Botulism	Foodborne: 12–72 h (range, 2 h to 8 d) Inhalational: 12–80 h	Usually none. If foodborne, possibly nausea, vomiting, abdominal cramps, diarrhea	Afebrile, ptosis, diplopia, dysphonia, dysphagia, symmetric descending paresis or flaccid paralysis; generally normal mental status; progresses to airway obstruction and respiratory failure	Nasal swab (if obtained immediately after inhalation exposure), serum, gastric aspirate, stool, food sample when indicated	Specialized labs: mouse bioassay for toxin

Brucellosis	Very variable, 5-60 d	Fever (often intermittent), headache, chills, heavy sweats, arthralgias	Systemic illness, may become chronic with fever and weight loss; may have suppurative lesions; bone and joint lesions common	Blood, serum, bone marrow, tissue	Culture, serology, PCR
Equine encephalitides (eastern, western, Venezuelan)	Venezuelan: 2-6 d Others: 5-15 d	Nonspecific: sudden onset of malaise, fever, rigors, severe headache, photophobia, myalgias of legs and back	Fever, headache, stiff neck, nausea, vomiting, sore throat, diarrhea lasting several days and often followed by prolonged period of weakness and lethargy; CNS symptoms might develop	Serum, CSF	Viral culture, serology, PCR
Pneumonic plague	1-6 d	Nonspecific: high fever, cough, chills, dyspnea, headache, hemoptysis, nausea, vomiting, diarrhea	Fulminant pneumonia, often with hemoptysis, rapid progression of respiratory failure, septicemia, shock Hemoptysis can help distinguish from inhalational anthrax	Blood, sputum, lymph node aspirate, serum	Gram, Wright, or Wayson stain; culture Specialized labs: serology, DFA, PCR

(Continued)

INFECTIOUS DISEASES 10

TABLE 10-4
RECOGNIZING ILLNESSES POSSIBLY DUE TO BIOTERRORISM—cont'd

Disease	Incubation Period	Early Symptoms	Clinical Syndrome	Diagnostic Samples	Diagnostic Tests
Q fever	10-40 d	Fever, headache, chills, heavy sweats, arthralgias	Self-limited febrile illness lasting 2 d to 2 wk; can manifest like atypical pneumonia (*Legionella*)	Serum, sputum	Serology; culture difficult
Ricin (toxin from castor bean oil)	18-24 h	Inhalation: fever, weakness, cough, hypothermia, hypotension, cardiac collapse	In high doses, short incubation and rapid onset suggestive of chemical agent	Blood, tissue	Serology, IHC, staining of tissue
Smallpox	12 d (range, 7-17 d)	Nonspecific: fever, malaise, headache, prostration, rigors, vomiting, severe backache	Maculopapular, vesicular, then pustular lesions all at the same developmental stage in any one location; begins on face, mucous membranes, hands, and forearms; can include palms and soles	Vesicular or pustular fluid, pharyngeal swab, scab material, serum	Specialized labs: PCR, viral culture, electron or light microscopy, serology

Staphylococcal enterotoxin B	Inhalation: 3-12 h; Ingestion: minutes to hours	Inhalation: fever, chills, headache, myalgias, cough, nausea; short incubation and rapid onset suggestive of chemical agent	Inhalation: dyspnea, retrosternal pain can develop; Ingestion: nausea, vomiting, diarrhea	Inhalation: serum, urine; Ingestion: stool, vomitus	Specialized labs: Ag-ELISA, Ab-ELISA, serology
Tularemia	3-5 d (range, 1-14 d)	Nonspecific: fever, fatigue, chills, cough, malaise, body aches, headache, chest discomfort, GI symptoms	Pneumonitis, ARDS, pleural effusion, hemoptysis, sepsis; ocular lesions, skin ulcers, oropharyngeal or glandular disease possible	Serum, urine, blood, sputum, pharyngeal washing, fasting gastric aspirate, other	Gram stain, culture; DFA or IHC staining of secretions, exudates, or biopsy specimens
Viral hemorrhagic fevers (Ebola, arenavirus, filoviruses)	2-21 d (varies by virus)	Fever, myalgias, petechiae, easy bleeding, red, itchy eyes, hematemesis	Febrile illness complicated by easy bleeding, petechiae, hypotension, shock	Serum, blood	Viral culture, PCR, serology

Ab, antibody; Ag, antigen.
Adapted from New York State Department of Health: Bioterrorism rapid response card. PDF available for download at http://www.health.state.ny.us/nysdoh/bt/pdf/rapid_response_card.pdf (accessed December 1, 2005).

INFECTIOUS DISEASES   10

TREATMENT AND PROPHYLAXIS OF BIOTERRORISM AGENTS

Agent	Treatment	Prophylaxis
Anthrax (cutaneous or inhalational)	Ciprofloxacin, doxycycline Inhalational: consider combination therapy of ciprofloxacin *or* doxycycline *plus* one or two other antimicrobials	Ciprofloxacin *or* doxycycline, ± vaccination If susceptible, consider PCN *or* amoxicillin
Botulism	Supportive care; ventilation might be necessary Administer trivalent equine antitoxin (serotypes A, B, E, available from CDC) immediately after clinical diagnosis	None
Brucellosis	Doxycycline *plus* streptomycin or rifampin Alternatives: ofloxacin *plus* rifampin; doxycycline *plus* gentamicin; TMP–SMX *plus* gentamicin	Doxycycline *plus* streptomycin or rifampin
Equine encephalitides (eastern, western, Venezuelan)	Supportive care: analgesics, anticonvulsants as needed	None
Pneumonic plague	Streptomycin, gentamicin Alternatives: doxycycline, tetracycline, ciprofloxacin, chloramphenicol	Tetracycline, doxycycline, ciprofloxacin
Q fever	Tetracycline, doxycycline	Tetracycline, doxycycline (might delay but not prevent illness)
Ricin	Supportive care; treatment for pulmonary edema; gastric decontamination for ingestion	None
Smallpox	Supportive care; cidofovir shown to be effective in vitro	Vaccination given within 3-4 d of exposure can prevent or decrease severity of disease
Staphylococcal enterotoxin B	Supportive care	None
Tularemia	Streptomycin, gentamicin; alternative: ciprofloxacin	Tetracycline, doxycycline, ciprofloxacin
Viral hemorrhagic fevers	Supportive care Ribavirin may be effective for Lassa fever, Congo–Crimean hemorrhagic fever, Rift Valley fever	Ribavirin may be effective for Lassa fever, Congo–Crimean hemorrhagic fever, Rift Valley fever

Adapted from New York State Department of Health: Bioterrorism rapid response card. PDF available for download at http://www.health.state.ny.us/nysdoh/bt/pdf/rapid_response_card.pdf (accessed December 1, 2005).

TABLE 10-6
INFECTION CONTROL PRECAUTIONS FOR BIOTERRORISM AGENTS

Agent	Precaution Category*	Personal Protective Equipment	Private Room
Anthrax	Standard Contact precautions for cutaneous and GI anthrax if diarrhea is not contained	Gloves when entering the room Gown if likely contact with patient, equipment, or environment	No
Botulism	Standard		No
Brucellosis	Standard		No
Pneumonic plague	Standard Droplet precautions until patient is on appropriate therapy for 72 h Contact precautions if draining buboes are present	Gloves when entering room Gown if likely contact with patient, equipment, or environment Surgical mask	No; cohort if necessary
Q fever	Standard		No
Smallpox	Standard, contact, airborne	Gloves, gown when entering room N95 respirator	Yes; negative pressure
Tularemia	Standard Contact precautions if lesions are present	Gloves when entering room Gown if likely contact with patient, equipment, or environment	No
Viral hemorrhagic fever	Standard and contact Airborne precautions in late stages	Gloves, gown when entering room N95 respirator	Yes; negative pressure
Venezuelan equine encephalitis	Standard		No

*For descriptions of precaution categories see Garner JS and the Hospital Infection Control Practices Advisory Committee: Guideline for isolation precautions in hospitals. *Infect Control Hosp Epidemiol* 17:53-80, 1996, and *Am J Infect Control* 24:24-52, 1996. Available at http://www.cdc.gov/ncidod/hip/ISOLAT/ISOLAT.HTM (accessed December 1, 2005).
Adapted from the New York State Department of Health: Bioterrorism rapid response card. PDF available for download at http://www.health.state.ny.us/nysdoh/bt/pdf/rapid_response_card.pdf (accessed December 1, 2005).

INFECTIOUS DISEASES 10

BIBLIOGRAPHY

Aguero-Rosenfeld ME: Laboratory aspects of tick-borne diseases: Lyme, human granulocytic ehrlichiosis and babesiosis. *Mt Sinai J Med* 70:197-206, 2003.
Arnow P, Flaherty J: Fever of unknown origin. *Lancet* 350:575, 1997.
Astiz ME, Rackow EC: Septic shock. *Lancet* 351:1501, 2000.
Bernard GR, Vincent JL, Laterre PF, et al., Recombinant Human Protein C Worldwide Evaluation in Severe Sepsis (PROWESS) Study Group: Efficacy and safety of recombinant human activated protein C for severe sepsis. *N Engl J Med* 344:699-709, 2001.

Bharti AR, Nally JE, Ricaldi JM, et al: Leptospirosis: A zoonotic disease of global importance. *Lancet Infect Dis* 3:757-771, 2003.

Blumberg HM, Burman WJ, Caisson RE, et al: American Thoracic Society/Centers for Disease Control and Prevention/Infectious Diseases Society of America: Treatment of tuberculosis. *Am J Respir Crit Care Med* 167:603-662, 2003.

Bochud PY, Calandra T: Pathogenesis of sepsis: New concepts and implications for future treatment. *BMJ* 326:262-266, 2003.

Brouqui P, Raoult D: Endocarditis due to rare and fastidious bacteria. *Clin Microbiol Rev* 14:177-207, 2001.

Cross AS, Opal SM: A new paradigm for the treatment of sepsis: Is it time to consider combination therapy? *Ann Intern Med* 138:502-505, 2003.

Flinders DC, De Schweinitz P: Pediculosis and scabies. *Am Fam Physician* 69: 341-348, 2004.

Fowler VG Jr, Sanders LL, Sexton DJ, et al: Outcome of *Staphylococcus aureus* bacteremia according to compliance with recommendations of infectious disease specialists: Experience with 244 patients. *Clin Infect Dis* 27:478-486, 1998.

Frieden TR, Sterling TR, Munsiff S, et al: Tuberculosis. *Lancet* 362:887-899, 2003.

Gayle A, Ringdahl E: Tick-borne diseases. *Am Fam Physician* 64:461-466, 2001.

Giessel BE, Koenig CJ, Blake RL Jr: Management of bacterial endocarditis. *Am Fam Physician* 61:1725-1732, 2000.

Gilbert DN, Moellering RC, Eliopoulos GM, Sande MA: *The Sanford Guide to Antimicrobial Therapy*, 34th ed. Hyde Park, VT, Antimicrobial Therapy, 2004.

Hotchkiss RS, Karl IE: The pathophysiology and treatment of sepsis. *N Engl J Med* 348:138-149, 2003.

Hughes WT, Armstrong D, Bodey GP, et al: 2002 Guidelines for the use of antimicrobial agents in neutropenic patients with cancer. *Clin Infect Dis* 34:730-751, 2002.

Humar A, Keystone J: Fortnightly review: Evaluating fever in travelers returning from tropical countries. *BMJ* 312:953, 1996.

Jasmer RM, Nahid P, Hopewell PC: Latent tuberculosis infection. *N Engl J Med* 347:1860-1866, 2002.

Kirkland KB, Wilkinson WE, Sexton DJ: Therapeutic delay and mortality in cases of Rocky Mountain spotted fever. *Clin Infect Dis* 20:1118-1121, 1995.

Kucik CJ, Martin GL, Sortor BV: Common intestinal parasites. *Am Fam Physician* 69:1161-1168, 2004.

Masters EJ: Rocky Mountain spotted fever. *Arch Intern Med* 163:769-774, 2003.

Minneci PC, Deans KJ, Banks SM, et al: Meta-analysis: The effect of steroids on survival and shock during sepsis depends on the dose. *Ann Intern Med* 141:47-56, 2004.

Mourad O, Palda V, Detsky AS: A comprehensive evidence-based approach to fever of unknown origin. *Arch Intern Med* 163:545-551, 2003.

Mylonakis E, Calderwood SB: Infective endocarditis in adults. *N Engl J Med* 345:1318-1330, 2001.

Murray HW, Pepin J, Nutman TB, et al: Recent advances: Tropical medicine. *BMJ* 320:490-494, 2000.

New York State Department of Health: Bioterrorism rapid response card. Available at http://www.health.state.ny.us/nysdoh/bt/pdf/rapid_response_card.pdf (accessed December 1, 2005).

Nolan CM, Goldberg SV, Buskin SE: Hepatotoxicity associated with isoniazid preventive therapy: A 7-year survey from a public heath tuberculosis clinic. *JAMA* 281: 1014-1018, 1999.

O'Grady NP, Barie PS, Bartlett JG, et al: Practice guidelines for evaluating new fever in critically ill adult patients. *Clin Infect Dis* 26:1042, 1998.

Olano JP, Walker DH: Human ehrlichiosis. *Med Clin North Am* 86:375-392, 2002.

Riedemann NC, Guo RF, Ward PA: The enigma of sepsis. *J Clin Invest* 112:460-467, 2003.

Sands K, Bates DW, Lanken PN, et al: Epidemiology of sepsis syndrome in 8 academic medical centers. *JAMA* 278:234-240, 1997.

Stanek G, Strle F: Lyme borreliosis. *Lancet* 362:1639-1647, 2003.

Steere AC, Coburn J, Glickstein L: The emergence of Lyme disease. *J Clin Invest* 113:1093-1101, 2004.

Suh KN, Kain KC, Keystone JS: Malaria. *CMAJ* 170:1693-1702, 2004.

Whitty CJ, Rowland M, Sanderson F, Mutabingwa TK: Malaria. *BMJ* 325:1221-1224, 2002.

AIDs = CD4 <200

OR Aids-defug illns

HIV–AIDS

Antoine Azar

DEFINITION AND TRANSMISSION

I. **AIDS results from infection with HIV, a retrovirus.** The management of HIV/AIDS and related illnesses is a rapidly evolving field of considerable complexity. Although current at the time of writing, the treatment guidelines outlined here are subject to change.

II. **HIV infects CD4$^+$/mm^3 lymphocytes (also known as helper T or T4 lymphocytes) and causes their death.** Opportunistic infections, unusual malignancies, and various other disorders develop as immunity declines commensurate with progressive CD4$^+$ cell loss. The virus actively replicates in all stages of infection. The diagnosis of AIDS is given to HIV$^+$ persons who have a CD4 count <200 cells/mm^3 of blood or an AIDS-indicator condition as defined by the CDC. HIV-1 is pandemic and causes AIDS worldwide. HIV-2 is found primarily in West Africa and is less virulent in producing AIDS compared to HIV-1.

III. **Highly Active Antiretroviral Therapy (HAART) is credited for greatly improving survival of persons living with HIV/AIDS.**

IV. **High-Risk Behavior and Modes of Transmission.** The HIV virus is transmitted by the exchange of infected body fluids, such as blood, cervicovaginal secretions, and semen. High-risk behavior includes:

A. **Unprotected sexual (vaginal, rectal, or oral) intercourse** with multiple partners, a high-risk partner (commercial sex worker, IV drug user, men who have sex with men), or an HIV$^+$ partner.

B. IV drug use or exchanging sexual intercourse for drugs.

C. **Receiving blood products before 1985.**

D. **Artificial insemination** (transmission has occurred in women who were artificially inseminated).

E. **There is no evidence implicating** an insect vector in the transmission of HIV. Likewise, living with an HIV$^+$ person or even using the same toothbrush is not considered a risk for contracting HIV–AIDS.

V. **Perinatal and Vertical Transmission. HIV can be transmitted in utero, during delivery, or by breastfeeding,** which results in a perinatal transmission rate of 15% to 30% in the absence of chemoprophylaxis. Risk factors include advanced maternal HIV disease (low CD4$^+$ cell count), infant exposure to maternal blood, prolonged duration of ruptured membranes, maternal vitamin A deficiency, increased quantity of HIV virus in maternal blood at delivery, and acute maternal HIV infection. HIV$^+$ mothers in the United States should not breastfeed in order to prevent HIV transmission to babies through breast milk. See later for details about perinatal diagnosis and prophylaxis of HIV transmission.

POSTEXPOSURE PROPHYLAXIS

I. **Table 11-1 (needle-stick exposure/percutaneous exposure) and Table 11-2 (mucus membrane exposure)** give CDC recommendations for postexposure prophylaxis (PEP).

II. Although infected transfusions almost always transmit HIV, **health care workers who are exposed to infected blood via a percutaneous injury acquire infection only three times per 1000 exposures, and the infection risk after exposure of mucous membrane to tainted blood is approximately 0.9 per 1000 exposures.** The transmission risk is increased with deep injury, visible blood on the device, needle placement in a vein or artery, large-bore hollow needle, or a source with late-stage HIV infection (high viral load).

III. **The source patient should be tested for presence of HIV antibodies (keeping within the limits of state regulations), as well as for HBV and HCV.** If the source is HIV+, determine stage of HIV disease, viral load, HIV medication history, and antiretroviral resistance information if possible. The health care worker should have HIV serology checked at the time of injury and repeated at 6 weeks and at 3 and 6 months after exposure. **If the source is HIV+, PEP should be initiated as soon as possible, preferably within 1 to 2 hours of exposure; the interval after which PEP is no longer beneficial is not known.** HIV PEP and further testing of the health care worker is unnecessary if the source is HIV−.

IV. **The National Clinician's Postexposure Prophylaxis Hotline (PEPline) provides around-the-clock advice,** 7 days a week, at telephone number 888–448–4911.

V. **A basic two-drug PEP regimen** consists of two nucleoside analogue reverse transcriptase inhibitors (NRTIs): zidovudine (ZDV) 600 mg daily in 2 or 3 divided doses and lamivudine (3TC) 150 mg bid. These are available in combination as **Combivir.** An **expanded three-drug regimen** is the basic regimen in addition to **one** of the following: indinavir 800 mg q8h, nelfinavir 750 mg tid or 1250 mg bid, efavirenz 600 mg qhs, or abacavir 300 mg bid.

VI. **PEP should be continued for 4 weeks when the HIV status of the source is either HIV positive or unknown but high risk.** PEP has many side effects and is not without risk. Discussions of the pros and cons should be initiated with the prospective recipient. Consider seeking expert consultation in the following situations: delayed exposure report (>24-36 hours), unknown source (stuck with needle from unknown source), possible pregnancy, HIV+ source having a virus resistant to antiretroviral therapy, or toxicity from the initial PEP regimen.

VII. **Nonoccupational exposure.** The CDC now recommends PEP in the setting of needle exposure and high-risk sexual exposure within 48 to 72 hours of exposure and continued for 28 days. **Figure 11-1, Box 11-1** and **Table 11-3** give details.

(text continued on p. 493)

TABLE 11-1
RECOMMENDED HIV POSTEXPOSURE PROPHYLAXIS FOR NEEDLE-STICK EXPOSURE/PERCUTANEOUS EXPOSURE

Type of Exposure	Infection Status of Source*				
	HIV-Positive Class 1	HIV-Positive Class 2	Unknown HIV Status	Unknown Source	HIV Negative
Not severe: solid needle, superficial injury	Basic 2-drug PEP	Expanded 3-drug PEP	Generally, none; consider 2-drug PEP[†] for source with HIV risk factors[§]	Generally, none; consider 2-drug PEP[†] in settings where exposure to HIV-infected persons is likely	None
More severe: large bore, deep puncture, visible blood on device, needle in patient's artery or vein	Expanded 3-drug PEP	Expanded 3-drug PEP	Generally, none; consider 2-drug PEP[†] for source with HIV risk factors[§]	Generally, none; consider 2-drug PEP[†] in settings where exposure to HIV-infected persons is likely	None

Note: See text for recommended drug regimens.

*Status definitions: *HIV-positive, class 1:* asymptomatic HIV infection or known low viral load (<1500 RNA copies/mL); *HIV-positive, class 2:* symptomatic HIV infection, AIDS, acute seroconversion, or known high viral load. If drug resistance is a concern, obtain expert consultation. Initiation of PEP should not be delayed pending expert consultation, and, because expert consultation alone cannot substitute for face-to-face counseling, resources should be available to provide immediate evaluation and follow-up care for all exposure; *unknown HIV status:* e.g., deceased source person with no samples available for HIV testing; *unknown source:* e.g., needle from a sharp disposal container.

[†]PEP is optional and should be based on an individualized decision between the exposed person and the physician.

[§]If PEP is offered and taken and the source is later determined to be HIV negative, discontinue PEP.

Adapted from US. Public Health Service: *MMWR Recomm Rep* 50(RR-11):1-52, 2001.

HIV–AIDS   11

TABLE 11-2
RECOMMENDED HIV POSTEXPOSURE PROPHYLAXIS FOR MUCOUS MEMBRANE EXPOSURE AND NONINTACT SKIN EXPOSURE

Type of Exposure	HIV-Positive Class 1	HIV-Positive Class 2	Unknown HIV Status	Unknown Source	HIV Negative
			Infection Status of Source*		
Small volume: few drops	Consider 2-drug PEP[†]	Basic 2-drug PEP	Generally, none; consider 2-drug PEP[†] for source with HIV risk factors[§]	Generally, none; consider 2-drug PEP[†] in settings where exposure to HIV-infected persons is likely	None
Large volume: major blood splash	Basic 2-drug PEP	Expanded 3-drug PEP	Generally, none; consider 2-drug PEP[†] for source with HIV risk factors[§]	Generally, none; consider 2-drug PEP[†] in settings where exposure to HIV-infected persons is likely	None

Note: See text for recommended drug regimens. For skin exposures, follow-up is indicated only if there is evidence of compromised skin integrity (e.g., dermatitis, abrasion, or open wound).

*Status definitions: *HIV-positive, class 1:* asymptomatic HIV infection or known low viral load (<1500 RNA copies/mL); *HIV-positive, class 2:* symptomatic HIV infection, AIDS, acute seroconversion, or known high viral load. If drug resistance is a concern, obtain expert consultation. Initiation of PEP should not be delayed pending expert consultation, and, because expert consultation alone cannot substitute for face-to-face counseling, resources should be available to provide immediate evaluation and follow-up care for all exposure; *unknown HIV status:* e.g., deceased source person with no samples available for HIV testing; *unknown source:* e.g., needle from a sharp disposal container.

[†]PEP is optional and should be based on an individualized decision between the exposed person and the physician.

[§]If PEP is offered and taken and the source is later determined to be HIV negative, discontinue PEP.

Adapted from US. Public Health Service: *MMWR Recomm Rep* 50(RR-11):1-52, 2001.

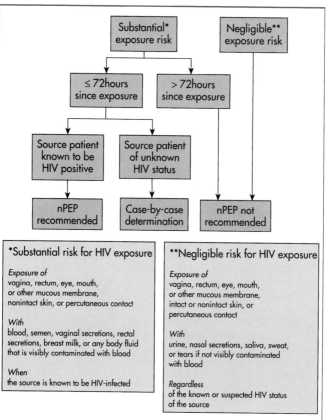

FIG. 11-1

Algorithm for evaluation and treatment of possible nonoccupational HIV exposures. nPEP, non-occupational postexposure prophylaxis.

From Smith DK, Grohskopf LA, Black RJ, et al: MMWR Recomm Rep 54(RR-2): 1-20, 2005.

> ## BOX 11-1
>
> ### ANTIRETROVIRAL REGIMENS FOR NONOCCUPATIONAL POSTEXPOSURE PROPHYLAXIS OF HIV INFECTION
>
> #### PREFERRED REGIMENS
>
> **NNRTI Based**
>
> Efavirenz* plus lamivudine or emtricitabine plus zidovudine or tenofovir
>
> **Protease-Inhibitor Based**
>
> Lopinavir/ritonavir (coformulated as Kaletra) plus lamivudine or emtricitabine plus
>   zidovudine
>
> #### ALTERNATIVE REGIMENS
>
> **NNRTI Based**
>
> Efavirenz plus lamivudine or emtricitabine plus abacavrir or didanosine or
>   stavudine[†]
>
> **Protease-Inhibitor Based**
>
> Atazanivir plus lamivudine or emtricitabine plus zidovudine or stavudine or abacavir
>   or didanosine or tenofovir plus ritonavir (100 mg/day)
>
> Fosamprenavirplus lamivudine or emtricitabine plus zidovudine or stavudine or
>   abacavir or tenofovir or didanosine
>
> Fosamprenavir/ritonavir[§] plus lamivudine or emtricitabine plus zidovudine or
>   stavudine or abacavir or tenofovir or didanosine
>
> Indinavir/ritonavir[§‡] plus lamivudine or emtricitabine plus zidovudine or stavudine or
>   abacavir or tenofovir or didanosine
>
> Lopinavir/ritonavir (coformulated as Kaletra) plus lamivudine or emtri plus stavudine
>   or abacavir or tenofovir or didanosine
>
> Nelfinavir plus lamivudine or emtri plus zidovudine or stavudine or abacavir or
>   tenofovir or didanosine
>
> Saquinavir (hgc or sgc)/ritonavir[†] plus zidovudine or stavudine or abacavir or
>   tenofovir or didanosine
>
> **Triple NRTI**
>
> Abacavir plus lamivudine plus zidovudine (only when an NNRTI- or protease
>   inhibitor-based regimen cannot or should not be used)

hgc, hard-gel saquinavir capsule (Invirase); NNRTI, non-nucleoside reverse transcriptase inhibitor; NRTI, nucleoside reverse transcriptase inhibitor; sgc, soft-gel saquinavir capsule (Fortovase).
*Efavirenz should be avoided in pregnant women and women of childbearing potential.
[†]Higher incidence of lipoatrophy, hyperlipidemia, and mitochondrial toxicities associated with stavudine than with other NNRTIs.
[§]Low-dose (100 mg-400 mg) (ritonavir). See Table 11-5 for doses used with specific protease inhibitors.
[‡]Use of ritonavir with indinavir might increase risk for renal adverse events.
From Smith DK, Grohskopf LA, Black RJ, et al: Antiretroviral postexposure prophylaxis after sexual, injection-drug use, or other nonoccupational exposure to HIV in the United States: recommendations from the U.S. Department of Health and Human Services. *MMWR Recomm Rep* 54(RR-2):1-20, 2005.

TABLE 11-3

RECOMMENDED LABORATORY EVALUATION FOR NONOCCUPATIONAL POSTEXPOSURE PROPHYLAXIS (nPEP) OF HIV INFECTION

Test	Baseline	During nPEP*	4-6 Weeks after Exposure	3 Months after Exposure	6 Months after Exposure
HIV antibody	E, S[†]		E	E	E
CBC with differential	E	E			
Serum liver enzymes	E	E			
BUN/creatinine	E	E			
STD screen[‡]	E, S	E[§]	E[§]		
Hepatitis B serology	E, S		E[§]	E[§]	
Hepatitis C serology	E, S			E	E
Pregnancy test	E	E[§]	E[§]		
HIV viral load	S		E[¶]	E[¶]	E[¶]
HIV resistance testing	S		E[¶]	E[¶]	E[¶]
CD4+ T lymphocyte count	S		E[¶]	E[¶]	E[¶]

*Other specific tests might be indicated depending on the antiretrovirals prescribed. Literature pertaining to individual agents should be consulted.
[†]HIV antibody testing of the source patient is indicated for sources of unknown serostatus.
[‡]Gonorrhea, chlamydia, syphilis.
[§]Additional testing for pregnancy, STDs, and hepatitis B should be performed as clinically indicated.
[¶]If determined to be HIV infected on follow-up testing; perform as clinically indicated once diagnosed.
E, exposed patient; S, source.
Adapted from Smith DK, Grohskopf LA, Black RJ, et al: *MMWR Recomm Rep* 54(RR-2):1-20l 2005.

HIV/AIDS BY ORGAN SYSTEM

Use the following list to help to identify an illness in a patient with HIV–AIDS who has symptoms referable to a particular organ system.

I. Cardiopulmonary Disease.

A. Dilated cardiomyopathy, pulmonary hypertension, endocarditis (IV drug use).

B. Pulmonary diseases. Pneumonia caused by *Pneumocystis*, pyogenic bacteria, mycobacteria, fungi (*Histoplasma, Coccidioides, Cryptococcus, Aspergillus*), *Nocardia*, viruses (CMV, varicella zoster, influenza, other respiratory viruses); Kaposi's sarcoma; non-Hodgkin's lymphoma; lymphoid interstitial pneumonitis.

II. Gastrointestinal Disease.

A. Oral and esophageal diseases including gingivitis, thrush, ulcers (aphthous, HSV, CMV, drug-induced), oral hairy leukoplakia, esophagitis (candida, CMV, HSV), Kaposi's sarcoma, and non-Hodgkin's lymphoma.

B. Intestinal disease

1. **Bacteria:** *Salmonella, Shigella, Campylobacter, Clostridium difficile; Mycobacterium avium* complex (MAC).

2. **Parasites:** *Cryptosporidia, Isospora, Cyclospora, Entamoeba, Giardia.*

3. **Viruses:** CMV, HSV, HIV (enteropathy).

4. **Neoplasms:** Kaposi's sarcoma, non-Hodgkin's lymphoma, anogenital carcinoma, condylomata acuminata.

C. **Hepatobiliary and pancreatic disease**

1. Many AIDS-related infections and neoplasms can affect the hepatobiliary system.

2. **Hepatitis:** hepatitis B and C viruses; less commonly, hepatitis A and D viruses; antiretroviral drugs

3. **Pancreatitis:** drugs (ddl, ddC, d4T, sulfonamides, pentamidine, erythromycin, INH, rifampin), hypertriglyceridemia (secondary to protease inhibitors).

4. **AIDS cholangiopathy:** RUQ pain, fever, cholestasis, and findings of sclerosing cholangitis and papillary stenosis. About 20% to 40% are idiopathic; other causes include *Cryptosporidium*, microsporidia, CMV, and *Cyclospora*. ERCP or HIDA-scan is useful in diagnosis.

III. **Ophthalmologic Disease.**

A. **Cornea disease** including ulcerative keratitis, dry eye, herpes simplex keratitis, zoster ophthalmicus, microsporidia.

B. **Retina and choroid diseases** including microvasculopathy (cotton-wool spots, retinal hemorrhages), CMV retinitis, acute retinal necrosis, progressive outer retinal necrosis, syphilis, toxoplasmosis, pneumocystis choroidopathy, cryptococcosis, mycobacterial infection, intraocular lymphoma, candidiasis, and histoplasmosis.

C. **Drug-associated ocular toxicity** including didanosine-associated retinal depigmentation or optic neuritis and rifabutin-associated uveitis.

D. **Neuro-ophthalmic disorders** including disk edema (papilledema), optic neuropathy, and cranial nerve palsies.

E. **Orbital disorders** including orbital lymphoma and infections.

IV. **Neurologic Disease.**

A. **Primary HIV syndromes** including encephalopathy, dementia, aseptic meningitis, spinal vacuolar myelopathy, distal sensory polyneuropathy, mononeuropathy multiplex (exclude CMV), polyradiculopathy (exclude CMV and HCV), and neuromuscular weakness syndrome.

B. **Opportunistic viral illnesses:** CMV, HSV, varicella-zoster virus, JC virus (progressive multifocal leukoencephalopathy), and adenovirus.

C. **Nonviral infections:** *Toxoplasma*, fungi (*Cryptococcus*, *Coccidioides*, *Histoplasma*), tuberculosis, and syphilis.

D. **Neoplasms:** primary CNS lymphoma and metastatic non-Hodgkin's lymphoma.

E. **Cerebrovascular complications:** infarction, hemorrhage, and vasculitis.

F. **Antiretroviral toxic neuropathy** (usually a distal sensory neuropathy).

G. **Inflammatory demyelinating polyneuropathy.**

V. **Gynecologic Disease.**

A. **Typical STDs.** Gonorrhea, chlamydia, trichomoniasis, syphilis, and bacterial vaginosis correlate with lower CD4$^+$ counts. Genital herpes is more severe and frequent in HIV-infected patients, and it has atypical recurrences with progressive immunosuppression.

B. **Pelvic inflammatory disease.** Recurrent PID is more common in HIV⁺ women, who are more likely to require surgical intervention than are women with PID in the general population.

C. **HPV, CIN, and cervical cancer.**

1. Abnormal cervical cytology is 10- to 11-fold more common among HIV⁺ women and is associated with the presence of HPV and degree of immunosuppression.

2. **The 2001 consensus guidelines for screening women infected with HIV suggest the following:**

a. Obtain a Pap smear during initial evaluation. Liquid-based media are preferred because of better sensitivity and ability to check for HPV on collected specimens. If the initial Pap smear is normal, a follow-up Pap should be obtained in 6 months to rule out false-negative results. If the initial two Pap smear results are normal, Pap should then be repeated on a yearly basis. More frequent Pap smears should be done in women with a prior abnormal Pap smear, HPV infection, and symptomatic HIV infection.

b. If either the initial or follow-up Pap smear reveals ASCUS, ASCH, atypical glandular cells, SIL (low grade or high grade), or squamous cell carcinoma, then further work-up is required, including colposcopy and directed biopsy.

c. Colposcopy is not indicated for HIV-infected women with normal Pap smears.

D. **Breast cancer screening with mammograms.** Follow the standard guidelines for the general population. Breast cancer risk is not increased by HIV.

VI. **Hematologic Disease.**

A. **Anemia.** HIV, marrow-infiltrating tumor or infection, drug-induced marrow suppression or hemolysis, parvovirus B19, or B_{12}/folate or iron deficiency.

B. **Thrombocytopenia.** HIV-associated immune thrombocytopenia (idiopathic thrombocytopenic purpura), drugs, thrombotic thrombocytopenic purpura (TTP).

C. **Neutropenia.** HIV or drugs.

VII. **Kidney Disease.** HIV-associated nephropathy or immune-mediated glomerulonephritis, IgA nephropathy, HCV-related mixed cryoglobulinemia, TTP, nephrotoxic drugs (e.g., pentamidine, foscarnet, amphotericin B, tenofovir), and urolithiasis especially with indinavir (indinavir stones not visible on noncontrast CT).

HOW TO DIAGNOSE HIV INFECTION

I. **Background.** While obtaining informed consent for HIV testing, it is important to first discuss with the patient the implications of a positive test, including insurance and work or school ramifications. Many HIV⁺ persons still face substantial public intolerance. Confidentiality in

11

HIV–AIDS

diagnosis and treatment are therefore useful for HIV+ persons. Post-test counseling is also recommended to include information on high-risk behavior and retesting for seronegative patients, behavior to prevent transmission, strategies for health protection with a compromised immune system, and the necessity of contact tracing for HIV+ patients.

II. **Diagnostic Tests.**

A. **Screening ELISA,** an enzyme immunoassay, is the standard for detection of antibodies against HIV (sensitivity is 99.9%; specificity is >99%). **A positive screening test requires confirmation by Western blot or another confirmatory method.** ELISA is often positive at approximately 10 to 14 days following the time of infection, but it can take 3 to 4 weeks to become positive. **Virtually all patients have positive ELISA and Western blot within 6 months of infection.** With an indeterminate Western blot result, repeat serologic testing is generally advocated at 1, 2, and 6 months. **HIV RNA testing is not generally used for confirmatory testing** because false-positive rates (2%-9%) and negative rates are problematic, but it is commonly used for diagnosing acute HIV infection, a condition in which plasma viral RNA load is high but ELISA and Western blot results are negative or equivocal.

B. **Alternative antibody-based tests. Rapid testing** quickly gives **screening results** that must be confirmed for antibodies against HIV in saliva, serum, plasma, or finger-stick whole blood (specimen type used varies among the multiple commercial products available). It is especially useful for occupational exposures, women who present in labor and lack prior testing, and persons who are less likely to return for the test results (e.g., emergency department). The rapid **OraQuick** test does not require special training or equipment, has no restrictions on where it can be performed, and produces results in 20 minutes. **OraSure** is an inexpensive kit for easy collection of saliva for HIV antibody testing. The test may be anonymous or confidential, and the results are available by phone or fax in 3 days. The kit can be ordered by calling 800–Ora–Sure. The sensitivity and specificity of the rapid and OraSure tests are >99%.

C. **HIV RNA** is quantified in plasma using a commercially available method of PCR, branched-chain DNA (bDNA), or nucleic acid sequence-based amplification (NASBA). The assays differ in lower and upper limits of RNA detection. Quantitative HIV RNA detection is useful in diagnosing acute HIV and neonatal infections, determining prognosis, assessing transmission risk, and monitoring treatment effectiveness.

D. **Other viral detection methods.** Testing for HIV p24 antigen in plasma is a relatively inexpensive but insensitive method for diagnosing acute HIV infection. Culturing HIV is possible but impractical.

E. **Resistance testing** with genotypic or phenotypic assays is a newer molecular technique for detection of resistance to antiretroviral drugs to assist in HIV therapy selection. It is routinely used in chronically infected patients who are failing HIV therapy or are pregnant and in acute HIV infection.

III. **The diagnosis in neonatal HIV infection is complicated** by findings of positive ELISA and Western blot results in uninfected neonates for up to 18 months because of transfer of maternal HIV antibodies across the placenta.

A. **For a child younger than 18 months who is known to be HIV seropositive (ELISA plus Western blot) or born to an HIV⁺ mother, the diagnosis is confirmed with positive results on two separate determinations with one or more of the following tests:**

1. **Culture,** very good but expensive; 48% sensitive at birth and 75% sensitive at 3 months. It can take 4 to 6 weeks.

2. **PCR** or other technique for demonstrating viral RNA in the blood. This is highly sensitive and specific, is reasonably priced, and requires a small sample of whole blood. Accuracy is 84% at birth and 98% to 100% at 1 month of age.

3. **p24 antigen** (a major core protein of the HIV virus) can be found in more than half of HIV-infected infants during the first year of life but in substantially fewer babies during the first months of life and in only 10% of infected newborns

B. **For a child 18 months of age born to an HIV-infected mother or any child infected by blood, blood products, or other known modes of transmission,** the diagnosis of HIV is confirmed under the following conditions: HIV-antibody positive by screening assay and confirmatory test (Western blot or IFA) or meets any of the criteria listed for younger children.

INITIAL PRESENTATION OF HIV INFECTION

I. Patients with HIV–AIDS can present during any phase of the disease from acute conversion to full-blown AIDS with an AIDS-defining illness.

II. **The acute phase of HIV infection occurs soon after exposure and can manifest as a flulike or mononucleosis-like illness** with fever, sweats, fatigue, adenopathy, diarrhea, arthralgias, rash, headache, and occasionally thrombocytopenia. HIV infection can manifest with epistaxis or even seborrheic dermatitis. There may also be an acute drop in the CD4⁺ lymphocyte count with an occasional opportunistic infection. **High levels of viremia are present during the initial conversion.**

III. **AIDS-related complex (ARC) comprises lymphadenopathy, fever, and malaise in the absence of opportunistic infections.**

11

HIV-AIDS

Biopsy specimens of lymph nodes show a nonspecific hyperplasia. Normal lymph node architecture is gradually destroyed with time. HIV-infected persons are no longer capable of generating effective immune response and replace CD4+ cells already lost to this infection.

INITIAL EVALUATION OF THE HIV-POSITIVE PATIENT

I. **Initial laboratory data should include** hepatitis B surface antigen and core antibody and hepatitis A and hepatitis C antibodies; CD4+ count and HIV RNA load; CBC with differential, platelet count, and VDRL or RPR plus FTA if VDRL is positive; PPD (0.5 mm is considered positive in HIV+ patients); liver and renal function tests; electrolytes, fasting glucose, and lipid profile; urine screen for gonorrhea and chlamydia; toxoplasma and CMV IgG antibodies; chest x-ray if patient is symptomatic; G6PD (TMP–SMX and other drugs can cause hemolysis in these patients); and Pap smear and wet mount for *Trichomonas* in women.

II. Ongoing HIV replication leads to immune system damage and progression to AIDS. Disease progression tends to differ among HIV-infected persons. This virus is always harmful, and true long-term disease-free survival without clinically significant immune dysfunction is unusual. Asymptomatic phase is characterized by gradual decline of CD4+ count and, often, lymphadenopathy.

III. **Antigenic stimulation (intercurrent infections, parasites, etc.) of CD4+ cells hastens viral replication and cell death.**

IV. **There is some evidence that repeated exposure to different strains of the HIV virus shortens the time to the development of AIDS.** Therefore it is important to practice safe sex even if one's partner is also HIV positive.

MANAGEMENT OF HIV INFECTION

I. **Immunize.** Patients should be fully immunized, including pneumococcal vaccine, tetanus, influenza, and hepatitis B if not already immune, **but do not give live-attenuated vaccines to these patients. The following vaccines are live: BCG, measles, MMR, mumps, OPV, rubella, oral typhoid, varicella, and yellow fever.** If foreign travel is being considered, practitioners should consult the CDC Web page (www.cdc.gov).

II. **Ongoing Evaluation.** Schedule a follow-up at 2 to 4 weeks to discuss questions, lifestyle changes, and support systems and to deal with emotional issues and suicidal ideation (rates of suicide are increased in HIV+ patients).

III. **Initiation of antiretroviral therapy is based on** CD4+ counts, clinical manifestations, viral RNA load, and evidence of clinical benefit. Draw CD4+ counts at the same time each visit, due to diurnal variation.

Vr pre tx + G 1, 2+ then
40 3 mos
a fin

TABLE 11-4

INDICATIONS FOR THE INITIATION OF ANTIRETROVIRAL THERAPY (ARV) IN THE CHRONICALLY HIV-INFECTED PATIENT*

Clinical Category	CD4 T-Cell Count	Plasma HIV RNA	Recommendation
Symptomatic (e.g., AIDS, thrush, unexplained fever, other opportunistic infection)	Any value	Any value	Treat
Asymptomatic	<200/mm^3	Any value	Treat
Asymptomatic	200-350/mm^3	Any value	Treatment should usually be offered; discuss pros and cons with patient
Asymptomatic	>350/mm^3	≥100,000/mL	Most experts recommend deferring therapy, but some experts treat
Asymptomatic	>350/mm^3	<100,000/mL	Defer therapy

*The optimal time to initiate therapy is unknown among persons with asymptomatic disease and CD4$^+$ T-cell count >200 cells/mm^3. This table provides general guidance rather than absolute recommendations for an individual patient. All decisions regarding initiating therapy should be made on the basis of prognosis as determined by the CD4$^+$ T-cell count and level of plasma HIV RNA, the potential benefits and risks of therapy, and the willingness of the patient to accept therapy. Adapted from U.S. Department of Health and Human Services: http://www.aidsinfo.nih.gov/Guidelines/GuidelineDetail.aspx?MenuItem=Guidelines&Search=Off& GuidelineID=7&ClassID=1.

Table 11-4 gives the current criteria for starting antiretroviral therapy. **Box 11-2** contains the recommended regimens for HAART. **Table 11-5** lists antiretroviral agents and gives their dosing and side effects. **Adherence to therapy is crucial;** the virologic failure rate is >50%, with <95% adherence.

IV. **Laboratory Testing in Initiating and Monitoring ARV Therapy.**
A. **Viral RNA** load measures the magnitude of HIV replication and is associated with the rate of CD4$^+$ depletion. It correlates with the risk of disease progression and can be followed as a measure of response to antiretroviral therapy. Viral RNA should be obtained at the time of diagnosis of HIV and every 3 to 4 months in an untreated patient. It should be measured immediately before and every 4 to 8 weeks after initiation of antiretroviral therapy, then every 2 to 4 months to monitor success of therapy. Avoid measurements within 4 weeks of systemic infection or immunization because these can transiently increase the viral RNA.

BOX 11-2

RECOMMENDED* ANTIRETROVIRAL AGENTS FOR TREATMENT OF ESTABLISHED HIV

PREFERRED REGIMENS

International AIDS Society (United States)

2 NRTI + 1 PI ± low-dose ritonavir (100-400 mg)

2 NRTI + 1 NNRTI

3 NRTI

U.S. Department of Health and Human Services

Efavirenz plus (lamivudine or emtricitabine) plus (zidovudine or tenofovir DF)

Lopinavir/ritonavir plus (lamivudine or emtricitabine) plus zidovudine

CONTRAINDICATED REGIMENS OR COMBINATIONS

Monotherapies (except ZDV therapy in pregnancy)

2 NRTIs (rapid resistance)

Combinations of d4T plus ZDV, d4T plus ddI, d4T plus ddC, ddC plus ddI, ddC plus 3TC, emtricitabine plus 3TC (virologically undesirable or overlapping toxicities)

Atazanavir plus indinavir (additive hyperbilirubinemia)

Tenofovir plus 3TC plus (either ddI or abacavir) or emtricitabine (high rate of virologic nonresponse)

Ampenavir plus fosamprenavir (no benefit)

Amprenavir solution plus ritonavir solution (toxic)

Nevirapine (women CD4+ > 250, men CD4+ > 500) (toxic)

*Recommendations are based on strong evidence of clinical benefit and/or sustained suppression of plasma viral loads. There are many other alternative regimens.

NNRTI, non-nucleoside reverse transcriptase inhibitor; NRTI, nucleoside reverse transcriptase inhibitor; PI, protease inhibitor.

B. CD4+ count indicates the extent of immune damage. It helps to establish the risk of developing opportunistic infections and should be measured at the time of diagnosis and every 2 to 3 months.

C. Fasting blood glucose and lipid profile should be measured every 3 to 6 months while on therapy.

V. Treatment regimen failure is classified as virologic, immunologic, and clinical; there are many causes including adherence, toxicity, resistance, and pharmacokinetics. Careful evaluation of the patient for the underlying etiology and resistance testing are necessary before changing the drug regimen.

A. Virologic failure. HIV RNA >400/mL at 24 weeks or >50/mL at 48 weeks or viral rebound with repeated detection of HIV RNA >400/mL after initial suppression.

B. Immunologic failure. Failure to increase CD4 count by 25% to 50% from baseline over the first year or to decrease to below baseline. Mean increases in CD4+ counts are approximately 150 cells/mm^3 over the first year.

C. Clinical failure. Occurrence of HIV-related events after at least 3 months on therapy.

INFECTIONS IN AIDS PATIENTS

Remember, AIDS patients get the usual organisms too and have an increased incidence of *Haemophilus influenzae, Streptococcus pneumoniae,* salmonella sepsis, etc. Do not focus only on the opportunistic organisms. Always pursue a definitive diagnosis but treat broadly in life-threatening conditions until you have isolated an organism. AIDS patients might not mount a WBC response and might not run a fever with infections. Maintain a high clinical suspicion.

I. Opportunistic Infections.

A. Occurrence of opportunistic infections and noninfectious complications is based on decreasing CD4⁺ count.

1. **CD4⁺/mm³ >500:** recurrent vaginal candidiasis, lymphadenopathy, myopathy, aseptic meningitis.

2. **CD4⁺/mm³ 200 to 500:** herpes zoster, oral candidiasis, pulmonary TB, cervical intraepithelial neoplasia, anemia, Kaposi's sarcoma, lymphoma.

3. **CD4⁺/mm³ <200:** *Pneumocystis carinii* pneumonia, extrapulmonary TB, disseminated histoplasmosis and coccidioidomycosis, AIDS dementia complex, AIDS-related wasting, cardiomyopathy, progressive multifocal leukoencephalopathy.

4. **CD4⁺/mm³ <100:** cryptosporidiosis, toxoplasmosis, nonhealing HSV ulcers, candidal esophagitis.

5. **CD4⁺/mm³ <50:** CMV disease, disseminated MAC, primary CNS lymphoma.

B. Primary prophylaxis (Table 11-6) is indicated against certain opportunistic infections, and recommendations are based on the CD4+ count.

1. **Strongly recommended prophylaxis** by CD4⁺ count (see Table 11-6):

a. CD4⁺/mm³ <200: pneumocystis.

b. CD4⁺/mm³ <100: toxoplasma.

c. CD4⁺/mm³ <50: MAC.

2. **Not routinely recommended prophylaxis** but may be considered in selected patients (Table 11-6):

a. CD4⁺/mm³ <100: histoplasma.

b. CD4⁺/mm³ <50: CMV, cryptococcus.

C. Secondary prophylaxis after treatment of an acute infection. Secondary prophylaxis or chronic suppression is required after the initial episode of certain diseases **(Table 11-7). Prophylaxis for opportunistic infections can be discontinued in some situations** when the CD4⁺ count has been stable and elevated for several months. **Table 11-8** summarizes the criteria to start, discontinue, and restart prophylactic medications.

D. Management of Opportunistic Infections.

1. ***Pneumocystis carinii (P. jiroveci)*** is the presenting infection in 50% of those with AIDS. Clinically patients have subacute, nonproductive cough, tachypnea, and hypoxia (cardinal signs); may have clear lungs or only wheezes.

(text continued on p. 518)

HIV–AIDS   11

TABLE 11-5
ANTI-HIV DRUGS

Drug	Forms	Dose	Adjust Dose*
NUCLEOSIDE OR NUCLEOTIDE REVERSE TRANSCRIPTASE INHIBITORS			
Zidovudine [(AZT, Retrovir)	100 mg cap 300 mg tab 10 mg/mL syrup	300 mg q12h	Renal, hepatic
Lamivudine (3TC, Epivir)	150, 300 mg tabs 10 mg/mL oral soln	150 mg q12h <50 kg: 2 mg/kg q12h	Renal
Stavudine (d4T, Zerit, Zerit XR)	15, 20, 30, 40 mg caps 37.5, 50, 75, 100 mg XR caps 1 mg/mL oral soln	>60 kg: 40mg (100 mg XR) q12h <60 kg: 30 mg (75 mg XR) q12h	Renal, hepatic
Didanosine (ddI, Videx, Videx EC)	25, 50, 100, 150, 200 mg buffered tabs 125, 200, 250, 400 mg EC cap	>60 kg: 200 mg q12h or 400 mg qd (400 mg qd EC) <60 kg:125 mg q12h or 250 mg qd (250 mg qd EC)	Renal; consider hepatic
Zalcitabine (ddC, Hivid)	0.375, 0.75 mg tabs	0.75 mg q8h	Renal; consider hepatic

*Adjust dose for renal or hepatic insufficiency. Contact pharmacist for specific dosing requirements.
†Rare, but life threatening.

Diet Restriction	Adverse Effects	Monitoring	Comments
None	Nausea, vomiting, headache, bone marrow suppression (anemia and/or neutropenia), loss of muscle tissue, insomnia; lactic acidosis†	CBC with differential, LFTs	Also available as: Combivir (3TC/AZT 150/300 mg), 1 tablet q12h Trizivir (3TC/AZT/ABC 150/300/300 mg), 1 tablet q12h
None	Nausea, headache, low WBC, peripheral neuropathy, hair loss (rare); lactic acidosis†	CBC, creatinine, LFTs	Also available as: Combivir (3TC/AZT 150/300 mg, 1 tablet q12h
None	Peripheral neuropathy, stomach upset, pancreatitis, liver damage; lactic acidosis†	Serum amylase and lipase, creatinine, LFTs	Avoid combination with ddI in pregnancy
Empty stomach; contains buffer, separate from some other meds.	Peripheral neuropathy, pancreatitis, diarrhea, nausea; lactic acidosis†	Serum amylase and lipase, LFTs, electrolytes	Chew or crush tablets before swallowing. Must have two tablets for each dose to get adequate buffer for absorption. Alcohol may exacerbate toxicity. Avoid combination with d4T in pregnancy. EC capsule should be swallowed whole
Avoid Al- and Mg-containing antacids	Peripheral neuropathy, pancreatitis, stomatitis; lactic acidosis†	CBC, serum amylase and lipase, LFTs, glucose, creatinine	Likely to be withdrawn from the market in 2006 in the United States

11

HIV–AIDS

(continued)

TABLE 11-5
ANTI-HIV DRUGS—cont'd

Drug	Forms	Dose	Adjust Dose*
Abacavir (ABC, Ziagen)	300 mg tabs 20 mg/mL oral soln	300 mg q12h	Possibly hepatic
Tenofovir (TDF, Viread)	300 mg tabs	300 mg qd	Renal
Emtricitabine (FTC, Emtriva)	200 mg caps 10 mg/mL syrup	200 mg qd or 240 mg oral solution/d	Renal
NON-NUCLEOSIDE REVERSE TRANSCRIPTASE INHIBITORS			
Nevirapine (NVP Viramune)	200 mg tab 50 mg/5 mL oral soln	200 mg qd × 14 d, then 200 mg q12h	Hepatic
Delavirdine (DLV Rescriptor)	100, 200 mg tabs	400 mg q8h	Considered hepatic
Efavirenz (EFV, Sustiva)	50, 100, 200 mg caps 600 mg tab	600 mg qhs	Caution with hepatic; no specific dose recs

*Adjust dose for renal or hepatic insufficiency. Contact pharmacist for specific dosing requirements.
†Rare, but life threatening.

Diet Restriction	Adverse Effects	Monitoring	Comments
None Alcohol increases drug level by 41%	Hypersensitivity reaction, nausea, vomiting, diarrhea, anorexia, insomnia; increase in blood glucose, LFTs, CPK triglycerides; lactic acidosis[†]	LFTs, glucose, triglycerides	If hypersensitivity reaction occurs, *stop immediately; do not rechallenge* Criteria: skin rash or 2 or more of: Fever Nausea, vomiting, or abdominal pain Severe tiredness, achiness, or generally ill feeling Sore throat, shortness of breath, cough
Take with food	Asthenia, headache, nausea, vomiting, diarrhea; lactic acidosis[†]	Creatinine	Contraindicated with CrCl <60 mL/min
None	Hyperpigmentation	LFTs	Testing for hepatitis B is recommended before beginning therapy; hepatitis B may be exacerbated when emtricitabine is discontinued.
None	Rash, increased AST/ALT, hepatitis	LFTs	Dose escalation to lower risk of rash
1 h apart from antacids Take with acidic beverage if patient has achlorhydria	Rash (less frequently than with nevirapine), increased AST/ALT, headache	LFTs, creatinine, CBC	May make slurry in ≥3 oz water and drink immediately (not with 200-mg tabs) Experimental: 600 mg q12h
Take on empty stomach	Insomnia, difficulty concentrating, dizziness, drowsiness, unusual dreams, rash, nausea, vomiting, diarrhea, increased AST/ALT	LFTs, creatinine, CBC, lipids	CNS effects less noticeable if taken at bedtime Patient should avoid becoming pregnant (teratogenic in monkeys)

11

HIV–AIDS

(continued)

TABLE 11-5
ANTI-HIV DRUGS—cont'd

Drug	Forms	Dose	Adjust Dose*
PROTEASE INHIBITORS			
Indinavir (IDV, Crixivan)	200, 333, 400 mg caps	800 mg q8h If taken with ritonavir [800 mg plus ritonavir 100 or 200 mg] q12h	Hepatic
Ritonavir (RTV, Norvir)	100 mg caps 600 mg/7.5 mL oral soln	600 mg q12h as booster for other protease inhibitors 100 mg-400 mg divided into 1 or 2 doses	Caution with hepatic; no specific dose recs
Saquinavir (SQV, Fortovase soft-gel cap)	200 mg cap 500 mg cap	1200 mg q8h	Caution with hepatic; no specific dose recs
Nelfinavir (NFV, Viracept)	250 mg caps Powder 50 mg/g 625 mg caps	750 mg q8h, or 1250 mg bid	Caution with hepatic; no specific dose recs

*Adjust dose for renal or hepatic insufficiency. Contact pharmacist for specific dosing requirements.

Diet Restriction	Adverse Effects	Monitoring	Comments
Best on empty stomach; may take with low-fat, low-calorie, low-carb snack	Nausea, rash, nephrolithiasis, headache, asthenia, blurred vision, dizziness, metallic taste, hyperglycemia, thrombocytopenia, hyperlipidemia, increased indirect bilirubin	Lipids, LFTs, bilirubin, glucose	Drink ≥48 oz of water per day
Take with food, if possible	Nausea, vomiting, diarrhea, asthenia, paresthesias, taste perversion, hepatitis, triglyceride increase >200%, AST/ALT elevation, elevated CPK and uric acid, hyperglycemia, hyperlipidemia	Lipids, LFTs, bilirubin, CPK, glucose	Dose escalation if using without another PI: Days 1-2: 300 mg q12h Days 3-5: 400 mg q12h Days 6-13: 500 mg q12h Days 14: 600 mg q12h Refrigerate caps unless stored at <77°F and used within 30 days Use low doses (100-400mg): boost other PIs
Take with full meal (high-fat preferred)	Stomach upset, gas, abdominal pain, nausea, diarrhea, headache, elevated AST/ALT, hyperglycemia, hyperlipidemia	Lipids, LFTs, bilirubin, glucose, lipids	**RTV 100 mg plus SQV 1000 mg bid no longer recommended unless boosted by ritonavir** Invirase is a hard-gel cap with lower bioavailability
Take with food (high-fat meal preferred)	Diarrhea, hypoglycemia, increased LFTs	Lipids, LFTs, bilirubin, glucose	May take CaCO$_3$ with each dose to help alleviate diarrhea

11

HIV–AIDS

(continued)

TABLE 11-5
ANTI-HIV DRUGS—cont'd

Drug	Forms	Dose	Adjust Dose*
Amprenavir (APV, Agenerase)	50 mg 15 mg/mL oral soln	1400 mg bid	Hepatic
Lopinavir/ Ritonavir (LPV/r, Kaletra)	133 mg LPV + 33 mg RTV caps 80 mg LPV + 20 mg RTV/mL oral soln	400/100 mg (3 caps or 5 mL) bid Alternative: LPV 800 mg plus RTV 200 mg qd (qd dosing only for drug naive patients).	Hepatic
Atazanavir (ATV, Reyataz)	100, 150, 200 mg caps	400 mg qd	Hepatic
Fosamprenavir (FPV, Lexiva)	700 mg tabs	1400 mg bid	Hepatic
Tipranavir (TPV, Aptivus)	150 mg caps	500 mg bid with RTV 200 mg bid (not to be used unboosted)	Hepatic

FUSION PROTEIN INHIBITORS

Enfuvirtide (T20, Fuzeon)	90 mg/mL vials	90 mg (1 mL) SQ bid	None

*Adjust dose for renal or hepatic insufficiency. Contact pharmacist for specific dosing requirements.
Note: This chart is not all-inclusive. Please refer to manufacturer labeling for additional information.
caps, capsules; carb, carbohydrate; CrCl, creatinine clearance; EC, enteric coated; max, maximum; recs, recommendations; soln, solution; tabs, tablets.

Diet Restriction	Adverse Effects	Monitoring	Comments
Avoid high-fat meal Separate at least 1 h from antacids Avoid large quantity vitamin E	Nausea, vomiting, rash, fatigue, depression, oral/perioral paresthesias, headache, hyperglycemia, hyperlipidemia	Lipids, LFTs, bilirubin, glucose	Potential for sulfa cross allergy
Take with food	Nausea, vomiting, diarrhea, asthenia, elevated AST/ALT, hyperlipidemia	Lipids, LFTs, glucose	Oral soln contains 42% alcohol; possible disulfiram reaction
Take with food	Increased indirect bilirubin, prolonged PR interval, increased AST/ALT, hyperlipidemia, hyperglycemia	Glucose, bilirubin, LFTs	Many drug interactions (check label) Dosage adjustment required for combination therapies (tenofovir and/or efavirenz)
None	Skin rash; elevated ALT/AST; GI intolerance, headache, fatigue		Many drug interactions Dosage adjustment required for combination therapies (ritonavir and/or efavirenz)
Take with food	Hepatotoxic	LFTs	Sulfonamide moiety, increased hepatotoxicity in those with hepatitis B or C; many drug interactions
None	Insomnia, injection site reactions, anorexia, myalgia, eosinophilia		Increased incidence of pneumonia during clinical trials

11

HIV-AIDS

TABLE 11-6
PROPHYLAXIS TO PREVENT FIRST EPISODE OF OPPORTUNISTIC DISEASE IN ADULTS AND ADOLESCENTS INFECTED WITH HIV

Pathogen	Indication	First Choice	Alternatives
STRONGLY RECOMMENDED AS STANDARD OF CARE			
Pneumocystis carinii*	CD4+ count <200/µL, oropharyngeal candidiasis, *or* unexplained fever × 2 wk	TMP–SMX 1 DS PO qd TMP–SMX 1 SS PO qd	Dapsone 50 mg PO bid *or* 100 mg PO qd Dapsone 50 mg PO qd *plus* pyrimethamine 50 mg PO q1wk *plus* leucovorin 25 mg PO q1wk Dapsone 200 mg PO *plus* pyrimethamine 75 mg PO *plus* leucovorin 25 mg PO q1wk Aerosolized pentamidine 300 mg q1mo via Respirgard II nebulizer Atovaquone 1500 mg PO qd TMP–SMX, 1 DS PO tiw
Mycobacterium tuberculosis, isoniazid-sensitive†	TST reaction ≥5 mm *or* prior positive TST result without treatment *or* contact with patient with active tuberculosis	Isoniazid 300 mg PO *plus* pyridoxine 50 mg PO qd × 9 mo *or* isoniazid 900 mg PO *plus* pyridoxine 100 mg PO biw × 9 mo Rifampin 600 mg *plus* pyrazinamide 15–20 mg/kg PO qd × 2 mo	Rifabutin 300 mg PO qd *plus* pyrazinamide 20 mg/kg PO qd × 2 mo Rifampin 600 mg PO qd × 4 mo

M. tuberculosis, isoniazid-resistant	Same as for isoniazid-sensitive; high probability of exposure to isoniazid-resistant tuberculosis	Rifampin 600 mg *plus* pyrazinamide 15-20 mg/kg PO qd × 2 mo	Rifabutin 300 mg *plus* pyrazinamide 20 mg/kg PO qd × 2 mo Rifampin 600 mg PO qd × 4 mo Rifabutin 300 mg PO qd × 4 mo
Multidrug (isoniazid and rifampin) resistant	Same as for isoniazid-sensitive; high probability of exposure to multidrug-resistant tuberculosis	Choice of drugs requires consultation with public health authorities	None
Toxoplasma gondii‡	IgG antibody to *T. gondii* and CD4+ count <100/μL	TMP–SMX 1 DS PO qd	TMP–SMX 1 SS PO qd Dapsone, 50 mg PO qd *plus* pyrimethamine, 50 mg PO q1wk *plus* leucovorin, 25 mg PO q1wk Atovaquone 1500 mg PO qd ± pyrimethamine 25 mg PO qd *plus* leucovorin 10 mg PO qd
Mycobacterium avium complex†	CD4+ count <50/μL	Azithromycin 1200 mg PO q1wk Clarithromycin 500 mg PO bid	Rifabutin 300 mg PO qd Azithromycin 1200 mg PO q1wk *plus* rifabutin 300 mg PO qd
Varicella-zoster virus	Significant exposure to chickenpox or shingles for patients who have no history of either condition or, if available, negative antibody to VZV	VZIG 5 vials (1.25 mL each) IM, administered within 96 h of exposure, ideally within 48 h	

(continued)

HIV–AIDS 11

TABLE 11-6

PROPHYLAXIS TO PREVENT FIRST EPISODE OF OPPORTUNISTIC DISEASE IN ADULTS AND ADOLESCENTS INFECTED WITH HIV—cont'd

Pathogen	Indication	First Choice	Alternatives
USUALLY RECOMMENDED			
Streptococcus pneumoniae‡	CD4+ > 200/mm³ CD4+ < 200/mm³	23-valent polysaccharide vaccine, 0.5 mL IM	None
Hepatitis B virus	All susceptible (anti-HBc-negative) patients	Revaccinate q3-5yr Hepatitis B vaccine: 3 doses	None
Influenza virus	All patients (annually before flu season)	Inactivated trivalent influenza virus vaccine: one annual dose (0.5 mL) IM	Oseltamivir 75 mg PO qd (influenza A or B) Rimantadine 100 mg PO bid Amantadine 100 mg PO bid (influenza A only)
Hepatitis A virus	All susceptible (anti-HAV-negative) patients, chronic liver disease, and chronic hepatitis C	Hepatitis A vaccine: 2 doses	None
NOT ROUTINELY INDICATED			
Bacteria	Neutropenia	G-CSF 5-10 mg/kg SQ qd × 2-4 wk or GM-CSF 250 mg/m² IV over 2 h qd × 2-4 wk	None
Cryptococcus neoformans	CD4+ <50/mm³	Fluconazole 100-200 mg PO qd	Itraconazole 200 mg PO qd
Histoplasma capsulatum§	CD4+ <100/mm³, endemic geographic area	Itraconazole capsule 200 mg PO qd	None

| Cytomegalovirus¶ | CD4+ count <50/µL and CMV antibody positivity | Oral ganciclovir 1 g PO tid | None |

*Prophylaxis should also be considered for persons with a CD4+ <14%, with a history of an AIDS-defining illness, and possibly with CD4+ counts >200 but <250 cells/µL. TMP-SMX also reduces the frequency of toxoplasmosis and some bacterial infections. Patients receiving dapsone should be tested for G6PD deficiency. A dose of 50 mg qd is probably less effective than 100 mg qd. Efficacy of parenteral pentamidine (e.g., 4 mg/kg/mo) is uncertain. Fansidar (sulfadoxine–pyrimethamine) is rarely used because of severe hypersensitivity reactions. Patients taking therapy for toxoplasmosis with sulfadiazine–pyrimethamine are protected against *Pneumocystis carinii* pneumonia and do not need additional prophylaxis against PCP.

†Directly observed therapy is recommended for isoniazid, 900 mg biw; isoniazid regimens should include pyridoxine to prevent peripheral neuropathy. Rifampin should not be administered concurrently with protease inhibitors or NNRTIs. Rifabutin should not be given with hard-gel saquinavir or delavirdine; use caution when coadministered with soft-gel saquinavir. Rifabutin may be administered at a reduced dose (150 mg qd) with indinavir, nelfinavir, or amprenavir; at a reduced dose of 150 mg qod (or 150 mg tiw) with ritonavir; or at an increased dose (450 mg qd) with efavirenz. Information is lacking regarding coadministration of rifabutin with nevirapine. Exposure to multidrug-resistant tuberculosis might require prophylaxis with two drugs; consult public health authorities. Possible regimens include pyrazinamide plus either ethambutol or a fluoroquinolone.

‡Protection against toxoplasmosis is provided by TMP-SMX, dapsone plus pyrimethamine, and possibly by atovaquone. Atovaquone may be used with or without pyrimethamine. Pyrimethamine alone probably provides little, if any, protection.

§Vaccination can be offered to persons who have a CD4+/mm³ <200, although the efficacy is probably diminished. Revaccination ≥5 yr after the first dose is considered optional, as is revaccination sooner if the initial vaccination was administered when the CD4+/mm³ was <200 and the CD4+/mm³ has increased to >200 while on HAART. Certain authorities are concerned that vaccinations might stimulate the replication of HIV.

‖In a limited number of occupational or other circumstances, prophylaxis should be considered; a specialist should be consulted.

¶Acyclovir is not protective against CMV. Valacyclovir is not recommended because of an unexplained trend toward increased mortality observed among persons with AIDS who were being administered this drug for prevention of CMV disease.

anti-HBc, antibody to hepatitis B core antigen; TST, tuberculin skin test.

Modified from Kaplan JE, Masur H, Holmes KK; USPHS; Infectious Disease Society of America: *MMWR Recomm Rep* 51(RR-8):1-52, 2002.

TABLE 11-7

PROPHYLAXIS TO PREVENT RECURRENCE OF OPPORTUNISTIC DISEASE (AFTER CHEMOTHERAPY FOR ACUTE DISEASE) IN ADULTS AND ADOLESCENTS INFECTED WITH HIV

Pathogen	Indication	First Choice	Alternatives
I. RECOMMENDED FOR LIFE AS STANDARD OF CARE			
Pneumocystis carinii	Prior *P. carinii* pneumonia	TMP–SMX 1 DS PO qd TMP–SMX 1 SS PO qd	Dapsone 50 mg PO bid or 100 mg PO qd Dapsone 50 mg PO qd plus pyrimethamine 50 mg PO q1wk *plus* leucovorin 25 mg PO q1wk Dapsone 200 mg PO *plus* pyrimethamine 75 mg PO *plus* leucovorin 25 mg PO q1wk Aerosolized pentamidine 300 mg every month via Respigard II nebulizer Atovaquone 1500 mg PO qd TMP–SMX 1 DS PO tiw
*Toxoplasma gondii**	Prior toxoplasmic encephalitis	Sulfadiazine 500-1000 mg PO qid *plus* pyrimethamine 25-50 mg PO qd *plus* leucovorin 10-25 mg PO qd	Clindamycin 300-450 mg PO q6-8h *plus* pyrimethamine, 25-50 mg PO qd *plus* leucovorin, 10-25 mg PO qd Atovaquone 750 mg PO q6-12h ± pyrimethamine 25 mg PO qd *plus* leucovorin 10 mg PO qd
Mycobacterium avium complex†	Documented disseminated disease	Clarithromycin 500 mg PO bid *plus* ethambutol 15 mg/kg PO qd ± rifabutin 300 mg PO qd	Azithromycin 500 mg PO qd *plus* ethambutol 15 mg/kg PO qd ± rifabutin 300 mg PO qd
Cytomegalovirus	Prior end-organ disease	Valganciclovir 900 mg PO qd Ganciclovir 5-6 mg/kg/d IV 5-7 days weekly or 1000 mg PO tid	Cidofovir 5 mg/kg IV qowk with probenecid 2 g PO 3 h before the dose followed by 1 g PO 2 h after the dose, and 1 g PO 8 hours after the dose (total of 4 g)

		Foscarnet 90-120 mg/kg/day IV; For retinitis, ganciclovir, sustained-release implant q6-9mo *plus* ganciclovir 1.0-1.5 g PO tid or valganciclovir 900 mg PO qd	Fomivirsen 1 vial (330 µg) injected into the vitreous, then repeated q2-4wk *plus* ganciclovir 1.0-1.5 g PO tid or valganciclovir 900 mg PO qd
Cryptococcus neoformans	Documented disease	Fluconazole 200 mg PO qd	Amphotericin B 0.6-1.0 mg/kg IV q1wk-tiw; Itraconazole, 200 mg PO qd
Histoplasma capsulatum	Documented disease	Itraconazole capsule 200 mg PO bid	Amphotericin B 1.0 mg/kg IV q1wk
Coccidioides immitis	Documented disease	Fluconazole 400 mg PO qd	Amphotericin B 1.0 mg/kg IV q1wk; Itraconazole 200 mg PO bid
Salmonella species (non-typhi)‡	Bacteremia	Ciprofloxacin 500 mg PO bid for ≥2 mo	Antibiotic chemoprophylaxis with another active agent
RECOMMENDED ONLY IF SUBSEQUENT EPISODES ARE FREQUENT OR SEVERE			
Herpes simplex virus	Frequent/severe recurrences	Acyclovir 200 mg PO tid or 400 mg PO bid; Famciclovir 250 mg PO bid	Valacyclovir 500 mg PO bid
Candida (oropharyngeal or vaginal)	Frequent/severe recurrences	Fluconazole 100-200 mg PO qd	Itraconazole solution 200 mg PO qd
Candida (esophageal)	Frequent/severe recurrences	Fluconazole 100-200 mg PO qd	Itraconazole solution 200 mg PO qd

*Pyrimethamine-sulfadiazine confers protection against PCP and toxoplasmosis; clindamycin-pyrimethamine does not.

†Certain multidrug regimens are not well tolerated. Drug interactions (e.g., with clarithromycin and rifabutin) can be problematic; rifabutin has been associated with uveitis, chiefly when administered at daily doses of >300 mg or concurrently with fluconazole or clarithromycin. During pregnancy, zithromycin is recommended instead of clarithromycin because clarithromycin is teratogenic in animals.

‡Efficacy of eradication of *Salmonella* has been demonstrated only for ciprofloxacin.

Adapted from Centers for Disease Control and Prevention: *MMWR Morb Mortal Wkly Rep* 49:185-189, 2000.

HIV–AIDS 11

TABLE 11-8

CRITERIA FOR STARTING, DISCONTINUING, AND RESTARTING OPPORTUNISTIC INFECTION PROPHYLAXIS FOR ADULTS WITH HIV

Opportunistic Illness	Initiate Primary Prophylaxis	Discontinue Primary Prophylaxis	Restart Primary Prophylaxis	Initiate Secondary Prophylaxis	Discontinue Secondary Prophylaxis	Restart Secondary Prophylaxis
Pneumocystis carinii pneumonia	CD4+/mm³ <200 or oropharyngeal cadidiasis	CD4+/mm³ >200 for ≥3 mo	CD4+/mm³ <200	Prior *Pneumocystis carinii* pneumonia	CD4+/mm³ >200 for ≥3 mo	CD4+/mm³ <200
Toxoplasmosis	IgG antibody to toxoplasma and CD4+/mm³ <100	CD4+/mm³ >200 for ≥3 mo	CD4+/mm³ <100-200	Prior toxoplasmic encephalitis	CD4+/mm³ >200 sustained (e.g., ≥6 mo) and completed initial therapy and asymptomatic for toxoplasmosis	CD4+/mm³ <200
Disseminated *Mycobacterium avium* complex	CD4+/mm³ <50	CD4+/mm³ >100 for ≥3 mo	CD4+/mm³ <50-100	Documented disseminated disease	CD4+/mm³ >100 sustained (e.g., ≥6 mo) and completed 12 mo MAC therapy and asymptomatic for MAC	CD4+/mm³ <100

Cryptococcosis	None	NA	NA	Documented disease	CD4+/mm³ >100-200 sustained (e.g., ≥6 months) and completed initial therapy and asymptomatic for cryptococcosis	CD4+/mm³ <100
Histoplasmosis	None	NA	NA	Documented disease	No criteria recommended for stopping	NA
Coccidioidomycosis	None	NA	NA	Documented disease	No criteria recommended for stopping	NA
Cytomegalovirus retinitis	None	NA	NA	Documented end-organ disease	CD4+/mm³ >100-150 cells/µL sustained (e.g., ≥6 mo) and no evidence of active disease, regular ophthalmic examination	CD4+/mm³ <100-150 cells/µL

NA, not applicable.

Modified from Kaplan JE, Masur H, Holmes KK; USPHS; Infectious Disease Society of America: Guidelines for preventing opportunistic infections among HIV-infected persons—2002.
Recommendations of the U.S. Public Health Service and the Infectious Diseases Society of America. *MMWR Recomm Rep* 51(RR-8):1-52, 2002.

HIV–AIDS 11

a. A symmetric interstitial pneumonitis pattern is common on radiograph, but the **chest x-ray is negative in 10% to 20% of patients.** Occasionally, cavitary lesions are seen.

b. Diagnosis is by seeing the organism in the sputum, especially by immunofluorescent techniques. Bronchoscopy with bronchoalveolar lavage yields the diagnosis in 95% of cases.

2. *Pneumocystis* pneumonia

a. If patient is not acutely ill with Po_2 >60 mm Hg: TMP–SMX 10 to 15 mg/kg PO or IV bid or tid based on the TMP component for 21 days. Rash and fever are common in AIDS patients taking TMP–SMX, but you can continue drug if reaction is not severe.

b. If acutely ill with Po_2 <60 mm Hg or A-a gradient >35, add prednisone 40 mg PO bid for 5 days (15-30 minutes before TMP–SMX dose), then 40 mg qd for 5 days, followed by 20 mg PO qd until completion of treatment. This reduces the rate of respiratory failure and mortality, although it increases the rate of herpes zoster. It is important to get a definitive diagnosis if you are going to use steroids, because prednisone can worsen TB.

c. **Alternative regimens** include TMP 5 mg/kg PO tid plus dapsone 100 mg PO qd × 21 days; atovaquone 750 mg PO bid × 21 days; clindamycin 600 mg PO or IV tid plus primaquine 15 to 30 mg base PO qd × 21 days; pentamidine 3 to 4 mg/kg per day IV × 21 days (reserved for severe cases); trimetrexate IV plus leucovorin (PO or IV) with or without dapsone (leucovorin should continue for 3 days longer than trimetrexate). Patient may have clinical and radiographic worsening during the first 3 to 5 days of therapy, but usually there is improvement within 7 to 10 days. **Do not change TMP–SMX on the assumption that therapy has failed until after at least 5 days of treatment.**

d. Mortality is 100% in untreated patients and 15% to 20% in treated hospitalized patients.

3. Mucosal candidiasis/esophagitis

a. **Diagnosis.** Candidiasis manifests with oral curdlike lesions or dysphagia, odynophagia. **Patient may have esophageal disease without oral disease.**

b. **Therapy**

(1) **Oral candidiasis:** nystatin 100,000 U/mL swish and swallow 5 mL or 500,000 U tablets PO q6h, or clotrimazole troches 10 mg 5 times per day dissolved in mouth, or fluconazole 100 mg PO. Alternative is itraconazole 100 to 200 mg oral solution PO qd or amphotericin IV. Treat until symptoms resolve (usually 10-14 days).

(2) **Esophageal candidiasis:** fluconazole 200 to 800 mg PO or IV qd for 14 to 28 days, or itraconazole 200 mg PO qd. Alternatives are amphotericin B IV, voriconazole 200mg/d, or caspofungin IV. For refractory cases, perform endoscopy with cultures, and change therapy (increase fluconazole dose or use another alternative drug). Secondary prophylaxis for chronic suppression is indicated in case of recurrence.

4. **Cytomegalovirus**
a. **Manifestations**
   (1) **Retinitis** may be asymptomatic, or patient can present with decreased vision, floaters, scotomata, or field defects. Diagnosed by funduscopic exam. Fluffy white infiltrates associated with central pallor, surrounding retinal hemorrhage, and perivascular sheathing are seen ("cottage cheese and ketchup").
   (2) **CNS infection,** mononeuritis, esophagitis, colitis. Same treatment as for retinitis, but efficacy is not as good.
   (3) **Hepatitis.** No treatment recommended.
b. **Treatment.** Both ganciclovir and foscarnet are fairly toxic. Ganciclovir is associated with myelosuppression and foscarnet is associated with nephrotoxicity and hypocalcemia.
   (1) **Vision-threatening lesion.** Intraocular ganciclovir implant q6-8mo plus valganciclovir 900 mg PO bid × 14 to 21 days, then 900 mg daily.
   (2) **Peripheral lesions.** Oral valganciclovir (same doses as above). Alternative regimens include ganciclovir 5 mg/kg IV q12h for 14 to 21 days followed by valganciclovir 900 mg/day; foscarnet 60 to 90 mg/kg IV Q8-12h × 14 to 21 days followed by 90 to 120 mg/kg q12h.
   (3) **Continue maintenance therapy for CMV retinitis.** Valganciclovir 900 mg qd with or without intraocular implants q6-8mo (see Table 11-7 on when to stop).
5. *Toxoplasma gondii* is the most common cause of CNS mass lesion in AIDS.
a. **Diagnosis.** Infection manifests with frequent headache, focal neurologic defects, altered mentation, fever, and seizures. **CT/MRI show ring-enhancing lesions**, usually multiple and bilateral.
b. **Treatment.**
   (1) Pyrimethamine 200 mg PO once for induction, then 50 to 75 mg PO qd plus sulfadiazine 1 to 1.5 g PO q6h plus leucovorin 10 to 20 mg/d. Use this regimen for at least 6 weeks. Give dexamethasone 4 mg IV or PO q6h for mass effect.
   (2) Alternative regimens include pyrimethamine plus leucovorin (same doses), **in addition to one of the following:** clindamycin 600 PO or IV q6h; atovaquone 1500 mg PO bid; azithromycin 900 to 1200 mg PO qd; or clarithromycin 500 mg PO bid. Bactrim (5mg/kg bid based on TMP) is another alternative.
   (3) Use maintenance therapy to prevent recurrence (see Tables 11-6 and 11-7).
6. **Herpes zoster (varicella-zoster virus)**
a. **Diagnosis.** Herpes manifests with grouped vesicles over one or more dermatomes. Consider immunosuppression in any patient who presents with zoster in more than one dermatome.

b. **Treatment**
  (1) Famciclovir 500 mg PO tid or valacyclovir HCl 1000 mg PO tid; acyclovir 800 mg PO 5 times a day for 7 to 10 days. For severe disease, acyclovir 10 mg/kg per day IV q8h.
  (2) Resistance can develop; if the patient has been treated previously with acyclovir, you might have to use foscarnet 120 to 200 mg/kg per day for 14 to 26 days.
  (3) Most benefit is achieved if therapy is begun within 24 hours of onset.
  (4) Use gabapentin, tricyclics, carbamazepine, lidocaine patch, or narcotics for pain relief.

7. **Cryptococcal meningitis**
  a. **Diagnosis.** Meningitis with headache, fever, delirium, nausea, and vomiting. Only one third have meningismus or photophobia. Rarely patients present with seizures.
  b. CSF usually shows mildly elevated protein, normal or slightly low glucose, and few lymphocytes.
  c. Detect organism in CSF by India ink, cryptococcal antigen, or fungal culture; serum cryptococcal antigen is positive in >95%.
  d. Do head CT before LP because of high incidence of mass lesions in AIDS patients, to avoid transtentorial herniation.
  e. **Treatment.** Amphotericin B 0.7 mg/kg per day IV plus flucytosine 100 mg/kg per day PO for 2 weeks. Follow with fluconazole 400 mg PO qd or itraconazole 200 mg PO bid for 8 weeks or until CSF is sterile. Continue maintenance therapy until adequate immune reconstitution (see Tables 11-6 and 11-7).

8. **Bacterial infections** (only in selected patients). For neutropenia, start G-CSF 5 to 10 μg/kg SQ qd or GM-CSF 250 μg/m^2 IV over 2 hours.

9. *Mycobacterium tuberculosis* (see Chapter 10 for details of diagnosis and treatment).
  a. Because *M. tuberculosis* is more virulent than *Pneumocystis*, it often occurs at an earlier stage of HIV infection than *Pneumocystis*.
  b. Of those with TB, extrapulmonary disease develops in 70% of patients with preexisting AIDS and 45% of those with HIV infection.
  c. Incidence is inversely associated with baseline CD4+ count. Among those who have disease, it is most likely reactivation rather than from a recent exposure.
  d. CXR shows perihilar adenopathy and cavitary lesions; there may be effusions. Miliary TB can mimic pneumocystis on CXR.
  e. Do not initiate treatment simultaneously with anti-TB and antiretrovirals if the patient is not already on antiretroviral therapy.
  f. Do not use nebulized pentamidine in those with TB because of the possibility of transmission of the disease to others.

10. *Mycobacterium avium-intracellulare/M. avium* complex (MAI/MAC)
  a. Can manifest as diarrhea, fever, night sweats, and generalized wasting.
  b. Can generally be cultured from blood or stool.

c. Treatment regimens include clarithromycin 500 PO bid or azithromycin 500 to 600 mg PO qd plus ethambutol 15 mg/kg/day PO. Consider a third drug if CD4$^+$ <50 or MAC load is high: rifabutin 300 mg PO qd, ciprofloxacin 500 to 750 mg PO bid, levofloxacin 500 mg PO qd, or amikacin 10 to 15 mg/kg IV qd.

II. AIDS-Associated Diarrhea.

A. General. From 30% to 50% of AIDS patients in the United States have diarrhea at some point during their illness. Because the causes of diarrhea in these patients are protean, empiric therapy is almost never indicated. It is important to try to identify the organism. A general approach includes good history, physical exam, and stool. It may be necessary to proceed to colonoscopy (culture and biopsy for CMV, *Mycobacterium*, adenovirus, and herpes simplex) or esophagogastroduodenoscopy (culture for CMV and *Mycobacterium*). General supportive measures are also indicated, including fluids and antimotility drugs, unless the patient has fecal leukocytes or abdominal pain. Test stool for

1. Culture and sensitivity (need to culture for *Salmonella* species (100 times more common than in the normal population), *Shigella flexneri*, and *Campylobacter jejuni*.
2. O&P × 3 and *Cryptosporidia* and *Giardia* antigens.
3. *C. difficile* toxin.
4. Acid-fast stains and in advanced disease chromotrope-based stains × 2.

B. Dietary and drinking water precautions

1. Avoid raw meat (sushi, etc.) and raw eggs. Cook meat thoroughly. Do not use cracked eggs. Thaw frozen meat in the refrigerator or microwave, not at room temperature.
2. Listeriosis is a rare disease; however, it may be contracted by eating hot dogs and cold cuts from delicatessen counters. These foods should be reheated before consumption.
3. Avoid drinking water from lakes or rivers because of the risk of cryptosporidiosis and giardiasis. Even accidental ingestion while swimming carries a risk.

C. Specific causes of AIDS-associated diarrhea

1. Cryptosporidium

a. Transmitted by fecal–oral route. Causes 10% to 30% of chronic diarrhea in AIDS patients.
b. Manifests with chronic voluminous watery diarrhea and abdominal pain, anorexia, nausea, and malabsorption.
c. Modified acid-fast stain, or direct immunofluorescence antibody on the stools. Diagnosis can also be made by biopsy of colon or small bowel.
d. **The only treatment that controls persistent infection is HAART with immune reconstitution.** Some antimicrobials are used but are not consistently effective: paromomycin 1000 mg PO bid or 500 mg qid, azithromycin 1200 mg PO qd, nitazoxanide 500 mg PO bid, atovaquone 750 mg PO bid. Supplemental benefit from octreotide 50 to 500 μg SQ q8h or 1 μg/h IV.

e. Cryptosporidiosis resolves spontaneously in most patients with CD4$^+$ >100 in 2 to 8 weeks.

2. *Giardia lamblia.* See Chapter 5.

3. *Isospora*

a. *Isospora* constitutes 1% to 3% of AIDS diarrhea in the United States (higher elsewhere).

b. Symptoms are similar to those of *Cryptosporidium*, but the patient gets an associated eosinophilia.

c. Diagnosed by acid-fast stain of stool; may require several stool specimens.

d. Treatment is by TMP–SMX 1 DS PO qid or 2 DS PO bid × 10 days. Alternative regimens include pyrimethamine 50 to 75 mg PO qd plus leucovorin 5 to 10 mg PO qd × 10 days, or ciprofloxacin 500 mg PO bid × 10 days. Chronic suppression needed: TMP–SMX 1 to 2 DS PO qd or tiw, or sulfadoxine–pyrimethamine (Fansidar) once weekly

4. Microsporidia, including *Enterocytozoon bieneusi, Septata intestinalis.*

a. An excellent screening test is fluorescence with calcofluor. Diagnose by duodenal biopsy and electron microscopy, or stain formalin-fixed stool with Giemsa or chromotrope-based technique and use light microscopy.

b. Mainstay treatment is HAART to achieve CD4$^+$ >100. Albendazole 400 mg PO bid until CD4$^+$ > 200 has been used for *S. intestinalis.*

5. CMV

a. Incidence of chronic diarrhea in AIDS is 15% to 40%. Biopsy of colon is needed for diagnosis.

b. There is no good treatment for CMV diarrhea, but you can try ganciclovir or foscarnet (see protocol above).

c. May cause necrosis and perforation.

6. *Histoplasma capsulatum*

7. *Mycobacterium avium* complex. Diarrhea is usually associated with disseminated disease. See section on mycobacterial disease.

8. AIDS-associated enteropathy comprises villous atrophy, malabsorption, and lactase deficiency in the absence of an identifiable pathogen after extensive work-up. Antiretroviral drugs may improve symptoms.

9. Bacterial disease. See Chapter 5.

10. HSV

a. May have proctitis, esophagitis, or genital and perianal lesions.

b. Manifests with tenesmus, constipation, dysphagia, and anorectal pain.

c. Treatment is acyclovir 400 mg tid qd × 7 to 10 days. Alternatively, famciclovir HCl 500 mg bid or valacyclovir 1 g bid × 7 to 10 days. Longer durations are required for severe mucocutaneous disease.

d. Chronic suppression with acyclovir 400 mg bid if there is recurrence.

III. **Syphilis.**
 A. **Penicillin is recommended for treatment in all HIV-infected patients at all stages of syphilis.** Skin testing is advised to confirm allergy, though the utility in immunocompromised patients is questionable. For HIV-infected patients who are penicillin allergic, the CDC recommends desensitization and then treatment with PCN. **Alternative treatments are suboptimal.**
 B. **Some experts suggest an LP for all HIV patients with syphilis.** If there is CSF pleocytosis or positive CSF VDRL test, treat for neurosyphilis. Patients may also have elevated CSF total protein.
 C. **See Chapter 8 for treatment regimens for primary, secondary, and latent syphilis.**
 D. Treatment for neurosyphilis is aqueous penicillin G 18 to 24 million units IV qd × 10 to 14 days divided q3-4h or continuous, with or without benzathine penicillin G 3 million units weekly for 3 weeks after IV course. Alternative outpatient treatment is procaine penicillin 2.4 million units IM qd plus probenecid 500 mg PO qid × 10 to 14 days.
 E. **For treatment failure, evaluation of CSF is indicated** (if not already done). If the CSF is normal, the penicillin dose is the same as that for latent syphilis. Follow-up study for treatment failure includes clinical and serologic evaluation at 1 month and then 2, 3, 6, 9, and 12 months after treatment.

AIDS-ASSOCIATED WEIGHT LOSS AND WASTING

 I. Weight loss and tissue wasting are major problems in the AIDS patient for several reasons, including HIV-induced hypermetabolic state, anorexia, eating difficulties from oral and esophageal disease, diarrhea and malabsorption, hypogonadism, and infection.
 II. **Treatment** consists of exercise and increased dietary protein, as well as some hormones or hormone-like drugs.
 III. **Dronabinol (Marinol),** one of the active ingredients in marijuana, is widely used by patients with AIDS to improve their appetite; some evidence indicates that it may be effective. It can cause side effects such as confusion, emotional lability, or hallucinations. **Short-term use of marijuana has also been used by HIV+ patients.**
 IV. **Megestrol acetate** 400 to 800 mg daily has been associated with a significant weight gain in patients with AIDS-associated wasting, but it seems to be mostly from gaining fat and therefore is being used less. Megestrol may be associated with adrenal suppression and should not be discontinued abruptly.
 V. **Anabolic steroids** (nandrolone, testosterone, and oxandrolone) have resulted in a significant weight gain in AIDS patients.
 VI. Some less frequently used appetite stimulants include thalidomide, recombinant human growth hormone, insulin-like growth factor-1 and omega-3 fatty acids (e.g., fish oil) supplementation.

11

HIV-AIDS

NEUROPSYCHIATRIC DISEASE

I. **General.** About 60% of patients with AIDS have some neuropsychiatric manifestations of the illness. This may be because macrophages and monocytes carry the HIV into the CNS. The virus may also gain direct access because many CNS components are CD4+. It is critical to ascertain that neurologic manifestations are not attributable to infectious causes (e.g., *Toxoplasma*, CMV) or CNS lymphoma before attributing symptoms to the direct effects of the AIDS virus. Persons with HIV–AIDS are undergoing a major stress, and psychologic support is critical to the successful management of their illness. Drug therapies are helpful, but social and psychologic support is important to their overall care.

II. **AIDS Dementia Complex** (AIDS encephalopathy, HIV-associated dementia, HIV-associated cognitive motor complex).

A. **AIDS dementia complex is defined by** progressive dementia, psychomotor retardation, focal motor abnormalities, behavioral changes, and short-term memory deficits. Cognitive decline is subacute, with a course of at least 6 months. Motor slowing generally shows symmetric involvement of arms and legs.

B. **It can manifest as** headache and problems of coordination, apathy, and affective blunting. Later manifestations include inappropriate behavior, emotional lability, seizures, aphasia, and psychotic manifestations.

C. **Patients with advanced cases develop global cognitive deterioration**, incontinence, sensory loss, and visual disturbances.

III. **Testing.**

A. Useful tests include the Symbol Digit Modalities Test and Parts A and B of the Trail Making Test, which test psychomotor function. The HIV Dementia Scale is a reliable and quantitative scale superior to the Mini-Mental State Exam and the Grooved Pegboard in identifying HIV dementia, and it can be used to follow response to HAART.

B. **Brain imaging is not diagnostic, but it is critical to rule out alternative diagnoses,** such as *Toxoplasma*, CNS lymphoma, and progressive multifocal leukoencephalopathy. The most common abnormality reported on CT scans of these patients is cerebral atrophy. MRI is best at demonstrating degeneration; the most common white matter lesions are diffuse over a wide area, typically in the centrum semiovale and periventricular white matter. Less commonly, there is localized involvement, with patchy or punctate lesions. Magnetic resonance spectroscopy is a promising means of detecting HIV brain involvement.

C. **CSF examination is important to rule out meningitis.** CSF should be tested for syphilis, cryptococcal antigen, and CMV (by PCR). In patients with AIDS dementia complex, CSF shows few mononuclear cells, slightly elevated protein, and normal glucose; oligoclonal bands may be found (but are not specific).

D. EEG is not particularly helpful.

E. Look for other causes of delirium and dementia in patients with HIV once HIV-related disease has been ruled out. The most common are affective disorders. See Chapters 9 and 18 for details.

IV. Treatment

A. AIDS-related dementia responds to some degree to HAART.

B. Some experimental agents have been investigated in small clinical trials to treat AIDS dementia, including CPI-1189, nimodipine, memantine, lexipafant, and peptide-T. The most promising results were seen with selegiline.

C. Agitation secondary to delirium may be treated with lorazepam 0.5 mg IV slow push.

D. Treat psychotic symptoms with haloperidol 0.5 to 1 mg PO qid.

E. Depression can be treated with standard antidepressants. Some patients respond rapidly to methylphenidate 5mg every AM up to 20 to 60 mg divided tid. Patients may be sensitive to anticholinergic side effects late in HIV illness. MAO inhibitors are contraindicated.

F. AIDS patients can develop a manic syndrome related to the use of ganciclovir, zidovudine, and fluoxetine, which may respond to lithium. Treat agitation as above.

G. Anxiety can be treated with standard drugs.

DERMATOLOGIC MANIFESTATIONS

I. Cutaneous Infections.

A. Viral

1. **Herpes simplex** produces oral or genital lesions. Severe disseminated disease can occur, as well as chronic herpetic ulcers. Treat with acyclovir 400 mg PO tid or 5 to 10 mg/kg IV q8h for severe disease. Maintenance dose is acyclovir 400 mg PO bid, indicated for six or more recurrences per year.

2. **Herpes zoster.** Preferred treatment is valacyclovir 1g PO tid × 7 to 10 days. Use acyclovir 30 mg/kg per day IV for severe disease.

B. Fungal

1. **Dermatophytosis (tinea):** fungi of the genera *Trichophyton, Microsporum*, and *Epidermophyton*.

2. **Yeasts** and mucosal candidiasis: treat with systemic antifungals (see section on candidiasis).

3. **Rarely:** histoplasmosis and cryptococcosis (in disseminated disease).

C. Bacterial

1. **Bacterial folliculitis,** impetigo. The most common agent is *Staphylococcus aureus*.

2. **Mycobacterial infections.** Treatment involves systemic antibiotics (see previous section on Mycobacteria).

3. **Bacillary angiomatosis** (caused by *Bartonella* species). Treat with erythromycin 500 mg PO qid until lesions resolve or doxycycline 100 mg PO bid.

11

HIV–AIDS

II. **Cutaneous Neoplasms.**

A. **Kaposi's sarcoma.** Human herpesvirus-8 (HHV-8) has been implicated as the causative agent of this skin neoplasm. Clinically it appears as purplish macules, papules, plaques, and nodules, usually asymptomatic, on legs, face, oral cavity, and genitalia. Therapy includes observation, cryotherapy, laser surgery, excisional surgery, radiation therapy, or systemic chemotherapy. HAART significantly reduces the incidence of Kaposi's sarcoma and tumor burden.

B. **Lymphoma cutis.** Skin is rarely involved; usually B cell in origin.

C. Possible increased incidence of melanoma, basal cell carcinoma, and squamous cell carcinoma.

D. **Oral hairy leukoplakia** is caused by EBV. It manifests as a well-demarcated verrucous plaque with an irregular, corrugated, or hairy surface, most commonly on the lateral or inferior surface of the tongue or on the buccal and soft palatal mucosa. Unlike *Candida*, it cannot be scraped off. It is usually asymptomatic.

III. **Inflammatory Dermatitides.**

A. **Seborrheic dermatitis**, psoriasis, eczematous dermatitis, and folliculitis. See Chapter 17 for treatment options. Avoid methotrexate.

B. **Pruritus, prurigo, and eosinophilic folliculitis** are extremely common and extremely debilitating, with 3- to 5-mm edematous follicular papules and pustules. Treatment is often unsatisfactory: antihistamines, potent topical fluorinated corticosteroids (such as clobetasol propionate bid), or phototherapy with natural sunlight or UVB radiation.

C. Cutaneous eruption of HIV manifests as erythematous nonpruritic macules soon after infection.

AIDS AND PREGNANCY

I. **Probability of perinatal transmission is directly related to viral load at the time of delivery.** The probability of perinatal transmission is 20% to 28% without treatment, 8% to 11% with AZT monotherapy, and 1% to 2% with HAART therapy. Elective C-section should be offered at 38 weeks for women with viral loads that are likely to be >1000/mL at delivery to reduce the risk of perinatal transmission. The treatment and monitoring guidelines for pregnant women are similar to those for the general population. HAART is also recommended for any pregnant woman with a viral load >1000/mL, irrespective of $CD4^+$ counts, in order to prevent perinatal transmission. With viral load <1000/mL and $CD4^+$ is >350, AZT monotherapy may be given. Include AZT in the regimen when possible. Avoid efavirenz (teratogenic in the first semester), hydroxyurea (teratogenic), and d4T + ddI combination (severe lactic acidosis).

A. **ACTG 076 trial protocol.** Start AZT at 300 mg PO bid or 200 mg PO tid at 14 weeks of gestation and continue throughout the remainder of the pregnancy. During labor, give AZT IV 2 mg/kg for the first hour, then a continuous infusion of 1 mg/kg per hour until delivery. Postpartum, give the infant 2 mg/kg PO (or 1.5 mg/kg IV) q6h for a total of 6 weeks.

B. **Nevirapine** is at least as effective as AZT. Give the mother a single 200-mg dose at delivery, and give the infant one dose of 2 mg/kg. Avoid if CD4$^+$ is >250 because of hepatotoxicity.

II. **Breastfeeding.** Risk of HIV transmission is 10% to 16%, greatest in the first 4 to 6 months. Risk is increased with the presence of mastitis, cracked nipples, prolonged breastfeeding, or breast abscess. Breastfeeding should therefore be discouraged.

III. **HIV$^+$ women have higher rates of preterm delivery, low birth weight, and stillbirths** (data from developing countries). HIV$^+$ women should be counseled about their options regarding pregnancy. Information about contraception, prenatal care, and abortion services should be provided.

IV. **Procedures that increase the likelihood of direct fetal exposure to maternal blood should be minimized during the antepartum and intrapartum periods.** Examples include amniocentesis, fetal scalp electrode placement, and fetal scalp pH measurements.

V. **Prophylaxis of Opportunistic Infections during Pregnancy.** HIV in pregnancy presents a special dilemma in which the health care provider must carefully weight the risks and benefits. Unfortunately, there are very few data in this area of medicine. Listed below are generally accepted guidelines.

A. Try to limit drug exposures during the first trimester, the most critical period for organogenesis.

B. **PCP prophylaxis is important** with CD4$^+$ <200. Although animal studies have shown TMP–SMX to be associated with cleft palate, retrospective human studies have shown no increased risk of congenital malformations. Aerosolized pentamidine and dapsone are believed to be safe during pregnancy; however, pyrimethamine should be used with caution.

C. **Preventive therapy should be instituted in pregnant women who have a positive PPD test or who are exposed to persons with active tuberculosis.** Treatment with isoniazid should be deferred until after the first trimester and, when started, should be given with pyridoxine 25 to 50 mg PO bid, given the risk of peripheral neuropathy. Experience with rifampin and rifabutin is limited.

AIDS IN THE PEDIATRIC PATIENT

Perinatal transmission accounts for the vast majority of HIV infection in children in the United States. For infants who are born to HIV$^+$ mothers, AZT should be started beginning 8 to 12 hours after birth at a dose of 2 mg/kg PO q6h; AZT should be continued for a total of 6 weeks if HIV PCR turns out to be negative. Compared with adults, children have more rapid disease progression and a different pattern of primary and secondary HIV-related manifestations. Because the normal range for the number of CD4+ T cells changes with age, so does the number that defines immunodeficiency, and CD4% is often used instead. Additionally, all infants born to an HIV-positive mother should have PCP prophylaxis started at 4 to 6 weeks, regardless of the CD4+ count, and continued to 12 months unless the child is proved to be HIV negative.

BIBLIOGRAPHY

Aberg JC, Gallant JE, Anderson J, et al: Primary care guidelines for the management of persons infected with human immunodeficiency virus: Recommendations of the HIV Medicine Association of the Infectious Diseases Society of America. *Clin Infect Dis* 39:609-627, 2004

Abrams DI, Hilton JF, Leiser RJ, et al: Short-term effects of cannabinoids in patients with HIV-1 infection: A randomized, placebo-controlled clinical trial. *Ann Intern Med* 139:258-266, 2003

Centers for Disease Control and Prevention: Management of possible sexual, injecting-drug-use or other nonoccupational exposure to HIV, including considerations related to antiretroviral therapy. Public Health Service Statement. *MMWR Recomm Rep* 47(RR-17):1-14, 1998.

Centers for Disease Control and Prevention; Health Resources and Services Administration; National Institutes of Health; HIV Medicine Association of the InfectiousDiseases Society of America: Incorporating HIV prevention into the medical care of persons living with HIV. Recommendations of CDC, the Health Resources and Services Administration, the National Institutes of Health, and the HIV Medicine Association of the Infectious Diseases Society of America. *MMWR Recomm Rep* 52(RR-12):1-24, 2003.

Clavel F, Hance AJ: HIV drug resistance. *N Engl J Med* 350:1023-1035, 2004.

Clifford DB: AIDS dementia. *Med Clin North Am* 86:537-550, 2002.

Masur H, Kaplan JE, Holmes KK, et al: Guidelines for preventing opportunistic infections among HIV-infected persons—2002. Recommendations of the U.S. Public Health Service and the Infectious Diseases Society of America. *Ann Intern Med* 137(5 Pt 2):435-478, 2002.

Mylonakis E, Paliou M, Lally M,et al: Laboratory testing for infection with the human immunodeficiency virus: Established and novel approaches. *Am J Med* 109: 568-576, 2000.

Nduati R, John G, Mbori-Ngacha D, et al: Effect of breastfeeding and formula feeding on transmission of HIV-1: A randomized clinical trial. *JAMA* 283:1167-1174, 2000.

Paterson, DL, Swindells S, Mohr J, et al: Adherence to protease inhibitor therapy and outcomes in patients with HIV infection. *Ann Intern Med* 133:21-30, 2000.

Pinkerton SD, Martin JN, Roland ME, et al: Cost-effectiveness of postexposure prophylaxis after sexual or injection-drug exposure to human immunodeficiency virus. *Arch Intern Med* 164:46-54, 2004.

Strang P: The effect of megestrol acetate on anorexia, weight loss and cachexia in cancer and AIDS patients. *Anticancer Res* 17(1B):657-662, 1997.

Tuomala RE,Shapiro DE, Mofenson LM, et al: Antiretroviral therapy during pregnancy and the risk of an adverse outcome. *N Engl J Med* 346:1863-1870, 2002.

U.S. Department of Health and Human Services: Aids Info Clinical Guidelines: Guidelines for the Use of Antiretroviral Agents in HIV-Infected Adults and Adolescents—October 6, 2005. Available at http://www.aidsinfo.nih.gov/Guidelines/GuidelineDetail.aspx?MenuItem=Guidelines&Search=Off&GuidelineID=7&ClassID=1 (accessed December 28, 2005).

U.S. Public Health Service: Updated U.S. Public Health Service Guidelines for the Management of Occupational Exposures to HBV, HCV, and HIV and Recommendations for Postexposure Prophylaxis. *MMWR Recomm Rep* 50(RR-11):1-52, 2001.

Yeni PG, Hammer SM, Carpenter CC, et al: Antiretroviral treatment for adult HIV infection in 2002: Updated recommendations of the International AIDS Society—USA Panel. *JAMA* 288:222-235, 2002.

Pediatrics

Tracy Shaw and Mark A. Graber

NEWBORN NURSERY

I. **Normal Body Temperature.**
A. **Observe and maintain a normal body temperature. Rectal temperatures provide the only accurate noninvasive method of measuring temperature.** Hyperthermia or hypothermia warrants further investigation.
B. **If hyperthermia,** consider sepsis or intracranial bleed.
C. **If hypothermia,** consider sepsis, hypoglycemia, hypothyroidism, and heat loss caused by environmental conditions.

II. **Initial Gastrointestinal and Genitourinary Function.**
A. **Approximately 70% of newborns pass meconium and urine in the first 12 hours of life,** 25% between 12 and 24 hours and the other 5% between 24 and 48 hours.
B. **If meconium is delayed,** look for meconium plug, sepsis, narcotic exposure, Hirschsprung's disease, hypothyroidism, cystic fibrosis (CF), or imperforate anus.
C. **If infant is anuric or oliguric,** think about dehydration, sepsis, renal abnormalities, or obstruction.

III. **Monitor weight and head circumference.** Weight initially drops (not >10%) and is usually regained by 2 weeks. Head circumference may decrease or increase (not >1 cm) as a result of initial trauma or molding of labor, or both.

IV. **Red Reflex.** The pupil should be black on direct examination, and red when examined through an ophthalmoscope. If the red reflex looks pale or white, suspect retinoblastoma or congenital cataract.

V. **Newborn Prophylaxis.**
A. **Eyes.** Erythromycin 0.5% ointment to prevent gonorrheal conjunctivitis or *Chlamydia trachomatis* ophthalmia neonatorum.
B. **Vitamin K** 0.5 to 1 mg IM to prevent hemorrhagic disease. Avoid products containing benzyl alcohol because they can be toxic to the newborn.
C. **Hepatitis.**
1. **For those born of a hepatitis B–negative mother.** Give hepatitis B vaccine routinely at birth (within 12 hours) and at 1 and 6 months. Use thimerosal free vaccine.
2. **If mother hepatitis B positive (positive HepBsAg).**
a. Clean newborn of HepBsAg-positive mother thoroughly (use alcohol).
b. Give hepatitis B immune globulin 0.5 mL IM and hepatitis B vaccine ASAP.
c. Repeat hepatitis B vaccine at 1 and 6 months.

    d. Do a hepatitis B screen at 9 months; if negative, give fourth dose of vaccine; if positive, monitor for chronic active or carrier state.

  D. AIDS. See Chapter 11 for information about diagnosis, treatment, and prophylaxis of the newborn born to an HIV-positive mother.

VI. Bathing. Once the body temperature is stabilized, the infant may be bathed with **warm standing water.** Avoid running water to prevent burns. Immersion above the umbilicus should be avoided until the umbilical stump has fallen off.

VII. Umbilical Cord Care. Keep dry. Apply an antiseptic agent such as triple dye (Brilliant Green, Crystal Violet, and proflavine hemisulfate) or alcohol to avoid colonization and infection with *Streptococcus, Staphylococcus*, and *Clostridium* species and coliforms. The use of alcohol and triple dye is variable depending on your practice setting. The cord generally separates by the end of the second week but may not do so until the third week of life. Delayed separation may be normal or may be attributable to sepsis or poorly functioning leukocytes (especially leukocyte adhesion deficiency syndrome).

VIII. Screening Laboratory Tests.

  A. Metabolic Screen. Should be done at 24 hours of age or later. Phenylketonuria, hypothyroidism, galactosemia, etc., as required by state law or indicated (e.g., CF if delayed meconium stool). If screening is done before 24 hours of age, it may miss some diseases, and screening should be repeated at 7 to 10 days. Depending on the test being used, antibiotics may interfere with screening. Thus, repeat the test when the patient is off of antibiotics. **Newer tests obviate the need for repeat screening after antibiotics, so check your state's recommendations.**

  B. Hematologic. Hemoglobin and hematocrit at birth and at 12 months. Screening for glucose-6-phosphate dehydrogenase (G6PD) deficiency is best done when the infant is about 2 months of age. Sickle cell in patients of African descent and thalassemia in those of Mediterranean descent will be detected on the hemoglobinopathy portion of the neonatal screen (some states may not have a hemoglobinopathy test).

  C. Urinary and meconium drug screening. Obtain if there is maternal history of drug abuse or if a baby's clinical exam could be consistent with withdrawal. (See neonatal withdrawal syndrome below.)

  D. Glucose screening. Screen all babies who are large for gestational age, small for gestational age, or born to mothers with diabetes, or any baby who has signs consistent with hypoglycemia. Repeat regularly until glucose is stable (>40 mg/dL). Warm the infant's heel, and draw capillary blood samples from the side of the heel using finger-stick test strips for glucose. See section on hypoglycemia, later, for further information on diagnosis and management.

  E. Bilirubin. Transcutaneous bilirubinometry should be used to screen suspect neonates for jaundice. If value is above 17 mg/dL, serum bilirubin should be measured. The transcutaneous bilimeter is affected by factors such as gestational age, birth weight, and skin pigmentation.

F. ABO incompatibility. Perform blood type and direct Coombs' test (use cord blood) on every infant born to a mother with type O blood or those with Rh-negative mothers.

IX. Neonatal Nutrition. See section on pediatric wellness, later.

NEONATAL JAUNDICE

I. Jaundice is visible when a baby has a serum bilirubin level that exceeds 5 mg/dL. Generally jaundice is visible first on the head and progresses to the feet. It resolves in the opposite pattern, with the feet clearing first. Hyperbilirubinemia is categorized as either physiologic or non-physiologic.

II. Physiologic Hyperbilirubinemia.

A. Usually not present in first 24 hours of life.

B. Rarely increases by more than 5 mg/dL in 1 day.

C. Peaks at 48 to 72 hours of life in full-term infants and 4 to 5 days in premature infants.

D. Serum bilirubin does not exceed 13 mg/dL in the full-term infant and 15 mg/dL in the preterm infant.

1. Direct bilirubin fraction is generally ≤2 mg/dL.

2. Physiologic jaundice disappears by 1 week in full-term infants and by 2 weeks in premature infants.

E. Any infant who does not meet the preceding description has nonphysiologic hyperbilirubinemia and should be worked up.

III. Nonphysiologic Hyperbilirubinemia: Divided into direct and indirect.

A. Those with primarily elevated direct (conjugated) bilirubin. Defined as a direct (conjugated) bilirubin >15% of total. Liver is functional.

1. **Infections,** including sepsis, perinatally acquired viral infections, including hepatitis, and intrauterine viral infections (hepatitis B, TORCHS [*TO*xoplasmosis, *R*ubella, *C*ytomegalovirus, *H*erpes simplex, *S*yphilis]).

2. **Metabolic abnormalities,** including Rotor's syndrome and Dubin-Johnson syndrome, α_1-antitrypsin deficiency, galactosemia, tyrosinosis, CF, hereditary fructose deficiency.

3. **Anatomic abnormalities,** including biliary atresia and Alagille's syndrome (ductopenia), and obstructions, as with a choledochal cyst.

4. **Cholestasis** from CVN/TPN, antibiotics (especially ceftriaxone).

B. Those with primarily elevated indirect (unconjugated) bilirubin. Two basic mechanisms:

1. **From increased production of bilirubin (therefore hemolysis or hematoma breakdown).**

a. **With positive direct Coombs' test** (mother's antibodies on child's cells): Isoimmunization (Rh, ABO, minor blood group), erythroblastosis fetalis.

b. **With negative Coombs' test and RBC morphologic abnormalities:** Spherocytosis, thalassemias, G6PD deficiency, elliptocytosis.

PEDIATRICS 12

c. **Extravascular blood:** Cephalohematoma, severe bruising, cerebral and pulmonary hemorrhage.

d. **DIC, other hemolytic anemia.**

e. **Polycythemia** resulting from delayed clamping of cord, twin–twin transfusion, maternal–fetal transfusion, cord milking.

2. **From delayed excretion of bilirubin.**

a. **Inherited disorders of bilirubin metabolism,** including Crigler-Najjar syndrome, Gilbert's disease, Dubin-Johnson syndrome, Rotor's syndrome.

b. **Hypothyroidism and prematurity.**

IV. **Breast Milk Jaundice.**

A. **General.** One in every 200 infants has prolonged unconjugated hyperbilirubinemia. Serum bilirubin may reach maximum concentration (15-25 mg/dL) during the second to third week. Etiology is unknown. However, one theory is that there is a component in breast milk that can interfere with bilirubin conjugation. Kernicterus has not been reported with breast milk jaundice.

B. **Diagnosis.** Requires the exclusion of all other causes of elevated unconjugated bilirubin in a breastfed infant.

C. **Treatment options:** Observe; discontinue breastfeeding and substitute formula; alternate feedings of breast milk and formula; discontinue breastfeeding and start phototherapy; and continue breastfeeding and start phototherapy.

D. **Comment on therapy.** Although any treatment option is reasonable, it is believed that any interruption of breastfeeding is undesirable unless very severe hyperbilirubinemia is present (total serum bilirubin >25 mg/dL). Observe, and continue breastfeeding while phototherapy is initiated.

V. **Treatment of Hyperbilirubinemia from Any Cause (Table 12-1).**

A. **Treat the underlying disorder.**

B. **Ensure adequate hydration, caloric intake, and stooling (bilirubin is excreted in stool).**

C. **Prophylactic phototherapy** is indicated for infants showing a rapid rise in bilirubin (>1 mg/dL per hour) and as a temporizing measure when one is contemplating exchange transfusion.

D. **Conjugated bilirubin does not cause kernicterus.**

E. **Phototherapy.** The number of banks of phototherapy lights used is determined by the infant's total bilirubin level, the rate of rise of the total bilirubin, and the anticipated course of the underlying cause of the hyperbilirubinemia. "Bili blankets" are an option for the patient who has a borderline elevated bilirubin. Serum bilirubin usually decreases by 2.5 to 3 mg/dL per day and 1 to 2 mg/dL in first 4 to 6 hours of phototherapy. Bilirubin level should be followed every 12 hours. Phototherapy should be discontinued when the bilirubin reaches levels of about 13 mg/dL. Bilirubin levels should be rechecked again 12 hours after discontinuation to assess for recurrence.

TABLE 12-1
MANAGEMENT OF UNCONJUGATED HYPERBILIRUBINEMIA
IN THE TERM NEWBORN

Age (h)	Consider Phototherapy at TSB (mg/dL)*	Phototherapy at TSB (mg/dL)	Exchange Transfusion at TSB (mg/dL) if Phototherapy Fails†	Exchange Transfusion and Intense Phototherapy
<24‡	—	—	—	—
25-48	>12	>15	>20	>25
49-72	>15	>18	>25	>30
>72	>20	>25	>30	—

*Phototherapy at these TSB levels is a clinical option, meaning that the intervention is available and may be used on the basis of individual clinical judgment.
†Intensive phototherapy should produce a decline in TSB of 1-2 mg/dL within 4 to 6 hours, and the TSB level should continue to fall and remain below the threshold level for exchange transfusion. If this does not occur, it is considered a failure of phototherapy.
‡Term infants who are clinically jaundiced at age 24 h are not considered healthy and require further evaluation. They might require phototherapy or exchange transfusion but must be evaluated for underlying illness.
TSB, total serum bilirubin.

12

PEDIATRICS

RESPIRATORY DISORDERS IN THE NEWBORN

I. **Respiratory Distress Syndrome and Hyaline Membrane Disease.**
A. **Characteristics.**
1. **Most common in preterm infants because of surfactant deficiency.** Higher incidence with maternal diabetes, acute asphyxia, meconium aspiration, and in second twin.
2. **Prevention and diagnosis of preterm labor is paramount;** if delivery is imminent, steroids can be used to hasten lung maturity (betamethasone 12.5 mg IM q24h × 48 h or dexamethasone 6 mg q6h for 4 doses).
B. **Clinical findings.**
1. **Shortly after birth.** Tachypnea (respiratory rate >60 per minute), grunting, retractions, flaring, and cyanosis.
2. **Radiographs.** Ground-glass reticulogranular appearance, air bronchograms.
C. **Treatment.**
1. **Rule out infection;** use antibiotics as needed.
2. **Respiratory support** (endotracheal intubation, mechanical ventilatory support) and metabolic support.
3. **Exogenous surfactant (doses differ by preparation) is very effective in treating hyaline membrane disease.** Currently recommended drugs include beractant (Survanta), 4 mL/kg by endotracheal tube (ET) q6h for four doses, or colfosceril (Exosurf), 5 mL/kg by ET q12h for two to four doses. Nitric oxide has also been used with some success. Pediatric consult suggested.

4. *Postnatal* use of corticosteroids to treat lung prematurity is associated with significant adverse physical and neurologic deficits and little or no long-term benefit.

II. Transient Tachypnea of the Newborn.

A. **Characteristics.** Diagnosis of exclusion. **It is important to rule out sepsis as a possible etiology for respiratory distress.** More common in C-section deliveries and precipitous deliveries. Pathophysiology is the delayed clearance of lung fluid.

B. **Presentation.** Tachypnea, minimal respiratory distress.

C. **Radiographs.** Fluid in fissures, pleural effusion, streaky parenchymal changes.

D. **Management.** Short-term oxygen supplementation. This is a self-limited illness that will resolve spontaneously in 24 to 48 hours.

III. Meconium Aspiration Syndrome.

A. **Characteristics.**

1. **Caused by** the presence of thick meconium in the distal airways, causing a valvelike mechanism that obstructs air movement.

2. Meconium aspiration can occur in a stressed neonate in utero or at the time of delivery. Deep fetal gasping causes the aspiration of the meconium-mixed amniotic fluid into the lungs.

B. **Radiographs.** Thick infiltrates, air entrapment, pneumothorax.

C. **Preventive management. Although traditional, suctioning the nose and oropharynx at the perineum and intubation/suctioning after delivery have been shown to confer no benefit and may cause lower Apgar scores** (see Vain et al., 2004; Wiswell et al., 2000). However, this remains a widespread practice.

D. **Treatment. Management is complex, and a neonatologist should be consulted.** Treatment requires pulmonary support, as well as management of asphyxia-related effects on CNS and cardiovascular, renal, and GI systems. High-frequency ventilation, nitric oxide, and ECMO are being used with good results. Small studies suggest that surfactant may also be helpful.

IV. Spontaneous Pneumothorax.

A. **Spontaneous pneumothorax occurs in 1% to 2% of live births. It is symptomatic only in 1/1500 live births.**

B. **Symptoms include** tachypnea, minimal retractions, grunting, nasal flaring, cyanosis. May notice diminished air entry on affected side, shifting of cardiac impulse, muffled heart tones.

C. **Radiographs.** Pneumothorax seen on radiograph.

D. **Treatment.** Supportive; spontaneous resolution is common. Consider 100% oxygen therapy for 8 to 12 hours (only in full-term infants in whom retinopathy of prematurity will not be a problem). If not resolving, consider chest tube or pneumocentesis with a needle.

V. Bradycardia and Apnea Spells.

A. **Types. Bradycardia may be a primary cardiac event. The following refers only to noncardiogenic bradycardia and apnea spells.**

Neonates normally have 3-second pauses in respiratory effort (periodic breathing).

1. **Central.** No respiratory effort for 15 seconds because of arrest of respiratory drive. May have secondary bradycardia. May be secondary to CNS disorder.
2. **Obstructive.** Cessation of gas exchange in the lungs because of obstruction to air flow. May be infectious, functional (poor tone or coordination of pharyngeal muscles), or structural (e.g., tracheomalacia).

B. **Causes.** Prematurity, hypoxia, idiopathic, anatomic abnormalities (choanal atresia), maternal drugs (especially narcotics), infections, metabolic imbalances, temperature instability, seizures, hematologic, cardiovascular, genetic, and CNS disorders. GE reflux, trouble coordinating swallow, and palate malformations can all contribute to apnea. In the older child, consider breath-holding spells.

C. **Clinical characteristics, work-up, and treatment.**

1. **Document the duration, frequency,** state of consciousness; temporal relationship to feeding, sleep, stooling; seizure activity as well as obstetric history (such as maternal fever, meconium). Gestational age is especially important. Apnea and bradycardia from prematurity usually resolve by a corrected gestational age of 35 to 36 weeks.
2. **Physical exam** should include temperature, BP, gestational age, eye position (as an indication of a CNS disorder), pupillary dilation, muscle tone, dysmorphic features, respiratory effort, murmur, skin changes.
3. **Lab tests.** Blood glucose, electrolytes, differential CBC, drug levels, TSH, T_4, sepsis work-up, CXR, ABGs, head US (for CNS bleed), EEG.

D. **Treatment.**

1. **Apnea monitor and address underlying factors.** Teach CPR to parents and caregivers. Any individual spell generally resolves with stimulation.
2. **Ventilatory support.** Consider low-flow O_2, 4 to 6 cm of CPAP.
3. **For neonatal apnea.** Caffeine citrate 20 mg/kg PO or IV (contains 10 mg caffeine and 10 mg citrate) followed by 5 to 7 mg/kg qd, started 24 hours after first dose. Maintain serum caffeine levels at 5 to 25 mg/mL. Theophylline has also been used, but caffeine is preferred. Continue treatment for 5 to 7 days. Observe in hospital off treatment for 5 to 7 days. If the patient has no further episodes of neonatal apnea, he or she may be discharged with an apnea monitor if appropriate.

NEONATAL INFECTIONS

I. **Thrush.** Oral candidiasis; peaks at 14 days of life.
A. **Clinically.** White plaques on erythematous base over oral mucosa, tongue.
B. **Treatment.** Nystatin suspension 100,000 U/mL, 1 to 2 mL swabbed over affected areas qid × 7 d, or 1 mL PO qid × 7 d. Mycostatin cream to maternal areola and nipple if breastfed infant. Continue for 2 to 3 days after visual evidence of *Candida* infection resolves.

II. Neonatal Bacterial Sepsis.

A. General comments. Neonatal bacterial sepsis is associated with 10% to 40% mortality rate and significant morbidity, especially neurologic sequelae of meningitis. Infants <1 month of age are immunologically deficient and are predisposed to serious infections.

B. Predisposing factors. Prolonged rupture of membranes (>18 hours), premature labor, premature delivery <35 weeks, maternal fever, UTI, foul lochia, chorioamnionitis, IV catheters (in infant), intrapartum asphyxia, and intrauterine monitoring (pressure catheter or scalp electrode). Also, maternal group B streptococci (GBS) colonization, a mother who is GBS positive and has received less than two doses of intrapartum antibiotics, and maternal history of a previous child with invasive GBS disease are all risk factors for sepsis in the infant.

C. Organisms.

1. **Early infection (0-4 days of age).** GBS and *Escherichia coli* account for 60% to 70% of infections. Also *Listeria* (rare in United States), *Klebsiella, Enterococcus, Staphylococcus aureus* (uncommon), *Streptococcus pneumoniae*, group A streptococci.

2. **Late infection (5 days of age or older).** *S. aureus*, GBS, *E. coli, Klebsiella, Pseudomonas, Serratia, Staphylococcus epidermidis, Haemophilus influenzae.*

D. Signs and symptoms. Presentation may be subtle; thus, any febrile neonate (temp >38°C) must have a septic work-up. Fever may be absent, so watch for following symptoms.

1. **The presentation may include** irritability, vomiting, poor feeding, poor temperature control, lethargy, apneic spells, and hypoglycemia.

2. **May progress to** respiratory distress, poor perfusion, abdominal distention, jaundice, bleeding, petechiae, or seizures.

3. **Bulging fontanel is a very late sign of neonatal meningitis, and Brudzinski's sign or Kernig's sign is rarely found.**

E. Work-up.

1. **Includes LP** for cell count, protein, glucose, and culture. Consider sending CSF for viral studies.

2. UA, CBC (remember neutropenia or thrombocytopenia are also suggestive of infection) and repeat in 5 hours; CXR and C-reactive protein.

3. **Cultures** of blood, catheterized urine (or suprapubic tap), and any other site as indicated. Latex agglutination test for pneumococcus, *E. coli, H. influenzae*, GBS, and meningococci in blood, urine, and CSF is done even though the usefulness is questionable. **Negative latex agglutination tests do not rule out infection, but positive results may help guide therapy.**

F. Associated lab findings. Hypocalcemia, hypoglycemia, hyponatremia, and DIC.

G. Treatment.

1. Should be tailored to age of onset, clinical setting, and initial findings.

2. **There should be NO DELAY in antibiotic therapy.** Begin empiric therapy after cultures are obtained or before cultures if any delay is anticipated. There are isolates of *S. pneumoniae* that are resistant to penicillin and cephalosporins. **Add vancomycin with or without rifampin to these regimens until sensitivities are known when pneumococcal meningitis or pneumococcal sepsis is suspected.** Never use rifampin alone because resistance can rapidly develop.

3. **Empiric early (0-4 days of age).** Ampicillin 50 mg/kg per day (100 mg/kg per day in meningitis) divided q12h IV and gentamicin 5 mg/kg per day divided q12h IV. Or cefotaxime 50 mg/kg q12h plus ampicillin as above (preferred by some authors). Ceftriaxone is an alternative to cefotaxime.

4. **Empiric late (5 days of age or older).** Depends on cause (e.g., MRSA outbreak requires vancomycin). General guidelines include ampicillin 100 to 200 mg/kg per day divided q6h plus cefotaxime 150 mg/kg per day IV q8h, or ampicillin-gentamicin as above. Ceftriaxone 100 mg/kg per day IV q12h is an alternative to cefotaxime.

5. **Repeat cultures in 24 to 48 hours.** In meningitis, repeat LP every day until clear.

6. **Other.** Hemodynamic, respiratory, hematologic, metabolic, and nutritional support and surveillance are critical. Shock may require volume expansion; respiratory depression may require supplemental oxygen or artificial ventilation (see Chapter 2, Emergency Medicine).

CONGENITAL INFECTIONS

I. **Maternal Diagnostic Screening.**

A. Screen early for antibody to rubella, syphilis, and hepatitis B.

B. **Offer HIV testing to all pregnant women.** Perform serologic tests as indicated for HSV, CMV, HIV. Obtain viral cultures as indicated for HSV, rubella, CMV, enterovirus.

II. **Congenital Infections.** Congenital infections should be suspected in those infants who are premature or have IUGR, failure to thrive, hepatomegaly (elevated direct bilirubin), lethargy, thrombocytopenia, anemia, rashes, or seizures. See specific entities, later.

III. **Laboratory Studies for Suspected Congenital Infections.**

A. **TORCHS** titers on baby and mother (draw serum before any blood transfusion if possible). See below for discussion of specific entities.

B. **Obtain IgM antibodies from baby as well as acute and convalescent IgG titers from baby and mother. IgM does not cross the placenta and therefore indicates a reaction of the infant to infection.**

C. **Viral cultures** (HSV, rubella, CMV, enterovirus). Culture or PCR of CSF may be useful in HSV.

PEDIATRICS 12

D. Tzanck smear of vesicles in HSV (infant or mother).

E. Urine cytology and culture for CMV.

F. Dark-field exam of lesions or umbilical cord scraping in syphilis.

G. Send placenta to pathology lab for culture and microscopy.

H. General screening labs including LFTs, electrolytes, glucose, CBC, and clotting studies.

IV. Specific Agents.

A. Toxoplasmosis.

1. **Epidemiology.** Caused by *Toxoplasma gondii*. Fetus is infected by transplacental passage during maternal parasitemia. Infection occurs through ingestion of sporulated oocysts in cat feces or ingestion of poorly cooked meat. Fifty percent of the infants born to mothers who seroconvert during pregnancy will become infected. The later in pregnancy maternal infection occurs, the more likely transmission to the fetus will occur (first trimester, 17%; second trimester, 25%; and third trimester, 65% transmission). However, infections transmitted earlier in gestation are more likely to cause severe fetal effects (abortion, stillbirth, or severe disease with teratogenesis). Those transmitted later are more apt to be subclinical.

2. **Postnatal diagnosis.** Isolation of organism from placenta. ELISA detects specific IgG and IgM; comparison with mother's serum is necessary because maternal IgG will cross the placenta. PCR can also be used to make the diagnosis. **Use caution in interpreting IgM tests. There is a wide variability in the validity of the findings. A reference lab should be used to confirm a positive IgM result. Contact the FDA (301-594-3060) for details.**

3. **Clinical findings.**

   a. **Only 10% are symptomatic. Most of those who acquire *Toxoplasma* in utero are asymptomatic.**

   b. Maculopapular rash, generalized lymphadenopathy, hepatosplenomegaly, thrombocytopenia, signs of active CNS infection (e.g., CSF pleocytosis, CSF hypoglycemia, elevated CSF protein, and, in some instances, microcephaly, cerebral calcifications, seizures, and motor abnormalities), chorioretinitis, and pneumonitis. Infants with untreated congenital toxoplasmosis and generalized or neurologic abnormalities at presentation almost uniformly develop mental retardation, seizures, and spasticity.

4. **Prevention and treatment.**

   a. Avoid changing cat litter and eating raw and poorly cooked meat during pregnancy.

   b. It is not likely that prenatal treatment of the **mother** prevents adverse fetal outcomes, although this is still a matter of debate. However, some physicians choose to treat the mother prenatally with spiramycin (available from the FDA). If documented **fetal infection** is noted in the **prenatal** period (by amniotic PCR), consider treatment with pyrimethamine and sulfadiazine.

c. **Treat infant for clinically, serologically, or maternally apparent disease** with pyrimethamine and sulfadiazine for 1 year. Folinic acid should be given to prevent bone marrow suppression. A year of treatment allows the infant to become immunocompetent and will reduce neurologic sequelae compared with a shorter course of treatment. A pediatric infectious disease consultation should be obtained.

d. **Corticosteroid for ocular disease and CNS infection** (high level of CSF protein): Add prednisone 1.5 mg/kg per day PO divided q12h until CSF protein is normal and/or ocular inflammation resolves.

B. Cytomegalovirus.

1. Epidemiology.

a. **Most common congenital infection** (up to 2.5% incidence), with 95% asymptomatic.

b. Vertical transmission (from maternal primary or reactivated disease) may occur transplacentally or at birth in the genital tract. CMV may also be acquired postnatally by ingestion of CMV-positive breast milk. Infected infants are contagious.

2. Clinical findings.

a. Sensorineural deafness, mental retardation.

b. Cytomegalic inclusion disease, with jaundice, hepatosplenomegaly, petechial-purpuric rash, microcephaly, and cerebral calcifications.

3. Diagnostic tests. Virus isolated from urine, pharynx, WBC, CSF, human milk, cervical secretions. CMV IgM titers can be obtained. PCR has been used to detect virus as well.

4. Treatment. Evidence suggests that ganciclovir given postnatally may reduce incidence of retardation and other sequelae (but efficacy limited). Consider a pediatric infectious disease or neurology consultation.

C. Herpes simplex.

1. Epidemiology. Most HSV type 2 transmission occurs at birth through direct contact with open lesions (5% transmission in recurrent lesions, 50% in primary). Probably 20% or more of women have had HSV-2 and carry the virus. Many women are asymptomatic shedders at the time of delivery, and these patients account for most neonatal infections.

2. Clinical findings.

a. Average incubation 6 days; can be up to 20 days.

b. Disseminated disease may mimic fulminant sepsis with seizures, jaundice, hepatitis, encephalitis, DIC, or pneumonia. If untreated, up to 90% mortality rate.

c. Local mucocutaneous disease may be mild. Conjunctivitis, keratitis, or chorioretinitis can result in vision loss and blindness.

3. Prevention and treatment.

a. **Any active lesions during pregnancy should be cultured to confirm disease. Active disease at delivery mandates C-section.** Routine use of PCR to identify asymptomatic shedders is not yet standard of care.

b. **Recurrent maternal HSV. If vaginal delivery occurs over active lesions *or* membranes ruptured for >4 hours in a mother with a known**

12

PEDIATRICS

reactivation of HSV (even if membranes ruptured for >4 hours before C-section), the infection rate to the neonate is 1% to 3%.** Consider surface screening cultures from infant nose and rectum in 24 to 48 hours, and educate the parents about the signs and symptoms of early herpes infection. Treat if symptoms develop or the culture is positive.

c. **Primary maternal HSV. If vaginal delivery occurs over active lesions *or* membranes ruptured for >4 hours in a mother with primary HSV (e.g., the first outbreak ever), then the risk to the infant is 40%; therefore, you should treat empirically with acyclovir** 20 mg/kg per dose IV q8h × 14 d after cultures and CSF for PCR have been obtained. If the infant is symptomatic or has skin lesions after birth, surface cultures and CSF for PCR should be obtained, and the infant should be treated with acyclovir 20 mg/kg per dose × 14 d. Infected mother and infant should be kept in contact isolation.

D. Rubella.

1. **Epidemiology.** Nonvaccinated or rubella-susceptible mother acquires infection while pregnant. Teratogenicity is the greatest in the first trimester, less in second, none in third. Infants may be contagious.

2. **Presentation.** Retinopathy, cataracts, patent ductus arteriosus, pulmonary artery stenosis, deafness, thrombocytopenia with "blueberry-muffin" skin lesions.

3. **Treatment.** Supportive only. Immunize children and nonpregnant women of childbearing age. Immune globulin given to mother does not prevent prenatal infection.

E. Parvovirus B19 (fifth disease/erythema infectiosum).

1. **Epidemiology.** Transmission from mother infected during pregnancy occurs in one fourth to one third of cases. The second-trimester fetus is particularly vulnerable.

2. **Presentation.** Hemolytic anemia or aplastic anemia with hydrops secondary to high-output CHF or myocarditis. Generally, if the pregnancy continues to term, the resulting infant is healthy.

3. **Treatment.** Weekly US of mother after documented infection looking for evidence of hydrops for 10 to 12 weeks. Intrauterine transfusions have been used with success.

4. **Prevention.** Because most pregnant women have had inapparent infection and because of the low risk to the fetus, routine exclusion from schools, day care, etc., is not recommended for pregnant women. In addition, individuals who manifest symptoms are no longer infectious.

F. Syphilis.

1. **Epidemiology.** High probability that infected mother will transmit the disease. Treponemes cross placenta in all trimesters.

2. **Presentation.**

a. Fifty percent are asymptomatic. Clinical picture can be benign to fatal.

b. Findings include SGA, jaundice, recurring rashes, anemia, hepatosplenomegaly, "snuffles" (a serous rhinitis), meningitis, condylomata lata, and osteochondritis, usually of humerus or tibia.

3. **Diagnosis and treatment.**

a. **Suspect strongly in** infants of mothers who are seropositive and are untreated or inadequately treated; had no decrease in antibody titers after treatment; had poor follow-up during pregnancy; were treated with a nonpenicillin regimen, such as erythromycin; and were treated <1 month before delivery.

b. **Evaluate with** physical exam, VDRL, RPR, FTA-ABS, CSF analysis, dark-field microscopy of fluids of vesicular lesions or of condylomata lata, long bone radiographs.

c. **Treat if** there is a fourfold greater titer of antibody in the infant than in the mother, abnormal CSF (reactive VDRL, cells in the CSF, elevated CSF protein), evidence of active disease by exam (e.g., rash) or radiologic evidence of disease.

d. **Treatment.** Procaine penicillin G 50,000 U/kg IM qd × 14 d or aqueous penicillin G 50,000 U/kg IV q8-12h × 14 d.

e. **Follow-up titers.** Measure at 1, 2, 3, 6, and 12 months to ensure that they are falling. Titer should revert to negative at 6 months. HIV testing should be considered.

G. **HIV.** See section on treatment of newborn, and Chapter 11.

H. **Enterovirus.**

1. **Characteristics.** Enteroviruses (coxsackievirus, hepatitis A virus, echovirus, and poliovirus) are prevalent during warmer months and are transmitted to the fetus transplacentally or during the postpartum period.

2. **Treatment.** Supportive measures for enterovirus infection. Hepatitis A immunoglobulin 0.5 mL should be given at birth if appropriate.

I. **Gonorrhea and chlamydia.**

1. **Prevention.** Diagnosis and treatment of maternal gonococcal and chlamydial infections will prevent most neonatal infections. Both infections are transmitted intrapartum by direct contact. Culture the mother's endocervix initially and at 36 weeks if indicated.

2. **Clinical findings.** Both can cause conjunctivitis at 2 to 12 days. Obtain chlamydial, viral, and bacterial cultures of any purulent conjunctival discharge with Gram stain and Giemsa stain of conjunctival scraping for *Chlamydia*. For documented disease, obtain blood and CSF cultures and treat for systemic disease.

3. **Disseminated *gonorrhea* typically involves arthritis and meningitis.** Treat all **asymptomatic** infants of culture-positive mothers with a single dose of ceftriaxone 50 mg/kg IM (maximum, 125 mg). If **symptomatic** and evidence of disease or positive culture of blood or CSF, then ceftriaxone 25 to 50 mg/kg per day IV or IM qd × 7 to 10 d (100 mg/kg per day divided bid × 10-14 d for meningitis).

4. ***Chlamydia* may produce pneumonia at about 3 weeks with the insidious onset of tachypnea, cough, and no fever.** Conjunctivitis is often present but may be absent. Interstitial infiltrate and hyperinflation may be present on CXR. Diagnose chlamydia with nasopharyngeal culture or seropositivity. Topical treatment has minimal efficacy even for

isolated conjunctival disease because of colonization of other sites. Treat with PO or IV erythromycin 50 mg/kg per day divided q6h × 2 to 3 wk. Trials with azithromycin are currently underway.

NEONATAL HEMATOLOGIC DISORDERS

I. **Polycythemia.** Hyperviscous blood from increased Hct, which can cause stasis resulting in venous congestion or thrombosis. Increased incidence with IUGR, Down syndrome and other chromosomal abnormalities, congenital hypothyroidism or congenital adrenal hyperplasia, maternal diabetes, and maternal smoking. May also be a response to chronic in utero hypoxia with secondary increase in RBC mass. Finally, it may be caused by increased blood volume from cord milking or twin-to-twin transfusion.

A. **Clinical diagnosis.** Usually presents by 2 to 72 hours with plethora, acrocyanosis, poor peripheral perfusion, respiratory distress, or irritability. May be confused with cyanotic congenital heart disease, hypoglycemia, seizures.

B. **Lab diagnosis. Venous** Hct >65% (capillary Hct is usually 4%-7% higher); thrombocytopenia may occur.

C. **Complications.** Majority do well; stroke is the most common lasting complication, but there can be CHF, oliguria, gangrene, or necrotizing enterocolitis.

D. **Treatment.**

1. **If Hct 65% to 70% and asymptomatic:** Observation is an option but consider fluid therapy. Repeat a venous Hct q6h until the level is falling, generally by 24 hours.

2. **If Hct >70% or symptomatic:** Do partial exchange transfusion through umbilical vein using FFP or 5% albumin in saline.

Volume of exchange = ([observed Hct − desired Hct] × [0.9] × [weight in kg])/observed Hct

3. **Do not merely phlebotomize!** This can cause shock and worsen the situation. Watch for hypoglycemia or hypocalcemia.

NEONATAL METABOLIC DISORDERS

I. **Hypoglycemia is defined as** serum glucose <40 mg/dL at term, or <30 mg/dL in a premature infant. Use a level of 40 mg/dL to begin looking for cause and treating in all patients.

A. **Causes.** Neonatal gluconeogenesis is underdeveloped and easily disrupted. Be aware of hypoglycemia in SGA and postdate infants, and in infants with a history of asphyxia, hypothermia, sepsis, prematurity, hypermetabolism (e.g., erythroblastosis), if mother is diabetic (hyperinsulinism), or if there was maternal ingestion of oral hypoglycemics or of β-agonists. May also be secondary to sepsis.

B. Diagnosis. Have a high index of suspicion. Clinical signs: pale, cool, irritable, jittery, poor feeding, apnea, seizures; or may be asymptomatic. Routinely screen as described in the newborn nursery section, earlier, and recheck if any clinical suspicion of hypoglycemia.

C. Treatment should be given for 48 hours before tapering with frequent monitoring as follows:

1. **Stable,** age ≥34 weeks, and blood glucose >30 mg/dL: 15 to 30 mL D_5W PO or IV and then advance to breastfeeding or formula. Check glucose q2-3h until three normal readings.

2. **Unstable, or age <34 weeks,** or blood glucose <30 mg/dL: $D_{10}W$ 2 mL/kg × 10 min and then 2 to 4 mL/kg per hour IV. Consider adding ¼ normal saline to avoid electrolyte abnormalities. Advance to PO while continuing IV, follow serial glucose level and taper off IV. Remember that the highest concentration of glucose that can be infused in a peripheral catheter is 12.5%. If a more concentrated solution is required, a central catheter will have to be placed. An umbilical venous catheter can be used in an emergency.

3. **If no IV access attainable, glucagon** 0.1 mg/kg IM/SQ/IV (up to 1 mg) q30min will raise glucose for 2 to 3 hours but **depletes glycogen stores and is not effective when stores are not present (e.g., SGA).** NG feeding is another option.

II. Hypocalcemia. Serum calcium ≤8 mg/dL; it is usually associated with asphyxia, SGA, premature infant, or diabetic mother. Hypocalcemia is usually transient.

A. Diagnosis. Hypotonia, apnea, poor feeding, jitters, seizures, serum calcium <8 mg/dL.

B. Treatment. Usually resolves in a few days; no need to treat asymptomatic infant.

1. **If asymptomatic and wish to treat.** Give 5 to 10 mL/kg per day of 10% solution of calcium gluconate either PO in feedings or by continuous IV over 24 hours.

2. **If symptomatic.** Give 1.0 to 1.5 mL/kg of calcium gluconate 10% IV with a maximum of 5 mL in premature infants or 10 mL in a full-term infant. Should get a maximum of 1 mL/min. Can repeat if still symptomatic and then initiate treatment as in (1), above.

3. **Consider low magnesium level or congenital hypoparathyroidism if persistent.**

III. Neonatal Withdrawal Syndrome. Passive addiction to drugs by maternal use. Estimated incidence of 10% of urban births. Narcotics, and stimulants (such as cocaine) most common. These infants have an increased risk of sudden infant death syndrome (SIDS).

A. Diagnosis.

1. **Narcotics.** Jittery, irritable, large appetite, vomiting, hypertonicity, and sneezing. Usually presents within first 72 hours of life.

2. **Cocaine.** Lethargy, hypotonia, and poor feeding. Look for IUGR and cerebral infarctions. Usually presents within the first 72 hours.

12

PEDIATRICS

3. **Methadone.** Poor feeding, seizures, irritability. Presents at 2 to 4 weeks of life because of the long half-life of methadone.
B. **Treatment.** For all, swaddling and frequent high-caloric feedings are helpful. Neonatal Narcotic Abstinence Scales are available. These scales provide an objective system that helps you determine when pharmacologic treatment is necessary. For narcotics, use tincture of opium (10 mg/mL morphine) diluted 1:25 in water, 2 drops/kg q4-6h to control symptoms; monitor closely. Alternatively, may use phenobarbital 5 mg/kg per day divided q8h or q12h IV, IM, or PO. Taper either regimen gradually over 1 to 3 weeks.

NEONATAL GASTROINTESTINAL DISORDERS

I. **Vomiting and Regurgitation.** See section on vomiting, diarrhea, and dehydration later in chapter for additional discussion.
A. **General comments. Regurgitation of the first few feedings is common. Eighty percent infants <3 months of age regurgitate formula at least once a day;** this is not an indication for medications or a change in formula if the child is gaining weight appropriately. Bilious vomiting usually represents a surgical cause of obstruction.
B. **Cause.**
1. **Nonbilious.** Benign overfeeding, gastroenteritis, reflux, necrotizing enterocolitis, CNS lesion with increased ICP, pyloric stenosis, metabolic or electrolyte disorders, drugs, sepsis, other entities discussed elsewhere.
2. **Bilious.** Malrotation with or without a volvulus, atresia, stenosis, or other congenial anomalies.
C. **Evaluation.**
1. **History.** In infants, need to determine how much is being fed (overfeeding), relation to position (reflux), choking or coughing with feeding (achalasia, tracheoesophageal fistula), timing of emesis in relationship to feeds.
2. **Exam and lab tests.** Evaluate state of hydration (see section on dehydration, later). Look for site of infection. Perform abdominal and rectal exam for obstruction or imperforate anus. Obtain radiologic studies as indicated, including Gastrografin if indicated.
a. **If child <2 months of age, consider US for pyloric stenosis** if the history or exam is compelling. Gastrografin study is alternative.
b. **If neonatal,** consider congenital abnormalities such as duodenal or esophageal atresia, Hirschsprung's disease, volvulus, malformation.
c. **Reye's syndrome.** Generally occurs after viral illness and presents with intractable vomiting, elevated liver enzymes, decreased mental status, prolonged PT, and elevated serum ammonia. See section on vomiting, later.
d. Consider elevated ICP as a cause of isolated vomiting.

3. **Treatment.** See dehydration section. Also consider antiemetics such as prochlorperazine or trimethobenzamide if cause is benign. If there is bilious vomiting, consider a surgical emergency. Make infant NPO, place an NG tube to suction, obtain abdominal films, and consult pediatric surgery.

II. Meconium Plug Syndrome.

A. General comments. Obstruction of the colon with meconium or mucus. More common in premature, infants of diabetic mothers, and those with acute illness. Can be early presentation of CF or Hirschsprung's disease.

B. Signs and symptoms. Difficulty passing stools, normal results on rectal exam.

C. Management. Rectal stimulation with digital exam or glycerin suppository. See constipation section.

III. Necrotizing Enterocolitis.

A. Causes. Unclear, more common in premature infants (80%), SGA, maternal preeclampsia, cyanosis, exchange transfusions, umbilical catheterization, polycythemia. Precipitated by enteral feeding, ischemia, and bacteria.

B. Prognosis. Mortality rate of 20% to 40%.

C. Signs and symptoms. Baby has abdominal distention, lethargy, bloody stools, ileus, vomiting. It can progress to DIC, apnea, shock, perforation. Onset may be gradual or fulminant.

D. Diagnosis. Abdominal radiograph shows distended loops of bowel, air–fluid levels, pneumatosis intestinalis, free air. Requires full sepsis work-up, including stool and CSF cultures, CBC, electrolytes, and enzymes. Also obtain INR/PTT, ABG, etc.

E. Treatment. Surgical consult mandatory.

1. NPO, nasogastric tube to suction, IV fluids.
2. Supportive treatment of acidosis, shock.
3. Surgery indicated if perforation, peritonitis, acidosis.
4. Begin broad-spectrum antibiotics (e.g., ampicillin and gentamicin) after cultures done. If resistant organisms known in hospital, cover with other antibiotics as required. Add anaerobic coverage (clindamycin or metronidazole) if perforation is suspected.

FEEDING AND SUPPLEMENTATIONS

I. Breastfeeding.

A. Breastfeeding should be recommended to all pregnant and postpartum mothers (except those who are HIV positive) and should provide adequate nutrition for the first 5 to 9 months. Human colostrum immediately after delivery is the optimal first feeding. Normal, term babies are born fully hydrated, and supplementation of the first breastfeeding is not required.

B. Information and encouragement must be provided. References, such as those to the local chapter of La Leche League, may prove valuable.

C. **Feeding on demand should be encouraged,** with recognition that there is a large variety in normal feeding patterns. Typically, infant feeding intervals average every 2 to 3 hours in the first few weeks. Newborns should not go longer than 4 to 5 hours between feedings.

D. **The supply of breast milk is adequate if the infant is satisfied after each nursing period, has six to eight wet diapers a day, sleeps 2- to 4-hour intervals, and gains weight according to the growth chart.**

E. **Attention to sore nipples should be provided early** before severe pain with cracking and abrasions occur. Exposing nipples to air and varying the infant feeding position are recommended; avoid drying soaps. Check the infant for thrush and treat both mother's nipples and infant if present.

F. **Engorgement can be very uncomfortable for the mother.** The mother should be encouraged to nurse or pump often, every 2 to 3 hours. If engorgement is severe, it can cause difficulty with the infant latching on. In this case, recommend manual expression before feeding.

G. **Maternal fatigue and psychosocial factors should be addressed.** Mothers should be encouraged to sleep when their infant sleeps.

H. **Mastitis.** Mastitis is an infection of the breast usually secondary to a blocked milk duct.

1. **Exam.** Reveals a hot, swollen, tender, and erythematous breast; mastitis is most commonly secondary to *S. aureus*.

a. **Treatment is by use of antistaphylococcal antibiotics** such as dicloxacillin, amoxicillin–clavulanate, cephalexin, or clindamycin. If there is MRSA in the community, consider doxycycline, TMP–SMX for outpatients, or vancomycin for inpatients. Mastitis can usually be treated in an outpatient setting; however, if patient is febrile or looks ill, consider admission for IV antibiotics.

b. **The mother should continue to breastfeed or use a breast pump. This is critical and will help resolve the infection.**

c. Local care, including hot packs, may be helpful.

I. **Drugs and breast milk.** Drugs concentrated in breast milk tend to be weak bases (e.g., metronidazole, antihistamines, erythromycin, or antipsychotics and antidepressants). Check the breastfeeding recommendations of every drug before approving its use in the nursing mother.

J. **Failure to thrive in the breastfed infant.**

1. Infant causes include inadequate intake or increased caloric need.

2. Maternal causes include poor milk production because of inadequate diet (especially fluids), illness and fatigue, or poor letdown because of smoking, drugs, or psychological reasons.

II. **Formula Feeding.**

A. There is *no* causal link between the early introduction of cow's milk and the development of diabetes.

B. In cases of preference or inability to breastfeed, commercial infant formulas can provide adequate nutrition. Most are cow's milk based and contain lactose. Lactose-free, soybean-based formulas are available for infants with primary lactase deficiency (watery, guaiac-negative stools, gas), galactosemia, secondary lactase deficiency from GI insult (e.g., from viral gastroenteritis), and cow's milk protein allergy (generally have diarrhea with blood and failure to thrive). However, remember that some children who are allergic to cow's milk protein will also be allergic to soy protein.

C. Most formulas contain 20 kcal/oz, osmolality of 300 to 400 mOsm, and calorie breakdown of 7.2% to 18% protein, 30% to 54% fat, and 40% to 50% carbohydrate.

D. An on-demand schedule of feeding should be encouraged. Most newborns will typically take 2 to 3 ounces every 2 to 3 hours and should not be allowed to go greater than 5 hours between feedings. It is important to inform the parents to avoid overfeeding by being aware of satiety clues from the infant.

E. Reflux and occasional diarrhea are not in themselves indications for switching formula and do not support the diagnosis of formula allergy.

III. Dietary Advancement.

A. Solids may begin to be added between 4 and 6 months of age, typically when the infant's hunger is no longer satisfied by milk alone or it is convenient in the family's schedule. Infants should have considerable head control before any solid foods are introduced.

1. New foods should generally be introduced at the rate of one new food every 5 to 7 days. In this manner, if an infant has an allergic reaction to a food it will be easier to identify which food is the culprit.

2. Generally, cereal is started first, followed by fruits and vegetables and then meats. Infants typically show an interest in self-feeding at 6 to 8 months of age. Zwieback toast and crackers are typically offered first for the self-feeder. A spoon can typically be introduced between 10 and 12 months. By the end of the second year of life, infants should not require feeding assistance.

3. **The introduction of cow's milk should be delayed until 12 months of age.** Cow's milk given as primary food source before 12 months of age is associated with an increased incidence of iron-deficiency anemia believed to be secondary to occult GI blood loss.

IV. Toddler Feeding. Toddlers typically eat three meals as well as one or two snacks a day. Many toddlers will resist eating certain foods or insist on eating one or two favorite foods for long periods of time. It is advisable to avoid struggles and offer a variety of foods, leaving the choices to the child. Vitamin supplements are rarely necessary. Toddlers typically have varying appetites. They will eat well at some meals and hardly eat anything at other meals. This is to be expected.

V. Vitamin Supplementation.

A. Iron. *Note:* **Iron is toxic and should be stored out of the reach of infants and toddlers.**

1. Iron supplementation in breastfed infants is indicated for infants not receiving formula supplementation or iron-fortified cereal after 4 to 6 months of age.

2. Ferrous sulfate drops may be added at a dose of 1 to 2 mg of elemental iron/kg per day. An alternative is iron-fortified cereals, particularly when mixed with juice, because the vitamin C enhances iron absorption (two to three servings per day).

3. Premature infants should have supplementation with ferrous sulfate drops at a dose of 2 mg of elemental iron/kg per day at 2 months of age.

4. Bottle-fed infants should use an iron-fortified formula throughout the first year of life. Constipation should not be an indication to switch to a low-iron formula because there is no evidence that there is a causal relationship.

B. Vitamin D. Supplementation is currently recommended for all babies to prevent vitamin D deficiency and rickets. All babies should be getting 200 IU of vitamin D supplementation per day during the first 2 months of life. This can be stopped in formula-fed babies when they are taking at least 17 ounces of formula daily. Breastfed infants should continue to receive supplementation until they are weaned, and/or taking 17 ounces of infant formula or vitamin D–fortified milk daily.

C. Vitamin B$_{12}$. Be aware of vitamin B$_{12}$ deficiency in the children of strict vegetarian mothers.

D. Fluoride.

1. Dietary fluoride supplements are recommended by the American Academy of Pediatrics and American Dental Association for infants and young children without access to optimally fluoridated water. A dosage schedule based on age and water fluoride level has been recommended since 1979 **(Table 12-2).**

2. Although a new dosage schedule and guidelines have not been agreed on, there now is a general consensus that **breastfed infants in areas with fluoridated water usually do not need fluoride supplementation,** in part because very few infants are exclusively breastfed for extended periods.

PEDIATRIC WELLNESS

I. Immunizations. See Figure 24-10 for a schedule of recommended childhood immunizations. An updated schedule, along with a PDA version, can be obtained at **www.immunizationed.org.**

A. There is no link between standard childhood immunizations and autism or other neurologic or physical abnormalities!

TABLE 12-2
RECOMMENDED SUPPLEMENTAL FLUORIDE DOSAGE SCHEDULE

Age (y)	Fluoride Concentration in Water Supply		
	<0.3 ppm	0.3-0.7 ppm	>0.7 ppm
≤2*	0.25 mg	0 mg	0 mg
2-3	0.50 mg	0.25 mg	0 mg
3-13*	1.00 mg	0.50 mg	0 mg

*Recommended by the Council on Dental Therapeutics of the American Dental Association and the Committee on Nutrition of the American Academy of Pediatrics. The American Academy of Pediatrics recommends providing supplementation from 2 wk of age through at least 16 y of age.

B. **The measles–mumps–rubella (MMR) vaccine is safe in those with egg allergies and should not be withheld in this group.**

C. **Recommended vaccinations.** An afebrile URI is not a contraindication to vaccination. Antibody conversion rates are the same in this population as in the well population.

D. **If a patient misses a vaccination, start up where the patient left off.** *There is no need to restart the series!* For example, if a patient had a diphtheria–pertussis–tetanus (DPT) vaccine at 2 months but missed subsequent doses and shows up at 2 years of age, start at what would have been the fourth-month dose and continue the series from there. Therefore, the patient would get a 4th-month, 6th-month, 15th-month, and 4- to 6-year dose for a total of 5 doses by 6 years of age.

E. **Immunization side effects.**

1. **DPT vaccine.** Local reaction common, with erythema, tenderness, swelling. Mild systemic symptoms may occur, including low-grade fever, listlessness. Few children develop high fever. The relationship between DPT vaccine and neurologic symptoms has not been substantiated when cases are looked at critically. In any case, the acellular pertussis vaccine should allay any fears.

2. **MMR vaccine.** May have local reaction. Fever may occur and may be delayed, with onset between 5 and 7 days. A morbilliform rash may occur at the same time.

3. *H. influenzae* **vaccine.** Minimal reaction, including local reaction and low-grade fever.

4. **Poliomyelitis vaccine.** Adults may develop polio if given oral immunization, as may the immunosuppressed. For this reason, the IM (killed virus) polio vaccine is now recommended for all patients.

5. **Pneumococcal vaccine.** Local erythema, swelling, temperature up to 38.5°C (102°F).

II. **Growth and Development.**

A. **The caloric requirements for full-term infants** are 80 to 120 kcal/kg per day for the first few months of life and 100 kcal/kg per day to the 12th month of life. There is significant individual variation.

B. **The newborn infant can be expected to lose up to 10% to 15% of body weight in the neonatal period.** The birth weight should be regained by 10 to 14 days of life. The full-term infant generally doubles its birth weight by 4 months of age and triples it by 1 year.

C. **Fontanels and sutures.** Principal sutures should fuse by fifth to sixth month. Premature closure is termed *craniosynostosis* and may lead to neurologic abnormalities. Lateral fontanel closes by week 6 of life and posterior by 4 months of age. Anterior fontanel should start to shrink after 6 months of life and closes by 9 to 16 months.

D. **Sinuses.** Maxillary and ethmoid sinuses present at birth and enlarge during childhood. Sphenoid sinuses develop by 1 to 2 years and continue to enlarge during childhood, frontal sinuses by 2 to 6 years.

E. **See Figures 24-4 to 24-7 for growth charts.**

12
PEDIATRICS

III. Developmental Screening. See Table 24-4.

IV. Developmental Milestones. See Table 24-4.

V. Pediatrics: Failure to Thrive.

A. General comments. *Failure to thrive* is a general term used to describe a child who is failing to maintain growth above the third percentile for weight or height. Also suspect this in patients falling off their previously established growth curve. Typically, weight for height is the first parameter affected and later height and head circumference are affected. Psychosocial and parental factors are the most common causes, but many disease states can also prevent adequate growth. There are three major patterns of inadequate growth when one is comparing age to height, weight, and head circumference.

B. Decreased weight in proportion to height with a normal head circumference is the pattern most commonly seen. In the majority of these cases, there is inadequate caloric intake for social, economic, or physical reasons. Malabsorption and metabolic abnormalities can also be the cause.

C. A moderate decrease in weight compared to height with a normal or enlarged head circumference can signal a structural dystrophy, endocrine disorder, or other congenital reason for low weight and short stature.

D. Small head circumference with low weight for height may indicate a CNS defect or IUGR.

E. Evaluation.

1. **A thorough history and physical exam** focusing on diet, feedings, mother–child interaction, signs of neglect, signs of physical abuse, or obvious physical illness such as diarrhea or chronic infection; **a complete calorie count should be done to ensure adequate caloric intake.**

2. **Initial screening lab tests include** CBC, UA, electrolytes, sedimentation rate, serum glucose, stool for ova, parasites, and guaiac test. Depending on the clinical situation, serum lead levels, thyroid functions, and evaluation for adrenal disease may be important.

3. **The hallmark of evaluation is a period (1-2 weeks) under careful observation,** with appropriate physical stimulation and adequate caloric intake while growth parameters are being monitored. This typically requires hospitalization but may be accomplished elsewhere if close observation with objective data collection is possible. Usually this cannot be accomplished at home. To determine dietary need: **Caloric requirements = (120 kcal/kg [actual weight]/day) × (ideal weight/actual weight).** This is an approximation of calories required for catch-up growth. Consulting a dietitian may be helpful. An approach to evaluating a period of observation is found in **Table 12-3.**

SHORT STATURE

I. Definition. Subnormal height (usually less than third to fifth percentile) relative to other children of the same sex, age, and ethnicity. This contrasts with growth failure, which is a slow rate of growth regardless of stature.

TABLE 12-3

POSSIBLE APPROACHES FOR FAILURE TO THRIVE

Adequate Intake?	Weight Gain?	Most Likely Diagnoses	Treatment Plan
Yes	Yes	Feeding problem Neglect Inability to purchase food	Counseling and information Social services help
Yes	No	Malabsorption, CF, celiac sprue, parasitic infection, milk allergy	Stool: culture O&P, pH, reducing substances, 72-h stool fat, D-xylose test
		Hypermetabolic, chronic infection, malignancy, hyperthyroid	Thyroid function tests, CBC, ESR, CRP, LFTs
		Metabolic dysfunction, renal acidosis, hypercalcemia, diabetes, others such as inborn errors of metabolism	Serum pH, electrolytes, glucose, calcium, UA
No	No	Sucking or swallowing difficulties caused by neurologic disease, congenital anomaly	If nonorganic cause is definitely ruled out, begin to do further work-up and appropriate consultation
		Regurgitation: GI obstruction (e.g., pyloric stenosis), CSF pressure elevation, chronic metabolic disease	Neurologic work-up: head CT, consultation GI work-up: barium swallow, consultation Endocrine work-up: TSH, T_4, etc.

II. **Short Stature should be defined with parents' height being taken into account.** If the child is on the growth curve to reach projected height based on parents' heights, it is not considered short stature.

A. **For girls:** Approximate projected adult height = (mother's height + [father's height − 5 inches])/2.

B. **For boys:** Approximate projected adult height = ([mother's height + 5 inches] + father's height)/2.

III. **Causes.** May be a variation of normal (familial or constitutional); endocrine disorders including growth hormone deficiency, diabetes, and hypothyroidism; skeletal dysplasias; genetic syndromes including Turner's syndrome and Prader-Willi syndrome; malnutrition; chronic disease; lysosomal storage disorders; and psychosocial deprivation. Precocious puberty or elevated levels of androgens and estrogens will prematurely mature bones causing epiphyseal closure and short stature.

IV. **History.** Should include a family history (parental heights, relatives with short stature, genetic syndromes), perinatal insults, hypopituitarism, social and nutritional components. Review of systems should include respiratory and GI systems.

V. Physical Exam. Should include examination of sexual development, nutritional status, disproportionate body segments (seen in chondromalacias), and observation for stigmata of genetic syndromes.

VI. Laboratory Tests. Should be considered in those more than 3 standard deviations below the mean and whose history and physical exam do not reveal a cause. Consider CBC for evidence of anemia, inflammation, infection, malignancy, and bone marrow suppression; electrolytes, BUN, UA to assess renal status; ESR to screen for inflammatory bowel disease and other chronic inflammatory disorders; karyotype, particularly in girls to evaluate for Turner's syndrome; thyroid studies and calcium, phosphorus, and alkaline phosphatase to screen for rickets.

VII. Assess Growth Hormones. Draw insulin-like growth factor (IGF)-I and IGF-II and IGF-binding protein. Additional studies may include insulin infusion and induced hypoglycemia, which should lead to an increase in serum growth hormone if system is functioning properly. This test should generally be done under the supervision of an endocrinologist.

VIII. Hand and Wrist Radiographs to determine bone age. Delay is seen in hypopituitarism, constitutional delay, chronic disease, Turner's syndrome, and hypothyroidism. It may also be delayed in psychosocial dwarfism, gonadal dysgenesis, and primordial dwarfism. The bone age is normal in cases of familial short stature. Delayed bone age is hopeful because growth potential is still maintained and child may still reach normal adult stature with resolution of the underlying cause.

CRYING AND COLIC

I. General Comments. About one fifth of infants are described as having colic. This is described as inconsolable crying often accompanied by drawing up of the legs and gaseous distention of the abdomen. It may occur around the clock but more commonly occurs at a predictable time in the evening. Colic starts by 3 weeks of age, and the peak occurs by 6 weeks of age and may include about 3 hours of crying a day. The severity declines and by 3 months of age normal crying patterns are reestablished.

II. Contributing Factors. Contributing factors may include formula, aerophagia, too small a hole in a bottle nipple, various foods in the diet of the mother of breastfed infants.

III. Treatment.

A. After an exam to rule out other causes for irritability and crying (especially otitis, other infectious causes, intussusception, hairs around the penis, fingers, or toes, corneal abrasion, etc.), the parents should be advised on the anticipated course and management. The importance of never shaking a baby should be stressed. An alternative caregiver should be identified if the parents feel at the limit of their ability to cope. In addition, there is good evidence that behavioral interventions (beyond simple emotional support) can be of benefit (Wolke et al., 1994).

B. Rocking the child, cuddling, swaddling, taking child for a car ride, or using a child swing may be beneficial. Elimination of cruciferous vegetables and chocolate from a breastfeeding mother's diet may be helpful but has not been proven in a blinded study. Changing formulas to soybean milk or a hydrolyzed milk formula may help in some cases.

C. A well-done, blinded study showed that 2 mL of 12% sucrose/distilled water solution helped mitigate colic that did not respond to stimuli reduction, etc. Others have used a 30% solution. Sucrose causes endorphin release in the child and the analgesic effect of sucrose (and glucose) has been demonstrated in other studies as well (see Carbajal et al., 1999). Making the solution using Pedialyte or other rehydration solution ensures that the infant gets a proper electrolyte balance.

D. There is no evidence that simethicone works for infantile colic. Dicyclomine has some benefit but also many side effects.

SAFETY AND ACCIDENT PREVENTION

I. SIDS Prevention. SIDS is the leading cause of death in infants 1 to 12 months of age. To reduce risk, infants should be placed to sleep on their back or side on a firm surface with no pillows or other compressible objects in the bed. **Allowing the child to use a pacifier in bed also seems to reduce the incidence of SIDS.** This is especially true in children who sleep on their stomach (which should nonetheless be avoided). Avoiding smoking in the house may also be helpful. Sleeping in the same bed with an infant should be discouraged because it, too, can contribute to SIDS.

II. Table 12-4 shows age-specific safety recommendations.

INFECTIONS

Table 12-5 describes common childhood infectious diseases.

I. Approach to the Febrile Child. Fever may be a marker of sepsis, localized infection, occult bacteremia, or benign illness. **A note on the approach suggested below:** This is considered a prudent approach. However, many have questioned the need for such a stringent approach in the age of the pneumococcal vaccine. Specifically, there is no good cutoff of the WBC count that reliably differentiates septic/bacteremic patients from those who have a viral illness.

A. General considerations.

1. **Temperature should be taken rectally.** Axillary and tympanic temperatures are not adequate in the small child.

2. **The degree of elevation of the temperature does correlate with the likelihood of bacteremia, especially if >40°C. However, those with a low-grade fever can be septic, and those with high temperatures can have a benign course.**

TABLE 12-4

AGE-SPECIFIC SAFETY RECOMMENDATIONS

AGE	DEVELOPMENTAL RISK	SAFETY RECOMMENDATIONS
Prenatal/ newborn	Completely dependent, can squirm into position of suffocation or off a surface	Crib safety, car seat use, smoke detectors in home, water heater set to 120°F (50°C), SIDS prevention
4 months	Beginning to reach, roll over, take solids	Constant supervision in bathtub, prevention of ingestion and aspiration, caretaker need for choking first aid training, toy safety
6 months	Begin to crawl, pull to stand	Poison control number, walker dangers
12 months	Walking, stair and furniture climbing	Water safety including constant supervision in bathtub, poisoning prevention, continuation of car seat use
Toddler	Can learn to climb out of crib	Matches, electrical hazards, knives/kitchen hazards, fall precautions
Preschool	Increased initiative and desire to imitate adults can lead to more accidents	Traffic safety, matches/fire hazards, supervised play
School age	Increasing autonomy	Water safety, bicycle safety, fire and burn prevention
Preteen/teen		Drugs, alcohol, cigarettes, sports safety, safe sex practices, driving

3. **The response to antipyretics cannot be used as a guide to differentiate septic children from those with viral illnesses.** Responders to antipyretics may be septic, whereas those who do not respond may have a mild illness.

4. **In those older than 2 to 3 months of age, clinical appearance is the best indicator of severity of illness. Children younger than 2 to 3 months of age may not manifest signs of systemic illness.**

5. Even though they will look ill, children 3 months to 2 years of age may not manifest the "typical" localizing symptoms of their underlying illness (e.g., no meningeal signs with meningitis).

6. **Blood cultures are of limited usefulness in determining which patients should be treated because results are delayed 48 to 72 hours.** A single blood culture may miss up to 50% of bacteremic children, and if cultures are appropriate, two cultures should be done with the largest volume of blood possible (at least 6 mL total). In addition, most bacteremic children will clear the bacteremia spontaneously.

7. **Teething is related to fever,** but look for other sources in the ill-appearing child.

TABLE 12-5
COMMON PEDIATRIC INFECTIOUS DISEASES AND EXANTHEMS

Disease	Etiologic Agent	Incubation	Prodrome	Signs and Symptoms	Isolation	Treatments and Comments
Chickenpox (varicella)	Varicella	10-21 d	Minimal	Mixture of macules, papules, vesicles in all stages of development; spreads from trunk to extremities for 5-20 d	Until all lesions are crusted Infectious 2 d before appearance of lesions	Symptomatic or acyclovir*
Fifth disease (erythema infectiosum)	Parvovirus B19	6-14 d	None	Maculopapular rash on face with circumoral pallor (slapped cheek) and spreading to extremities; rash lasts a few days to a few weeks and is brought out by warmth Arthritis can develop, esp. in adults	Avoid pregnant women, otherwise not needed	Symptomatic
Herpangina	Coxsackievirus, herpesvirus	?	None	High fever, vomiting, ulcers of oral mucosa for 5-6 d	2-6 d	Symptomatic
Kawasaki's disease (mucocutaneous aneurysms, lymph node syndrome)	Probable infectious agent not yet discovered	?	Unknown	Fever, adenopathy, inflamed mucosa (pharyngitis, cracked lips, etc.), polymorphous maculosquamous rash, conjunctivitis	?	Can have cardiac involvement with artery aneurysms

(Continued)

TABLE 12-5
COMMON PEDIATRIC INFECTIOUS DISEASES AND EXANTHEMS—cont'd

Disease	Etiologic Agent	Incubation	Prodrome	Signs and Symptoms	Isolation	Treatments and Comments
Meningococcal meningitis	*Neisseria meningitidis*	1-7 d	URI, fever, headache, diarrhea	Most common younger than 1 y Meningitis; purpuric or petechial rash; septic arthritis	Until 24 h after first antibiotic dose	See meningitis in text
Mononucleosis	Epstein–Barr virus, CMV, toxoplasmosis, primary HIV	2-8 wk	None	Fatigue, anorexia, exudative tonsillitis, lymphadenopathy, splenomegaly Macular rash not unusual with amoxicillin use	Avoid saliva contact for 3 mo	See section on mononucleosis in Chapter 20
Roseola infantum (exanthema subitum)	Human herpesvirus types 6 and 7	1-15 d	3-4 d of sustained high fever, child generally-looks well	Fine pink rash begins at fever defervescence and lasts 2 d; seen from age 6 mo to 3 y	Unknown	Fever control, can have aseptic meningitis
Rubella, German measles, 3-day measles	Rubivirus	14-21 d	Lymphadenopathy, fever, headache, malaise	Maculopapular appears on face and rapidly spreads to trunk and proximal extremities; lasts 1-3 d; postauricular and suboccipital lymphadenopathy	Communicable discrete rash from 7 d before until 5 d after rash appears	Symptomatic

Rubeola (measles)	Rubeola virus	10-12 d	High fever, cough, coryza, conjunctivitis for 3 d	Koplik's spots appear 1 or 2 d before maculopapular rash; rash is confluent and spreads from hairline to face and then body; lasts 4-5 d	From fifth day of incubation to fifth day after rash appears	Symptomatic care of cough, coryza, conjunctivitis
Periodic fever, aphthous stomatitis, pharyngitis, adenopathy syndrome	Unknown			Recurrent fever, exudative tonsillitis, malaise, cervical adenopathy, 2/3 with aphthous stomatitis; patient looks well between episodes	Unknown	Prednisone 2 mg/kg × 1
Whooping cough (pertussis)	Bordetella pertussis	5-10 d; 21 d max.	1-3 wk of cough, coryza, and occasional emesis	Short paroxysmal cough ending with inspiratory "whoop"	5-10 d with treatment	Erythromycin; culture nasopharynx

*Some authors would treat the second and subsequent children in a family who develop chickenpox with acyclovir. The second and subsequent cases in a family tend to be more severe than the first case because of a higher initial viral load. Acyclovir reduces duration of illness by 24-48 h and must be started within the first 24 h of the illness to be effective. Adults and adolescents with chickenpox may be better candidates for acyclovir because they tend to have more consequences.
Adapted from Driscoll CE, Bope ET: *The Family Practice Desk Reference*, 3rd ed. St. Louis, Mosby, 1996.

PEDIATRICS 12

8. **Fever may be treated with acetaminophen** 15 mg/kg q4-6h or ibuprofen 10 mg/kg q6-8h, or both. Rectal acetaminophen must be dosed at 25 to 35 mg/kg q6h to achieve adequate serum levels. Acetaminophen and ibuprofen have comparable efficacy; acetaminophen is less toxic. Tepid bathing does not add much to the efficacy of these drugs. Sponging with alcohol may lead to toxicity and is never indicated. Aspirin should be avoided because of the risk of Reye's syndrome.

B. **History.** Should focus on the duration and height of the fever; associated symptoms such as vomiting and diarrhea, rash (especially petechiae), behavioral changes, and parental estimation of the degree of illness. Known exposures should be reviewed as well as an immunization and travel history.

C. **Physical exam.** Should begin with a careful consideration of the general appearance. Careful observation and analysis of the vital signs, state of hydration, and peripheral perfusion are required. Attention should be paid to tachypnea out of proportion to fever, which may indicate pneumonia. A complete exam should be performed, including a musculoskeletal exam for septic arthritis and osteomyelitis, neurologic exam, and skin exam. An oxygen saturation should be obtained in the ill-appearing child.

D. **Approach to the febrile child without an obvious source of infection varies with age:**

1. **For a child <8 weeks of age with any degree of fever greater than 38°C (100.4°F).**

a. **The exam and clinical signs and symptoms do not correlate well with seriousness of illness in these children and are unreliable indicators of severity of disease.** Three percent to 10% of febrile children in this age group will have a bacterial illness, usually transient bacteremia. This rate is reduced now that pneumococcal vaccine is being used.

b. **Any febrile child of this age without an identifiable focus of disease should have a complete septic work-up, including CBC, blood cultures, LP with CSF Gram stain, culture, glucose and cell count, UA, and C&S.** The WBC count is an insensitive indicator of bacterial illness but can be used to separate febrile children into high-risk and low-risk categories. Those with a WBC count of <5000/mm^3 or >15,000/mm^3 are in the high-risk group. Some authors suggest a CXR as well, but in a child without pulmonary or respiratory symptoms the yield is very low. However, 12% of those with isolated rhinorrhea will have a positive CXR.

c. **Decide if patient has a high risk or a low risk. A low-risk infant is considered:**

(1) Age 28 to 90 days and previously healthy.
(2) Nontoxic appearing.
(3) No apparent site of focal bacterial infection, except for otitis.
(4) Good social situation.
(5) WBC count of 5000 to 15,000 with a band count below 1500.
(6) Normal urinalysis with fewer than 5 WBCs/HPF.

(7) If diarrhea is present, there should be fewer than 5 WBCs/ HPF in the stool.

d. **Admit all patients who look toxic or ill or are <28 days of age and cover with ceftriaxone (50-75 mg/kg qd, not greater than 2 g) until cultures available.**

e. **Admit and treat patients with an identifiable illness requiring hospitalization** such as meningitis, pneumonia, or UTI (see specific sections for treatments).

f. **Admit all high-risk infants** (WBC count >15,000/mm^3 or <5000/mm^3, inability to follow up for social reasons, abnormal UA, WBCs in stool) even if no source evident, and treat as for sepsis with ceftriaxone while awaiting cultures.

g. **Patients who are at low risk (see c, above) and appear well can be treated as an outpatient** with ceftriaxone 50-75 mg/kg IM (not greater than 2 g) while awaiting culture results, and should be followed up in 24 hours. If cultures are positive, treat as appropriate. If cultures are negative and patient is afebrile and looks well, can follow up closely. If the child remains febrile, cover with ceftriaxone until cultures final.

2. **Children 3 months to 2 years of age.**

a. Many authors will treat children up to 3 months of age as above.

b. Four percent of febrile children in this age group will have occult bacteremia with *S. pneumoniae* or *H. influenzae*, though most of these children will clear the bacteremia spontaneously and have no sequelae.

c. **Those with a WBC count >15,000/mm^3 or <5000/mm^3 are at a higher risk of sepsis, but this should not be used as an absolute guide because children with any WBC count can be septic.**

d. **Non–toxic-appearing children with a temperature of <39°C may be observed** with lab testing addressed to the clinical picture.

e. **For those who are toxic appearing but with a temperature of <39°C,** a complete physical exam should be done and lab examination should be addressed to findings. Blood cultures should be done in those considered at high risk for sepsis (generally look ill). Do not forget a UA.

f. **Those with a temperature of >39°C should have** a CBC, blood culture, UA, and urine culture. LP should be done if indicated clinically. If WBC count >15,000/mm^3 or <5000/mm^3, cover with ceftriaxone 50 to 75 mg/kg IM (not greater than 2 g) and see patient back the next day.

II. **Bacterial Meningitis.** See Chapter 9 for CSF findings in various CNS infections.

A. **Bacterial meningitis must be suspected in any febrile child or any child with mental status changes.** Prompt diagnosis and treatment are paramount to successful outcome. Viral (or aseptic) meningitis is more common, seldom needs more than supportive care, and rarely causes significant sequelae. Antibiotics must be started within one-half hour of presentation if meningitis is suspected.

PEDIATRICS 12

B. **Epidemiology.** There is an increased frequency among rural, African-American, and Native American populations. Most common organisms are:

1. **Less than 1 month:** GBS, *E. coli*, *Listeria*.

2. **HSV encephalitis commonly presents from 2 to 4 weeks of age.** Thirty percent to 40% of infants with HSV encephalitis will not have vesicular skin lesions. These infants can present with seizures, lethargy, poor feeding, bulging fontanelle, or temperature instability.

3. **Greater than 1 month.** *H. influenzae* type B (especially in toddlers), *Neisseria meningitidis*, *S. pneumoniae*.

4. *H. influenzae*, *N. meningitidis*, and *S. pneumoniae* are respiratory tract–borne pathogens, *Listeria* species are most commonly food borne (e.g., hot dogs and prepared meats).

C. **Clinical signs and symptoms.**

1. **Triad of nuchal rigidity (may be absent in those <2 years of age), fever, and headache is present in only two thirds of patients. However, one part of the triad is always present. Kernig's and Brudzinski's signs are present only in 9%,** so meningitis should never be ruled out based only on the absence of these clinical signs.

2. Nonspecific signs of irritability, lethargy, poor feeding, nausea, and vomiting are more commonly the presentation in younger children. Check for bulging fontanel in the neonate (a late sign).

3. Most common neurologic sign is altered mental status. Focal neurologic deficits are uncommon.

4. Generalized signs include erythematous (early) or petechial (later) rash and endotoxin-mediated hypotension in meningococcal sepsis.

D. **Laboratory findings.**

1. **Do not delay LP and CSF examination to do a CT scan unless focal neurologic signs or papilledema suggestive of increased ICP are present. If any of these is present, get a head CT first (but start antibiotics before CT).** Send CSF for CBC, glucose, protein, culture, and Gram stain. Look for leukocytosis, high protein, and low glucose. See Table 24-7 for normal CSF fluid analysis. Do not delay antibiotics if an LP is not possible. See Chapter 9 for characteristic findings in bacterial versus viral meningitis.

2. General sepsis work-up including CBC, UA, and CXR (if indicated) should be done. Perform latex agglutination test on serum and urine and send blood, CSF, and urine cultures. However, a negative latex agglutination test does not rule out an infectious disease and should be used only to guide the choice of antibiotics.

3. Monitor electrolytes, oxygen saturation, serum glucose, C-reactive protein, serum osmolality, and INR/PTT.

E. **Treatment.**

1. **Stabilize** with proper airway management (if needed) and IV access. Evaluate and institute needed therapy for dehydration, hypotension, hypoxia, electrolyte abnormalities, SIADH, hypoglycemia, or DIC.

2. **Give empiric IV antibiotics** immediately according to most likely organism for age. Do not await culture results. However, changing antibiotics to reflect sensitivities once available is prudent. **Vancomycin should be added to all of the following regimens in those with LP-proven meningitis until cultures and sensitivities are available!**

a. **Dexamethasone** 0.15 mg/kg q6h × 4 d likely improves outcome when given together with antibiotics; this is true for both pneumococcal and *H. influenzae* meningitis. To be effective, however, steroids should be started before or just after first dose of antibiotics.

b. **Neonate <7 days:** Ampicillin 200 to 400 mg/kg per day divided q12h plus gentamicin 4 to 5 mg/kg/ divided q12h, or ampicillin plus cefotaxime 50 mg/kg per dose q12h. A gentamicin trough should be checked before the second dose, and should be <1.

c. **Neonate >7 days:** Ampicillin 200 to 400 mg/kg per day divided q12h plus gentamicin 2.5 mg IV q12h, or ampicillin plus cefotaxime 50 mg/kg per dose divided q8h. A gentamicin peak level can be obtained 30 minutes after the infusion to help determine dosing interval. Trough should be <1 before the second dose.

d. **Age 1 to 3 months:** Ampicillin 300 mg/kg per day divided q6h plus cefotaxime 200 mg/kg per day divided q6h, or ceftriaxone 100 mg/kg as a single dose or divided q12h. Consider the addition of vancomycin until sensitivities are available.

e. **Age >3 months and <6 years:** Cefotaxime 200 mg/kg per day divided q6h, or ceftriaxone 100 mg/kg per day as a single dose or divided q12h, or ampicillin 300 mg/kg per day divided q6h plus chloramphenicol 100 mg/kg per day divided q6h. Consider the addition of vancomycin until sensitivities are available.

f. **Age >6 years:** Ceftriaxone 100 mg/kg per day as a single dose or divided q12h. Consider addition of vancomycin while waiting for culture and sensitivities.

g. **Duration of therapy:** 14 to 21 days for GBS or gram-negative bacteria; 10 days for others.

VOMITING, DIARRHEA, AND DEHYDRATION

I. Vomiting.

A. Overview. Forceful ejection of gastric contents as opposed to passive reflux. Most common cause is gastroenteritis. In infants, consider GE reflux, overfeeding, anatomic obstruction, and systemic infection. In children, consider systemic infection, toxic ingestion, appendicitis, Reye's syndrome, and pertussis. Consider elevated ICP as a cause of isolated vomiting.

B. Evaluation.

1. History. Assess pattern and severity as well as accompanying dehydration/malnutrition. If neonatal, consider congenital abnormalities such as duodenal or esophageal atresia, Hirschsprung's disease, volvulus, malformation. In infants, assess how much is being fed

12

PEDIATRICS

(overfeeding), relation to position (reflux), choking or coughing with feeding (achalasia, tracheoesophageal fistula).

2. **Reye's syndrome.** Reye's syndrome generally occurs after viral illness and presents with intractable vomiting, elevated liver enzymes (but normal bilirubin), decreased mental status (encephalopathy), prolonged PT/INR, and elevated serum ammonia and hypoglycemia. Treatment includes glucose (at least 0.4 mg/kg per hour) to maintain normal serum glucose, fluid and electrolytes at one-half maintenance (correct shock first), neomycin 100 mg/kg per day PO q6h, vitamin K 5 to 10 mg IV for coagulopathy or FFP for acute bleeding, and management of elevated ICP. Some would add lactulose to this regimen.

3. **Pyloric stenosis.** Occurs at <2 months of age and presents with intractable vomiting after feeds. Most common in first-born boys, may have severe electrolyte disturbance depending on duration. Diagnosis is by US or "string sign" on upper GI film (barium or Gastrografin contrast passing through a narrowed pylorus). Treatment is surgical, although recent studies indicate that nitric oxide may be helpful. **Pyloric stenosis does not produce bilious vomiting. Midgut volvulus must be considered if there is bilious vomiting.**

C. **Exam and lab tests.** Evaluate state of hydration (see section on dehydration, later). Look for site of infection. Perform abdominal and rectal exam for obstruction or imperforate anus. Obtain radiologic studies as indicated. If child is <2 months of age, consider US or upper GI for pyloric stenosis.

D. **Treatment.** See dehydration and oral rehydration sections, later. Also consider antiemetics such as ondansetron, metoclopramide, prochlorperazine, and trimethobenzamide. Although classically avoided in children, antiemetics can reduce vomiting and aid recovery. There are few adverse reactions.

II. **Diarrhea** (see Chapter 5).

A. **Overview.** There are numerous causes of acute and chronic diarrhea. Infectious causes include viruses (rotavirus most common), bacteria (*Salmonella, Shigella, Campylobacter* most common), parasites (*Giardia* and *Cryptosporidium* most common), localized infection elsewhere, antibiotic-associated (antibiotic side effect, as well as *Clostridium difficile*), and food poisoning. Noninfectious causes include overfeeding (particularly of fruit juices), irritable bowel syndrome, celiac disease, milk protein intolerance, lactose intolerance after infectious diarrhea, CF, and inflammatory bowel.

B. **Evaluation.**

1. **History.** Acute versus chronic. Volume, frequency, character of stools, presence of blood or mucus. Associated symptoms (e.g., vomiting, fever, malaise). Epidemiologic data (travel, day care, family history).

2. **Exam.** Estimate dehydration (see section on dehydration, later). Examine for other infectious process or source. Determine if nutritional status is compromised. Neurologic symptoms, mental status changes, or seizures suggest *Shigella* or rotavirus.

3. **Lab tests.** Culture is indicated for acute bloody or guaiac-positive diarrhea. Fecal leukocytes and RBCs are not sensitive or specific enough to be useful in the diagnosis of infectious diarrhea; there is a high frequency of false-negative test results. Obtain O&P for prolonged diarrhea or as indicated. Conduct studies for chronic disease as appropriate. An ELISA test is available for rotavirus (Rotazyme). See Chapter 5.

C. **Treatment.**

1. **Acute diarrhea with dehydration in the absence of vomiting is treated with large amounts of osmotically balanced clear liquids** such as Pedialyte, Ricelyte, or the WHO rehydration formula until rehydration is complete. See dehydration and oral rehydration section.

2. **There is abundant evidence that early reinstitution of a lactose-free general diet will decrease the duration and severity of diarrhea.** Foods provided should be the same as those in the child's normal diet with the exclusion of high-sugar foods such as apple juice, which may cause an osmotic diarrhea, and milk products with lactose. Breastfed infants should continue to nurse without restrictions; lactose-free soybean formulas may be used in those who are bottle fed.

3. Avoid the use of antiperistaltic agents in infants and children.

4. **Most episodes of diarrhea do not benefit from antimicrobial therapy.** Bacterial diarrhea should be treated appropriately after culture results are available, although many would treat heme-positive diarrhea presumptively once cultures have been obtained. Caution should be used in the treatment of diarrhea caused by *Salmonella* species because this may prolong the carrier state. However, antibiotics should be used for *Salmonella* in infants <3 months of age or in patients with symptoms of toxicity, metastatic foci, or *Salmonella typhi* infection. See Chapter 5. Avoid treating enterohemorrhagic *E. coli* (0157:H7) with antibiotics because it may increase the risk of hemolytic uremic syndrome (see Wong et al., 2000).

5. Diarrhea with vomiting is treated as for vomiting until patient is able to tolerate oral feedings.

6. Racecadotril (acetorphan), an antisecretory agent, has been used successfully in children as young as 3 months with watery, heme-negative diarrhea (see Salazar-Lindo et al., 2000).

III. **Dehydration.**

A. **Clinical assessment.**

1. **Clinical observation (Table 12-6).** Clinical signs and symptoms are neither sensitive nor specific (only about 75% sensitive), so have a high index of suspicion for dehydration given the proper history.

2. **Laboratory diagnosis.** BUN/creatinine ratio of >20 is 92% sensitive but only 33% specific for dehydration. Serum bicarbonate, urine specific gravity, etc., are all poor predictors of dehydration.

3. **Degree of dehydration.** Because it is clinically very difficult to determine the percentage dehydration, the WHO has suggested categorizing patients as having "none," "some," or "severe," rather than trying to predict a percentage.

12

PEDIATRICS

CLINICAL SIGNS ASSOCIATED WITH VARIOUS DEGREES OF DEHYDRATION*

Dehydration (%)	Clinical Observation
5-6	Heart rate (10%-15% above baseline value)
	Slightly dry mucous membranes
	Concentration of the urine
	Poor tear production[†]
7-8	Increased severity of above signs
	Decreased skin turgor
	Oliguria
	Sunken eyeballs[†]
	Sunken anterior fontanel[†]
>9	Pronounced severity of above signs
	Decreased blood pressure
	Delayed capillary refill (>2 sec)
	Acidosis (large base deficit)

*Categorization as "none," "some," or "severe" is preferable because laboratory and physical findings are not sensitive or specific.
[†]These signs may be less sensitive indicators of dehydration than the others are.

4. **In hypotonic dehydration (Na <130 mEq/L) all manifestations appear with less fluid deficit,** whereas in hypertonic dehydration (Na >150 mEq/L) the circulating volume is relatively preserved, and so circulatory disturbances are seen later.
5. **Calculation of electrolyte deficits.** See section C. below and **Table 12-7**.
B. **Oral rehydration. There is no role for weak tea, flat soda, Jell-O (gelatin) water, etc.**
1. **The concept of gut rest, that is, stopping oral intake for several hours before refeeding, has been found to have several negative effects,** such as increased intestinal permeability and worsening of starvation and dehydration. Studies have shown that stool production is actually less with early refeeding.
2. Oral rehydration is appropriate in most cases of mild to moderate dehydration.

COMPOSITION OF INTRACELLULAR AND EXTRACELLULAR FLUID

Ion	Intracellular (mEq/L)	Extracellular (mEq/L)
Na^+	20	145
K^+	150	3-5
Cl^-	—	110
HCO_3^-	10	20-25
PO_4^-	110-115	5
Protein	75	10

Dehydration for <3 days: 80% ECF and 20% ICF losses. Dehydration for >3 days: 60% ECF and 40% ICF losses.

3. Currently only two fluids meet the recommendations of the WHO and the American Academy of Pediatrics for the rehydration phase of the treatment of diarrhea—Rehydralyte (Ross) and the WHO-ORS product (oral rehydration solution). These are the only two products that contain the 75 to 90 mEq/L of sodium recommended for rehydration. **A simple alternative for making a rehydration solution is to mix half a teaspoon of table salt and 8 teaspoons of sugar in 1 L of water. However, this solution neither replaces potassium nor contains bicarbonate.** One also needs to be sure that the parent is able to mix the solution properly. One can make a more complicated but more complete solution by adding 8 teaspoons of table sugar, half a teaspoon of salt, half a teaspoon of sodium bicarbonate (baking soda), and a third of a teaspoon of potassium chloride (e.g., "light salt products") to 1 L of water.

4. **Oral rehydration should be accomplished over 4 hours.** The dose for mild dehydration is 50 mL/kg, or 100 mL/kg for moderate dehydration. If vomiting is occurring, the child may be given frequent small doses of the rehydration fluid and then subsequent maintenance fluids by using a teaspoon or a small oral syringe to provide a rate of approximately 5 mL/min.

5. **For replacement of ongoing losses, it is recommended that a fluid with a lower sodium content than the rehydration fluid be used.** Pedialyte (Ross) or Ricelyte (Mead Johnson) are examples of appropriate maintenance fluids. Other solutions, such as weak tea, dilute or full-strength soft drinks, Jell-O (gelatin) water, tap water, apple juice, are contraindicated and may lead to hyponatremia. Alternatively, the rehydration fluid may be given along with other low-sodium fluids, such as breast milk or formula. Replacement of ongoing losses is advised at a rate of 10 mL/kg or $\frac{1}{2}$ to 1 cup of ORS for each diarrheal stool.

C. **Intravenous rehydration.**

1. **Formulas for calculating electrolyte deficits.**

a. **Sodium deficit** (mEq total) = (125 [or desired serum Na] – current serum Na) × 0.6 × weight (kg).

b. **Potassium deficit** (mEq total) = (desired serum K [mEq/L] – measured serum K) × 0.25 × weight (kg).

c. **Chloride deficit** (mEq total) = (desired serum Cl [mEq/L] – measured serum Cl) × 0.45 × weight (kg).

2. **Correction of free-water deficit in hypernatremic dehydration.** Free-water deficit = 4 mL/kg for every mEq that the serum Na exceeds 145 mEq/L.

3. **Maintenance requirements for fluids and electrolytes.**

a. Fluid maintenance.

(1) **Weight <10 kg:** 100 mL/kg per day.

(2) **Weight 11 to 20 kg:** 1000 mL + 50 mL/kg per day for every kg over 10 kg.

(3) **Weight >20 kg:** 1500 mL + 20 mL/kg per day for every kg over 20 kg.

(4) **Adult:** 2000 to 2400 mL/day.

4. Total body water: 60% of body weight.
5. Maintenance electrolyte requirements.
a. Na: 3 mEq/kg per day, or 3 mEq/100 mL of H_2O.
b. K: 2 mEq/kg per day or 2 mEq/100 mL of H_2O (adult: 50 mEq/day).
c. Cl: 3 mEq/100 mL of H_2O.
d. Glucose: 5 g/100 mL of H_2O.
6. Replacement of ongoing losses.
a. **Table 12-8 gives the composition of various body fluids.**
b. **NG losses usually replaced with D$_5$ 1/2NS with 20 mEq/L of KCl.**
c. **Diarrhea usually replaced with D$_5$ 1/4NS with 40 mEq/L of KCl.**
D. **General principles in treating dehydration.**
1. **Weigh the child.**
2. Be sure to add ongoing losses to maintenance fluids and electrolytes.
3. **If moderately or severely dehydrated, give an initial fluid bolus of 20 mL/kg of NS over 20 minutes.** Repeat bolus if response is inadequate. If poor response after three fluid boluses, that is, poor perfusion, no urine output, abnormal vital signs, may need CVP or PCWP to guide fluid resuscitation.
4. In hypotonic or isotonic dehydration, calculate the total fluids and electrolytes (maintenance plus deficit replacement) for the first 24 hours, give half over the first 8 hours and the other half over the next 16 hours. In hypertonic dehydration, correct the fluid and electrolyte deficits slowly over about 48 hours.
5. Do not add potassium to IV until urine output is established. Diabetic ketoacidosis may be an exception, where correction of hyperglycemia and acidosis may lead to rapid development of hypokalemia (see Chapter 6).
6. **Increase maintenance fluids by 12% for each degree Celsius of fever.**
E. **Hypotonic dehydration** (Na <125 mEq/L).
1. Symptomatic earlier than in isotonic or hypertonic dehydration. Therefore, use weight loss of 3% = mild, 6% = moderate, and 9% = severe dehydration as a guide.
2. Hypotonic dehydration usually results from replacing losses (vomiting and diarrhea) with low-solute fluids, such as dilute juice, cola, weak tea.

TABLE 12-8				
ELECTROLYTE COMPOSITION OF VARIOUS BODY FLUIDS				
Fluid	Na$^+$ (mEq/L)	K$^+$ (mEq/L)	Cl$^-$ (mEq/L)	Protein (g/dL)
Gastric	20-80	5-20	100-150	—
Pancreatic	120-140	5-15	40-80	—
Small bowel	100-140	5-15	90-130	—
Bile	120-140	5-15	80-120	—
Ileostomy	45-135	3-15	20-115	—
Diarrhea	10-90	10-80	10-110	—
Burns	140	5	110	3-5

3. Lethargy and irritability are common, and vascular collapse can occur early.
4. **Therapy.** Calculate total fluid and electrolyte needs according to the maintenance and deficit replacement formulas in section C.
a. Do not try to raise serum Na more than 10 mEq/L (that is, if the current serum Na is 125, use 135 as the desired serum Na level in the calculation) in first 24 hours.
b. To calculate the milliequivalents of Na needed in each liter during the first 24 hours of therapy: mEq of Na per liter of IV fluid = total Na needed in the first 24 hours divided by total volume of fluid needed (concentration of Na in normal saline = 154 mEq/L).
c. Usually D_5 1/2NS or D_5 NS is used. Potassium can be added after urine output is established. Give half of the calculated total fluid and electrolyte requirements for the first 24 hours over the first 8 hours and the other half over the subsequent 16 hours.
F. **Severe, symptomatic hyponatremia.** See Chapter 6.
G. **Isotonic dehydration** (Na = 130-150 mEq/L).
1. Symptoms are less dramatic than in hypotonic dehydration.
2. Use estimate (loss of weight): 5% = mild, 10% = moderate, 15% = severe dehydration.
3. Calculate total maintenance + deficit replacement fluids and electrolytes for first 24 hours.
4. Treatment is similar to that for hypotonic dehydration: give half of first 24 hours' needs in first 8 hours, and give the remaining half over the next 16 hours.
5. Usually can use D_5 1/4NS or D_5 1/2NS; may add potassium after urine output established.
6. Remember to estimate and replace ongoing losses.
H. **Hypertonic dehydration.**
1. Usually occurs as a result of using inappropriately high solute load as replacement, renal concentrating defect with large free-water losses, heat exposure with large insensible losses, etc.
2. Typical symptoms include thick, doughy texture to skin (tenting is uncommon), shrill cry, weakness, tachypnea, intense thirst.
3. Shock is a very late manifestation. If severe dehydration or shock is present, the patient may need up to three boluses of 20 mL/kg NS over the first hour.
4. Free-water deficit (mL) is estimated to be 4 mL/kg × ([actual serum Na (mEq/L) − 145 mEq/L]).
5. Replace the free-water deficit slowly over 48 hours. Aim to decrease the serum Na by about 10 mEq/L per day. Reducing serum sodium more rapidly can have severe repercussions, such as cerebral and pulmonary edema.
6. Usual replacement fluid is D_5 1/4NS or D_5 1/2NS.
7. If Na >180 mEq/L, may need dialysis.

PEDIATRICS 12

CONSTIPATION AND ENCOPRESIS

I. **Overview.** Infrequent passage of dry, hard stools. Causes can be organic (Hirschsprung's disease, anal stenosis, anal stricture, drugs, dehydration, neuromuscular disease) or functional (voluntary withholding). Beyond the neonatal period, 90% to 95% of constipation is functional.

II. **Causes.**

A. **In newborn must rule out anatomic and congenital causes** such as rectal or colonic atresia, myelomeningocele, absent abdominal muscles, CF, Hirschsprung's disease.

B. **In older children, cause usually functional or dietary.**

1. **Dietary.** Lack of dietary bulk, excessive intake of cow's milk, early introduction of cow's milk.

2. **Stool retention.** Painful defecation caused by fissure, rectal abscess, etc., or conflicts in toilet training. Voluntary withholding results in decreased rectal sensation and rectal distention and subsequent loss of defecation urge. Stooling around impaction with soiling is known as *encopresis* if noted after normal toilet training age of 4 to 5 years.

3. **Other causes of constipation.** Narcotics, antidepressants and other anticholinergics, overuse of laxatives, hypothyroidism, hypokalemia.

III. **Evaluation.**

A. **History.** Age of onset. Parent expectation of stool pattern. Stool consistency, size, frequency, soiling, abdominal pain, anorexia, tenesmus. Infants should pass meconium in first 24 hours.

B. **Exam.** Palpable abdominal mass. Rectal exam reveals hard stool present with dilated ampulla. Anal fissure may be present.

C. **Lab tests as appropriate.** Abdominal flat plate will show stool filling the colon. Administer barium enema to demonstrate atresia. Obtain rectal biopsy for Hirschsprung's disease. Measure thyroid function, electrolytes, and calcium as indicated.

IV. **Treatment.**

A. **Simple constipation in infants treated with lactulose** 2.5 to 10 mL/24 h, divided tid or qid. Add fruit and fruit juices to diet if older than 4 months. Karo syrup (corn syrup) 15 to 20 mL per 8 oz of formula can be helpful. Previous concerns about the possibility of botulism are unfounded. A glycerin suppository may stimulate the passage of a stool. Changing to Carnation Good Start formula may be helpful with constipation.

B. **In older children, clear impaction** using pediatric enema or cathartic (e.g., bisacodyl suppositories). Polyethylene glycol (GoLYTELY, MiraLax) may also be used. Give 40 mL/kg over 6 hours. Increase dietary fiber (prunes, figs, raisins, beans, bran, fresh fruits, and vegetables) or use a psyllium supplement. Limit milk if excessive by history. Avoid hypotonic and phosphate enemas, which can cause electrolyte abnormalities and seizures.

C. Encopresis (soiling with impaction).

1. Usually starts as a functional voluntary withholding but progresses to decreased urge to defecate because of rectal enlargement and loss of sensation of full rectum.

2. Counseling of patient and parents on cause of soiling. Outline plan to help patient resolve problem.

3. Clear rectum of impaction before starting treatment.

4. Start milk of magnesia (<1 year of age, 0.5 mL/kg per day; 2-5 years, 5-15 mL/day; 6-12 years, 15-30 mL/day; >12 years, 30-60 mL/day), or mineral oil (do not use if <5 years of age) 5 to 30 mL, and increase until having soft stools. Polyethylene glycol (e.g., Miralax) is also being used for this indication. Mix 17 g, or one capful, into 8 oz of fluid. Start with 1 g/kg per day divided bid. The dose can be adjusted with a goal of one or two soft stools per day. Lactulose 5 to 10 mg PO bid can also be used. Continue treatment for 2 to 6 months while rectal size and sensation return to normal.

5. When decreasing dose of laxative, start toilet-sitting regimen, that is, sitting for 15 minutes after each meal. Consider reward system appropriate to age.

6. Implement dietary changes as above.

GASTROINTESTINAL BLEEDING IN CHILDHOOD

I. Surgical Causes.

A. If <1 year of age, think of anal fissure (43%), intussusception (39%), duodenal-gastric ulcer (15%), gangrenous bowel (9%), Meckel's diverticulum (3.8%).

B. If >1 year of age, think of polyps (50%), ulcers (14%), anal fissure (12.5%), esophageal varices (10.5%), intussusception (9%), hemorrhoids (0.8%).

II. Medical Causes.

A. Hematologic abnormalities. Hemophilia, iron deficiency, thrombocytopenia, vitamin K deficiency.

B. Systemic causes. Milk allergy, infectious diarrhea, Henoch-Schönlein purpura, scurvy, uremia.

C. Drugs. NSAIDs, iron poisoning.

D. Swallowed blood. From nose bleed, maternal blood from breastfeeding, etc.

E. To differentiate swallowed maternal blood (e.g., breastfeeding) from neonatal blood. Take vomitus, stool, etc., and mix with 5 to 10 parts of water. Centrifuge to remove debris and decant the pink supernatant (if not pink, will not work). Mix 1 mL of 0.25 (1%) sodium hydroxide with 5 mL of supernatant. Read color change in 2 minutes. If remains pink, blood is of fetal origin. If it turns brown-yellow, blood is of adult origin. It is helpful to run a control of the infant's blood.

12

PEDIATRICS

STRIDOR AND DYSPNEA

The differential diagnosis of stridor and dyspnea is listed in Table 12-9.

I. Epiglottitis.

A. Definition. Infection of the epiglottis and of the aryepiglottic folds and surrounding soft tissues. Becoming less common since use of *H. influenzae* vaccine. Is more common in adults, in whom it presents as a severe sore throat with drooling, neck tenderness.

B. Cause. Almost always by *H. influenzae* type B. Other causes: β-hemolytic streptococci, *S. aureus*, and *S. pneumoniae*.

C. Clinical presentation. May occur at any age, with a peak incidence at 2 to 7 years. Presents with sudden onset of high fever, respiratory distress, severe dysphagia, drooling, muffled voice, and a toxic appearance. Stridor, if present, may be mild compared with croup. Often there is little or no coughing. Child typically prefers being upright in "sniffing" position.

D. Lab tests. Invasive procedures and examinations should be avoided until after airway is secured. CBC and blood and epiglottic cultures may then be obtained. Radiographs of lateral area of neck shows characteristic swollen epiglottis (thumb sign). **Never send a child suspected of having epiglottitis to be radiographed without being accompanied by someone who can emergently manage the airway. A radiograph is an adjunct to clinical diagnosis and need not be done.**

E. Treatment.

1. **Do not move, upset, or lay child down unless prepared to manage obstructed airway.**

2. **Airway.** In an emergency, **a bag-valve-mask can buy time.** Consider a needle cricothyrotomy. Top of size 3 ET fits on Luer-lock needle, allowing for easy bagging. Controlled intubation by an experienced operator is preferred. Tracheostomy is acceptable if unable to intubate. The patient usually can be safely extubated in 48 to 72 hours after appropriate antibiotics are started. Airway must be secure.

3. **Antibiotics.** Initiated once artificial airway secure. Cefotaxime 50 to 200 mg/kg per day divided q6h or ceftriaxone 75 mg/kg qd are the first-line drugs, with TMP–SMX as a second-line agent.

4. **Admission to ICU.** Use proper sedation during period of intubation. Antibiotics continue for 7 to 10 days after extubation.

II. Croup (Laryngotracheobronchitis).

A. Definition. A syndrome of airway swelling in the glottic and subglottic area, of viral origin.

B. Causes. Parainfluenza virus types 1 and 3 responsible for majority of cases; remainder RSV, influenza virus, and adenovirus.

C. Clinical presentation. Age usually 6 months to 6 years. Symptoms of the common cold usually precede onset. Brassy cough (seal bark), hoarseness, and inspiratory stridor are characteristic. If severe may

TABLE 12-9
DIFFERENTIAL DIAGNOSIS OF STRIDOR AND DYSPNEA

	Viral			
	Laryngotracheitis	Bacterial Tracheitis	Retropharyngeal Abscess	Epiglottitis
Cause	Parainfluenza Influenza RSV	Viral prodrome *plus* Staphylococci Streptococci *Haemophilus influenzae* Enteric pathogens	β-Hemolytic streptococci Anaerobes	*H. influenzae* Staphylococci Streptococci
Age	3 mo to 3 y	3 mo to 3 y	6 mo to 3 y	2-7 y
Clinical characteristics	Low-grade fever Coryza Barking cough Hoarse voice Winter/spring peak	Improving croup then sudden increase: temperature, work of breathing, stridor No drooling Fall/winter peak	Initial URI Dysphagia, refusal to feed Drooling, toxic appearance, stridor	Sudden onset of high fever, dysphagia, stridor, drooling No cough Unnecessary (thumb sign)
Radiograph	Unnecessary (steeple sign unreliable)	Detached pseudomembrane may give soft tissue shadow	Radiograph shows retropharyngeal soft tissue density and air-fluid level	
Treatment	Cool mist, epinephrine, steroids	Intubation, antibiotics	Surgical drainage, antibiotics	Intubation, antibiotics

include retractions, decreased air entry, and cyanosis. The course is usually benign, but can progress to obstruction.

D. May be resolved by presentation to office or ED from exposure to cool air.

E. Must differentiate from epiglottitis and bacterial tracheitis, which require emergent management. See Table 12-9.

F. Classification.

1. **Very mild.** Intermittent stridor, present when awake or excited, goes away when sleeping.

2. **Mild.** Continuous stridor when awake or asleep not audible without stethoscope.

3. **Moderate.** Continuous stridor audible without stethoscope and may be accompanied be sternal retractions.

4. **Severe.** Continuous stridor with evidence of respiratory failure (cyanosis, altered mental status).

G. Lab tests. Usually not indicated and may induce further agitation with respiratory compromise. If in doubt and no need for emergent airway management, AP radiograph of neck may show subglottic narrowing (steeple sign).

H. Management.

1. Calm the child on the parent's lap and provide cool, humidified air.

2. Provide oxygen if saturation <95%.

3. Reassess status after 15 to 30 minutes.

4. If classified as mild, consider discharge with instructions for cool mist humidifier.

5. If moderate classification:

a. The traditional treatment has been nebulized racemic epinephrine, 2.25% solution, 0.5 mL diluted in 3 mL of saline.

b. **Nebulized epinephrine, 5 mL diluted 1:1000, has been shown to be as safe as, at least as good as, and perhaps superior to racemic epinephrine.** May repeat prn.

c. **There is no rebound effect from epinephrine, but patients may return to their pretreatment state.**

d. **Steroids.** Generally those who need nebulized epinephrine should also be treated with dexamethasone 0.3-0.6 mg/kg per dose IM or PO, up to 10 mg. Although not standard of care, nebulized budesonide 1 mg given twice at 30-minute intervals is effective in **mild to moderate** croup and may prevent the need for systemic steroids. However, up to now, it has not been compared with dexamethasone in any trial. Dexamethasone can also be used in moderate croup if desired.

e. Continuation of cool, humidified air may also be helpful.

f. **Disposition.** Patients may be discharged with instructions for cool mist humidifier if, after 3 to 6 hours of observation, they require no further treatment with epinephrine and their croup is mild. If patient remains in the moderate classification, hospitalization with epinephrine or racemic epinephrine prn and dexamethasone 0.25 to 0.5 mg/kg per dose q6h for two to four doses.

6. **If in severe classification, the decision to intubate should be left to experienced personnel and, when feasible, be performed in the OR.**

III. **Foreign Body Aspiration.** See Chapter 2.

IV. **Bronchiolitis.**

A. **Epidemiology.** Illness of young children and infants. Most serious in first 2 years of life. RSV principal agent. Also associated with parainfluenza, adenovirus, influenza virus, rhinovirus. The majority occur during winter but can occur any season.

B. **Clinical presentation.** Rhinorrhea, sneezing, coughing, low-grade fever. Onset of rapid breathing and wheezing. Signs of respiratory distress in severe cases: nasal flaring, tachypnea, prolonged expiratory phase, retractions.

C. **Lab tests.** CBC usually within normal limits. Blood gas, O_2 saturation levels, as appropriate. Perform nasal wash for RSV culture and antigen assay. CXR can be normal but occasionally shows air trapping and peribronchial thickening.

D. **Treatment.**

1. **Indications for hospitalization.** Use clinical judgment. Some suggested criteria include <6 months of age, resting respirations over 50 to 60, Po_2 <60 mm Hg, pulse oximetry <95%, apnea, unable to tolerate oral feedings.

2. **Supportive measures.** Antipyretics, IV fluids, humidified O_2, nebulized bronchodilators (albuterol 2.5 mg/3 mL of NS repeated prn). Epinephrine, 5 mL of 1:1000, by nebulizer is safe and effective as an alternative. Steroids are ineffective. However, they continue to be widely used in doses similar to those for asthma. One controlled clinical trial has been published (see Schuh et al., 2002) that showed that a dose of 1 mg/kg of dexamethasone given early in the course of the illness resulted in decreased hospitalization from bronchiolitis. This study is controversial, and follow-up studies are needed.

3. **Ribavirin aerosol. Ribavirin is of questionable efficacy and may actually be detrimental.** The use of ribavirin even in severely ill patients is at the discretion of the physician. If croup or bronchiolitis secondary to RSV, consider use of ribavirin in high-risk groups:
   - Congenital heart disease
   - Chronic lung disease (such as bronchopulmonary dysplasia)
   - Infants <6 weeks of age
   - Neurologic disorders
   - Immunosuppressed
   - Severely ill infants.
   - Pao_2 <65 mm Hg or Sao_2 <90%
   - Increasing Pco_2

12

PEDIATRICS

4. **Intubation and mechanical ventilation as indicated.**
5. **RSV immunoglobulin (RSV-IVIG) 750 mg/kg IV q30d can prevent RSV infection and hospitalization in those children with severe underlying illness such as bronchopulmonary dysplasia or prematurity.** An alternative is Synagis (palivizumab), an RSV immunoglobulin that can be given IM (15 mg/kg per dose IM every month). Use with caution in those with thrombocytopenia or coagulation defects because of IM bleeding.

LIMP AND JOINT PAIN

I. **Joint Pain.**
A. Will have pain on weight bearing or refusal to bear weight. Pain on passive motion of joints involved with arthritis.
B. Determine if true arthritis (versus just joint pain) by exam, presence of fever, number of joints involved.

II. **Limp.**
A. Hip joint disease often felt as knee pain in children.
B. Examine shoes and feet (look for tiny pebble in shoe bottom, etc.).
C. **General approach to the child with a limp.**
1. **A conservative approach indicated because very few children without systemic symptoms or true arthritis have any significant disorder.** If pain persists or you suspect an acute arthritis, diagnostic evaluations can include a CBC with differential, ESR, ASO titer, rheumatoid factor, throat and urine cultures, US for joint effusion, and radiographic studies of the hips. Perform arthrocentesis if there is any clinical suspicion of a septic joint or an effusion by US.
D. **Differential diagnosis and approach.**
1. **Transient tenosynovitis (irritable hip).**
   a. Most common cause of limp (well over 90% in some series).
   b. Frequently follows URI or streptococcal infection.
   c. May have joint effusion but not true arthritis.
   d. ESR—normal or mildly elevated.
   e. Generally resolves within 24 to 48 hours with rest and ibuprofen-acetaminophen. Close follow-up is indicated.
2. **Septic hip joint. A true emergency (see also Chapter 7).**
   a. Generally febrile with elevated ESR, WBC >18,000/mm^3, but lab values may be normal and may overlap with those of other illnesses.
   b. Will generally look sick and hold hip in flexion and external rotation.
   c. Effusion present on US but may also have effusion with transient tenosynovitis (71%). Joint tap is diagnostic.
   d. Relatively sudden onset and rapid course.
   e. Treat with antistaphylococcal antibiotics. Requires orthopedic consultation and surgical intervention.

3. **Legg-Calvé-Perthes disease (aseptic necrosis of the femoral head).**
   a. Most common between 5 and 10 years of age.
   b. Slow, insidious onset of limp and hip pain, which is progressive. Have limitation of motion of the hip.
   c. Diagnosis by radiography of affected hip (see lucency of femoral head and eventually sclerosis and destruction of femoral head). Bone scan may reveal abnormalities earlier than a plain radiograph.
   d. Treatment requires consultation with orthopedics and includes rest, anti-inflammatories, and casting for more severe cases.

4. **Slipped capital femoral epiphysis.**
   a. Generally seen in overweight teenagers, especially boys who are prepubertal.
   b. May have insidious onset of pain but can also follow acute trauma.
   c. May be pain with passive motion. Patient will hold hip in external rotation.
   d. Diagnosis by frog-legged radiographs of both hips.
   e. Treatment is by orthopedic referral and surgical fixation.

5. **Osgood-Schlatter disease.**
   a. Characterized by pain over the tibial tubercle, which is usually unilateral. May have swelling over the area of pain.
   b. Usually occurs in active children between 10 and 15 years of age.
   c. Treatment is rest, NSAIDs, and local heat.

6. **Diskitis.**
   a. An inflammatory process of the disk or disks (usually L3-L5), which may be infectious in cause (staphylococcal primarily).
   b. Presents with refusal to walk or limp, low-grade fever, and "tripod posturing"—leaning back with back extended onto outstretched arms when sitting.
   c. Generally have pain over involved disk area but may also have pain on straight-leg raising, hip motion.
   d. ESR almost always elevated, but CBC may be normal. Disk space may be narrowed on radiograph. Bone scan will show inflammatory focus.
   e. Treatment is generally supportive with anti-inflammatories, but may need antibiotics. Orthopedic consultation recommended.

7. **Juvenile rheumatoid arthritis.**
   a. Defined as presentation of rheumatoid arthritis before 16 years of age.
   b. See Chapter 7, Rheumatology, as well.
   c. Still's disease in 20%, which is JRA plus fever, thrombocytopenia, splenomegaly, generalized adenopathy.
   d. Onset in one or a few joints in 40%.
   e. Polyarticular onset similar to adult onset in 40%.
   f. Complete remission in 75%.

8. Rheumatic fever: see Chapter 7.

9. Sickle cell crisis in appropriate populations (see Chapter 6).

10. Other arthritides including manifestation of ulcerative colitis, Crohn's disease, etc. Diagnosis by looking for and finding symptom complex.

NOCTURNAL ENURESIS

I. Definition. Involuntary loss of urine during sleep. Nocturnal enuresis is a disorder of delayed maturation and generally cannot be officially diagnosed until the child is at least 5 years of age.

II. Primary Enuresis. Wetting that proceeds more or less continuously for at least 1 year without prior dry spells.

III. Secondary Enuresis. The child has been dry at least for 1 year before wetting the bed.

IV. Epidemiology. Most often primary, affects 10% to 20% of children 5 to 6 years of age; 1% of adults are affected. Tends to be familial; affects the child's self-esteem. Only 1% to 4% are attributable to uropathies. Etiology theories: "organic" (deficiency in the nocturnal production of ADH, obstructive sleep apnea, need to rule out other organic causes), "psychological," "sleep stage," and "failure to learn control." The definite cause is yet undetermined.

V. Evaluation. History: developmental milestones (assess delay in neurologic development), voiding history, toilet training, social history, child rearing, family milestones. Obtain history of UTI, medical and surgical problems, medications, diet. Exam: gait, posture, spine exam may be important in diagnosing neurologic abnormalities. Abdominal mass, bladder size, UA, and culture to look for UTI, obstruction with overflow. If child is diurnal and nocturnal wetter, a renal and bladder US should be done. If there is history of UTI, should do VCUG.

VI. Management.

A. Motivate the child to establish control!

B. Pharmacotherapy. DDAVP 1 or 2 sniffs qhs. Oxybutynin 1 to 5 mg qhs (used in daytime also for day wetting); imipramine less effective (25-50 mg qhs 6-12 years of age, 50-75 mg qhs >12 years). Also must be aware of the risks of overdose of imipramine. Enuresis often recurs when the medication is discontinued.

C. Behavioral (most successful). Self-monitoring, motivation and responsibility training, charting of success and failure nights, bladder training, enuresis alarms, nocturnal awakenings; avoid diapers. Enuresis alarms or pagers have been found to be the most effective form of therapy for enuresis.

D. Diet. Avoid caffeine, liquids before bedtime. May use DDAVP on sleepovers, travel.

BIBLIOGRAPHY

Carbajal R, Chauvet X, Couderc S, Olivier-Martin M: Randomised trial of analgesic effects of sucrose, glucose, and pacifiers in term neonates. *BMJ* 319:1393-1397, 1999.

Lucassen PLBJ, Assendelft WJ, Gubbels JW, et al: Effectiveness of treatments for infantile colic: Systematic review. *BMJ* 316:1563-1569, 1998.

Markestad T: Use of sucrose as a treatment for infant colic. *Arch Dis Child* 76:356-357, 1997.

Salazar-Lindo E, Santisteban-Ponce J, Chea-Woo E, Gutierrez M: Racecadotril in the treatment of acute watery diarrhea in children. *N Engl J Med* 343:463-467, 2000.

Schuh S, Coates AL, Binnie R, et al: Efficacy of oral dexamethasone in outpatients with acute bronchiolitis. *J Pediatr* 140: 27-32, 2002.

Vain NE, Szyld EG, Prudent LM, et al: Oropharyngeal and nasopharyngeal suctioning of meconium-stained neonates before delivery of their shoulders: Multicentre, randomised controlled trial. *Lancet* 364:597-602, 2004.

Wiswell TE, Gannon CM, Jacob J, et al: Delivery room management of the apparently vigorous meconium-stained neonate: Results of the multicenter, international collaborative trial. *Pediatrics* 105:1-7, 2000.

Wolke D, Gray P, Meyer R: Excessive infant crying: A controlled study of mothers helping mothers. *Pediatrics* 94:322-332, 1994.

Wong CS, Jelacic S, Habeeb RL, et al: The risk of the hemolytic-uremic syndrome after antibiotic treatment of *Escherichia coli* O157:H7 infections. *N Engl J Med* 342:1930-1936, 2000.

12

PEDIATRICS

Gynecology

Lauri Lopp and Kelly Skelly

CONTRACEPTIVES

Table 13-1 lists the percentage of women experiencing an unintended pregnancy during the first year of typical use and the first year of perfect use of contraception.

I. **Combined Oral Contraceptive Pill.**

A. **Mechanism of action.** The OCP suppresses ovulation through inhibition of the hypothalamic–pituitary–ovarian axis. It also alters the cervical mucus, retards sperm entry, and discourages implantation into an unfavorable endometrium. **OCPs may be less effective in obese patients (two additional pregnancies per 100 patient-years) but are still more effective than many other methods** (see Table 13-1).

B. **Risks and adverse effects** include hypertension, thromboembolism, stroke, myocardial infarction (especially in smokers), gallstone formation, hepatocellular adenomas or cancer, and growth of fibroids. Minimally increases risk of breast cancer, might increase risk of cervical cancer. Possible higher risk of HIV due to intercourse without condoms.

C. **Side effects** include nausea, breast tenderness, weight gain, decreased libido, leg cramping, headache, bloating, acne, spotting. Depression and migraines can worsen or improve.

D. **Absolute contraindications** include pregnancy; history of thromboembolic disease, stroke or TIA; focal or severe migraine; ischemic heart disease; severe hypertension; history of breast cancer or estrogen-dependent neoplasms; hepatic dysfunction or tumor; porphyria; current prolonged immobilization or recent surgery on legs; diabetes with end-organ damage; and smoking in patients older than 35 years. Ask about family history of venous thromboembolism; if positive, consider screening for factor V Leiden, etc. (see Chapter 4).

E. **Relative contraindications** include postpartum less than 3 weeks, lactation, active gallbladder disease, active mononucleosis, undiagnosed abnormal vaginal bleeding, light smoking in patients older than 35 years, and long-term use of drugs decreasing the efficacy of the pill (rifampin, rifabutin, griseofulvin, phenytoin, phenobarbital, topiramate, carbamazepine, ampicillin, doxycycline, tetracycline). See later for pill management with antibiotics, etc.

F. **Noncontraceptive benefits of oral contraceptives** include more regular menses, decreased menorrhagia, decreased dysmenorrhea, increased iron stores, treatment of irregular menses secondary to anovulation; improvement in hirsutism; protection from benign breast disease, functional ovarian cysts, PID, ectopic pregnancy, epithelial ovarian cancer, and endometrial carcinoma. Also increases bone mineral density.

TABLE 13-1
CONTRACEPTIVE EFFICACY*

Method	Typical Use (%)	Perfect Use (%)
No method	85	85
Oral contraceptive pills	5	
Combination OCP		0.1
Progestin-only OCP		0.5
Depo-Provera	0.3	0.3
Norplant and Norplant-II	0.05	0.05
Copper-T 380A (Paraguard)	0.8	0.6
Progesterone IUD (Progestasert)	2.0	1.5
Condom	18.5	9.8
Female condom (Reality)	21	5
Male condom	14	3
Spermicide alone	26	6
Diaphragm	20	6
Cervical cap, parous women	40	26
Cervical cap, nulliparous women	20	9
Sponge, parous women	40	20
Sponge, nulliparous women	20	9
Lactational amenorrhea	2	
Periodic abstinence	25	
Periodic abstinence, calendar method		9
Periodic abstinence, ovulation method		3
Periodic abstinence, symptothermal		2
Periodic abstinence, postovulation		1
Withdrawal	19	4
Female sterilization	0.5	0.5
Male sterilization	0.15	0.10

*Percentage of women experiencing an unintended pregnancy during the first year of typical use and the first year of perfect use of contraception.
Adapted from Hatcher RA, Trussell J, Stewart F, et al: *Contraceptive Technology*, 18th rev ed. New York, Argent, 2004.

G. Benefits in special situations. Patients desiring less-frequent menses for convenience reasons or women with polycystic ovarian disease (PCOS), severe dysmenorrhea, PMS, or amenorrhea can prolong their cycle by taking two or three consecutive packages of active pills followed by 7 days of inactive pills or by using a 3-month oral contraceptive pill that is in one package. These regimens allow withdrawal bleeding (and minimize the risk of endometrial cancer). However, the long-term effects of this regimen have not been well studied.

H. Perimenopausal use of oral contraceptives. Perimenopausal women who still have menses can safely use oral contraceptives if they are nonsmokers without other contraindications. Well-controlled hypertension not exacerbated by contraceptives may be acceptable. **To determine menopausal status, ask about hot flushes during the placebo week and check the FSH on the sixth or seventh day of the placebo week.**

When the patient is menopausal, discuss symptom management after stopping the contraceptives.

I. **Managing the patient taking the pill**

1. **When starting OCPs, exclude pregnancy** and supplement with alternative contraception during the first month. Recommend the use of condoms with OCPs to reduce risk of STDs and HIV.

2. **Starting regimens.** Start active pills day 1 after the start of menses. Many women choose to start on the Sunday after the start of their menses for convenience. For postpartum nonbreastfeeding women, start OCP during week 4 after delivery. OCPs can be started the day after an induced or spontaneous abortion. For those who have had major surgery or leg surgery, do not start OCPs until the patient has been ambulatory for 2 weeks.

3. **Pills can be taken cyclically (21 active followed by 7 placebo pills) or as an extended-cycle regimen (84 active followed by 7 inactive pills).**

4. **Missed pill.** If a pill is missed, it should be taken as soon as possible and the next dose should be taken as usual. If two pills are missed, take two pills together on 2 consecutive days to catch up. Alternative contraception should be used for 7 days.

5. **If taking antibiotics or other interacting medication for a short time** (United Kingdom National Guidelines), use another form of birth control for the duration of the (antibiotic) treatment and for 7 days afterwards. If this 7 days extends into the next month, the patient should start the active pills without taking the placebo (i.e., skip menses).

6. **Breakthrough bleeding.** Breakthrough bleeding is not uncommon during the first 3 months of OCP use. **Generally, breakthrough bleeding in the first 10 days of the cycle is due to inadequate estrogen, whereas breakthrough at other times in the cycle is due to inadequate progesterone.** For heavy bleeding in the first 7 days of the cycle, treat with conjugated oral estrogen 1.25 mg or estradiol 2.0 mg PO qd for the first 7 days of the cycle while continuing the contraceptive medication. If breakthrough bleeding continues, consider changing to oral contraceptives with additional progesterone or estrogen depending on when in the cycle the problem occurs.

7. **Amenorrhea is usually due to excess progestin effects.** Consider adding conjugated estrogen for the first 7 days of the cycle or change to a higher-estrogen or lower-progesterone OCP.

8. **Third-generation progestins.** Three progestogens—desogestrel, norgestimate, and gestodene—that have low androgenicity, minimal metabolic effects, and good cycle control are available. They are useful for acne and hirsutism. However, they are more expensive, and **there is some evidence that the risk of thromboembolic disease may be slightly increased (2 per 10,000 woman-years) with desogestrel and gestodene (Ortho-Cept and Desogen).**

II. **Transdermal Contraceptive Patch.** Mechanism of action, benefits, risks, and adverse effects are the same as for the combined oral contraceptive.

GYNECOLOGY 13

Place patch (e.g., Ortho-Evra) on the skin once weekly for 3 weeks followed by a patch-free week. This delivers 20 μg ethinyl estradiol and 150 μg norelgestromin daily. **This is more estrogen than with other estrogen-based contraceptives, but to date there is no evidence of an increase in thromboembolic disease compared with other estrogen contraceptives.**

III. **Contraceptive Vaginal Ring.** Mechanism of action, benefits, risks, and adverse effects are the same as for the combined oral contraceptive. Place the ring (Nuvaring) intravaginally for 3 weeks of every 4 weeks. This provides daily dosages of 15 μg ethinyl estradiol and 120 μg etonogestrel daily with efficacy results of ovarian suppression similar to those for oral contraceptives.

IV. **Progestin-Only Contraceptives.**

A. **Types of progestin-only contraceptives**

1. **Progestin-only OCPs ("minipills")** are less effective than combination pills except in women who are breastfeeding full-time. Because they must be taken at the same time every day to be effective, they are less suitable for patients who might have irregular work schedules or are prone to missing doses (e.g., adolescents). They have no adverse effect on lactation.

2. **Injectable medroxyprogesterone acetate** (Depo-Provera) is given 150 mg IM every 3 months. Some women (especially obese women) require higher doses because of higher levels of circulating estrogens. Most women have irregular bleeding for up to a year and then become amenorrheic. Return to fertility can be delayed up to 10 months due to persistence of the depot medication. **Because of bone loss, Depo-Provera should not be used for longer than 2 years unless other contraceptive options are inadequate.**

3. **Progestin implants** are no longer available in the United States. This subcutaneous insertion of six Silastic capsules contains levonorgestrel for slow release, providing contraception for 5 years. Removal is recommended any time up until 5 years after implants were placed. Fertility usually returns within 2 months after removal.

B. **Advantages and disadvantages of progestin-only contraceptives.**

1. **Advantages.** Because of their reduced potential to cause clotting abnormalities, progestin-only methods (minipill, Depo-Provera, Norplant) are useful in women with risk factors for cardiovascular disease, such as smokers, women older than 35 years, and diabetic patients.

2. **Absolute contraindications.** Pregnancy, abnormal vaginal bleeding of unknown etiology, progestin-sensitive breast cancer. **Medroxyprogesterone can accelerate the development of breast cancer (acts as a promoter) and decreases bone density.**

3. **Relative contraindications.** Manufacturers of progestin-only methods continue to list estrogen-related contraindications despite the absence of estrogen in the contraceptives. See combined OCP above for list.

Exercise caution when using phenytoin, carbamazepine, primidone, phenylbutazone, rifampin, or rifampicin.

4. **Side effects** include breast tenderness, weight gain, and possible depression.

V. Intrauterine Devices.

A. Mechanism of action is primarily through inhibition of sperm migration, ovum transport, and fertilization. **IUDS are no longer thought to be a significant abortifacient, although occasionally implantation fails to occur.**

B. Safety. Currently available IUDs are considered safe and have very low complication rates in properly selected patients. Patient selection is extremely important to avoid increasing the risk of infection and infertility. The ideal candidate is a parous woman in a mutually monogamous relationship with no history of PID.

C. Duration. Copper-T 380A (ParaGard) is replaced after 10 years. Progesterone-T IUD (Progestasert) is replaced annually. Mirena, a levonorgestrel IUD, lasts 5 years.

D. Other uses. Progestasert and Mirena offer effective treatment for severe menorrhagia.

E. Absolute contraindications include current, recent (within 3 months), or recurrent endometritis, PID, or STD; pregnancy; anatomically distorted uterine cavity; and known or suspected HIV infection. For Progestasert and Mirena, progestin-sensitive neoplasm.

F. Relative contraindications include any history of gonorrhea or chlamydia, multiple sexual partners or a partner with multiple other partners, undiagnosed abnormal vaginal bleeding, known or suspected uterine or cervical malignancy, and previous problems with an IUD (pregnancy, expulsion, perforation, pain, heavy bleeding). Copper allergy and Wilson's disease have been suggested as reasons to select one of the hormonal IUDs even though the amount of copper released by the ParaGard is likely less than that of a daily diet. Use of an IUD in nulliparas is controversial.

G. Adverse effects include PID after insertion and uterine perforation during insertion. For Paraguard, spotting, heavy menstrual flow, and dysmenorrhea. For Progestasert and Mirena, spotting and amenorrhea.

H. Special notes

1. **Expulsions.** The patient should check that the string is palpable each month after her menses. Between 2% and 10% of women expel their IUD within the first year.

2. **Ectopic pregnancy.** The absolute rate of ectopic pregnancy is reduced with the IUD because of its high contraceptive efficacy. However, when accidental pregnancy does occur, there is an increased incidence of ectopic pregnancy, which is highest with the Progestasert.

VI. Spermicides containing nonoxynol-9 destroy sperm cell walls and provide some protection against STDs but may increase the risk of HIV transmission. When used alone, the failure rate is relatively high. When spermicides are used with a condom, the failure rate is comparable to that of oral contraceptives and much better than for either spermicides or condoms alone. May cause vaginal irritation.

VII. Barrier Devices (Male condom, female condom, diaphragm, cervical cap, intravaginal sponge). These methods (especially male condoms) decrease the risk of STDs when used properly. Adverse effects include latex allergy and increased risk of UTI with diaphragm.

A. Condoms. Efficacy of condoms is improved when used with vaginal spermicide. Patient education is important to promote proper use. Remember that natural "skin" condoms are less effective at preventing transmission of HIV.

B. Diaphragm and cervical cap. Proper fitting is important. Carefully review product instructions with the patient: comfort with touching oneself, proper insertion technique, and correct use of contraceptive cream/jelly is required for maximum efficacy. Have the patient demonstrate insertion and removal in the office before prescribing. The cervical cap is not recommended for use in parous women. The diaphragm is a risk factor for UTIs.

C. Contraceptive sponge. Available without a prescription. Not recommended for parous women.

VIII. Lactational Amenorrhea. Full or nearly full breastfeeding (supplements given for less than 5%-15% of feeding episodes) is 98% effective for contraception during the first 6 months postpartum but is not reliable after 6 months. **Women who do not wish to become pregnant should use an additional contraceptive method during the entire postpartum period** but especially if bottle-feeding is increased.

IX. Periodic Abstinence during presumed fertile times requires long periods of abstinence. Highest failure rates are in women with irregular cycles.

X. Sterilization.

A. Both female and male sterilization are effective and permanent forms of birth control.

B. Female sterilization has a high initial cost and is performed under local or general anesthesia. It is associated with an increased risk of ectopic pregnancy should pregnancy occur. When performed immediately following delivery or abortion, the health risks are minimized. Failure can occur due to pregnancy at the time of sterilization, tube reanastomosis, fistula formation, equipment failure, or surgical error. Overall failure rate in 10 years is up to 3.2% with laparoscopic procedures. Surgical reversibility is limited and expensive, so sterilization should be considered permanent. Careful patient counseling beforehand is essential.

C. Male sterilization costs less than half as much as female sterilization and is less invasive. The procedure is performed under local anesthesia. A waiting period after vasectomy is required to clear the reproductive tract of sperm.

TABLE 13-2
OPTIONS FOR POSTCOITAL CONTRACEPTION*

Brand	Pills per Dose
Plan B: levonorgestrel (most effective, best tolerated)	1 pill
Levlen	4 light-orange pills
Lo/Ovral	4 white pills
Triphasil	4 yellow pills
Preven	2 pills
Tri-Levlen	4 yellow pills
Ovral	2 white pills
Alesse	5 pink pills
Ovrette	20 yellow pills
Nordette	4 light-orange pills

*All regimens are 2 doses, 12 h apart.
Adapted from Hatcher RA, Trussell J, Stewart F, et al: *Contraceptive Technology*,
18th rev ed. New York, Argent, 2004.

XI. **Emergency Contraception.**
A. **All female patients of reproductive age should be made aware of postcoital contraception (Table 13-2).** This knowledge does not increase the likelihood of high-risk behavior. A course of high doses of oral contraceptives begun within 72 hours of unprotected intercourse decreases the risk of pregnancy by 74%. Only RU-486 (mifepristone) has been shown to be effective after 72 hours; other regimens are unstudied but may be effective. Consider prescribing an antiemetic (e.g., prochlorperazine, metoclopramide), because nausea and vomiting are common side effects.
B. **Regimens.** See Table 13-2 for high-dose contraceptive regimens. **Mifepristone (RU-486) and levonorgestrel are the two most effective; levonorgestrel is as effective as mifepristone 10 mg within 48 hours. Although not approved for this indication, levonorgestrel 1.5 mg as a single dose is as effective as 0.75 mg taken 12 hours apart.** Mifepristone doses as low as 10 mg have been effective up to 5 days after unprotected intercourse.
C. For the drugs in Table 13-2, women should be instructed to take one dose as soon as possible after unprotected intercourse and a second dose 12 hours later. An antiemetic should be taken 1 hour before each dose. If a dose is vomited, the patient should contact the health care practitioner to obtain an additional dose. Patients should avoid unprotected intercourse and if there is no menses within 3 weeks, return for a pregnancy test.

VAGINAL, VULVAR, AND RELATED CONDITIONS

I. **Vestibulitis.** Inflammation, pain, and tenderness probably due to up-regulated nerve supply in the vestibular area.
A. **Etiology.** Although the true etiology is unknown, vulvar vestibulitis syndrome is strongly associated with candidal infection.

B. **Clinically** there is entry dyspareunia, erythema, and point tenderness of the vestibule, primarily at the base of the hymenal remnant.

C. **Treatment** may include long-term oral antifungal therapy, tricyclic antidepressants, topical estrogen, anesthetics or steroids, injectable steroids, or, more controversially, surgery. Mycolog-II (triamcinolone acetonide, nystatin) is often very effective.

II. **Vulvovaginitis.** All types of vaginitis can produce vulvar itch, irritation, dyspareunia, or dysuria. Evaluation includes history, exam, microscopic exam of secretions with saline and KOH (wet prep obtained from vaginal vault), and vaginal pH. Consider a UA to rule out UTI, and check cervical cultures for gonorrhea and chlamydia if indicated. Obtain a Pap smear if not done recently.

A. **Candidal vaginitis**

1. **Etiology.** *Candida albicans*, other *Candida* species (such as *glabrata*), *Torulopsis* species, other yeasts. Not generally sexually transmitted, although in refractory cases treatment of the partner may be needed. Precipitating factors include systemic antibiotic therapy, pregnancy, high-dose estrogen oral contraceptives, and tight-fitting undergarments. Recurrent infections can occur in uncontrolled diabetes and immunosuppression (HIV, corticosteroid use). Asymptomatic colonization does not require treatment.

2. **Discharge** is nonmalodorous, is thick and white, looks like cottage cheese, and adheres to vaginal walls.

3. **Diagnostic tests.** Wet mount: pseudohyphae or budding yeast cells. Wet mount is insensitive (65%-80%); if wet mount is negative, consider empiric treatment for typical pruritus without a watery discharge. Vaginal pH is normal (<4.5). Reserve fungal cultures for recurrent/resistant cases.

4. **Treatment**

a. **Vaginal suppositories** can be used at bedtime for 3 days: clotrimazole 200 mg, miconazole 200 mg, or terconazole 80 mg. Single-dose treatments are also available (e.g., miconazole 1200 mg).

b. **Vaginal creams** are used at bedtime for 7 days: clotrimazole 1% 5 g, miconazole 2% 5 g, or terconazole 0.4% 5 g.

c. **Oral.** One dose of fluconazole 150 mg PO is effective. Itraconazole 200 mg PO qd × 3 days may also be used.

d. **Recurrent or resistant cases** may require 10 to 14 days of topical or oral therapy, followed by suppressive therapy with clotrimazole 500 mg vaginal suppository or fluconazole 100 mg PO once weekly. Clotrimazole and miconazole are available OTC; terconazole is prescription and should be reserved for resistant disease. Encourage cotton underwear, avoid lubricants, avoid pantiliners, and evaluate the patient for diabetes and other immunosuppressing illnesses.

e. **In pregnancy,** use creams for 7 days and avoid oral therapy.

B. **Bacterial vaginosis**

1. **Etiology.** Bacterial vaginosis is much more common than previously thought. Polymicrobial (*Gardnerella vaginalis, Mycoplasma hominis,*

Prevotella, Mobiluncus, Bacteroides, etc.). Not generally considered sexually transmitted but is less common in virginal women. Treatment of male partner(s) does not reduce the rate of recurrence (although condom use does). **It is less common in women who are on OCPs than women who are not.** Bacterial vaginosis can lead to premature delivery, chorioamnionitis, and postpartum endometritis; however, it is not clear that treatment prevents these complications.

2. **Discharge.** Thin, white or dull gray, homogeneous malodorous discharge that adheres to the vaginal walls.
3. **Diagnostic tests.** Three of four criteria: Elevated pH (>4.5), positive whiff or amine test when KOH is applied to vaginal secretions, clue cells seen on saline wet mount, homogeneous discharge noted.
4. **Treatment**
a. **Oral: metronidazole** 500 mg PO bid for 7 days or 2 g PO as single dose; clindamycin 300 mg PO bid × 7 days.
b. **Vaginal: metronidazole** 0.75% gel 5 g per vagina bid × 5 days or clindamycin 2% cream per vagina qhs × 7 days.
c. **Pregnancy.** During the first trimester avoid oral therapy; use vaginal metronidazole (avoid vaginal clindamycin—higher rate of preterm delivery), but treatment probably does not prevent preterm labor. After the first trimester, use metronidazole 250 mg PO bid for 7 days or 2 g PO as a single dose, or use clindamycin PO as above.

C. Trichomonas vaginitis
1. **Etiology** is *Trichomonas vaginalis*, a sexually transmitted protozoan.
2. **Discharge** is copious, yellow-gray or green, foamy, and malodorous.
3. **Diagnostic tests.** Elevated pH (>4.5). Presence of mobile, flagellated organisms and leukocytes on wet mount.
4. **Treatment**
a. **Metronidazole** 2 g PO as a single dose, or 500 mg PO bid × 7 days. **Treat partner as well.** Vaginal metronidazole is not effective. For multiple treatment failures (reinfection excluded) use metronidazole 2 g PO qd × 3 to 5 days.
b. **Pregnancy.** During the first trimester, use clotrimazole 100 mg vaginal tabs qhs for 2 weeks. Then re-treat in the second trimester with the 7-day metronidazole regimen.

D. Contact irritant/allergic vaginitis. Itching, burning, soreness, variable discharge, with or without erythema. By definition, an evaluation for other etiologies is negative.
1. **Etiology.** Obtain a careful history to identify the offending agent, such as menstrual pads, chemicals (soaps, laundry detergent, spermicides, perfumes, feminine hygiene products, etc.), latex condoms, antifungal creams.
2. **Treatment.** Avoid the irritant; use bicarbonate sitz baths, topical vegetable oil. Avoid corticosteroids, which cause burning and atrophy.

E. Atrophic vaginitis predominantly occurs in postmenopausal women; it can also occur during lactation or with progesterone-only contraceptives.

GYNECOLOGY **13**

1. **Clinically,** epithelium has few rugae and is inflamed and dry, producing itching, dyspareunia, spotting, and urinary symptoms. Patients may have significant vaginal hemorrhage, especially elderly women. Vaginal pH is generally 5 to 7. Wet mount may show increased cocci and coliforms, small round parabasal cells, PMNs, and absence of lactobacilli.

2. **Treatment is estrogen,** either oral HRT or topical estradiol 0.01% cream 2 to 4 g daily for 1 to 2 weeks, then half the dose for 1 to 2 weeks, and maintenance dose 1 g one to three times per week. Another option is conjugated estrogen cream 2 to 4 g daily (3 weeks on, 1 week off) for 3 to 6 months. If estrogen is contraindicated, patient may use glycerin/mineral oil preparations (Replens) symptomatically. If symptoms do not resolve with hormone or antifungal therapy, biopsy is indicated.

F. **Chronic purulent vaginitis** has been reported. It is an exudative vaginitis with purulent discharge and an elevated vaginal pH due to replacement of normal flora with gram-positive cocci. Occasionally there is a spot-like vaginal rash. Responds to clindamycin cream.

III. **Cervical Infections.** Most commonly *Neisseria gonorrhoeae* and *Chlamydia trachomatis*.

A. **Symptoms range** from none to mucopurulent cervicitis; patient may have associated urethritis or infection of Bartholin's glands.

B. **Evaluation.** Pelvic exam: Look for purulent yellow or green cervical discharge, check for >10 WBC/HPF on cervical smear, and check Gram stain for gram-negative intracellular diplococci (GC). Cervical cultures for GC/chlamydia should be done. Consider a Pap smear if none has been done recently.

C. **Collecting specimens.** Collect cervical culture for gonococcus culture first, because this organism will be found in the mucus. Endocervical cells are needed to culture for *Chlamydia*, which is intracellular. For both specimens use an endocervical swab held in the cervix for 30 seconds. Twirling the *Chlamydia* swab will increase yield. See Chapter 8 for treatment.

D. **Routine screening is recommended in high-risk groups such as sexually active teens and women younger than 25 years or with new or multiple sexual partners.** DNA-based screening tests of vaginal secretions or urine specimens are also available.

IV. **Urethritis.** Causes for urethritis with negative UA include low colony-count UTI (up to 30% of culture-proven UTIs have a negative UA), *N. gonorrhea, C. trachomatis, Mycoplasma* species, *Ureaplasma urealyticum, T. vaginalis*, herpes simplex, *Candida*, interstitial cystitis, contact sensitivity (to soaps, feminine hygiene products, latex condoms, spermicides, etc.). PCR of voided urine can detect *Chlamydia*. See Chapter 8 for more information.

V. **Proctitis and proctocolitis** can also be caused by sexually transmitted infections such as *N. gonorrhoeae, C. trachomatis*, and HSV when receptive anal intercourse or oral–anal contact is practiced.

VI. **Syphilis, Genital Herpes Simplex, and other STDs.** See Chapter 8.

PELVIC INFLAMMATORY DISEASE

I. **General.** PID is an infection that can involve the uterus, fallopian tubes, ovaries, and pelvic cavity and can produce tubo-ovarian abscesses.

II. **Pathogenesis.** PID is usually sexually transmitted but can occur after uterine instrumentation. It is often polymicrobial, with ascending infection initiated by *N. gonorrhoeae* or *C. trachomatis* and secondary infection by other organisms including *Mycoplasma* species, *U. urealyticum, Bacteroides, Enterobacteriaceae, Streptococci*, gram-negative enterics, and other anaerobes.

III. **Predisposing Factors.** Multiple sexual partners, nonbarrier contraceptive use (especially IUD), transvaginal instrumentation of cervix and uterus, recent menstrual period, douching, current STD infection, and history of PID.

IV. **Diagnosis.**

A. **Differential diagnosis.** Appendicitis, ectopic pregnancy, septic abortion, endometriosis, hemorrhagic corpus luteum, ovarian cyst, adnexal torsion, inflammatory bowel disease, mesenteric lymphadenitis, pyelonephritis, or other intra-abdominal processes. See discussion of acute abdomen in Chapter 15 for a more complete discussion of abdominal and pelvic pain.

B. **Evaluation.** Abdominal and complete pelvic exam. Obtain UA, CBC, pregnancy test, Gram stain of cervical discharge, and appropriate cultures: endocervix, rectum, urethra, blood, and peritoneal fluid as indicated. Obtain Pap smear if none recently.

C. **Criteria for diagnosis**

1. **Primary criteria for treatment:** Uterine tenderness *or* adnexal tenderness *or* cervical motion tenderness and no other pathology that explains the symptoms. **The primary criteria alone are sufficient to treat for PID!!**

2. **Secondary criteria used to confirm the diagnosis:**

a. Temperature greater than 38.5°C (101°F).

b. Abnormal vaginal discharge (mucopurulent).

c. Adnexal mass on bimanual exam or ultrasonography.

d. WBC >10,500/mm^3.

e. Elevated ESR or CRP.

f. Endocervical Gram stain with gram-negative intracellular diplococci, positive rapid assay for *Chlamydia*, or other documentation of GC or *Chlamydia* infection.

g. Diagnostic laparoscopy or endometrial histology.

V. **Treatment. Because of the risk of infertility, treat all patients meeting the primary criteria presumptively while awaiting cultures even if no secondary criteria are met.**

A. **Outpatient therapy** if temperature is less than 38°C, WBC less than 11,000/mm^3, minimal signs of peritonitis, active bowel sounds, able to tolerate PO medication, and good compliance likely. **Note that fluoroquinolone-resistant gonorrhea is becoming more common and**

fluoroquinolones should not be used if this is a problem locally (certainly in Asia or California or people infected in these locations).

1. **Ofloxacin 400 mg PO bid for 14 day or levofloxacin** 500 mg daily for 14 days *plus* metronidazole 500 mg PO bid for 14 days. Alternative: Ofloxacin as above *plus* clindamycin 450 mg PO qid for 14 days or ceftriaxone 250 mg IM once *plus* doxycycline 100 mg PO bid for 14 days with or without metronidazole. Reevaluate in 48 to 72 hours. May also elect IV therapy.
2. **Single-dose azithromycin is not adequate therapy for chlamydia in the setting of PID.**
B. **Inpatient therapy** if suspected abscess, pregnancy, temperature greater than 38°C, WBC greater than $11,000/mm^3$, patient is unable to take PO medication, peritonitis, no response to oral antibiotics within 48 hours, unclear diagnosis, or inability to comply with outpatient treatment and follow-up. Some authorities admit all adolescents with PID.
1. **Cefotetan** 2 g IV q12h plus doxycycline 100 mg IV/PO q12h or cefoxitin 2 g IV q6h plus doxycycline 100 mg IV/PO q12h until improvement. Follow with doxycycline 100 mg PO bid to complete 14 days.
2. **In IUD-related infection,** suspected abscess, or procedure-related infection: Remove IUD; clindamycin 900 mg IV q8h plus gentamicin loading dose 2 mg/kg IV followed by gentamicin 1.5 mg/kg q8h until improvement. (Adjust gentamicin dose in renal insufficiency. Can also use single daily gentamicin dosing.) Adding ampicillin 1 g IV q6h to clindamycin and gentamicin appears to improve efficacy in the setting of abscess. Alternative: ofloxacin 400 mg IV q12h plus metronidazole 500 mg IV q8h. Follow as outpatient with doxycycline 100 mg PO bid or clindamycin 450 mg PO qid to complete 14 days; follow-up in 7 days.
VI. **Complications.** Infection rarely remains confined to fallopian tubes, and peritonitis is common. Acute complications include rupture of tubo-ovarian abscess, adnexal torsion, Fitz-Hugh-Curtis syndrome (perihepatic GC) and septicemia. Long-term complications include an increased risk of ectopic pregnancy (6-10 ×), infertility (20%), and bowel obstruction secondary to adhesions.

BARTHOLIN'S GLAND

I. **General.** Bartholin's glands are pea-sized organs situated at the 5 and 7 o'clock positions of the vaginal introitus. When normal they are nonpalpable. A Bartholin gland can become enlarged from cystic dilation, abscess, or adenocarcinoma (generally in women younger than 40 years).
II. **Cystic dilation of the Bartholin duct** can result from trauma or inflammation. These cysts are usually asymptomatic, and in women younger than 40 years they generally do not require treatment. Symptomatic cysts can be treated with placement of a Word catheter for 4 weeks or marsupialization. In women older than 40 years there is a

small incidence of adenocarcinoma in Bartholin's gland, which can be evaluated with drainage and selective biopsy. Try to avoid surgical treatment during pregnancy for uninfected cysts.

III. Bartholin's gland abscess is a polymicrobial infection accompanied by severe dyspareunia, vulvar pain, difficulty walking or sitting, erythema, edema, and possibly cellulitis of the surrounding tissue.

A. Etiology includes *B. fragilis, N. gonorrhoeae, Bacteroides* species, *Peptostreptococcus, E. coli, Proteus*, and *Klebsiella*.

B. Treatment includes hot soaks, pain medication, and antibiotics if surrounding cellulitis is present. Abscesses may spontaneously rupture and drain after 4 or 5 days or may require surgical drainage. A GC culture should be obtained (present in 20%). Antibiotics should be directed against gram negative species and anaerobes (e.g., amoxicillin–clavulanate or metronidazole plus TMP–SMX). IV combinations include metronidazole plus gentamicin, amoxicillin–clavulanate, etc.

C. Further management. Abscesses tend to recur after simple incision and drainage, so placement of a Word catheter for 4 to 6 weeks or marsupialization is recommended. The gland should be excised if the abscess reforms on multiple occasions.

GYNECOLOGY 13

ABNORMAL VAGINAL BLEEDING, MENSTRUAL PROBLEMS, AND SECONDARY AMENORRHEA

See also the discussion of endometrial abnormalities later.

I. Terminology. Menorrhagia is heavy or prolonged bleeding. **Metrorrhagia** is intermenstrual bleeding, spotting, or breakthrough bleeding. **Menometrorrhagia** is heavy irregular bleeding. **Polymenorrhea** is menstrual interval less than 21 days. **Oligomenorrhea** is menstrual interval greater than 35 days. **Amenorrhea** is absence of menstrual bleeding.

II. Evaluation.

A. History. Ascertain bleeding history (timing, duration, flow, presence of clots, number of pads used). Obtain menstrual and obstetric history, sexual history, drug and medication use, familial bleeding disorders and bleeding tendencies, contraceptive use, postcoital bleeding (may indicate cervicitis, cervical polyp), galactorrhea, headaches (e.g., from prolactinoma), visual disturbances, menopausal symptoms, change in weight, diet, exercise, stressors.

B. Physical exam. Look for obesity or low body weight, acne, hirsutism, and cushingoid habitus. Do thyroid exam, check skin for petechiae and ecchymoses. Do breast exam; pelvic exam noting vaginal or cervical lesions, uterine size and shape, adnexal masses. Exclude rectal source of bleeding. Obtain Pap if none done recently.

C. Initial lab tests. Pregnancy test, CBC (for anemia, platelet count), free T_4/TSH, GC and *Chlamydia* cultures if sexually active. As indicated: PT, PTT, FSH, and LH (elevated ratio of FSH/LH greater than 3:1

suggests PCOS; see discussion below), prolactin, UA (for microscopic hematuria) and androgens (testosterone, DHEA-S), 24-hour urinary free cortisol, liver/kidney function tests. Pelvic ultrasound of palpable mass. Consider endometrial biopsy especially patient is if older than 35 years or is obese with more than 12 months anovulatory bleeding.

III. Causes.

A. Dysfunctional uterine bleeding is usually associated with anovulatory cycles and patchy asynchronous sloughing of estrogen-stimulated endometrium due to tonic hormone levels rather than cyclically fluctuating gonadotropins and sex hormones. Common causes include puberty, perimenopause, stress, weight loss (anorexia, athletes), PCOS, and simple obesity. In obesity and PCOS, chronic anovulation results in long-term unopposed estrogen exposure, increasing the risk of endometrial hyperplasia or carcinoma. Failure to establish regular menses at puberty or prolonged absence of regular cycles from weight loss can lead to loss of bone mass. (Female athlete's triad: anorexia nervosa, anovulation, osteoporosis.)

B. Other endocrinopathies include hypothyroidism or hyperthyroidism, hyperprolactinemia, androgen-producing adrenal disorders.

1. Hyperprolactinemia is most commonly caused by microadenoma of the pituitary but may also be due to hypothyroidism or antipsychotics or other medication. Patient may have headaches or visual symptoms. Check TSH and free T_4. High-resolution CT of the sella turcica or MRI are the imaging studies of choice. Refer appropriately if imaging is abnormal or, if normal, follow prolactin every 6 months and CT or MRI every 1 to 2 years.

2. Microadenomas can be treated with bromocriptine, pergolide, or cabergoline (all about 90% effective). Prolactin level should respond in 2 to 3 weeks. Consider tapering or withdrawing drugs after patient has had normal prolactin for 1 year. Some will recur but many remain normal.

C. Structural lesions: cervical polyps, endometrial polyps, leiomyomas. Submucosal fibroids are present in a significant fraction of women with postmenopausal bleeding.

D. Malignant lesions: vaginal or cervical neoplasm; endometrial hyperplasia or carcinoma; estrogen-producing ovarian neoplasms.

E. Coagulopathies. Most common is von Willebrand's disease. Also consider leukemia and thrombocytopenia (see Chapter 6).

F. Pregnancy-related bleeding can be caused by ectopic pregnancy, threatened abortion, molar pregnancy, abruptio placentae, placenta previa, implantation of blastocyst.

G. Infections: chlamydia, chronic cervicitis, chronic endometritis.

H. Miscellaneous: atrophic vaginitis, bleeding during ovulation, hormone contraceptive–related breakthrough bleeding, IUD use, some herbal drugs (ginseng), foreign object, trauma, severe organ dysfunction (renal, liver).

IV. **Treatment.**

A. **Ovulatory menorrhagia** (heavy menstrual bleeding). NSAIDs will decrease menstrual bleeding. Treat with maximum dose of NSAID (ibuprofen, naproxen, etc.) beginning 1 or 2 days before menses. Combination oral contraceptives are another option to decrease menstrual bleeding. In refractory cases, consider progestin IUD (Progestasert, Mirena).

B. **Acute management of dysfunctional uterine bleeding**

1. **Severe bleeding requiring inpatient therapy** (symptomatic, Hb <10, hypotension, etc.) may require IV fluid resuscitation and blood transfusion. Use conjugated estrogen 25 mg IV q4h until bleeding abates or for 12 hours followed by conjugated estrogen 1.25 mg PO qd for 7 days. Antiemetics will help with nausea. After 7 days of estrogen, induce withdrawal bleed with medroxyprogesterone acetate 10 mg PO qd for 7 to 10 days. On day 5 of withdrawal bleeding begin low-dose OCP. Options for refractory hemorrhage include intrauterine tamponade with inflatable catheter, D&C, endometrial ablation, hypogastric artery ligation or embolization, and hysterectomy.

2. **Major bleeding not requiring inpatient therapy.** May use conjugated estrogen 1.25 mg or estradiol 2.0 mg PO qd for 7 to 10 days (for severe bleeding, dose q4h initially for 24 h). Prescribe antiemetics. Follow with medroxyprogesterone acetate 10 mg PO qd for 7 to 10 days, then low-dose OCPs.

3. **Moderate bleeding.** Use any combined progestin–estrogen OCP, one active pill qid for 7 days (1.5 packs, avoid placebo pills). Prescribe antiemetics. Expect cessation of flow in 12 to 24 hours. Heavy withdrawal flow with cramping will start 2 to 4 days after regimen is completed. On day 5 of withdrawal flow, begin daily low-dose combination OCP or use medroxyprogesterone acetate 10 mg qd for 10 days each month for at least 3 months.

4. **Mild bleeding.** Use medroxyprogesterone acetate 5 to 10 mg PO qd for 10 to 14 days to induce a coordinated withdrawal bleed ("medical curettage"). Expect heavy but limited bleed to begin within 5 days afterward. If withdrawal bleed does not occur, further work-up is indicated. After the induced withdrawal bleed, if spontaneous cycles do not resume, treat as next for long-term management. Persistent abnormal bleeding requires reevaluation.

5. **Long-term management of dysfunctional uterine bleeding.** If regular cycles do not resume, induce cycles with combined OCPs, especially if contraception is needed. Alternatively, use medroxyprogesterone acetate 5-10 mg qd for 10 days monthly (or at least every 3 months). Either treatment prevents endometrial hyperplasia.

6. **Management of perimenopausal bleeding.** Work-up is usually not needed for a single anovulatory cycle. Determine menopause status by checking an FSH and treat as per dysfunctional uterine bleeding above. Avoid long-term OCP use in smokers over 35, but they may be used in

GYNECOLOGY 13

nonsmoking, healthy patients premenopausally to prevent dysfunctional uterine bleeding (see section on contraception above for contraindications). Recurrent irregular bleeding should be evaluated with an endometrial biopsy or D&C to exclude endometrial hyperplasia or carcinoma. This can be followed by hysteroscopy looking for other organic lesions (polyps, submucosal fibroids) if bleeding continues.

7. **Management of postmenopausal bleeding.** Mild spotting may be observed on initiation of HRT. Otherwise, postmenopausal bleeding always requires complete evaluation for endometrial hyperplasia or carcinoma, with endometrial biopsy or D&C followed by hysteroscopy if bleeding continues. Alternatively, an endovaginal ultrasound showing an endometrial stripe of less than 5 mm excludes endometrial carcinoma with sensitivity close to 100% and specificity 75% (although in the editors' opinion, an endometrial biopsy should be done if there is any question). Biopsy is required if stripe is 5 mm or greater. The specificity is markedly reduced in women on HRT because of the resulting increase in endometrium. The same contraindications for OCPs should be considered. For bleeding due to atrophic endometrium, start HRT, or if already on HRT increase the estrogen component by 50% to 100% for 3 months. For bleeding due to proliferative endometrium, start HRT, or if already on HRT increase the progestin component by 50% to 100%.

8. **Less-common therapies.** Persistent bleeding may require prolonged therapy. Depending on the underlying problem, some possible treatments include progestin IUD (chronic illness, renal failure), desmopressin (coagulopathies, renal failure), and GnRH agonists (blood dyscrasias, renal failure, transplant patients).

V. Secondary amenorrhea is defined as absence of menses for at least 3 to 6 months in a previously menstruating woman. Primary amenorrhea (patient has never menstruated) has a different differential and work-up.

A. Causes include pregnancy and hypothalamic anovulation. Hypogonadotropism or hypothalamic-related amenorrhea manifests with a low LH (<0.5 IU/mL), which can be the result of weight loss, anorexia, or stress. Also recent discontinuation of hormonal contraceptives, physiologic menopause, premature ovarian failure, hyper- or hypothyroidism, hyperprolactinemia, PCOS, ovarian or adrenal tumor, uterine outflow tract abnormality. Failure to maintain an adequate weight (e.g., in anorexia or the female athlete) is an important cause of secondary amenorrhea.

B. History and exam as above for abnormal vaginal bleeding. Consider endometrial biopsy if patient is amenorrheic for longer than 12 months.

C. Initial lab tests. Pregnancy test in all reproductive-age patients with amenorrhea, regardless of reported sexual history or tubal ligation. Serum prolactin, TSH/free T_4. (May elect to check FSH and LH as well with initial labs.) If serum prolactin is high, see discussion of hyperprolactinemia above.

D. If pregnancy test is negative, evaluation begins with a progestin challenge test. Give medroxyprogesterone acetate 10 mg qd for 5 days.

Withdrawal bleeding within 7 days indicates ovaries are secreting estrogen and rules out premature ovarian failure.

E. Diagnosis and further evaluation depend on above results.

1. Positive progestin challenge. Expected withdrawal bleed indicates sufficient endogenous estrogen is present. If patient has a normal prolactin level and no galactorrhea, pituitary tumor is effectively ruled out.

a. **Differential includes** hypothalamic (idiopathic, e.g., stress, weight loss) anovulation or PCOS or ovarian or adrenal tumors if hirsute.

b. **Treatment in those with idiopathic anovulation and PCOS.** Induce cycles with combined OCPs, especially if contraception is needed. Alternatively, use medroxyprogesterone acetate 10 mg qd for 10 days, monthly or at least every 3 months to prevent endometrial hyperplasia. If fertility is desired, treat with clomiphene citrate. See also section on PCOS.

2. Negative progestin challenge. No withdrawal bleeding and normal prolactin level indicates either insufficient estrogen or outflow tract abnormality.

a. **Next step** is estrogen/progestin challenge test: Give conjugated estrogen 1.25 mg PO qd for 21 days, with medroxyprogesterone acetate 10 mg qd during the last 5 days.

b. **Positive estrogen/progestin challenge test.** Expected withdrawal bleed occurs. Check FSH and LH more than 2 weeks after challenge test.

(1) **FSH and LH high** indicates premature ovarian failure. Evaluate for systemic causes and start hormone replacement if appropriate. (See section on menopause.)

(2) **FSH and LH normal or low** indicates pituitary or hypothalamic dysfunction. Evaluate for pituitary tumor and start hormone replacement. (See section on menopause.)

c. **Negative estrogen/progestin challenge test: no withdrawal bleed occurs.** May repeat once to confirm result. Differential includes Asherman's syndrome (uterine synechiae) if history of D&C; other outflow tract abnormalities.

ENDOMETRIAL ABNORMALITIES

See also the previous section on abnormal uterine bleeding.

I. Endometritis.

A. Puerperal endometritis (see Chapter 14).

B. Acute endometritis is a component of PID (see earlier discussion of PID).

C. Chronic endometritis is often asymptomatic except for intermenstrual bleeding, menorrhagia, or postcoital bleeding. Patients may complain of a dull, heavy discomfort.

1. Diagnosis is made by endometrial biopsy showing inflammation with plasma cells. Culture endometrial and cervical specimens for chlamydia and gonorrhea. Check wet mount for bacterial vaginosis.

2. Treatment. Doxycycline 100 mg PO bid for 10 days. If bacterial vaginosis is also present, include anaerobic coverage as well.

3. **IUD-associated chronic *Actinomyces* infection can occur** or *Actinomyces* may be noted on routine Pap smear. Remove IUD.
4. Tuberculous endometritis is rare today.

II. Endometrial Polyps.

A. Bleeding due to polyps may respond to hormone therapy or NSAIDs.

B. Malignant transformation is rare but can occur.

C. Polypectomy can be done at the time of diagnostic hysteroscopy.

III. Endometrial Hyperplasia and Adenocarcinoma.

A. Spectrum. Hyperplasia may be simple (including cystic hyperplasia), complex (adenomatous without atypia), or atypical (atypical adenomatous). **Atypical hyperplasia progresses to adenocarcinoma in about 25% of cases.**

B. Signs and symptoms of endometrial hyperplasia and adenocarcinoma. Most women present with prolonged, heavy, or intermenstrual bleeding and are older than 40 years or postmenopausal. The probability that postmenopausal bleeding is caused by an endometrial carcinoma increases with the patient's age. The presence of atypical glandular cells (AGCUS) on a Pap smear also suggests an endometrial problem. Women receiving hormone replacement therapy who have regular withdrawal bleeding in response to exogenous progestins do not require scheduled monitoring with endometrial biopsy.

C. Risk factors include chronic anovulation (as in PCOS), obesity (increased conversion of androstenedione to estrone by adipose tissue aromatase), unopposed exogenous estrogen use, diabetes mellitus, nulliparity, late menopause, and hypertension.

D. Diagnosis. Diagnose with office endometrial biopsy, D&C, or hysteroscopy. In postmenopausal women, a transvaginal pelvic ultrasound can effectively exclude hyperplasia or cancer if the endometrial stripe measures less than 5 mm; however, many women have a thicker endometrial stripe and require biopsy.

E. Treatment

1. **Simple hyperplasia.** The risk of malignancy is low. Treatment is with progesterone, induction of regular endometrial shedding, D&C, or observation.
2. **Complex hyperplasia.** Risk of malignancy is slightly higher. Treatment is with intermittent or continuous progestin.
3. **Atypical hyperplasia.** Often total abdominal hysterectomy and bilateral salpingo-oophorectomy is performed. High-dose progestin therapy is an alternative in poor surgical candidates or if fertility is desired, but endometrial surveillance is necessary to watch for progression to cancer.
4. **Endometrial carcinoma.** Total abdominal hysterectomy and bilateral salpingo-oophorectomy plus adjuvant radiation. Should be coordinated with GYN oncology.

DYSMENORRHEA

I. Characteristics and Etiology.

A. Primary dysmenorrhea is defined as menstrual pain in the absence of pelvic pathology, resulting from excessive prostaglandin production. The onset is usually before age 20. Pain is crampy and spasmodic in the lower abdomen or back and begins within a day of onset of flow, lasts 24 to 72 hours, and may be associated with headache, fatigue, nausea, vomiting, diarrhea, thigh pain, and dizziness. Primary dysmenorrhea usually improves after childbirth.

B. Secondary dysmenorrhea is defined as menstrual pain associated with pelvic pathology. Secondary dysmenorrhea usually has an onset after age 20, progresses with age, and is less characteristically timed with menses. Causes include endometriosis, leiomyomas, endometrial cancer, IUD use, polyps, PID, cervical stenosis, ovarian cysts, imperforate hymen or other obstructive malformation, and uterine synechiae.

II. Evaluation.

A. History. Past menstrual history, need for contraceptives, family history, review of systems, effect on daily activities or work, and psychologic effect.

B. Exam. Pelvic exam; rectovaginal exam for uterosacral nodules.

C. Lab tests. Not usually necessary. If indicated by H&P, consider Pap smear, cultures, wet mount. Endometrial biopsy, ultrasonography, or laparoscopy may be useful, especially in diagnosing secondary dysmenorrhea.

III. Treatment.

A. Primary

1. Reassurance

2. **NSAIDs.** Ibuprofen 400 to 800 mg PO tid; naproxen 500 mg PO bid. Mefenamic acid 500 mg initially and then 250 mg PO tid may be especially effective. Start 3 days before expected menses and continue until flow stops. Reassess the need for medications in 1 year.

3. **Combination OCPs.** Three-month trial; continue if effective.

4. If no response, look for organic cause. Consider laparoscopy.

B. Secondary. Treat underlying cause.

PREMENSTRUAL SYNDROME

I. General. PMS is a constellation of physical, emotional, and behavioral symptoms occurring during the second half of the menstrual cycle (luteal phase, 7 to 10 days before menses), with resolution of symptoms soon after flow begins. There must be a symptom-free interval of at least 1 week during the first half (follicular phase) of the menstrual cycle to diagnose PMS. PMS affects 90% of women minimally and 10% severely. It affects primarily those in late 20s to

13

GYNECOLOGY

early 30s without racial, socioeconomic, or other demographic predilection. Hysterectomized patients can still experience PMS if at least one ovary is present.

II. **Diagnosis is clinical.** DSM-IV criteria for premenstrual dysphoric disorder are listed in **Box 13-1.**

III. **Variability in symptoms can be wide.** PMS may be diagnosed even if all criteria for PMDD are not met. Additional symptoms such as flatulence, constipation, diarrhea, sore throat, palpitations, urinary symptoms, dizziness, and others may be present.

IV. **Symptom calendar is helpful in documenting cyclicity and in monitoring response to therapy.**

V. **Causes** are multifactoral including physiologic changes and psychosocial factors (e.g., coexisting stressors).

VI. **Treatment.**

A. **Validation.** The symptoms are not "all in her head." Consider support groups.

B. **Regular aerobic exercise** helps both mood and somatic symptoms.

C. **Psychological therapy.** Stress management, relaxation therapy, and supportive psychotherapy.

D. **Diet.** Limit salt (fluid retention), caffeine (breast tenderness), alcohol, and fat. Increase complex carbohydrates and fiber. Consider vitamin B_6 50 mg PO tid, keeping in mind risk of peripheral neuropathy.

E. **Medications**

1. **Breast symptoms may respond to bromocriptine** 2.5 mg qhs or danazol 200 mg/day or bid.

BOX 13-1

DSM-IV CRITERIA FOR PREMENSTRUAL DYSPHORIC DISORDER (PMDD)

Five or more of the following symptoms, present for the majority of the past year and start the week before menses and resolve within a few days after menses, are required for a diagnosis of PMDD.

- At least one of the following:
  - Feeling sad, hopeless, or self-deprecating
  - Feeling tense, anxious, or on edge
  - Lability of mood with frequent tearfulness
  - Persistent irritability, anger, and increased interpersonal conflict
- Any number of the following:
  - Decrease in usual activities
  - Difficulty concentrating
  - Fatigue or lethargy
  - Changes in appetite (especially binging)
  - Hypersomnia or insomnia
  - Subjective feeling of being overwhelmed or out of control
  - Physical symptoms such as bloating, joint or muscle pain, breast tenderness, weight gain

2. **Antidepressants.** SSRIs (fluoxetine, sertraline, etc.) may be titrated to effect. Clomipramine 25 to 75 mg/day is also effective. Use only during the luteal phase if possible, but all month if necessary.
3. **Antianxiety medication** such as buspirone 5 to 10 mg PO tid is useful where anxiety predominates. Benzodiazepines have also been used but are addictive and should be used very cautiously. SSRIs have an antianxiety affect.
4. **Calcium** 1000 to 1200 mg daily (divide bid) or magnesium 400 IU PO qd during the luteal phase have both been shown to be effective in placebo-controlled trials.
5. **Diuretics.** Spironolactone 25 mg tid or qid during luteal phase (12 days before menses). Best for those with weight gain, bloating, and edema.
6. **Prostaglandin inhibitors.** Ibuprofen 400 to 800 mg tid, naproxen 500 mg PO bid, or mefenamic acid 500 mg tid 10 days before period through day 2 of menses have been shown to reduce the intensity of both the physical and emotional symptoms.
7. **Cycle suppression with oral contraceptives or Depo-Provera. Rarely, GnRH agonists are used.**
8. **Progesterone** 100 to 400 mg PO bid; vaginal or rectal suppository 200 to 400 mg/d during luteal phase. Medroxyprogesterone acetate 10 to 20 mg PO qd is another possibility.

CHRONIC PELVIC PAIN

See Chapter 15 for acute abdominal and pelvic pain.

I. **Characteristics.** Unpleasant sensation or discomfort in the lower abdomen or pelvis with a duration longer than 6 months, causing enough physical or psychological suffering to impair the quality of life. Patients usually report incomplete relief by most previous treatments, significantly impaired function at home or at work, signs of depression, pain out of proportion to pathologic condition, and altered family roles. **Many have a history of past sexual abuse.** In 5% of cases no identifiable somatic source of pain can be found.

II. **Sources of Noncyclic Pain.**

A. **Gynecologic disorders:** pelvic inflammatory disease, pelvic adhesions, and cervical stenosis.

B. **Musculoskeletal disorders:** Poor posture, scoliosis, unilateral standing habits, lumbar lordosis, leg-length discrepancy, abnormal gait, abdominal wall trigger points, history of low back trauma, and levator syndrome of pain/pressure in the perirectal area.

C. **Gastrointestinal tract disorders:** irritable bowel syndrome, chronic constipation, and diverticulitis.

D. **Urinary tract disorders:** chronic urethritis, detrusor instability, recurrent cystitis, and interstitial cystitis. Other unusual diagnoses may also provide a source of pain.

GYNECOLOGY 13

III. **Sources of Cyclic Pain.** Mittelschmerz, primary and secondary dysmenorrhea, endometriosis, adenomyosis, cervical stenosis, IUD, leiomyomas, PMS, obstructive uterine/vaginal malformation in adolescents.

IV. **Psychosocial factors.** Major depression or anxiety disorders, somatoform disorders, sexual or physical abuse, dissociation disorders, PTSD, marital stress, spouse response to patient's pain, familial model of handling pain.

V. **History.** Take a comprehensive history of the pain including cyclicity, association with sexual activity, pinpoint pain (trigger point), and associated GI (e.g., irritable bowel) or urologic symptoms including bowel and urinary habits. A pain diary may be helpful. Take a detailed sexual history including physical or sexual abuse. Screen for depression (Beck Depression Inventory, see Chapter 18), psychological response to pain and its effect on lifestyle, family, and friends, and previous abdominopelvic surgical procedures or episodes of PID.

VI. **Evaluation.**

A. **Physical examination** focuses on the abdomen and pelvis. The examiner should probe for abdominal wall trigger points and evaluate for musculoskeletal disorders and tenderness of the bladder, urethra, and other pelvic organs.

B. **Lab tests.** UA and urine culture, stool guaiac, Pap smear, cervical cultures. Laparoscopy, endoscopy, colonoscopy, barium enema if indicated. Patient-assisted laparoscopy under local anesthesia can provide "pain mapping."

VII. **Management.** If a pathologic cause of chronic pelvic pain is ruled out, provide symptomatic relief. Focus on breaking the biopsychosocial cycle of pain and disability. Try to manage rather than eliminate the pain (which is usually unlikely).

A. **Analgesics.** Use **scheduled dosing** of an NSAID (ibuprofen, naproxen) because prn dosing increases attention to pain. Avoid narcotics, which exacerbate dysmotility syndromes and are addictive.

B. **Trigger points can be injected** with 5 to 10 mL bupivacaine 0.25% to 0.5% (may mix with 40 mg triamcinolone). Repeat this every 2 to 4 weeks at first, followed by successively longer intervals until the nidus of pain resolves. Alternatives include TENS, acupuncture, and physical therapy.

C. **Antidepressants.** Low doses of tricyclic antidepressants (imipramine, amitriptyline, doxepin 10 to 25 mg, titrate to 75 mg if needed) taken at bedtime will decrease pain intensity, promote sleep, and reduce depressive symptoms. May exacerbate constipation. For treatment of major depression, consider using an SSRI in addition, or increasing the tricyclic. See Chapter 18 for further information.

D. **Functional bowel disorders.** Use daily psyllium supplements (6 g daily or more) with increased dietary fiber to reestablish normal bowel motility. Psychotherapy may be helpful. Use antispasmodics (dicyclomine) only after thorough GI evaluation.

E. **Psychological therapies.** Cognitive behavior therapy to control pain: relaxation techniques, stress management, and pain-coping strategies. Psychotherapy for mood disorders, eating disorders, abuse survivors, etc. Marital/family counseling, sex therapy, substance abuse treatment as indicated.

F. **Ovarian cycle suppression for cyclic pain.** Monophasic oral contraceptives, medroxyprogesterone acetate either injectable (Depo-Provera 150-300 mg q3mo) or oral (10-30 mg qd).

G. **Antibiotics if evidence of chronic endometritis, (positive cultures or endometrial biopsy), or for urethritis with pyuria.** See appropriate section for management.

H. **Surgical management.** Diagnostic laparoscopy, lysis of adhesions, uterine suspension, uterosacral nerve ablation, presacral neurectomy, hysterectomy (high recurrence rate of pain).

POLYCYSTIC OVARIAN SYNDROME

I. **General. New diagnostic criteria are based on a 2003 consensus meeting and require two out of three of the following: oligomenorrhea and/or anovulation, clinical and/or biochemical signs of hyperandrogenism, and polycystic ovaries by ultrasound.** This must occur in a patient in whom other etiologies are excluded (see differential diagnosis later).

II. **History.** Menstrual irregularities, usually of teenage onset (patients often state that they never have had regular menses), hirsutism, acne, family history of PCOS (50% chance of first-degree female relatives being affected), or type 2 diabetes.

III. **Physical.** The patient with PCOS is traditionally described as obese and with acne and excess body hair. However, not all patients with PCOS have these manifestations, and those with PCOS may be thin and have a fair complexion. Patients may have palpably enlarged ovaries. Virilization is uncommon (deepened voice, etc.)

IV. **Laboratory Evaluation.** Work-up menstrual irregularities as described under abnormal vaginal bleeding and secondary amenorrhea. LH/FSH ratio greater than 2 or 3 suggests PCOS. Testosterone and DHEA-S levels may be mildly elevated. Consider endometrial biopsy at any age for prolonged amenorrhea or oligomenorrhea, and especially if the patient is older than 35 years. Evaluate for T2DM if appropriate.

V. **Differential Diagnosis.** For hirsutism: late-onset adrenal hyperplasia, androgen-producing ovarian or adrenal tumors, Cushing's syndrome, drug-induced, idiopathic hirsutism. For menstrual irregularities, see discussions of abnormal vaginal bleeding and secondary amenorrhea.

GYNECOLOGY 13

VI. Sequelae.
A. Gynecologic: infertility, amenorrhea, dysfunctional uterine bleeding, increased risk of endometrial cancer, possible increased risk of breast cancer. Metformin may restore fertility.
B. Dermatologic: hirsutism, alopecia, acne.
C. Cardiovascular: lipid changes, increased risk of cardiovascular disease.
D. Endocrine: increased risk of insulin resistance leading to diabetes mellitus.
VII. Treatment. It is important that women with PCOS have menstrual periods at least every 3 or 4 months to reduce the risk of endometrial carcinoma.
A. Obesity. Weight loss may reduce hirsutism and reverse menstrual irregularities, infertility, and insulin resistance.
B. Menstrual irregularity and endometrial protection. Treat menstrual irregularity with medroxyprogesterone or OCPs if pregnancy is not desired. If pregnancy is desired, consider metformin or clomiphene.
C. Hirsutism. Weight loss, depilation, and electrolysis. Oral contraceptives may improve hirsutism (especially those with norgestimate). An alternative is Depo-Provera up to 400 mg IM every 3 months or medroxyprogesterone acetate 30 to 40 mg PO daily. **Spironolactone** is an antialdosterone diuretic and an antiandrogen that can be used alone or with hormones. Give up to 100 to 200 mg PO daily (or in two divided doses) initially, and reduce to maintenance dose of 25 to 50 mg qd after results are obtained. Monitor for hyperkalemia and use with effective contraception: Spironolactone could feminize a male fetus. Second-line agents have more adverse effects: flutamide, finasteride.
D. Insulin resistance. Metformin is useful to reduce insulin resistance, promote weight loss, induce ovulation, and prevent diabetes. Additionally, both rosiglitazone and pioglitazone can be used in women who don't tolerate metformin and are not seeking fertility.

PAP SMEARS AND CERVICAL DYSPLASIA

I. Pap Smear Schedule.
A. Women should have a **first Pap smear** 3 years after initiation of sexual intercourse but no later than age 21.
B. Annual Pap smears should be performed for women who are younger than 30 years, are immunocompromised (for HIV Pap 6 months apart × 2 after diagnosis, then annually), have DES exposure, or have a history of CIN 2 or CIN 3.
C. Women older than 30 years should have a Pap smear
1. Every 2 to 3 years if they have three consecutive exams with negative cervical cytology.
2. Every 3 years if cytology and HPV testing are both are negative and if they are low risk, in a mutually monogamous relationship,

have no STDs and no HPV, do not smoke, and have no DES exposure.

D. Women who have had hysterectomy that was not done for malignancy and women older than 70 years who have had three negative Pap smears **no longer need Pap smears.**

II. Abnormal Pap Smears. Patients should be aware that Pap smears are not 100% accurate, yet they provide the best way to screen for cervical cancer and precancerous lesions. New liquid-based cytology has increased sensitivity and increased specificity. Approach is dictated by Pap smear findings.

A. Pap reads "no endocervical cells present." Pap test is considered inadequate and should be repeated soon for high-risk patients (multiple partners, history of STDs, HPV, DES exposure, cervical dysplasia, or smoking). If patient is low risk, repeat within 6 months to 1 year.

B. Pap reads "unsatisfactory for evaluation." Repeat the Pap.

C. Pap reads "ASCUS" (atypical squamous cells of undetermined significance). Often reactive/reparative changes noted. Look for causative agent on wet mount or cultures and treat only if a specific organism is identified. Follow-up Pap as below.

1. **ASCUS.** HPV (human papillomavirus) reflex test is done. If HPV positive, proceed to colposcopy and endocervical Pap smear. If HPV negative, repeat Pap test every 6 months for 2 years, until four consecutive negative Pap results are obtained, then return to yearly Paps. Proceed to colposcopy at 1 year if ASCUS is persistent. Immediate colposcopy is indicated if the patient is not able to comply with follow-up Pap smears.

2. **ASC-H (favor high grade).** Proceed to colposcopy and endocervical Pap smear after the first abnormal Pap smear.

3. **ASCUS in a postmenopausal patient.** Atrophic cells may look like dysplastic cells. If atrophic, use intravaginal estrogen cream for 4 to 6 weeks and repeat the Pap smear. If still abnormal, proceed to colposcopy.

D. Pap reads "LGSIL/LSIL (low-grade squamous intraepithelial lesion, which encompasses HPV and CIN 1). Proceed to colposcopy and endocervical Pap smear. Repeat Pap every 6 months and repeat colposcopy for persistent ASCUS with HPV or greater dysplasia. For postmenopausal women, prescribe intravaginal estrogen cream for 4 to 6 weeks and repeat cytology 1 week after therapy.

E. Pap reads "HGSIL/HSIL" (high-grade squamous intraepithelial lesion, which encompasses CIN 2, CIN 3, CIS). Proceed to colposcopy and endocervical Pap smear.

F. Pap reads "AGCUS" (atypical glandular cells of undetermined significance)

1. **Reported as "AGCNOS."** Proceed to colposcopy with endocervical curettage. Include endometrial sampling if patient is older than 35 years or has abnormal bleeding.

2. **Reported as "atypical endometrial cells."** Do endometrial sampling.

3. **Reported as "AGC–FN (favor neoplasia.)"** Gynecology referral for cold-knife conization.

G. **Other indications for colposcopy.** Visible lesion (even if Pap is normal), squamous cell carcinoma, adenocarcinoma, HPV infection (cervical or external genitalia), persistent inflammation.

III. **All Women Should Have a Yearly Bimanual Pelvic Exam.**

IV. **Rectal exam** is done on women older than 50 for hemoccult testing and assessing for rectal masses (but a single negative stool does not count as colon cancer screening!).

V. **Colposcopy.**

A. **Colposcopy is satisfactory** if entire squamocolumnar junction (SCJ) is seen.

B. **Treatment** is based on cytology result of endocervical PAP smear, biopsy result, and if the entire SCJ is seen.

1. **If colposcopy is satisfactory, biopsy CIN 1 and do endocervical Pap smear for LGSIL.** Repeat Pap in 6 months, repeat colposcopy if greater than LGSIL. Repeat colposcopy with plan to treat if persistent at 12 months. Treat with ablation only if endocervical Pap smear is negative, the entire lesion is seen, and the entire transition zone can be destroyed; otherwise use LEEP excision.

2. **If colposcopy is unsatisfactory,** use LEEP as diagnostic excisional method.

3. **If colposcopy biopsy confirmed CIN 2 or CIN 3,** excise with LEEP.

4. **Follow-up**

a. If margins are LEEP positive, follow-up in 6 months with colposcopy and cytology.

b. If margins are LEEP negative, repeat cytology every 6 months until there are three consecutive negative Pap results.

INFERTILITY

I. **General.** Involuntary infertility is defined as the inability to conceive after one year of unprotected intercourse. Infertility affects 10% to 15% of couples. The use of medical services for infertility has increased because of delayed childbearing and an increased incidence of STDs and PID. Prevalence of infertility not significantly increasing.

A. **Average time to conception** is 3 months: 25% of normal couples conceive in the first cycle, 85% within 1 year.

B. **Acknowledge the emotional nature of the problem** and define infertility as a couple's shared concern. Inquire about partner responses.

II. **Common Major Problems.** Absolute infertility factors include azoospermia and bilateral tube obstruction. Other factors are anovulation (15%), male factors (35%), tubal and pelvic disease (35%), or a combination of these. Less common problems include cervical problems or immune infertility. Smoking decreases female fertility.

III. **Diagnostic Evaluation.**

A. **Thorough history and physical examination** of both male and female. Ask about menstrual history, obstetric history, previous children, prior contraceptives used, history of STDs or PID, pelvic surgery, cervical treatments, medications or herbs used. Determine coital frequency, sexual practices, and impotence or dyspareunia. Postcoital douches or lubricants such as K-Y or petroleum jelly can be spermicidal; therefore, recommend vegetable oil.

B. **Preconception evaluation to address risk factors before conception** (recommend daily prenatal vitamin for adequate folate). See Chapter 14.

C. **Semen analysis.** Because 35% of couples have some component of male factor infertility, a semen analysis should be one of the initial tests done. Collect after a 2- or 3-day period of abstinence in a glass container. Male causes for infertility include testicular disorders, varicocele, hypospadias, ductal obstruction, endocrine abnormalities, retrograde ejaculation, and genetic disorders (e.g., Klinefelter's syndrome).

1. **Normal semen analysis.** The 2001 criteria include sperm concentration of greater than 48×10^6/mL, sperm motility greater than 63%, normal morphology greater than 12%. Older WHO criteria include volume greater 2 mL, sperm count greater than 2×10^6/mL, motility greater than 50% with forward progression, normal morphology greater than 30% normal forms, WBC less than 10^6/mL.

2. **If semen analysis is normal,** look for female factors causing infertility.

3. **If pyospermia is present** (>1 million WBC/mL), search for and treat infections of urethra, epididymis, or prostate.

4. **If otherwise abnormal, repeat in 2 months.** If abnormalities persist, refer to urologist for further evaluation.

D. **Ovulation assessment**

1. **Symptoms of ovulation** (such as Mittelschmerz, PMS), length and regularity of menstrual cycle.

2. **Basal body temperature charting.** Should see a 0.4°F to 0.6°F (0.2°C-0.3°C) rise the day after ovulation that is sustained 11 to 16 days until menstruation due to progesterone production. To maximize the chances of conception, advise coitus every 36 to 48 hours from 4 days before ovulation until 2 days after. Temperature rise is often too late with ovulation to be useful.

a. **LH surge** precedes ovulation by 38 hours and can be detected by urinary testing kits. Test is positive when LH is greater than 40 IU/L. Clinical utility is estimated at 85%.

3. **Evaluate and treat menstrual abnormalities.**

a. **Amenorrhea.** Rule out premature ovarian failure (FSH >40 mg/mL and estradiol <40 pg/mL in the same sample).

b. **Oligomenorrhea with hirsutism or galactorrhea.** Suspect PCOS. Assess for hyperprolactinemia, and, if present, work up to exclude pituitary cause. If idiopathic hyperprolactinemia, treat with bromocriptine 2.5 mg qhs until BBT demonstrates ovulation. Dose can be increased

GYNECOLOGY 13

by 2.5 mg every 3 days until prolactin is normal with maximum daily dose 15 mg divided bid. If no ovulation in 2 to 3 months, add clomiphene. Hypothyroidism can be associated with hyperprolactinemia and should be evaluated and treated.

c. **Luteal phase defect** is described as poor production of progesterone or poor endometrial response to progesterone stimulation. Diagnosis by endometrial biopsy or serum progesterone levels is inexact. Fertile women may have a luteal phase defect, but it is more common in infertile women.

d. Endometrial biopsy is considered normal if assigned date from histology exam is within 2 days of actual date of ovulation determined by serum LH surge to be day 14.

e. Serum progesterone level on day 18 to 24 after onset of menses. Normal concentration is 6 to 25 ng/mL. If abnormal, recheck. (One value is not enough for diagnosis.)

E. Uterine factors. Hysterosalpingography, hysteroscopy, and pelvic ultrasound to evaluate for uterine septum, submucosal or cornual fibroid, polyps, synechiae, fibroids.

F. Tubal factors. Major infertility due to endometriosis, PID, ectopic pregnancy, adhesions from nontubal abdominopelvic surgery, IUD use. Hysterosalpingography and laparoscopy assess for tubal patency and identify uterine anomalies, fibroids, and synechiae. Laparoscopy is gold standard. Perform 2 to 6 days after end of menses and before ovulation to minimize possibility of disrupting pregnancy.

G. Endometriosis is diagnosed by laparoscopy if no cause is found after work-up as outlined

H. Infections of cervix. Ureaplasma and mycoplasma. Culture cervical mucus; treat both partners with doxycycline 100 mg PO bid for 7 days.

I. Cervical factors. Postcoital testing (testing relation with sperm and cervical mucus) has limited validity and is rarely used. Often leads to more testing and procedures and doesn't increase rates of pregnancy.

IV. Treatment.

A. Lifestyle change: cigarette smoking cessation, weight loss, decrease caffeine (2 cups of coffee per day max), decrease alcohol consumption.

B. Timed intercourse. To maximize the chances of conception, advise coitus every 36 to 48 hours from 4 days before ovulation until 2 days after.

C. Urinary ovulation kits to measure LH surge: LH surge precedes ovulation by 38 hours. The test is positive when the LH is higher than 40 IU/L. Conception is most likely with intercourse 24 to 48 hours before ovulation.

D. Idiopathic hyperprolactinemia. Bromocriptine 2.5 mg qhs until basal body temp demonstrates ovulation. Dose can be increased by 2.5 mg every 3 days until prolactin is normal, with maximum daily dose 15 mg divided bid. If no ovulation in 2 to 3 months, add clomiphene. Hypothyroidism can be associated with hyperprolactinemia and should be evaluated and treated.

E. **PCOS and insulin resistance.** Metformin 500 mg tid or 850 mg bid in combination with clomiphene has been shown in three randomized, controlled trials to induce ovulation.

F. **Ovulation induction if documented defect is found.**

1. **Clomiphene citrate** 50 mg qd for days 5 to 9 after either induced or spontaneous menses. Monitor for ovulation with BBT or ovulation kits to allow timing of intercourse. If ovulation fails to happen, in the next cycle the dose can be increased to 100 mg qd for the next cycle then by 50 mg each cycle to a maximum dose of 250 mg qd. **Side effects** include ovarian enlargement (14% women), cyst formation, pain, bloating and hot flushes (10%-20%), visual symptoms (1%-2%), mood swing, depression, headache. Five percent to 10% of patients have multiple gestation. Advise coitus every other day, for 1 week, beginning 5 days after the final dose of clomiphene (LH surge occurs 5-12 days after clomiphene administration).

2. **If ovulation does not occur** on maximal doses of clomiphene, or if a short luteal phase is noted, a single dose of **HCG 10,000 IU IM** should only be given when transvaginal ultrasound shows leading follicle 18 to 20 mm in diameter. Ovulation occurs 36 to 44 hours after injection.

3. **Human menopausal gonadotropins (HMG) menotropins or recombinant FSH** used for hypothalamic–pituitary insufficiency in clomiphene-resistant patients. Multiple gestations occur at rates higher than those with other ovulation regimens, and close monitoring of follicle production is required. Consultation is recommended (high cost and complication of therapy).

4. **For luteal phase defect:** supplemental vaginal progesterone suppositories 25 mg bid starting 3 days after ovulation. Continue until menses; if pregnancy occurs, continue until week 10 when placental progesterone is sufficient to support pregnancy.

5. **Unexplained infertility and male factor infertility** are treated in specialized centers with intrauterine insemination of washed sperm or in vitro fertilization (IVF), which encompasses gamete intrafallopian transfer (GIFT), intracytoplasmic sperm injection (ICSI), and other techniques. Success rates are generally around 50% after up to 6 cycles in women under 35.

ENDOMETRIOSIS

I. **Definition.** Endometriosis is the presence of functioning endometrial tissue outside its normal location. **Most common sites** (by decreasing frequency) are ovaries, anterior/posterior cul-de-sac, posterior broad ligament, uterosacral ligament, uterus, fallopian tubes, sigmoid, appendix, and round ligament. It can also occur elsewhere including breast, pancreas, urethra, lung (cyclic hemoptysis), and diaphragm. It is estrogen dependent (occurs during active reproductive period) and generally regresses after menopause or oophorectomy.

13

GYNECOLOGY

II. **Pathogenesis.** Several factors can play a role: retrograde transport and implantation of shed endometrial tissue, metaplastic transformation of "coelomic" peritoneum (theory that pelvic organs derived from cells lining peritoneal cavity), lymphatic or hematogenous dissemination, immunologic defects, genetic predisposition. and transplantation during pelvic surgery.

III. **Evaluation.**

A. **History**

1. **The most common symptoms associated with pelvic endometriosis are** dysmenorrhea (66%), deep dyspareunia (33%), infertility (60%), and low back pain or chronic pelvic pain that worsens with menses. Patient may have premenstrual spotting and menorrhagia. Dysmenorrhea often precedes menses and lasts throughout the period.

2. **Less common symptoms include** dyschezia (painful defecation), diarrhea, intermittent constipation, cyclic abdominal pain, dysuria, urinary frequency, and hematuria.

3. **One third of women with endometriosis are asymptomatic, and even extensive disease may be asymptomatic.**

B. **Physical examination**

1. Fifty percent of women with endometriosis have a normal clinical examination.

2. Findings will be accentuated in early menses and include tenderness when palpating posterior fornix, a fixed, tender, retroverted uterus or adnexa, tender nodules along the uterosacral ligaments (with obliteration of the cul-de-sac); nodules on the back of the uterus and cervix; unilateral or bilateral fixed asymmetric adnexal masses. Rectovaginal exam is important to assess the posterior uterus and cul-de-sac.

3. Up to 10% of teens with endometriosis have congenital outflow tract obstruction.

C. **Diagnostic aids**

1. **Optimal diagnosis is by direct visualization through laparoscopy.** Clinical diagnosis may be wrong 30% to 40% of the time. Laparoscopy will help assess stage of disease (views site and severity of involvement) and tubal patency.

2. **Ultrasound** may be helpful with a large pelvic mass but cannot visualize small implants or differentiate types of cystic lesions.

IV. **Classification and Management.** Medical treatment of endometriosis cannot restore fertility (see section on infertility) but may help with pain or dyspareunia. Pain recurs after treatment is stopped in 53%.

A. **Minimal disease.** Isolated implants and no significant adhesions. Treatment is expectant management, NSAIDs, or oral contraceptives.

B. **Mild disease.** Superficial implants less than 5 cm together, scattered on peritoneum and ovaries. No significant adhesions. Diagnosis will be suspected but not confirmed, because laparoscopy is usually not indicated. Treatment includes observation, NSAIDs and:

1. Combination oral contraceptives, given for at least 6 months. Response rate is 75%.
2. Depo-Provera 150 mg IM every 3 months. Return to fertility may be delayed after discontinuation.

C. Moderate disease. Multiple implants (superficial and invasive), peritubal and periovarian adhesions. Diagnosis should be confirmed by laparoscopy prior to initiating therapy.

1. **GnRH analogues** inhibit pituitary gonadotropins and suppress estrogen production, help relieve pain, and reduce size of endometrial implants. They do not enhance fertility. Nasal **nafarelin** 400 to 800 mg PO daily, **goserelin** 3.6 mg monthly SQ, **leuprolide** 3.75 mg IM monthly for 3 to 6 months. Side effects: hot flushes, vaginal dryness, decreased libido, insomnia, breast tenderness, depression, headaches, transient menstruation, loss in bone density. Response rate is 90%.
2. **Pseudomenopause.** Danazol and GnRH analogues together. **Danazol** is a synthetic androgen that suppresses gonadotropins, causes amenorrhea, and inhibits endometriotic implants. Side effects include atrophic vaginitis, weight gain, fluid retention, migraines, dizziness, fatigue, depression, decreased HDL, acne, hirsutism, and voice changes. Prescribe danazol 200 or 400 mg PO bid for up to 6 months. Begin on first day of menstruation. Patient must use a barrier contraceptive the first month; female fetuses may be adversely affected. Response rate is 84% to 92%.
3. **Pseudopregnancy.** Continuous oral contraceptives: use a standard monophasic formulation. Side effects as per OCP. Patient takes one active pill every day continuously, beginning on the third day of menstruation. When breakthrough bleeding occurs, increase to two pills daily for 5 days, then return to a single pill daily. May use up to 3 or 4 pills daily, although nausea may limit therapy. Maintain amenorrhea for 6 to 9 months; 80% of patients will experience improvement of symptoms.
4. **Progestin therapy** provides partial or complete relief in 80%. It involves inhibition of endometriotic tissue by causing decidualization and atrophy and inhibits ovarian hormone production. **Side effects** include breakthrough bleeding, depression, irritability, and lipid changes. Initiate therapy during menses. Progestins appear to be as effective as other treatments.
a. **Depo-Provera** 100 to 150 mg IM monthly and continued for 6 months to produce prolonged amenorrhea. Return to fertility may be delayed after discontinuation.
b. **Medroxyprogesterone** 10 mg PO tid or norethindrone acetate 5 mg daily for 6 months are alternatives.
5. **Conservative surgery to laparoscopically remove extrauterine endometrial tissue** is often performed at the time of laparoscopic

diagnosis. You may also use pharmacotherapy 6 weeks before to 3 to 6 months after surgery. Recurrence rate is 19% over 5 years.

D. Severe disease. Multiple superficial and invasive implants, large ovarian endometriomas, and firm/dense adhesions.

1. **GnRH agonists** are used for this stage as well (see moderate disease).
2. **Aromatase inhibitors,** currently under investigation, inhibit prostaglandin E2, thereby decreasing positive feedback cycle of estrogen production.
3. **Conservative laparoscopy** for excision, fulguration, or laser vaporization of implants and adhesions. Offers 80% to 90% pain relief but 40% recurrence at 10 years.
4. **Definitive laparoscopic surgery** (future pregnancy not desired). Hysterectomy and bilateral oophorectomy. Recurrence rate is 10% over 10 years.

ADNEXAL MASSES

I. **Overview.** Ovaries are influenced by hormonal changes. Ovaries usually measure $3.5 \times 2 \times 1.5$ cm in the premenopausal patient and $1.5 \times 0.7 \times 0.5$ cm after menopause.

II. **Differential Diagnosis Based on Age.**

A. **Premenarcheal.** Most common adnexal mass is ovarian cyst, which occurs in 2% to 5% of prepubertal girls. Ovarian masses are at high risk for malignancy (germ cell tumors). In girls younger than 15 years, approximately 80% of ovarian tumors are malignant.

B. **Adolescents.** Most common masses are physiologic cysts (follicular, corpus luteum, and theca lutein) related to normal ovarian activity. Usually unilocular, thin walled, and smaller than 8 to 10 cm in diameter. Appendiceal abscess commonly occurs in this age group. Also consider imperforate hymen, blind uterine horn, benign cystic teratomas, paratubal cyst, ectopic pregnancy, uterine masses, and gastrointestinal conditions.

C. **Established menses.** Incidence of pelvic masses is 5% to 18%. Adnexal masses are less likely to be malignant in reproductive-aged women. Most common are physiologic or functional cysts, ectopic pregnancy, PID (tuboovarian abscess), endometrioma, benign and malignant ovarian neoplasms, neoplasms metastatic to the ovary (breast or GI cancers), PCOS, myomas, fibroids (25% in this age group), endometrioma (chocolate, complex cysts on ultrasound).

D. **Postmenopausal.** From 30% to 60 % of ovarian masses in women older than 50 years are malignant. Ovarian mass in a postmenopausal woman is considered malignant until proved otherwise. Malignant adnexal masses include ovarian masses, metastatic lesions from breast and gastrointestinal tract, and fallopian tube carcinomas. Nonmalignant causes are similar to those in patients of reproductive age.

III. Evaluation.

A. History

1. **Ovarian neoplasms are often clinically silent, except for nonspecific "pressure" symptoms including urinary frequency, constipation, and pelvic heaviness.**

2. Take gynecologic history including menses and STDs, sexual history including contraceptives, obstetric history, surgical history. Review of systems including bowel and bladder function and endocrine symptoms.

3. Family history of reproductive cancers (breast, uterine, ovarian) from both sides of family is critical because some ovarian tumors are familial (e.g., *BRCA* gene).

4. Multiparity, late menarche, early menopause, and the use of OCPs have all been shown to be protective against ovarian surface epithelial cell tumors.

5. Large tumors can cause increased abdominal girth and may be confused with pregnancy.

6. Midcycle pain in premenopausal women indicates possible follicular or corpus luteum cysts.

7. Dyspareunia may be related to a ruptured cyst or endometriosis.

8. Sudden onset of severe pain with nausea and vomiting suggests ovarian torsion, degenerating leiomyoma, or perforation, infarction, or hemorrhage from an ovarian neoplasm.

9. Dysmenorrhea and menorrhagia occur with endometriosis or leiomyomas, and pain with fever is often PID, appendicitis, or diverticulitis.

B. Physical exam

1. Look for virilization, adenopathy; breast, abdominal, and pelvic exams including rectovaginal exam after woman has emptied bladder.

2. **Benign tumors are characteristically unilateral,** cystic, and mobile and do not cause ascites.

3. **Malignancies are usually solid, fixed,** and nodular and often cause ascites.

C. Diagnostic evaluation. Ultrasonography (transvaginal and transabdominal) will help characterize the mass. Transabdominal is better tolerated, helpful in visualizing abdominal processes. Transvaginal gives better resolution of pelvic structures with less artifact, does not require a distended bladder.

1. **Ultrasound** tells whether mass is cystic or solid, and whether smooth surface, **internal septae, papillae, excrescences, or ascites** (latter four suggesting malignancy). **Large cysts greater than 10 cm in diameter and solid tumors are more likely to be malignant and require immediate evaluation and probable excision. Ultrasound is suggested for all ovarian masses because of limited reliability of physical exam.**

2. **Labs.** Check pregnancy test. Obtain CBC if there is bleeding or if infectious disease is suspected, FSH and LH if virilization is present. CA-125 is recommended for postmenopausal women with ultrasound suspicious for malignancy. AFP, LDH, and HCG are recommended for premenarchal adolescent girls with solid ovarian masses suggestive of germ cell tumors. Additional tests indicated by history and physical exam.

GYNECOLOGY 13

IV. **Treatment of Ovarian Masses.** Evaluation and treatment are based on the patient's age and reproductive status.

A. **Premenarcheal.** For functional cysts, serial ultrasound examinations every 4 to 8 weeks. Ultrasound-guided aspiration or laparoscopic surgery should be considered for enlargement or failure of a cyst to resolve in 3 to 6 months. Solid or complex mass requires surgical assessment and consultation with a gynecologic oncologist.

B. **Adolesents.** For cysts less than 10 cm on ultrasound, observe for up to 3 months with or without administration of OCPs. Evaluate monthly by bimanual or ultrasound examination. If fluid-filled cyst increases in size, is greater than 10 cm, or causes symptoms, laparoscopic cystectomy is recommended. Cyst sent for pathologic examination.

C. **Premenopausal**

1. If an easily palpable, smooth, mobile ovarian mass **less than 6 cm diameter** is felt, it may be observed with repeat pelvic exam in 6 weeks if the clinical picture is consistent with a benign functional cyst. **Any mass 6 cm or greater should be evaluated by ultrasound.**

2. **If ultrasound demonstrates a simple ovarian cyst less than 6 cm in diameter,** observe with repeat clinical exam and ultrasound in 6 to 8 weeks. If the cyst persists but decreases in size, it may be observed through another cycle. Oral contraceptives are sometimes used for 1 or 2 months to suppress ovarian function and prevent further cyst formation.

3. **If an ovarian mass persists, is greater than 6 cm, or increases in size during 2 months, surgical excision is indicated to exclude neoplasm.**

D. **Postmenopausal women.** Ovarian masses have a high risk of malignancy (surface epithelial or stromal tumors). Proceed to full evaluation without a period of observation.

1. Asymptomatic women with pelvic examination not suspicious for malignancy, normal Pap smear, and normal CA 125 concentration, and a simple unilateral cyst on ultrasound that is less than 3 cm in diameter can be followed with serial ultrasounds (3, 6, 9, and 12 months, then annually) and CA 125 levels. Most of these cysts resolve in 12 to 24 months.

2. Cysts greater than 3 cm should be examined by exploratory surgery.

3. Symptomatic women with elevated serum CA 125, ascites, suspicion of metastatic disease, a family history of breast or ovarian cancer in a first degree relative, or nonsimple cyst on ultrasound should undergo laparotomy by a gynecologic oncologist.

PEDIATRIC GYNECOLOGY

I. **General.** Gynecologic problems of infancy and childhood are uncommon before the onset of puberty; however, when present, they must be appropriately evaluated. Always consider child abuse and if suspected, document the exam carefully and report to the appropriate authorities.

Consultation with a specialist in pediatric gynecology may be helpful in cases with legal ramifications.

II. **Common Disorders of Infancy and Childhood.**

A. **Vulvovaginitis** is the most common complaint.

1. **Symptoms.** Soreness, pruritus, discharge, and burning.

2. **Exam.** Microscopic exam of vaginal secretions, UA, and possible vaginal cultures. Recurrent or refractory infections of foul-smelling, bloody discharge require vaginoscopy to exclude foreign body or tumor.

3. **Causes.** Nonspecific polymicrobial infection secondary to poor hygiene or foreign body, lack of labial development, unestrogenized thin mucosa, bubble baths, shampoos, obesity, tight clothing (tights, blue jeans), chronic masturbatory activity leading to vulvar irritation, sexual abuse, primary infections (*Candida, Gardnerella, Trichomonas*, gonorrhea, syphilis, herpes, etc.), **pinworms,** respiratory pathogens transmitted by hand *(S. pyogenes, S. aureus, H. influenzae, S. pneumoniae, N. meningitidis*, and *B. catarrhalis*), lichen sclerosus et atrophicus may also occur. Neoplasms are rare.

4. **Treatment**

a. Remove foreign body, if present, with warm saline irrigation or bayonet forceps. Obtain vaginal and urine cultures and treat concurrent infection.

b. Treat specific infections. **Candidiasis:** see discussion earlier in this chapter. **Bacterial vaginosis and *Trichomonas* vulvovaginitis:** metronidazole 35 to 50 mg/kg per day up to 750 mg divided tid for 7 days. **Gonorrhea:** ceftriaxone 125 mg IM, azithromycin 10 mg/kg PO (max 1 g). **UTI:** TMP–SMX. **Scabies and pediculosis pubis:** see Chapter 10. Suspect sexual abuse if bacterial vaginosis, *Trichomonas*, gonorrhea, or chlamydia is present.

c. Educate about perineal hygiene.

B. **Pinworms** *(Enterobiasis vermicularis)*. May cause vulvovaginitis or rectal itching. Girls often have vaginal pain that wakes them. See Chapter 10 for diagnosis and treatment.

C. **Diaper dermatitis** (primary contact irritant dermatitis)

1. **Caused by** irritants in urine, producing red, papulovesicular, shiny rash sparing skin folds; may fissure.

2. **Treat with** good hygiene and protection with zinc oxide or white petroleum jelly, frequent diaper changes allowing skin to dry fully. Treat secondary infections caused by *Streptococcus, Staphylococcus*, or *Candida* organisms.

D. **Labial adhesions**

1. Related to low estrogen levels, poor hygiene, and vulvar irritation. Usually asymptomatic but may interfere with urination, leading to dysuria and recurrent vulvar and vaginal infections.

2. Treat with good hygiene and topical estrogen cream bid for 7 to 10 days, which will lyse adhesions. Use surgical intervention only as a last resort.

E. **Neonatal vaginal bleeding** can occur at 3 to 5 days, representing withdrawal of transplacental estrogens. No treatment except reassurance of parents.

13

GYNECOLOGY

F. Polyps. Vaginal polyp may also manifest with chronic discharge. Benign polyps involving the vagina and hymenal area are rare.

G. Ectopic ureter. An ectopic ureter can cause chronic vulval irritation and wetness.

H. Urethral prolapse

1. Prolapse of estrogen-dependent distal urethral mucosa forming painful, friable mass at vaginal orifice. Catheter passed through center enters bladder.

2. Treat initially with topical estrogens and antibiotic creams. If urinary retention is present or lesion is large and necrotic, surgical excision may be required.

I. Systemic illness. Vaginal symptoms including vesicles, discharge, fistulae, ulcers, and inflammation have been associated with measles, chickenpox, Kawasaki disease, scarlet fever, Stephens–Johnson syndrome, mononucleosis, and Crohn's disease among others.

J. Rare but serious disorders of infancy and childhood

1. **Sarcoma botryoides** (embryonal carcinoma of vagina) manifests as bloody vaginal discharge most commonly in 2- to 5-year-olds with polypoid growth, which may look like a cluster of grapes involving hymen, lower urethra, or anterior vaginal wall.

2. **Ovarian tumors.** (Refer to pediatric section of prior adnexal masses section.) Symptoms include pain, mass, pressure; can cause vaginal bleeding or the precocious development of secondary sex characteristics if hormonally active. Requires complete evaluation by experienced gynecologist.

MENOPAUSE

Physiology

I. Definition. Menopause is the physiologic cessation of menses due to diminished ovarian function. By definition, the diagnosis is made after 6 months of amenorrhea. **Menopause is a clinical diagnosis and does not require laboratory studies.**

II. Clinical Features. Average age is 51 years; 95% of women become menopausal between 45 and 55 years of age. Symptoms begin in premenopausal years and progress as estrogen and progesterone levels decrease.

A. Vasomotor symptoms include hot flushes and night sweats. Atrophic symptoms include vaginal dryness, pruritus, irritation, and dyspareunia; urinary frequency, dysuria, incontinence, and increased incidence of cystitis.

B. Emotional symptoms include lability, irritability, depression, and insomnia. Increased risk of coronary artery disease.

C. **Osteoporosis.** About 50% of postmenopausal bone loss occurs in the first 7 years, and resultant hip and vertebral fractures are a major cause of increased morbidity and mortality.

III. **Initial Assessment.**

A. History including family history.

B. Physical exam highlighting breast and pelvic exam.

C. Pap smear at baseline. See "Pap Smears and Cervical Dysplasia" above for Pap recommendations.

D. Mammogram at baseline and annually.

E. **FSH measurement.** If the patient is clearly menopausal, with amenorrhea 3 to 6 months and/or compatible vasomotor symptoms, confirmation with serum FSH is not necessary. If the clinical picture is unclear, check FSH. For women on oral contraceptives, look for hot flushes during the placebo week or check FSH on the 6th or 7th placebo day.

F. Endometrial biopsy is not necessary before beginning HRT unless there are risk factors such as abnormal vaginal bleeding, history of prolonged anovulation, history of unopposed estrogen use, obesity, or diabetes.

GYNECOLOGY 13

Hormone Replacement Therapy

I. **Risks and Benefits of HRT.**
Recent data from the Women's Health Initiative, revealed no cardiovascular benefit from unopposed estrogen or combined estrogen/progestin therapy but rather revealed risks. HRT is still appropriate in some circumstances. Discuss the risks and benefits with each patient.

A. **Benefits**

1. **In the short term (months),** estrogen effectively controls perimenopausal vasomotor and psychologic symptoms. There are few risks for short-term use beyond venous thromboembolism and endometrial stimulation.

2. **In the long term (years),** estrogen can help prevent advancement of osteoporosis, decrease frequency of fractures, and help atrophic vaginal symptoms.

3. **Treatment for 5 years can decrease hip and vertebral fractures (NNT = 228) and risk for colon cancer (NNT = 1667). Treatment also improved quality of life in the Women's Health Initiative subjects.**

B. **Risks**

1. **Treatment for 5 years can increase the risk of CAD (NNH = 1428), invasive breast cancer (NNH = 1250), stroke (NNH = 1250), thromboembolic disease (NNH = 555), and pulmonary embolism (NNH = 1250).**

2. **Endometrial hyperplasia or carcinoma** risk doubles if estrogen is used alone. This risk depends duration and dose. Cyclic estrogen alone still increases risk of hyperplasia. When progestin is added, in cyclic or continuous regimen, risk of these cancers is lower than in patients not treated with hormones.

3. **Gallbladder disease risk increases.** The Nurses' Health Study found that women on estrogen therapy were at increased risk for cholecystectomy compared with nonusers.
4. **Bronchospasm.** Estrogen possibly causes worsening of bronchospasm.
5. **Ovarian cancer.** The Women's Health Initiative found a nonsignificant increase in ovarian cancer risk, but this risk was small and not considered a major factor for whether to use therapy or not.

C. **Contraindications** include unexplained vaginal bleeding, active liver disease or chronically impaired liver function, carcinoma of the breast, endometrial carcinoma, recent vascular thrombosis, or past history of thromboembolic disease with previous hormone therapy.

D. **Relative contraindications** include hypertension, uterine leiomyomas, migraine headaches, familial hyperlipidemia, hypertriglyceridemia, endometriosis, gallbladder disease, or close family history of venous thromboembolism.

II. **Regimens of Hormone Replacement.**

A. As a result of the Women's Health Initiative, the **primary indication for estrogen (unopposed or combined with progestin) is for control of menopausal symptoms.** The FDA requires labels on all estrogen and estrogen–progestin products warning of the risk of heart disease, stroke, and cancer.

B. **Estrogen therapy should be used for the shortest duration possible, taking into account symptoms (hot flushes, sleep, sexual function), patient age, and quality of life.**

C. Endometrial hyperplasia and cancer can occur 6 months after unopposed estrogen therapy. Therefore, progestin should be added in women who have not had hysterectomy.

D. **Continuous combined estrogen/progesterone**

1. **Estrogen component.** Try to use low-dose conjugated estrogen (e.g., Premarin 0.3 mg PO qd or estradiol 0.5 mg PO qd).
2. **Progestin component.** Medroxyprogesterone acetate 2.5 mg PO qd or micronized progesterone 100 mg PO qd. Micronized progesterone may have fewer side effects.
3. **Two lower-dose combined conjugated estrogen preparations** (low-dose Prempro: 0.45 mg conjugated estrogen/1.5 mg medroxyprogesterone acetate; and Prempro 0.3 mg/1.5 mg) approved by the FDA for treating menopausal symptoms and preventing osteoporosis. Low-dose unopposed Premarin 0.45 mg has also been approved for menopausal symptoms.

E. **Cyclic combined estrogen–progesterone**

1. **Estrogen component.** Daily dose same as above. Cyclic regimens using only 25 days of estrogen each month produced vasomotor symptoms.
2. **Progestin component.** Medroxyprogesterone acetate 2.5 mg PO qd or micronized progesterone 200 mg PO qd for 10 to 14 days each month. Micronized progesterone may have fewer side effects.

F. Unopposed estrogen for hysterectomized patients. Daily estrogen dose is the same as above. Occasionally a patient with a uterus will elect unopposed estrogen due to intolerance of progesterone. If so, annual endometrial sampling is imperative, and periodic withdrawal or progestin use to induce menses every 3 to 6 months is recommended.

G. Vaginal estrogen (cream, tablets, or rings) is an effective therapy for genitourinary symptoms. It is an option for all postmenopausal women except breast cancer patients. It can be administered long-term as systemic absorption is low when appropriate doses are used.

H. Selective estrogen receptor modulators (SERM)

1. **Raloxifene 60 mg/d or a bisphosphonate is used for primary prevention of osteoporosis (preferred over standard estrogen). SERMs do not improve vasomotor symptoms.** Antiresorptive effects of raloxifene are less than those of bisphosphonates, so SERMS are reserved for those who can't tolerate bisphosphonates (alendronate and risedronate).

2. **Effects** are estrogenic in bone and lipid metabolism and antiestrogenic in endometrial and breast tissue. Raloxifene preserves bone density and decreases osteoporotic fractures without increasing the risk of endometrial or breast cancer. Raloxifene's effect on lipids and the cardiovascular system are being investigated.

3. **Side effects** include increased hot flushes, leg cramps, and increased risk of venous thromboembolism (work-up before starting raloxifene if there is a family history of venous thromboembolism).

III. Managing Vaginal Bleeding on Combined HRT.

A. Breakthrough bleeding occurs in 80% to 90% of patients on cyclic HRT (daily estrogen [continuously] with 2.5 mg medroxyprogesterone on days 1 to 13 or 14 of each month). Bleeding is often light and after last dose of progestin, but bothersome.

B. About 40% to 60% have bleeding on continuous HRT during the first 6 months. Breakthrough bleeding is more common in women who recently had periods.

C. Evaluation. Endometrial biopsy if irregular bleeding continues longer than 6 months. See management of postmenopausal bleeding above.

D. Treatment options. In a continuous regimen, double the baseline daily progestin dose (from 2.5 to 5 mg of medroxyprogesterone) or consider changing to a cyclic regimen. Consider endometrial ablation, progestin IUD, or hysterectomy.

IV. Special Considerations.

A. Libido. Women with persistently decreased libido despite HRT may benefit from addition of methyltestosterone (e.g., Estratest).

B. Endometriosis. Women with a history of endometriosis who have had a hysterectomy should be given progestin in addition to estrogen to prevent adenocarcinoma developing from residual pelvic and intra-abdominal endometrial implants.

C. Bisphosphonates are used for preventing and treating osteoporosis.

GYNECOLOGY 13

V. Cessation of Hormone Replacement Therapy. Many women eventually discontinue hormone replacement after short-term or long-term therapy. Abrupt withdrawal of estrogen at any age results in hot flushes, which are often severe. Taper medication to avoid recurrence of vasomotor symptoms. Decrease the estrogen and progestin by one pill per week until the taper is completed. If patient is unable to tolerate 6-week taper, taper over 12 weeks, making change every 2 weeks.

VI. Alternative Treatments.

A. Other treatments are available for what were HRT indications. Osteoporosis should be treated with bisphosphonates; cardiovascular risk modified with lipid-lowering agents and aspirin; hot flushes treated with progesterone, venlafaxine, clonidine, naloxone, or methyldopa; and vaginal atrophy treated with topical estrogen cream (although high doses may have systemic effects) or hydrating agents (e.g., Replens).

B. Phytoestrogens (those in soy, etc.) have been popularized for herbal treatment of menopausal symptoms. Doses large enough to effect symptomatic relief are likely to also produce estrogen-related side effects such as endometrial stimulation.

SEXUAL ASSAULT

I. Rape-Trauma Syndrome.

A. Acute phase may last for hours to days and is characterized by a distortion or paralysis of the individual's coping mechanism. Generalized body pain, eating and sleeping disturbances, vaginal discharge, itching and rectal pain, depression, anxiety, and mood swings may be present.

B. Delayed or organizational phase is characterized by flashbacks, nightmares, phobias, and a need for reorganization of thought processes, as well as the gynecologic and menstrual complaints noted above. This phase can occur months or years after the event. Mood disorders and post-traumatic stress syndrome may develop.

C. Counseling should be phase specific.

II. Child Sexual Abuse.

A. Babies, children, handicapped people, and the elderly can be victims of sexual assault. A high index of suspicion is needed for diagnosis.

B. Symptoms

1. **Behavioral:** anxiety, sleep disturbances, withdrawal, somatic complaints, increased sex play, inappropriate sexual behavior, school problems, acting-out behavior, self-destructive behavior, depression, low self-esteem.

2. **Physical:** unexplained vaginal or rectal injuries, unexplained vaginal or rectal bleeding, bruising, bites, scratches, pregnancy, sexually transmitted disease, recurrent vaginal infections, pain in the anal or genital area, recurrent atypical abdominal pain.

C. Physical findings

1. **Colposcopy** allows a detailed magnified inspection of the vulva to search for physical signs of abuse that may have escaped detection by unaided examination. However, most findings are visible to the naked eye. **Take pictures and document any findings well. Videocolposcopy is the standard of care.**
2. **Nonspecific.** Redness of external genitalia, increased vascular pattern of the vestibule and labia, presence of purulent discharge from the vagina, small skin fissures or lacerations in the area of the posterior fourchette, and agglutination of the labia minora after trauma.
3. **Specific findings.** Recent or healed lacerations of the hymen and vaginal mucosa may indicate abuse. An enlarged hymenal opening of 1 cm or more is nonspecific. Proctoepisiotomy and indentations in the skin indicating teeth marks (bite marks) or laboratory confirmation of a venereal disease may indicate abuse.
4. **Definitive findings.** Any presence of sperm.

III. Prophylactic Therapy after Rape. Treat presumptively for chlamydia and gonorrhea (for doses, see Chapter 8). The patient should be instructed to return for repeat STD testing in 3 to 4 weeks. The patient should be counseled about possible HIV infection and offered prophylactic therapy (see Chapter 11). HIV serologic analysis should be obtained at the time of assault and repeated in 6 months. If the patient is at risk for pregnancy, a postcoital contraceptive regimen should be offered (see section on contraception), and a pregnancy test should be performed during the return visit. If the patient becomes pregnant, she should be counseled about all available options. Arrange for follow-up medical care and counseling.

OSTEOPOROSIS

I. Overview.

A. Bone mass peaks at age 30 and gradually declines thereafter. Bone loss accelerates after menopause to 1.5% per year, then slows again after 10 to 15 years.

B. Osteoporosis. Decreased bone mass with normal ratio of mineral to matrix. A bone mineral density (BMD) T score below 2.5 SD (below the mean for young adults) is considered osteoporosis. **When comparing BMD, the patient's T score is compared to the normal T score of a young adult at maximum bone density. For children, the Z score is used, which compares bone density to age-normal bone density.**

C. Osteopenia is decreased bone mass with a T score between 1 and 2.5 SD (below the mean for young adults).

D. Risk factors for osteoporosis include exercise-related amenorrhea, time since menopause, corticosteroid use, thin body habitus, sedentary lifestyle, inadequate calcium or vitamin D intake, family history of osteoporotic fractures, white or Asian race, high alcohol consumption, smoking, hyperthyroidism, chronic kidney or liver disease,

GYNECOLOGY **13**

and long-term therapy with corticosteroids, thyroid hormone, anticonvulsants, or heparin. **Discuss these risk factors with all patients.**

E. Protective factors include obesity, diabetes mellitus, thiazide diuretic use, and possibly statins.

F. Fractures resulting from osteoporosis include hip fractures (with 5%-20% mortality rate within 3 months), vertebral compression fractures (causing loss of height, kyphosis, and resulting pulmonary, GI, and bladder problems), Colles' fracture, and tooth loss.

G. Whom to screen? Different organizations have different recommendations regarding osteoporosis screening.

1. **AAFP: Menopausal women with one or more risk factors** for osteoporosis regardless of age.

2. **U.S. Preventive Services Task Force: All women older than 65 years** regardless of risk factors.

II. Diagnosis.

A. Radiographs show osteopenia only after there is 20% to 30% bone loss.

B. DEXA scan is the most accurate method of measuring BMD. Measure BMD when it will make a significant difference in decision to start a bisphosphonate or raloxifene.

C. Osteoporotic fractures are often the first indication of osteoporosis.

D. Differential diagnosis. Once osteoporosis is diagnosed, consider whether there is an underlying condition that might be causing osteoporosis: hyperparathyroidism, chronic renal failure, multiple myeloma, leukemia, lymphoma, hyperthyroidism, excessive thyroid replacement, hypercortisolism, metastatic cancer, or paraneoplastic syndrome.

III. Prevention.

A. Calcium intake. Adolescents and reproductive-age women producing endogenous estrogen require 1000 mg of calcium daily through diet or supplements. Postmenopausal women require 1500 mg daily if not taking estrogen or raloxifene. Calcium should be taken with meals in doses up to 500 mg. Calcium carbonate is cheapest, although calcium citrate is better absorbed.

B. Vitamin D intake of 400 IU (800 IU after age 70) through fortified milk, multivitamin, or supplement is required for absorption of calcium. Deficiency is especially common in winter in the higher latitudes, and in institutionalized patients.

C. Exercise. Regular weight-bearing exercise such as walking, running, weight training, aerobics, or any other weight-bearing sport improves bone density.

D. Quit smoking and avoid excessive alcohol use.

E. Minimize corticosteroid and thyroid hormone use as much as possible. If on chronic steroids, vitamin D and calcium with or without alendronate or risedronate should be considered.

F. Alendronate 5 mg PO qd or 35 mg PO once a week is used for **prevention** of osteoporosis in postmenopausal women as is **risedronate** 5 mg/day.

G. Modify the home environment to identify and eliminate factors predisposing to falls.

IV. Treatment is recommended for women without risk factors who have BMD that is 2 SD below the mean and in women with risk factors who have BMD that is 1.5 SD below the mean.

A. Bisphosphonates or selective estrogen receptor modulators (raloxifene).

B. Bisphosphonates are effective monotherapy and have a small additive effect when given with HRT (see related risks in HRT section). They are also useful in corticosteroid-related osteoporosis.

1. **Alendronate** (10 mg PO qd or 70 mg PO q1wk, just as effective) reduces risk of vertebral fractures by 90% and nonvertebral fractures by 30% to 50% in established osteoporosis. To prevent esophageal ulceration, it must be taken in the morning with 8 oz water at least $1/2$ hour before any other foods or fluids are taken. Patient must remain upright until after first meal.

2. **Risedronate** is the most potent bisphosphonate and also has lowest incidence of GI side effects. It is approved for osteoporosis in a dose of 5 mg/d for both prevention and treatment.

3. **Etidronate** is an alternative. Given cyclically, 400 mg PO qd for 2 weeks, followed by 12 weeks without the drug. It is probably as effective as alendronate.

4. **Calcitonin** 1 spray in alternating nostrils each day is expensive but effective in increasing BMD. It relives the pain of vertebral compression fractures.

5. **Thiazide diuretics,** in patients needing an antihypertensive, increase bone mass and have an additive effect with estrogen.

6. **Fluoride,** although it increases bone density, increases hip fracture risk, so it is no longer used.

7. **Raloxifene** 60 mg PO daily in those not tolerating bisphosphonate.

C. Treat all patients with vitamin D, exercise, calcium, etc., as noted above in prevention.

ECTOPIC PREGNANCY

Ectopic pregnancy is potentially life threatening but often misdiagnosed. It must be suspected in any woman with vaginal bleeding and lower abdominal pain. Ruptured ectopic pregnancy is a true medical emergency.

I. General Information.

A. Risk factors include history of ectopic pregnancy, PID, tubal or pelvic surgery, infertility, endometriosis, anatomic anomalies, DES exposure, cigarette smoking, and older age. IUDs do not increase the absolute risk of ectopic pregnancy, but accidental pregnancies with an IUD are more

GYNECOLOGY **13**

likely to be ectopic than intrauterine. Fertility treatment leads to a heterotopic pregnancy (intrauterine with coexistent ectopic pregnancy) in up to 3% of patients.

B. Differential diagnosis includes early intrauterine gestation with implantation bleeding, spontaneous abortion, ruptured functional ovarian cyst, appendicitis, PID, and other gynecologic and abdominal conditions causing pain. (See Chapter 15 for further information about the acute abdomen.)

II. Evaluation.

A. Symptoms include abdominal pain (98%), amenorrhea (65%), and vaginal bleeding/spotting (80%), with or without symptoms of early pregnancy. **Not all patients report amenorrhea or vaginal bleeding!** Patients may have nausea, vomiting, dizziness, syncope, hypovolemic shock, referred shoulder pain, tenesmus, and low-grade fever. Usually occurs 6 to 8 weeks after LMP.

B. Exam. Check vital signs. Blood pressure and pulse may be normal even with significant intraperitoneal bleeding! **Pelvic exam may be normal;** only 50% have palpable adnexal mass. Uterus may be enlarged secondary to deciduation or blood. Cervical motion tenderness may be found as well as doughy cul-de-sac secondary to bleeding. Marked abdominal tenderness with guarding and rebound suggests ruptured or bleeding ectopic pregnancy. When an acute abdominal emergency or hemorrhagic shock is suspected, immediate surgical consultation is indicated.

C. Lab tests include pregnancy test. Urine pregnancy test may miss a very early ectopic pregnancy (limit 50 mIU/mL). A serum quantitative β-HCG is sensitive to 5 mIU/mL. If possible, a quantitative serum HCG should be done. Obtain CBC, type and screen, and transvaginal ultrasound.

III. Correlation of Ultrasonography with the Serum Quantitative HCG.

A. β-HCG less than 1500 mIU/mL. Ultrasonography might not show evidence of a gestational sac. If patient is stable and ultrasound is negative, she can be followed up as discussed below. But do not assume a benign course if the β-HCG is low. If an ectopic pregnancy is present, it can still rupture.

B. β-HCG greater than 1500 mIU/mL. If β-HCG is higher than 1500 mIU/mL and the sonographer is reasonably skilled, an intrauterine pregnancy should be detectable by transvaginal ultrasonography in 95% of cases. **If an intrauterine sac is not visible with a serum β-HCG greater than 1500 mIU/mL, suspicion of ectopic pregnancy is markedly increased.**

C. β-HCG greater than 3500 mIU/mL. The adnexal gestation is often not visible until the β-HCG is 3500 to 6500 mIU/mL.

D. β-HCG greater than 6000 mIU/mL with no visible intrauterine gestational sac is presumptive evidence of an ectopic implantation.

IV. **Follow-up.**

A. **For the patient in whom the diagnosis of ectopic pregnancy cannot be proved or ruled out on the first visit,** if the patient is stable and reliable and if ultrasonography does not exclude ectopic pregnancy, obtain serial quantitative β-HCG every 48 hours and follow clinical exam. The β-HCG should approximately double in 48 hours. In an unreliable patient, treat as presumed ectopic pregnancy.

B. **If β-HCG rises by more than 66% in 48 hours,** the pregnancy is continuing; repeat the ultrasound when the β-HCG is greater than 1500 mIU/mL to differentiate between ectopic and intrauterine pregnancy. If result is still indeterminate, follow-up in another 48 hours with repeat quantitative β-HCG and ultrasound. If the β-HCG is not rising or is falling, the pregnancy is likely nonviable and D&C should be done to look for chorionic villi.

C. **Culdocentesis** is used rarely due to transvaginal ultrasonography. Hemoperitoneum (greater than 5 mL of nonclotting blood) in combination with a positive pregnancy test is 99% predictive of a ruptured ectopic pregnancy.

D. **Serum progesterone** levels are not very helpful.

V. **Treatment.**

A. **Primary treatment is surgical.** Tube-sparing surgical techniques such as laparoscopic salpingostomy allow preservation of fertility with little increased risk for recurrent ectopic pregnancy.

B. **Methotrexate injection is a nonsurgical treatment** for ectopic pregnancies of less than 3.5 cm with no fetal heart motion. The effect of methotrexate treatment on future fertility needs more study; fertility may be preserved but recurrent ectopic pregnancies may be more common.

C. **Rhogam.** If ectopic pregnancy or spontaneous abortion is confirmed, give Rh prophylaxis to Rh-negative women.

GYNECOLOGY 13

BIBLIOGRAPHY

ACOG Committee on Practice Bulletins: ACOG Practice Bulletin: Clinical management guidelines for obstetrician–gynecologists. Number 45, August 2003. Cervical cytology screening. *Obstet Gynecol* 102:417-427, 2003.

Ailawadi RK, Jobanputra Katraria M: Treatment of endometriosis and chronic pelvic pain with letrozole and norethindrone acetate. A pilot study. *Fertil Steril* 81:290-296, 2004.

Anderson GL, Limacher M, Assaf AR, et al: Effects on conjugated equine estrogen in postmenopausal women with hysterectomy: The Women's Health Initiative randomized controlled trial. *JAMA* 291:1701-1712, 2004.

Davey DD: Cervical cancer screening: Will human papillomavirus testing replace cytology? *J Low Genit Tract Dis* 8:6-9, 2004.

Genant HK, Lucas J, Weiss S, et al: Low-dose esterified estrogen therapy: Effects on bone, plasma estradiol concentrations, endometrium, and lipid levels. Estratab/Osteoporosis Study Group. *Arch Intern Med* 157:2609-2615, 1997.

Goldie SJ, Kim JJ, Wright TC: Cost-effectiveness of human papillomavirus DNA testing for cervical cancer screening in women aged 30 years or more. *Obstet Gynecol* 103:619-631, 2004.

Guzick DS, Overstreet JW, Factor-Litvak P, et al: Sperm morphology, motility, and concentration in fertile and infertile men. *N Engl J Med* 345:1388-1393, 2001.

Holt VL, Cushing-Haugen KL, Daling JR: Oral contraceptives, tubal sterilization, and functional ovarian cyst risk. *Obstet Gynecol* 102:252-258, 2003.

Hulley S, Grady D, Bush T, et al: Randomized trial of estrogen plus progestin for secondary prevention of coronary heart disease in postmenopausal women. Heart and Estrogen/progestin Replacement Study (HERS) Research Group. *JAMA* 280:605-613, 1998.

Jick H, Jick SS, Gurewich V, et al: Risk of idiopathic cardiovascular death and nonfatal venous thromboembolism in women using oral contraceptives with differing progestagen components, *Lancet* 346:1589-1593, 1995.

Lahteenmaki P, Haukkamaa M, Puolakka J, et al: Open randomised study of use of levonorgestrel releasing intrauterine system as alternative to hysterectomy. *BMJ* 361:1122-1126, 1998.

Nestler JE, Jakubowicz DJ, Evans WS, Pasquali R: Effects of metformin on spontaneous and clomiphene-induced ovulation in polycystic ovary syndrome. *N Engl J Med* 338:1876-1880, 1998.

Rapp SR, Espeland MA, Shumaker SA, et al: Effect of estrogen plus progestin on global cognitive function in postmenopausal women: The Women's Health Initiative Memory Study: A randomized controlled trial. *JAMA* 289:2663-2672, 2003.

Saslow D, Runowicz CD, Solomon D, et al: American Cancer Society guideline for the early detection of cervical neoplasia and cancer. *J Low Genit Tract Dis* 7:67-86, 2003.

Stricker T, Navratil F, Sennhauser FH: Vulvovaginitis in prepubertal girls. *Arch Dis Child* 88:324-326, 2003.

Tenore JL: Ectopic pregnancy. *Am Fam Physician* 61:1080-1088, 2000.

Wassertheil-Smoller S, Hendrix SL, Limacher M, et al: Effect of estrogen plus progestin on stroke in postmenopausal women. Women's Health Initiative: A randomized control trial. *JAMA* 289:2673-2684, 2003.

Yen S, Shafer M, Moncada J, et al: Bacterial vaginosis in sexually experienced and non–sexually experienced young women entering the military. *Obstet Gynecol* 102:927-933, 2003.

Obstetrics

Barcey T. Levy and David A. Bedell

PRECONCEPTION CARE

Preconception care and counseling should be offered to all women of childbearing age to prevent congenital anomalies and maximize maternal health. Thirty percent to 50% of pregnancies are unplanned.

I. **Prepregnancy prophylaxis with proven benefits** include folic acid supplementation (can prevent neural tube defects), tight glucose control in DM, rubella immunization in unimmunized women, smoking and alcohol cessation, and identification and control of genetic and chronic health conditions (HTN, thyroid disease, maternal hyperphenylalaninemia, antiphospholipid antibody syndrome, etc.).

II. **Prepregnancy Advice.**

A. Give patient advice on proper nutrition, exercise, smoking cessation, abstinence from alcohol and drugs, protection from radiation (x-rays) and chemical exposures in the workplace, health care and environment, and information on prescribed and OTC drugs (to avoid teratogenicity).

B. Determine Pap smear status and appropriate treatment, infection control (STD protection and treatment, rubella, varicella, tuberculosis, HIV, toxoplasmosis and hepatitis immunity/exposure status), and psychosocial counseling for planning a pregnancy.

C. Assess risk of congenital disease (α- and β-thalassemias, Tay-Sachs, cystic fibrosis, sickle cell, etc.) and order appropriate tests based on risk.

D. Advanced maternal age leads to increased risks of infertility, fetal anomaly, preeclampsia, gestational diabetes, and stillbirth.

E. Offer rubella and varicella vaccines if appropriate and recommend avoiding pregnancy for 3 months after vaccination, because these are live-attenuated vaccines.

GENERAL PRENATAL CARE

I. **History at Initial Evaluation.**

A. **Menstrual history.** Focus on cycle length and regularity, characteristics of previous two menses, and previous methods of contraception. **Establish dates carefully** based on first day of LMP and size of uterus **(Table 14-1 and Box 14-1)**. Obtain ultrasound if in doubt. Ultrasound dating is most accurate between 7 and 14 weeks.

B. **Obstetric history.** Determine dates of all pregnancies, including terminations and spontaneous abortions, as well as duration, complications, and outcomes of pregnancy and labor. Particular note should be made of preeclampsia, gestational diabetes, shoulder dystocia, premature labor, premature rupture of membranes (PROM),

TABLE 14-1
UTERINE SIZE FOR DATING

| Weeks of Gestation | Size (cm) per US* | | Fruit Model | Sports Ball Model |
	Length	Width		
5 wk or less	7.6-9.8	2.9-4.3	Small unripe pear	Hardball
6 wk	7.3-9.1	3.6	Small juice orange	Softball†
8 wk	8.8-10.8	4.8	Large navel orange	
12 wk	11.7-14.2	6.9	Grapefruit	

*Increases with parity.
†Actually between 6 and 8 weeks' size.
Adapted from Margulies R, Miller L: *Obstet Gynecol* 98:341-344, 2001.

placenta previa, and postpartum hemorrhage. Check type of delivery: normal spontaneous vaginal delivery (NSVD), forceps or vacuum, and cesarean section (indicate, type of uterine incision). Obtain records if in doubt. Get weight, sex, and Apgar scores of live-born infants, neonatal complications, and number of living children.

C. Medical history. Check previous and chronic health problems, recent illnesses, STDs, medications, family history and genetic history, and previous surgeries (especially gynecologic surgeries) and transfusions.

D. Medications. Ask about medications, including OTC and supplements, and assess for possible teratogenicity using a comprehensive drug reference such as *Drugs in Pregnancy and Lactation*.

E. Habits: Tobacco, alcohol, other recreational drugs, diet, activity, caffeine.

F. Social history: Occupational hazards, support network, whether the father of the child is involved, whether pregnancy is wanted or unwanted, expectations, potential stresses, and need for social or financial services. Screen for domestic violence or sexual assault.

II. Physical Exam.

A. General physical exam. Pay particular attention to height, weight, BP, thyroid gland, dentition, heart, breasts, deep tendon reflexes, and signs of underlying heart disease.

B. Pelvic exam

1. **External.** Look for evidence of condylomata acuminata. It often spreads during pregnancy, and infants are at slight risk for laryngeal papillomas

BOX 14-1

GESTATION DATING CRITERIA

First day of last menstrual period: Use gestational age wheel, or add 7 days and subtract 3 months

Uterine size (early bimanual exam): See Table 14-1

Ultrasound: First trimester ± 1 week, second ± 2 weeks, third ± 3 weeks

Fetal heartbeat by office Doppler*: By 12 weeks (earlier in thin patients)

Sense fetal movement*: By 18 weeks (multiparas recognize it earlier)

*Lack of fetal heartbeat or quickening at expected date should make one consider US. Heartbeat and quickening can appear several weeks earlier than expected.

or anogenital warts, which are not prevented by C-section. Podophyllin is contraindicated during pregnancy, but cryotherapy, laser, and TCA may be used. Also look for and culture lesions suspicious for herpes simplex.

2. **Vaginal and cervical.** Look for evidence of condylomas and herpes. Examine vaginal discharge and evaluate for *Candida, Trichomonas*, and bacterial vaginosis if symptomatic; culture cervical discharge for gram-negative intracellular diplococci (GC) and *Chlamydia*. Treat GC and *Chlamydia* should be treated; other vaginal infections if symptomatic. Rule out cervical anomalies. Pap smear should be obtained if patient has not had one in the last 6 months.

3. **Bimanual exam.** Rule out adnexal abnormalities. Determine uterine size: 8 weeks is 2 × normal; 10 weeks is 3 × normal; 12 weeks is 4 × normal; 16 weeks is halfway to umbilicus; 20 weeks is at umbilicus. Use fundal height to calculate weeks of gestation: 1 week is 1 cm from pubic symphysis to fundus. See Table 14-1.

III. **Laboratory Evaluation at First Prenatal Visit.**

A. **Routine.** Pap smear, CBC, ABO blood group, Rh type, antibody screen (indirect Coombs'), VDRL test, rubella antibody titer, and hepatitis B surface antigen; UA and culture to screen for bacteriuria. Treat asymptomatic bacteriuria to prevent pyelonephritis during pregnancy. Urine should also be screened for protein and glucose by dipstick at each visit. Offer HIV testing. Many states require HIV testing because AZT administered during pregnancy substantially decreases risk of transmission of HIV to infant (see Chapter 11).

B. **When indicated,** perform cervical culture for GC and *Chlamydia*, toxoplasmosis antibody test, sickle cell preparation or hemoglobin electrophoresis in all previously unscreened African-American women, tuberculin skin testing, HIV antibody testing, and CMV titers.

IV. **Labs During Pregnancy.**

A. **Every visit.** Dipstick urine for protein and glucose.

B. **10 to 13 weeks.** Chorionic villus sampling when indicated.

C. **14 to 20 weeks.** Amniocentesis when indicated.

D. **15 to 20 weeks**. Serum triple-screen (α-fetoprotein, β-HCG, and estradiol). See below.

E. **24 to 28 weeks.** One-hour blood glucose screen after 50 g of oral glucose, urine culture.

F. **28 to 32 weeks.** Hematocrit.

G. **26 to 28 and 36 weeks.** Rh antibody screening if indicated.

H. **36 Weeks** Group B *Strep* culture (vaginal and rectal). Consider GC, *Chlamydia*, and herpes rescreening in high-risk women. Repeat hematocrit if indicated.

V. **Expected Weight Gain.**

A. **First trimester** should gain 2 to 5 lb total.

B. **After first trimester** should gain 3/4 to 1 lb per week.

C. **Average total weight gain** should be 25 to 35 lb for patient of average weight prior to pregnancy.

Prenatal Patient Education

I. Nutrition in Pregnancy.

A. Caloric requirements are 30 to 35 kcal/kg per day plus 300 kcal/day. Requirements are higher in adolescents and multiple gestations.

B. Calcium

1. **Requirements** are 1200 to 1500 mg of elemental calcium per day.

2. **Calcium sources** are milk (300 mg calcium in 8 oz glass or 1 cup yogurt); generic calcium carbonate (260 mg Ca/650 mg tablet); Tums regular strength (200 mg Ca/500 mg chewable tablet); calcium gluconate chewable (45 mg Ca/500 mg tablet).

C. Iron

1. **Requirements** are 30 mg of elemental iron per day.

2. **Additional requirements.** If the pregnant woman is iron deficient or has a multiple-gestation pregnancy, she should take 60 to 100 mg of elemental iron per day. If her Hb is below 10, she requires 200 mg/day.

3. **Iron supplements:** ferrous sulfate 65 mg of elemental Fe per 324 mg tablet (20% elemental iron); ferrous fumarate 106 mg Fe/325 mg tablet (33% elemental iron); ferrous gluconate 38 mg Fe/325 mg (11.6% elemental iron).

D. Folic acid

1. **Requirements** are 0.8 mg/day. Most prescription prenatal vitamins contain 1 mg of folate. OTC prenatal vitamins contain 0.8 mg of folic acid.

2. **Sources** include green leafy vegetables, broccoli, mushrooms, and liver.

3. **Adequate folate before conception has been shown to reduce the risk of NTDs.**

4. **If patient has prior history of NTD or family history of NTD,** recommend 4 mg/day for at least 3 months before conception and during the first trimester.

II. Activity.

A. Work. If occupation presents no greater risk than those encountered in routine living, the woman may continue to work until the onset of labor. If physical demands are high, there is a higher risk of preterm delivery, especially if the patient is already at higher risk for preterm delivery. Patient may resume working 4 to 6 weeks after an uncomplicated delivery.

1. **Working during pregnancy should be limited or is contraindicated** in women with vaginal bleeding, short (<3 cm) or dilated cervix before 36 weeks, uterine malformation, pregnancy-induced hypertension (PIH), fetal growth restriction (FGR), multiple gestation, prior preterm birth, polyhydramnios, or maternal problems associated with poor placental perfusion. Bed rest may be indicated if there is a suspicion of FGR, preeclampsia, or preterm labor (PTL).

2. **Pregnant women should avoid exposure** to lead, ethylene oxide, ionizing radiation, and organic solvents. Pregnant health care workers

should minimize exposure to anesthetic gases, infectious agents, antineoplastic drugs, and organic solvents. Pregnant women may work in operating rooms equipped with gas scavenging systems and adequate ventilation.

B. Exercise. Women in good health should be encouraged to engage in regular, moderate-intensity physical activity during a normal, uncomplicated pregnancy. Scuba diving and exercising in the supine position pose increased risk for pregnant women. Skiing can pose increased fall risk, and jogging can increase stress on joints. Individual prepregnancy abilities and fitness should be taken into account. Swimming or other water exercise may be preferred because large muscle groups are exercised with relative protection of joints. Women need to pay attention to hydration and avoid overheating. Exercise is contraindicated in women with PIH, PROM, PTL, incompetent cervix, vaginal bleeding, or FGR.

C. Other. There are no routine restrictions on sexual relations, other than comfort and position. Caution should be used if any of the conditions listed above apply.

III. Habits and Miscellaneous.

A. Alcohol increases the risk of second-trimester abortion, mental retardation, and behavior and learning disorders. There is a 10% to 30% risk of fetal alcohol syndrome in offspring of women who drink three to five drinks per day. Risks with lesser consumption are unknown.

B. Tobacco increases the risk of low birth weight, premature labor, spontaneous abortion, stillbirth, and birth defects.

C. Crack cocaine or other illicit drug use is associated with perinatal addiction, preterm labor, and cognitive and psychologic difficulties in the infant. Cocaine abuse during pregnancy is associated with a significant increase in the incidence of abruptio placentae.

D. Caffeine. About one cup of coffee a day (100 mg caffeine a day) does not increase the risk of spontaneous abortion or FGR. Higher doses are not well studied.

E. Seatbelts. Seatbelts should be worn so that the belts do not directly cross the gravid uterus: lap belt low over hips and under uterus, shoulder belt above uterus and between the breasts.

F. Medications. In general, no medications should be used without checking with a physician.

1. FDA classification of medication with regard to adverse fetal effects

a. **Category A.** Controlled studies in women fail to demonstrate a risk to the fetus in the first trimester (and there is no evidence of a risk in later trimesters).

b. **Category B.** Animal studies have not demonstrated a fetal risk, but there are no controlled studies in pregnant women or adverse effects shown in animal studies have not been reproduced in human studies (e.g., penicillin).

c. **Category C.** Either studies in animals have revealed adverse effects on the fetus and there are no controlled studies in women, or studies in women and animals are not available.

d. **Category D.** There is evidence of human fetal risk, but benefits may be acceptable despite the risk if the drug is needed in a life-threatening situation (e.g., carbamazepine).

e. **Category X** includes drugs with proven fetal risks that outweigh any benefits. These drugs are contraindicated in women who are or who might become pregnant.

2. **Confirm the category of all medications in pregnancy before prescribing or recommending them to your patient.**

3. **Drugs that are used in pregnancy with no known adverse effect at the usual dose** (some are class B):

a. Antihistamines (B: cetirizine, chlorpheniramine, clemastine, cyproheptadine), decongestants (e.g., pseudoephedrine).

b. Some antibiotics (penicillin, ampicillin, cephalosporins, erythromycin), nonquinine antimalarials, metronidazole vaginal gel (B), metronidazole (B) (avoid in first trimester if possible, though one study showed no teratogenicity), tuberculostatics (INH, PAS, and rifampin).

c. General anesthetics, acetaminophen, steroids.

d. Accidental use of clomiphene, bromocriptine, birth control pills, and vaginal spermicides have shown no adverse effects.

G. Infections. Avoid children with viral illnesses, especially if the pregnant woman is not immune to rubella or CMV. Avoid direct contact with cat litter and eating raw meat to minimize contact with *Toxoplasma gondii* (toxoplasmosis).

H. Domestic violence. Screen all pregnant women for domestic violence. Violence often escalates with pregnancy. It affects 0.9% to 20% of pregnant women in the United States. Ask direct questions, for example, "Have you been hit, pushed or kicked in the last year?"

I. Potential problems. Advise patient to contact her physician if she experiences vaginal bleeding, leakage of fluid, fever, persistent nausea or vomiting, burning on urination, severe abdominal pain, severe headache or visual disturbance, persistent RUQ pain, peripheral edema, decrease in fetal movement. (Generally after quickening, one should expect four or more fetal movements per hour or at least 10 discrete movements in 2 hours.)

Rh Screening and Rho(D) Immunoglobulin

I. Protocol for Routine Rh Screening and Administration of Rho(D) Immunoglobulin.

A. Initial visit. Draw blood for ABO group, Rh type, and antibody screening (indirect Coombs' test).

B. **If patient is Rh negative,** repeat antibody screen at 26 weeks, and if no antibody is detected, give 300 μg Rho(D) immunoglobulin IM. You may give Rho(D) immunoglobulin before knowing antibody result. If antibody is detected, see discussion of additional Rho(D) later.

C. **After delivery,** check fetal ABO/Rh type. If infant is Rh positive, mother receives 300 μg Rho(D) immunoglobulin IM within 72 hours of delivery; if infant is Rh negative, no additional doses are needed. One vial suppresses immunity to approximately 30 mL of whole blood (15 mL of Rh(+) packed RBCs).

II. **Additional Rho(D) Immunoglobulin Requirements.**

A. If at any time during pregnancy a fetal–maternal hemorrhage is suspected, perform a Kleihauer–Betke (acid elution) test. If the test is positive, the mother should receive 10 mg Rho(D) immunoglobulin per milliliter of fetal blood calculated to have entered the maternal circulation. **However, the Kleihauer–Betke test is not 100% sensitive, and so if there is trauma and a suggestion of fetal–maternal hemorrhage, presumptive use of Rho(D) is indicated.**

B. A 50-μg dose of Rho(D) immunoglobulin is indicated for an Rh-negative woman after a first trimester terminated or spontaneously aborted pregnancy. **There is no harm in giving 300 μg, which is more readily available.**

C. A 300-μg dose of Rho(D) immunoglobulin is indicated for the Rh-negative woman who undergoes amniocentesis or a spontaneous or induced abortion or who has an ectopic pregnancy.

D. The Kleihauer–Betke test should be performed after delivery if a larger than usual fetal–maternal hemorrhage may have taken place, as with abruptio placentae. Some institutions now use a flow cytometry methodology to quantitate fetal–maternal transfusion with greater sensitivity and more accuracy. More than the standard 300-μg dose may be required (which protects only up to 15 mL of Rh-positive red blood cells).

III. **Isoimmunization.**

A. If the patient is Rh negative and the antibody screen is positive *before* Rho(D) immunoglobulin administration, obtain an antibody titer and paternal blood type and Rh antigens. Alloimmunization to other erythrocyte antigens (e.g., c, C, e, E, Kell, Duffy) also occurs and is followed in a similar fashion.

B. Antibody titers are repeated each month until 24 weeks, then every 2 weeks. **Antibody titers aren't helpful if the mother has had a previously affected infant.**

C. If the titer reaches a critical value (8-32, depending on antigen and institution), refer to a specialist for more invasive testing (e.g., amniocentesis, fetal blood sampling, and/or fetal middle cerebral artery Doppler velocimetry). These infants are at risk for erythroblastosis fetalis and hemolytic disease of the newborn.

14

OBSTETRICS

Prenatal Diagnosis of Congenital Disorders

   I. Overview. Major congenital anomalies occur in 3% of live-born infants at term and represent the leading cause of infant mortality in the United States. Family history should be obtained to evaluate the risk of congenital disease. All women should be offered serum AFP/quadruple screen. A patient's attitude toward termination should not influence the screening/counseling. Knowledge of fetal abnormality can facilitate psychologic adjustment and aid in the care of the fetus.
  II. Methods of Screening and Diagnosis.
   A. AFP/quadruple screen. Offer to all pregnant women at 15 to 20 weeks (see below).
   B. Chorionic villus sampling at 10 to 12 weeks (fetal loss rate is 0.5% to 1.5%). Association with increase in limb defects is controversial and may not exist.
   C. Early amniocentesis performed between 12 and 15 weeks with 1% to 2% fetal loss rate.
   D. Second-trimester amniocentesis at 15 to 20 weeks, with 0.5% to 1% fetal loss rate.
   E. Fetal ultrasound.

α-Fetoprotein and Quadruple Screen

   I. Overview.
   A. The measurement of AFP, estriol, and HCG (triple screen) or AFP, estriol, HCG, and inhibin A (quadruple screen) in maternal serum at 15 to 20 weeks of gestation is used as a screening test for fetal structural abnormalities and chromosomal abnormalities (trisomy 21). Levels depend on maternal weight and gestational age. **Because proper interpretation depends on fetal age, women with abnormal values should be referred for ultrasound to confirm gestational age and to evaluate for neural tube defects and other structural abnormalities.**
   B. In the United States, the incidence of NTDs is roughly 1 per 1000 live births. The incidence of Down's syndrome increases dramatically with maternal age; at age 25 the risk is 1:1500 and by age 35 the risk is 1:300. The patient should be counseled regarding the use of this test because the false positive rate for Down's syndrome is 7%, and the detection rate is 81%. **Incidence also increases with increasing paternal age,** although the link is less well defined.
  II. If ultrasound dating confirms the patient's dates but no diagnostic structural abnormalities are seen (i.e., the triple/quadruple screen is abnormal), the patient should be referred for amniocentesis.
 III. Risks. Psychologic stress, false-positive results, false reassurance, and potential fetal trauma secondary to amniocentesis.
 IV. Causes of an Elevated AFP. Underestimated gestational age; open NTDs (meningomyelocele, anencephaly); fetal nephrosis and

cystic hygroma; fetal GI obstruction, omphalocele, gastroschisis; prematurity, low birth weight, FGR; abdominal pregnancy; multiple fetuses; fetal demise.

V. Causes of a Low AFP. Overestimated gestational age, missed abortion, molar pregnancy, chromosomal abnormalities (including Down's syndrome).

VI. Trisomy 21 (Down's syndrome) also causes a low estriol, elevated HCG, low AFP, and low inhibin.

Fetal Surveillance

I. Obstetric Ultrasound.

A. Indications. Value of routine screening ultrasound is questionable. Utility includes:

1. To determine location and viability of pregnancy.
2. To determine gestational age.
3. To measure and monitor fetal growth (identify macrosomia or intrauterine growth restriction).
4. To identify multiple-gestation pregnancies.
5. To detect fetal anomalies (nearly 100% sensitive for detection of NTD).
6. To detect oligohydramnios or polyhydramnios (if size greater or less than dates).
7. To demonstrate placental abnormalities (e.g., abruption, placenta previa).
8. To identify maternal uterine and pelvic anomalies.

B. Timing depends on the indication for ultrasound.

1. Estimated date of conception: the earlier, the better (first trimester ultrasound gives EDC ± 5-7 days; second trimester EDC ± 10-14 days; third trimester EDC ± 3 weeks).
2. Fetal anomalies might not become apparent until after 16 to 20 weeks.
3. Presentation when ready for external version or delivery.

II. Nonstress Testing (NST).

A. Timing depends upon indication; however, a nonreactive NST prior to 28 weeks has poor predictive value.

B. Indications. High-risk pregnancies including hypertension, diabetes mellitus, multiple gestation, suspected oligohydramnios or FGR, known placental abnormality, maternal heart or kidney disease, hemoglobinopathy, postdated pregnancies, previous unexplained fetal demise, and maternal perceptions of decreased fetal movement.

C. Equipment. External fetal heart rate monitor and uterine contraction monitor.

D. Interpretation.

1. **A reassuring NST** requires two fetal heart rate accelerations of 15 bpm or more lasting at least 15 seconds during a 20-minute period.
2. The **NST is nonreactive** when the criteria for a reassuring NST are not met in 40 minutes (give mother juice or a snack after 20 minutes).

14

OBSTETRICS

Acoustic stimulation, a contraction stress test, or a biophysical profile (BPP; see later) is then indicated. Late decelerations or repetitive (3 in 20 min) or prolonged (≥1 min) variable decelerations on the NST require further evaluation or expeditious delivery.

3. **Follow-up testing** depends on severity of indication for the test. Early surveillance for mild conditions are usually done weekly, whereas hospitalized patients often require daily or continuous monitoring. A reactive test predicts about 5 days of fetal well-being but can't predict unforeseeable events (e.g., cord accident or abruption).

III. **Fetal Acoustic Stimulation.**
   A. **Indication.** Nonreassuring NST or nonreassuring fetal heart rate tracing in labor.
   B. **Equipment.** A mechanical diaphragm to transmit a sound through the maternal abdomen.
   C. **Interpretation.** Reassuring when fetal heart rate acceleration (15 bpm for 15 sec) is generated in response.

IV. **Contraction Stress Test.**
   A. **Indication.** Follow-up of a nonreassuring NST.
   B. **Procedure.** Use nipple stimulation or intravenous oxytocin (see induction of labor) to produce three contractions of 40 seconds' duration in 10 minutes.
   C. **Interpretation.** Lack of fetal heart rate deceleration associated with contractions is reassuring.

V. **Biophysical Profile.**
   A. **Indications.** May be used as early as 26 to 28 weeks for surveillance of a complicated or high-risk pregnancy. Usually used to assess a fetus after a nonreassuring NST.
   B. **Procedural details.** Real-time ultrasound coupled with an NST.
   C. **Interpretation.** Five parameters: fetal breathing movements; gross body movements, fetal muscle tone, amniotic fluid volume (look for pocket of amniotic fluid that measures 2 cm in two perpendicular planes), reactivity of fetal heart rate. Each component of the BPP is given a score of 0 (parameter absent) or 2 (parameter present). A score of 8 or 10 is reassuring, 6 is equivocal, and 4 and lower is abnormal. If amniotic fluid volume is low, further evaluation is needed regardless of total score.

VI. **Amniotic Fluid Index** is the sum of the diameter of the largest pocket of amniotic fluid in each of the four quadrants. Normal values depend upon gestational age (>5 is normal late in pregnancy). Some practitioners use NST plus AFI (modified biophysical profile) for surveillance in late second and third trimester.

VII. **Amniocentesis.**
   A. **Indications**
   1. **Advanced maternal age** (35 years of age or older).
   2. **Previous pregnancy** resulting in the birth of a child with a chromosome abnormality.

3. **Down's syndrome or other chromosome abnormality** in either parent or close family member or if either parent is a carrier of a genetically transmitted disease (e.g., Duchenne's muscular dystrophy, hemophilia, metabolic disease).

4. **NTD** in either parent or a first-degree relative or previous child born with an NTD.

5. **Abnormal serum AFP/triple screen.**

6. **To detect isoimmunization.**

7. **To determine fetal lung maturity** (i.e., risk of early delivery).

a. **Lecithin-to-sphingomyelin (L/S) ratio.** If L/S is >2.0, there is a low risk of respiratory distress secondary to prematurity.

b. **Phosphatidylglycerol** first appears at 35 weeks' gestation and increases in concentration until 40 weeks. If present, it provides reassurance of fetal lung maturity.

B. **Timing.** Identification of inherited disorders in women at risk is done at 14 to 18 weeks of gestation. Determination of fetal lung maturity is done when weighing the risk of early delivery against risk of not delivering.

Nausea and Vomiting of Pregnancy

I. **Cause.** Unknown. Probably not related to serum HCG levels, but other hormones have been implicated (estradiol, thyroxine).

II. **Hyperemesis Gravidarum.**

A. The incidence of hyperemesis gravidarum (severe nausea and vomiting causing ketosis and dehydration requiring hospitalization) is increased in multiple gestation and molar pregnancies. Therefore, ultrasound is advisable in cases of hyperemesis gravidarum.

B. Exclude organic causes: disorders of GI tract, gallbladder, pancreas, hepatitis, and urinary infection. Recent data suggest an association with *Helicobacter pylori*, but this has not yet been proved, and treatment for *H. pylori* is not yet standard of care. Elevation of serum transaminases and mild jaundice can be observed; these return to normal after adequate hydration and nutrition. Hyperemesis gravidarum has a 26% recurrence rate in subsequent pregnancies.

III. **Outpatient Management.**

A. Reassurance that condition improves with time, usually by end of first trimester. Avoid environmental triggers, especially strong odors.

B. Avoid medications whenever possible.

C. Advise patient to arise slowly and to keep soda crackers at the bedside to eat before rising.

D. Omit iron supplementation until nausea resolves.

E. Eat frequent, small meals and protein snacks at night.

F. **Antiemetics**

1. Monotherapy: vitamin B_6 (pyridoxine; category A) 10 to 25 mg, tid or qid.

2. Add doxylamine succinate (Unisom; category A) 25 mg, 0.5 to 1 tablet PO qAM and qPM. This can be used in conjunction with pyridoxine, and dosage can be adjusted according to the patient's symptoms.
3. Add promethazine 12.5 to 25 mg q4h PO or PR (Phenergan; category C); or dimenhydrinate (Dramamine; category B) 50 to 100 mg q4-6h PO or PR, not to exceed 400 mg/d (not to exceed 200 mg/d if on doxylamine); or diphenhydramine (Benadryl) 25 to 50 mg PO q6-8h.
4. Phosphorylated carbohydrate (Naus-A-Way, Emetrol, Nausetrol) 15 to 30 mL PO on arising and q3h prn for nausea.
5. Meclizine 25 to 100 mg PO bid to qid.
6. See below for other pharmacological agents also used in difficult out-patient cases.

IV. Inpatient Management.
A. Inpatient management is required for those with severe symptoms, weight loss, dehydration, ketones in urine, or high urine specific gravity. Correct hypovolemia, ketosis, and electrolyte imbalances with IV fluids. Use oral fluids as tolerated. **Monitor fluid intake and output.** Give IV fluids and IV thiamine daily for 2 to 3 days.
B. Antiemetics as above; also consider phenothiazines: prochlorperazine (Compazine; class C) 5 to 10 mg q4h IM/PO or 25 mg PR bid, droperidol (Inapsine) and promethazine (Phenergan). Metoclopramide (Reglan; class B) 5 to 10 mg q8h IM/PO. Ondansetron (Zofran; class B) has also been used in extreme cases of nausea and vomiting of pregnancy without adverse fetal effects.
C. Parenteral nutrition for prolonged vomiting.
D. Psychotherapeutic measures, stimulus control, biofeedback, and imagery can also be helpful.
E. Steroids and erythromycin have also been used with good effect in some studies. These are a last resort; steroids may increase malformations.

SPECIAL PRENATAL CARE

Fetal Growth Restriction

I. Definition. FGR is defined as a fetus weighing less than the tenth percentile for gestational age.
A. Symmetric FGR (intrinsic). Normal head circumference–to–abdominal circumference ratio; caused by genetic disease or fetal infection and has a poor prognosis.
B. Asymmetric FGR (extrinsic). Increased head circumference–to–abdominal circumference ratio; caused by placental insufficiency and has good prognosis with appropriate treatment.
II. Risk Factors.
A. Chronic maternal disease including chronic maternal hypertension, PIH, diabetes, cyanotic heart disease, collagen vascular disease,

severe maternal anemia, renal disease, multifetal pregnancy, maternal thrombophilic disorder, etc.

B. Fetal genetic disorders or fetal malformations; consider fetal karyotyping.

C. Intrauterine infections including rubella, herpes, toxoplasmosis, syphilis, CMV, and varicella.

D. Previous history of small-for-gestational-age baby, smoking, or drug or alcohol abuse.

E. Abnormalities of the placenta or placental blood flow.

III. Diagnosis. Be suspicious when the fundal height does not exhibit the predicted 1 cm/wk growth between 20 and 36 weeks of gestation. A lag in fundal height by 4 cm mandates ultrasonographic evaluation; otherwise, consider ultrasound on a clinical basis. Serial ultrasonic scanning may confirm the diagnosis.

IV. Management. FGR makes the pregnancy high risk. Close antepartum surveillance is required: serial US, weekly biophysical profile, and/or umbilical artery Doppler velocimetry. The decision about when to deliver the infant is complex. These patients should be referred or managed in consultation with a perinatologist.

V. Outcomes. Stillbirth, oligohydramnios, and intrapartum fetal acidosis are common complications. Neonatal complications include persistent fetal circulation, meconium aspiration syndrome, hypoxic ischemic encephalopathy, hypoglycemia, hypocalcemia, hyperviscosity, and defective temperature regulation.

14

OBSTETRICS

Hypertension, Preeclampsia, and Eclampsia

I. Definitions.

A. Pregnancy-induced hypertension (PIH) is the development of hypertension (DBP >90 mm Hg or SBP >140) during pregnancy without proteinuria.

B. Preeclampsia is defined as the new development of hypertension accompanied by proteinuria after 20 weeks' gestation. Preeclampsia traditionally has been divided into mild and severe forms.

1. Criteria for severe preeclampsia are new onset of hypertension and proteinuria plus one of the following:

a. BP >160/110 (on 2 occasions at least 6 hours apart with patient on bed rest).

b. Proteinuria (>5 g/24 h or 3+ or 4+ on urine dipstick).

c. CNS dysfunction (severe headache, blurred vision, altered mental status, scotomata).

d. Evidence of liver capsule distention (RUQ pain, nausea, vomiting).

e. Oliguria (<500 mL/24 h).

f. Lab abnormalities (serum transaminase higher than 2 times normal or platelets <100,000/mm^3).

g. Pulmonary edema, cyanosis, or cerebral vascular accident.

h. Intrauterine growth restriction.

2. **Preeclampsia is mild if patient has all of the following:**
   a. Mild hypertension (BP >140/90, but <160/110).
   b. Mild proteinuria (300 mg to <5 g/24 h).
   c. No criterion for severe preeclampsia.

   C. Eclampsia is the occurrence of a seizure that is not attributable to other causes in a preeclamptic patient.

II. Risk factors. First pregnancy (especially if <20 y), mother older than 35 years, multiple gestation, malnutrition, high BMI, family history of PIH, preeclampsia with previous pregnancy, chronic hypertension, DM, antiphospholipid antibody syndrome, and underlying vascular, renal, or connective tissue disease. Suspect molar pregnancy if gestational hypertension occurs early in gestation.

III. Evaluation of PIH and Preeclampsia.

   A. History. Document risk factors and any symptoms outlined above.

   B. Physical. Document edema (particularly of the hands and face), BP changes, volume status, retinal changes, neuro exam, hyperreflexia, clonus, and RUQ tenderness.

   C. Initial laboratory studies.

   1. **Blood tests:** CBC, electrolytes, BUN and creatinine, uric acid may be elevated (>5.5 ng/dL) before there are other signs or symptoms of preeclampsia; LFTs (elevated AST, ALT, LDH), and coagulation studies (elevated PT, PTT, and elevated fibrinogen degradation products). If patient is in labor, send a blood type and screen.

   2. **Urine:** 24-hour urine for creatinine clearance, total protein.

IV. Complications of Preeclampsia. Eclamptic seizures; HELLP syndrome (hemolysis, elevated liver function tests, low platelet count); hepatic rupture; DIC; pulmonary edema; acute renal failure; placental abruption; intrauterine fetal demise (IUFD); cerebral hemorrhage; cortical blindness; retinal detachment.

V. Management of PIH and Preeclampsia.

   A. Outpatient management. Home bed rest, home blood pressure monitoring, weight, and urine protein checks are helpful. Antepartum surveillance (NST) should begin early. Ultrasound exams should be performed periodically to ensure adequate amniotic fluid and to monitor for fetal growth restriction.

   B. Hospital management

   1. **Indications.** No improvement of mild preeclampsia or gestational hypertension with home bed rest or severe preeclampsia.

   2. **Orders.** Bed rest with bathroom privileges. The goal of IV fluids is to replace urine output and insensible losses. Periodic deep tendon reflex and neurologic checks.

   3. **Laboratory evaluation and weights** performed daily to every other day. Antepartum surveillance including daily fetal movement count, daily NSTs, and weekly amniotic fluid determinations by ultrasound is essential. Monitor symptoms such as headache, vision disturbances, and epigastric pain.

4. **Delivery is treatment of choice.** Delivery should be accomplished when the fetus is mature but may be required early if maternal health is in danger or if there is evidence of fetal distress. Delivery is indicated when the patient meets criteria for severe preeclampsia. Betamethasone 12 mg IM should be given twice, 24 hours apart, to stimulate fetal lung maturation. Giving repeat doses weekly if pregnancy is prolonged is controversial and not recommended by ACOG because studies have shown possible risk greater than benefit. Electronic FHR monitoring during labor is indicated.

5. **Antihypertensive therapy** is indicated only if BP is persistently >160/110. Aim for a DBP 90 to 100 mm Hg. Avoid overcorrection, because normal blood pressures can cause placental hypoperfusion.

a. Diuretics and ACE inhibitors are contraindicated during pregnancy.

b. Acute management: hydralazine (category C) IV 5-mg bolus and infusion.

c. Long-term medications (if the fetus is immature) include methyldopa (Aldomet; category B), atenolol (category D), and labetalol (category C).

6. **Anticonvulsant therapy.** Seizure prophylaxis is indicated in all preeclamptic patients during labor and delivery and for a minimum of 24 hours postpartum. Seizures may occur in the absence of hyperreflexia, and increased DTRs may be present in the normal population; therefore, hyperreflexia is not a useful predictor of who will have a seizure.

a. Drug of choice for seizure prophylaxis is magnesium sulfate (category B).

b. The loading dose is 4 to 6 g $MgSO_4$ IV over 20 minutes and continued at 2 g/h.

c. To treat active seizures, $MgSO_4$ 1 g/min IV until seizures are controlled, up to 4 to 6 g maximum. If this fails, see Chapter 2 for management of status epilepticus.

d. Continue $MgSO_4$ therapy at least 24 hours postpartum. Twenty-five percent of seizures occur postpartum. Monitor urine output postpartum and stop therapy if urine output is >200 mL/h for 4 consecutive hours. Watch for postpartum hemorrhage because $MgSO_4$ can relax the uterus.

7. **Managing magnesium therapy**

a. Monitor urine output (100 mL in 4 h), deep tendon reflexes, and serum levels. Therapeutic magnesium level is 4 mEq/L, but because it takes 12 to 18 hours to equilibrate, serum levels of $MgSO_4$ are of dubious value.

b. Magnesium toxicity. Loss of reflexes and drowsiness herald magnesium toxicity. At levels of 10 to 12 mEq/L and greater, muscle weakness, respiratory paralysis, and cardiac depression can occur.

c. To treat magnesium toxicity, 10 mL 10% calcium gluconate (or calcium chloride) may be administered by IV push in the event of magnesium toxicity, or the magnesium infusion can be turned off for 1 to 2 hours.

VI. **Prevention of Preeclampsia.** No evidence-based preventive measures have been found.

OBSTETRICS 14

VII. Chronic Hypertension Superimposed on Pregnancy.

A. Risks

1. **Maternal.** The risk to the mother is the same as in the nonpregnant state. However, in the presence of superimposed preeclampsia (20%), there is increased maternal mortality, often from intracranial hemorrhage.
2. **Fetal.** There is an increased incidence of perinatal death, FGR, and fetal distress.

B. Management

1. **Treatment of chronic hypertension can decrease maternal and, to some extent, fetal morbidity.** Appropriate medications include methyldopa, hydralazine, and β-blockers.
2. **During pregnancy, it is _not_ appropriate to use**
   a. Sympathetic ganglion blockers (orthostatic hypotension)
   b. Diuretics (aggravation of volume depletion)
   c. ACE inhibitors (associated with fetal defects and neonatal renal failure)
3. **Laboratory evaluation is performed early in pregnancy.**
4. **Obstetric visits** are scheduled every other week from 24 to 30 weeks, and weekly thereafter.
5. **Early ultrasound** is obtained for dating and then repeated periodically to look for evidence of FGR.
6. **Prenatal surveillance** (NSTs) should begin at 34 weeks.
7. **Timing the delivery.** The pregnancy should not be allowed to go beyond 40 weeks. Delivery may be required earlier if there is evidence of FGR or fetal distress or if hypertension cannot be controlled by bed rest and medication.
8. **Intrapartum monitoring** is required during labor.
9. If there is evidence of FGR, cesarean section is preferable to a prolonged induction.
10. Complicated cases or women with superimposed preeclampsia should be handled at an appropriate referral center.

Group B Streptococcal Infection

I. **Risk factors for Neonatal Sepsis.** Intrapartum chorioamnionitis, maternal group B streptococcal (GBS) colonization in the rectum or vagina, prolonged rupture of membranes, and prolonged monitoring with an internal pressure catheter or fetal scalp lead.

II. **Vertical Transmission of GBS.** GBS is the number one cause of neonatal sepsis and meningitis in the United States. Infection occurs in 2 or 3 neonates per 1000 live births. Maternal colonization can be transient, and 20% to 25% of pregnant females are carriers at any given time. In addition to threatening the life of the neonate, GBS is also an important risk factor for development of chorioamnionitis in the mother, thereby increasing morbidity and the rate of intrapartum complications.

III. **Screening.**

A. **Women with a previous GBS-affected pregnancy, positive urine culture during this pregnancy, or delivering prior to GBS screening and prior to 37 weeks should be given prophylactic antibiotics.**

B. **Culture all other women** (rectal and vaginal swab) at 35 to 37 weeks. Patients positive for GBS should be given intrapartum antibiotic prophylaxis. Sensitivities should be requested for penicillin-allergic patients.

C. **Treatment.** Goal is antibiotics at least 4 hours prior to delivery.

1. **Penicillin G** 5 MU IV and then 2.5 MU q4h until delivery. Penicillin G is the preferred antibiotic because of its efficacy and narrow spectrum.

2. **Ampicillin** 2 g IV followed by 1 g q4h until delivery.

3. **For penicillin allergy,** clindamycin 900 mg IV q8h, cefazolin 2 g IV followed by 1 g q8h, or erythromycin 500 mg IV q6h may be given until delivery.

D. **Unscreened patients.** Provide antibiotic prophylaxis to:

1. Women with history of **previous GBS-affected neonate** or GBS bacteriuria during this pregnancy or when labor starts prior to 37 weeks.

2. If **membranes have been ruptured for ≥18 hours** (≥12 hours in some institutions).

3. Intrapartum **temperature 38.0° C** (100.4° F) or higher.

IV. **Care of the Infant of a Mother Who Has Had GBS Prophylaxis.**

A. **Any infant with symptoms or signs of GBS must have a full work-up** (CBC, CRP, blood culture, CXR for pulmonary symptoms, LP if indicated). Such infants should be treated until culture results are negative.

B. **Infants born at less than 35 weeks** of gestation without signs of GBS infection should get a limited work-up (CBC with differential, CRP, and blood culture). Antibiotics depend on lab results and level of clinical suspicion.

C. **For infants delivered after 35 weeks without symptoms,** approach is stratified based on duration of labor after administration of antibiotics.

1. If duration of labor after **antibiotics is less than 4 hours,** infant should have CBC, CRP, blood culture, and 48 hours of observation.

2. If duration of labor after **antibiotics is at least 4 hours,** observation for 48 hours is indicated.

Gestational Diabetes Mellitus

I. **Potential Morbidity.**

A. Infants born to diabetic mothers have five times the normal risk of respiratory distress syndrome, an increased risk of congenital anomalies (especially with first-trimester hyperglycemia), and increased risk of neonatal hypoglycemia, hypocalcemia, and jaundice.

B. The mother has increased risk of preeclampsia, infection, postpartum bleeding, shoulder dystocia, and cesarean section (secondary to macrosomia).

II. Evaluation.

A. Glucose challenge test (GCT)

1. **Timing.** A GCT is performed as a routine screen for GDM in all pregnancies at 24 to 28 weeks of gestation in the United States.
2. If there are risk factors or signs or symptoms of GDM (e.g., BMI >35, prior history of GDM), consider screening at the first prenatal visit. Repeat at 24 to 28 weeks if the initial test is negative.
3. **Procedure.** A blood glucose level is obtained 1 hour after a 50-g oral glucose load.
4. **Interpretation.** A level of 140 mg/dL or greater is abnormal, although some centers use lower values. Some also adjust cutoff if the patient has high pretest probability.

B. Glucose tolerance test (GTT)

1. **Indication.** Follow-up of an abnormal GCT result.
2. **Procedure.** The patient must eat a diet containing at least 150 g of carbohydrate for 2 days. Draw a serum glucose level after an overnight fast. The patient then ingests 100 g of glucose solution. Serum glucose levels are then obtained at 1, 2, and 3 hours after ingestion.
3. **Interpretation (Box 14-2).** If two or more of these readings are abnormal, the patient needs treatment for GDM.

C. Management of gestational diabetes

1. **Diet adjustment** is the mainstay of therapy.
   a. Caloric intake should be 30 to 35 kcal/kg per day. Intake should be reduced to 24 kcal/kg per day if the patient is obese.
   b. Avoid sweetened beverages, sweets, candy, and other fast-acting carbohydrates.
   c. Exercise has shown added benefit along with diet therapy.
2. **Obstetric surveillance**
   a. **Early ultrasound** for accurate gestational dating.
   b. **Follow clinically every 2 weeks** until 36 weeks and then weekly.
   c. **Blood sugar monitoring.** Home glucose monitoring initially 5 times a day: fasting (goal <100 mg/dL), 1 to 2 hours postprandially

---

BOX 14-2

UPPER LIMITS OF NORMAL SERUM GLUCOSE LEVELS WITH 3-HOUR GTT

Test is given after 3 days of unrestricted diet (>150 g carbohydrates/day) and activity. Give 100-g oral glucose load after overnight fast. Two or more abnormal values indicate gestational diabetes.

Fasting: 95 mg/dL

1 hour: 180 mg/dL

2 hours: 155 mg/dL

3 hours: 140 mg/dL

(goal <140 mg/dL) and at bedtime (goal <140 mg/dL). Review home monitoring at each visit and periodically check a glucose level in the office. If the patient does not successfully control blood sugar with diet and exercise, she will need insulin. Consider referral to high-risk OB. Late in pregnancy, loss of glycemic control may be managed with oral agents. Studies suggest that glyburide throughout pregnancy is as efficacious as insulin in treating GDM, and without increased teratogenicity. Metformin is also being studied for prevention and treatment of GDM, with initial results being favorable.

d. **Check for ketonuria** daily to make sure there has been adequate calorie consumption.
e. **Obtain an ultrasound if macrosomia is suspected.** If the estimated fetal weight is >4000 g at term, consider C-section.
f. **Fetal surveillance** (NST) is indicated for patients whose blood glucose is not controlled by diet.
g. Weigh risks and benefits of cervical ripening and induction at or before 40 weeks.
h. Amniocentesis is helpful in documenting fetal lung maturity before early C-section, because infants of diabetic mothers have delayed lung maturity.

3. **Postpartum**
a. Infants need glucose monitoring (e.g., 1, 2, 4, 8, 24 hours after delivery) until they are feeding well.
b. Women with gestational diabetes should have a 75-g oral GTT checked 6 weeks postpartum to rule out persistent carbohydrate intolerance. Warn that approximately 35% of women with gestational diabetes develop diabetes later in life. Encourage prudent diet and exercise.

Trauma and Pregnancy

I. **Differential.** Retrospective study in a tertiary referral center showed etiology of trauma in pregnancy: 54% motor vehicle accidents, 22% domestic violence, 21% falls, and 1.3% burn, puncture, or assault. Up to 50% of falls cause some degree of abruption.
A. **Physical or sexual abuse.** Abused women tend to present late for prenatal care. Generally, abuse continues and can worsen during pregnancy. Abused patients have an increased risk for preterm labor, chorioamnionitis, and LBW infants. Asking direct questions, such as "Has anyone hit, slapped, or kicked you?" is the best way of screening for abuse.
B. **Serious injuries have the greatest risk of obstetric complications,** although there are case reports of fetal death after minimal trauma resulting in force to the uterus, especially after 35 weeks. Most common sequelae are preterm labor, spontaneous abortion, and placental abruption.

14

OBSTETRICS

II. **Management.**

A. **Treatment of pregnant woman.** ABCs of evaluating and stabilizing the mother take priority. Deflect uterus away from great vessels by placing wedge under right hip or tilt table laterally. Once the mother has been stabilized, consider fetus. **If mother is Rh negative, give RhoGAM.**

B. **Evaluation of fetus**

1. Trauma increases the risk of placental abruption and fetomaternal hemorrhage. Monitoring fetal heart rate and maternal contractions are the best way to assess for significant abruption. Ultrasound is less sensitive and MRI is not generally practical (although very sensitive). Monitoring for approximately 4 hours is sufficient if the fetal tracing is normal (reactive with good beat-to-beat variability, contractions <6/h, and no fetal decelerations with contractions), and no ominous signs (rupture of membranes, vaginal bleed, contractions, or uterine tenderness) are noted.

2. If contractions are not detected or occur less than every 10 minutes and monitoring of the fetus is normal, abruption is unlikely. Twenty percent of women with contractions more frequent than every 10 minutes have associated abruption.

C. **Patient education.** Women should be instructed to return for abdominal cramps, increasing pain, or vaginal bleeding.

PRENATAL CARE FOR PATIENTS AT RISK FOR PRETERM LABOR

I. **Risk factors** for preterm labor include history of preterm birth, infection, placental pathology, occupational fatigue, extremes of reproductive age, substance abuse, and significant life stressors.

II. **Management.** Frequent visits during weeks 16 to 32, a second-trimester urine culture for asymptomatic bacteriuria (regular retesting for high-risk women—i.e., sickle cell trait, history of recurrent UTIs, DM, or renal disease), treatment of periodontal disease, cervical exam for cervical length (or US for cervical length assessment), monitoring uterine activity, and reinforcing warning signs for preterm labor (abdominal cramping, pressure, backache, increased vaginal discharge, fluid leak, regular uterine contractions).

Early Antepartum Hemorrhage

I. **Definition.** Vaginal bleeding earlier than 20 weeks of gestation.

II. **Differential Diagnosis of Early Vaginal Bleeding.**

A. **Spontaneous abortion**

1. **Incidence** of spontaneous abortion is 15% to 25% of clinically recognized pregnancies.

2. **Causes.** Fetal abnormalities incompatible with life (chromosomal and other), defective implantation, maternal infection, and uterine and cervical anomalies.

3. **Evaluation**
   a. **History** suggestive of pregnancy (missed period or periods, nausea, vomiting, breast tenderness) followed by cramping and spotting or bleeding, often with passage of tissue. All patients should be evaluated to rule out an ectopic pregnancy. Remember patients must be seen within 48 hours for RhoGAM if mother is Rh negative.
   b. **Exam** including stability of vital signs, orthostatic vital signs, pelvic exam looking for open or closed cervical os, presence of tissue, other causes of vaginal bleeding (such as cervical eversion, polyp, infection, vaginal lesion, ectopic fetus). Size uterus. Check for fetal heart tones with Doppler if 10 to 12 weeks.
   c. **Lab tests**
      (1) **Urine pregnancy test** is positive in only 75% of cases, so a negative pregnancy test does not rule out spontaneous abortion.
      (2) **CBC, blood type, and antibody screen** in all patients for Rh status. RhoGAM is indicated for all Rh-negative, antibody-negative women.
      (3) **Uterine ultrasound** or pathologic exam of tissue if indicated.
      (4) **Serial quantitative HCG** should increase by at least 60% in 48 hours. Mean doubling time is 1.4 to 2.1 days. If HCG does not rise or drops, it is likely that the pregnancy is nonviable.
   d. **β-HCG levels and transvaginal US findings.** (Table 14-2)
B. **Threatened abortion.** Vaginal bleeding with or without cramps but with a cervix that is long and closed, with a uterus appropriate for gestational age. Roughly 50% progress to inevitable abortion.
C. **Inevitable abortion.** Persistent cramps, moderate bleeding, and open cervical os. Do not confuse with an incompetent cervix, which is a painless cervical dilation not associated with cramping and is potentially treatable.
D. **Incomplete abortion.** The same symptoms as an inevitable abortion but with some retained products of conception in the uterus or cervical canal. There is ongoing cramping and excessive vaginal bleeding. Speculum examination reveals a dilated internal os and tissue present within the endocervical canal or vagina. Bleeding may be heavy and clots may be mistaken for products of conception.
E. **Complete abortion.** The entire conceptus is expelled, and cramping and bleeding abate or resolve completely. On examination, the uterus is firm and is smaller than one would expect for gestational age.
F. **Missed abortion.** Products of conception retained 3 or more weeks after fetal death. Signs and symptoms of pregnancy abate; pregnancy test becomes negative. Brownish vaginal discharge (rarely frank bleeding) occurs. Cramping is rare. The uterus is soft and irregular. Ultrasound exam rules out live pregnancy.
G. **Septic abortion.** Any of the above scenarios and a temperature greater than 38° C (100.5° F) with no other source of fever. Septic abortion is associated with (but does not require) IUD use or instrumentation during abortion. Abdominal and uterine tenderness are present as well as purulent discharge and possibly shock.

14

OBSTETRICS

H. Ectopic pregnancy. See Chapter 13.

I. Molar pregnancy (hydatidiform mole)

1. Placenta undergoes trophoblastic proliferation and typically resembles a cluster of grapes. Occurs more often in women younger than 20 or older than 40 years and almost always causes some degree of vaginal bleeding.

2. Hydatidiform moles are associated with hyperemesis gravidarum and the onset of preeclampsia before the third trimester. The uterus is larger than expected for gestational age in 50% of the cases. Ovarian enlargement may occur secondary to thecal lutein cysts. Ultrasound findings typically show a "snowstorm" pattern. Nearly 20% of hydatidiform moles progress to gestational trophoblastic tumor.

3. **Treatment** is immediate evacuation of mole and subsequent meticulous follow-up for detection of persistent trophoblastic proliferation or malignant change.

J. Cervical insufficiency (previously incompetent os, incompetent cervix). History of recurrent second-trimester fetal loss. Generally painless or lower abdominal pressure. Value of cerclage is debated.

III. Treatment of Bleeding

A. Ensure adequate circulating volume. Treat with IV normal saline or lactated Ringer's. Consider transfusion if Hb is less than 8 g/dL or patient is unstable.

B. Threatened abortion. Bed rest if possible; use acetaminophen for discomfort, nothing in the vagina (no tampons, douches, intercourse). Consider ultrasound for gestational sac, cardiac activity, or to rule out ectopic pregnancy; positive cardiac activity >90% predicts continued pregnancy. Consider monitoring quantitative β-HCG; a rise of less than 66% in 48 hours predicts abortion or ectopic implantation.

C. Incomplete or inevitable abortion. Hospitalize patient if she is hypovolemic, anemic, or carrying gestation greater than 12 weeks.

TABLE 14-2

CORRELATION OF β-HCG AND ULTRASOUND FINDINGS

β-HCG Level	Ultrasound Examination
>1500 mIU/mL	Should see intrauterine gestational sac
>1500 mIU/mL and rising or plateaued	If no intrauterine gestational sac, then ectopic implantation is very likely
Falling β-HCG	Failed pregnancy (arrested pregnancy, blighted ovum, tubal abortion, resolving ectopic pregnancy)
<1500 mIU/mL	If US is negative, repeat both tests in 3 days (β-HCG should double every 1.5 to 2 days until 6-7 weeks' gestation)
After 3 days: β-HCG should at least double	Intrauterine pregnancy should be demonstrated at 1500 mIU/mL
If β-HCG does not double	If US is negative, then pregnancy is nonviable (ectopic or intrauterine destined to abort)

Tissue visible in os should be gently removed with ring forceps to allow contraction of uterus, but minimize manipulation to decrease risk of infection. Patients with incomplete abortion (tissue passed with continued bleeding) often require suction curettage or D&C. Consider oxytocin drip as an alternative (20 IU in 1000 mL crystalloid solution at 50 to 100 mL/h). If unsuccessful, proceed with D&C.

D. Complete abortion. Discharge home if vital signs stable, Hb documented to be stable, and bleeding decreased. Consider methylergonovine (Methergine) 0.2 mg PO tid for 3 days if diagnosis is certain or after uterine evacuation.

E. Missed abortion. Obtain CBC with differential, platelet count, PT and PTT, and DIC (see Chapter 6) panel if indicated. Outpatient management may be considered if conceptus is retained for less than 4 weeks, if weekly fibrinogen levels are obtained, and if the patient is monitored closely for DIC. Hospitalize if there are signs of infection or DIC or if the fetus has been retained longer than 4 weeks. Fibrinogen levels less than 150 mg/dL call for immediate evacuation of the uterus.

F. Septic abortion. Obtain CBC, UA, culture of discharge from uterus, blood cultures, CXR for diagnosis of septic emboli and to rule out free air from perforation, and abdominal radiograph to evaluate for uterine foreign body. Obtain electrolytes and ABG. Organisms include both anaerobes and aerobes (*Bacteroides, Streptococcus, Enterobacter, Chlamydia, Clostridium*). Hospitalize, treat sepsis, D&C, IV antibiotics: doxycycline plus cefoxitin or imipenem or ticarcillin, or clindamycin plus third-generation cephalosporin or gentamicin. Discharge to home on oral doxycycline or clindamycin.

G. Long-term management. Give RhoGAM to Rh-negative women. Provide emotional support. Traditional but not well-founded recommendation is to wait 3 months before attempting conception. Having a single spontaneous abortion does not increase the risk of aborting the next pregnancy. Evaluate couple for habitual abortion if the woman has had two or more successive spontaneous abortions. If the patient is a habitual aborter, obtain antiphospholipid antibody titers. Obtain fetal tissue for karyotyping if possible.

Late Antepartum Hemorrhage

I. Definition. Vaginal bleeding that occurs after 20 weeks' gestation. Late antepartum hemorrhage is one of the leading causes of antepartum hospitalization, maternal morbidity, and operative intervention. Fetuses also have a higher rate of prematurity and perinatal death than in pregnancies without bleeding.

II. Differential Diagnosis.

A. Placenta previa is implantation of the placenta over the internal cervical os.

OBSTETRICS 14

1. **Incidence.** Occurs in 1 of 200 third-trimester pregnancies (0.5%). The diagnosis of placenta previa is very common in the second trimester, but more than 95% of these will have resolved by delivery. Routine later pregnancy US in low-risk or unselected populations is not recommended.

2. **Classification.** Placenta previa may be marginal, partial, or total depending on how much of the placenta is over the cervical os. "Low-lying placenta" is a subjective assessment that the placenta is close to, but does not cover, the internal os.

3. **Risk factors.** Previous cesarean, previous uterine instrumentation, high parity, advanced maternal age, smoking, and multiple gestations.

4. **Diagnosis.** Vaginal bleeding is typically bright red and painless. The blood loss is not massive but tends to recur and become heavier as the pregnancy progresses. Diagnosis may be made by ultrasound. A gentle speculum exam is permissible. Digital vaginal examination is contraindicated in patients with vaginal bleeding, unless the placental location is precisely known or in a double-setup situation when delivery is desirable and can be rapidly accomplished by C-section.

B. Placental abruption is premature separation of the placenta from the uterine wall.

1. **Incidence.** Placental abruption occurs in 1% to 2% of all pregnancies. Severe abruption is rare.

2. **Classification.**

a. **Mild.** Slight vaginal bleeding (<100 mL), no FHR abnormalities are present, no evidence of shock or coagulopathy.

b. **Moderate.** Moderate vaginal bleeding (100-500 mL) and uterine hypersensitivity with or without elevated tone. Mild shock and fetal distress may be present.

c. **Severe.** Extensive vaginal bleeding (>500 mL), tetanic uterus, and moderate to profound maternal shock are present. Fetal demise and maternal coagulopathy are characteristic.

3. **Diagnosis.** The diagnosis of placental abruption is clinical. Patients often present with abdominal pain that varies from mild cramping to severe pain. Patients with posterior placental abruption may complain of back pain. Active laboring women without abruption or chorioamnionitis should not have pain between contractions. Although dark vaginal bleeding (or bloody amniotic fluid) is present in 80% of cases, bleeding may be concealed in the remainder (that is, retroplacental bleeding). Thus, the maternal hemodynamic situation might not be explained by observed blood loss. Pain and increased uterine tone are typically present. Ask patient about trauma (including domestic violence), presence of pain and contractions, rupture of membranes, and risk factors including hypertension and preeclampsia.

4. **Risk factors** include prior history of abruption, maternal hypertension, cigarette, alcohol, or cocaine use, increasing maternal age, and/or multiparity. Abruption may be associated with premature rupture

of membranes, blunt abdominal trauma, and twin gestation after delivery of first infant.

C. Uterine rupture is very rare. It can mimic severe abruption. An abdominal film may show free intraperitoneal air or an abnormal fetal position. Rupture is accompanied by persistent fetal bradycardia. Emergent C-section and hysterectomy are required.

D. Other.

1. **Vasa previa** (velamentous insertion of the cord). Delivery should be by scheduled C-section. If pregnancy is allowed to progress to term, spontaneous rupture of membrane or amniotomy should be averted because it could lead to fatal bleeding for fetus and possibly mother.

2. Cervical dilation with loss of mucus plug can be confused with other causes of vaginal bleeding or cervical or vaginal lesions (polyps, condylomas, cancer, trauma to the vagina or cervix).

III. Physical Exam. Include assessment for circulatory instability (including orthostatic pulse and blood pressures), trauma, and assessment of fundal height, uterine tenderness, estimated fetal weight, and fetal lie. The patient should have continuous fetal heart rate and contraction monitoring.

IV. Laboratory Evaluation. CBC, type and cross, coagulation studies, urinalysis, and ultrasound.

V. Management of Placenta Previa and Placental Abruption.

A. Placenta previa

1. If pregnancy is 37 weeks or greater, or if fetal lung maturity has been documented, a cesarean section is indicated unless only a minimal degree of placenta previa is present.

2. If bleeding is sufficient to jeopardize the mother or fetus despite transfusion, cesarean section may be indicated regardless of gestation.

3. In the preterm gestation, expectant management is indicated in patients with no observed bleeding, reactive nonstress test, and stable hematocrit, who are compliant with instructions. Most patients require inpatient observation. Corticosteroids may be indicated to help fetal lung maturation. Physical activity is restricted. Placement of cervical cerclage for symptomatic placenta previa can reduce the risk of delivery before 34 weeks or the birth of a baby weighing less than 2 kg (evidence category C). Nothing is allowed in the vagina, including examining fingers. The hematocrit is maintained at 30% or greater. Preterm labor can be managed with magnesium sulfate. There does not appear to be any increased morbidity or mortality associated with the use of tocolytic therapy for preterm third-trimester bleeding in a controlled tertiary care setting (evidence category B). Once 36 to 37 weeks of gestation is reached with fetal lung maturity demonstrated by amniocentesis, the patient is readied for elective double-setup examination. If operative delivery is indicated, regional anesthesia is preferable to general because of increased intraoperative blood loss and need for blood transfusion with general anesthesia.

14

OBSTETRICS

4. **Check for fetal bleeding.** To 5 mL of tap water add 6 drops of 10% KOH in two test tubes. Add 3 drops of maternal blood to one tube and 3 drops of vaginal blood to the other. The maternal blood will turn green-yellowish-brown after 2 minutes. If fetal red blood cells are present, the solution will turn pink. Immediate delivery is indicated.

5. Remember that placenta accreta can complicate placenta previa in women with a history of previous C-section. Hemorrhage can necessitate hysterectomy.

B. Placental abruption

1. Occasionally a small separation occurs without further problem. These patients have no uterine symptoms. Observation is required with fetal heart rate monitoring, serial labs, and ultrasound, but if no fetal distress occurs within the next 48 hours, the patient may be sent home.

2. **If placental abruption is mild and the fetus is immature, expectant management may be indicated,** with fetal heart rate monitoring and serial laboratory and ultrasound examination. **In all other cases, delivery is indicated.** A vaginal delivery is preferred when fetal distress is not present or when the fetus is no longer viable. A C-section is indicated if fetal distress is present. A C-section is also performed when there is a threat to the mother's life or a failed trial of labor.

3. **Shock must be treated with adequate replacement of fluids and packed red blood cells;** NS or Ringer's lactate should be used. Urine output must be maintained at 25 to 30 mL/h. A central venous pressure line or Swan–Ganz catheter will assist in monitoring hemodynamic status. See section on shock in Chapter 2.

4. **Coagulopathy should be treated with fresh frozen plasma.** One unit of FFP increases the fibrinogen concentration by 25 mg/dL. Platelet transfusion is required if the count is less than 50,000. Heparin is not used in DIC secondary to placental abruption. See section on DIC in Chapter 6.

LABOR

Preterm Labor

I. Definition.

A. Uterine contractions between 20 and 37 weeks of gestation (at least three in 30 min) with associated cervical change. Discrimination from "false labor" is difficult. Postponement of treatment until cervical change occurs may lower the chances of success.

B. Preterm deliveries occur in more than 11% of all pregnancies. PTL and preterm premature rupture of membranes (PPROM) are common causes of preterm delivery.

II. Causes. Often unknown. Several factors have been associated with preterm labor.

A. **Maternal factors.** Infections (systemic, vaginal, urinary tract, amnionitis), uterine anomalies, fibroids, retained IUD, cervical incompetence, overdistended uterus (polyhydramnios, multiple gestation), rupture of membranes, race (African Americans disproportionately high).

B. **Fetal factors.** Congenital anomalies, intrauterine death.

C. **Teach patients warning signs:** uterine contractions, backache, bleeding, leaking of fluid, and increased vaginal discharge.

III. **Management.** Determine whether the patient is in labor, membrane status, gestational age of fetus, and underlying risk factors that might require evaluation and management.

A. **Initial examination**

1. **Estimate fetal weight and age** by ultrasound if necessary.

2. **Document FHR** and uterine activity with external monitoring.

3. **Perform sterile speculum exam** to rule out rupture of membranes.

a. Exam will show **pooling** of fluid in vaginal vault.

b. **pH determination.** Amniotic fluid typically turns Nitrazine paper blue. Contamination with vaginal–cervical mucus, blood, semen, or urine can lead to false positives.

c. **Fern test.** Allow a sample of fluid to air dry on a glass or slide. Examination of amniotic fluid under the microscope reveals a classic "fern" pattern.

4. **Pelvic examination.** Attempt to limit to one examiner and use sterile technique. Obtain cervical cultures for group B streptococci, chlamydia, and gonorrhea; do rapid group B streptococci antigen testing if available. If membranes are not ruptured, get vaginal fluid to check for bacterial vaginosis or trichomonas, which can be associated with PTL. If membranes are ruptured, you can used pooled amniotic fluid to determine fetal maturity by looking at the L/S ratio and PG levels; otherwise amniocentesis may be necessary.

5. **Obtain cath UA and culture.**

6. **Consider fetal-fibronectin assay.** Swab posterior vagina **if digital exam of vagina or intercourse have not been performed within 24 hours.** Fetal fibronectin helps maintain placental attachment to the decidua. It is normally present early in pregnancy and then decreases so that none is detectable by 20 weeks. It then reappears shortly before the onset of labor. Can be combined with transvaginal US of cervical length to help predict those who have increased risk of spontaneous preterm birth.

B. **Tocolysis**

1. **Contraindications:** Evidence of fetal distress, fetal anomalies, abruptio placentae, placenta previa with heavy bleeding, severe maternal disease.

2. **Risks of treatment.** If membranes are ruptured, there is increased risk of cord prolapse and amnionitis. Fetal mortality is increased if labor is suppressed when there is FGR. Mother may experience tachycardia, nervousness, or pulmonary edema secondary to medication.

3. Tocolysis most likely will be **ineffective if labor is well established or if the cervix is dilated to 4 cm** or more. Preparation should be made to deliver in the optimal setting. Up to now there have been no large-scale controlled clinical trials demonstrating that tocolytics delay delivery.

4. **β-Adrenergic receptor agonists** can inhibit uterine contractility but only prolong gestation for about 48 hours. To a large extent, the goal of tocolysis is to arrest labor long enough for exogenous steroids to stimulate fetal surfactant production so as to prevent the pulmonary complications of preterm birth.

a. **Protocol**
   (1) Bed rest in left lateral decubitus position. Effective alone in 50% of patients.
   (2) Sedation (100 mg of secobarbital or 50 mg of hydroxyzine).
   (3) Hydration, but avoid large boluses (should not exceed 500 mL).
   (4) Antibiotics are controversial. Do not use for more than 2 days, to limit incidence of resistance.
   (5) FHR and uterine activity monitoring.
   (6) Steroids accelerate fetal lung maturation (betamethasone or dexamethasone 12.5 mg IM q24h for 48 hours).

b. **Drug therapy (tocolytics)**
   (1) **Terbutaline.** Infusion should be titrated on an individual basis so as to maximize inhibition of uterine activity and minimize maternal side effects. Alternative to infusion is 0.25 mg SQ q20-60 min until contractions have subsided. Short-term tocolytic therapy with IV β-mimetics will stop or delay labor for up to 7 days, but there is no improvement in neonatal outcomes (evidence category A). Oral terbutaline does not result in either pregnancy prolongation or reduction in the incidence of recurrent PTL (evidence category E). A single dose of subcutaneous terbutaline is effective in temporarily stopping preterm contractions and results in shortest hospital stay of several methods tested, including IV fluids and observation (evidence category A).
   (2) **Magnesium sulfate.** $MgSO_4$ also decreases uterine contractility, but despite its widespread use it is ineffective in preventing preterm birth (evidence category D).
   (3) **Others.** Prostaglandin synthetase inhibitors (such as indomethacin), calcium channel blockers, aminophylline, and progesterone are under investigation.

Premature Rupture of Membranes

I. Definitions.
A. **"Premature" rupture of membranes (PROM)** occurs if there is a delay of greater than 1 hour until onset of labor.
B. **"Preterm premature" rupture of membranes (PPROM)** occurs before 37 weeks of gestation.

II. Diagnosis.

A. History of fluid gush per vagina. Urine leakage can sometimes be confused with the rupture of membranes.

B. Sterile speculum exam. See discussion of initial exam above under "Preterm Labor."

1. **Equivocal cases** can be evaluated by fetal-fibronectin assay, intrauterine injection of indigo carmine, or ultrasound for severe oligohydramnios.

2. **Cervical digital examinations should be avoided** (increases risk of chorioamnionitis), unless patient is in labor and delivery is inevitable! Evaluate cervix visually with sterile speculum. Check for cord prolapse.

III. Management.

A. PROM at term. Most sources recommend induction and delivery within a range of 24 to 36 hours after admission. Recent data question the dictum that infection rates go up at 24 hours, however.

B. Preterm PROM.

1. Fetal maturity must be considered. Manage expectantly until the fetus is mature unless chorioamnionitis (see below) or fetal distress develops or labor cannot be inhibited with tocolysis (see above).

2. Positive cervical cultures should be treated, but they do not necessitate induction without other signs of chorioamnionitis or fetal distress. Follow maternal and fetal vital signs, including temperature every 6 to 8 hours. Check WBC as indicated and perform regular fetal surveillance. Antibiotics have been shown to prolong pregnancy and decrease infant morbidity (ampicillin plus erythromycin). A single course of corticosteroids to hasten fetal lung development (see protocol above) should be given if prior to 32 weeks and signs of chorioamnionitis are absent.

C. Deliver if there is amnionitis. Signs include maternal or fetal tachycardia, maternal fever, uterine tenderness, foul cervical discharge, uterine contractions, leukocytosis, and presence of leukocytes or bacteria in amniotic fluid. If fetal lung maturity is confirmed at 32 weeks or later, then risk of delivery is less than expectant management.

Postdate Pregnancy

I. Definitions.

A. Prolonged pregnancy. Greater than 40 weeks of gestation.

B. Postdate pregnancy. Greater than 42 weeks (>294 d after the first day of LMP).

C. Postmature pregnancy. Greater than 42 weeks with evidence of placental dysfunction.

II. Etiology.

A. Most common is error in estimating EDC based on LMP, which often leads to overestimation of duration of gestation because of physiologic variations in the length of the follicular phase.

OBSTETRICS 14

B. Risk factors. History of prior prolonged gestation (50% risk), primiparity, anencephaly, or fetal endocrinopathy. Maternal age older than 35 years is protective.

III. Potential Morbidity.

A. Maternal

1. **Birth trauma** secondary to macrosomic infant because of shoulder dystocia.

2. **Operative delivery.** Secondary infection and hemorrhage are more common with postdate pregnancies.

B. Neonatal. Fetal distress, labor dysfunction, hemorrhage, meconium aspiration syndrome, polycythemia, hyperbilirubinemia, hypoglycemia, and anoxic organ damage are more common among postterm deliveries (compared with term).

IV. Management. Delivery should be accomplished by 42 weeks.

A. Antepartum fetal surveillance with NST and amniotic fluid index assessment should be done at 40 and 41 weeks and twice weekly thereafter. The Cochrane Collaboration demonstrated no advantage to allowing pregnancy to continue beyond 41 weeks.

B. Indications for immediate delivery include ripe cervix, decreased amniotic fluid, large fetus (abdominal circumference), nonreactive NST, and presence of meconium in fluid. Pregnancies complicated by hypertension and diabetes should be induced at or near term.

C. Ultrasound is notoriously inaccurate for estimating fetal weight. Depending on the cutoff used, positive predictive values for macrosomic infants are disappointingly low in nondiabetic patients. A prophylactic cesarean policy for US-diagnosed fetal macrosomia would require more than 1000 cesareans to avert one brachial plexus injury. One maternal death would occur for every 3.2 brachial plexus injuries prevented.

D. Evidence does not support induction of labor for suspected macrosomia. However, if induction is felt to be prudent, cervical ripening can be accomplished using PGE_2 gel or insert. PGE_2 gel (1 mg placed intracervically) has been shown to decrease the amount of oxytocin needed to establish labor and to decrease rate of cesarean section in labor induced for medical indications before 41 weeks of gestation. Decreased amniotic fluid leading to variable decelerations and meconium staining may be managed with amnioinfusion (see later). Nasopharyngeal aspiration at the perineum and endotracheal aspiration may be performed once the baby is born to prevent meconium aspiration, although the benefit is questionable. Anticipate shoulder dystocia.

Evaluation of Labor (Box 14-3)

I. Collect the information listed in Box 14-3 on admission to labor and delivery.

II. Pelvic Exam.

> **BOX 14-3**
>
> **ADMISSION INFORMATION FOR LABOR AND DELIVERY**
>
> | | |
> |---|---|
> | Gravida/para | Dating by US or by LMP |
> | Complications | Weight gain during pregnancy |
> | Blood type | Contraction onset, duration, frequency |
> | Rho(D) administered? | Membranes intact or ruptured |
> | Hb/HCT | Fetal movement |
> | Coexisting medical problems? | Fetal position |
> | VDRL, rubella, GBS status | Fundal height |
> | LMP and EDC | Auscultate fetal tones |

14

OBSTETRICS

A. Inspection
1. Look for herpetic lesions, condylomata, and lacerations.
2. **Speculum examination.** Perform sterile speculum exam to rule out rupture of membranes.
B. Palpation of the cervix
1. **Dilation of the cervical os.** Dilatation may range from 0 to 10 cm.
2. **Effacement.** The degree of thinning of the cervix. The cervix may range from 3 cm long (thick or with no effacement) to paper thin (100% effaced). In primiparas, effacement often precedes dilation. Simultaneous effacement and dilation is seen in multiparas.
3. **Palpation of the presenting part**
a. **Identification.** Head, foot, buttock, other.
b. **Station.** Station is described as the relationship of the fetal presenting part to the level of the ischial spines in the maternal pelvis. Station may range from −3 to +3. Zero station (engagement) occurs when the lowermost presenting part is palpable at the level of the ischial spines. Always assess station by both abdominal method and pelvic method to avoid errors caused by caput.
c. **Position.** Position is described as the orientation of the presenting part in regard to the maternal pelvis. Vertex presentation with the occiput positioned either to the right or left anteriorly is the most common.

Normal Labor and Dysfunctional Labor

I. Normal Phases of Labor.
A. Latent phase. Slow rate of dilation, less than 0.6 cm/h. Mean time in latent phase is 8.6 hours for nulliparas, with 95% reaching active phase by 20 hours. It is important not to admit women too early in labor because of increased risk of interventions and more diagnoses of complicated labor.
B. Active labor. Generally once the cervical os reaches 3 to 4 cm. Dilation usually is at least 1.2 cm/h in primiparas and 1.5 cm/h in multiparas. **Active labor is divided into three phases.**

1. **Acceleration.** Dilation rate >0.6 cm/h.
2. **Maximum slope of dilation.** Cervix >5 cm or rate >1.2 cm/h for nulliparas and >1.5 cm/h for multiparas.
3. **Deceleration.** Cervix >9 cm, not completely effaced.

II. Problems with the Progression of Labor. Active management of labor requires recognition of nonprogressive labor. This can be done by graphing the progress of labor (rate of cervical dilation vs. time), monitoring cervical change frequently, especially in early labor (every hour or two), and maintaining the continuity of the examiner to minimize subjective differences.

A. Prolonged latent phase is defined as longer than 20 hours in nulliparas and longer than 14 hours in multiparas.

1. **Causes** include unripe cervix, false labor, sedation, and uterine inertia.
2. **Management** includes observation and need for oxytocin stimulation. Avoid amniotomy. Good prognosis for vaginal delivery.

B. Protracted active phase. Rate of dilation once women enter the active phase is less than 1.2 cm/h in nulliparas and less than 1.5 cm/h in multiparas.

1. **Causes** include fetal malpositions (occiput posterior), CPD, hypotonic uterine contractions, and anesthesia.
2. **Management** includes amniotomy and oxytocin stimulation to increase dilation and shorten labor more than amniotomy alone, or expectant management.

C. Secondary arrest of cervical dilation is cessation of dilation for longer than 2 hours. High incidence of CPD; often requires a cesarean section.

D. Failure of descent is arrest of descent during second stage. High incidence of CPD; often requires cesarean section.

E. Malposition, especially persistent OP position, contributes to dystocia. May be more frequent with epidural use. Maternal position change and manual rotation by provider may help fetus rotate.

F. Protracted descent in nulliparas is less than 1 cm/h and in multiparas is less than 2 cm/h. Causes include CPD, full bladder, and macrosomia. Inadequate pushing because of anesthesia can also cause this disorder. Some advocate waiting until the fetal head is at the introitus in women with epidural anesthesia.

G. Precipitous labor is dilation faster than 5 cm/h in nulliparas and faster than 10 cm/h in multiparas. **Complications** include trauma to birth canal, fetal distress, and postpartum hemorrhage.

H. With adequate contractions as documented with intrauterine pressure catheter, if no change in dilation (active phase) or station (second stage), consider obstetric consult.

I. Patient education, cautious use of induction, use of doulas, and/or alternative pain control options may help prevent dystocia.

Intrapartum Monitoring and Management

Electronic fetal heart rate monitoring may be performed by means of external Doppler or by direct scalp lead when membranes are ruptured.

I. **Indications.** Structured intermittent auscultation (q15-30min during active labor and q5-15min in second stage) or continuous electronic fetal monitoring are recommended for uncomplicated pregnancies. Continuous or more intensive intermittent monitoring is indicated with any high-risk pregnancy.

II. **Interpretation.** Use a systematic approach, such as the ALSO mnemonic or DR C BRAVADO (**Table 14-3**):

A. **D**etermine **R**isk: Is this fetus at high risk (e.g., meconium, FGR)?

B. **C**ontractions (external pressure transducer shows frequency; an intrauterine pressure catheter is needed to measure strength).

1. **Frequency** (every 3-5 min desired). Watch for hyperstimulation (lack of uterine relaxation between contractions, coupling, or tripling).

2. **Strength** should be 50 to 75 mm Hg lasting 45 to 90 seconds. One measure of adequacy is Montevideo units (sum of amplitude of all contractions in a 10-min period ≥200 mm Hg).

C. **B**aseline Fetal Heart **RA**te.

1. **Normal** is 120 to 160 bpm.

2. **Tachycardia** is >160 bpm. **Cause** can be fetal hypoxia, maternal fever, maternal hyperthyroidism, or parasympatholytic or sympathomimetic drugs.

3. **Bradycardia** is <120 bpm. **Cause** can be fetal asphyxia, anesthetics, or fetal cardiac conduction defect. Usually benign if good variability is present.

D. **V**ariability.

1. **Short-term variability.** Beat-to-beat variation is normally 5 to 10 bpm.

2. **Long-term variability.** Waviness of the FHR tracing, which normally has a frequency of 3 to 10 cycles per minute and an amplitude of 10 to 25 bpm.

3. **Decreased variability.** Variability may be decreased by fetal sleep cycles, CNS depression secondary to hypoxia or drugs, parasympatholytic agents, extreme prematurity, or congenital anomalies. Loss of variability

14

OBSTETRICS

TABLE 14-3

INTERPRETATION OF VARIABLE DECELERATIONS

Benign	Ominous
Rapid descent and recovery	Late start (compared to contraction), slow recovery
Good baseline variability	Decreased variability
Acceleration at start and end ("shoulders" or M shape)	Loss of "shoulders"
Intermittent or isolated variables	Baseline tachycardia
	Increased severity of variables

is associated with a high incidence of fetal acidosis and low Apgar
scores.

4. **Sinusoidal pattern.** A smooth sine wave 2 to 5 times per minute of
about 10 bpm amplitude. Variability is absent! **A sinusoidal pattern is
ominous and indicates need for immediate intervention.**

E. **Accelerations.** Reassuring if associated with fetal movement. May be
compensatory before or after deceleration.

F. **Decelerations.**

1. **Early decelerations** mirror uterine contractions (beginning and ending
with the contraction) and are associated with fetal head compression.
The FHR rarely falls below 100 bpm. Benign if other FHR
abnormalities are absent.

2. **Late decelerations** are transient but repetitive deceleration of the FHR
observed to occur late in the contraction phase. These reach their
lowest point after the peak of the contraction and return to baseline
rate after the contraction is over. Recurrent late decelerations can
indicate uteroplacental insufficiency or fetal hypoxia and are considered
ominous.

3. **Variable decelerations** are characterized by variable duration, shape,
and timing in relation to contraction and intensity. This is a reflex
pattern, typically secondary to umbilical cord compression. May benefit
from amnioinfusion. **Mild:** FHR >80 bpm and <30 seconds' duration.
Moderate: FHR drops to 70 to 80 bpm and last 30 to 60 seconds.
Severe: FHR <70 bpm and last >60 seconds.

4. **Prolonged decelerations.** Isolated decelerations >120 seconds
can be seen with maternal hypotension, maternal hypoxia, tetanic
contractions, prolapsed umbilical cord, fetal scalp procedures (vagal),
and paracervical or epidural anesthesia. A prolonged deceleration
after severe variable deceleration can signal impending fetal
demise.

G. **Overall Assessment.** Includes risk associated with this pregnancy,
expected time to delivery, FHR assessment, and patient's current
physical capabilities and preference. Remember FHR tracing has
poor specificity (many normal fetuses have FHR tracings that are
ominous).

III. **Management of Ominous FHR Pattern or Fetal Distress.**

A. **Turn patient onto left side** to alleviate vena cava compression.

B. **Discontinue intravenous oxytocin** and with hyperstimulation consider
terbutaline.

C. **Apply 100% oxygen** to mother by face mask.

D. **Correct maternal hypotension or hypertension.**

E. **Vaginal examination to rule out prolapsed cord.**

F. **Fetal scalp stimulation.** Stimulate fetal scalp; if this stimulates FHR
acceleration of 15 bpm lasting 15 seconds, this is reassuring
(corresponds with a scalp pH ≥7.22). This is a diagnostic maneuver,
not therapeutic.

TABLE 14-4

INTERPRETATION OF FETAL SCALP pH

Fetal Scalp Blood pH	Interpretation	Management
≥7.25	Normal	Continue FHR monitoring and re-sample if appropriate
7.20-7.24	Preacidotic	Consider re-sampling and continue FHR monitoring
≤7.19	Fetal acidosis	Re-sample in 5 to 10 minutes and prepare for immediate delivery if low scalp pH is confirmed

G. **Consider fetal scalp blood sampling** for pH determination **(Table14-4)** except in cases of maternal fever, where a normal pH doesn't have as good a predictive value.

H. **With prolonged bradycardia** unresponsive to other maneuvers or late decelerations with fetal acidosis (pH <7.20), proceed with immediate delivery (vacuum/forceps-assisted or C-section).

Amnioinfusion

I. **Definition.** Amnioinfusion is a procedure in which a physiologic solution (such as normal saline) is infused into the uterine cavity to replace the amniotic fluid. The goal is to maintain the amniotic fluid index (AFI) between 8 and 12 cm.

II. **Indications.**

A. **Correcting variable decelerations** caused by cord compression.

B. **Reduce fetal distress caused by meconium** staining of fluid.

C. **Correction of oligohydramnios.**

III. **Technique.**

A. **Perform a vaginal exam** to determine presentation and dilation and to rule out cord prolapse. Obtain informed consent.

B. **Catheter.** Double-lumen catheter to monitor contractions while at the same time giving fluid.

C. **Infusate.** Normal saline, lactated Ringer's (like amniotic fluid) at body temperature. Room temperature fluid can cause fetal bradycardia if infused rapidly.

D. **Methods.** Give 250 mL to 500 mL initially, then 50 to 60 mL/h maintenance. Small risk of uterine rupture if efflux of infusate is blocked.

E. *Note:* Resting tone will be increased while the infusion is running, but elevated baseline tone prior to infusion is a contraindication.

IV. **Efficacy.**

A. **Oligohydramnios.** Lower rate of C-section for fetal distress and higher umbilical artery pH at birth compared to those in patients not receiving amnioinfusion.

B. **Moderate to thick meconium.** Decreased rate of operative delivery, increased average 1-minute Apgar scores, less meconium aspirated from below neonate's vocal cords, and a lower incidence of meconium aspiration syndrome compared to that in patients not treated with amnioinfusion.

Induction of Labor

I. Indications and Contraindications.

A. Indications include pregnancy-induced hypertension, premature rupture of membranes, chorioamnionitis, postdate pregnancy, FGR, isoimmunization, other evidence of hostile intrauterine environment, diabetes mellitus, other selected maternal diseases, or fetal demise.

B. Contraindications include placenta previa, cord presentation, floating presenting part, abnormal fetal lie, active genital herpes, invasive cervical carcinoma, pelvic structural deformities, prior and classic uterine incision. Oxytocin stimulation would be relatively contraindicated in conditions that predispose to uterine rupture (high parity, advanced maternal age, fetopelvic disproportion, uterine overdistention, prior uterine scar).

II. Induction Methods. Assess the inducibility of the cervix using Bishop score **(Table 14-5).** Determine route of induction.

A. Amniotomy

1. Cervix should be dilated enough to allow reaching the membranes with the amniotomy hook. The **fetus should be vertex with the presenting part well engaged** and well applied to the cervix. The umbilical cord should not be palpable.

2. Membranes are hooked, and a gentle tug should cause release of amnionic fluid. Assess fluid for presence of meconium.

3. **Monitor fetal heart tones** before and after the procedure.

4. **Risks** include cord prolapse, injury to fetal part (unlikely with amnio hook).

B. Dinoprostone (PGE$_2$)

1. **Indicated for cervical ripening** if Bishop score is <5 (see Table 14-5).

TABLE 14-5
BISHOP SCORING SYSTEM

Feature	Cervix Score			
	0	1	2	3
Position	Posterior	Midposition	Anterior	—
Consistency	Firm	Medium	Soft	—
Effacement (%)	0-30	40-50	60-70	≥80
Dilation (cm)	Closed	1-2	3-4	≥5
Station	−3	−2	−1	+1, +2

Bishop score of >9 indicates induction should be successful.

Modified from Romney SL, Gray MJ, Little AB, et al (eds): *Gynecology and Obstetrics: The Health Care of Women.* 2nd ed. New York, McGraw-Hill, 1981.

2. **Cervidil** (10 mg dinoprostone [PGE$_2$], a small vaginal pessary, aka "Barbie tampon on a string"). Placed in the posterior fornix. Monitor for 120 minutes after insertion. Releases 0.3 mg/h over 12 hours. Patients remain supine for 2 hours after insertion. Requires continuous fetal monitoring ($150/hour). Can easily remove if hyperstimulation occurs. Cost is $159 per insert. *Do not drop on the floor!* May start oxytocin after 30 minutes after removal.

3. **Prepidil** (0.5 mg dinoprostone/3-g syringe) Administered intracervically. Monitor for 2 hours. If no contractions after 2 hours, may be up walking or sent home. May repeat after 6 hours. No more than 3 doses in 24 hours. If hyperstimulation, reposition mother, provide oxygen; may need terbutaline. May start oxytocin 6 hours after last dose. Cannot wash out or wipe it away! Acquisition cost ~ $145/gel—do not drop on the floor! Risks: hyperstimulation and uterine rupture.

C. **Misoprostol** (Cytotec; PGE$_1$) —*not* **to be used for VBACs!**

1. Currently not FDA-labeled for cervical ripening but meta-analysis compared use of intravaginal misoprostol with dinoprostone, oxytocin, and placebo. Misoprostol has lower rate of cesarean section, higher incidence of vaginal delivery within 24 hours, and reduced need for oxytocin augmentation.

2. Most common dose **is 25 μg (one-quarter of a 100 μg tablet!)** inserted into the posterior vaginal fornix when Bishop score is <6. May be used every 4 hours up to 6 doses. Continuous fetal monitoring is recommended for 3 hours after dose. Do not use if there is already uterine hyperactivity, active labor, or nonreassuring FHR pattern. In case of PROM near term, may use 25 μg every 6 hours. If hyperstimulation occurs, terbutaline 0.25 mg SQ is given. If SROM occurs, at least 2 hours should elapse before redosing. If uterine activity remains minimal, another dose may be given. May start oxytocin 4 hours after last dose. Cost is 75 cents for a 100-μg tablet.

3. **Risks.** Hyperstimulation, possible increased meconium staining, uterine rupture.

D. **Foley catheter** (dilates and softens cervix).

1. Document placenta position. Use 14 F with 30 mL balloon. Insert using sterile speculum so that balloon is above the cervical os. Inflate balloon with sterile saline. Tape under traction to inner thigh. Procedure results in gradual dilation and effacement of cervix over 6 to 12 hours.

2. Start oxytocin if patient is not in labor after extrusion of Foley. This procedure is sometimes used in combination with Prepidil.

E. **Oxytocin administration.**

1. You can use oxytocin to ripen the cervix, but often it is used after one of the above methods of cervical ripening. Low-dose or high-dose regimens may be used (ACOG category C). Local preferences and protocols should be followed.

14

OBSTETRICS

2. **Close monitoring** of the parturient and fetus is essential. Most hospitals have written protocols available. Set-up for C-section should be immediately available.

3. Place 10 units of oxytocin in 1000 mL D_5NS or D_5LR. Begin with a **low dose of oxytocin: 0.5 to 2 mU per minute**. You may consider starting **high-dose oxytocin: 6 mU/min.** (Each milliliter of the above solution contains 10 mU).

4. **Advancing dose.** There are various protocols regarding the rate for increasing the dose and the maximum dose. If little uterine response is observed, the dose can be increased by 1 to 2 mU/min (low dose) or 1 to 6 mU/min (high dose) every 30 minutes. Most patients respond to rates of 20 mU/min or less. The faster the increase, the more likely the risk of hyperstimulation. The rate of administration is held steady when a good labor pattern (contractions every 2-3 min lasting 60-90 sec with an intrauterine pressure of 50-60 mm Hg and a resting tone of 10-15 mm Hg) is achieved. Ideally you want 150 to 250 Montevideo units:

Montevideo units = (number of contractions/10 min)
        × (Average peak of contraction − Average baseline of contraction)

5. If at any point the FHR indicates distress, place the patient on her left side, administer oxygen, and discontinue oxytocin. Reinstituting oxytocin requires reassessment of the situation.

OBSTETRIC ANESTHESIA AND ANALGESIA

I. **Overview.** Pain during first stage of labor is attributable to uterine contractions and cervical dilation. During the second stage, pain occurs from distention and stretching of pelvic structures and the perineum. Pain is conducted along the paracervical or inferior hypogastric plexus.

II. **Systemic Narcotics.**

A. Meperidine 25 mg IV or nalbuphine (Nubain) 10 mg IV provide transient pain relief. Caution is needed near delivery because of fetal respiratory depression.

B. **Maternal complications** include drowsiness, nausea, vomiting, decreased gastric motility, respiratory depression.

C. **Fetal complications** include decreased reactivity of FHR, respiratory depression, CNS depression, and impaired temperature regulation. Naloxone (0.01 mg/kg) can be administered to depressed newborn as IV bolus or IM for counteracting the effect of narcotics.

III. **Local Anesthesia.**

A. **Pudendal block** provides analgesia to vaginal introitus and perineum. It is usually used in the second stage of labor.

B. **Paracervical block** provides analgesia during active phase of labor. Blocks pain caused by uterine contractions.

C. **Lumbar epidural anesthesia**
1. Associated with prolonged labor and an increased risk of chorioamnionitis.
2. Contraindications include maternal fever, preexisting CNS disease, severe hypertension, hypotension, hypovolemia, and coagulopathy. **Causes elevated temperature in the newborn but no increase in sepsis.**
IV. **Psychologic Methods of Pain Relief.** Lamaze classes aid in preparation; hypnosis, acupuncture, whirlpool use, maternal position change, and biofeedback are also used.

VAGINAL DELIVERY

Episiotomy

I. **Overview.** Episiotomy is a deliberate incision in the perineum used to facilitate vaginal delivery. Stretching of the vaginal tissues manually can prevent the need for episiotomy and minimize the risk of tears.
II. **Types.**
A. **Midline episiotomy** gives good anatomic results, is easy to repair, and has low incidence of postpartum pain or dyspareunia. **However, it increases the risk of a third- or fourth-degree laceration compared to patients without an episiotomy.**
B. **Mediolateral episiotomy** is less likely to extend through the sphincter but more likely to cause pain during healing, dyspareunia, or excessive blood loss. Good anatomic results are more difficult to obtain.

Normal Spontaneous Vaginal Delivery

I. **Cardinal Movements** (for vertex presentation).
A. **Engagement** occurs late in pregnancy for primigravidas and at the onset of labor for multigravidas.
B. **Flexion** of the neck so that the smallest diameter possible presents. If the neck does not flex, it may actually extend during labor, producing a brow or face presentation.
C. **Descent** is progressive, with thinning of the cervix and lower uterine segment. It depends on the force of contractions and on the configuration of the pelvis and presenting part.
D. **Internal rotation** occurs during descent. Vertex rotates from transverse to either posterior or AP to pass the ischial spines.
E. **Extension** occurs as the head distends the perineum and the occiput passes beneath the symphysis.
F. **External rotation** occurs after delivery of the head, with the head rotating back to a transverse position as the shoulders internally rotate to an anteroposterior position.
II. **Management of Vertex Delivery.**
A. **Preparations for delivery** should be made when the presenting part begins to distend the perineum, sooner for multigravidas.

(Local or pudendal anesthesia can be administered at this time.) Episiotomy (if needed) is not performed until delivery is imminent. Episiotomy likely increases the risk of third- and fourth-degree tears.

B. Delivery of the head

1. **Control** so that there is no forceful, sudden expulsion that can produce injury. As the vertex appears beneath the symphysis, the perineum is supported by direct pressure from a draped hand over the coccygeal region (Ritgen's maneuver). This will protect the perineum and assist in extension of the head as the vertex passes the symphysis.

2. As the head is delivered, it will rotate to a transverse position, at which time the baby should be **checked for the presence of umbilical cord about the neck.** If present, the cord should be gently slipped over the infant's head (or double clamped and cut if this cannot be done easily).

3. The **mouth and nose should be cleared of secretions with a bulb syringe** or DeLee suction trap.

C. Delivery of the shoulders. Shoulders should be rotated to an AP position in the pelvic outlet as the head externally rotates. Gentle traction downward on the head will assist in bringing the anterior shoulder beneath the symphysis. Gentle elevation of the infant's head toward the symphysis will release the posterior shoulder.

D. Delivery of the body. The rest of the body will generally deliver spontaneously and quickly after delivery of the shoulders. Care must be taken to control the delivery of the body to prevent unnecessary injury.

E. Immediate care of the infant includes double clamping and cutting of the umbilical cord. **Do not milk the cord because this causes hyperviscosity syndrome.** The clamp closest to the umbilicus should be just distal to the skin, or longer if you anticipate a need for an umbilical line. A clear airway must be ensured and body temperature should be maintained by drying and wrapping or by placing the baby under a radiant heater or in skin-to-skin contact with the mother's chest.

III. Forceps Delivery. Forceps are generally used to shorten the second stage of labor when that is in the best interest of the mother or the fetus. A fully dilated cervix and experienced physician are required. Advantages must be weighed against the increased risk of maternal lacerations.

A. Indications

1. **Prolonged second stage**
   a. >3 hours in a primigravida with regional anesthesia.
   b. >2 hours in primigravida without regional anesthesia.
   c. >2 hours in multigravida with regional anesthesia.
   d. >1 hour in multigravida without regional anesthesia.

2. **Fetal distress**

3. **Maternal exhaustion**

B. Requirements

1. Fetal head is engaged and in vertex-face presentation.

2. Position of head is known exactly.

3. Membranes have ruptured.

4. Cervix is fully dilated.

a. No clinical evidence of cephalopelvic disproportion.

b. Appropriate anesthesia.

C. Definitions

1. **Outlet forceps.** The fetal scalp is visible at the introitus. The head is at or on the perineum, and the sagittal suture is in the AP plane or rotated up to 45 degrees.

2. **Low forceps.** The leading point of the skull is at least at +2 station.

3. **Midforceps.** The leading point of the skull is engaged but is above +2 station. (Midforceps delivery should be attempted only in extreme situations while simultaneously preparing for C-section.)

D. Selection of forceps

1. **Simpson forceps** are good for a primigravida with prolonged second stage (molded fetal head).

2. **Elliot** is better if the mother is a multigravida and the fetal head is less molded.

3. **Tucker–McLane** has a sliding lock and is good for an asynclitic fetal head.

4. **Kielland** has minimal pelvic curve and is often used for rotation.

5. **Piper** is used in breech extractions.

IV. Vacuum extraction is a safe, effective alternative to forceps delivery. A term, vertex fetus is required. Delivery should not be one that will require rotation or excessive traction. Prior scalp sampling is a contraindication.

A. Advantages. Simpler to apply with fewer mistakes in application. Less force is applied to fetal head. Less anesthesia is necessary (local anesthetic may suffice). No increase in diameter of presenting head. Less maternal soft-tissue injury. Less fetal injury. Less parental concern.

B. Disadvantages. Traction is applied only during contractions. Proper traction is necessary to avoid losing vacuum. Possibly longer delivery than with forceps. Small increase in incidence of cephalohematomas.

C. Technique

1. Ascertain that the cervix is fully dilated and the head is in low or outlet position.

2. Wipe the head clean, spread the labia, and compress and insert the cup. Apply pressure inward and downward until contact is made with the fetal scalp. The cup should be placed over the posterior fontanel.

3. Sweep a finger around the cup to make sure no maternal tissue is within the cup. Raise suction pressure to 100 mm Hg, and recheck the location of the cup.

4. With the onset of a contraction, raise suction pressure to a range of 380 to 580 mm Hg. (Negative pressure should not exceed 600 mm Hg.) Apply traction perpendicularly to the cup, in line with the maternal axis.

5. Should the cup be dislodged, check the fetal scalp before reapplying the cup.
6. When the contraction subsides, reduce the suction pressure to 100 mm Hg.
7. As the head crowns, an episiotomy may be cut but likely increases the risk of third- and fourth-degree tears. Traction is then changed to a 45-degree angle upward as the vertex clears the symphysis.
8. Suction is released and the cup is removed after delivery of the fetal head.
9. The procedure should be discontinued if extraction is not achieved after 10 minutes at maximum pressure, if extraction is not achieved within 30 minutes of initiation, if the cup disengages three times, if the fetal scalp sustains trauma, or if no progress is made after three pulls.

Breech Presentation

I. Overview.
A. Incidence is 25% of all pregnancies at 28 weeks of gestation and 3% to 4% of all pregnancies at or beyond 34 weeks of gestation.
B. Cause includes low birth weight, placenta previa, uterine and fetal anomalies, contracted pelvis, and multiple fetuses.
C. Treatment. Consider external cephalic version (optimal timing at about 37-38 weeks). Otherwise recommend C-section.
II. Types of Breech.
A. Frank. Thighs and hips flexed, knees extended; 65% of cases are frank.
B. Complete. Thighs and hips flexed, one or both knees flexed; 10% of cases are complete.
C. Incomplete or footling. One or both thighs extended, one or both knees below the buttocks; 25% of cases are incomplete or footling.
III. Vaginal Delivery of Breech Presentation. Only perform if it is impossible to provide a timely, safe cesarean delivery. Recent studies support cesarean delivery of all breech singleton presentations.

Shoulder Dystocia

I. Incidence. Directly related to fetal size: <2500 g 0.15%; 2500 to 4000 g 0.3% to 1%; 4000 to 4500 g 5% to 7%.
II. Diagnosis. Suspect shoulder dystocia if you suspect macrosomia (gestational diabetes, history of large infants, large maternal size, prolonged gestation) or if second stage is prolonged. Consider C-section. If the head pulls back against the perineum after delivery (turtle sign) shoulder dystocia is very likely. Fifty percent are unanticipated and in normal birth weight infants.

III. Management.

A. Downward traction on the fetal head while the mother pushes.

B. Call for appropriate help if assistance is not immediately available. Consider episiotomy for maneuvers that require reaching into the vagina.

C. McRobert's maneuver. The mother's thighs are hyperflexed, bringing her feet "to her ears."

D. Suprapubic pressure. Have an assistant apply constant CPR-like pressure on the posterior aspect of the anterior shoulder of the fetus. This causes the shoulder to move under the symphysis pubis.

E. Ruben II maneuver. Insert the fingers of one hand into the vagina behind the anterior shoulder and push through the shoulder toward the opposite maternal hip.

F. Woods' screw maneuver. Insert opposite hand anterior to the posterior shoulder and rotate it toward the symphysis. This may be done in combination with the Rubin II maneuver.

G. Reverse Woods' screw maneuver. Place hands on opposite sides of the fetal shoulder from Ruben II and the Woods' screw and push in opposite direction (always through the shoulder).

H. Remove the posterior arm. Grab and pull out the posterior arm, which allows the anterior shoulder to collapse.

I. Roll the patient to "all fours." With gentle traction downward, the posterior shoulder is delivered first.

J. If all else fails:

1. Fracture the clavicle by putting upward and outward pressure on the midportion of the clavicle.

2. Perform the Zavanelli maneuver by putting the head back into the pelvis and performing a C-section.

3. Perform symphysiotomy by cutting the fibrous cartilage of the symphysis pubis transcutaneously.

Vaginal Birth after Cesarean Section

I. Definition. Attempted vaginal delivery in a woman who has undergone previous cesarean section.

II. Decision to Attempt VBAC.

A. Institutional reasons. Must have facilities and personnel for emergency C-section available during entire labor. VBAC reduces health care cost and maternal morbidity and mortality.

B. Personal reasons. Patient prefers a vaginal delivery.

C. Contraindications include a history of previous classic, T-shaped, or unknown uterine incision, multiple gestation, an estimated birth weight >4000 g, or a nonvertex presentation.

D. Probability of success depends primarily on the indication of the previous C-section. When the primary C-section was for breech position, abruption, placenta previa, cord accident, antepartum hemorrhage, hypertensive disorder, or fetal distress, there is a 74% to 94% rate of success.

14

OBSTETRICS

When the primary C-section was for cephalopelvic disproportion (CPD), or failed induction, there is a 35% to 77% rate of success.

III. Risks. In addition to the usual risk of delivery, other risks include:

A. Uterine rupture. Estimated at 0.5% to 1.5% with 1 in 10 of these affecting the well-being of the baby (anything from fetal distress to fetal death). Incidence is increased if prior C-section was classic.

B. Cesarean section. There is increased risk of C-section morbidity after failed VBAC relative to elective C-section.

IV. Management.

A. Preparation

1. **Type and screen** for two units of packed cells; intravenous line should be inserted.

2. **The anesthesiologist, surgeon, and physician caring for the newborn infant must be notified in advance and be available.**

B. Labor

1. **Electronic fetal monitoring** is recommended.

2. **Oxytocin may be cautiously used** to augment labor, and close monitoring of uterine contractions (using intrauterine pressure catheter) is necessary. **Oxytocin must be titrated with great care in a VBAC. Avoid prostaglandins and misoprostol!**

3. The same expectations of normal progression during labor should be applied to patients with a prior C-section.

4. An experienced physician should be in attendance throughout labor and delivery.

5. **Postpartum.** Manual exploration of the uterus after delivery of the placenta is indicated to assess scar integrity.

CESAREAN SECTION

I. Indications.

A. Maternal and fetal. Cephalopelvic disproportion, failed induction or progression of labor, abnormal uterine contraction pattern.

B. Maternal

1. **Maternal diseases.** Eclampsia or preeclampsia with noninducible cervix, diabetes mellitus (if macrosomic infant precludes vaginal delivery), cardiac disease, cervical cancer, active herpes genitalis. One double-blind clinical trial showed that acyclovir suppression (400 mg PO tid) given after 36 weeks of gestation significantly reduces the need for cesarean section by preventing a herpetic outbreak at term.

2. **Previous uterine surgery.** Classic cesarean section (vertical uterine incision), previous uterine rupture, or full-thickness myomectomy. If there is any question about the type of incision made during a previous cesarean section, the operative report for that delivery must be obtained so that incision type can be known with certainty. This should be done shortly after the first prenatal visit, not when the patient presents in labor! Some centers require cesarean for any woman with a previous

cesarean, due to the risk of uterine rupture with VBAC. It is prudent to follow local norms.

3. **Obstruction to the birth canal** including fibroids and ovarian tumors.

C. **Fetal.** Fetal distress, cord prolapse, fetal malpresentations.

D. **Placental.** Placenta previa (unless marginal) and abruptio placentae.

II. **Risks.**

A. **Maternal risks** include infection, hemorrhage, injury to urinary tract, adverse reactions to anesthesia, and prolonged recovery.

B. **Fetal risks** depend on gestational age and indications for C-section. There is less birth trauma, although injury can be sustained during operative delivery. There is increased incidence of respiratory distress syndrome.

III. **Antibiotic Prophylaxis.** There is reduced incidence of endometritis, wound infection, UTI, and fever post-op with a single dose of antibiotic (e.g., ceftriaxone, cefotetan) prior to caesarean delivery.

AFTER DELIVERY

General Postpartum Care

I. **Examples of Orders after Routine Vaginal Delivery.**

A. **Immediately postpartum**

1. **Pitocin** 10 units IM.

2. **Bed rest,** and vitals q15 min for 1 hour postpartum.

3. **Ice pack to perineum** immediately postpartum prn.

B. **Thereafter**

1. **Ambulate** as soon as possible.

2. **Diet.** General or other.

3. **Vital signs.** q4h.

4. **Tucks** to perineum prn.

5. **Sitz baths** tid and hs prn.

6. **IV (if present).** Discontinue when vital signs are stable and uterine bleeding is normal.

7. **Bladder catheterization** if unable to void in 6 to 8 hours.

8. **CBC** postpartum day 2.

9. **Administer Rho(D)** immunoglobulin if indicated.

10. **Medications**

a. **Vitamins.** Continue prenatal vitamins; additional $FeSO_4$ if anemic.

b. **Pain.** Acetaminophen 650 mg PO q4-6h prn or ibuprofen 400 to 600 mg PO q4-6h for cramping pain. Narcotics as needed (but be careful if breastfeeding).

c. **Bowels.** Docusate sodium 100 mg PO bid; milk of magnesia 30 mL PO qd prn; bisacodyl 10 mg PO or PR prn.

II. **Physical Examination.**

A. **Monitor uterine changes.** The fundus should be firm and at or below the umbilicus. Gradual involution occurs over the next 6 weeks.

OBSTETRICS 14

B. Lochia (uterine drainage) is initially red or bloody, gradually becoming serosanguineous. By 2 to 3 weeks it should be white. Tampons are contraindicated.

C. Breasts are examined for signs of infection and presence of milk. Colostrum is present initially. Milk production should occur by the third to fifth day in primiparas, sooner in multiparas. Breastfeeding should initially not be allowed for longer than 15 minutes on each breast per feeding to help prevent soreness.

D. Legs should be examined for evidence of thrombophlebitis and edema.

III. Parent Education.

A. Newborn care, including bathing, cord care, signs of infection, etc.

B. Breastfeeding and prevention of lactation or engorgement if applicable.

IV. Discharge Instructions.

A. Give rubella vaccination, if indicated, before discharge.

B. Instruct regarding signs of puerperal infection, postpartum hemorrhage, and mastitis.

C. Counsel on avoidance of intercourse and tampons for 4 weeks.

D. Contraception counseling. OCPs can be started during week 4, if desired. Low-dose or progestin-only pills and Depo-Provera have less influence on lactation.

E. Give nutrition counseling, especially if breastfeeding.

F. Medications. Vitamins, iron, stool softener, when appropriate. Counsel on medications to avoid during breastfeeding.

G. Discuss need for rest, possible stresses that can occur with new infant at home, possibility of postpartum depression.

V. Follow-up Exam.

A. Postpartum check at 4 to 6 weeks.

B. Newborn checkup typically at 1 to 2 weeks.

Postpartum Hemorrhage

I. Definition. Postpartum hemorrhage is most often defined as a blood loss greater than 500 mL in the first 24 hours after delivery. However, blood loss after spontaneous vaginal delivery is often up to 600 mL and between 1 and 1.5 L after instrumental or operative delivery. Therefore, clinical experience is necessary to determine when bleeding is occurring too rapidly, occurring at the wrong time, or unresponsive to appropriate treatment. Blood loss will be less well tolerated if the patient has not had the normal expansion of blood volume during pregnancy, as in cases of preeclampsia.

II. Risk Factors. Multiparity (>5 births), previous postpartum hemorrhage or C-section, manual removal of the placenta, placental abnormality (e.g., abruption, accrete, etc.), polyhydramnios, prolonged labor or third stage, precipitant labor, difficult forceps delivery, prolonged oxytocin administration, breech extraction.

III. **Etiology.** Four Ts:
A. **Tone:** 70%, uterine atony.
B. **Trauma:** 20%, cervical, perineal or vaginal lacerations, pelvic or vulvar hematomas, uterine rupture or inversion.
C. **Tissue:** 10%, retained or invasive placenta.
D. **Thrombin:** 1%, coagulopathies.
IV. **Management.**
A. **Uterine massage** (simultaneous assessment for atony; if atony is present proceed with management of atony, below).
B. **Vaginal exam** may reveal evidence of laceration (generally bright red blood) or atony (darker blood). **Inspect cervix** if bleeding is from higher up and not due to atony.
C. **Reliable IV access** must be obtained with two large-bore IVs.
D. **Monitor vital signs** and maintain circulatory status with fluids.
E. **Managing uterine atony**
1. **Uterine massage.** Bimanual uterine massage.
2. **Oxytocin** 10-20 U IM or 40 U/L at 250 mL/h IV if no contraindications.
3. **Methergine** 0.2 mg IM is contraindicated if patient has hypertension, preeclampsia, or hypersensitivity.
4. **Prostaglandin F_2** (Hemabate) IM or intramyometrially 0.25 mg q15min up to 8 doses. PGF_2 is contraindicated if patient has active cardiac, renal, pulmonary, or hepatic disease.
F. **Managing trauma.** Identify lacerations and/or hematoma, and repair. Consider uterine inversion and uterine rupture.
G. **Managing tissue problems**
1. **Retained fragments.** If delivered, inspect placenta for missing cotyledons (these can be extracted manually, with ring forceps or via blunt curettage).
2. **Trapped placenta.** If the placenta is low in the uterus and the uterus is firm, consider trapped placenta. Brandt maneuver (suprapubic pressure and firm traction on the cord) often is successful.
3. **Retained placenta or invasive placenta** requires uterine exploration and manual removal. Identify the cleavage plane between the uterus and the placenta and advance your hand, separating them. If cleavage plane can't be identified, there is either a contraction ring (which requires more force), uterine relaxation, or invasive placenta (usually requires emergency hysterectomy).
H. **Management of clotting problems.** Most patients with coagulation problems are identified prior to delivery. Severe preeclampsia, sepsis, amniotic fluid embolism, intrauterine fetal demise, and placental abruption are associated with DIC but rarely with an acute coagulopathy. A low platelet count often identifies patients with a risk of coagulation problems. Check a coagulation profile (PT, PTT, fibrinogen level, and fibrin split products). Treat the underlying disease. See Chapter 6 for further details.

I. Persistent bleeding. Draw CBC, type and cross, and coagulation profile (PT, PTT, fibrinogen level, and fibrin split products) in cases of worrisome bleeding or symptomatic hypovolemia. BP and pulse abnormalities are very late and worrisome signs.

Puerperal Fever

I. Definition. Temperature >38.5° C (>101° F) in first 24 hours or >38.0° C (>99° F) for two consecutive days in the 9 days following delivery.

II. Differential Diagnosis

A. Endometritis

1. **Etiology** is polymicrobial, with a mixture of aerobic and anaerobic organisms. In particular, high fever within the first 25 hours after delivery may be caused by gram-negative sepsis, group B streptococcal disease, clostridial sepsis, or toxic shock syndrome. Infections 2 days to 6 weeks postpartum may be secondary to *Chlamydia*.

2. **Risk factors.** C-section (20 times greater than vaginal delivery), chorioamnionitis, prolonged rupture of membranes or premature labor, multiple vaginal exams, retained products, manual exploration of the uterus, low socioeconomic status.

3. **Diagnosis** is clinical: fever, leukocytosis, uterine tenderness, foul-smelling vaginal discharge. Cultures of the cervix, placenta, or retained tissue and blood can help identify the causative organism.

4. **Treatment**

  a. **Treatment is empiric** unless a culture comes back positive. If *Chlamydia* is isolated or suspected based on late presentation, add doxycycline or azithromycin to the regimen.

  b. There is no consensus on the safest and most effective antibiotic regimens, only that the antibiotic must have a broad spectrum. Antibiotics are usually continued for 4 or 5 days and for 24 to 48 hours after defervescence.

  c. **Gold standard** is gentamicin (2 mg/kg IV loading dose, followed by 1.5 mg/kg IV q8h) with clindamycin (900 mg IV q8h). Alternative is daily dosing with gentamicin 5 mg/kg daily and clindamycin 2700 mg daily.

  d. **Newer regimens** (second- or third-generation cephalosporins, semisynthetic penicillins).

    (1) Cefoxitin 1 to 2 g IV q6-8h or cefotetan 2 g IV q12h.

    (2) Ampicillin/sulbactam 1.5-3 g IV q6h.

    (3) Piperacillin 4 g IV q6h.

  e. **If no response** (maximum temperature not dropping within 48 hours of initiating therapy), add ampicillin 2 g IV q6h.

B. Pelvic abscess. Suspect if patient develops a pelvic mass or has persistent fever and pain despite therapy for aerobic bacteria. Abscess often develops 5 or more days after delivery. Must add therapy for anaerobic bacteria and consider surgical or percutaneous drainage.

C. **Septic pelvic thrombophlebitis.** Symptoms include spiking fevers with or without pain despite antibiotic therapy. The patient may have a tender palpable mass. Patient may have a diagnostic response with improvement of symptoms after beginning intravenous heparin and antibiotics. CT and MRI have been used to diagnose this illness.

D. **Wound infection.** Presentation includes fever, a tender erythematous or fluctuant incision, and drainage of pus or blood. It usually occurs after the fifth postoperative day. Risk factors include intrapartum cesarean section, emergent abdominal delivery, use of electrocautery, placement of open drains, obesity, and diabetes.

E. **Pulmonary atelectasis.** See Chapter 15 for a discussion of pulmonary atelectasis and fever.

F. **Deep vein thrombosis.** Symptoms include fever and lower extremity pain, swelling, and pallor. Traumatic delivery, cesarean section, delay in the resumption of ambulation, and varicose veins all increase likelihood for DVT formation. See Chapter 4.

G. **Pyelonephritis.** Often accompanied by fever, malaise, flank pain, costovertebral angle tenderness, and pyuria. Risk factors include occult bacteriuria, bladder trauma, and Foley catheterization.

H. **Mastitis.** Suggested by fever and swollen, tender breast. Typically occurs 3 to 4 weeks after delivery. Breastfeeding and contact with a carrier of *Staphylococcus aureus* are the two prime risk factors.

Postpartum Dyspnea

Consider pulmonary embolism/amniotic fluid embolism (see Chapter 4) and CHF due to postpartum cardiomyopathy. Etiology is unknown and treatment is the same as usual CHF treatment.

BIBLIOGRAPHY

American Academy of Family Physicians: ALSO Educational Materials. Available at http://www.aafp.org/x837.xml (accessed December 29, 2005).

Briggs GG, Freeman RK, Yaffe SJ (eds): *Drugs in Pregnancy and Lactation: A Reference Guide to Fetal and Neonatal Risk*, 7th ed. Philadelphia, Lippincott Williams & Wilkins, 2005.

Committee on Obstetric Practice: ACOG committee opinion: Antenatal corticosteroid therapy for fetal maturation. *Obstet Gynecol* 99(5 Pt 1):871-873, 2002.

Niebyl JR, Simpson JL, Gabbe SG (eds): *Obstetrics: Normal and Problem Pregnancies*, 4th ed. New York, Churchill Livingstone, 2002.

Guinn DA, Atkinson MW, Sullivan L, et al: Single vs weekly courses of antenatal corticosteroids for women at risk of preterm delivery: A randomized controlled trial. *JAMA* 286:1581-1587, 2001.

Jones GC, Macklin JP, Alexander WD: Contraindications to the use of metformin. *BMJ* 326:4-5, 2003.

Smaill F, Hofmeyr S: Antibiotic prophylaxis for cesarean section. *Cochrane Database Syst Rev* 3:CD000933, 2002.

Kremer CJ, Duff P: Glyburide for the treatment of gestational diabetes. *Am J Obstet Gynecol* 190:1438-1439, 2004.

Livingston JC, Llata E, Rinehart E, et al: Gentamicin and clindamycin therapy in postpartum endometritis: The efficacy of daily dosing versus dosing every 8 hours. *Am J Obstet Gynecol* 188:149-152, 2003.

Marcovici I, Scoccia B: Postpartum hemorrhage and intrauterine balloon tamponade: A report of three cases. *J Reprod Med* 44(2):122-126, 1999.

Margulies R, Miller L: Fruit size as a model for teaching first trimester uterine sizing in bimanual examination. *Obstet Gynecol* 98:341-344, 2001.

Scott LL, Sanchez PJ, Jackson GL, et al: Acyclovir suppression to prevent cesarean delivery after first-episode genital herpes. *Obstet Gynecol* 87:69-73, 1996.

Wald NJ, Huttly WJ, Hackshaw AK: Antenatal screening for Down's syndrome with the quadruple test. *Lancet* 361:835-836, 2003.

Warner MW, Salfinger SG, Rao S, et al: Management of trauma during pregnancy. *Am J Surg* 74:125-128, 2004.

General Surgery

Mark A. Graber

WOUND MANAGEMENT

I. **General Principles.** The goal of wound management is primarily restoration of function, which requires minimizing risk of infection and repair of injured tissue with a minimum of cosmetic deformity.

II. **Significant History.**

A. **Mechanism of injury**

1. **Blunt trauma.** Split- or crush-type injuries will swell more and tend to have more devitalized tissue and a higher risk of infection.

2. **Sharp trauma.** Clean edges, low cellular injury, and low risk of infection.

3. **Bite injury.** See Chapter 2.

B. **Contaminants.** Wound contact with manure, rust, dirt, etc. will increase risk of infection. Wounds sustained in barnyards or stables are considered contaminated with *Clostridium tetani*.

C. **Time of injury.** After 3 hours, the bacterial count in a wound increases dramatically. Wounds may be closed primarily up to 18 hours out; clean well and use clinical judgment when choosing which wounds to close. For cosmetic reasons, wounds up to 24 hours old on the face may be closed after good cleaning. The blood supply in this area is much better and the risk of infection therefore much less. Again, use clinical judgment! The risk of infection may be reduced in wounds by use of tape closures (such as Steri-Strip tape).

D. **Tetanus status (Table 15-1).** Note that the new Tetanus/Diphtheria/Pertussis vaccine should be used in adults when updating tetanus immunization (Tdap).

E. **Other medical illnesses.** Diabetes, chemotherapy, steroids, peripheral vascular disease, and malnutrition may delay wound healing and increase the risk of infection.

III. **Physical Exam.**

A. **Vascular injury.** Direct pressure is the first choice for controlling bleeding. If a fracture is involved, immobilization will help control bleeding. Do not clamp vascular structures until it is determined whether it is a significant vessel needing repair. If the anatomy is suspect for injury to major vascular structures, obtain angiogram and consider surgical consult. Capillary refill should be checked distally. Bleeding on the scalp is best controlled by suturing the wound. For extremities, inflating a blood pressure cuff above systolic pressure assists in wound inspection and repair. However, be careful not to cause ischemic injury to the extremity.

B. **Neurologic injury.** Check distal muscle strength and sensation. Always check sensation before administering anesthesia. For hand and finger lacerations, check two-point discrimination, which should be <5 mm at the fingertips. A crush injury may also decrease two-point discrimination.

TABLE 15-1

TETANUS STATUS

Last Tetanus Booster	Clean Wound	Dirty Wound
Unknown or never immunized	0.5 mL of tetanus toxoid. Repeat immunization at 6 wk and 6 mo to 1 y	0.5 mL of tetanus toxoid; repeat immunization at 6 wk and 6 mo to 1 y 250 U of human tetanus immune globulin
>5 y to <10 y	None (consider 0.5 mL of tetanus toxoid)	0.5 mL of tetanus toxoid
10 y	0.5 mL of tetanus toxoid	0.5 mL of tetanus toxoid

This may take several months to recover. A lacerated nerve may be repaired immediately or have repair delayed. Loss of sensation may be the first sign of a developing compartment syndrome. See Chapter 2 for a full discussion of compartment syndrome.

C. **Tendons.** Can be evaluated by inspection, but individual tendons must also be tested for full range of motion and full strength. Patients with a lacerated tendon may still have digit motion secondary to intrinsic muscles, so always compare strength with the uninvolved side.

D. **Bones.** Check for open fracture or associated fractures. X-ray if any question. An open fracture is an indication for surgical debridement and repair except in the case of a distal phalanx fracture secondary to a nail bed injury, where copious irrigation and oral antibiotics are acceptable treatment if the injury can be watched carefully for infection.

E. **Foreign bodies.** Inspect and x-ray the area. Remember that wood or low-lead glass may not show on radiograph. Wound markers can be used during radiography, and views obtained in two planes can help localize the object for recovery. Glass may penetrate at an angle and be buried deeper than it appears to be. **US is very sensitive at picking up foreign bodies if radiograph is questionable or there is strong clinical suspicion.**

F. **A hand wound sustained in a fight as a result of punching someone in the mouth is a high-risk injury; these wounds frequently penetrate a joint (especially the second MCP joint). These wounds need to be thoroughly explored and will need operative repair if the joint is violated.**

IV. **Repair.**

A. **Wound healing**

1. **Collagen formation.** Peaks at day 7. The wound has 15% to 20% of full strength at 3 weeks and 60% of full strength at 4 months. Epithelialization occurs in 48 hours under optimal conditions. The wound is then completely sealed.

2. **Scar formation.** Requires 6 to 12 months for a mature scar. The smallest scar will be formed when the wound not under tension. Scars should not be revised until 12 months have passed.

B. Anesthesia

1. **Topical anesthesia.** LAT and TAC can be used alone or can be used to greatly decrease the pain of infiltration.

a. **LAT:** 4% lidocaine, 1:2000 epinephrine (also known as adrenaline), and 0.5% tetracaine, 5 mL on cotton ball and placed in wound.

   (1) Works as well as TAC and does not need to be locked up as controlled substance, takes 10 to 30 minutes to work, and is cheaper than TAC ($3.00 versus $35.00 per dose).

   (2) **Precautions.** Avoid use on face or near mucous membranes (absorption through mucous membranes may cause seizures). Avoid LAT in areas where epinephrine would be contraindicated, as on distal digits, tip of nose, ears, and penis.

b. **TAC:** 0.5% tetracaine, 1:2000 epinephrine (also known as adrenaline), 11.8% cocaine; requires approximately 30 minutes for onset of action. Put 5 mL on a cotton ball and then place in wound. Same precautions as with LAT.

2. **Local.** Use 27- or 30-gauge needle and infiltrate slowly and through the open wound edge, avoiding the intact skin. This decreases the pain of infiltration. The addition of bicarbonate to lidocaine before infiltration has been shown significantly to decrease the pain of injection (9 mL of lidocaine and 1 mL of bicarbonate).

a. **Lidocaine** (0.5%-2%) is most frequently used, with onset 2 to 5 minutes, duration 60 minutes. Can use 3 to 5 mg/kg with not more than 300 mg total (in adults). **Avoid using lidocaine with epinephrine on distal extremities** such as the ears, fingers, toes, and penis. However, if lidocaine with epinephrine is accidentally injected into a finger, do not panic. **It is very rare to get a complication, and lidocaine with epinephrine is routinely used for digital blocks outside of the United States.**

b. **Bupivacaine** (Marcaine) has onset 2 to 5 minutes, duration of hours, and is the longest lasting of the local anesthetics (approximately 8 hours). IV administration may cause serious arrhythmias.

c. **For "caine" allergies,** use diphenhydramine diluted to 1%. Mix 5% diphenhydramine 1:4 mL with NS to make a 1% solution. Onset of anesthesia takes longer and does not last as long as with lidocaine. Stronger solutions may cause tissue necrosis.

3. **Regional anesthesia.** Especially good for fingers, hands, feet, toes, mouth, and face. See Chapter 21 for common blocks.

C. Wound prep

1. **Debridement.** Devitalized tissue should be removed; avoid taking healthy tissue. High-pressure irrigation is the most effective means of cleansing a wound. Can use a 35-mL syringe with a 19-gauge needle and normal saline. Scrubbing does not cleanse the wound as well, and using any disinfectant in the wound damages healthy cells needed for healing.

2. **Skin disinfection.** Can be performed with povidone–iodine solution or chlorhexidine. Avoid getting these solutions in the wound because they impede wound healing. Shaving the area increases the risk of infection.

15

GENERAL SURGERY

Hair can be clipped in the area if necessary. Never shave eyebrows because they are needed for alignment of the wound and may not grow back.

D. Wound closure

1. **Avoid primary closure of infected and inflamed wounds, dirty wounds, human and animal bites (dog bites without crushed tissue are an exception; see Chapter 2, Emergency Medicine), neglected and severe crush wounds.**

2. Tape closure (with Steri-Strips or others). Strips carry a lower risk of infection than suturing does and may be a consideration for higher-risk wounds.

3. **Open wound care.** Keep the wound debrided but moist. Gentle washing of the wound two to three times per day will remove bacterially contaminated secretions (showers or water picks are appropriate for this). Dress with saline-moistened gauze. **Note: the classic "wet to dry" dressing is not helpful beyond the time that the wound must be debrided. Keeping the healing wound moist will promote healing.** Avoid iodine dressings because they damage healthy tissue and will slow granulation. When clean granulation tissue is apparent, secondary closure may be considered or can change to dry, sterile, packing material.

4. **Suturing.** The two types of sutures are: absorbable and nonabsorbable. Precision-point cutting needles and small-sized suture (5-0 or 6-0) should be chosen for skin when a cosmetic closure is important, as on the face. A conventional cutting needle is used for routine skin closure; 4-0 or 3-0 nylon may be used on extremities. A noncutting needle should be used for subcutaneous tissue. Extensor tendons are slow healing and should have a permanent suture of small size chosen (e.g., polypropylene). Depending on your practice situation, a surgical consultation should be considered for tendon repair. The majority of subcutaneous or dermal suturings may be performed with an intermediate-duration absorbable suture. However, some wounds require permanent sutures (e.g., stainless steel wires in sternotomy; **Table 15-2**).

5. **Staples.** Can be used on the scalp and abdomen with good result. However, avoid use on face, hand, or other areas where structures such as tendons and nerves may become entrapped by the staples.

6. **Glue** (Octyl-cyanoacrylate, e.g., Dermabond) can be used to close wounds once bleeding has stopped. Avoid use on palms and soles, which are areas of high moisture. Tissue glues are less effective in high-stress areas such as over knee and elbow joints.

7. **Dressings.** Consider antibiotic ointment on face and torso. Antibiotic ointment should be avoided on distal extremities for more than 24 to 48 hours because it may lead to maceration and delayed wound healing. Immobilize if motion of a joint is going to increase skin tension. Keep the wound dry for 24 hours, after which time most wounds do not require a dressing.

8. **Facial wounds** should have crusts soaked off and bacitracin or other ointment applied qid to reduce scar formation.

TABLE 15-2
SUTURE MATERIALS AND CHARACTERISTICS

Suture	Strength	Inflammatory Reaction	Ease of Use	Infection Resistance	Comments
NONABSORBABLE SUTURES					
Nylon monofilament	+++	++	+++	+++	Good for skin closure Use two throws on the first knot
Polypropylene (Prolene) monofilament	++++	+	+	++++	Good for skin More difficult to use than nylon
Silk	+	++++	++++	++	Has fallen out of favor Used mostly intraorally
ABSORBABLE SUTURES					
Gut or chromic gut	++	+++	++	+	Rarely used Can almost always be replaced by Dexon or Vicryl
Dexon (polyglycolic acid braided polymer)	++++	+	++++	++++	A good choice for subcutaneous and intraoral sutures
Vicryl (polyglactin 910 braided polymer)	++++	+	++++	+++	Same as above

Adapted from Barkin R, Rosen P (eds): *Emergency Pediatrics*. St. Louis, Mosby, 1986.

9. **Antibiotics.** There is no medical indication for using prophylactic antibiotics in routine, noncontaminated skin wounds. Consider antibiotic use for patients prone to endocarditis, patients with hip prostheses, lymphedema, or contaminated foot wound, diabetic patients, or others with peripheral vascular disease. See Chapter 2 for antibiotic choices for bite wounds.

V. Follow-up Care.

A. Risk of infection is highest at 24 to 48 hours, so all wounds should be rechecked.

B. General guidelines for suture removal:

1. **Face,** 3 to 5 days, with tape or glue reinforcement after suture removal if desired.

2. **Scalp,** 7 to 10 days; trunk, 7 to 10 days; arms, 7 to 10 days; legs, 10 to 14 days; joints, dorsal surface, 14 days.
3. Increase length for diabetic or steroid-dependent patients who may require several weeks to heal.

PREOPERATIVE CARDIAC RISK ASSESSMENT

I. Approximately 8 million surgeries per year are performed in the United States on patients with known or suspected cardiac disease. Preoperative evaluation can help stratify risk.

A. **The Goldman index.** Useful in predicting cardiac events in an unselected, random group of patients. However, it does not work well when applied to subgroups, such as all those with known heart disease. The type and extent of surgery anticipated needs to be taken into account when one is interpreting the results of the Goldman index. **Table 15-3** shows the Goldman index, **Table 15-4** lists risks, and **Table 15-5** lists preoperative characteristics and testing required. (This approach is suggested by Mangano and Goldman, 1995.)

B. **Functional status.** If patient can walk up stairs while carrying a load (functional status class I and II), has a low Goldman index, and has no known cardiac disease, there is a very low risk of cardiac complications.

C. **Electrocardiography.** Ischemia on a resting ECG (Q waves, T-wave inversions, etc.) is suggestive of a worse outcome. However, exercise

TABLE 15-3
GOLDMAN INDEX

Factor	Definition	Number of Points
Ischemic heart disease	MI within 6 mo	10
Congestive heart failure	S_3 gallop, JVD	11
Cardiac rhythm	Rhythm other than sinus or premature atrial contractions on first preoperative ECG or >5 premature ventricular contractions per minute at any time before surgery	7
Valvular heart disease	Significant aortic stenosis	3
General medical status	Po_2 <60 mm Hg, Pco_2 >50 mm Hg, K^+ <3.0 mmol/L, bicarbonate <20 mmol/L, BUN >50 mg/dL, creatinine >3.0 mg/dL, abnormal AST, signs of chronic liver disease, patient bedridden from noncardiac causes	3
Age	>70 y	5
Type of surgery	Intraperitoneal, intrathoracic, aortic	3
	Emergency surgery	4

Class I, 0-5 points; class II, 6-12 points; class III, 13-25 points; class IV, >25 points.
Modified from Mangano DT, Goldman L: Preoperative assessment of patients with known or suspected coronary disease. *N Engl J Med* 333:1750-1756, 1995.

TABLE 15-4

RISK OF MAJOR CARDIAC COMPLICATIONS OF DIFFERENT PATIENT GROUPS USING THE GOLDMAN INDEX

Goldman Index Class	Unselected Patients >40 Years (%)	Patients with Known Coronary Disease or Other High-Risk Patients (%)	Unselected Patients Undergoing Minor Surgery (All Patients) (%)
I	1.2	3	0.3
II	3.0	11	1
III	12	30	~2.8
IV	48	75	~19

Modified from Mangano DT, Goldman L: Preoperative assessment of patients with known or suspected coronary disease. *N Engl J Med* 333:1750-1756, 1995.

tolerance appears to be more important than resting ECG changes in predicting outcomes. So, if functional status is good (class I or II), a graded exercise stress test (GXT) need not be done. Reserve GXT for recent-onset chest pain and unclear functional status.

D. Echocardiography. Should be reserved for those who would need an echocardiogram even if they were not having surgery, such as those with murmurs that have not been previously evaluated and those with CHF of unknown cause (diastolic versus systolic versus valvular, etc.). Stress echocardiography can substitute for the GXT.

E. Radionuclide ventriculography–determined ejection fraction has not been shown to be useful in determining risk for infarction perioperatively. Note, however, evidence of CHF is taken into account in the Goldman index (S_3 gallop, JVD) and in functional status (class).

F. Thallium scanning. Thallium scanning is highly sensitive at selecting those who will have postoperative cardiac problems. Specificity is a problem (53%-80%) unless restricted to a high-risk group. The use of thallium scanning should be restricted to those individuals who cannot exercise (therefore the functional status of these patients cannot be determined) and those whose risk cannot be determined by clinical criteria.

G. History of MI. If <3 weeks ago, has 25% mortality rate; do urgent procedures only. At 3 months, 10% mortality; at 6 months, 5% mortality. At 1 year, same risk as asymptomatic patient with cardiac disease.

II. β-Blockers reduce perioperative ischemia in those undergoing noncardiac surgery who have known coronary artery disease or a high risk of coronary artery disease (two or more risk factors). Atenolol started preoperatively and continued until discharge from the hospital decreases overall mortality at 2 years. Most of the lower mortality is attributable to lower cardiac mortality in the 6 to 8 months after surgery. Others have used bisoprolol with similar results.

III. Note that cardiac revascularization has not been shown to benefit mortality outcome in clinically stable patients even with 70% or greater coronary artery stenosis (see McFall et al., 2004). Whether we should even stress test these patients is now a matter of controversy.

TABLE 15-5

PATIENT CHARACTERISTICS AND PREOPERATIVE TESTING REQUIRED

Characteristics of Patient	Preoperative Diagnostic Testing	Special Perioperative Treatment
No known cardiac disease, good functional status, class I or II (can walk up steps carrying groceries or similar load) on the Goldman index	None except routine ECG and CXR if indicated	None
Known stable coronary artery disease and good functional status (class I or early class II)	None except routine ECG and CXR if indicated	Conservative treatment*
Known coronary artery disease, functional status unclear	Noninvasive testing[†]	If test is negative, conservative treatment*
		If test is positive, aggressive medical therapy[‡] or angiography; then retest
		If retest is positive, aggressive medical treatment[‡] and repeat test
		If retest now negative, use conservative treatment*
		If retest still positive, consider more aggressive treatment and repeat noninvasive test
		If still positive, consider coronary angiography and revascularization (e.g., PTCA) if indicated (see note above)
		Outcomes are no better with revascularization than without in the stable patient.
Known coronary artery disease, poor cardiac functional status	None except routine ECG and CXR if indicated	Aggressive medical treatment[‡] or angiography if indicated

For patients with no or few risk factors[§] no other evaluation or treatment is required. For patients with multiple risk factors,[§] noninvasive testing[†] is indicated. If testing is negative, conservative treatment.* If testing is positive, aggressive medical[‡] therapy or angiography.

Modified from Mangano DT, Goldman L: Preoperative assessment of patients with known or suspected coronary disease. *N Engl J Med* 333:1750-1756, 1995.

*Continue cardiac medications on postoperative ECG day 1, after any suspect perioperative events, and before discharge.

[†]Exercise stress testing if patient can exercise. If patient cannot exercise, use stress echocardiogram, dipyridamole–thallium scan, or ambulatory monitor for ischemia.

(Continued)

TABLE 15-5
PATIENT CHARACTERISTICS AND PREOPERATIVE TESTING REQUIRED—cont'd

Characteristics of Patient	Preoperative Diagnostic Testing	Special Perioperative Treatment
Coronary artery disease and either class III or IV on Goldman cardiac risk index	None	Aggressive medical treatment[‡] or angiography
Poor *noncardiac* functional status, no known coronary artery disease or status unclear[§]	Stratified by risk factors[‡]	Stratified by risk factors[‡]

[‡]Aggressive medical treatment, including medication intensification and addressing risk factors (e.g., smoking), followed by repeat noninvasive testing.

[§]Risk factors include age >70 y, DM, CHF, important arrhythmias, known vascular disease, and need for aortic, abdominal, or thoracic surgery.

PREOPERATIVE PULMONARY EVALUATION

I. **Postoperative Pulmonary Complications** are up to 4.3 times more frequent in smokers.

II. **Smoking.** Patients should stop smoking at least 8 weeks before surgery. Paradoxically, patients who quit less than 8 weeks before surgery may have increased risks. For patients with a symptomatic exacerbation of COPD, surgery should be delayed if possible and aggressive management with usual agents before surgery is recommended. In addition, a 2-week course of corticosteroids may be helpful.

III. **Preoperative Spirometry** has a variable predictive value. Clinical status seems to be a better predictor of outcome.

IV. See section on orders for postoperative pulmonary treatment.

PREOPERATIVE LABORATORY EVALUATION

I. **A Complete History and Physical Examination will uncover most abnormalities, and preoperative lab testing can be targeted to those in whom it is indicated.** One guideline suggests that the minimal preoperative test requirements are an ECG and determination of creatinine and glucose in apparently healthy patients 40 to 59 years of age; an ECG, CXR, and determination of the CBC, creatinine, and glucose in patients ≥60 years of age; and no testing for apparently healthy patients <40 years of age. Other literature would suggest the approach in **Table 15-6** in the healthy patient who is having an elective procedure.

PREOPERATIVE MANAGEMENT OF ANTICOAGULATION

See Table 6-3 for preoperative management of anticoagulation.

TABLE 15-6
PREOPERATIVE TESTING

Test	Routine Use Indicated?	Indications
Coagulation studies (PT/INR, PTT)	No	Stigmata liver disease, hepatic coagulopathy, possible DIC, anticoagulation, alcohol abuse
Bleeding time	No	Unreliable test; very subjective, no longer used
CBC	No	Possible hematologic or infectious process, significant blood loss predicted
Electrolytes	No	Diuretic use; hepatic, renal, or cardiac disease; possible dehydration by history or physical
Glucose	No	Diabetic pts, obese pts, pts undergoing vascular procedures, other reason for increased glucose (e.g., steroids)
BUN/Cr	No	Age >60 y; history of renal, cardiac, or vascular disease
Urinalysis	No	Symptomatic pts, diabetic pts, pregnant pts
Pregnancy	No	If indicated by history
Liver enzymes	No	Historical or physical evidence of liver disease
ECG and CXR	No	As indicated by history and physical

PREOPERATIVE CARE, EVALUATION, AND ORDERS

I. Admit Orders. *Note:* Supplemental oxygen (80% by nonrebreather mask) during and for 3 hours after surgery can reduce wound infections.

A. Admit to ward or primary physician.

B. Diagnosis and planned procedure.

C. Condition.

D. Vital signs. Obtain for elective procedure every shift; for emergency procedure as dictated by condition.

E. Allergies. Medications (especially antibiotics), foods, dressing materials (such as tape), etc.

F. Activity. Bed rest if unstable vital signs or other indication; otherwise encourage activity to avoid DVT, muscle atrophy, pneumonia.

G. Nursing. Neurologic checks, monitoring lines (CVP, Swan-Ganz), preoperative teaching, PCA pump, pulmonary toilet, etc.

H. Diet/NPO. Determined by rest of medical history and the preparation required for surgery. Period of NPO before surgery depends on age of patient and anesthesia class. Canadian Anesthesiologists' Society recommends only 3 hours of NPO in healthy patients (anesthesia class I and II). Stomach volumes are actually larger in patients who have a prolonged fast. Anesthesia class III and IV patients should be NPO at least 6 to 8 hours.

I. Intake and output. Fluids for rehydration (NS), maintenance and correction of electrolyte imbalance. Blood products if needed.

Monitoring of fluids and fluid status (CVP/Swan-Ganz, Foley). **Swan-Ganz may increase mortality, however, as demonstrated in several studies.**

J. Special tests. As indicated by diagnosis (e.g., endoscopy before colorectal surgery for cancer).

K. Special medications

1. Patient's routine medications; change medications to IM or IV as needed.
2. Mupirocin to nares preoperatively reduces rate of wound infection.
3. Increased steroids preoperatively if steroid dependent. Stress doses: hydrocortisone succinate 100 mg IV q6-8h.
4. **Pain medications** as needed.
5. **Antibiotics** as indicated for infection and sepsis or prophylaxis of endocarditis, indwelling hardware or graft placement.
   a. Preoperative antibiotics are most effective when given within 2 hours before surgery. Cefotaxime 1 g IV or cefoxitin 2 g IV has been shown to reduce infection rates for intra-abdominal surgery and should be used. **There is no evidence that continuing prophylactic antibiotics postoperatively is helpful.** However, antibiotics should be continued if there is active infection or contamination.
   b. For cardiac valvular disease, history of artificial valve, etc., use additional prophylactic antibiotics as recommended by the American Heart Association (see Chapter 3).
6. **Prep for surgery.** Bowel preps, DVT prophylaxis (see next section for DVT prophylaxis recommendations), and antiseptic shower and hair clipping, if indicated **(shaving surgical area may increase infection rate).**
7. **Premedication** by anesthesia to lower anxiety, lower secretions, and interact with narcotics for sedation.

L. Lab tests. See previous section for suggested routine lab tests.

II. Medical History of Major Importance.

A. Neurologic disorders. Some anticonvulsants are PO only. May need to change medications if patient will be NPO for long period of time.

B. Hematologic disorders

1. **Positive sickle cell screen.** Needs Hb electrophoresis. If majority is Hb S, will need partial exchange transfusion before surgical procedure (see Chapter 6).
2. **Clotting disorders.** May need evaluation, treatment (see Chapter 6).
3. **Anemia.** Ideally, Hct >30%, with Hb >10 g at surgery. No evidence that anemia contributes to surgical morbidity in the well-hydrated, hemodynamically stable patient with a Hb >7 g.

C. Integument disorders. If possible, avoid operating when there are active skin infections present. Chronic skin disorders should be optimally controlled for postoperative healing. For those who form keloids, may need to consider different closure techniques.

15

GENERAL SURGERY

D. Nutritional status

1. For elective or semielective surgery, consider optimizing nutritional status if patient has chronic disease.
2. **Obesity.** Weight loss to improve cardiopulmonary status and decrease problems with healing.

E. Cardiac. See preoperative cardiac evaluation, earlier.

F. Pulmonary. COPD. Optimize pulmonary toilet and use incentive spirometry to encourage lung expansion. See section on preoperative pulmonary evaluation, earlier.

III. Operative Note.

A. Preoperative diagnosis.

B. Postoperative diagnosis.

C. Procedure or operation performed.

D. Surgeon, assistants.

E. Anesthesia. General endotracheal, general mask, spinal, epidural, regional block, local, etc., include specific agent used.

F. Findings.

G. Specimen. Frozen section if obtained, pathologic and microscopic characteristics, etc.

H. Estimated blood loss.

I. Intraoperative fluids and blood products administered.

J. Drains and tubes placed.

K. Complications.

L. Patient's condition and disposition.

POSTOPERATIVE CARE

I. Orders.

A. Admit to ward, ICU, or recovery room.

B. Diagnosis. Operation.

C. Vital signs. Every 30 minutes for first few hours and then reduce as stable.

D. Allergies.

E. Activity. Bed rest until fully awake; up walking that night or next morning depending on surgery. Up to chair qid if unable to ambulate.

F. Diet. NPO until nausea resolves or resumption of bowel activity as determined by bowel sounds, passing gas, or having bowel movement. Start with clear liquids and advance as tolerated.

G. Pulmonary. Deep breathing and incentive spirometry. Deep breathing has been shown significantly to reduce the rate of respiratory complications such as pneumonia. Intermittent or continuous positive-pressure breathing (CPAP) can also reduce postoperative pulmonary complications, but is more expensive and should be used only in those unable or unwilling to take deep breaths or use incentive spirometry. **Pain management is critical for good pulmonary function (deep breathing, etc.).**

H. Intake and output
1. Record I&O every shift or more frequently if patient's condition is unstable.
2. IV fluids. With surgeries involving third spacing, replace with isotonic solutions for first 24 hours. NG losses should be replaced with 0.45 NS, and if in exceptionally large amounts, replace losses milliliter for milliliter. Maintenance fluids should generally be 0.2 NS in children or D_5 1/2NS in adults. Potassium is normally included in replacement solutions but is excluded from maintenance solutions until normal renal function is established. **Colloids do not provide any survival benefit and are expensive.** See later for evaluation of postoperative oliguria.
3. Instructions for care of all tubes and drains, including a Foley catheter and NG tube. NG tube should be connected to low intermittent suction and irrigated frequently to ensure patency. **Remove Foley and other tubes as soon as possible. Prolonged indwelling catheters predispose to infection.**

I. Nursing.
1. Encourage turning, coughing, deep breathing, and incentive spirometry.
2. Dressing changes.
3. Parameters to notify doctor, such as urine output (<0.5 mL/kg per hour), fever, hypertension or hypotension, tachycardia or bradycardia, inability to void within 8 hours of surgery, or unusual drainage on dressings, tachypnea, or bleeding.
4. Specify neurologic or vascular checks.

J. Medications
1. **Pain medications.** PO or IV. Patient-controlled analgesia (PCA) provides better analgesia, and patients generally require less narcotic than with IM or PRN IV treatment; there is little indication for IM pain medications. Adequate doses of pain medications improve mobility and decrease complications such as respiratory and thromboembolic problems. PRN orders provide worse pain management than do standing orders. If cannot use PCA, use scheduled IV doses of morphine (e.g., 2-5 mg/h IV).
2. **There is no evidence that hydroxyzine or promethazine HCl (Phenergan) have an opiate-sparing effect. In fact, promethazine may have an antianalgesia effect. They are, however, sedatives.**
3. **Tramadol (Ultram) has been shown to be ineffective in postoperative pain.**
4. **Propoxyphene–acetaminophen combinations have not been shown to be any better than acetaminophen alone.**
5. Hydrocodone combinations (e.g., Lortab, Vicodin) are as effective or more effective than codeine combinations (Tylenol #3 and others) and have fewer GI and CNS side effects. In addition, 10% of patients cannot metabolize codeine to its active form (morphine). Oxycodone (Percodan and others) is also effective.
6. **PCA is the preferred modality but will not work in the patient with dementia.**
   a. **Morphine.** Bolus with 2 to 10 mg over 20 to 30 minutes. Use PCA pump that delivers 1-mg aliquots with an initial lockout time of about

5 to 15 minutes (therefore 4-12 mg/h). Generally start at 10-minute lockout and adjust from there. **Localized urticaria at the infusion site is not a contraindication to the use of morphine. Morphine simply releases histamine, which can cause a localized reaction.**

b. **Meperidine.** Bolus with 20 to 100 mg over 20 to 30 minutes and then PCA pump that delivers 10-mg aliquots with a lockout time of 5 to 20 minutes. Generally start at 10-minute lockout and adjust from there. **Meperidine is metabolized to normeperidine, which can cause agitation and seizures, especially in the elderly. It can also cause serotonin syndrome in those on SSRIs. Morphine is preferred.**

7. **If using IM:**
a. Morphine: 0.05 to 0.1 mg/kg IM q3-6h.
b. Meperidine: 0.5 to 1.0 mg/kg IM q3-6h.

8. **Antiemetics.** First consider if medications may be causing nausea, if NG tube is plugged, or if this is postanesthetic nausea. Trimethobenzamide (Tigan) and promethazine (Phenergan) tend to be less effective than the following options:
a. **Prochlorperazine** (Compazine and others) 5 to 10 mg IV q6h. May cause hypotension and dystonic reactions.
b. **Metoclopramide** (Reglan and others) 5 to 10 mg or more (up to 30 mg) IV q6h. May cause dystonic reactions.
c. **Haloperidol** 1.25 to 5 mg IV. May be sedating but is an excellent antiemetic
d. **Ondansetron** (Zofran) 4 mg IV over 15 minutes (good but expensive). **May rarely cause dystonic reactions!** Alternatives include granisetron, dolasetron.
e. Watch for dystonic reactions and confusion with all of the above. Diphenhydramine 25 to 50 mg IV/IM or benztropine 1 to 4 mg IV/IM can be used to counteract dystonia.

9. **Antibiotics.** For infection.
10. Routine medications that need to be renewed.
11. PRN medications such as laxatives, sleeping medications, and antacids.

K. **Special tests, such as follow-up CXRs or serial ECGs.** ECG should be performed on postoperative day 1 for high-risk patients.
L. **Lab.** Follow-up CBC for possibility of hemorrhage or for large amount of blood loss. If patient continues on IV fluid, check daily electrolytes.
M. **See later for postoperative DVT prophylaxis.**
N. **Adequate nutrition is critical to good wound healing.** Start oral feedings as soon as possible by feeding tube if necessary. If oral feeding is not feasible, start parenteral nutrition. A dietary consult on all hospitalized patients should be considered. Up to 70% of surgical patients have inadequate nutrition.

II. **Postoperative Fever.** Fever at 24 to 48 hours postoperatively most commonly blamed on atelectasis, but **atelectasis does not cause fever.** Do not ignore other causes of fever **(Box 15-1)!**

BOX 15-1

CAUSES OF POSTOPERATIVE FEVER BY TIME OF ONSET

IMMEDIATE (WITHIN HOURS OF SURGERY)

Preexisting infection

Transfusion reaction (see Chapter 6) or reaction to drugs

Tissue trauma (including head trauma), either before surgery or from surgery
(the more extensive the surgery, the more likely there is to be postoperative fever);
fever is from the release of cytokines, etc.

Malignant hyperthermia within 30 minutes of anesthesia induction *but* may be
hours out

Aspiration pneumonitis (not pneumonia; see Chapter 4)

Thyroid storm

These causes of fever generally resolve within 3 days to 1 week (head trauma) after
surgery.

ACUTE (>2-3 HOURS BUT WITHIN FIRST WEEK AFTER SURGERY)

Nosocomial infections, community-acquired infection

Intubation-related pneumonia

Aspiration pneumonitis

Line-related infection

UTI, especially if chronic indwelling or urologic manipulation

Surgical site infection generally >1 wk as cause of fever, but may occur in first
week, especially in outpatients with early ambulation, discharge; but group A
Streptococcus and *Clostridium* infections can occur within hours of surgery

Less likely, but also consider pancreatitis, alcohol withdrawal, PE, MI,
thrombophlebitis, gout

Fat emboli from long bones, liposuction

SUBACUTE (>1 WEEK AFTER SURGERY)

IV-related and central catheter–related infection

Antibiotic-associated diarrhea

Drug fever: β-lactams, sulfa, heparin, etc.

Thromboembolic disease: DVT, PE

Wound infection: *Staphylococcus*, enteric organisms, and *Streptococcus*

A. Occurs in 50% of surgeries and 75% of orthopedic cases.

B. Postoperative fever usually noninfectious > UTI > pulmonary.

C. Fat embolism syndrome: Triad of hypoxia, mental status changes, and petechial rash.

1. **Associated with** closed pelvic and long bone fractures (up to 20% risk), "overzealous" reaming of femoral canal during surgery, trauma, liposuction. Also can be seen independent of surgery with pancreatitis, DM, osteomyelitis, panniculitis, bone tumor lysis, steroid therapy, sickle cell disease, fatty liver, infused lipids.

2. **Develops** 24 to 72 hours after insult (range, 12 hours to 2 weeks).

3. **Symptoms include** ARDS-like syndrome, mental status changes, petechial rash (30%-50%) on head, neck (generally above axilla). Eye findings, which are found in 50%, include cotton-wool spots and streak hemorrhages.

15

GENERAL SURGERY

4. **Lab findings** include thrombocytopenia, anemia, fat in urine (50%).
5. **Consider TTP in differential diagnosis** (see Chapter 6, Hematologic, Metabolic, and Electrolyte Disorders).

III. Postoperative Oliguria.

A. Oliguria (see also discussion of renal failure in Chapter 8) is defined as urine output <30 mL/h or 1 mL/kg per hour in children. Postoperative oliguria can be divided into:

1. **Prerenal azotemia.** Caused by decreased glomerular filtration rate secondary to poor kidney perfusion. This can occur with hypotension, hemorrhage, GI fluid loss, excessive renal loss (e.g., diuretics), CHF, and third spacing (among other causes). The BUN/Cr ratio is >20 with prerenal disease.

2. **Acute tubular necrosis.** Often develops postoperatively when there is one of the following: preexisting renal disease, long periods of hypotension, use of nephrotoxic agents, septicemia, or hemolysis. (See Chapter 8 for a detailed discussion of diagnosis and management.)

3. **Other causes of decreased urine output.**
a. Reflex spasm of voluntary sphincter because of pain or anxiety.
b. Medications such as anticholinergics and narcotics.
c. Detrusor atony as a result of surgery and manipulation (especially after retroperitoneal or pelvic surgery).
d. Preexisting partial bladder outlet obstruction such as an enlarged prostate.
e. Mechanical obstruction such as an expanding hematoma or fluid collection, or occluded Foley catheter.

B. Diagnosis. Look for signs of hypovolemia such as decreased skin turgor or dry mucous membranes, tachycardia, hypotension. If patient cannot or has no desire to urinate several hours postoperatively, consider oliguria secondary to hypovolemia. A palpable bladder is a sign of urinary retention.

C. Treatment. Relieve pain. If condition permits, standing or sitting may facilitate voiding.

1. **Hypovolemia.** Treat hypovolemia with boluses of NS (250-mL aliquots) until maintaining urine output at 30 to 60 mL/h in adults and 0.5 to 1 mL/kg per hour in children. Diuretics will worsen prerenal azotemia.

2. **Mechanical obstruction.** If mechanical obstruction, such as enlarged prostate, consider intermittent catheterization. If the patient already has a Foley catheter, irrigate it to assess for obstruction. There is no need to release urine gradually from the bladder. Drainage of even 1 L of urine is not associated with hypotension, etc.

IV. Postoperative Ileus.

A. Maintain NPO with NG suction; check electrolytes, including calcium and potassium. Avoid anticholinergics, narcotics (unless needed for pain), and calcium channel blockers.

B. If prolonged, consider pancreatitis, peritonitis, intra-abdominal abscess, pneumonia, free blood in the peritoneum.

C. For adynamic ileus with colonic distention (cecal diameter ≥9 cm, also known as Ogilvie's syndrome), neostigmine 2 mg IV will frequently lead to prompt resolution of the problem. An alternative is colonoscopy with decompression.

D. Chewing gum at least tid postoperatively may speed resolution of ileus.

POSTOPERATIVE DVT PROPHYLAXIS

I. **General.** Untreated, 40% to 50% of those with hip surgery will develop a DVT postoperatively; 16% will develop DVT even with the best prophylaxis. If not given prophylaxis, 15% to 30% of those with abdominal surgery will develop a DVT; DVT prophylaxis after surgery is cost effective. See Chapter 6 for details about peri-operative management of anticoagulation.

II. **Options for DVT Prophylaxis. Only LMWH and pneumatic compression stockings have been shown to reduce the incidence of pulmonary embolism.**

A. **Enoxaparin,** 30 mg SQ bid started within 24 hours after surgery. Alternative is 40 mg SQ qd starting 12 hours before surgery. Subcutaneous LMWH is the most effective form of prophylaxis and has fewer complications than unfractionated heparin. Continue until patient is ambulatory or up to 14 days. May have delayed excretion with renal failure. Reduce dose to 30 mg SQ qd if creatinine clearance is less than 30 mL/min.

B. **Dalteparin,** 2500 anti-factor Xa IU SQ qd starting 1 to 2 hours before abdominal surgery and continuing for 5 to 10 days postoperatively. Must be adjusted for renal function. Use with caution in renal and hepatic disease.

C. **Heparin** (unfractionated), 5000 units SQ q12h.

D. **Intermittent pneumatic compression.** Effective and has few side effects.

E. **Warfarin.** Less effective than LMWH and has greater bleeding complications.

F. **Aspirin**. Not very effective in postsurgical DVT prophylaxis, and other choices, especially enoxaparin, are preferred.

G. **Graduated compression stockings.** Effective only in low-risk patients.

ABDOMINAL PAIN

Although classic surgical teaching has been that pain medication may mask the correct diagnosis in abdominal pain, this is not supported by the literature. In fact, if anything, the diagnosis is clarified by judicious pain relief, which results in fewer unnecessary surgeries.

I. **History.**

A. The area of the pain, including its origin and pattern of radiation, time of onset, nature, and associated symptoms, will frequently make the diagnosis (Table 15-7). A menstrual history should be obtained.

B. **Associated symptoms**

1. Weight loss, which might indicate malignancy or malabsorption.
2. Vomiting, as with a small bowel obstruction or volvulus.

TABLE 15-7

ABDOMINAL PAIN BY MAIN LOCATION

Diagnosis	Usual Pain Location	Diagnostic Studies	Pain Radiation and Comments
UPPER QUADRANTS/MIDEPIGASTRIC			
Cardiac disease (see also Chapters 2 and 3)	Can manifest as epigastric pain	ECG and enzymes to rule out cardiac disease	Can be confused with esophageal reflux
Cholecystitis, choleithiasis, choledocholithiasis, and cholangitis	RUQ	US	Back, right scapula, midepigastric; sudden onset with associated nausea; can be related to ingestion of food
Duodenal ulcer or gastric ulcer (see Chapter 5)	Midepigastric/LUQ	UGI or endoscopy Usually historical (see Chapter 5)	Radiation to back if posterior ulcer; peritonitis/sudden onset of severe abdominal pain with perforation. *Many are asymptomatic until rupture!*
Fitz-Hugh-Curtis syndrome	RUQ and signs of PID	Perihepatitis: elevated liver enzymes, associated with gonorrhea	Right shoulder and back
Hepatitis (see Chapter 5), subphrenic abscess, hepatic abscess	RUQ	US, CT, elevated liver enzymes, jaundice	Right shoulder
Pancreatitis (see Chapter 5)	Midepigastric region	Elevated amylase, lipase, WBC Pts with chronic pancreatitis might have normal amylase and lipase CT scan or US shows edema	Radiates to back; pt may have peritonitis
Splenic hematoma or enlargement	LUQ pain	US or CT	Hypotension; peritonitis if ruptured
SMA syndrome	Midepigastric pain, especially after eating	Upper GI may show duodenal outlet obstruction, US shows increased blood velocity in SMA MRA/angiogram usually not necessary	Usually thin pts with a midepigastric bruit

LOWER QUADRANTS

Aortic aneurysm (see Chapter 2)	Periumbilical, especially into back flanks; May be colicky	US or CT	Can manifest as epigastric or back pain, flank/hip pain; Rule this out in the proper age group if history suggests renal stones; Hypotension if ruptured; Pt may present with peritoneal signs
Appendicitis	Early periumbilical; Late RLQ	CT or US may show abscess, enlarged appendix	May be generalized with persistent obstruction
Cecal volvulus	RLQ pain with sudden onset.	Seen on flat plate radiograph as RUQ distended bowel	Generally elderly pts
Crohn's disease or ulcerative colitis	RLQ but may be LLQ	ESR, ANCA, endoscopy (see Chapter 5)	Diarrhea (bloody in ulcerative colitis), cramps, elevated ESR
Cystitis (see Chapter 8)	Suprapubic pain	UA	
Diverticulitis	Generally LLQ, very rarely RLQ	Clinical diagnosis (LLQ pain, diarrhea, vomiting, fever), CT scan is most sensitive test	May be generalized
Epiploic appendagitis	Left midabdomen caused by torsion of an epiploic appendage; generally afebrile	Normal or mildly elevated WBC count; Diagnose by CT scan	Age usually 20s-60s. Generally self-limited disease, resolves in 3 d to 2 wk
Mesenteric adenitis	RLQ	Diagnosis of exclusion	Pain secondary to enlarged mesenteric nodes from streptococcal pharyngitis
Gynecologic disease (see Chapter 13)	Pain in pelvis, either adnexal area	Pregnancy test, cervical cultures, US	Radiation to groin, may radiate to right shoulder if free intraperitoneal bleeding
Ovarian torsion, mittelschmerz, ruptured ovarian cyst	Sudden-onset colicky lower abdominal pain	Pregnancy test, cervical cultures, US	May have marked cervical motion tenderness

(Continued)

GENERAL SURGERY 15

TABLE 15-7

ABDOMINAL PAIN BY MAIN LOCATION—cont'd

Diagnosis	Usual Pain Location	Diagnostic Studies	Pain Radiation and Comments
PID (see Chapter 13)	Gradual onset, fever, constant aching pain, vaginal discharge	Pregnancy test, cervical cultures, US	Marked cervical motion tenderness
Pneumonia (see Chapter 4)	May mimic appendicitis	CXR	Cough, etc.
Urolithiasis or nephrolithiasis (see Chapter 8)	Either flank	Noncontrast CT is most sensitive modality	May radiate to labia or testicles; may mimic AAA
GENERALIZED (SOME MAY LOCALIZE)			
Acute intermittent porphyria	Diffuse and especially into back	24-h urine for ALA, PGB, porphyrins Screening urine for PGB is also available	Colicky abdominal pain that is intermittent may be associated with dark urine Associated psychiatric or neurologic symptoms, including sensory changes, paresthesias, psychosis Exacerbated by medications (esp estrogens, alcohol, sulfonamides), menstruation, weight loss May be photosensitive
Hemolysis (see Chapter 6)	Back and costovertebral angle pain	Reticulocyte count, serum free hemoglobin, LDH, peripheral smear, haptoglobin	G6PD deficiency, transfusion reactions, paroxysmal nocturnal hemoglobinuria
Intussusception	Cramping abdominal pain with asymptomatic periods Mental status changes are common and may have periods of lethargy	Air enema (has replaced barium for this indication) is often curative (see text)	Generally age 2 wk to 2 y

Large bowel ischemia	Bloody currant jelly stools are a late sign Few have palpable sausage-shaped mass in RLQ	Patients generally >60 y
	Acute-onset lower abdominal pain followed within 24 h by bloody diarrhea or blood per rectum	Clinical diagnosis, colonoscopy
Meckel's diverticulum	Below or left of umbilicus	May be recurrent, with rectal bleeding or intestinal obstruction
Mesenteric thrombosis	Sudden onset of severe generalized abdominal pain without peritoneal signs and out of proportion to physical findings May have antecedent history of bowel angina (postprandial abdominal pain)	Patients generally >50 y with a history of other vascular disease, low-flow states (e.g. CHF, hypovolemia) Must rule out urolithiasis, AAA, perforated ulcer, etc. May have elevated serum phosphate, serum lactate, amylase, acidosis CT scan may show bowel edema Angiography is diagnostic
Metabolic disease such as DKA, Addison's disease	Pain may be diffuse, with associated nausea, vomiting; may have guarding	
Spontaneous bacterial peritonitis	Generalized with peritoneal signs	Paracentesis Usually in alcoholics or those with indwelling dialysis catheters

AAA, abdominal aortic aneurysm; PGB, porphobilinogen; SMA, superior mesenteric artery.

GENERAL SURGERY 15

3. Diarrhea and constipation, which might indicate inflammatory bowel disease, cancer, obstipation, malabsorption.
4. Melena or blood per rectum: check with Hemoccult. If negative, consider foods (Kool-Aid, beets) or medicines (iron). **Iron supplementation should not give a heme-positive test on stool.**
C. **Jaundice.** Consider pancreatic cancer (painless), hepatitis, hemolysis (sickle cell, G6PD deficiency, transfusion reaction: see Chapter 6), alcoholic hepatitis, choledocholithiasis, primary biliary cirrhosis.
D. **Urinary symptoms.** Dysuria, frequency, urgency, hematuria. Renal problems often present as a complaint of abdominal pain. Consider urolithiasis, UTI, testicular torsion.
E. **Sexual activity,** last period, birth control, history of sexually transmitted disease, vaginal discharge, spotting or bleeding. Consider ectopic pregnancy, PID, ovarian torsion, ruptured ovarian cyst.
F. **Past medical history: Medical problems that can present as abdominal pain** include DKA, hypercalcemia, Addison's disease, pneumonia, cardiac disease, herpes zoster, back/disk disease, and acute-angle glaucoma, among others. History should include other major illnesses, prior surgeries, prior studies performed for evaluation of abdominal problems, family history of any similar complaints.
G. **Medications. An amazing array of medications can be responsible for abdominal pain.** Examples include digoxin, theophylline, steroids, tetracycline/alendronate (esophageal ulcers), NSAIDs, analgesics, antipyretics, antiemetics.
II. **Physical Examination.**
A. **Vital signs.** Observe for signs of shock, elevated temperature.
B. **Abdominal exam**
1. **Inspection.** Scaphoid appearance or distention, point of most severe pain, hernia, scars.
2. **Auscultation.** High-pitched bowel sounds are suggestive of an obstructive process. Absent bowel sounds are suggestive of an ileus.
3. **Palpation and percussion.** Muscle rigidity (voluntary/involuntary), localized tenderness, masses, pulsation, hernias, peritoneal irritation (rebound: cough or jumping also may elicit "rebound"), involuntary guarding, obturator sign (pain on internal and external rotation of hip), psoas sign (pain on straight leg raising by using obturator muscle, may indicate abscess, etc. irritating the psoas), Murphy's sign (RUQ pain when breathing in and pressing over the liver), liver dimension and spleen dimension.
4. **CVA tenderness**
5. **Pelvic exam** in women (see later).
6. **Rectal exam.** To rule out GI bleeding, prostatitis, etc. The absence of rectal tenderness does not preclude the diagnosis of appendicitis, nor does it make the diagnosis of appendicitis (sensitivity and specificity both in the 50% range). The rectal examination should be used to add to your entire clinical picture.

7. Look for signs of pregnancy (nausea, breast tenderness, and urinary frequency).

III. Laboratory.

A. CBC with differential and urinalysis is routinely done on most cases of abdominal pain.

B. Electrolytes, BUN, creatinine with vomiting or diarrhea.

C. Glucose and calcium to rule out DKA and hypercalcemia, respectively.

D. LFTs and liver enzymes; amylase and lipase for upper abdominal pain.

E. Other studies as indicated: CXR (upright) for pneumonia or free air **(upright CXR is the best radiograph for free air).** Abdominal flat plate and upright for bowel obstruction, ileus, free air, abnormal calcification. US or CT to look for peritoneal fluid. ECG for acute MI, ischemia, or arrhythmias. Paracentesis may be important with fluid in the abdomen (e.g., to rule out spontaneous bacterial peritonitis).

F. Pelvic US or CT. Transvaginal US may be more helpful as an initial test in the reproductive-age woman because it is better at detecting gynecologic disease (e.g., ectopic pregnancy, ovarian torsion, ovarian cysts). Be sure to check blood flow to both ovaries to rule out ovarian torsion. CT is the test of choice in the diagnosis of appendicitis, diverticulitis, mesenteric ischemia, abdominal aneurysm.

G. Pregnancy test *on all reproductive-age women unless status post-hysterectomy.* Sexual history is often unreliable in the emergency setting and up to 3% of tubal ligations fail! Urine pregnancy test may very rarely miss very early ectopic pregnancies. Serum HCG is very sensitive and picks up virtually all pregnancies.

IV. Special Considerations in the Reproductive-Age Woman.

A. Pelvic exam. Complete vulvar and vaginal exam, cervix (dilation, tissue at os, lesions, motion tenderness), uterine size and tenderness, and adnexa (masses, tenderness, unilateral or bilateral). Obtain cultures for gonococcus and *Chlamydia*, wet mount.

B. Culdocentesis. Less useful with the advent of accurate US and CT. Culdocentesis will be positive with any intraperitoneal bleeding (e.g., ectopic pregnancy, bleeding corpus luteum cyst, ruptured liver adenoma, ruptured spleen, peptic ulcer). The absence of fluid is nondiagnostic and does not help in differentiating the cause of pain.

C. Partial differential diagnosis of pelvic pain.

1. **Ectopic pregnancy** (see Chapter 13), appendicitis, pyelonephritis, ovarian cysts, spontaneous abortion (see Chapter 14), PID (see Chapter 13), ovarian torsion, mittelschmerz, dysmenorrhea, endometriosis, uterine fibroids, ureteral stone, cystitis, diverticulitis, inflammatory bowel disease, IBS, bowel obstruction, inguinal hernia, among other causes.

2. Sudden onset is suggestive of ovarian or testicular torsion, mittelschmerz, urolithiasis, ruptured corpus luteum cyst, ruptured ectopic pregnancy. More gradual onset is suggestive of appendicitis, PID, abscess, etc.

GENERAL SURGERY 15

V. Initial Treatment.

A. Decide whether to admit and observe, discharge, operate. Serial exams may clarify the diagnosis.

B. Keep NPO until diagnosis is clear.

C. IV fluids: Decide on expected fluid losses and current level of hydration.

D. NG tube for vomiting, bleeding, or obstruction.

E. Foley catheter to monitor fluids.

F. Use judicious amounts of pain medication; it will help you clarify the diagnosis!

G. Serial labs may be helpful, especially CBC, cardiac enzymes.

APPENDICITIS

I. Overview. Appendicitis is a common cause of abdominal pain. However, the presentation is not always classic and a high index of suspicion is necessary. Affects any age group but is rare in infants, most common in adolescence and young adult years. Generally occurs from obstruction of the appendiceal lumen by lymphoid hyperplasia or a fecalith.

II. Clinical Presentation.

A. History. Classic history is that of periumbilical or epigastric pain that migrates to RLQ. Pain may be felt in flank (retrocecal appendix, pregnancy), testicle (retroileal appendix), or bladder (up to 20% present with dysuria). Anorexia, nausea, and vomiting may occur after the onset of pain. Anorexia is present only in 50% to 75% of cases. Presentation is more likely to be atypical in very young, very old, and pregnant patients. Maintain a high index of suspicion in any patient with abdominal pain.

B. Physical exam. Fever is found only in 15%. High temperature is not common unless perforation has occurred. Abdominal exam reveals RLQ pain, possibly with rebound or guarding. Psoas sign (pain on active elevation of the legs) may be present, as may be the obturator sign (pain on internal and external rotation of the hip). **Rectal exam, only 54% sensitive and 53% specific for appendicitis, does not add anything to the diagnosis and is mandatory only in infants.** Pelvic exam should be performed to rule out other illness (e.g., PID).

C. Lab tests. CBC with differential and UA should be obtained in all patients, and a pregnancy test in all reproductive-age women. Obtain cervical or urethral culture if indicated. Mild to moderately elevated WBC count with left shift is typical, but WBC count is normal in 10%. UA may show ketonuria or a few RBCs or WBCs, but the presence of significant hematuria or pyuria is suggestive of urinary tract as source of pain.

III. Management.

A. Classic presentation. Consultation with surgeon for appendectomy. Pain relief may help clarify the situation (small doses of IV morphine). Patient should be kept NPO after arrival at ED or clinic and hydrated IV.

B. **Unclear presentation.** The history and physical exam are more reliable indicators of appendicitis than is the WBC count. Surgeon should be consulted for suspected appendicitis if history and exam suggest the diagnosis. If minimal findings are present on exam, consider observation for several hours with repeated exams (including vital signs and temperature) and CBC q4h during observation period. CT has replaced US in questionable cases of appendicitis. It is unclear if CT reduces unnecessary surgery; **CT need not be done on those with obvious appendicitis.**

C. If going to the operating room, the patient should receive IV antibiotics within 2 hours of procedure (e.g., cefoxitin).

GALLBLADDER DISEASE

I. **Overview.** Cholelithiasis is found in 10% of the population. Choledocholithiasis, biliary colic, and acute cholecystitis are less common. The incidence of cholelithiasis increases with age and is more common in women. Other predisposing factors include obesity, pregnancy, DM, and chronic hemolytic states.

II. **Evaluation of the Gallbladder.**

A. **Laboratory tests,** including LFTs, amylase/lipase for evidence of pancreatic involvement. WBC count if symptoms acutely present. An elevated alkaline phosphatase is possibly the most sensitive and specific indicator of biliary disease. However, the ALT and AST may become elevated before the alkaline phosphatase.

B. **Plain radiographs** are not helpful because only about 15% of stones are radiopaque.

C. **US** should be the initial exam to evaluate for cholelithiasis. Can visualize stones and evaluate biliary ducts and pancreas. Obesity and overlying abdominal gas decrease the quality of the exam. Overall sensitivity is 90%, specificity 85%. CT has a lower sensitivity.

D. **Oral cholecystogram** is performed by having patient ingest 3 g of iopanoic acid about 12 hours before study. Failure of the gallbladder to opacify indicates gallbladder disease. Is not reliable in setting of significant hyperbilirubinemia or acute cholecystitis and has largely been replaced by US.

E. **Radionuclide hepatobiliary scan** (e.g., hydroxy iminodiacetic acid [HIDA] scan) can be used when there is a consideration of acute cholecystitis, biliary outlet obstruction, or sphincter of Oddi spasm. Failure of gallbladder to visualize when there is the presence of radioisotope in common bile duct 4 hours after injection indicates dysfunction of the gallbladder such as cholecystitis or outlet obstruction (e.g., tumor, choledocholithiasis).

F. **Endoscopic retrograde cholangiopancreatography (ERCP)** may also be used to define the anatomy of the biliary tree and may be a better choice than radionuclide scanning in many situations. This is especially true if consideration is being given to laparoscopic surgery and a common duct stone needs to be ruled out.

G. Endoscope-guided US. Not commonly available but sensitive at picking up common duct stones.

III. Asymptomatic Cholelithiasis.

A. Course. Eighty percent of gallstones are asymptomatic, with a small percentage becoming symptomatic each year (10% at 5 years, 15% at 10 years, 18% at 15 years). Stones are composed of bile salts, cholesterol (80% in the United States are cholesterol stones), phospholipids, or unconjugated bilirubin. Calcification may occur and results in about 15% of the stones becoming radiopaque.

B. Management. Asymptomatic patients do not require surgery. Previously, diabetes was considered an indication for cholecystectomy in the asymptomatic patient, but this recommendation has been changed. Consider surgery for those asymptomatic individuals with calcified gallbladder, those with particularly large stones (>3 cm), and those who are at a high risk for gallbladder cancer (Pima Indians and others). See later for medical management.

IV. Biliary Colic.

A. Caused by intermittent obstruction of the cystic duct by gallstones. History will generally include episodes of epigastric and RUQ pain, which may radiate to back. Pain is usually constant, is abrupt in onset, and subsides slowly. Nausea is commonly associated. Attacks may be precipitated by ingestion of fatty foods. Consider also choledocholithiasis (stone in common duct). **Spasm of the sphincter of Oddi can cause symptoms similar to cholelithiasis and is more common after cholecystectomy.** This may respond to SL NTG or PO nifedipine. Diagnosis is by HIDA scan or ERCP, during which sphincter pressures can be measured.

B. Physical exam will reveal absence of fever, possible RUQ or midepigastric tenderness without rebound. Gallbladder may be palpable and the patient may have a positive Murphy's sign (sudden increase in pain with palpation of RUQ during deep inspiration).

C. Laboratory evaluation. CBC with differential should be obtained and consider amylase and lipase. WBC count should not be significantly elevated. LFT results may be normal or slightly elevated.

D. Treatment. Analgesics and antiemetics (prochlorperazine, metoclopramide) should be provided acutely. **Morphine has traditionally been avoided. However, there is no evidence that morphine is problematic in biliary colic.** Although generally not a good choice for pain, ketorolac 15 to 30 mg IV is useful for biliary colic. Meperidine is a less desirable option than morphine. If pain resolves, further evaluation may be obtained as convenient in the next few days, with the patient instructed to avoid fatty foods. Cholecystectomy should be performed electively.

E. Elective surgery is appropriate treatment. Common duct stones can be cleared using ERCP.

V. **Acute Cholecystitis.**

A. **Ninety-five percent of those with cholecystitis will have cholelithiasis.**

B. **Presentation** is similar to biliary colic (nausea, vomiting, abdominal pain, RUQ tenderness) with the additional features of fever, leukocytosis, mild elevation of bilirubin, elevated alkaline phosphatase. Murphy's sign may be present.

C. **US** only 50% sensitive for cholecystitis (but will pick up stones and dilated ducts). US may miss pericolic fluid collections, etc. HIDA scan is diagnostic modality of choice.

D. **Treatment.** Consultation with surgeon is required. Antibiotics are indicated for acute cholecystitis. A third-generation cephalosporin plus metronidazole, or ampicillin–sulbactam (Unasyn), will cover the most common organisms. There are advantages and disadvantages to early or delayed surgery, although early surgery generally results in lower morbidity and shorter hospitalizations. Surgeon will ultimately need to decide based on the particular features of the case. **Regardless of timing of surgery, ERCP should be done to clear common duct stones, emergently if possible.**

E. **Percutaneous US-guided cholecystostomy.** For critically ill patients who are not currently good surgical candidates, this is a less invasive procedure to temporize until the patient has recovered from the acute illness.

VI. **Biliary Sludge.**

A. **General.** May be a cause of RUQ pain. Also implicated in 31% of nonalcoholic pancreatitis and 74% of "idiopathic" pancreatitis (e.g., alcohol, gallstones, metabolic problems, drugs have been excluded). Predisposing factors include prolonged CVN, fasting, pregnancy, rapid weight loss, transplantation, and ceftriaxone use.

B. **Diagnosed** on US, but the sensitivity is only about 55%, whereas endoscopic US has a sensitivity of 98%.

C. **Course is variable.** The majority remain asymptomatic. Of those with symptoms at time 0, 50% become asymptomatic and 20% remain symptomatic over 3 years. Of those asymptomatic at time 0, 10% to 15% become symptomatic over 3 years and another 5% to 15% develop stones.

D. **Treatment.** If symptomatic, treatment can be medical (see below) or by cholecystectomy.

VII. **Medical Management of Cholelithiasis.**

A. **Surgical therapy is considered the treatment of choice for cholelithiasis.** However, in patients in whom this is not practical, other modalities may be used.

B. **Cholesterol stones** may be dissolved using ursodeoxycholic acid. About 70% of cholesterol stones will respond. However, stones tend to recur when ursodeoxycholic acid is discontinued.

15

GENERAL SURGERY

C. **Lithotripsy** can be used to fragment stones, which are then passed spontaneously. ERCP may help with stone removal, and use of ursodeoxycholic acid may prevent recurrence.

D. **ERCP** with sphincterotomy may assist in passing stones.

ILEUS AND BOWEL OBSTRUCTION

I. **Classification.**

A. **Mechanical obstruction.** Complete or partial physical blockage of intestinal lumen (Box 15-2).

B. **Simple obstruction.** Implies one obstruction point.

C. **Closed-loop obstruction.** Blockage at two or more points.

D. **Paralytic (adynamic) ileus.** Impairment of muscle function (e.g., after abdominal surgery, trauma, peritonitis, spinal injury, pneumonia, hypokalemia, uremia, pancreatitis), intestinal parasitic infection.

BOX 15-2

DIFFERENTIAL DIAGNOSIS OF ILEUS, SMALL AND LARGE BOWEL OBSTRUCTION

DIFFERENTIAL DIAGNOSIS OF ILEUS

Chemical irritants (e.g., blood)

Drugs (e.g., anticholinergic)

Heavy metal poisoning

Hypokalemia

Hypoperfusion/ischemia

Pancreatitis or any retroperitoneal irritation

Pelvic inflammatory disease

Peritonitis

Pneumonia

Postsurgical

Sepsis

Spinal trauma

CAUSES OF SMALL BOWEL OBSTRUCTION (REPRESENTS 85% OF BOWEL OBSTRUCTIONS)

Adhesions (60%)

Hernia (15%)

Neoplasm (15%)

Intussusception

Gallstone ileus

Superior mesenteric artery syndrome

CAUSES OF LARGE BOWEL OBSTRUCTION (REPRESENTS 15% OF BOWEL OBSTRUCTIONS)

Colon cancer (65%)

Diverticulitis (20%)

Volvulus (5%)

Miscellaneous

E. **Strangulating obstruction.** When obstructing mechanism occludes mesenteric blood supply. Hard to diagnose presurgically.

II. **Small Bowel Obstruction.**

A. **Clinical manifestations**

1. **Cramping abdominal pain.** Crescendo–decrescendo pattern. Continuous pain is suggestive of strangulation.

2. **Vomiting.** Earlier in high obstruction. Feculent vomiting, caused by bacterial overgrowth, may be seen especially with distal obstruction.

3. **Distention, obstipation, high-pitched or absent bowel sounds.**

B. **Work-up**

1. CBC with differential, electrolytes.

2. Supine and upright abdominal radiographs with stepladder pattern of air-fluid levels and no colonic gas are suggestive of obstruction. CT is more sensitive for obstruction and may demonstrate the cause. Start with a plain film, however.

3. History and physical exam may point to a particular cause such as adhesions or obstipation.

C. **Treatment**

1. Fluid and electrolyte resuscitation and supportive care.

2. If partial obstruction with patient passing gas, may treat with NG tube. This may relieve vomiting and decompress distention.

3. Surgical intervention is indicated if obstruction does not resolve with conservative treatment.

III. **Large Bowel Obstruction.**

A. **Clinical manifestations**

1. **Cramping pain, little vomiting** (less with competent ileocecal valve, vomitus rarely feculent), constipation and obstipation, distention (severe), loud borborygmi, and little loss of electrolytes.

B. **Work-up**

1. Electrolytes, glucose, BUN/Cr, UA, and CBC, other labs as indicated.

2. Colonoscopy or flexible sigmoidoscopy may reveal obstructive lesion.

3. Radiograph will reveal gas-filled colon with absence of gas beyond obstruction.

C. **Treatment**

1. NG tube.

2. IV fluids and appropriate monitoring. Antibiotics only if suspect perforation or abscess formation.

3. Sigmoidoscopy may reduce a sigmoid volvulus.

4. Surgical intervention if above measures not successful in relieving obstruction.

IV. **Intussusception.**

A. **General**

1. Intussusception is the most common cause of bowel obstruction in those 3 months to 6 years of age. Intussusception is rare before 3 months and most commonly occurs between 4 and 12 months of age. Male-to-female ratio is 4:1.

2. Less than 10% have a "lead point," but lead points may include polyps, sarcoma, Henoch-Schönlein purpura.
3. Ileocecal valve area is the most commonly involved.

B. Clinical presentation

1. Main presenting symptom is intermittent, inconsolable crying with asymptomatic periods. **Frequently have mental status changes with lethargy between episodes of abdominal colic.**
2. **Vomiting** will develop 6 to 12 hours after onset of colicky pain. Eventually will vomit bilious material.
3. **Currant jelly stools are a late finding** after venous stasis and bowel wall necrosis. Generally pale and shocky by this point.
4. **Abdominal exam may be negative.** "Sausage-shaped mass" in only two thirds.
5. **Rule out other causes of pain** such as bone injury, hairs around fingers, toes, penis, otitis media, corneal abrasion.

C. Diagnosis

1. US and CT have been used successfully to diagnose intussusception.
2. Plain film may be negative.
3. Early lab test data are not helpful. Fever and elevated WBC count are late findings.
4. Only about 70% have guaiac-positive stool.
5. Barium or air enema is diagnostic and therapeutic.

D. Treatment

1. **Barium or air enema successful in 75% if caught early,** but only 25% successful if it has been over 1 or 2 days. Air enema preferred because of risk of barium peritonitis if perforation.
2. Surgical intervention if this does not work
3. Admit for 24 hours if reduced with enema. About 25% will recur.

BIBLIOGRAPHY

Brogan GX Jr, Giarrusso E, Hollander JE, et al: Comparison of plain, warmed, and buffered lidocaine for anesthesia of traumatic wounds. *Ann Emerg Med* 26: 121-125, 1995.

Cummings P, Del Beccaro MA: Antibiotics to prevent infection of simple wounds: A meta-analysis of randomized studies. *Am J Emerg Med* 13:396-400, 1995.

Daneman A, Alton DJ, Ein S, et al: Perforation during attempted intussusception reduction in children—a comparison of perforation with barium and air. *Pediatr Radiol* 25:81-88, 1995.

Dixon JM, Elton RA, Rainey JB, Macleod DA: Rectal examination in patients with pain in the right lower quadrant of the abdomen. *BMJ* 302:386-388, 1991.

Engoren M: Lack of association between atelectasis and fever. *Chest* 107:81, 1995.

Ernst AA, Marvez-Valls E, Nick TG, Weiss SJ: LAT (lidocaine-adrenaline-tetracycline) versus TAC (tetracaine-adrenaline-cocaine) for topical anesthesia in face and scalp lacerations. *Am J Emerg Med* 13:151-154, 1995.

Forbes JA, Bates JA, Edquist IA, et al: Evaluation of two opioid-acetaminophen combinations and placebo in postoperative oral surgery pain. *Pharmacotherapy* 14:139-146, 1994.

Glazier HS: Potentiation of pain relief with hydroxyzine: A therapeutic myth? *Ann Pharmacother* 24:484-488, 1990.

Goswick CB: Ibuprofen versus propoxyphene hydrochloride and placebo in acute musculoskeletal trauma. *Curr Ther Res* 34:685-692, 1983.

Greenfield SM, Webster GJ, Vicary FR: Drinking before sedation: Preoperative fasting should be the exception rather than the rule. *BMJ* 314:162, 1997.

Hale DA, Molloy M, Pearl RH, et al: Appendectomy: A contemporary appraisal. *Ann Surg* 225:252-261, 1997.

Hall JC, Tarala RA, Tapper J, Hall JL: Prevention of respiratory complications after abdominal surgery: A randomised clinical trial. *BMJ* 312:148-152, 1996.

Houry S, Georgeac C, Hay JM, et al: A prospective multicenter evaluation of preoperative hemostatic screening tests. *Am J Surg* 170:19, 1995.

Kirks DR: Air intussusception reduction: "The winds of change" [review]. *Pediatr Radiol* 25:89-91, 1995.

LoVecchio F, Oster N, Sturmann K, et al: The use of analgesics in patients with acute abdominal pain. *J Emerg Med* 15:775-779, 1997.

Mangano DT, Goldman L: Preoperative assessment of patients with known or suspected coronary disease. *N Engl J Med* 333:1750-1756, 1995.

Mangano DT, Layug EL, Wallace A, Tateo I: Effect of atenolol on mortality and cardiovascular morbidity after noncardiac surgery. *N Engl J Med* 335:1713-1720, 1996.

McFall EO, Ward HB, Moritz TE, et al: Coronary-artery revascularization before elective major vascular surgery. *N Engl J Med* 351:2795-2804, 2004.

Narr BJ, Hansen TR, Warner MA: Preoperative laboratory screening in healthy Mayo patients: Cost effective elimination of tests and unchanged outcomes. *Mayo Clin Proc* 66:155-159, 1991.

Nyman MA, Schwenk NM, Silverstein MD: Management of urinary retention: rapid versus gradual decompression and risk of complications. *Mayo Clin Proc* 72:951-956, 1997.

Pace S, Burke TF: Intravenous morphine for early pain relief in patients with acute abdominal pain. *Acad Emerg Med* 3:1086-1092, 1996.

Ransohoff DF, Gracie WA: Treatment of gallstones. *Ann Intern Med* 119:606-619, 1993.

Rao PM, Rhea JT, Rattner DW, et al: Introduction of appendiceal count: Impact on negative appendectomy and appendiceal perforation rates. *Ann Surg* 229:344-349, 1999.

Scholer SJ, Pituch K, Orr DP, Dittus RS: Use of the rectal examination on children with acute abdominal pain. *Clin Pediatr (Phila)* 37:311-316, 1998.

Stubhaug A, Grimstad J, Breivik H: Lack of analgesic effect of 50 and 100 mg oral tramadol after orthopaedic surgery: A randomized, double-blind, placebo and standard active drug comparison. *Pain* 62:111-118, 1995.

Sunshine A, Olson NZ, Zighelboim I, et al: Analgesic oral efficacy of tramadol hydrochloride in postoperative pain. *Clin Pharmacol Ther* 51:740-746, 1992.

Orthopedics

Scott Frisbie

General note: *There are no good studies of the use of ice and heat for strains, sprains, etc. Continue to recommend these treatments but realize there is no "proper" way to do them and efficacy is likely limited.*

LOW BACK PAIN

I. **Overview.** Approximately 80% of the general population will have at least one episode of low back pain during their lifetime. Back pain lasting at least 2 weeks affects approximately 14% of adults each year. Most cases (90%) resolve within 6 weeks and 40% in 2 weeks; 5% of cases of low back pain become chronic.

II. **Clinical Features.**

A. **Mechanical causes** account for up to 98% of cases of back pain.

1. **Disk injury.** Herniation of the nucleus pulposus usually occurs posteriorly. May impinge on nerve roots, particularly at the L4-L5-S1 level. Typically pain increases with coughing, sneezing, riding in a car, or flexing the trunk and includes radicular symptoms and signs. Associated bowel or urinary abnormalities constitute a surgical emergency (cauda equina syndrome).

2. **Degenerative changes in facet joints** result in nerve root impingement at the foramina. Patient has sudden attacks lasting for a few days with symptom-free intervals. Typically pain is worse with trunk extension.

3. **Spondylosis** is defined as degenerative changes in vertebral bodies and disks. This can cause a nerve root impingement.

4. **Spondylolisthesis** is a bilateral pars interarticularis defect that allows slippage of one vertebra anteriorly in relationship to the vertebral body below it. About 80% occur at L5-S1.

5. **Spondylolysis** is a unilateral or bilateral defect in the pars interarticularis that is generally the result of repeated lumbar stress and hyperextension, but it can occur secondary to a congenital deformity. It generally occurs in younger patients (18 years old to mid-twenties) and occurs in 6% of the population. It is much more common in gymnasts. Pain is worse with extension and better with flexion. Can cause spondylolisthesis.

6. **Vertebral body fracture** occurs after trauma or spontaneous "wedge" fractures in elderly persons with osteoporosis or those using steroids (see Chapter 13 for a discussion of osteoporosis-related fractures).

7. **Spinal stenosis.** Irritation during activity results in pain in one or both extremities while walking (pain similar to claudication). Pain is relieved with rest, exacerbated with back extension (so worse going down hills), and relieved with flexion (so better going uphill). Common in the elderly.

8. **Myofascial or soft-tissue injury or disorder.** Patient may have history of trauma, heavy work, or unusual activity.

9. **Arachnoiditis and postoperative scarring**
10. **Children younger than 10 years:** diskitis (see Chapter 12), tumor, AV malformations, and osteomyelitis. **Older than 10 years:** spondylolisthesis, herniated disks, juvenile kyphosis (Scheuermann's disease, an osteochondritis that leads to wedging of the vertebrae and kyphotic posture), overuse syndrome, tumor, spondylolysis.
11. **Sacroiliitis** is inflammation of SI joints. Pain is exacerbated with pressure on sacroiliac joint (although this is nonspecific for sacroiliitis).

B. **Systemic disorders**
1. **Malignancy**
a. **Primary tumors.** Multiple myeloma is most common.
b. **Metastatic disease.** About 85% are from the breast, prostate, lung, kidney, and thyroid. Most cause lytic lesions with the exception of prostate and thyroid cancer, which cause sclerotic lesions. About 30% bone loss is required before lytic changes are visible on radiographs.
C. **Miscellaneous.** Osseous, disk, or epidural infection; spondyloarthropathy; metabolic bone disease, including osteoporosis; vascular disorders such as atherosclerosis or vasculitis.
D. **Neurologic causes**
1. **Myelopathy** from intrinsic or extrinsic processes.
2. **Lumbosacral plexopathy,** especially in diabetes, causes diffuse or patchy weakness of involved lower extremity. Additionally gluteal weakness (abduction and extension) and sensory loss (tibial, femoral, peroneal nerves).
3. **Neuropathy,** including mononeuropathy and inflammatory demyelinating diseases.
4. **Myopathy,** including myositis and metabolic causes.
E. **Referred pain**
1. **GI disorders** such as pancreatitis and perforated ulcer.
2. **GU disorders,** including nephrolithiasis, prostatitis, and pyelonephritis.
3. **Gynecologic disorders,** including ectopic pregnancy and pelvic tumors.
4. **Abdominal aortic aneurysm**
5. **Hip/pelvis pathology**
III. **Evaluation.**
A. **Physical examination**
1. **Standing.** Palpate for tenderness or muscle spasm (poor interrater reliability). Test the mobility of the lumbar spine with flexion, extension, and lateral flexion. Observe the patient's gait and have the patient walk on toes (foot plantar flexion test S1) and heels (foot dorsiflexion test L5).
2. **Straight leg raising.** With the patient sitting, flex hip followed by passive extension of the knee. A positive test is radicular pain below the level of the knee (e.g., pain or paresthesias down the leg, not back pain or thigh pain from muscle stretching) at less than 60 degrees. However, positive straight leg raise is not specific for disk disease. "Crossover" pain with radicular symptoms in the leg not lifted is very specific for disk disease.

3. **Reflexes.** Patellar reflex tests the L4 root; Achilles tendon reflex tests the S1 root (L5-S1 disk). Babinski's sign, if present, indicates disorder above the lumbar region such as cord tumor or CVA.

4. **Sensation/motor**

a. The dermatomal chart (see Figures 24-7 and 24-8) gives a description of radicular sensory findings.

b. Check hip abduction (L5 motor), perianal sensation (S3-S5; also controls anal and urethral sphincter tone), hip extension (L5 motor). Saddle anesthesia and decreased anal sphincter tone indicate a surgical emergency (cauda equina).

B. **Laboratory and imaging studies**

1. **Lumbar spine films** are not necessary in most patients. Plain films should be obtained if symptoms last more than 6 weeks; if there is suspicion or history of malignancy; or if the patient is using steroids, is over 50 years of age, has a history of trauma, has neurologic deficits, or is younger than 20 years of age. There is no need to obtain radiographic evaluation for history consistent with muscle strain.

2. **CT/MRI.** Patients suspected of having infectious or neoplastic causes of low back pain should have an imaging study such as a bone scan, CT, or MRI.

3. **If severe symptoms persist for 6 weeks** despite conservative therapy, and disk herniation or another surgically correctable disorder is suspected, then CT or MRI imaging may be useful. Electromyogram and nerve conduction velocity can be used to evaluate suspected nerve root involvement.

4. **X-rays, CT and MRI scans, myelograms, and other tests may be abnormal in asymptomatic patients.** Thus, interpretation of these tests in the patient with low back pain must be made with the entire clinical presentation in mind. This point was illustrated in a study in which MRI was performed in asymptomatic persons and the following abnormalities were found:

a. Disc bulges in 52% (a bulge is a symmetric expansion of the disc beyond the border of the adjacent vertebra).

b. Disc protrudes in another 27% (a protrusion is an asymmetric expansion of the disc) and extrudes in 1% (an extrusion is asymmetric with a wider head than neck).

c. Among asymptomatic patients over 50 years of age, 75% to 80% had disc bulges located in at least one spinal level and 30% had disc protrusions located in at least one level.

C. **Lab tests**

1. **Differential CBC with ESR and biochemical screening** (calcium, phosphate, alkaline phosphatase) should be performed when a systemic cause for back pain is suspected.

2. **Immunoelectrophoresis of serum and urine samples** allows diagnosis of most cases of myeloma (Bence Jones proteins).

IV. **Treatment.**

A. **Acute back pain** (no longer than 6 weeks).

16

ORTHOPEDICS

1. **There is no difference in outcome** when a family physician, a chiropractor, or an orthopedic surgeon treats patients with acute back pain. Therapy by a family physician is the most cost-effective.
2. **Regardless of the method of treatment,** 40% of patients are better within 1 week, 60% to 85% in 3 weeks, and 90% in 2 months. Poor prognostic factors include more than three episodes of back pain, gradual onset of symptoms, and prolonged absence from work.
3. **Bed rest should be kept to a minimum** and early mobilization encouraged. This is true in both back strain and radicular disease. If symptoms recur or considerable pain develops in relation to a specific activity or level of activity, the patient should temporarily limit that activity for several days but should not cease all activity.
4. **Analgesia.** NSAIDs provide pain relief and decrease inflammation but have side effects. Acetaminophen provides analgesia but has no anti-inflammatory properties and may be used with or instead of NSAIDs. Narcotics should be used short term as needed. Muscle relaxants such as cyclobenzaprine or diazepam work mostly by sedating patients and preventing activity. However, they probably have little effect on muscle spasm. Other options for muscle spasm include baclofen and tizanidine; baclofen causes occasional weakness as a side-effect, something that is absent with tizanidine. Carisoprodol (Soma) is metabolized into meprobamate, a Schedule IV anxiolytic, and should be avoided.
5. **Physical therapy.** Although classically several modes have been used to hasten resolution of back pain, most physical therapy modalities have no effect when rigorously tested. Traction, local application of heat and cold, ultrasound, and corsets have been shown to have no effect. Proper lifting, strengthening, and weight loss may prevent recurrence. TENS may provide short-term symptomatic relief but has no proven long-term benefit. Acupuncture may also be of help.
6. **Epidural steroid injections.** These have been used classically, but several randomized trials show that there is no overall long-term benefit, although there may be a temporary lessening of pain.
7. **Rehabilitation exercises.** The main benefit of exercises involving trunk extensors, abdominal muscles, and aerobic conditioning is that they promote early mobilization, which is critical in treating acute back pain. The specific exercise does not matter as much as the mobilization.
8. **Back support belts are ineffective** in preventing back pain.
B. **Chronic back pain**
1. Once back pain has been established for more than 1 year, the prognosis is poor. Mild analgesia should be used. Avoid chronic reliance on narcotics if possible (although addiction rates are low with chronic pain). If depression is encountered, it should be treated. Tricyclic antidepressants and norepinephrine reuptake inhibitors (e.g., venlafaxine, duloxetine) have the additional advantage of being effective for pain (which other SSRIs are not). Other modalities for chronic pain include carbamazepine, gabapentin, and topiramate (although in the editors' opinion they are overused). Physical modalities include TENS or

acupuncture with electrical stimulation. Both are effective but for a limited time.

2. **Surgery.** At 1 year, patients who have surgery for disk disease have no better outcome than those who are treated conservatively. Choose your surgical patients well.

C. **Indications for admission and referral.** Cauda equina syndrome (urinary retention, sphincter incontinence, and saddle anesthesia), severe neurologic deficits (foot drop, areflexia, gastrocnemius–soleus or quadriceps weakness), progressive neurologic deficit, or multiple nerve root involvement. A post-void residual of less than 100 mL effectively rules out cauda equina syndrome. MRI is still the standard of care.

SHOULDER PAIN

I. **Overview.** Most shoulder problems are attributable to overuse and trauma. The shoulder is composed of one articulation, the scapulothoracic, and three true joints: the sternoclavicular, acromioclavicular, and glenohumeral. The rotator cuff muscles are the supraspinatus, infraspinatus, teres minor, and subscapularis. They provide dynamic stabilization of the humoral head in the glenoid. Additional static stabilization is provided by the joint capsule and labrum.

II. **Rotator Cuff Syndrome.**

A. **Stage I** rotator cuff syndrome

1. This is a **rotator cuff tendinitis** caused by forceful or repetitive overhead motion, typically in those 25 years of age or younger.

2. **Pain** is noted over the anterior aspect of the shoulder and is maximal when the arm is raised from 60 to 120 degrees of elevation.

3. **Treatment** consists of avoiding aggravating positions and activities, applying ice packs, and taking NSAIDS.

B. **Stage II** rotator cuff syndrome

1. This usually occurs in patients 25 to 40 years of age with multiple previous episodes. In addition to inflammation of the rotator cuff, some permanent fibrosis, thickening, or scarring is present. Calcific deposits may be noted within the rotator cuff on radiographs. Lithotripsy has been used successfully to break up calcific deposits.

2. Initial treatment is the same as that for stage I. If treatment is unsuccessful, the subacromial bursa can be injected with corticosteroids. If symptoms persist, referral to an orthopedist for a surgical consult should be considered.

C. **Stage III** rotator cuff syndrome

1. This is a partial thickness or complete tear of the rotator cuff tendon, usually the supraspinatus tendon, and usually occurs after 40 years of age. The patient may relate feeling a sudden pop in the shoulder and then suffer severe pain. The patient notes increasing weakness when trying to abduct and externally rotate the arm. The diagnosis is confirmed by MRI or a shoulder arthrogram.

2. Treatment is usually surgical repair within 6 weeks, depending on whether there is significant loss of function and other factors such as comorbidities. Many elderly patients have progressive rotator cuff loss over the years as a result of the aging process.

III. Adhesive Capsulitis (Frozen Shoulder).

A. Clinical features. This chronically stiff and painful shoulder may begin without any significant injury. The cause is prolonged immobilization from either protracted use of a sling or disuse because of pain in the arm. Shoulder motion is limited in one or more directions, with pain occurring at the limits of motion. Both passive and active range of motion are limited. There is a higher incidence in diabetic patients.

B. Treatment involves extended, aggressive physical therapy and NSAIDs or mobilization under anesthesia. Corticosteroid injection may provide some improvement. Symptoms can take 2 years to improve significantly.

IV. Tendinitis and Bursitis.

A. Clinical features. The supraspinatus and long head of the biceps are especially susceptible. The primary symptom is a painful, aching shoulder of rather nondescript type. With supraspinatus tendinitis, the pain is aggravated when attempting shoulder abduction and external rotation against resistance. With bicipital tendinitis, pain is aggravated when the patient flexes forward against resistance, and there is pain with palpation of the long head of the biceps.

B. Treatment

1. Initial conservative treatment is generally NSAIDs, ice, and rest for 5 to 7 days. This may be accompanied by physical therapy for mobilization followed by strengthening. Ultrasound may be useful in calcific tendinitis but is not as effective for other cases.

2. Most recalcitrant shoulder conditions can be relieved by injection of 2 to 5 mL of 1% bupivacaine and 40 to 60 mg of triamcinolone into the affected area (e.g., subacromial bursa or tendon region). Tendon rupture can occur but is generally secondary to return to significant activity because patients feel better after treatment.

V. Acromioclavicular Injuries. Clinical features usually result from a direct blow or fall on the tip of the shoulder.

A. Grade I (sprain). Partial tear of the joint capsule without joint deformity and minimal ligamentous disruption and instability. AC joint films (with and without weights) are normal. Treatment includes ice, pain medication, a sling for comfort, and early mobilization.

B. Grade II (subluxation). Complete tear of the acromioclavicular ligaments. The AC joint is locally tender and painful with motion. The distal end of the clavicle may protrude slightly upward. Stress radiograph of the AC joint with the patient holding a 10-pound weight in both hands reveals widening of the joint. Treatment is symptomatic in the same manner as the grade I injury but usually requires a longer period of immobilization (2 to 4 weeks).

C. **Grade III (dislocation).** Complete tear of the acromioclavicular and coracoclavicular ligaments with pain on any attempt at abduction. There is an obvious "step-off" on physical examination. Radiographs show superior displacement of the clavicle and complete dislocation of the joint with weights. Conservative treatment with a sling is appropriate, provided the patient understands that permanent deformity can result. Patients usually return to normal function. Surgical treatment is important if symptomatic treatment fails or if it will interfere with the patient's life (as in an athlete or person who does heavy work).

VI. **Glenohumeral Dislocations.**

A. **Clinical features**

1. Ninety-five percent are anterior, most commonly subcoracoid and then subglenoid. The usual mechanism is forced abduction and external rotation. Patients complain of severe pain and usually hold the arm in tightly against the body. The shoulder appears flattened laterally and prominent anteriorly. The acromion process is prominent, and so the shoulder appears to be squared off.

2. Check for associated injuries, including proximal humeral fractures, avulsion of the rotator cuff, and injuries to the adjacent neurovascular structures. Axillary nerve injury is most common and is associated with decreased active contraction of the deltoid muscle and hypesthesia over the deltoid. Think about grand mal seizures or electrical shock as an etiology in those with posterior dislocations.

B. **Radiographs taken in two planes** (AP and lateral scapula or axillary views) will confirm the dislocation and should be done to rule out fracture if mechanism is suggestive.

C. **Treatment.** The dislocation should be reduced as soon as possible. Adequate analgesia and relaxation can be obtained by a 20 mL intra-articular injection of 1% lidocaine. Narcotics (e.g., IV morphine, fentanyl) and muscle relaxants (e.g., diazepam) are useful as well.

1. **External rotation method (Hennipen technique).** The patient is placed supine, with the arm adducted against the body and the elbow flexed to 90 degrees. The examiner holds the elbow in position and externally rotates the shoulder. No pressure is applied to the forearm to force external rotation. If necessary, the arm can be abducted while in external rotation. Reduction usually occurs silently, unnoticed by the patient. This method has the lowest rate of complications.

2. **Modified Stimson reduction.**

a. Analgesia or relaxation as noted above. The patient is placed prone on a table with the injured shoulder hanging free.

b. Weight (up to 5-7 kg [10-15 lb]) is suspended from the wrist, and the patient is left for 5 to 15 minutes.

c. Further manipulation is often required, consisting of gentle internal and external rotation with downward traction.

d. Other reduction techniques include traction–countertraction and scapular manipulation.

16

ORTHOPEDICS

D. Postreduction care
1. **Postreduction radiographs** are obtained to ensure good relocation. Neurovascular status must be documented before and after reduction.
2. **Classically, the patient's arm is immobilized** in a sling-and-swathe dressing for 6 weeks, although recently early mobilization was found to be superior. Immobilization in external rotation shows promise for reducing future dislocations.
3. Early orthopedic follow-up care is recommended. Recurrent dislocation or subluxation is common and can require surgical repair.

ELBOW

I. **Lateral Epicondylitis (tennis elbow).**
A. **Clinical features.** Tennis elbow is a very common inflammatory process of the extensor origin of the lateral epicondyle. It may be secondary to overuse or repetitive use. Pain at the lateral epicondyle, with referred pain to the extensor surface of the forearm, is typical. The pain is exacerbated by resisted extension of the wrist or fingers.
B. **Treatment** includes avoiding exacerbating activities, NSAIDs, hot and cold modalities, and stretching. Occasionally immobilization of the wrist in a volar splint is required. Local steroid injection, iontophoresis, or orthopedic referral may be advised in recalcitrant cases. There is a trend toward recurrence in patients treated with steroids.
II. **Medial Epicondylitis.**
A. **Clinical features.** Medial epicondylitis results from repeated flexion activities of the wrist and fingers. Pain is at the medial epicondyle and exacerbated by resistant flexion of the fingers.
B. **Treatment** is the same as for lateral epicondylitis.
III. **Radial Head Subluxation (nursemaid's elbow).**
A. **Clinical features**
1. The mechanism is a sudden pull on the extended pronated elbow of a child less than 4 years of age (for example, when one picks up a child by the forearm or swings the child). The child holds the arm in pronation and usually refuses to move it. There is pain on supination and palpation of the radial head.
2. Although radiographic findings are usually normal, be sure to rule out undisplaced supracondylar fracture. Often the subluxation spontaneously reduces from x-ray positioning.
B. **Treatment is firm supination of the forearm,** flexing the elbow gently to 90 degrees with pressure over the radial head. Reduction is achieved with a palpable click over the radial head, and the pain is immediately relieved. The patient should resume full activity within several minutes of reduction, although some are hesitant. It can take an hour or so to resume full activity.
C. **Prolonged symptoms after reduction** of a presumed nursemaid's elbow should suggest a different diagnosis.

IV. Little Leaguer's Elbow.

A. Clinical features. This injury results from overuse of an adolescent's pitching elbow. On exam there is tenderness over the medial humoral epicondyle and mild swelling. An acute syndrome with sudden onset also occurs from avulsion of a fragment of bone from the medial humeral epicondyle.

B. Treatment is rest for 3 to 6 weeks followed by rehabilitation. Loose bodies and locking elbow require referral.

V. Olecranon Bursitis. *Note:* The same treatment and diagnostic modalities hold true for prepatellar and anserine bursitis.

A. Clinical features

1. There is tenderness and swelling over the olecranon bursa. Olecranon bursitis may be secondary to trauma (e.g., lying on carpet with elbows propped up while watching TV).

2. May be infectious (>80% staphylococcal). Traumatic bursitis often leads to infectious bursitis.

B. Diagnosis. Differentiate infectious from sterile bursitis. Tap the bursa and evaluate Gram stain, cell count, crystals, and culture.

C. Treatment

1. Perform serial aspiration until the bursa fluid is sterile. Start oral antistaphylococcal antibiotics (e.g., dicloxacillin, amoxicillin–clavulanate, cephalexin, vancomycin IV [if hospitalized] or ciprofloxacin plus rifampin) if an infectious etiology is likely. Antibiotic therapy for 2 to 3 weeks or 5 days after fluid sterilization is usually sufficient.

2. Indications for hospitalization and/or intravenous antibiotic (nafcillin or cefazolin) therapy for septic bursitis include the presence of overwhelming local infection, signs of systemic toxicity, or comorbid conditions (e.g., immunosuppression, diabetes).

3. If the etiology is not infectious, treat with NSAIDS, aspiration, and compression dressings. Occasionally, an olecranon bursa must be opened surgically.

VI. Cubital Tunnel Syndrome.

A. Clinical features

1. The ulnar nerve passes through the "cubital tunnel" whose boundaries are the ulnar collateral ligament of the elbow, the medial border of the trochlea, the medial epicondylar groove, and the arcuate ligament. The nerve can be compressed due to the superficial course from approximately 10 cm proximal to the tunnel to 5 cm distal. This can occur acutely secondary to a direct trauma or chronically due to prolonged direct pressure over the nerve or with activities that maintain prolonged elbow flexion putting a sustained stretch on the nerve (such as lying on the floor watching television with the elbows flexed or driving). Previous injury causing scar tissue or osteophytes to encroach on the course of the nerve can also lead to an ulnar neuritis. Repetitive overhead activity such as baseball pitching can also lead to an instability of the nerve within the groove, causing repetitive subluxation that chronically

16

ORTHOPEDICS

irritates the nerve. Similar findings may be present distally where the ulnar nerve passes through Guyon's canal in the palmar wrist/hand. This occurs commonly in cyclists and keyboard operators. Treatment is similar with the exception that local corticosteroid injection is often beneficial when conservative measures fail, whereas steroids are not indicated in cases of cubital tunnel syndrome.

2. The patient may present initially with pain, sensory changes, and/or paresthesias along the ulnar nerve distribution distally (fourth and fifth fingers); some occasionally complain of symptoms radiating proximally. Later findings can include weakness of hand intrinsics and grip strength, progressing finally to obvious atrophy of hand intrinsics and the hypothenar eminence.

3. EMG and nerve conduction studies may be helpful in assessing the extent of injury, but they are usually not necessary to make an initial diagnosis and initiate treatment. Radiographic studies are indicated in patients with past elbow trauma or repetitive overhead use by athletes and workers.

B. Treatment

1. Treatment begins with elimination of the offending activity and protection from direct pressure and limiting elbow flexion to avoid stretching or subluxing the nerve. NSAIDs may be most beneficial in acute cases where inflammation is causing symptoms of entrapment.

2. Surgical intervention for decompression or transposition should be reserved for those with late symptoms that fail to improve with 12 to 16 weeks of conservative management.

WRIST AND HAND

I. Ganglion Cyst.

A. Clinical features. Ganglion cyst is the most commonly noted nodule in the hand. Typical locations include the dorsal aspect of the lunate, radial volar aspect of the wrist, dorsal aspect of the hand, and palmar aspect of the fingers near the MCP joints. It is typically accentuated with extreme flexion or extension of the wrist.

B. Treatment. These are usually asymptomatic, and patient reassurance is sufficient. If the cyst is symptomatic and small, aspiration of the cyst contents may be performed with an 18-gauge needle. Steroid injection adds nothing. About one third resolve with aspiration, and it is unlikely that multiple aspirations will help if there is no resolution after the first aspiration. Most resolve over time. Orthopedic referral may be considered for surgical removal, but even this has a limited efficacy.

II. Carpal Tunnel Syndrome.

A. Clinical features. The symptoms are a result of median nerve dysfunction secondary to increased pressure within the carpal tunnel. **The causes include overuse, ganglion cyst, amyloid, synovial proliferation, pregnancy, rheumatoid arthritis, diabetes, and hypothyroidism among others.** Typical symptoms are pain, paresthesia, hypesthesia, or numbness in the median nerve distribution of the hand, usually in the thumb, index, middle, and radial aspect of the ring finger. Nocturnal paresthesia and pain are characteristic.

1. **Tinel's sign,** which is a painful sensation of the fingers induced by percussion of the median nerve at the level of the palmar wrist, may be positive, but specificity is only 54% and sensitivity is only 50%.
2. **Phalen's sign,** keeping both wrists in a palmar-flexed position, may reproduce symptoms. Sensitivity varies from 10% to 88% depending on the study; it has an 80% specificity.

B. **Treatment**

1. The patient without thenar atrophy can be treated with conservative therapy, which includes a resting splint with the wrist in neutral position and NSAIDs. Neutral position splints are more effective than "cock-up" splints that hold the wrist in slight extension. Steroid injections of the carpal tunnel may be effective in cases recalcitrant to conservative measures.
2. Symptoms are not always classic, and radial nerve syndrome and ulnar neuropathy can produce similar paresthesias, sensory changes, and weakness. However, these should be in a different myotomal and dermatomal distribution. Radial nerve symptoms may also hurt at the elbow and be confused with lateral epicondylitis.
3. If EMG and nerve conduction studies show an impaired conduction of the median nerve at the wrist, or the carpal tunnel symptoms do not improve in 6 weeks, or if there is evidence of thenar muscle weakness or atrophy, surgical referral is indicated.

III. **de Quervain's Tenosynovitis.**

A. **Clinical features**

1. Pain on movement of the thumb. This is an overuse injury in which the tendon sheath of the abductor pollicis longus and the extensor pollicis brevis becomes inflamed, causing a stenosis that restricts the tendon(s) gliding through the sheath. The patient complains of pain at the radial styloid and some swelling and occasionally a "catching" sensation when trying to extend the thumb.
2. On exam there is exquisite point tenderness over the radial styloid, particularly with full thumb flexion into the palm and ulnar deviation of the wrist (Finkelstein's test). There is often soft tissue crepitus with active thumb ROM due to the stenosis/triggering.

B. **Treatment.** Initial treatment is conservative, with a thumb spica wrist splint, NSAIDs, and hot and cold packs for 2 to 4 weeks. If conservative treatment fails, consider corticosteroid injection with continuation of the conservative measures and physical therapy referral. Iontophoresis has gained some favor as a second-line treatment before injection. Failure of these modalities is indication for referral to a hand surgeon.

IV. **Trigger Finger.**

A. **Clinical features.** A nodule forming in the flexor tendon causes inflammation of the flexor pulleys on the palmar surface of the hand, resulting in a stenosis that restricts motion. The finger may snap or "trigger" when an attempt is made to extend the joint. This can cause locking in flexion. It occurs most commonly in the long or ring finger and has a higher incidence in persons with diabetes, rheumatoid arthritis, carpal tunnel, or de Quervain's. There may be a palpable painful nodule in the distal palmar surface.

B. Treatment. NSAIDS can be tried but are generally ineffective. A corticosteroid injection is typically the first-line treatment. If symptoms fail to resolve within 3 or 4 weeks of injection, a second injection may be tried. After two failures with injections, referral for surgical release should be made. Early referral should be considered for patients with rheumatoid arthritis or diabetes.

V. Mallet Finger (acute)

A. Clinical features

1. Mallet finger is an **injury resulting from forced flexion of the distal tip of a finger.** The result is a stretching or rupture of the tendon of the extensor digitorum profundus or avulsion of part of the distal phalanx with the tendon attached. It commonly occurs with basketball and baseball injuries.

2. Exam reveals swelling, tenderness, DIP joint held in flexion with patient unable to extend it.

B. Treatment

1. Splint the finger in extension across the DIP joint, leaving the PIP joint free to allow continued function. Splint for 6 to 12 weeks with absolutely no flexion; longer times are required for injuries when the diagnosis has been delayed.

2. Operative repair is necessary for the minority of cases that don't respond to splinting.

VI. Fingertip Infections.

A. Paronychia is an infection under the nail fold. Treatment consists of warm soaks, antistaphylococcal antibiotics (e.g., cephalexin, amoxicillin–clavulanate; doxycycline or TMP–SMX for community-acquired MRSA) for 5 to 10 days and drainage using a No. 11 blade or 18-gauge needle guided along the nail into the site.

B. Felon is infection in the digital pulp. Treatment consists of drainage and packing as well as antistaphylococcal antibiotics. Closely monitor treatment response.

C. Herpetic whitlow is usually from direct inoculation of the finger with herpes 1 or herpes 2. Patient has local pain and swelling, followed by clear vesicles. Do not I&D. They resolve spontaneously in 3 to 4 weeks.

VII. Proximal Interphalangeal Joint Dislocation.

A. Mechanism is usually a hyperextension injury, with the base of the middle phalanx displaced dorsally and proximally.

B. Reduction may be done without anesthesia or with a metacarpal block. Neurovascular check should be performed prior to reduction.

1. Hyperextend the dislocated segment and then push with the thumb straight distally on the base of the dorsally displaced phalanx. As the base of the middle phalanx engages the joint surface, the direction of force changes to an arc to follow the phalanx into slight flexion. The examiner usually feels a sense of giving way as the joint reduces.
2. Obtain a postreduction x-ray to rule out avulsion fractures. Check active extension. Splint in full extension for 3 weeks, then begin exercises to restore range of motion.

HIP

I. Bursitis.

A. Clinical features. Bursitis of the hip largely involves the trochanteric bursa. Patients present with a history of pain with walking, running, or climbing. They may also complain of pain when lying on the affected side and sometimes of lower back pain. There is tenderness over the greater trochanter.

B. Treatment. NSAIDs are often ineffective. The most effective treatment is corticosteroid injection into the bursa. Palpate the bursa and inject triamcinolone 40 mg with 5 mL of bupivacaine into the tender area. Pain is usually relieved immediately but can recur until the anti-inflammatory takes effect.

II. Other Causes of Hip Pain. Stress and pathologic and occult fractures of the hip are not uncommon. CT or MRI of the hip should be considered in the patient who has acute or subacute onset of hip pain and cannot ambulate and in whom the radiograph is negative.

KNEE

I. Overview.

A. The majority of knee injuries in adults are ligamentous. However, a bloody effusion after injury often indicates bone injury.

B. Determination of radiographs. Only 5% to 10% of persons with knee trauma have a fracture. Guidelines have been established to help determine who should have a radiograph. Use clinical judgment, however.

C. Ottawa knee rules are 97% sensitive and 27% specific for fracture. X-ray patients who have any one of the following:

1. Age 55 or older.
2. Tenderness at head of fibula.
3. Isolated tenderness of patella.
4. Inability to flex knee to 90 degrees.
5. Inability to walk four weight-bearing steps in the ED or office.

D. Pittsburgh decision rules are 99% sensitive and 60% specific for fracture. X-ray anyone who has blunt trauma or fall as mechanism of injury *plus either* age >55 or <12 years *or* inability to walk four weight-bearing steps in the ED or office.

ORTHOPEDICS   **16**

II. Ligamentous Injuries.

A. Collateral ligament injury

1. Collateral ligament injury is **typically caused by direct trauma** to the contralateral side of the knee or excessive indirect force to the knee in a varus or valgus manner.

2. The patient may have noted **pain and a tearing sensation** at the time of injury. In case of medial collateral ligament injury, there may be tenderness along the distal femur extending to the joint line. Medial collateral ligament injuries are more commonly associated with meniscus tears.

3. **Valgus and varus tests** provide assessment of the collateral ligaments. With the knee in 30 degrees of flexion, the collateral ligaments can be isolated. In full extension the ACL and PCL act as secondary stabilizers.

4. **Grade I sprains** are caused by microtears of the ligament and have pain but no laxity on stress exam. **Grade II sprains** are a partial macrotear of the ligament with the presence of significant laxity but with an endpoint remaining. A **grade III sprain** is a complete tear of the ligament with no endpoint distinguishable on examination.

5. **Treatment** of isolated grade I and II injuries involves conservative measures, such as ice application for 15 to 20 minutes tid, elastic wrap compression, elevation for the first 24 to 72 hours, crutches with limited weight bearing, rest with an immobilizer or hinged brace for 7 to 14 days, and NSAID therapy. Lateral ligament requires 4 to 6 weeks with a brace. Prompt initiation of physical therapy should be included in initial treatment. Grade III injuries can be treated nonoperatively, but an orthopedic referral is recommended to assess the need for surgical intervention.

B. Anterior cruciate ligament injury

1. **History** is a twisting injury accompanied by a pop or tearing feeling and a subsequent effusion. "Did you or someone else hear a pop?" Suspect ACL tear (80%), meniscal injury (15%), rarely fracture, or other. Significant effusion is seen in less than 24 hours. In general, if effusion appears within 12 hours, suspect ACL or patella dislocation/subluxation. If an effusion appears in 12 to 24 hours, suspect meniscal injury. A hemarthrosis is found in 75% of cases. Suspect an intra-articular fracture if fat droplets are seen in the aspirate even if plain films are negative. ACL tear is frequently associated with a medial meniscal tear and medial collateral ligament injury (terrible triad).

2. **The Lachman test** is performed with the patient supine and the knee bent at 30 degrees and involves anterior displacement of the tibia on the femur. The femur is held stable and the tibia is translated anteriorly. Exam by an experienced practitioner is as or more sensitive for ACL injury than MRI.

3. **Always assess distal neurovascular status** because these structures are not uncommonly damaged, requiring emergent surgical intervention.

4. **Treatment** for partial or complete rupture should be supervised by an orthopedist. Treatment of acute injuries depends on the severity. Patients without associated meniscal, collateral ligament, or posterior cruciate

ligament injury should be treated initially by immobilization of the knee for comfort and crutches, ice, compression, and elevation. Early mobilization, reduction of effusion, and strengthening are key to both surgical and nonsurgical treatment. Injuries involving multiple ligaments and/or cartilage should be seen early by an orthopedist.

C. Posterior cruciate ligament injury

1. **Most injuries are the result of direct trauma to the proximal tibia** when the flexed knee is decelerated rapidly, as in a dashboard injury. In an isolated tear there is often limited effusion, because the PCL is extracapsular. The posterior drawer and tibial sag tests are used. In the posterior drawer test, the knee is flexed 90 degrees and posterior displacement of the tibia on the femur is attempted. In the tibial sag test, the knee is flexed to 90 degrees with the hip at 45 degrees, and the tibia is displaced posteriorly on the femur.

2. **Isolated tears** should be managed conservatively with physical therapy and quadriceps strengthening. If radiographs reveal displaced bone avulsions, PCL injury might require surgical fixation. Orthopedic referral is recommended for consideration of surgical repair.

D. Meniscal tears

1. **Clinical features**

a. The medial meniscus is injured more often than is the lateral. More than one third of meniscal injuries are associated with an ACL tear and may also be associated with MCL injuries.

b. Patients complain of pain at the time of injury that persists and interferes with weight-bearing activity. The most consistent physical finding is tenderness to palpation along the joint line. Patients often complain of the knee "locking" or "catching," which may be attributable to pain or a physical inability to extend the knee because the torn meniscus prevents extension or flexion like a door stop. Effusion may develop over 12 to 24 hours and is typically not bloody and is synovial fluid only.

c. Clinical indications of a meniscal tear include joint line tenderness, mild to moderate effusion, and a positive McMurray test. In the McMurray test, the knee is fully flexed. To test for lateral meniscal tears, apply a valgus force with the leg externally rotated; to test for medial meniscal tears, apply a varus force with the leg internally rotated. While maintaining rotation and the varus or valgus force, extend the knee with a firm controlled movement. A painful click or catch signifies a positive McMurray test.

2. **Diagnosis.** If there are any diagnostic doubts, patients should be referred for evaluation by MRI or to an orthopedist for consideration of arthroscopy.

3. **Treatment.** The knee should be immobilized as needed for comfort. Ice, compression, partial weight-bearing with crutches, quadriceps exercises, active non–weight-bearing range of motion, and NSAIDs can be used. If the knee remains locked or if symptoms of pain, giving way (a sense that the knee is going to collapse), and swelling persist, orthopedic referral should be made for surgical intervention.

16

ORTHOPEDICS

E. Anterior knee pain
1. **Clinical features.** There are multiple etiologies including patellofemoral maltracking, medial plica (redundant folds of synovium) inflammation, patellar tendonitis or bursitis, and pes anserine bursitis to name a few. Most manifest as anterior knee pain that is worse after prolonged sitting with the knee flexed, or on climbing or descending stairs or slopes. Patients may complain of some snapping, popping, or crepitus about the patella.
2. **Radiographs of the knee** are usually negative. However, lateral displacement of the patella on a Merchant view may be present with maltracking.
3. **Treatment.** Decreased activity or cross-training, NSAIDs, ice, and appropriate exercises including those that strengthen the medial quadriceps and stretch the hamstrings are useful (e.g., straight leg raising with the ankle and hip externally rotated).
F. Patellar dislocations
1. **Clinical features**
a. Patients complain of the **knee giving way or popping out.** The patella may still be dislocated when the patient is seen, but many spontaneously reduce. An effusion (hemarthrosis) may be present. The medial retinaculum is tender.
b. **Apprehension test.** Displace the patella laterally; patients feel as though the patella is going to dislocate and will be very apprehensive.
c. Between occurrences the patella is observed to have considerable lateral mobility, particularly during active extension. The patellar ligament may be noted to angulate laterally from the axis of the quadriceps muscle.
2. **Reduction.** Encourage the patient to relax the quadriceps and push the patella medially back into place. If the patient is unable to get the patella over the lateral femoral condyle, push the patella anteriorly while passively flexing the knee (the patella usually reduces by 30 degrees of flexion). If the effusion is tense, aspiration may reduce discomfort. Plain films should be taken before and after reduction.
3. **Postreduction care.** Adequate immobilization is obtained with the use of a knee immobilizer for 6 weeks. Have patients fully weight bearing as well as performing quadriceps isometric exercises while immobilized. After immobilization, patients are placed on partial weight bearing while quadriceps strengthening is initiated. Rehabilitation needs to include the vastus medialis, which operates only in the last 15 degrees of extension. Resume full weight bearing when flexion to 30 degrees is painless. An elastic knee support may add some patellar stability during strenuous activity. Multiple dislocations should be evaluated by an orthopedist.
4. All patients with a knee (not patella) dislocation should have a lower-extremity angiogram. There is a high risk of arterial injury.
G. Prepatellar bursitis. See the discussion of olecranon bursitis.
H. Iliotibial band syndrome is commonly seen in runners and bicyclists. It is an overuse syndrome that manifests with tenderness over the

lateral femoral condyle with an otherwise negative knee exam. Treatment is rest, ice, NSAIDS, and stretching.

I. **Quadriceps tendon rupture** is rupture of the tendon connecting the quadriceps to the patella. Patients note pain superior to the patella, inability to walk, and inability to extend the knee. The examiner will note a palpable defect in the area of the patellar tendon and limited ability to extend knee, especially last 10 degrees.

ANKLE

I. **Ankle Strain.**

A. **Clinical features.** The most common ligament injured is the anterior talofibular ligament with a mechanism of plantar flexion with inversion. A history of popping or a painful snap with ankle injury can indicate a significant ligament injury.

B. **Radiography.** The Ottawa ankle rules **(Fig. 16-1)** have been developed and validated to determine who needs a radiograph. Using these rules, an occasional fracture will be missed. However, these are generally of

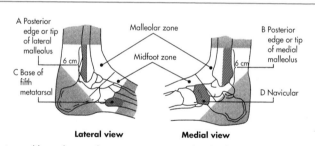

An ankle radiographic series is required only if there is any pain in the malleolar zone and any of these findings is present:
- Bone tenderness at A
- Bone tenderness at B
- Inability to bear weight both immediately and in the ED

A foot radiographic series is required only if there is any pain in midfoot zone and any of these findings is present:
- Bone tenderness at C
- Bone tenderness at D
- Inability to bear weight both immediately and in the ED

FIG. 16-1

Ottawa ankle rules. *(From Stiell IG, Greenberg GH, Wells GA, et al: JAMA 275: 611-615, 1996.)*

no clinical significance (as with an avulsion injury). They apply only to patients older than 17 years who have a clear mental state.

C. Treatment

1. In most ankle sprains, treatment includes external support such as the application of an air splint or posterior splint, application of ice, and elevation. NSAIDs or acetaminophen with or without hydrocodone or codeine can be used for pain control.

2. The patient should be allowed to bear weight as tolerated using crutches or a cane if necessary. Early mobilization and weight bearing hasten resolution. Patients with recurrent problems of instability or an acute grade III problem should be referred to an orthopedist for evaluation and the possibility of reconstructive surgery.

3. About 10% to 30% have chronic problems from the sprain. A sprained ankle that is not improving may represent an occult fracture, a syndesmosis injury (ligamentous disruption between tibia and fibula, diagnosed by MRI), osteochondral injury of the talus (patients will have continued joint pain, effusion), etc.

II. Nontrauma Ankle Pain. Tarsal tunnel syndrome is compression of the tibial nerve in the tarsal tunnel. The patient presents with pain and numbness both anterior and posterior to the medial malleolus as well as pain and numbness of the sole of the foot. Symptoms are exacerbated by dorsiflexion and eversion of the ankle. Patients with advanced cases may have weak toe flexion. Treatment includes NSAIDS, rest, and immobilization; surgery is required for a space-occupying lesion.

HEEL PAIN AND FOOT PAIN

I. Plantar Fasciitis.

A. Clinical. Pain over the heel/plantar fascia on weight bearing. The pain is especially severe in the morning and after protracted sitting. Passive dorsiflexion of the toes with foot eversion may exacerbate the pain. There may be associated pes planus. Note that pain on palpation is in the distal portion of the heel and over the plantar fascia and not on the center of the heel itself.

B. Radiographs are generally not indicated. Radiographs might show a calcaneal spur, but such a spur is incidental and not the cause of the fasciitis.

C. Differential includes herniated calcaneal fat pad, among others. This should not worsen with toe dorsiflexion **(Table 16-1).** Additionally, calcaneal fat pad pain is maximally tender over the calcaneus, and pain can last for 6 months or more; plantar fasciitis, however, is more tender distal to the heel.

D. Treatment includes NSAIDs, soaks, and rest. For plantar fasciitis, consider orthotics to correct pes planus and a soft rubber heel cup (e.g., Tuli's heel cup). Patient should stretch the fascia (lean forward against wall with heel on the ground) and wear nighttime dorsiflexion splints.

TABLE 16-1
DIAGNOSIS OF HEEL PAIN

Diagnosis	Location of Pain	Worse When?	Comments
Calcaneal apophysitis	Posterior heel	Exercise	Age 12-15 before fusion of apophysis
Calcaneal periostitis	Plantar aspects of heels and lateral borders, may be bilateral	Worse in morning	If bilateral, consider systemic rheumatic disease (e.g., Reiter's)
Distal tibial tarsal tunnel syndrome	Superior to the origin of the plantar fascia	Worse with activity	May have sensory findings (e.g., numbness), pain worse with dorsiflexion, inversion
Painful heel pad syndrome	Localized to heel pad	Exercise	Seen especially in runners from breakdown of fibrous septae that compartmentalize fat in the heel. May last for 6 months.
Piezogenic papules	Medial inferior aspect of heel	Standing	May see tender papules on weight bearing. These are fat pads herniated laterally
Plantar fasciitis	Tender over origin of plantar fascia (and more distal than other causes of heel pain)	With weight bearing, especially after prolonged sitting (e.g., in morning)	Spurs *do not* cause plantar fasciitis
Achilles tendinitis and rupture	Posterior heel over Achilles tendon	With foot motion	For Achilles rupture: Have patient lie prone with feet over edge of bed. Squeeze calf. If foot does not move, it confirms Achilles rupture.

ORTHOPEDICS   16

Injection of corticosteroids is indicated for plantar fasciitis if there is no improvement with conservative treatment and rest for 4 to 6 weeks. Complete resolution can take 10 to 12 months. Lithotripsy is a new option, but the efficacy is not yet clearly documented. Surgery is rarely indicated.

II. Metatarsalgia.

A. Metatarsalgia is pain on weight bearing in the anterior foot with tenderness over the plantar aspects of the metatarsal heads. Pain is exacerbated with wearing high-heeled shoes. It is increasingly common as patients age, with loss of the normal foot fat pads. Treatment is NSAIDs and a metatarsal pad that restores the normal convex contour of the foot and takes the pressure off of the metatarsal heads. These are available at most drug stores or from orthotics makers.

B. Differentiate from Morton's neuroma, a neurofibrillary tangle between the metatarsals, especially metatarsals 2-3 and 3-4. Pain is described as burning and is exacerbated with squeezing the anterior foot to compress the metatarsals together. Treatment is avoidance of extension of the toes and pain management. Surgical therapy has a good outcome and is often required.

ROTATIONAL DEFORMITIES OF THE LOWER EXTREMITY

I. In-Toeing (Pigeon Toes).

A. Internal tibial torsion. Observation of gait reveals forward facing knees with feet pointing toward the midline.

1. **To diagnose,** place patient on knees and observe the foot angle. Normally, the toes are pointed away from each other at an angle of 30 degrees (toes are pointed outward). With internal tibial torsion, the toes of the affected side are pointed inward. Also, with legs dangling over a table, the lateral malleolus is anterior to the medial malleolus (the opposite of the normal foot).

2. **Internal tibial torsion typically resolves spontaneously** by age 4 years. Intervention does not change outcome unless there is underlying neuromuscular pathology or the patient is older than 8 years and has an altered gait.

B. Medial femoral torsion is the most common cause of in-toeing in children.

1. **Typically the child presents at age 3 to 4 years** with increasing in-toeing secondary to the alignment of the femur in the acetabulum and loss of normal lateral rotatory forces of infancy.

2. **Diagnose** by placing the child prone with knees flexed 90 degrees, then internally and externally rotating the hip. Internal rotation of greater than 70 degrees with limitation of external rotation suggests femoral torsion. Alternatively, watch the patient walk. If the patella faces forward, the diagnosis of femoral torsion is ruled out.

3. **No treatment is generally necessary** unless the gait is severely altered. Medial femoral torsion does not lead to increased incidence of arthritis.

C. **Metatarsus adductus** is a functional deformity where a flexible forefoot is adducted in relation to the hindfoot. The forefoot can be brought into a neutral position by gently straightening. A line bisecting the heel would pass between the second and third toes on a normal foot; past the third toe is characteristic of metatarsus adductus. It typically resolves by 3 months. Parents can do gentle stretching with diaper changes, but there is no change in outcome. If it persists beyond 3 or 4 months, referral should be made. Unilateral metatarsus adductus is related to ipsilateral hip dysplasia.

D. **Metatarsus varus** is a rigid abnormality caused by subluxation of the tarsometatarsal joint with subluxation of the metatarsals. As opposed to metatarsus adductus, in which the foot is flexible, here the defect is relatively fixed. A prominent base of the fifth metatarsal, a convexity of the lateral border, and a deep crease of the plantar surface in addition to the fixed abnormality lead to the diagnosis. Referral for serial casting should be made with the diagnosis.

II. **Out-Toeing.**

A. **Physiologic out-toeing** is an external rotational contracture of the soft tissues surrounding the hip secondary to intrauterine forces. It generally resolves spontaneously with ambulation around 18 months.

B. **Lateral tibial torsion** manifests in the 3- to 5-year-old with increasing out-toeing. It can lead to knee pain. Severe torsion requires referral.

III. **Talipes Equinovarus (Clubfoot Deformity).**

A. The clubfoot has **significant plantar flexion,** the calcaneus seems to be drawn inward and upward, there is moderate forefoot adduction, and the foot can be placed in a neutral position by passive manipulation.

B. Clubfoot may be idiopathic or may be secondary and associated with neuromuscular conditions, spinal cord disorders, and constriction band syndromes.

C. The most appropriate form of treatment is **serial casting and manipulation** (Ponseti method). Specialty referral following early diagnosis in the first week of life provides the best opportunity for successful outcomes. Surgery is generally reserved for patients in whom conservative treatment fails.

FRACTURES

I. **Terms.**

A. **Closed fracture** is a fracture that does not communicate with the outside.

B. **Open fracture** is a fracture that communicates with the external environment.

C. **Comminuted fracture** consists of three or more fragments.

D. **Avulsion fracture** is a fragment of bone pulled from its normal position by a muscle contraction or resistance of a ligament.

E. **Greenstick fracture** is an incomplete, angulated fracture of a long bone, particularly in children.

ORTHOPEDICS **16**

F. Torus fracture is compression of the bone without cortical disruption. It is seen especially in the forearms of children.

II. Epiphyseal Plate Fractures. These are described using the Salter and Harris classification **(Fig. 16-2)**.

A. Salter I (approximately 6%)

1. Usually the result of a shearing force; can be associated with birth injury.
2. Most common in infants and young children.
3. High index of suspicion is necessary because spontaneous reduction can occur.

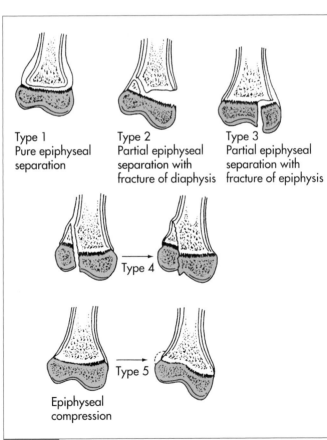

Type 1
Pure epiphyseal
separation

Type 2
Partial epiphyseal
separation with
fracture of diaphysis

Type 3
Partial epiphyseal
separation with
fracture of epiphysis

Type 4

Type 5

Epiphyseal
compression

FIG. 16-2

Salter and Harris classification of epiphyseal fractures.

4. Prognosis is excellent because epiphyseal blood supply is usually intact and growing cells of the epiphyseal plate are undisturbed.

B. Salter II (approximately 75%)

1. Most frequent in children older than 10 years.
2. Usually treated with closed reduction.
3. Prognosis is excellent because the blood supply is almost always intact.

C. Salter III (8%)

1. Commonly involves the lower tibial epiphysis.
2. Caused by an intra-articular shearing force.
3. Often requires open reduction.
4. Prognosis is good if the blood supply is intact and reduction is maintained.

D. Salter IV (10%)

1. Commonly involves lateral condyle of humerus.
2. Treated with anatomic reduction and internal fixation.
3. Prognosis is poor unless reduction is maintained.

E. Salter V (1%)

1. Results from a crush injury through the epiphysis to a portion of the epiphyseal plate.
2. Usually occurs in a joint that has only one plane of movement.
3. Most commonly seen in the knee and ankle.
4. Initial radiographs tend to be normal and so this fracture must be suspected from the mechanism of injury.
5. Results are poor, with premature cessation of growth.
6. Nontraumatic events causing a Salter V injury are metaphyseal osteomyelitis and epiphyseal aseptic necrosis.
7. Salter V can occur in conjunction with Salter I, II, and III fractures and not be recognized until growth arrest occurs.
8. Treat with 3 weeks of no weight bearing.

III. Repair of Fractures in General. A good general rule is that most bones join in 6 to 8 weeks; lower limb bones may take longer; fractures in children may take less time.

IV. Complications of Fractures in General.

A. Immediate complications, within the first few hours, include hemorrhage, damage to arteries, and damage to surrounding soft tissues. These may occur secondary to the initial trauma or compartment syndrome.

B. Early complications, within the first few weeks, include wound infection, fat embolism (see Chapter 15), shock lung, chest infection, DIC, and exacerbation of general illness. Patient may also have compartment syndrome, with the anterior compartment of the leg most commonly involved (see Chapter 2 for details of compartment syndrome).

C. Late complications, months and years later, include deformity, osteoarthritis of adjacent or distant joints, aseptic necrosis, traumatic chondromalacia, and reflex sympathetic dystrophy.

D. If a patient complains of pain after casting, assume a tight cast and possible compartment syndrome. Bivalve the cast including all layers of cotton, stockinet, etc., and wrap with an elastic wrap (Ace bandage). Consider recasting in several days.

V. Management of Some Specific Fractures.

A. Fracture of radial head

1. **Fracture is usually caused** by a fall onto an outstretched hand. Patients are reluctant to pronate the hand or to flex the elbow beyond 90 degrees. The only radiographic evidence may be an anterior or posterior fat pad sign. The posterior fat pad sign is more specific but less sensitive.

2. **Management** of nondisplaced fractures in those who can fully extend the elbow includes a sling and posterior elbow splint for 1 to 2 weeks with range-of-motion exercises after 1 week. Continue in the sling for another week and get a follow-up radiograph to document that no displacement has occurred with mobilization. If there is displacement of the radial head, the patient should be referred to an orthopedist for operative repair.

B. Radius fractures

1. In children, the most common injury is the torus (buckle) fracture, which occurs with a fall onto an outstretched hand. Radiographic findings may show only a slight cortical disruption on the lateral film. Treatment is a short-arm cast for 3 weeks.

2. In adults, the most common radial fracture is Colles' fracture, which is extra-articular and occurs 2.5 to 3 cm proximal to the articular surface of the distal radius. This fracture occurs with the hand dorsiflexed; the distal fracture segment is angulated dorsally and causes a "silver-fork" deformity. Reduction by traction and manipulation can be performed. After reducing the fracture, a plaster short-arm cast is applied for 5 to 8 weeks. If the fracture is nondisplaced, casting for 6 weeks without reduction is indicated.

C. Metacarpal fractures

1. **A boxer's fracture** is a fracture of the distal neck of the fifth metacarpal and is generally the result of punching something with a closed fist (generally a wall or refrigerator). Tenderness is localized to the injured metacarpal bone. Radiographs reveal a fracture of the involved metacarpal or subluxation at the carpometacarpal joint.

2. **Nondisplaced fractures of the base of the metacarpals are treated with immobilization** in a short-arm cast. Displaced fractures are reduced by traction with local pressure over the prominent proximal end of the distal metacarpal fracture. A follow-up radiograph is necessary within 7 days. If any instability is noted after reduction or the fracture is comminuted, the patient should be referred to an orthopedist for open reduction and internal fixation.

D. Finger fractures

1. Distal tip fractures are usually crush injuries to the tip of the finger. Protective splinting of the tip for several weeks is usually satisfactory.

2. Middle and proximal phalangeal fractures should be examined for evidence of angulation (by roentgenography) or rotation (by clinical examination),

which require reduction. Nondisplaced extra-articular fractures can be managed by 1 to 2 weeks of immobilization followed by dynamic splinting with buddy taping to the adjacent finger. Large intra-articular or displaced fractures are usually unstable and require orthopedic referral.

3. Small (25%) avulsion fractures of the middle phalangeal base occur with a hyperextension injury. These injuries are managed by 2 to 3 weeks of immobilization with up to 15 degrees of flexion at the PIP joint, followed by buddy taping for 3 to 6 weeks.

4. Unless there is a specific indication (e.g., avulsion of the distal extensor tendon) fingers should be splinted in a neutral position. The fingers should be positioned as though the patient is holding a baseball or tennis ball. Splinting the fingers in extension can lead to stiffness.

E. Hip fracture. Immediate or early repair is associated with better outcomes. Consider femoral nerve block for pain management; it is easy to do and effective (see Chapter 22 for details).

BIBLIOGRAPHY

Bigos SJ, Battie MC: The impact of spinal disorders in industry. In Frymoyer JW (ed): *The Adult Spine: Principles and Practice*. New York, Raven Press, 1991, p147.

Deyo RA, Tsui-Wu YJ: Descriptive epidemiology of low-back pain and its related medical care in the United States. *Spine* 12:264-268, 1987.

Greene WB (ed): *Essentials of Musculoskeletal Care*, 2nd ed. Rosemont, Ill, American Academy of Orthopedic Surgeons, 2001.

Hart LG, Deyo RA, Cherkin DC: Physician office visits for low back pain. Frequency, clinical evaluation, and treatment patterns from a U.S. national survey. *Spine* 20:11-19, 1995.

Jensen MC, Brant-Zawadzki MN, Obuchowski N, et al: Magnetic resonance imaging of the lumbar spine in people without back pain. *N Engl J Med* 331:69-73, 1994.

Klein BP, Jensen RC, Sanderson LM: Assessment of workers' compensation claims for back strains/sprains. *J Occup Med* 26:443-448, 1984.

Libetta C, Burke D, Brennan P, Yassa J: Validation of the Ottawa ankle rules in children. *J Accid Emerg Med* 16:342-344, 1999.

Stiell IG, Greenberg GH, Wells GA, et al: Prospective validation of a decision rule for the use of radiography in acute knee injuries. *JAMA* 275:611-615, 1996.

Tandeter HB, Shvartzman P: Acute knee injuries: Use of decision rules for selective radiograph ordering. *Am Fam Physician* 60:2599-2608, 1999.

Wigder HN, Cohan Ballis SF, Lazar L, et al: Successful implementation of a guideline by peer comparisons, education, and positive physician feedback. *J Emerg Med* 17:807-810, 1999.

16

ORTHOPEDICS

Dermatology

Wendy Shen

PRURITUS

I. **Overview.** Physiologic pruritus is a mild itch sensation due to trivial stimuli. Moderate-to-severe itchy sensations that cause damage and interfere with well-being are termed *pathologic pruritus*. Pruritus is mediated by histamine, prostaglandins, acetylcholine, kinins, and proteases. Common "itch spots" are located in warm areas where sweat is retained, especially the groin, foot, and scalp.

II. **Etiology.**

A. **Cutaneous causes**

1. **Exogenous causes**

   a. **Irritants:** most commonly fiberglass, wool, foreign bodies.

   b. **Infestations:** scabies, mites, pediculosis, jellyfish larvae.

   c. **Bites:** mosquitoes, fleas, etc.

   d. **Other:** lichen planus, nodular prurigo, dermatitis herpetiformis, eczema.

2. **Dermatoses:** fungal, bacterial, viral, herpes, miliaria, dry or chapped skin.

B. **Systemic causes**

1. **Drugs**

   a. Allergic reactions (e.g., penicillin, sulfa drugs).

   b. Vasoactive drugs (e.g., nicotinic acid, caffeine, alcohol).

   c. CNS drugs (e.g., morphine, cocaine, amphetamines, codeine).

2. **Endocrinopathy** (e.g., hypothyroidism, hyperthyroidism, diabetes mellitus, diabetes insipidus, hyperparathyroidism secondary to chronic renal failure).

3. **Hepatic disease** (e.g., obstructive biliary disease, cholestasis).

4. **Malignancy** (e.g., Hodgkin's disease, polycythemia rubra vera, leukemia, mycosis fungoides, Sézary syndrome, visceral neoplasia, carcinoid syndrome, multiple myeloma).

5. **Chronic renal failure.**

6. **Infection** (e.g., trichinosis, onchocerciasis, echinococcosis, focal infection).

7. **Miscellaneous:** gout, iron-deficiency anemia, primary amyloidosis, beriberi.

8. **Pregnancy.**

C. **Psychogenic causes** include pruritus secondary to psychosis, anxiety, or depression. Some patients have delusions of parasitosis, especially with methamphetamine abuse.

III. **Evaluation.** History should include details about any skin lesions preceding the pruritus; history of weight loss, fatigue, fever, malaise; recent emotional stress; and recent medications and travel. Physical exam should emphasize the skin and its appendages; look for xerosis, excoriation, lichenification, and hydration. Order lab tests as suggested by the physical exam, which can include CBC, ESR, fasting glucose, kidney and/or liver function tests, hepatitis panel, thyroid tests, stool for parasites, and CXR.

IV. Treatment.

A. Treat any underlying systemic disorder.

B. Nonsystemic treatment. Mild pruritus may respond to nonpharmacologic measures (e.g., avoiding irritants, using cool water compresses, trimming the nails to prevent scratching, behavior therapy).

C. Systemic symptomatic treatment includes H_1 blockers such as diphenhydramine or hydroxyzine or the nonsedating antihistamines (loratadine, cetirizine). Doxepin is the most potent H_1 blocker and can be used in recalcitrant cases. H_2 blockers such as cimetidine or ranitidine and tricyclic antidepressants (particularly doxepin and amitriptyline) may also be effective. Try oral prednisone as a last resort.

D. Topical symptomatic treatments include moisturizers, emollients, tar compounds, topical corticosteroids, topical anesthetics such as benzocaine or dibucaine, and pramoxine (alone or combined with menthol, petrolatum, or benzyl alcohol). Doxepin 5% cream (Zonalon) can be used to treat pruritus. It has a low potential for sensitization and is better tolerated than the oral form.

E. Other treatments include localized ultraviolet B phototherapy or intralesional injections of corticosteroid (e.g., with prurigo nodularis).

F. For pruritus secondary to cholestasis consider cholestyramine, phenobarbital, or naltrexone. Also consider rifampin 10 mg/kg per day for patients with primary biliary cirrhosis.

G. For pruritus secondary to renal disease consider dialysis, which may actually transiently increase pruritus, cholestyramine, or activated charcoal, 6 g/d for 6 weeks.

SKIN INFECTION

I. Bacterial Infections.

A. Impetigo

1. Impetigo is **usually caused by** group A β-hemolytic streptococci and/or coagulase-positive *Staphylococcus aureus*. Lesions appear as small vesicles with yellowish crusts or as purulent-appearing bullae, which may be localized or widespread on the skin and develop over days. There is often associated adenopathy but minimal systemic signs. Itching, pain, and tenderness can occur. Infection is moderately contagious.

2. **Treatment** is with mupirocin 2% ointment bid (although some staphylococci are becoming resistant) or systemic antibiotics (dicloxacillin 500 mg qid × 10 days, cephalexin 500 mg qid × 10 days, or erythromycin 500 mg qid × 10 days), daily bathing with antibacterial soap, use of alcohol "hand washes" on body, and attention to personal hygiene. Monitor for development of post-streptococcal glomerulonephritis. If community-acquired MRSA is prevalent or if patient is not responding

to the above, treatment with doxycycline or TMP–SMX should be considered.

B. Ecthyma

1. Ecthyma is considered a **deeper extension of impetigo** with the same etiology except that it may also be caused by *Pseudomonas* species. It is characterized by a hemorrhagic crust with erythema or induration that develops over weeks.

2. **Treatment** includes systemic antibiotics (as for impetigo) as well as debridement of the epidermis, which becomes necrotic. Scars may occur after healing. It usually occurs in debilitated patients, such as those with poorly controlled diabetes, but it can occur in anyone. Ecthyma gangrenosum is a variant that can cause systemic toxicity.

C. Erysipelas

manifests as a well-demarcated, tender, rapidly advancing erythematous plaque; there is pain associated with the lesion. The patient may have fever and leukocytosis. The usual organism is β-hemolytic streptococci. Treat as per cellulitis. Patients may have multiple recurrences, especially on a dependent extremity or after axillary dissection for breast carcinoma.

D. Cellulitis

1. Cellulitis is usually caused by group A β-hemolytic streptococci or *S. aureus;* it is a potentially suppurative inflammation of the dermis and subcutaneous tissue. It usually follows trauma, a break in the skin, or an underlying dermatosis.

2. Cellulitis manifests with local erythema, warmth, induration, and tenderness. The border is not well defined. There may be streaks of lymphangitis with involvement of the regional lymph nodes. Systemic symptoms are common, and bacteremia and septicemia may follow.

3. Treatment is with systemic antibiotics (if infection is mild, dicloxacillin or cephalexin 500 mg qid × 7-10 days; if infection is severe, nafcillin 1.5 g IV q4h or vancomycin 1.5 g/d initially, then switch to oral form). Alternative antibiotics include amoxicillin–clavulanate, erythromycin, clarithromycin, or azithromycin. If community acquired, MRSA is a consideration; use doxycycline 100 mg bid or TMP–SMX. Application of local heat, elevation, and immobilization can also help. For necrotizing fasciitis and synergistic gangrene, early wide surgical excision and debridement is necessary in addition to IV antibiotics. See also Chapter 2 for details on necrotizing fasciitis.

E. Erythrasma and related disorders

1. Superficial intertriginous skin infections caused by *Corynebacteria* organisms. It is often confused with fungal infection. Patient presents with skin color changes (e.g., reddish brown) and a slightly raised patch of affected skin. The bacteria produce porphyrins, so the skin is coral-pink under Wood's lamp.

2. Preferred treatment is oral erythromycin; topical clindamycin 2% is an alternative. Erythrasma responds to miconazole and clotrimazole, but the recurrence rate is high. These organisms also cause trichomycosis

17

DERMATOLOGY

axillaris and pitted keratolysis. The former leads to foul axillary odor and hyperhidrosis and the latter to painful burning of the feet with pits on calloused areas. Good hygiene, antiperspirants, and topical erythromycin are used to treat both. Botulinum toxin has recently been approved for use in axillary hyperhidrosis.

F. Folliculitis

1. Folliculitis (including sycosis barbae [barber's itch], pseudofolliculitis, and hot tub folliculitis) is a common problem with predisposing factors such as maceration, friction, and the use of irritant chemicals. It is usually caused by *S. aureus* but occasionally by *Klebsiella, Pseudomonas* (hot tub folliculitis), *Aerobacter*, or *C. albicans*. Lesion appears as a pustule with a central hair (follicle) with surrounding erythema. The patient may notice tenderness, pruritus, and pain. Particularly severe cases can result in scarring and destruction of the hair follicle.

2. Treatment includes antiseptic washes (e.g., pHisoDerm, pHisoHex, alcohol skin cleansers), which may also be used for prophylaxis. Systemic antibiotics such as dicloxacillin, cephalexin, or erythromycin 500mg qid for 7 to 10 days are an alternative. Mupirocin 2% ointment may be used for isolated areas. Use a fluoroquinolone (e.g., levofloxacin) to cover *Pseudomonas* for hot tub folliculitis. Complications can include cellulitis, furunculosis, and alopecia.

G. Furuncle (boil)

1. **Furuncle** is an acute, localized perifollicular abscess of the skin and subcutaneous tissue caused by coagulase-positive *S. aureus*, resulting in a red, hot, very tender inflammatory nodule that exudes pus from one opening. A **carbuncle** is an aggregate of connected furuncles and characteristically is painful and has a number of pustular openings. This can be an acute or chronic problem, with lesions commonly on areas of friction such as buttocks, axillae, breasts, and the nape of the neck.

2. Treatment involves systemic antibiotics (as for cellulitis), local heat, and rest. Incision and drainage is generally required. Prevention is often difficult. Improved personal hygiene, use of antibacterial soaps (e.g., pHisoHex, pHisoDerm) or alcohol skin washes, frequent hand washing, daily bathing, and change of clothing are important. Elimination of carrier states in the nose and perineum by the use of topical mupirocin and systemic antibiotics is often necessary.

H. Necrotizing fasciitis. See Chapter 2.

II. Viral Infections.

A. Warts (verruca vulgaris)

1. Warts are focal areas of epithelial hyperplasia caused by the human papilloma viruses. Lesions are most common on the hands, feet, anogenital area (condylomata), and face. They are infectious and autoinoculable. They are common in children, the elderly, and patients with immunologic deficiencies or atopic dermatitis.

2. Treatment is with keratolytic agents (salicylic acid–lactic acid–podophyllin preparations), immune modulation (imiquimod, IFN-α), cryotherapy, curettage, laser, or electrodesiccation. Duct tape applied for 6 days a

week followed by abrasion of the wart and repeating the cycle until the wart resolves is as effective as cryosurgery. Recurrences are common and no one treatment is uniformly effective. See also Chapter 8 for treatment of condylomata acuminata (genital warts). Cimetidine has been used to treat warts, but controlled trials show that there is no benefit.

B. Herpes simplex types 1 and 2 are DNA viruses. The early lesions are multiple 1-2 mm diameter yellowish, clear vesicles on an erythematous base. The vesicles can ulcerate and become quite painful. Classic type 1 herpes occurs around the mouth and type 2 occurs on the genitalia, but either type 1 or type 2 can occur anywhere.

1. **Diagnosis** can be made from clinical appearance, serologic antibody titers of acute and convalescent sera, Tzanck smear (Wright stain of material obtained from the base of the lesion showing multinucleated giant cells), and/or viral culture. A prodrome of pain, discomfort, or tingling is often reported a week to 10 days before the lesions appear.

2. **Clinical syndromes include**

a. **Gingivostomatitis.** Occurs periorally in children and young adults.

b. **Keratoconjunctivitis.** Ophthalmology consult is warranted. Usually heals without scarring.

c. **Vulvovaginitis.**

d. **Herpes gladiatorum.** Occurs on the head, neck, or shoulder. Common in wrestlers.

e. **Eczema herpeticum.** Occurs in those with underlying skin disorders, most commonly in atopic dermatitis, and in children more than adults. It consists of disseminated umbilicated vesicles confined to eczematous skin; lesions evolve into punched-out erosions that can become confluent.

f. **Hepatoadrenal necrosis and encephalitis** (see Chapter 9 for diagnosis and treatment of encephalitis).

g. **Herpetic whitlow.** Occurs on distal portion of fingers.

h. **Cold sores** (herpes labialis).

3. **Treatment** is symptomatic with cool compresses, analgesics, and topical drying agents (Burow's solution) for the oozing, weeping stages. **Topical acyclovir is no better than placebo and should be avoided. Docosanol (Abreva) is an over-the-counter topical product that is effective in reducing duration of symptoms and lesions.** Antivirals (e.g., acyclovir) have only a modest effect on recurrent genital herpes unless used prophylactically every day (see Chapter 8 for details). If used during the prodrome, antivirals can shorten duration of lesions, reduce severity of symptoms, and shorten length of viral shedding. Talk to patients about asymptomatic shedding of virus and the need for safer sex (e.g., use condoms).

C. Herpes zoster (shingles) is a reactivation of latent varicella zoster virus present in the sensory ganglia.

1. **Classic description** is that of grouped vesicles on an erythematous base in one unilateral dermatome. Thoracic nerve dermatomes are most commonly involved, followed by the major branches of the trigeminal nerve.

DERMATOLOGY 17

2. **Symptoms** consist of pain, dysesthesia, and pruritus. Healing requires 2 to 3 weeks, and the afflicted persons are infectious until the lesions have crusted over (may transmit chickenpox to those who are not immune). Persons of any age can be affected, but the disease is more common and more severe in the elderly.

3. **Diagnosis** is via clinical presentation, although Tzanck smear, biopsy, and viral culture may be performed.

4. **Treatment** is oral acyclovir 800 mg 5 times a day for 7 to 10 days, which is effective if treatment is initiated within 2 days of the onset of the rash. Alternatives include famciclovir 500 mg PO tid for 7 days and valacyclovir 1000 mg PO tid for 7 days. Steroids are ineffective. Capsaicin creams can be used for pain relief after the lesions have healed. Amitriptyline 25 to 150 mg qhs may be useful in treating postherpetic neuralgia. Other options include lidocaine patches (Lidoderm), carbamazepine, gabapentin, etc. Patients with recurrent herpes zoster, especially those with bilateral occurrence or when more than one dermatome is involved, may have a malignancy or be otherwise immunosuppressed.

D. Molluscum contagiosum is caused by a DNA pox virus.

1. Lesions appear as pearly papules up to 5 mm in diameter and have a central dimple (umbilication). Multiple lesions are usually present. The central core (molluscum body) can be expressed with a blade. The lesions are infectious and autoinoculation is common. Children are most commonly affected.

2. Spontaneous resolution can occur, but there is often an eczematous reaction before resolution. Treatment can be limited to simple superficial curettage without anesthesia. The removal of the molluscum body, application of 50% trichloroacetic acid, or liquid nitrogen cryotherapy are equally efficacious.

III. Fungal Infections (Dermatomycoses).

A. Candidiasis

1. Candidiasis is caused by *Candida albicans*. It is seen as thrush (see Chapters 11 and 12 for immunosuppressed patients and infants, respectively), diaper dermatitis, perineal infections, and intertriginous dermatitis. Diagnosis is by clinical exam, and microscopic examination of skin scraping in 10% KOH reveals yeast forms and budding hyphae.

2. Treat with topical imidazole (miconazole, clotrimazole) creams bid to affected areas for superficial fungal infections. See Chapter 13 for vaginal candidiasis. See Chapter 11 for recurrent mucocutaneous disease. Invasive disease can be treated with fluconazole 400 mg IV qd for 7 days and then PO for 14 days after the last positive blood culture. This dose may be doubled in patients who deteriorate. An alternative is amphotericin B (lipid formulations are better tolerated).

3. Patients who present with recurrent infections should be investigated for an underlying illness such as diabetes mellitus, hypoparathyroidism, Addison's disease, malignancies, or HIV. Use of steroids and antibiotics are also predisposing factors.

B. Dermatophytoses (tinea). These fungi, belonging to the genera *Trichophyton, Microsporum*, and *Epidermophyton*, infect the stratum corneum of epidermis, hair, and nails. Dermatophytoses are commonly referred to by the locus of infection: tinea unguium (nails), tinea pedis (foot, "athlete's foot"), tinea cruris (perineum, "jock itch"), tinea corporis (body, ringworm), tinea barbae (beard), tinea manus (hand), and tinea capitis (scalp and hair). Lesions can appear as grayish, scaling patches, which can be quite pruritic and can lead to autoinoculation or scalp alopecia. Skin scraping in 10% KOH will demonstrate fungal hyphae. Infected hairs when examined under black light fluoresce green-yellow. Treatment of selected areas is as follows:

1. **Tinea corporis** (body, ringworm), tinea cruris (perineum, jock itch), tinea pedis (foot, athlete's foot). Topical tolnaftate (Tinactin, OTC) or clotrimazole (Lotrimin) tid until clear, and then 1 to 2 weeks longer. For treatment failure, use the same regimen as per tinea capitis below.

2. **Tinea capitis** (scalp and hair) requires oral therapy. Micronized griseofulvin is usually used for up to 4 to 8 weeks. Itraconazole, fluconazole 6 mg/kg per day for 20 days *or* 6 to 8 mg/kg per *week* for 8 weeks, and terbinafine may work also. Adjunctive therapy includes selenium sulfide or shampoo every 2 or 3 days.

3. **Tinea unguium or onychomycosis** (nails). Griseofulvin 500 mg bid for 4 to 6 months or itraconazole 200 mg bid for 4 months (1 week on, 3 weeks off); the latter regimen is very expensive. An alternative is terbinafine 250 mg PO qd for 12 weeks or bid for 1 week of the month for 3 or 4 months. Success rates are about 75% but many recur (50%). The newer nail-paint preparations are expensive and have a very poor (12%!!) success rate.

C. Tinea (pityriasis) versicolor appears as slightly pigmented, superficial, and tan scaling plaques of various sizes, primarily on the neck, trunk, and proximal arms. With sun exposure, the infected regions do not tan and appear hypopigmented. They are usually caused by *Malassezia furfur*.

1. Diagnosis is via clinical exam and KOH preparations of skin scrapings.

2. Treatment can be with topical imidazoles twice daily or washing with zinc or selenium shampoos daily for 2 to 3 weeks. Although not FDA approved, ketoconazole 400 mg can be given as a single dose. Have the patient exercise to a sweat and not shower for at least 4 hours afterward. This treatment has up to a 97% success rate in a single dose. Alternatives are ketoconazole 200 mg PO qd for 7 days or either fluconazole or itraconazole 400 mg PO qd for 7 days.

17

DERMATOLOGY

ACNE

I. Overview. Acne commonly begins in adolescence with stimulation of the sebaceous glands by sex hormones, primarily androgens. Acne can be aggravated by drugs, steroids, cosmetics, comedogenic agents, and picking and squeezing. No convincing evidence indicates that diet, stress, or hygiene worsens acne. Acne has a predilection for the face, upper neck, chest, and back. In females with severe acne, consider polycystic ovarian disease (see Chapter 13), congenital adrenal hyperplasia, or Cushing's disease.

II. Types of Acne and Their Treatment.

A. Comedones

1. **Appear as** whiteheads and blackheads (closed and open comedones, respectively).

2. **Treatment** is with topical agents and takes a minimum of 2 weeks to show any improvement. Patient education is important because attempts to extrude blackheads or pustules may lead to deeper, potentially scarring lesions:

a. **Topical retinoids including tretinoin (Retin A)** is the treatment of choice. Begin with nightly application of 0.025% cream or 0.01% gel and increase concentration as necessary and as tolerated. Usually requires 3 to 5 months of therapy. Retin-A Micro (0.1% gel) is less irritating than 0.1% tretinoin cream. For those who do not tolerate tretinoin, other retinoids include adapalene (Differin) 0.1% and tazarotene (Avage) 0.1%. These are equally effective and more expensive but less irritating than tretinoin.

b. **Benzoyl peroxide,** available in 2.5%, 5%, and 10% strengths as lotions and gels, should be applied frequently enough (qd to bid) to produce drying and even scaling, but without significant irritation. Because it is an oxidizer, benzoyl peroxide can bleach clothing or other linens. Benzoyl peroxide in the morning can be alternated with topical tretinoin at bedtime.

c. Scrubbing the skin is counterproductive and should be discouraged.

d. **Azelaic acid.** First used as a treatment for hyperpigmentation, it has antibacterial and antikeratinizing properties. It is as effective as benzoyl peroxide and tretinoin and may be better tolerated. Comes as 20% cream applied bid. Use with caution in darker-skinned people.

e. **Oral contraceptives** with a low androgenic potency may be helpful (most OCPs will do).

B. Papulopustular acne

1. Has a significant inflammatory component with inflamed papules and pustules.

2. **Treatment** is as listed above for comedonal acne with the addition of antibiotics. As the inflammation decreases, the antibiotics can be tapered and discontinued.

a. **For less severe cases,** use topical erythromycin 2% to 4% solution, gel, or ointment applied bid; clindamycin 1% solution, gel, or lotion; or tetracycline 4% applied bid.

b. **Moderate-to-severe cases** require systemic antibiotics. Tetracycline 250 to 1000 mg qd, doxycycline 100 mg, erythromycin 500 to 1000 mg qd, or minocycline 50 mg to 150 mg qd are reasonable alternatives (higher doses should be divided). These must be taken for 6 weeks before efficacy can be ascertained. With improvement, the dose can be tapered gradually. *Note:* Do not administer tetracycline to pregnant women or to children under 12 years of age.

C. Nodulocystic acne

1. **Manifested by** comedones, inflammatory papules/pustules, and deep, inflamed nodules and cysts. Can result in scarring. Hypertrophic scars often form on the chest and back.

2. **Treatment** consists of two modalities in addition to the regimens previously mentioned.

a. **Corticosteroid.** Inject enough corticosteroid, triamcinolone 5 mg/mL, to cause the cyst to blanch. Some recommend needle drainage of the cyst first.

b. **Oral isotretinoin** (Accutane) 0.5 to 2 mg/kg per day with meals for a 4- to 5-month course, is usually highly effective but expensive. **It is absolutely contraindicated in pregnancy; thus, a negative pregnancy test must be obtained within 2 weeks of initiating treatment, and two forms of contraception must be used from 1 month before to 1 month after therapy.** Careful monitoring of liver function tests and serum lipid levels is required. Monitor for side effects as well (e.g., dry eyes, chapped lips, epistaxis, pruritus, alopecia, scaling on the palms and soles, inability to wear contact lenses, and pseudotumor cerebri). **Because of ongoing problems with birth defects, special registration is required in order to prescribe isotretinoin (available from the manufacturer, Roche).**

c. **Other therapies include** estrogen with low androgenic progesterone (e.g., Ortho-Cept, although any OCP will do) in the form of an oral contraceptive for girls unresponsive to antibiotics who are not a candidate for Accutane; spironolactone for a patient with evidence of androgen excess; or comedo extraction.

III. Other Acneform Eruptions.

A. Acne in the pediatric population

1. **Acne neonatorum** is seen with a positive family history. It occurs in children younger than 3 months and is usually self-limited.

2. **Acne of infancy** occurs in infants between 3 months and 2 years of age and there is usually a positive family history. Consider comedogenic agents, virilization, and candidiasis.

B. Acne secondary to chemical exposure (acne venenata, chloracne) is acne caused by chemical agents via contact in sensitive persons. Prognosis is good with avoidance. Examples are chlorinated hydrocarbons, insoluble cutting oils (impure paraffin–oil mixtures), and other petroleum products (crude petroleum, heavy coal tar distillates), and dioxin.

C. Acne medicamentosa is induction of acne or aggravation of preexisting acne by medications. Agents include phenobarbital, corticosteroids, isoniazid, iodides and bromides, and vitamins D and B_{12}.

17

DERMATOLOGY

ERYTHEMA NODOSUM

I. **Overview.** Erythema nodosum is an inflammatory panniculitis generally found on the anterior shins. It presents as painful, erythematous nodules and occasionally plaques. Most cases are in women between ages 20 and 45.

II. **Causes are protean and include** recent streptococcal throat infection (50% of the cases), oral contraceptives and multiple other medications, sarcoid, tuberculosis, coccidioidomycosis, histoplasmosis, Hodgkin's disease, inflammatory bowel disease, bacterial gastroenteritis, connective tissue disorders, and HIV, among others.

III. **Treatment.** Generally self-limited. Treat underlying etiology. Avoid systemic steroids because of risk of immunosuppression and extension of any fungal or other infection (e.g., TB) but use clinical judgment. NSAIDS may be useful for pain. Potassium iodide (360 mg to 900 mg divided tid) has been helpful in many cases. Colchicine (0.6 mg bid) may be helpful, as well as topical steroid under occlusion or intralesional steroids.

PAPULOSQUAMOUS DISEASES

I. **Significant Plaque Formation.**

A. **Psoriasis** is a common skin disorder affecting more than 1% of the population. Primary lesions are erythematous papules and plaques with gray-white, silvery scale. It usually occurs on extensor surfaces (elbows, knees, lumbosacral areas) and often only on the scalp (where it is difficult to differentiate from seborrheic dermatitis). Guttate psoriasis, which manifests as diffuse small plaques, especially on the trunk and extremities but excluding the palms and soles, can occur after an antecedent URI or streptococcal pharyngitis. Psoriasis can manifest Koebner's phenomenon (lesions can appear at sites of trauma, e.g., an excoriation, tattoo, burn). Removal of the scale often causes tiny bleeding points (Auspitz's sign). Nails manifest pitting and stippling, and distal and lateral onycholysis is common. Psoriatic arthritis can affect the DIPs and MCPs, but rheumatoid factor is usually negative.

1. **Treatment.** Topical corticosteroids can be helpful, as can keratolytics such as salicylic acid. Keeping areas moisturized with topical emollients or urea can be beneficial. Calcipotriene (Dovonex) 0.005% applied topically bid is a newer topical treatment for mildly to moderately severe psoriasis (but is not used on the face or groin, where it can cause irritant dermatitis). The efficacy of calcipotriene is comparable to mid-potency topical corticosteroids; however, it does not cause skin atrophy or tachyphylaxis. Treatment with topical crude coal tar formulas and daily exposure to UV light may also be used.

2. **Severe forms of psoriasis should be referred** to a dermatologist for other forms of treatment, including acitretin (Soriatane), cyclosporine (Sandimmune), isotretinoin (Accutane), methotrexate, hydroxyurea, inhibitors of EGFR kinase, other immunomodulatory drugs (etanercept, alefacept, efalizumab and infliximab), CO_2 resurfacing laser, electrodessication with curettage, or PUVA (psoralen photochemotherapy). Moreover, studies look promising using a new IL-2 fusion protein treatment.

B. **Lupus erythematosus (discoid type)** is characterized by extensive papules and plaques with adherent scaling, which later involute and scar centrally, leaving an annular or polycyclic pattern with irregular borders. It primarily affects the face and scalp, but other areas include nose, dorsa of forearms, hands, fingers, toes, and less frequently the trunk. The lupus band test (biopsy showing IgG deposits at the dermoepidermal junction) is positive in 90% of active lesions at least 6 weeks old and not recently treated with topical corticosteroids; however, the test is negative in burned-out (scarred) lesions and in normal skin. Treatment with antimalarial drugs (hydroxychloroquine 6.5 mg/kg/d), topical fluorinated corticosteroids, or intralesional corticosteroids (triamcinolone acetonide 3-5 mg/mL) helps control or clear the eruption. Only 1% to 5% develop SLE. Thalidomide has been used for persistent discoid lesions in patients with SLE.

DERMATOLOGY 17

II. **Nonconfluent Papules.**
A. **Lichen planus** is a pruritic eruption in which violaceous, flat, polygonal papules occur in linear, annular, or confluent groups.
1. Lesions of the mucous membranes appear as whitish, reticulated, lacy plaques of the buccal mucosa and may be painful (Wickham's striae). Lichen planus exhibits Koebner's phenomenon (lesions appear at sites of trauma, e.g., an excoriation, tattoo, burn).
2. Treatment of this chronic, idiopathic, self-limited disease is supportive, with topical corticosteroids (anti-inflammatory), systemic antihistamines (antipruritic), and occasionally intralesional corticosteroids (help to flatten large plaques). Short doses of alternate-day prednisone temporarily suppress active lesions. Vulvar lichen planus can occur in isolation. It can become chronic and has malignant potential. Referral to gynecology is warranted.

B. **Pityriasis rosea**
1. The cause may be viral, possibly human herpes virus 7 (HHV-7), although other studies refute this. It is characterized by occurrence of a herald patch, which is larger than other lesions. It is usually a bright red, round or oval, sharply demarcated plaque (2-5 cm) with scaly margins and central clearing. A few days to weeks later a generalized reaction occurs, frequently in a "fir tree" pattern. Pruritus may be severe.
2. Treatment is not indicated because the eruption is self-limited (usually clears in 4-10 wk and seldom recurs). Oral antihistamines (hydroxyzine or diphenhydramine) are used to alleviate the itching and a mild hydrocortisone cream may soothe the skin. New evidence suggests that

oral erythromycin used for 14 days is effective for some. Must differentiate this from secondary syphilis.

VESICULOBULLOUS LESIONS - PARTIAL DIFFERENTIAL

I. Vesicular Disease.

A. Dermatitis herpetiformis lesions consist of extremely itchy, tense, grouped herpetiform vesicles, usually 3 to 6 mm in diameter and occurring in a distinctive distribution over the elbows, knees, buttocks, upper back, and posterior scalp. Because of excoriation, round crusts are often the only visible sign of the disease.

B. The gold standard for diagnosis is biopsy with direct immunofluorescence of lesional or normal skin showing IgA deposits, usually in a granular pattern at the tips of dermal papillae. About 90% of patients have evidence of gluten-sensitive enteropathy on small-bowel biopsy. However, less than 10% of patients with dermatitis herpetiformis have GI symptoms that suggest celiac disease. Both skin and bowel disease regress after several months of a gluten-free diet (see also Chapter 5).

C. The mainstay of treatment is lifelong dapsone 100 mg PO daily (pruritus and new lesions stop in 24 hours). CBC should be monitored every 1 to 2 weeks for the first 3 months to detect agranulocytosis. Liver function tests should be performed regularly to detect idiosyncratic dapsone-induced hepatitis.

II. Bullous Diseases.

A. Bullous pemphigoid

1. Bullous pemphigoid is an autoimmune subepidermal disease with blisters that are tense, round, and well defined and usually occur on a pink, edematous, inflamed base. Before the bullae form, severely itchy urticarial plaques may be present for several weeks. Flexural areas and the lower legs are the sites of predilection.

2. Diagnosis is confirmed by biopsy of perilesional skin, which reveals many eosinophils and neutrophils in and below the bulla at the dermoepidermal junction. On electron microscopy, the split is seen at the level of the lamina lucida where the bullous pemphigoid antigen is found.

3. Control is usually achieved with a daily dose of 60 to 80 mg of prednisone initially, followed by fairly rapid tapering to 30 to 40 mg and then slower tapering. Dapsone, cyclophosphamide, or azathioprine are often added if there is difficulty tapering the steroid. Other options include mycophenolate mofetil or the combination of niacin plus doxycycline *or* tetracycline. The disease often remits in 1 to 2 years, and steroids can be stopped. Relapse occurs in only 10%.

B. Pemphigus vulgaris

1. Lesions begin around or in the mouth or on the scalp and can spread to any area. Primary lesions are flaccid, noninflamed bullae that break easily and leave large denuded areas, which then crust. Nikolsky's sign is positive (lateral pressure results in dramatic extension of blisters).

Lesions heal with temporary hyperpigmentation but without scarring. A pemphigus-like eruption has been reported with use of certain medications: penicillamine, captopril, piroxicam, penicillin, rifampin, and phenobarbital.

2. **Diagnosis is confirmed by biopsy** of the skin or oral mucosa adjacent to active blisters; in virtually 100% of pemphigus cases of all types, IgG and C3 are seen outlining the intracellular spaces of the epidermis.

3. **Therapy is high-dose steroids,** which dramatically reduces the mortality rate; referral to a dermatologist is suggested. A common approach is to start with prednisone 80 mg daily and increase the dose by 50% every 7 days until no new blisters form. If the dose nears 200 mg, then consider IV pulse therapy with steroids or plasmapheresis. After control is achieved, an immunosuppressive agent (most commonly azathioprine [Imuran] or cyclophosphamide [Cytoxan]) is added to allow steroid tapering.

C. Erythema multiforme

1. **Erythema multiforme** is an acute, self-limiting vascular skin reaction with a wide variety of causes. Early lesions are pink, edematous papules; some of these evolve into hallmark target lesions (flat, dull red macules with central clearing or vesicle formation). The distribution is symmetric, and lesions occur on the palms, soles, extensor extremities, and often on oral mucosa.

2. **Herpes simplex infection triggers most mild, recurrent cases.** More severe, widespread cases may be caused by other infectious agents, especially *Mycoplasma* species and viruses, and by medications, especially penicillins, sulfonamides, anticonvulsants, NSAIDs, topical steroids, topical aminoglycosides, and allopurinol. The lesions are often preceded by a prodrome of fever, malaise, myalgias, and upper respiratory symptoms.

3. Mild cases are self-limited over a 7- to 10-day period and might not require treatment. Suppressive doses of anti-herpes drug (see Chapter 8) may prevent recurrences associated with herpesviruses. For more severe or widespread disease, treatment involves prednisone.

D. Erythema multiforme variants

1. **Stevens–Johnson syndrome.** Severe mucosal erosions (mouth, vagina, etc.) accompanied by high fever and severe constitutional symptoms usually associated with extensive bullous erythema multiforme of the skin. Stevens–Johnson syndrome may be related to infections with herpesviruses or mycoplasma or a drug allergy. Ocular steroids might be required to prevent synechiae formation. Patient generally requires dermatology and/or burn unit care.

2. **Toxic epidermal necrolysis** is almost always drug induced (see drugs for erythema multiforme). It is manifested by a burning or painful eruption that predominates on the trunk and proximal extremities. Painful edematous erythema of palms and soles often develops. The initial presentation is followed by epidermal necrosis and sloughing of the skin and mucous membranes. Twenty percent to 100% of total

DERMATOLOGY 17

body surface area can be affected. The mortality rates are about 30%. Treatment is a short (2-3 weeks) course of prednisone, starting at 30 to 40 mg. Severe cases should be treated in a burn unit. Dermatology consult should be obtained.

WHITE LESIONS

I. White Patches and Plaques (Vitiligo).

A. Vitiligo is an idiopathic, circumscribed hypomelanosis of skin and hair. It might be an autoimmune disease and is associated with other autoimmune diseases including pernicious anemia, diabetes mellitus, and Addison's disease. Peak incidence is 10 to 30 years of age. It occurs in all races but is most cosmetically disfiguring in darker-skinned people. Affected persons develop white macules varying in size from 1 mm to large areas of the body, often in a symmetric pattern and at sites of repeated trauma, such as the bony prominences (malleoli, tip of the elbow, and necklace area).

B. Treatment of vitiligo is most appropriately managed by a dermatologist. Topical corticosteroids are the treatment of choice for patients with limited disease. Other treatment includes tacrolimus, pseudocatalase cream (reduces oxidative stress on the skin), PUVA photochemotherapy, and bleaching of normally pigmented skin. Immunomodulators such as cyclosporin and levamisole and vitamins such as vitamin B_{12} and folic acid plus sunlight are effective in some patients.

II. White Papules.

A. Milia are 1- to 2-mm, superficial, white-to-yellow, keratin-containing epidermal cysts, occurring multiply, located on the eyelids, cheeks, and forehead in pilosebaceous follicles and at sites of trauma (often the dorsal surface of the hands and over the knees). They are usually asymptomatic. Treatment consists of incision and expression of the white keratin plug.

B. Keratosis pilaris is a common condition of children and young adults that consists of clustered firm white papules approximately 1 mm in diameter formed at a follicular orifice. The lesions have a sandpaper feel on palpation and are usually asymptomatic, though sometimes they are associated with mild pruritus. Lesions are most common on the lateral arms, anterior thighs, and buttocks. Topical application of alpha hydroxy acids, such as glycolic acid and lactic acid, is quite effective.

OTHER DERMATITIDES

I. Allergic contact dermatitis (e.g., poison ivy, poison oak) is a pruritic, inflammatory reaction that progresses from erythema and irritation to a blistering, vesiculobullous exanthem. It is caused by a reaction to a sensitizing chemical (not necessarily a caustic agent) via a delayed cellular (type IV) hypersensitivity mechanism. The reaction requires a prior exposure.

A. Diagnosis. The location of the lesion often suggests the diagnosis. The eyelids are very sensitive and may react when other skin does not (e.g., to a perfume or new soap). Oleoresins (poison ivy, oak, and sumac) and a few chemicals (DNCB) will sensitize almost everyone. Other common agents are dyes/coloring agents, tanning chemicals, nickel, mercury, soaps, and perfumes. Common drugs include ethylenediamine, thimerosal, bacitracin, and sunscreen lotions. The patch test, in which a dilute solution of the suspected culprit is allowed to react with normal skin, is diagnostic.

B. Treatment consists of symptomatic care with wet to dry soaks of astringent solutions (Burow's solution) and antipruritics (e.g., diphenhydramine or hydroxyzine). Acetaminophen or ibuprofen will also help with pruritus. Oral corticosteroids are effective and indicated for treating severe cases involving large areas of the skin, swelling of the face or genitalia, or large areas of bullae. Steroids should be tapered over several weeks. **Poison ivy can be prevented by the use of Armor-All, a preexposure barrier available at drug stores. Postcontact prevention of poison ivy includes washing with soap and water and Tecnu (and others) which neutralize the sensitizing resin.**

II. Irritant Contact Dermatitis.

A. Etiology. Irritant contact dermatitis is caused by exposure to caustic agents. These cause a reaction consisting of irritation progressing to erythema and inflammation.

B. Treatment consists of thoroughly cleansing the affected region with cool water followed by supportive measures that include moisturizing lotions and antiseptic creams, systemic steroids, and antibiotics depending on the insult to the skin.

III. Seborrheic Dermatitis.

A. Seborrheic dermatitis is a common condition that is usually first noticed as dandruff. It affects the scalp, the center of the face, the anterior portion of the chest, and/or the flexural creases of the arms, legs, and groin (i.e., areas of the body that have high concentrations of sebaceous glands). It most commonly affects infants (ages 1-3 mo) and adults ages 30 to 60 years. It typically manifests as a greasy scale on the scalp, with erythema and scaling of the nasolabial folds and retroauricular skin. Seborrheic dermatitis is said to be associated with deficiencies of riboflavin, biotin, or pyridoxine and with various neurologic disorders (parkinsonism, CVA, epilepsy, CNS trauma, facial nerve palsy, and syringomyelia). New-onset severe seborrheic dermatitis may be associated with HIV.

B. Treatment for infants is a mild nonmedicated shampoo. In adults or for refractory infant cases, use a shampoo two or three times a week containing salicylic acid (X-Seb T, Sebulex), selenium sulfide (Selsun, Exsel), coal tar (DHS Tar, Neutrogena T-Gel, Polytar), or pyrithione zinc

17

DERMATOLOGY

(DHS Zinc, Danex, Sebulon). More severe cases may be treated with medicated shampoos (ketoconazole [Nizoral] 2% initially daily then tapered to once a week if possible). A new therapy is a topical form of γ-linoleic acid, borage oil, which is effective in infantile seborrheic dermatitis.

IV. Xerotic Eczema (Winter Itch, Asteatotic Eczema).

A. Xerotic eczema is a relatively common dermatitis that occurs in the winter and in the elderly and is characterized by dry, cracked, fissured skin and pruritus. Predisposing factors include old age; a genetic tendency for dry skin; too-frequent bathing; and dry, nonhumidified, heated rooms.

B. Treatment includes avoidance of overbathing with soap, room humidifiers, tepid-water baths using bath oils with liberal application of emollients after drying, medium-potency corticosteroids applied bid until eczema clears, and topical alpha-hydroxy acids (e.g., glycolic acid or lactic acid).

V. Eczema with Significant Excoriations.

A. Atopic dermatitis is caused by a genetic predisposition to react to environmental allergens with the development of a pruritic, inflammatory rash. Atopic dermatitis is associated with asthma, hay fever, and urticaria. Elevated levels of IgE have been associated with atopic dermatitis. The features vary with age. Atopic dermatitis commonly begins as infantile eczema, affecting the face, scalp, and upper extremities, often associated with food consumption (cheese, egg white, wheat, legumes, nuts). This may resolve or progress to involve the neck and the upper and lower extremities, especially the popliteal and the antecubital fossae. Vesiculation, oozing, and crusting are common, and lesions are very pruritic, manifesting lichenified, reddened skin due to excoriation. Stress may be a contributing factor in exacerbations.

B. Treatment is directed at relieving pruritus, controlling infection, and promoting healing. Vesicles and crusting are treated with wet-to-dry dressings of cool Burow's solution and oral antihistamines to relieve the pruritus. Topical corticosteroids and emollient creams can also be used once the lesions are clean. Use of steroids and emollients under occlusion may be helpful (e.g., under gloves or a PVC body suit at night). A course of antistaphylococcal antibiotics for 2 weeks may be helpful in acute exacerbations because many episodes seem to have an infectious trigger. A short course of systemic corticosteroids is not unreasonable; cyclosporine has been used in severe cases but should be prescribed under the direction of a dermatologist. Avoidance is important, and a trial of environmental control, elimination of specific foods, and skin testing for food and inhalant allergens might be useful.

VI. Stasis Dermatitis.

A. Stasis dermatitis is chronic dermatitis of the lower legs in people with chronic venous insufficiency. It is associated with mild pruritus, pain (if an ulcer is present), aching discomfort in the limb, swelling of the ankle, and nocturnal cramps. Lesions consist of erythematous scaling plaques with exudation, crusts, and superficial ulcers, particularly on the medial aspect of the ankle.

B. Treatment. Pressure dressings/stockings are critical to the successful treatment of stasis dermatitis and stasis ulcers. Pressures of at least 20 to 30 mm Hg are critical, and up to 50 mm Hg is used in some patients. Gradient stockings with higher pressures at the ankle are more effective. Knee length is generally as effective as thigh length. **Acute treatment** of stasis dermatitis consists of Burow's wet dressings and cooling pastes, topical corticosteroids, and systemic antibiotics if cellulitis is present. **Chronic treatment** of stasis dermatitis includes topical corticosteroids, **supportive stockings (Jobst, TEDs), compressive bandages,** and/or vein surgery; **an Unna boot (zinc oxide–impregnated gauze) can be placed for 72 hours to promote healing of skin and ulcers.** If ulcers are present, treatment includes keeping the area clean but moist (e.g. water-pick with saline bid, keep covered with Tegaderm), silver sulfadiazine or bacitracin, elevation of the leg; compressive bandages; supportive stockings; and/or surgery. Becaplermin (Regranex), a platelet-growth factor, has been used to promote ulcer healing but is expensive and of limited efficacy. Pentoxifylline may be beneficial in healing recalcitrant ulcers.

VII. Dyshidrotic Eczema.

A. Dyshidrotic eczema manifests with deep-seated, pruritic, tapioca-like vesicles on the palms, soles, or sides of the fingers. The differential diagnosis includes pustular psoriasis. Dyshidrosis can begin in childhood or adult life and may be an id reaction to skin infection elsewhere, especially to tinea.

B. Treatment is often unsatisfactory. Treatment of the vesicular stage includes Burow's wet dressings bid and/or "black cat" (10% crude coal tar in equal parts of acetone and flexible collodion) applied once daily. In moderate or severe disease, erythromycin or dicloxacillin 250 mg qid should be started because bacterial infection may be present even without obvious signs (crusts, tenderness, etc.). Additional measures include intermittent high-potency topical steroids or a burst of systemic steroids. Dietary restriction of certain metals (cobalt, nickel, or chromium) has been found to be successful in uncontrolled trials. PUVA is saved for severe refractory disease.

VIII. Other Eczematous Eruptions.

A. Nummular (discoid) eczema is a chronic pruritic, inflammatory dermatitis occurring in the form of coin-shaped plaques (4-5 cm in diameter). It is especially prevalent during the winter months and in atopic persons. Treatment includes topical corticosteroids, oral dicloxacillin or erythromycin for infection, crude coal-tar pastes, and skin moisturizers.

B. **Lichen simplex chronicus (neurodermatitis)** is a circumscribed area of lichenification caused by repeated physical trauma (rubbing and scratching). It occurs in the anogenital area and on the nuchal areas, arms, legs, and ankles. **Treatment.** Stop the rubbing and scratching with antiinflammatory agents (crude coal tar and topical corticosteroids) covered by continuous dry occlusive gauze dressings. Intralesional corticosteroids are effective for small, localized areas. Treatment is needed long term and may be unsatisfactory.

URTICARIA

I. **Overview.** Urticaria is a common disorder that affects 15% to 20% of the population at some time. Urticaria is characterized by a transient pruritic, patchy eruption that consists of lightly erythematous papules or wheals with raised borders and blanched centers involving the superficial skin layers; involvement of the deeper layers and/or the submucosa is called *angioedema*. Lesions vary considerably in size, from 2 mm to more than 30 cm, and may be circular or irregularly shaped. The most common site for urticaria is the trunk, although lesions can occur on any part of the body. Urticaria has been divided into major groups:
A. **Acute urticaria** is defined as hives persisting for less than 4 to 6 weeks (usually 2-3 d). It occurs with a higher incidence in atopic persons. Commonly identified causes include foods, drugs, and infections, but in more than half of patients there is no identifiable cause.
B. **Angioedema.** Acute attacks are manifested as large irregular areas of subcutaneous swelling. Cause is similar to urticaria but may also include hereditary angioedema (see below) or, commonly, ACE inhibitors.
C. **Chronic urticaria** attacks that persist for 6 weeks or more. Patients usually are not atopic.
II. **Types of Urticaria.**
A. **Idiopathic.** Largest category; about one third of acute and two thirds of chronic cases of urticaria are idiopathic.
B. **Physical.** Approximately 15% of cases are physical. There are several types:
1. **Dermatographism** is a reaction to firm stroking of the skin that occurs within 1 to 3 minutes and lasts 5 to 10 minutes. It is not true urticaria, although it may be severe enough to require medical attention.
2. **Cholinergic urticaria.** Exercise and/or sweating is the provocative agent. It is the cause of 10% of reactions, affects young people, and can last 6 to 8 years. Lesions appear as 1- to 2-mm wheals on a confluent erythematous base and are found on the trunk and arms with sparing of the palms, soles, and axillae.
3. **Cold urticaria** is an uncommon reaction to cold and/or rewarming after cold exposure (cold winds are an effective stimulus). It can also be caused by syphilis. Diagnose by exposure of the skin to an ice cube.

4. **Solar urticaria** is a rare reaction caused by exposure to light. It appears as pruritus and erythema, followed by urticaria. Onset is sudden and it occurs in any age group.

5. **Delayed pressure urticaria** is a rare reaction caused by sustained pressure.

6. **Aquagenic urticaria** is a rare reaction caused by contact with water.

7. **Localized heat urticaria** is a rare reaction caused by hot water.

C. **Immunologic.** Examples include anaphylaxis, serum sickness, and atopic persons with seasonal exacerbations. Some common antigens include foods (fish, nuts, berries, eggs) and insect stings (bees, wasps, hornets, yellow jackets). Drugs can induce urticaria, especially PCN and sulfonamides. Urticaria can also be caused by immune complexes seen in systemic rheumatologic diseases (SLE, Sjögren's syndrome, rheumatic fever, juvenile rheumatoid arthritis, chronic hepatitis B and C, necrotizing vasculitis, and polymyositis), cryoglobulinemias, serum sickness, neoplastic disorders, transfusion reactions, Epstein–Barr virus, and streptococcal infections.

D. **Hereditary angioedema** is a potentially fatal autosomal dominant disease caused by the functional absence of C1-esterase inhibitor. This enables vascular permeability and potentially fatal recurrent acute angioedema of the skin, mucosa, and airway. One retrospective survey of 58 patients found that 40% had died by asphyxiation; average age at death was 39.

1. Occasionally, patients present with acute abdominal symptoms mimicking a surgical abdomen. Serum levels of C2 are normal during asymptomatic periods but decreased during an attack. C4 and CH-50 are low all the time. Low C1-esterase inhibitor levels are diagnostic. However, there are nonfunctioning alleles of C1-esterase inhibitor, so some persons with the disease have normal levels; a functional assay should be performed if clinically indicated.

2. **Treatment.** Patients with hereditary angioedema should be pre-treated with fresh frozen plasma before painful procedures or procedures known to induce attacks. Additionally, they can be treated with fresh frozen plasma to abort an ongoing attack. C1-esterase inhibitor is currently investigational but should have FDA approval soon. Long-term therapy includes enough danazol to prevent acute attacks (200 mg tid or less).

E. **Infections.** Urticaria is occasionally associated with acute or chronic protozoan, parasitic, bacterial, or viral infections. Sources such as sinusitis, dental abscesses, periodontal disease, gallbladder infection, chronic bronchitis, chronic UTIs, and low-grade fungal (athlete's foot) or yeast (*Candida* vaginitis) infections should be investigated in persons with chronic urticaria.

F. **Infestations** are most commonly due to scabies, caused by the mite *Sarcoptes scabiei*. See the section on scabies in Chapter 10 for details.

G. **Urticaria pigmentosa** is an uncommon disease with focal dermal infiltration of tissue mast cells. There can be infiltrates in other organs, as well with representative organ system disease. It manifests as brown patches that form a wheal and flare upon stroking.

17

DERMATOLOGY

H. Miscellaneous

1. **Neoplastic disorders.** Carcinoma (colorectal, lung, ovarian, uterine, liver), choriocarcinoma, Hodgkin's disease, lymphoma, leukemia, or myeloma.

2. **Endocrinopathy.** Hypothyroidism or hyperthyroidism, hyperparathyroidism, diabetes mellitus, menopause.

3. **Arthropod assault** (insect bite). A papular lesion, usually from flea or red ant bite.

4. **Psychogenic.** A diagnosis of exclusion, but psychogenic and emotional factors are contributory or aggravating in at least one fourth of chronic urticaria patients.

III. Diagnostic Tests.

A. Acute urticaria. Laboratory tests generally are not needed.

B. Chronic urticaria. If physical agents have been excluded as a cause, then judicious use of the following laboratory, radiographic, and pathology studies may provide clues to the diagnosis of an occult systemic illness. However, extensive work-up is expensive and rarely yields results.

1. **Routine tests**

a. **Laboratory:** CBC, chemistry profile, ESR, T4, TSH measurements, UA and urine culture, ANA.

b. **Radiographic:** CXR, sinus films, dental films.

2. **Selective tests** include cryoglobulin, hepatitis and syphilis serology, rheumatoid factor, serum complement, serum IgE, IgM.

3. **Skin biopsy** (if the ESR is elevated, to exclude urticarial vasculitis).

IV. Treatment.

A. Treatment as for anaphylaxis if concurrent anaphylaxis. See Chapter 2.

B. Hereditary angioedema does not respond to typical therapy as outlined below. See section on hereditary angioedema for management.

C. Eliminate or limit exposure to the causative agent.

D. Treat any underlying disease that may be a causative factor.

E. Symptomatic care

1. **Antihistamines**

a. **Classic H_1 blockers** include chlorpheniramine (Chlor-Trimeton) 4 mg q4-6h, cyproheptadine (Periactin) 4 to 8 mg q6h, diphenhydramine (Benadryl) 25 to 50 mg q6-8h, hydroxyzine (Atarax, Vistaril) 25 to 50 mg q6-8h, and promethazine (Phenergan) 12.5 to 25 mg q12-24h. Hydroxyzine is believed to be one of the most effective agents, and diphenhydramine and chlorpheniramine are less expensive and OTC.

b. **Nonsedating H_1 blockers** include fexofenadine (Allegra), loratadine (Claritin), and cetirizine (Zyrtec). They are equally effective compared to classic agents, are less sedating, and have simpler dosing schedules.

c. **H_2 blockers** (e.g., cimetidine [Tagamet], ranitidine [Zantac]) may be added in patients who do not respond to therapy with H_1 antagonists alone.

TABLE 17-1

POTENCY OF TOPICAL CORTICOSTEROIDS

Group*	Concentration (%)†	Generic Name‡
I	0.05	Betamethasone dipropionate
II	0.01	Amcinonide
	0.05	Fluocinonide
	0.25	Desoximetasone
III	0.5	Triamcinolone acetonide
	0.1	Betamethasone valerate
IV	0.05	Flurandrenolide
	0.025	Fluocinolone acetonide
V	0.1	Betamethasone valerate
VI	0.01	Fluocinolone acetonide
	0.03	Flumethasone pivalate
VII	0.2	Betamethasone valerate
	1-2.5	Hydrocortisone

Note: Use rule of nines: for tid application, 9 g of cream covers 1% of skin area daily.

*Potencies decrease from group I (strongest) to group VII (weakest).

†Increasing the concentration increases the potency. At equal concentrations, potency decreases as the viscosity of the substance increases.

‡Brand name drugs are available in a variety of strengths and vehicles (such as ointment, solution, cream, lotion).

Adapted from Habif TP: Clinical dermatology: A color guide to diagnosis and therapy, 4th ed. St. Louis, Mosby, 2003.

    d. **Oral β-agonists,** such as terbutaline (Brethine, Bricanyl), may be a useful adjunct to antihistamines in chronic urticaria.

    e. **Doxepin** (Adapin, Sinequan) is a potent H_1 blocker with efficacy comparable to, or greater than, hydroxyzine's.

2. **Topical application of capsaicin** (Zostrix) or local anesthetic can suppress wheal-and-flare reactions in local heat urticaria.

3. **Stress-related urticaria** (adrenergic urticaria) may respond to propranolol.

4. **Cold urticaria** may respond to doxepin or especially cyproheptadine 4 mg PO tid.

5. **Corticosteroids.** Topical or systemic corticosteroids should be reserved for patients with refractory symptoms. **Table 17-1** lists potency of topical corticosteroids. Compared to placebo, a short course (prednisone 40 mg × 3-5 d) is quite effective at controlling symptoms.

6. **New therapies under study**

    a. **Leukotriene inhibitors** including zileuton 600 mg qid, zafirlukast (Accolate) 10 mg bid, and montelukast have some marginal benefit but may be worth a try if other modalities have failed.

    b. **Other agents and therapies** include ketotifen (Zaditen), cyclosporine (Sandimmune), UVB phototherapy, and plasmapheresis. Calcium channel blockers can also be used as an adjuvant for refractory urticaria.

BIBLIOGRAPHY

Asawanonda P, Anderson RR, Chang Y, Taylor CR:: Pendulaser carbon dioxide resurfacing laser versus electrodesiccation with curettage in the treatment of isolated, recalcitrant psoriatic plaques. *J Am Acad Dermatol* 42:660-666, 2000.

Ellis CN, Krueger GG: Treatment of chronic plaque psoriasis by selective targeting of memory effector T lymphocytes. *N Engl J Med* 345:248-255, 2001.

Leonardi CL, Powers JL, Matheson RT, et al: Etanercept as monotherapy in patients with psoriasis. *N Engl J Med* 349:2014-2022, 2003.

Metze D, Reimann S, Beissert S, Luger T: Efficacy and safety of naltrexone, an oral opiate receptor antagonist, in the treatment of pruritus in internal and dermatological diseases. *J Am Acad Dermatol* 41:533-539, 1999.

Pacor ML, Di Lorenzo G, Corrocher R: Efficacy of leukotriene receptor antagonist in chronic urticaria. A double-blind, placebo-controlled comparison of treatment with montelukast and cetirizine in patients with chronic urticaria with intolerance to food additive and/or acetylsalicylic acid. *Clin Exp Allergy* 31:1607-1614, 2001.

Syed TA, Hadi SM, Qureshi ZA, et al: Treatment of external genital warts in men with imiquimod 2% in cream. A placebo-controlled, double-blind study. *J Infect* 41:148-151, 2000.

Van Doorn R, Van Haselen CW, van Voorst Vader PC, et al: Mycosis fungoides: Disease evolution and prognosis of 309 Dutch patients. *Arch Dermatol* 136: 504-510, 2000.

Psychiatry

Alison C. Abreu and Oladipo Kukoyi

Mental health concerns are present in more than half of primary care visits. The physician is obligated to determine if and how much of a patient's symptoms are psychological versus physical. Primary care physicians must be attuned to the high prevalence of mental health conditions in the clinical setting while efficiently determining which symptoms require further evaluation and treatment and which symptoms are best treated by providing consistent, regular, and thoughtful primary care.

NOTATION OF PSYCHIATRIC ILLNESS

I. **Axis 1.** Major psychiatric diagnosis (e.g., depression, schizophrenia).
II. **Axis 2.** Personality disorders (see Table 18-6).
III. **Axis 3.** Medical conditions relevant to understanding a patient's psychiatric illness.
IV. **Axis 4.** Psychosocial and environmental contributors (divorce, homelessness, low mental function, etc.).

MOOD DISORDERS

Major Depressive Disorder

I. **Overview.** Lifetime risk as high as 12% for men and 26% for women. Prevalence of major depression in the primary care setting is 5% to 10% and minor depression (not meeting DSM-IV criteria for major depression) is present in 10% to 20%.
II. **Risk factors** include female gender, prior episodes of major depression, history of depressive illness in first-degree relatives, ongoing alcohol or other substance abuse, prior suicide attempts, age 18 to 45 years, medical comorbidity, decreased social support, stressful life events, being unmarried, and poverty.
III. **Clues to possible depression in a primary care setting** include fatigue, somatic complaints (e.g., headache, backache, chest pain, dyspepsia, and limb pain), anxiety symptoms, depressed mood, weight loss or gain, or insomnia. Diagnostic criteria are given in **Box 18-1.**
IV. **Symptoms.**
A. **Emotional:** dysphoria, irritability, anhedonia, withdrawal.
B. **Cognitive:** self-criticism, sense of worthlessness or guilt, hopelessness, poor concentration, memory impairment, delusions or hallucinations.
C. **Vegetative:** fatigue, decreased energy, insomnia, hypersomnia, anorexia, psychomotor retardation or agitation, impaired libido.
D. **Somatic:** aches and pains. Most patients in primary care with depression complain of pain or fatigue.

BOX 18-1

DIAGNOSTIC CRITERIA FOR DEPRESSION

DSM-IV criteria for a major depressive episode include at least five of the following symptoms present for at least 2 weeks that represent a change from previous level of functioning. The symptoms must cause clinically significant distress or impairment in functioning and must not be attributable to the effects of substance use, general medical condition, or bereavement.

- Depressed mood (most of day, almost daily)*
- Diminished interest or pleasure in all or most activities
- Significant weight loss or gain or decrease or increase in appetite nearly every day
- Insomnia or hypersomnia
- Psychomotor retardation or agitation (observable by others)
- Fatigue or decreased level of energy
- Feelings of worthlessness or inappropriate guilt
- Poor concentration or indecisiveness
- Recurrent thoughts of death or suicidal ideation

Note: At least one of the above symptoms must be either depressed mood or loss of interest or pleasure.
*In children and adolescents there may be an irritable mood.

V. Evaluation.
A. History. Further evaluation includes assessment of:
1. Time course and severity.
2. Any prior episodes, type of treatment, and level of recovery.
3. Any history of manic or hypomanic episodes.
4. Presence of any other major psychiatric disorders (e.g., alcohol dependence, personality disorder).
5. Psychotic symptoms such as paranoid delusions.
6. Any suicidal ideation, plan, or intent.
B. Examination. Mental state exam, including level of alertness, orientation, mood, affect, thought content (hallucinations, delusions, suicidal/homicidal ideation, if present), thought processes (logical, circumstantial, tangential, or illogical), psychomotor activity, speech, insight, and judgment. The Mini Mental State Exam can help identify a delirium or dementia. Beck and Geriatric Depression Scale are patient administered (see **Boxes 18-2 and 18-3,** respectively). Obtain an initial score, then repeat periodically to assess response to treatment.
C. Lab tests. Screen for medical causes of depressive symptoms (if suspected by history or physical examination). Lab tests may include complete blood count with differential, electrolytes, kidney and liver functions, thyroid studies, urine drug screen, etc.
VI. Treatment.
A. Hospitalization is indicated if serious suicidal ideation is present. Suicide risk is difficult to assess because no screening tool has high sensitivity, but ask about a plan, intent, access to the means, and

BOX 18-2

BECK INVENTORY FOR THE SCREENING OF DEPRESSION

Name:

Date:

On this questionnaire are groups of statements. Please read each group of statements carefully. Then pick out the one statement in each group that best describes the way you have been feeling the past week including today. Circle the number beside the statement you picked. If several statements in the group seem to apply equally well, circle each one. Be sure to read all the statements in each group before making your choice.

1. 0 I do not feel sad. 1 I feel sad. 2 I am sad all the time and can't snap out of it. 3 I am so sad or unhappy that I can't stand it.

2. 0 I am not particularly discouraged about the future. 1 I feel discouraged about the future. 2 I feel I have nothing to look forward to. 3 I feel that the future is hopeless and that things cannot improve.

3. 0 I do not feel like a failure. 1 I feel I have failed more than the average person. 2 As I look back on my life, all I can see is a lot of failures. 3 I feel I am a complete failure as a person.

4. 0 I get as much satisfaction out of things as I used to. 1 I don't enjoy things the way I used to. 2 I don't get real satisfaction out of anything anymore. 3 I am dissatisfied and bored with everything.

5. 0 I don't feel particularly guilty. 1 I feel guilty a good part of the time. 2 I feel quite guilty most of the time. 3 I feel guilty all of the time.

6. 0 I don't feel I am being punished. 1 I feel I may be punished. 2 I expect to be punished. 3 I feel I am being punished.

7. 0 I don't feel disappointed in myself. 1 I am disappointed in myself. 2 I am disgusted with myself. 3 I hate myself.

8. 0 I have not lost interest in other people. 1 I am less interested in other people than I used to be. 2 I have lost most of my interest in other people. 3 I have lost all of my interest in other people.

9. 0 I make decisions about as well as I ever could. 1 I put off making decisions more than I used to. 2 I have greater difficulty in making decisions than before. 3 I can't make decisions at all anymore.

10. 0 I don't feel I look worse than I used to. 1 I am worried that I am looking old or unattractive. 2 I feel that there are permanent changes in my appearance that make me look unattractive. 3 I believe that I look ugly.

11. 0 I can work about as well as before. 1 It takes an extra effort to get started to do something. 2 I have to push myself very hard to do anything. 3 I can't do any work at all.

12. 0 I can sleep as well as usual. 1 I sleep somewhat more/less than usual. 2 I sleep a lot more/less than usual. 3 I sleep most of the day.

13. 0 I don't get tired more than usual. 1 I get tired more easily than I used to. 2 I get tired from doing almost anything. 3 I am too tired to do anything.

14. 0 My appetite is no worse than usual. 1 My appetite is not as good as it used to be. 2 My appetite is much worse now. 3 I have no appetite at all anymore.

Continued

> **BOX 18-2—Cont'd**
>
> **BECK INVENTORY FOR THE SCREENING OF DEPRESSION**
>
> 15. 0 I don't feel I am any worse than anybody else. 1 I am critical of myself for my weaknesses or mistakes. 2 I blame myself all the time for my faults. 3 I blame myself for everything bad that happens.
> 16. 0 I don't have any thoughts of killing myself. 1 I have thoughts of killing myself but would not carry them out. 2 I would like to kill myself. 3 I would kill myself if I had the chance.
> 17. 0 I am no more worried about my health than usual. 1 I am worried about physical problems such as aches and pains or upset stomach or constipation. 2 I am very worried about physical problems, and it is hard to think of much else. 3 I am so worried about my physical problems that I cannot think of anything else.
> 18. 0 I don't cry any more than usual. 1 I cry more now than I used to. 2 I cry all the time now. 3 I used to be able to cry, but now I can't cry even though I want to.
> 19. 0 I have not noticed any recent change in my interest in sex. 1 I am less interested in sex than I used to be. 2 I am much less interested in sex now. 3 I have lost interest in sex completely.
> 20. 0 I am no more irritated now than I ever am. 1 I get annoyed or irritated more easily than I used to. 2 I feel irritated all the time now. 3 I don't get irritated at all by the things that used to irritate me.
> 21. 0 I haven't lost much weight, if any lately. 1 I have lost more than 5 pounds. 2 I have lost more than 10 pounds. 3 I have lost more than 15 pounds. (I am purposely trying to lose weight by eating less. Yes___ No___)
>
> Scoring: 0-9, normal; 10-15, mild depressive symptoms; 16-19, mild-moderate depressive symptoms; 20-29, moderate-severe depressive symptoms; 30, severe depressive symptoms.

ability to contract for safety; careful documentation is important, as always. Admission is also indicated if the patient is a danger to self or others, if there is a complicating medical condition, or if there is lack of a support system at home. Admission may be indicated if the patient is experiencing psychosis as a sign of severe depression.

B. **Medication (Table 18-1).** Most antidepressants are believed to be equally effective in equivalent therapeutic doses. Factors to consider in selecting a particular agent include cost, side-effect profile, antidepressants previously tried, and safety in overdose. Counsel patients that it can take more than a week before any effect from antidepressant medication is noticed, and they should expect a 6- to 8-week latent period before the full effect is seen at therapeutic doses. To prevent relapse, continue medication for at least 6 to 12 months after achieving remission. For recurrent depression, consider chronic therapy.

1. **Second-generation, but first-line, antidepressants**
a. **Selective serotonin reuptake inhibitors** (SSRIs: fluoxetine, sertraline, citalopram, etc.).

BOX 18-3

GERIATRIC DEPRESSION SCALE

This may be administered in oral or written format. If written, the answer sheet must have printed Yes/No after each question. The subject is instructed to circle the better response. If given orally, the question may need to be repeated to get a response of "yes" or "no." The GDS seems to work well with other age groups.

1. Are you basically satisfied with your life? N
2. Have you dropped many of your activities and interests? Y
3. Do you feel that your life is empty? Y
4. Do you often get bored? Y
5. Are you hopeful about the future? N
6. Are you bothered by thoughts that you just cannot get out of your head? Y
7. Are you in good spirits most of the time? N
8. Are you afraid that something bad is going to happen to you? Y
9. Do you feel happy most of the time? N
10. Do you often feel helpless? Y
11. Do you often get restless and fidgety? Y
12. Do you prefer to stay home at night, rather than go out and do new things? Y
13. Do you frequently worry about the future? Y
14. Do you feel that you have more problems with memory than most? Y
15. Do you think it is wonderful to be alive now? N
16. Do you often feel downhearted and blue? Y
17. Do you feel pretty worthless the way you are now? Y
18. Do you worry a lot about the past? Y
19. Do you find life very exciting? N
20. Is it hard for you to get started on new projects? Y
21. Do you feel full of energy? N
22. Do you feel that your situation is hopeless? Y
23. Do you think that most people are better off than you are? Y
24. Do you frequently get upset over little things? Y
25. Do you frequently feel like crying? Y
26. Do you have trouble concentrating? Y
27. Do you enjoy getting up in the morning? N
28. Do you prefer to avoid social gatherings? Y
29. Is it easy for you to make decisions? N
30. Is your mind as clear as it used to be? N

Scoring: Count 1 point for each depressive answer shown after each question. 0 to 10, normal; 11 to 20, mild depression; 21 to 30, moderate or severe depression.

(1) Consider starting at lower doses to improve tolerability, especially in the elderly or others sensitive to side effects. Titrate up as needed. **Side effects vary and may include nausea, anorexia, insomnia or mild sedation, sweating, headache, tremor, sexual dysfunction, and nervousness (including akathisia).**

(2) SSRIs are considered safe for patients with cardiovascular disease. These antidepressants are favored in post-MI depression because

TABLE 18-1
COMPARISON OF ANTIDEPRESSANTS

Drug	Common Dose Range (mg/d)*	Dosage Schedule	Side Effects			
			Orthostatic Hypotension	Anticholinergic†	Sedation	Weight Gain
TRICYCLIC ANTIDEPRESSANTS‡						
Amitriptyline (Elavil)	150-200	qhs	++++	++++	++++	+++
Desipramine (Norpramin)	50-300	qhs	++++	++	+++	+
Imipramine (Tofranil)	150-200	qhs	++++	+++	+++	++
Nortriptyline (Pamelor)	50-150	qhs	++	++	++	+
SEROTONIN-SPECIFIC REUPTAKE INHIBITORS (SSRIs)						
Fluoxetine§ (Prozac)	20-40	qAM	Minimal to neutral with regard to sedative, anticholinergic, and orthostatic hypotensive side effects; may cause mild weight loss in some persons. May cause akathisia if titrated up too rapidly. Also GI side effects, anorgasmia, decreased libido. Escitalopram has fewer GI side effects than does citalopram.			
Paroxetine (Paxil)	20-40	qAM or qhs				
Fluvoxamine (Luvox)	120-200	qhs or bid				
Citalopram (Celexa)	20-40	qAM or qhs				
Escitalopram (Lexapro)	10-20	qd				
Sertraline (Zoloft)	75-150	qAM or qhs				

SEROTONIN-NONSELECTIVE REUPTAKE INHIBITORS

Venlafaxine (Effexor)	75-225	qd-tid	0	±	+	0
Duloxetine	40-60	qd	0	±	+	0
DOPAMINE ACTIVE						
Bupropion (Wellbutrin)	150-450	bid-tid	0	+	+	—
(Wellbutrin SR)	300-400	qd-bid	0	+	+	—
OTHER						
Nefazodone (Serzone)	300-500	bid	±	±	+	0
Mirtazapine (Remeron)	15-60	qhs	±	0	+++	++
Trazodone (Desyrel)	50-400	qhs-tid	+++	++	++++	+

*Doses should be lowered in the elderly.

†Blurred vision, constipation, dry mouth, urinary retention.

‡Therapeutic ranges: amitriptyline, >120 ng/mL; desipramine, >125 ng/mL; imipramine, >225 ng/mL; notriptyline, 50-150 ng/mL.

§Fluoxetine can be dosed 60 mg PO weekly for those stable on 20 mg/d.

Adapted from Knesper DJ, Rba MB, Schwenk TL.: *Primary Care Psychiatry.* Philadelphia, WB Saunders, 1997.

they are not associated with increased risk of ventricular arrhythmia and have antiplatelet effects.

(3) All SSRIs are contraindicated with MAOIs; a "wash-out" period is required if switching from an SSRI to an MAOI.

(4) Taper short-acting SSRIs over 1 to 2 weeks to avoid flulike discontinuation symptoms.

(5) Several are now available in generic form.

(6) **Several studies show no benefit over placebo (especially paroxetine) in pediatric and teenage patients. Avoid in these groups and be aware of potential limited efficacy in other groups as well.**

b. **Bupropion** (Wellbutrin), a norepinephrine–dopamine reuptake inhibitor. Very low incidence of sexual dysfunction. Safe in patients with history of cardiac disease. It may be especially useful in those with prominent apathy. May be added to SSRI therapy for augmentation. Longer-acting formulations improve compliance with once- or twice-daily dosing. Contraindicated in patients with seizure disorder (lowers seizure threshold, risk of seizures 0.4%) or history of bulimia or anorexia nervosa. Also used for smoking cessation (Zyban).

c. **Serotonin and norepinephrine reuptake inhibitors (SNRIs)**

(1) **Venlafaxine (Effexor).** Similar in action and side-effect profile to SSRIs. Monitor for blood pressure elevation.

(2) **Duloxetine (Cymbalta).** Newly approved antidepressant that is similar to venlafaxine. Also approved for diabetic neuropathy. Approved in Europe for stress incontinence.

(3) **Mirtazepine (Remeron).** Sedating, useful for patients with comorbid sleep disturbance (give at bedtime). Often increases appetite.

(4) **Trazodone (Desyrel).** Rarely used as an antidepressant, but low doses (50-200 mg) are often used with other antidepressants as a sleep aid at bedtime. Risk of priapism is 1:6000.

2. Tricyclic antidepressants (TCAs)

a. Although no longer first line, this class of antidepressants is useful in certain circumstances. They are less expensive than the newer agents, they are often sedating and can help restore sleep, and they are useful in managing chronic or neuropathic pain. They are a poor choice in patients who may take an overdose, and they may be fatal in overdoses around 2000 mg or more in adults. In selecting a TCA, consider the patient's sedation requirements as well as ability to tolerate orthostatic hypotension, weight gain, and anticholinergic adverse effects (see Table 18-1). TCAs are usually taken qhs to take advantage of sedating effects. *Note:* Nortriptyline (Pamelor) has the lowest risk for orthostatic hypotension of all TCAs, making it a safer choice in the geriatric patient.

b. All TCAs can cause slowing of cardiac conduction. They are contraindicated in the first 6 weeks after an MI because of increased risk of ventricular arrhythmia. In patients with preexisting first-degree AV block, blood levels and ECG monitoring are recommended.

c. A therapeutic trial usually is considered >100 mg/d of amitriptyline or its equivalent for at least 3 weeks. There are therapeutic window plasma levels for nortriptyline, desipramine, and imipramine.

3. **MAOIs** (phenelzine, selegiline) are mainly used in depression refractory to the other treatments. Consider consulting a psychiatrist before starting because of the serious adverse effect profile and diet restrictions.

4. **Augmentation agents** (methylphenidate, lithium, T3 [Cytomel]). Consider adding a stimulant in the patient with prominent apathy, or for a more immediate effect while the traditional antidepressant takes effect. Stimulants can be very useful in a post-stroke patient failing rehabilitation. T3 or lithium can be added when the patient is getting partial but not complete symptom relief at therapeutic doses of the traditional antidepressant. See section below for more information about prescribing lithium.

C. **Psychotherapy or counseling.** Supportive therapy is a cornerstone of family medicine care and always part of depression treatment. Other types of psychotherapy, including cognitive behavior therapy and interpersonal psychotherapy, have been shown to be helpful in mild and moderate depression, alone or with medication. Studies indicate that patients who receive both psychotherapy and medication have improved outcomes compared to those who receive only one treatment type. Counseling is more likely to be effective if the patient desires this form of treatment.

D. **Electroconvulsive therapy** is the most effective and rapid method of treating severe major depression. It is indicated for patients with poor response to medications, poor tolerance of usual antidepressants, severe vegetative symptoms, or psychotic features. It is considered very safe and has few contraindications. The decision to administer ECT should be made by a psychiatrist.

Depression in Women

Women have a higher lifetime risk of depression than men.

I. **Depression and Pregnancy.** For a variety of reasons, pregnancy and the postpartum period are the most vulnerable times in a woman's life with regard to her risk of onset of depression. Untreated maternal depression can cause adverse cognitive and psychologic effects in the infant. It also has adverse implications for the mother's long-term mental health, maternal–infant bonding, her partner, and her other children.

A. **Factors contributing to postpartum depression are usually multifactorial:** There are changes in family, self-identification, employment, finances, marital relations, sexuality, hormones, and socialization that are inherent in having a child. Psychotherapy that targets some of these stressors (interpersonal psychotherapy) has been shown to be as effective as medication for treating postpartum depression. The highest risk time for "postpartum depression" is depression during pregnancy. Screening tools such as the Edinburgh

Postnatal Depression Scale (EPDS) can be used during pregnancy and following delivery to screen for high-risk patients.

B. Although TCAs appear to be safe for use during pregnancy and breastfeeding, some women prefer to minimize medication exposure. Fluoxetine has the most data concerning its use in pregnancy, and SSRIs are considered first-line treatment. During breastfeeding, sertraline and paroxetine confer the lowest detectable levels of medication in nursing infants. **Paroxetine (Paxil) is associated with an increase in birth defects and neonatal withdrawal. It should be avoided in pregnancy.** Data on other SSRIs is limited but fluoxetine appears safe.

II. Premenstrual Dysphoric Disorder (PMDD). See Chapter 13.

Bipolar Affective Disorder

I. Overview.

A. Lifetime prevalence is 2% to 5%. It affects males and females equally. Age of onset is usually late teens to mid-30s.

B. Bipolar affective disorder type 1 is characterized by one or more manic episodes or by mixed (manic and depressive) episodes. Persons affected often have a history of one or more episodes of depression. More than 90% of persons with a manic episode have future episodes of depression or mania.

C. Bipolar affective disorder type 2. Hypomanic episodes (not severe enough to meet criteria for mania) are the hallmark along with recurrent depression. Medication treatment is the same as in type 1 bipolar disorder.

II. DSM-IV Criteria for Manic Episode. A distinct period of abnormally and persistently elevated, expansive, or irritable mood lasting at least 1 week (or any duration if hospitalized). During this period, **the patient must exhibit at least three of the following (four if mood is only irritable):**

A. Grandiosity.

B. Decreased need for sleep.

C. Pressured speech or unusual talkativeness.

D. Racing thoughts or flight of ideas.

E. Distractibility.

F. Psychomotor agitation or increased goal-directed activity (social, work, school, or sexual).

G. Excessive involvement in pleasurable activities with a high potential for painful consequences (e.g., unrestrained buying sprees, sexual indiscretions).

H. Symptoms are not better accounted for by another general medical, mental, or substance abuse disorder.

I. Symptoms cause pronounced impairment of functioning, require hospitalization, or are associated with psychotic features.

III. Evaluation.

A. History. Interviews with family or friends are essential. Often a family history of affective disorders and/or alcoholism is present in first-degree relatives. In patient older than 40 years with a first manic episode, look for medical causes.

B. Examination. Evaluate for a medical cause, such as drug abuse or intoxication.

C. Laboratory tests. Tests are needed before starting lithium carbonate, carbamazepine, or valproate (see below under specific medications). Labs can also be used to rule out some causes of secondary mania, such as substance abuse, megaloblastic anemia, hyperglycemia and hypoglycemia, thyroid dysfunction, SLE, syphilis, HIV, medication (e.g., steroid) effect, and liver disease induced by alcohol or other substances.

IV. Treatment. Hospitalization is usually indicated for full manic syndromes, because the patient's well-being is at risk due to impaired judgment. This includes a risk of death from exhaustion. Consider ECT in medication nonresponders and pregnant women.

V. Medications.

A. Antipsychotics are often required initially for sedation or to control behavior or psychotic symptoms. All work well and have some mood-stabilizing properties, but only the newer ones (olanzapine, risperidone, aripiprazole, quetiapine, and ziprasidone) are FDA approved for treatment of bipolar mania. They should be used as an adjunct, except for olanzapine, which may be used alone. Symbiax (olanzapine plus fluoxetine) is FDA approved for treatment of mania. Injectable forms of typical and atypical antipsychotics are available for acute agitation and patients unable to take oral medications. Benzodiazepines are a useful adjunct for sedation.

B. Antimanic drugs (mood stabilizers).

1. **Lithium carbonate.** Best-studied and usually the drug of choice for mania, with response rates of 80%. Up to 3 weeks is generally needed at therapeutic blood levels before clinical effects are noted. Lithium is also effective in treating recurrent depression, both unipolar type and depression associated with bipolar illness. It is the only drug shown to be effective at reducing suicide risk.

   a. **Dose is 600 to 2400 mg/day.** Start with divided doses initially to minimize GI side effects, then change to single dose qhs to minimize potential tremor, polyuria, and kidney damage.

   b. **Monitor serum trough levels** (12 hours after last dose) at least twice weekly initially and then every 2 to 3 months for maintenance. In acute mania, 0.9 to 1.4 mEq/L levels are needed. Maintenance levels range from 0.4 to 0.8 mEq/L (elderly patients require the higher range).

   c. **Side effects** include polyuria, polydipsia, muscle weakness, tremor, GI upset or diarrhea, hypothyroidism, acne, weight gain, leukocytosis, and sedation. Psoriasis is also possible.

   d. **Toxicity can occur at serum levels just over the therapeutic range.** Mild toxicity symptoms are exacerbations of side effects listed above. More severe toxicity includes primarily neurologic manifestations

PSYCHIATRY **18**

(lethargy, confusion, coma, seizures, ataxia, dysarthria, nystagmus) and nephropathy. Nephrogenic diabetes insipidus and chronic renal failure may result.

e. **Lab monitoring.** Baseline tests before starting lithium include BUN and creatinine, pregnancy test, TSH/free T_4 (lithium may induce hypothyroidism), EKG for patient older than 40 years, and a CBC. During the first 6 months of lithium treatment, monitor BUN and creatinine every 2 to 3 months and thyroid function tests once or twice. Subsequently check creatinine and thyroid functions (q6-12mo) while patient is receiving maintenance lithium treatment.

f. **Warnings.** Avoid in pregnancy (especially first trimester) unless benefits outweigh risks. Lithium is associated with cardiac malformations (8%) and Ebstein's anomaly (2%) in infants exposed in utero. Dehydration and sodium-restricted diets may increase lithium levels and risk of toxicity.

g. **Drug interactions.** Any medication that can decrease renal clearance (e.g., NSAIDs); sodium-depleting diuretics should be used with caution.

2. **Valproic acid (Depakene, Depakote)** is a second-line treatment for mania. However, it is the preferred choice in rapid cycling and mixed mania. The usual starting dose is 15 mg/kg per day in two or more divided doses. Therapeutic blood level is not established for mania. Increase the dose until therapeutic response or adverse effects occur. Obtain baseline hematologic and hepatic tests. Instruct patients about potential symptoms of leukopenia and liver disease. Depakote may be less likely to produce GI side effects than Depakene. Avoid use in pregnancy unless benefits outweigh risks. One percent of infants exposed in utero develop neural tube defects. Concomitant administration of folic acid, 1 mg daily, may reduce risk to fetus.

3. **Carbamazepine (Tegretol) is another alternative** to lithium for treatment of mania. Dosage is 600 to 2000 mg/d for acute mania. Monitor for leukopenia and liver dysfunction. Avoid use in pregnancy unless benefits outweigh risks.

4. **Lamotrigine (Lamictal) is an anticonvulsant** recently FDA approved for bipolar affective disorder. It shows particular efficacy for preventing bipolar depression and is now considered first line. Dose should be titrated up slowly to 100 to 200 mg daily to prevent rare but potentially fatal Stevens–Johnson reaction. There are multiple drug interactions to be aware of, particularly with other anticonvulsants.

ANXIETY DISORDERS

I. **Overview.** Anxiety is defined as unpleasant and unwarranted feelings of apprehension sometimes accompanied by physiologic symptoms.

II. **Types.** Generalized anxiety disorder, panic disorder, agoraphobia, social or simple phobias, obsessive–compulsive disorder, and posttraumatic stress disorder.

III. Differential Diagnosis.

A. Psychiatric. Anxious depression, drug abuse or withdrawal (alcohol, benzodiazepines), stimulant use (caffeine, amphetamines), some personality disorders, akathisia in patients on antipsychotic medications.

B. Medical

1. **Cardiovascular** (e.g., angina, cardiac arrhythmias, MI).

2. **Respiratory** (e.g., asthma, COPD, hyperventilation, hypoxia, PE).

3. **Endocrine** (e.g., hypoglycemia, hyperthyroidism, menopause, pheochromocytoma, Cushing's syndrome).

4. **Neurologic** (e.g., delirium, multiple sclerosis, partial complex seizures, postconcussion syndrome, vestibular dysfunction).

5. **Drugs** (e.g., theophylline, bronchodilators, steroids, calcium channel blockers, neuroleptics, anticholinergics).

6. **Gastroesophageal reflux**

Generalized Anxiety Disorder

I. Overview. Generalized anxiety disorder is probably the most common anxiety disorder in primary care, with lifetime prevalence of 5%. Onset is gradual, with peak in the teen years. Patients are at high risk for other comorbid psychiatric disorders.

II. DSM-IV Diagnosis.

A. Excessive anxiety and worry about a number of issues, occurring on most days for at least 6 months.

B. Difficulty controlling the worry

C. The anxiety and worry are associated with at least 3 of the following 6 symptoms for the past 6 months:

1. Restlessness or feeling on edge.

2. Irritability.

3. Easy fatigability.

4. Difficulty concentrating.

5. Muscle tension.

6. Sleep disturbance.

D. Focus of the anxiety and worry does not relate to another major emotional disorder (e.g., depression).

E. Anxiety causes significant distress or impairment in functioning.

F. The symptoms are not attributable to substance use or a medical condition and are not present only during the course of a mood, psychotic, or developmental disorder.

III. Treatment.

A. Therapy

1. **Psychotherapy.** Many patients with mild symptoms can be treated with supportive counseling and education without need for medication.

2. **Other therapies.** Relaxation training and cognitive therapy.

PSYCHIATRY

18

B. **General measures** include regular exercise, adequate sleep, avoidance of caffeine and alcohol, and resolution of underlying stressors (e.g., credit counseling for financial burden).

C. **Medications**

1. **SSRIs.** Several have received FDA approval for treatment of GAD, and all are probably effective. Use in doses similar to those for panic disorder (see below). In select patients you may add a benzodiazepine for first several weeks of treatment, because it has a quicker onset of action and prevents the potential initial side effect of increased anxiety with SSRIs.

2. **Benzodiazepines** are usually for short-term use with no long-term efficacy proven. Use the lowest dose that alleviates anxiety. Drugs with longer half-lives may be easier to taper and reduce incidence of dependence. May cause rebound anxiety with taper or withdrawal. Good choices include clonazepam (Klonopin) and lorazepam (Ativan). Avoid alprazolam (Xanax).

3. **Venlafaxine (Effexor)** is FDA approved for GAD and considered an alternative to SSRIs. Duloxetine has similar properties and should perform similarly.

4. **TCAs** are also effective for GAD. Like SSRIs, they take at least 2 to 3 weeks to become effective. May concomitantly target sleep disturbance.

5. **β-Blockers.** Propranolol (Inderal) may help physical symptoms such as racing heart but has no effect on the psychic component of anxiety. Can also be used for performance anxiety.

6. **Buspirone** clinically appears less effective than other agents. Start 5 mg PO tid and increase to typical dose of 20 to 30 mg/d. Takes 2 weeks to be effective. Nonsedating and little abuse potential.

Panic Disorder

I. **Overview.** Estimated lifetime prevalence is 2% to 5%; it is more common in women. Patients with panic disorder are frequent users of the medical system. About one third of patients with panic disorder have comorbid major depression.

II. **DSM-IV Diagnosis.** Recurrent unexplained panic attacks (discrete periods of intense fear) **(Box 18-4).**

A. **At least one of the attacks** has been followed by 1 month (or more) of at least one of the following:

1. Concern about having future attacks
2. Worry about consequences of the attack
3. Change in behavior related to the attacks

B. **Panic attacks are not substance induced,** related to a general medical condition, or better accounted for by another mental illness.

C. During the attack at least four of the symptoms listed in Box 18-4 develop quickly and peak within 10 minutes.

BOX 18-4

SYMPTOMS OF PANIC ATTACKS

Palpitations or tachycardia

Trembling or shaking

Nausea or abdominal discomfort

Feeling dizzy, unsteady, or faint

Fear of losing control or going crazy

Derealization (feelings of unreality) *or*

Depersonalization (feeling detached from oneself)

Sweating

Feelings of dyspnea

Chest pain or discomfort

Fear of dying

Paresthesias

Flushing or chilling

Feelings of choking

III. Treatment.

A. Medications

1. **Serotonergic agents are the drugs of choice.** These include the SSRIs and SNRIs. Bupropion and buspirone have no role in the treatment of panic disorder. Start at lowest dose and increase after first week as tolerated (e.g., fluoxetine 10 mg PO qod for week 1, 10 mg qd for week 2, and then 20 mg qd for week 3). Monitor for initial worsening of anxiety secondary to drug side effect. It usually resolves with time, but consider a benzodiazepine short term to temporize anxiety symptoms until medication becomes effective.

2. **Tricyclic antidepressants** are also effective for panic disorder. Start at low end of the dose range and gradually increase dose as tolerated to target symptoms.

3. **Benzodiazepines** have a quicker onset of action than other drugs; use as a short-term adjunct to SSRIs if initial paradoxical anxiety arises. They may be used long term if patients fail treatment or are unable to tolerate SSRIs or TCAs.

B. Psychotherapy

1. **Supportive therapy** is always indicated.

2. **Cognitive behavior therapy** (CBT) is often very effective. Its efficacy is comparable to that of medication.

III. Agoraphobia is an intense fear of and resulting avoidance of places or situations from which escape may be difficult (or embarrassing). Furthermore, the person worries about having a panic attack in that setting. It often co-occurs with panic disorder. Treatment is the same as for panic disorder.

Social Phobias and Other Phobias

  I. **Overview.** Social phobia has a lifetime prevalence of 13%, with onset most common in the mid-teens. Other specific phobias are more common in females, and impairment is usually minimal.

 II. **DSM-IV Criteria.**

  A. Persistent fear of humiliation or embarrassment in certain social situations (social phobia) or irrational fear of other circumscribed stimuli (specific phobia).

  B. Exposure to the particular stimulus provokes anxiety, which may include a situationally bound panic attack.

  C. The person usually realizes that the fear is excessive.

  D. The fear results in avoidance of the stimulus that interferes with the patient's social environment or produces significant distress.

  E. The fear or avoidance is not attributable to substance use, a general medical condition, or another mental disorder.

III. **Treatment.**

  A. Systematic desensitization and exposure (for specific phobias) and cognitive behavior therapy (for social phobias).

  B. β-Blockers may be effective in treating performance-anxiety symptoms.

  C. Drugs used in generalized social phobias include SSRIs and SNRIs.

Obsessive–Compulsive Disorder

  I. **Overview.** Lifetime prevalence of OCD is 2.5%. Onset is usually in adolescence or early adulthood. This condition is frequently difficult to treat; consider psychiatric consultation to optimize management.

 II. **DSM-IV Diagnosis.** Obsessions or compulsions that significantly interfere with daily functioning because of distress or time consumption.

  A. **Obsessions are recurrent, persistent thoughts** that are experienced as intrusive and inappropriate. Examples include fear of contamination and constant worry about performing inappropriate or dangerous acts. The person recognizes the thoughts as a product of his or her own mind and attempts to ignore or suppress them.

  B. **Compulsions are repetitive, purposeful acts** performed in response to an obsession or according to certain rules. They include repetitive hand washing, checking rituals, organization rituals, and ritualistic counting. These are designed to neutralize or prevent discomfort. In general, they are recognized by the patient as unreasonable.

III. **Treatment** is generally not curative but can produce significant improvement.

  A. **Medications**

  1. **SSRIs.** Start at low dose and titrate to doses higher than those used for depression (e.g., fluoxetine [Prozac] start 20 mg daily; usual daily dose 40 to 80 mg). If a therapeutic trial with one SSRI fails, another one may be efficacious. Venlafaxine and duloxetine are alternatives.

2. **Clomipramine (Anafranil).** Start with 25 mg and titrate up to 150 to 250 mg daily. Give in divided doses with meals to minimize GI side effects or at bedtime to minimize sedation.

B. **Behavior therapy** uses exposure and response prevention to limit the dysfunction that results from the obsessions or compulsions.

Posttraumatic Stress Disorder

I. **Overview.** Lifetime prevalence is 1% to 14%. PTSD can occur at any age. Symptoms usually begin within 3 months after the inciting trauma.

II. **DSM-IV Diagnosis Criteria.** PTSD occurs in persons who experienced an extraordinarily distressing event (combat, sexual abuse or rape, natural disasters) involving self or others. In addition, the person's response includes intense fear or helplessness.

A. **PTSD is characterized by** persistent re-experiencing of the event in at least one of the following ways:

1. Intrusive, recurrent recollections of the event.
2. Recurrent distressing dreams of the event.
3. Sudden sense of reliving the experience (flashbacks, hallucinations).
4. Intense distress with exposure to symbols or representations of the event (e.g., anniversaries).

B. **Results in avoidant behavior** of stimuli associated with the trauma or decreased responsiveness to the external world (psychic numbing).

C. PTSD is **associated with** two or more symptoms of increased arousal (insomnia, irritability, anger, poor concentration, hypervigilance, or exaggerated startle).

D. **The disturbance lasts more than 1 month** and causes significant distress or functional impairment.

III. **Treatment.**

A. **Supportive therapy** that is appropriate for grief reaction.

B. **Group therapy** may be helpful.

C. **SSRIs are efficacious.** Prazosin, antipsychotics, mood stabilizers, and topiramate can be helpful adjuncts.

MEDICALLY UNEXPLAINED SYMPTOMS

I. **Overview.** Medically unexplained symptoms account for more than half of all visits to primary care. A variety of underlying causes can lead to medically unexplained symptoms, including failure to identify an existing medical process, patient misrepresentation of symptoms (e.g., malingering, factitious disorder), and most commonly, physical symptoms in response to psychologic stressors (e.g., somatization, conversion disorder).

II. **Somatization.**

A. **Somatization** includes a spectrum that ranges from exaggerated stress responses (e.g., anxiety-related headaches, a student who experiences a stomach ache before a test) to, at its most severe, somatization disorder.

18

PSYCHIATRY

Somatization is very common and often coexists with other psychiatric conditions, particularly depression, anxiety, and substance abuse/dependence.

B. Somatization disorder. History of multiple physical complaints starting before age 30 that interferes with functioning (work, home, etc.). Should have all of the following at some time: four pain complaints, two GI symptoms (bloating, cramps, etc.), one sexual symptom, and one neurologic symptom. Somatization disorder (in contrast to somatization) is rare.

C. Treatment. Once an appropriate work-up has ruled out medical pathology, patients with somatization are best managed in the primary care setting with frequent, regular clinic visits to reassess symptoms and provide reassurance, avoidance of emergency department care and multiple providers, and avoidance of unnecessary and potentially risky evaluations and treatments. Studies have shown this strategy can reduce costs and improve both patient and physician satisfaction.

III. Related Disorders.

A. Hypochondriasis. Patients are convinced that there is something serious or mortally wrong with them (e.g., cancer, MS, ALS) despite repeated negative evaluations.

B. Conversion disorder. Patients act out a stereotypical but physiologically unlikely scenario (e.g., pseudoseizure, paralysis, blindness). Disorder is often exacerbated during times of discrete stress (e.g., after an argument with a spouse).

C. Factitious disorder. Self-induced illness, e.g., purposeful hypoglycemia from insulin, poor wound healing from repeated, purposeful trauma. Common in health care professionals.

D. Malingering. Purposefully faking symptoms, generally to remove oneself from a situation (e.g., to get out of jail, to get disability). Common in antisocial personality disorder, drug abuse, etc.

SUBSTANCE-USE DISORDERS

I. Overview (Box 18-5, Table 18-2, and Table 18-3).

A. Epidemiology. Marijuana is the most commonly used illicit drug, with 10 million current users. One-third of the U.S. population has tried marijuana at least once. Cocaine is used by 2 million Americans. Substance use rates are highest in ages 18 to 25 years. Substance use is involved in 50% of all highway deaths and over 50% of domestic violence.

B. Substance-*dependence* DSM-IV criteria. Maladaptive pattern of substance use leading to significant impairment or distress with at least three of the following occurring within a 12-month period:

1. **Tolerance** (increased amount of substance required to produce desired effect).

BOX 18-5
DRUGS OF ABUSE
OPIOIDS
Heroin
Hydromorphone
Oxycodone
Methadone
Meperidine
HALLUCINOGENS
Phencyclidine (PCP)
Lysergic acid diethylamide (LSD)
Mescaline
Psilocybin
MDMA (3,4-methylenedioxymethamphetamine, "ecstasy")
DEPRESSANTS
Alcohol
Benzodiazepines
Barbiturates
Methaqualone
Meprobamate
Glutethimide
Ethchlorvynol
STIMULANTS
Cocaine
Amphetamines
CANNABINOIDS
Marijuana
Hashish

Adapted from Hyman SE, Tesar GE: *Manual of Psychiatric Emergencies*, 3rd ed. Boston, Little, Brown, 1994.

2. **Withdrawal syndrome,** or using a substance to relieve withdrawal symptoms.
3. **Substance taken in larger amounts** or over longer periods than intended.
4. **Persistent desire or unsuccessful attempts to cut down use.**
5. **Significant amount of time spent in obtaining, consuming, or recovering from the substance.**
6. **Important social or occupational activities reduced because of substance use.**
7. **Persistent use despite knowledge of social, psychologic, or physical problems** caused by its use.
C. Substance-*abuse* DSM-IV criteria (Box 18-6).
1. Maladaptive pattern of use leading to a significant impairment or distress with at least one of the following within a 12-month period:
a. Recurrent substance use resulting in a failure to fulfill major role obligations at work, school, or home.

TABLE 18-2
INTOXICATION AND OVERDOSE

Signs or symptoms	Opioids	Depressants	Stimulants	Hallucinogens	Phencyclidine (PCP)
Anxiety	−	+	+	+	+
Arrhythmia	−	−		−	−
Coma	+	+	−	+	+
Delirium	+	−	+	+	+
Diaphoresis	+	+	+	+	+
Euphoria	+	+	+	+	+
Hallucinations	−	−	+	+	+
Hypertension	+	−	+	+	+
Hyperthermia	−	−	+	+	+
Hypotension	+	−	−	−	−
Nausea and vomiting	+	−	+	+	+
Nystagmus	−	+	−	−	+
Pupils, dilated	−	−	+	+	−
Pupils, pinpoint	+	−	−	−	−
Reflexes increased	−	+	+	−	+
Respiratory depression	+	+	+	−	±
Seizures	−	−	+	+	+
Tachycardia	−	−	+	+	+
Tremor	−	−	+	+	+
Violent or bizarre behavior	−	+	+	+	+

Compiled from Hyman SE, Tesar GE: *Manual of Psychiatric Emergencies*, 3rd ed. Boston, Little, Brown, 1994.

TABLE 18-3
WITHDRAWAL

Signs or Symptoms	Opioids	Depressants	Stimulants
Anxiety	+	+	−
Depression	−	+	+
Fatigue	−	−	+
Hallucinations	−	+	+
Hypertension	+	+	−
Hypotension (orthostatic)	−	+	−
Insomnia	+	+	−
Nausea and vomiting	+	+	−
Pupils, dilated	+	−	−
Reflexes, hyperactive	−	+	−
Seizures	−	+	−
Tachycardia	+	+	−

Compiled from Hyman SE, Tesar GE: *Manual of Psychiatric Emergencies*, 3rd ed. Boston, Little, Brown, 1994.

    b. Recurrent use in situations where use is physically hazardous (driving while intoxicated).

    c. Recurrent substance abuse–related legal problems.

    d. Continued use despite knowledge of having a persistent/recurring social or interpersonal problem that is caused or worsened by the substance use.

  2. Symptoms have never met criteria for substance *dependence* for this class of substance.

Alcoholism

  I. Prevalence. Lifetime prevalence of alcohol abuse or dependence is 15% to 20% in men. Male alcoholics outnumber female alcoholics 5:1.

  II. Suspect alcohol abuse if any of the complaints in Box 18-6 are present.

  III. Complications of alcohol abuse are listed in **Box 18-7.**

  IV. Alcohol-Withdrawal Syndromes.

  A. Uncomplicated alcohol withdrawal begins 12 to 18 hours after cessation of drinking. Peaks between 24 and 48 hours. Untreated, subsides

BOX 18-6
SYMPTOMS AND SIGNS SUGGESTIVE OF ALCOHOL ABUSE

Chronic anxiety or tension

Chronic depression

Frequent falls or minor injuries

Headaches or blackouts

Insomnia

Legal or marital problems

Seizures

Vague GI problems

BOX 18-7

COMPLICATIONS OF ALCOHOL ABUSE

Cardiomyopathy

Dementia

Depression

Erectile dysfunction

Gastritis or peptic ulcer disease

Hypertension

Insomnia

Liver disease (cirrhosis, ascites)

Myopathy

Nutritional deficiencies

Pancreatitis

Peripheral neuropathy

---

within 7 days. Characterized by tremors, nausea, vomiting, tachycardia, and hypertension.

B. Alcohol seizures occur 7 to 38 hours after cessation of alcohol and peak at 24 to 48 hours. Phenytoin is not useful in preventing seizures. However, lorazepam 2 mg IV given after a first seizure will reliably prevent the majority of recurrent seizures.

C. Alcohol-induced psychotic disorder, with hallucinations. Onset is within 48 hours of cessation and may last 1 week or more. Characterized by unpleasant auditory hallucinations without evidence of delirium.

D. Alcohol-withdrawal delirium (delirium tremens). May begin 2 or 3 days after cessation and peak in 4 or 5 days. Typically lasts 3 days but can persist for weeks. Symptoms include mild fever, autonomic hyperarousal, and delirium. Important to monitor closely in the hospital because of risk of mortality if untreated.

V. Evaluation.

A. Screening with CAGE questions. Two positive questions have 85% sensitivity and 90% specificity in detecting problems with alcohol. One positive answer may be significant:

1. Have you ever felt you should **c**ut down on your drinking?
2. Have people **a**nnoyed you by criticizing your drinking?
3. Have you ever felt bad or **g**uilty about your drinking?
4. Have you ever had a drink first thing in the morning to steady your nerves or get rid of a hangover (**e**ye-opener)?

B. History. Ask about previous alcohol problems and about prior treatment for detoxification or in a rehabilitation program. Determine history of DWI (driving while intoxicated); history of public intoxication charges, fights while intoxicated, other legal complications, and family history of alcohol abuse.

C. Physical exam. Early findings may include hepatomegaly, tremor, or mild peripheral neuropathy. In later stages, sequelae such as pneumonia, hypertension, Wernicke's syndrome (ophthalmoplegia, ataxia, and confusion), Korsakoff's syndrome (amnesia, disorientation, impairment of recent memory, and confabulation), gynecomastia, and spider angiomas may occur.

D. Laboratory tests. Blood alcohol level, CBC, liver enzymes, PT/PTT, general screen. Consider other tests: hepatitis B and C, RPR, vitamin B_{12}, folate, Mg, amylase, UA, urine drug screen, stool guaiac, CXR, TB skin test, and HIV based on risk factors and clinical situation.

VI. Management.

A. Psychotherapy includes cognitive behavior therapy that stresses goal setting, self-monitoring, identifying antecedents to drinking, learning alternative coping skills, and social skills training. Total abstinence and relapse prevention are the goals.

B. Alcoholics Anonymous. Encourage patient to attend AA meetings.

C. Detoxification may be required if tolerance or withdrawal is present.

1. **Vitamins.** To prevent Wernicke–Korsakoff syndrome, give thiamine 50 to 100 mg IV or IM immediately and then 100 mg PO daily. Additional treatment includes folate 1 mg PO daily and multivitamin daily.

2. **Benzodiazepines** should be used to decrease withdrawal symptoms in medically unstable patients and as prophylaxis in patients with history of DTs. **The traditional "Librium taper" (chlordiazepoxide) has fallen out of favor** and a symptom-based regimen is preferred.

a. **In medically stable patients,** benzodiazepine treatment is necessary only if three of seven signs or symptoms of withdrawal occur: temperature >38.3° C, pulse >110 bpm, SBP >160 mm Hg, DBP >100 mm Hg, nausea, vomiting, or tremors. **Of course, be sure the patient does not have another illness such as sepsis, etc.**

b. **Diazepam (Valium)** 5 to 10 mg IV q5min until the patient is calm and comfortable is recommended. In patients with severe symptoms of withdrawal, up to 500 mg IV (yes, *500 mg;* this is not a typo) over 60 to 90 minutes may rarely be required. Patients may need no further doses because of the long half-life of diazepam. An alternative is lorazepam 1 to 2 mg IV q5min until symptoms are controlled.

c. Give additional doses when the patient becomes symptomatic. **Overall, this strategy reduces the total dose of benzodiazepines needed and reduces hospital stays significantly.**

d. **Oxazepam and lorazepam** are good choices in patients with significant liver disease because they are minimally metabolized by the liver.

3. **β-Blockers are sometimes used with benzodiazepines** to reduce autonomic nervous system hyperactivity. The drug masks symptoms of withdrawal, however, which complicates assessment.

4. **Avoid the antipsychotics, which can lower the seizure threshold and can reduce thermoregulation.** Use adequate doses of benzodiazepines. If benzodiazepines are unsuccessful, consider adding phenobarbital or propofol (realizing that respiratory support may be necessary).

PSYCHIATRY

18

D. Disulfiram (Antabuse). Controlled trials have not demonstrated benefits over placebo in achieving total abstinence or delaying relapse. May benefit some patients who remain employed, socially stable, and motivated. Advise patient to avoid all forms of alcohol (24 hours before starting disulfiram to 14 days after last dose) to prevent toxic and potentially fatal reaction. Dosage range 125 to 500 mg PO qhs.

E. Naltrexone (Revia). FDA approved for alcohol dependence to decrease risk for relapse. No disulfiram-like reactions as a result of ethanol ingestion. Average dose is 50 mg PO daily for 12 weeks. Naltrexone proved superior to placebo in measures of drinking including abstention rates (51% versus 23%), number of drinking days, and relapse (31% versus 60%). **However, at 1 year there is no difference from placebo.** Patients must be highly motivated to discontinue alcohol. Liver function tests prior to initiation then again at one month after initiation and periodically thereafter are recommended. Naltrexone should be avoided in patients with severe liver disease or hepatitis, before consulting a liver specialist.

F. Acamprosate (Campral) is likely more effective than naltrexone and is considered safer; there is no change in pharmacokinetics with liver disease. There is some benefit to using both drugs simultaneously.

ACUTE PSYCHOSIS

I. Definition. Acute psychosis is significant impairment of sense of reality (incoherence, looseness of associations, delusions, hallucinations, catatonic or disorganized behavior) that results in impairment of ability to communicate, emotional turmoil, and impaired cognitive abilities.

II. Differential Diagnosis.

A. Substance-induced (intoxication or withdrawal). For example, hallucinogens, amphetamines, cocaine, alcohol withdrawal, anticholinergic drugs, corticosteroids, and L-dopa.

B. Acute exacerbation or initial episode of chronic psychotic disorder (e.g., schizophrenia).

C. Major affective syndrome, anxiety disorder, manic episode in bipolar disorder, or personality disorder (cluster A, see Table 18-6).

D. Secondary to general medical condition. For example, temporal lobe epilepsy, CNS tumors, stroke, trauma, endocrine or metabolic disorders, infections, autoimmune disorders, vitamin deficiency, and toxins. **Suspect psychosis caused by a medical condition if:**

1. Delirium is present (clouding of the sensorium, see Chapter 9).
2. No personal or family history of psychotic disorder.
3. Age older than 35 years.
4. Rapid development of psychosis in a previously functioning person.

III. Laboratory Tests. May include CBC, UA, liver enzymes, electrolytes, calcium, BUN, Cr, TSH/free T_4, VDRL, and HIV. Also urine drug screen and occasionally heavy-metal screen and ceruloplasmin (Wilson's disease), urine for porphobilinogen (acute intermittent porphyria). Also perform head CT or MRI in selected patients.

IV. Treatment.

A. General. Antipsychotics are initially used to control behavior, including rapid tranquilization. Long-term treatment depends on the cause. Further history may need to be obtained from family or friends to evaluate baseline functioning. Hospitalization may be indicated for patient safety.

B. Rapid tranquilization (Table 18-4). Used to treat violent, assaultive, or extremely agitated patients. It is very useful in the emergency department as well as for inpatients. It is effective for treating symptoms regardless of the cause of the aggression (i.e., it works for agitation secondary to schizophrenia, mania, dementia, delirium, etc.). **Patients who have been tranquilized must have vital signs closely monitored.**

1. **For rapid sedation,** haloperidol 5 to 10 mg IM plus lorazepam 2 to 4 mg IM is an option for rapid chemical control. Midazolam (5 mg IM) is an alternative to lorazepam and may work more quickly. Oral medications are not as reliable and should be avoided if rapid sedation is needed. Injectable olanzapine and ziprasidone are now available; however, they are expensive and less effective for rapid sedation. Droperidol, while safe, has an FDA black box warning in the United States and should be avoided for this reason.

2. **Extrapyramidal symptoms** (e.g., parkinsonism, dystonic reactions [torticollis, facial grimacing, or oculogyric crisis], or akathisia [restlessness, pacing]) **can be treated** with diphenhydramine 25 to 50 mg IM or IV or benztropine (Cogentin) 1 to 2 mg IV or IM. Long term, these medications can be given PO. Vitamin E 1000 mg PO bid may help prevent the development of tardive dyskinesia, etc, but data are poor.

3. **Atypical antipsychotics** are useful in patients willing to take medications orally, but generally not the acutely psychotic and agitated patient. Risperidone 1 to 2 mg PO q4-6h, up to 8 mg/day, or olanzapine 5 to 10 mg PO q4-8h up to 30 mg/day are reasonable choices.

TABLE 18-4
RECOMMENDED ANTIPSYCHOTIC DOSE FOR RAPID TRANQUILIZATION

Drug	IM (mg)	Oral Concentrate (mg)
HIGH POTENCY		
Haloperidol (Haldol)	5	10
Fluphenazine (Prolixin)	5	10
Thiothixene (Navane)	10	20
Trifluoperazine (Stelazine)	10	20
LOW POTENCY		
Chlorpromazine (Thorazine)	50	100
Thioridazine (Mellaril)	NA	100

18

PSYCHIATRY

4. **Benzodiazepines.** Drug of choice for alcohol or benzodiazepine withdrawal (see alcohol abuse section earlier). May be used as an adjunct to antipsychotics for sedative effect, such as lorazepam (Ativan) 2 to 4 mg IM every 30 minutes to 2 hours up to 120 mg/24 h or midazolam 5 to 10 mg IM. Both of these drugs are absorbed when given IM.

SCHIZOPHRENIA AND OTHER PSYCHOTIC DISORDERS

I. **Prevalence.** Schizophrenia is the most common psychotic disorder, affecting 1% of the world's population, and has a strong familial tendency. One third to one half of homeless Americans have schizophrenia.

II. **DSM-IV Criteria.**

A. **Characteristic symptoms.** Two (or more) of the following, each present for a significant time during a 1-month period (or less if treated successfully):

1. Delusions.
2. Hallucinations.
3. Disorganized or catatonic behavior.
4. Disorganized speech.
5. Negative symptoms (e.g., flattened affect, alogia [poverty of speech or thought content], or avolition [inability to initiate and persist in goal-directed activities]).

B. **Social or occupational dysfunction.** Significant impairment in work, relationships, or self-care since onset of illness.

C. **Continuous signs of the disturbance** persist for at least six months.

D. **Exclusions.** Symptoms not attributable to a mood disorder or to the effects of a general medical condition or psychoactive substance.

III. **Differential Diagnosis.** Any condition that can produce acute psychosis (see previous section on acute psychosis).

IV. **Treatment.**

A. **First psychotic episode.**

1. **Consider atypical antipsychotics** such as risperidone or olanzapine as first choice. Although costly, these medications have fewer extrapyramidal side effects, which improves medication compliance. Other atypical antipsychotics include quetiapine, ziprasidone, and aripiprazole. Although highly effective, clozapine should be considered second line because of the frequent blood monitoring needed. The patient needs 6 to 8 weeks at a therapeutic dose for adequate trial. If no response consider switching to another atypical antipsychotic.

2. If the patient fails two atypical antipsychotics, **consider the typical antipsychotics** (haloperidol, etc.). Typical antipsychotics are chosen based on the side effects the patient will tolerate best (see examples in **Table 18-5**). If medication noncompliance is an issue, consider administration of medications under supervision or change medication to long-acting decanoate injections (haloperidol, fluphenazine, and the atypical risperidone).

TABLE 18-5

ANTIPSYCHOTIC DOSES AND SIDE EFFECTS FOR CHRONIC USE

Drug	Relative Potency (milligram equivalents)	Dose (mg/day)	Anticholinergic*	EPS†	Sedation	Orthostatic Hypotension
TYPICAL ANTIPSYCHOTICS						
Chlorpromazine (Thorazine)	100	100-2000	+++	++	++++	++++
Thioridazine (Mellaril)	100	100-600	++++	+	++++	++++
Trifluoperazine (Stelazine)	5	5-60	++	+++	+	++
Thiothixene (Navane)	5	5-60	++	+++	++	++
Fluphenazine (Prolixin)	4	5-30	++	++++	++	++
Haloperidol (Haldol)	4	2-100	+	++++	++	+
ATYPICAL ANTIPSYCHOTICS						
Risperidone (Risperdal)	1	1-6	±	+	+	++
Clozapine (Clozaril)‡	50	25-900	+++++	±	++++	++++
Olanzapine (Zyprexa)	2	5-20	±	±	++	+
Quetiapine (Seraquil)		75-800	±	±	++	++
Ziprasidone (Zeldox)	N/A					

Adapted from Bernstein JG: *Handbook of Drug Therapy in Psychiatry*, 3rd ed. St. Louis, Mosby, 1995.

*Dry mouth, constipation, blurred vision, urinary retention.

†Extrapyramidal side effects (dystonia, parkinsonism, akathisia, tardive dyskinesia).

‡Requires weekly WBC because of risk of agranulocytosis.

N/A, not applicable.

3. Patients should be maintained on their medications for 1 to 2 years. Drug therapy is usually managed in consultation with a psychiatrist. **Atypical antipsychotics have been associated with development of diabetes, hyperlipidemia, and obesity, so patients should be monitored with periodic assessment of blood pressure, weight, abdominal girth, serum glucose, and lipids.**

B. Relapsing psychosis requires long-term treatment with antipsychotics (see Table 18-5). Minimize dose of medication to help prevent long-term side effects such as tardive dyskinesia with typical agents and weight gain with atypical agents.

1. Supportive psychotherapy. Individual or family counseling is a helpful adjunct to reduce risk for relapse.

2. Community programs are beneficial in providing support, social skills training, and vocational rehabilitation. They may also be able to provide support services to help improve medication compliance.

3. Cognitive behavior therapy. Recent evidence supports the efficacy of CBT for reducing the positive symptoms of schizophrenia, such as delusions.

V. Adverse Reactions to Antipsychotics.

A. Neuroleptic malignant syndrome can occur at any point during the course of treatment; it is seen with atypical and typical antipsychotics. It includes symptoms of autonomic instability (which can progress to hyperthermia), altered mental status, stupor, and muscle hypertonicity. Death can occur. See section on neuroleptic malignant syndrome in Chapter 2 for treatment.

B. Tardive dyskinesia is involuntary movements of the tongue, face, mouth, or jaw associated with long-term administration of antipsychotics. Elderly women are at highest risk. May be irreversible. Patients should be made aware of this possible side effect, which occurs less when atypical antipsychotics are used. Benztropine and diphenhydramine can be used to reduce extrapyramidal symptoms. Vitamin E, 1000 U bid may help prevent extrapyramidal symptoms, although the most methodologically sound trials found no benefit.

C. Diabetes mellitus with the atypical antipsychotics. There have been numerous reports of the onset of diabetes and diabetic ketoacidosis with the use of atypical antipsychotics. The FDA now requires that each atypical antipsychotic include a black box warning on its package insert. Recent guidelines suggest periodic monitoring of weight, blood glucose, and lipids in patients maintained on chronic atypical antipsychotics. Aripiprazole and ziprasidone are considered weight and lipid neutral.

EATING DISORDERS

Anorexia Nervosa

I. Overview. Onset is usually in adolescence and affects females 10:1 over males. Prevalence in young women is up to 3.7%. Some patients also have episodes of binge eating or purging. Anorexia nervosa is a life-threatening disorder, with mortality greater than 10%.

II. Diagnosis.

A. Early signs may include withdrawal from family and friends, increased sensitivity to criticism, sudden increased interest in physical activity, and anxiety or depressive symptoms.

B. DSM-IV criteria

1. Refusal to maintain body weight over a minimal normal weight for age and height (e.g., weight <85% of expected).
2. Intense fear of becoming fat even though underweight.
3. Disturbed body image or denial of seriousness of current low body weight.
4. Absence of three consecutive menstrual periods.

C. Differential diagnosis includes hyperthyroidism, Addison's disease, diabetes, inflammatory bowel disease, depression, and pregnancy, among others.

D. Laboratory tests. Anorexia nervosa is not a laboratory diagnosis. However, a battery of tests should be performed to rule out medical complications of starvation. CBC, general screen including electrolytes, glucose, calcium, phosphate, BUN, Cr, Mg, liver and thyroid function tests, amylase (salivary amylase may be elevated in purging), carotene, UA, and ECG. Measures of nutrition include cholesterol/triglycerides, albumin, and prealbumin. Other useful tests include troponin if patient abuses ipecac (cardiomyopathy) or bone densitometry if patient has been amenorrheic for 6 months.

III. Potential medical complications.
Dry skin, hypothermia, bradycardia, hypotension, dependent edema, anemia, lanugo, infertility, osteoporosis, cardiac failure, and death (most commonly results from starvation, suicide, or electrolyte imbalances).

IV. Treatment.

A. Inpatient treatment. Indications for hospitalization may include any of the following:

1. Patient's weight 70% of ideal body weight or less.
2. Persistent suicidal ideation.
3. Need for withdrawal from laxatives, diet pills, or diuretics.
4. Failure of outpatient treatment.

B. Outpatient treatment

1. Treat the medical complications of starvation.
2. Nutritional counseling to establish a balanced diet, an expected rate of weight gain (up to 2 lbs per week), and a final goal weight.
3. Use behavioral techniques to reward weight gain.
4. Individual and group cognitive therapy to alter attitude towards food, enhance autonomy, and improve self-esteem.
5. Family therapy may also be useful.
6. Treat any associated mood disorder. Antidepressants have not been shown to improve weight restoration but may help maintain weight after it has been restored.

PSYCHIATRY

18

Bulimia Nervosa

I. **Overview.** Onset is usually in late adolescence or early adulthood and is more prevalent in females than in males. As many as 17% of college-aged women engage in bulimic behavior. Bulimics tend to be normal weight to slightly overweight. Associated dysphoria or depression is common. From 30% to 80% of bulimics have a history of anorexia nervosa.

II. **DSM-IV Criteria.**

A. **Recurrent episodes of binge eating** characterized by eating large amounts of food in a short period of time and lack of control over eating behavior.

B. **Regular inappropriate compensatory behavior** to prevent weight gain (e.g., use of self-induced vomiting, laxatives, diuretics, fasting, or excessive exercise).

C. Binge episodes and compensatory behavior both **occur on average twice a week** for at least 3 months.

D. **Persistent overconcern with body shape and weight.**

III. **Laboratory Tests.** No single lab test helps with the diagnosis; however, to check for complications, several tests should be performed: general screen including electrolytes, glucose, calcium, phosphate, BUN, Cr, Mg, and amylase.

IV. **Potential Medical Complications.** Complications include erosion of dental enamel, dental caries, parotitis, menstrual irregularity, laxative dependence, electrolyte disturbances, gastric rupture, cardiac arrhythmias, and chronic pancreatitis.

V. **Treatment should include** medical stabilization, routine monitoring of serum potassium and magnesium, education about medical complications, supportive and cognitive behavioral therapy, and nutrition counseling.

A. **Fluoxetine** 60 mg PO qAM has been shown to reduce the number of binge episodes and associated vomiting (start at 20 mg PO daily and titrate up). Fluoxetine is the only medication FDA approved for treatment of bulimia, although other SSRIs are likely as effective.

B. **Hospitalization** is necessary in a minority of patients (admission criteria are similar to those for anorexia nervosa except for weight loss).

ATTENTION DEFICIT DISORDER

I. **Overview.** The prevalence of ADHD in school-age children is 3% to 6%, with males outnumbering females. Onset is in childhood, with symptoms first being apparent in early grade school (by definition, by age 7). Contrary to previously held beliefs, approximately 65% have symptoms that persist into adulthood. Patients can have primarily inattentive, hyperactive, or mixed subtypes. Many patients with ADHD have a comorbid psychiatric disorder. **Note that there is no such thing as "adult-onset ADHD." By definition, symptoms must have been present since childhood.**

II. **Diagnosis** (Box 18-8).

III. **Diagnostic Tools.**

A. **Interview** with child's caregivers.

B. **Mental status exam** of the child.

C. **Physical exam** for general and neurologic health, a hematocrit drawn if the patient has a history of lead exposure, hearing and vision testing.

D. **Cognitive ability screen.**

E. **ADHD rating scales** (e.g., Conners forms) can be filled out by teacher and parent to assist in collecting objective assessments of attention and focus.

F. **School reports** on the patient.

BOX 18-8

CRITERIA FOR DIAGNOSIS OF ADHD

1. Some of the symptoms must be present before 7 years of age.
2. There is clear evidence of significant impairment in functioning that is present in two or more settings (e.g., work, school, and home).
3. The symptoms are not better accounted for by another disorder.

ATTENTION

At least 6 symptoms must be present for at least 6 months and evident in at least two situations (e.g., home, school, play).

- Avoids/dislikes work requiring sustained mental effort
- Fails to give close attention to detail
- Fails to sustain attention
- Has difficulty organizing
- Is easily distracted
- Is often forgetful
- Loses things
- Often doesn't follow through with instructions on work
- Seems to not listen when spoken to

HYPERACTIVITY/IMPULSIVITY

At least 4 symptoms must be present for 6 months.

- Blurts out answers to questions
- Fidgets
- Has difficulty playing quietly
- Has difficulty awaiting one's turn
- Intrudes on others
- Is often "on the go"
- Leaves seat in situations where seating is expected
- Often runs about in inappropriate settings
- Talks excessively

IV. Pharmacologic Treatment.

A. **Stimulants such as methylphenidate and dextroamphetamine are first-line treatment.** Response rate is 70% to 90%. *Reminder:* **A favorable response does not confirm the diagnosis of ADHD. Most patients feel better and perform better on these drugs!** Side effects include decreased appetite, headache, insomnia, jitteriness, stomach ache, and occasional dysphoria. Rare cases of amphetamine abuse have been reported. Dosage range for regular release methylphenidate is 0.3 to 0.6 mg/kg per dose given bid or tid. Dosage range for dextroamphetamine is 0.15 to 0.3 mg/kg per dose bid. Both medications come in sustained-release formulations along with regular release. **Cardiac arrest and myocardial infarction have been reported with these drugs.**

B. **Atomoxetine (Strattera)** is a recently approved medication that is the first nonstimulant approved for ADHD. It is also effective in adults. Onset of effect is delayed compared to stimulants and clinically it has not proved to be as effective as stimulants. It is a noncontrolled substance and can be dosed once or twice daily. Watch out for irritability. **An FDA warning about liver toxicity with atomoxetine has been issued.**

C. **Antidepressants such as imipramine and bupropion** are used in patients with ADHD and tic disorders. Tricyclic medications are known to be associated with prolongation of the QT interval; EKG monitoring is recommended.

D. **α-Adrenergic agents such as clonidine and guanfacine** are helpful for hyperactivity. The primary side effects are sedation and hypotension. Doses should be titrated slowly from 0.05 mg tid as a starting dose for clonidine. Avoid use in children with cardiovascular disease.

V. Nonpharmacologic therapies
include parental and patient psychoeducation, behavioral therapy, and supportive therapy. Multimodal therapy is most recommended.

PERSONALITY DISORDERS

I. Overview.

A. **DSM-IV definition of personality disorder** is an enduring pattern of inner experience and behavior that deviates markedly from the expectations of the individual's culture, is inflexible and pervasive, has an onset in early adulthood or adolescence, is stable over time, and leads to distress or impairment. The clinical manifestations of a personality disorder should not be better accounted for as a consequence of another mental disorder. Some personality disorders, such as borderline personality disorder, have a strong association with specific experiences during childhood (e.g., childhood sexual abuse).

B. **Personality disorders occur in at least 10% of the population.**

C. **Many people with personality disorders do not seek treatment on their own** and may minimize their personality problems.

TABLE 18-6
SYNOPSIS OF PERSONALITY DISORDERS

Personality Disorder	Characteristics	Complications
CLUSTER A: ODD OR ECCENTRIC		
Paranoid	Unwarranted mistrust and suspicion manifested by jealousy, questioning loyalty, tendency to be easily slighted, and bearing grudges	Delusions
Schizoid	Indifference to social relationships, few or no friends, emotional constriction, and preference for solitary activities	None
Schizotypal	Peculiar thoughts, appearance, perceptions, and behavior plus deficits in interpersonal relations	Transient psychosis under stress
CLUSTER B: DRAMATIC, EMOTIONAL, OR ERRATIC		
Antisocial	Chronic antisocial and irresponsible behavior starting before age 15 with conduct disturbance	Premature violent death, substance abuse
Borderline	Unstable relationships, impulsiveness, emotional instability, identity disturbance, inappropriate anger, self-mutilating behavior	Depression, substance abuse psychosis, suicide
Histrionic	Attention-seeking, seductive, immature, overreactive, and excitable self-dramatizing behavior	Conversion, somatization
Narcissistic	Grandiose sense of self-importance, exhibitionistic, lack of empathy, hypersensitivity to evaluation by others, high sense of entitlement, and preoccupation with success	Depression, psychosis
CLUSTER C: ANXIOUS OR FEARFUL		
Avoidant	Low self-esteem, timidity, hypersensitivity to rejection, and social withdrawal but desire for acceptance	Social phobia
Dependent	Submissive to others, low self-confidence, indecisiveness, fears abandonment, and dislikes solitude	Depression
Obsessive–compulsive	Rigid, perfectionistic, over-conscientious, restricted affect, preoccupation with details, inflexibility	OCD, hypochondriasis, depression

Adapted from Fuller AK, LeRoy JB: *South Med J* 86:431-432, 1993.

18 PSYCHIATRY

D. A brief description of personality disorders and their consequences is found in **Table 18-6.**

II. Treatment is guided by a patient's symptoms and may include psychotherapy (interpersonal, cognitive, behavioral, or psychodynamic) and/or pharmacologic therapy. Establish safeguards to protect patients from dangerous impulsive behavior (e.g., limit medication supply). Periods of hospitalization may be needed.

A. Cluster A Personality Disorders
1. Maintain honest, courteous relationship.
2. Acknowledge understanding of patient's inner feelings and need for privacy.
3. Avoid expressing too much warmth.
4. Outline plan for care to reassure.

B. Cluster B Personality Disorders
1. Develop sympathetic understanding relationship.
2. Be calm and firm.
3. Establish limits and define professional boundaries.
4. Communicate understanding of patient's strengths, vulnerabilities, and fears.
5. SSRIs may help reduce mood swings.

C. Cluster C Personality Disorders
1. Build an undemanding, trusting relationship.
2. Involve the patient in decision making.
3. Balance necessary restrictions with minor concessions.

BIBLIOGRAPHY

American Psychiatric Association: *Diagnostic and Statistical Manual of Mental Disorders*, 4th revised edition. Washington, DC, American Psychiatric Association, 2000.

American Psychiatric Association: *Diagnostic and Statistical Manual of Mental Disorders*, 4th ed, primary care version, 1st ed. Washington, DC, American Psychiatric Association, 1995.

American Psychiatric Association: Practice guideline for the treatment of patients with eating disorders (revision). *Am J Psychiatry* 157:1-39, 2000.

American Psychiatric Association: Practice guideline for the treatment of patients with major depressive disorder (revision). *Am J Psychiatry* 157:1-45, 2000.

American Psychiatric Association: Practice guideline for the treatment of patients with substance use disorders: Alcohol, cocaine, and opioids. *Am J Psychiatry* 152: 5-80, 1995.

Andreasen NC, Black DW: *Introductory Textbook of Psychiatry*, 2nd ed. Washington, DC, American Psychiatric Press, 1995.

Andreasen NC: Symptoms, signs, and diagnosis of schizophrenia. *Lancet* 346: 477-481, 1995.

Aquila R, Weiden PJ, Emanuel M: Compliance and the rehabilitation alliance. *J Clin Psychiatr* 60 (Suppl 19):23-27, 1999.

Blumenreich PE, Lippmann SB: Phobias: How to help patients overcome irrational fears. *Postgrad Med* 96:125-134, 1994.

Boyer W: Serotonin uptake inhibitors are superior to imipramine and alprazolam in alleviating panic attacks: A meta-analysis. *Int Clin Psychopharmacol* 10:45-49, 1995.

Bruce TJ et al: Social anxiety disorder: A common, underrecognized mental disorder. *Am Fam Physician* 60:2311-2320, 1999.

Bustillo JR, Lauriello J, Keith SJ: Schizophrenia: Improving outcome. *Harvard Rev Psychiatr* 6: 229-240, 1999.

Eddy MF, Walbroehl GS: Recognition and treatment of obsessive–compulsive disorder. *Am Fam Physician* 57:1623-1630, 1998.

Goldman HH (ed): *Review of General Psychiatry*, 4th ed. East Norwalk, Conn, Appleton & Lange, 1995.

Goldman LS, Genel M, Bezman RJ, Slanetz PJ: Diagnosis and treatment of attention-deficit/hyperactivity disorder in children and adolescents. Council on Scientific Affairs, American Medical Association. *JAMA* 279:1100-1107, 1998.

Guze B, Fernq HK, Szuba MP, Richeimer S (eds): *The Psychiatric Drug Handbook*, 2nd ed, St. Louis, Mosby, 1995.

Jibson MD, Tandon R: New atypical antipsychotic medications. *J Psychiatr Res* 32: 215-228, 1998.

Kaplan HI, Sadock BJ: *Pocket Handbook of Clinical Psychiatry*, 2nd ed. Baltimore, Williams & Wilkins, 1996.

Miller NS, Gold MS, Smith DE (eds): *Manual of Therapeutics for Addictions*. New York, Wiley-Liss, 1997.

Noyes R, Hoehn-Saric R: *Anxiety Disorders*. New York, Cambridge University Press, 1996.

Perry PJ, Alexander B, Liskow BI (eds): *Psychotropic Drug Handbook*, 7th ed. Washington DC, American Psychiatric Press, 1997.

Peterson CB, Mitchell JE: Psychosocial and pharmacological treatment of eating disorders: A review of research findings. *J Clin Psychol* 55:685-697, 1999.

Pliszka SR: The use of psychostimulants in the pediatric patient. *Pediatr Clin North Am* 45:1085-1097, 1998.

Sadock BJ, Sadock VA: *Kaplan and Sadock's Comprehensive Textbook of Psychiatry*, 7th ed. Philadelphia, Lippincott, Williams & Wilkins, 2000.

Thase ME: Do we really need all these antidepressants? Weighing the options. *J Practical Psychiatr Behav Health* 3:3-17, 1997.

Weiden PJ: Olanzapine: A new "atypical" antipsychotic. *J Practic Psychiatr Behav Health* 3:49-53, 1997.

PSYCHIATRY

18

Ophthalmology

Jennifer L. Jones

EYE EXAMINATION

I. **Definitions.** *Miosis* refers to constricted pupils; *mydriasis* refers to dilated pupils; *anisocoria* refers to pupils of different size.

II. **Pupils.** Assess pupil size, shape, reactivity, and accommodation (i.e., constriction when eyes cross nasally).

A. Anisocoria is normal in a proportion of the population, and baseline pupil size should be established before one looks for a cause. Causes include:

1. Cranial nerve III palsy (as from diabetes mellitus, multiple sclerosis), uncal herniation (comatose patient, other CNS signs and symptoms).

2. Horner's syndrome (interruption of sympathetic innervation of eye causing miosis, ptosis, ipsilateral decreased sweating [anhidrosis]; may be secondary to lung cancer, etc.).

3. Adie's syndrome (parasympathetic dysfunction at or distal to the ciliary ganglion from trauma, etc., leading to unilateral dilated pupil).

4. Ocular trauma or inflammation, prescription or OTC eye drops.

5. Argyll–Robertson pupil (pupils may be small, accommodating to near vision but not reacting to light or painful stimuli; seen with neurosyphilis or Lyme disease).

6. Common causes of weak reactivity include the problems aforementioned plus optic nerve and retinal disease. A dilated pupil is not indicative of pending herniation unless the patient is comatose.

B. **Swinging flashlight test** checks for relative afferent pupillary defect (RAPD).

1. Normal is constriction on direct light and constriction when the contralateral eye is stimulated (consensual reflex).

2. **The consensual constriction of a pupil with absence of the direct response indicates an afferent pupillary defect (i.e., visual loss in the eye with preserved brain function allowing consensual reflex).** May be caused by optic neuritis, ischemic optic neuropathy, chiasmal tumors, retinal artery or vein occlusion, retinal detachment, acute angle-closure glaucoma, optic tumors, orbital disease (affecting the optic nerve), etc. **RAPD is not caused by** hyphema, refractive error, cataracts, or vitreous hemorrhage.

III. **Ocular Motility.**

A. Check six cardinal positions of gaze, corneal light reflection, and the cover test. Cover each eye in turn as patient looks at an object about 20 ft (6 m) away. When the eye is covered, the uncovered eye should not move in a normal patient.

B. Common causes of motility and alignment abnormalities include congenital and childhood-onset strabismus, cranial nerve palsies (e.g., from diabetes), orbital trauma, Graves' disease, myasthenia gravis, stroke, or brain tumor.

IV. **Fluorescein Staining.** Moisten fluorescein paper and gently touch to inner surface of lower lid. Disrupted corneal epithelium will fluoresce under Wood's lamp or cobalt blue slit lamp. However, this test can miss up to 21% of defects. A dendritic defect will be highlighted in herpes simplex keratitis. Don't forget the usefulness of the slit lamp, if available.

V. Always check visual acuity and evert upper and lower lids to look for foreign body.

VI. **Pain with eye motion** may indicate optic neuritis, intraorbital infection, sinusitis, orbital cellulitis, injury (foreign body, corneal abrasion, etc.), Graves' disease, orbital myositis, sarcoid, thyroid disease, and infectious/inflammatory processes (lymphoma, etc.).

VII. **Topical Anesthetic.** Can be used to differentiate topical problems such as foreign body and corneal abrasions from deeper problems such as iritis and glaucoma. If pain resolves with topical anesthetic, this finding suggests, but does not prove, a superficial cause.

VIII. **Some Useful Drugs.**

A. **Mydriasis.** Cyclopentolate: maximum dilation at 25 to 75 minutes, lasting 6 to 24 hours; homatropine: maximum dilation is rapid, must be used tid or qid to maintain mydriasis; scopolamine: dilation at about 1 hour, must be used tid to qid.

B. **Miosis.** Pilocarpine in 0.25%, 0.5%, and 1.0%. Generally needed only once per day. See section on acute glaucoma for exception.

C. **Anesthesia.** Tetracaine 1%, proparacaine 0.5%. These cause corneal toxicity with repeated use. **Never** prescribe for home use.

THE RED EYE (TABLE 19-1)

I. **Conjunctivitis.**

A. **Overview.** Conjunctivitis is conjunctival erythema/injection caused by hyperemia of superficial vessels. Etiology includes infection, allergies, chemicals, and tear deficiency. It may be accompanied by itching, burning, or foreign-body sensation. Often discharge or drainage is present, and crusting of the eyelids can occur during sleep. Vision is generally not affected. If symptoms are particularly severe, consider gonococcal disease. If conjunctivitis is seen in a neonate, *Chlamydia* may be the culprit (usually 3 weeks of age).

B. **Viral** ("pink eye")

1. **Usually caused by adenoviruses,** although epidemics may involve coxsackievirus or enteroviruses. Symptoms include acute redness, serous or watery discharge, foreign-body sensation, and preauricular lymphadenopathy. Infection is usually self-limited but can last up to 2 weeks.

2. **Treatment. Antibiotics are not helpful and are not indicated.** Boric acid washes, which can be obtained OTC, often provide excellent symptomatic relief. Patients should throw away eyeliner, etc., which

TABLE 19-1
THE RED EYE

Sign or Symptom	Conjunctivitis Bacterial	Conjunctivitis Viral	Conjunctivitis Allergic	Corneal Injury or Infection	Iritis	Glaucoma
Vision	Normal	Normal	Normal	Decreased or greatly decreased	Decreased	Greatly decreased
Pain	–	–	–	+	+	+++
Photophobia	–	±	–	+	++	–
Foreign-body sensation	–	±	±	+	–	–
Itch	±	±	++	–	–	–
Tearing	+	++	+	++	+	–
Discharge	Mucopurulent	Mucoid	–	–	–	–
Preauricular adenopathy	–	+	–	–	–	–
Pupils	–	–	–	Normal or small	Small	Mid-dilated and fixed
Conjunctival hyperemia	Diffuse	Diffuse	Diffuse	Diffuse and ciliary flush	Ciliary flush	Diffuse and ciliary flush
Cornea	Clear	Sometimes faint punctate staining or infiltrates	Clear	Depends on disorder	Clear or slightly cloudy	Cloudy
Intraocular pressure	Normal	Normal	Normal	Normal	Decreased, normal, or increased	Greatly increased

OPHTHALMOLOGY 19

can be a reservoir for infection. OTC drops (e.g., artificial tears, oxymetazoline) may help as well. Oxymetazoline should not be used in children because of risk of toxicity.

C. Bacterial

1. **Symptoms** include acute redness with copious purulent discharge and severe morning crusting. Usually caused by *Staphylococcus* spp., *Streptococcus pneumoniae*, or *Haemophilus* spp. but may also be caused by *Moraxella* spp., gram-negative pathogens, or *Pseudomonas* (contact lens wearers).

2. **Treatment.** Antibiotics decrease length of symptoms, but most infections are self-limited. Treat with topical agents for 2 or 3 days *except* gonococcal and chlamydial infections, which should be treated topically and systemically. Antibiotic agents include sulfacetamide sodium (although some data are showing significant resistance to sulfonamides), erythromycin, fluoroquinolones, and bacitracin or gentamicin drops or ointment. Avoid neomycin because of a higher chance of hypersensitivity. If no corneal destruction, gonococcal infection is treated with ceftriaxone 1 g IM as well as topical agents. Refer if any evidence of corneal ulceration is noted. Treat *Chlamydia* with oral tetracycline, doxycycline, or erythromycin for 2 weeks, as well as topical agents.

D. Allergic

1. Often patient has a history of atopic problems including allergic rhinitis, asthma, and eczema. Watery, red, itchy eyes, mild eyelid swelling, without purulent drainage, but can see stringy mucoid discharge. May also see "chemosis," which is boggy edema of conjunctivae that gives the sclera a jelly-like appearance. Usually seen in late childhood or early adulthood and may be seasonal or perennial.

2. **Treatment.** Allergen avoidance; systemic treatment with antihistamines will help and is indicated if the patient has other allergic symptoms. If symptoms are isolated to the eye or not responsive to oral therapy, topical mast cell stabilizers (e.g., cromolyn, lodoxamide) are recommended for mild to moderate cases. Topical antihistamines can be used (e.g., levocabastine); NSAIDs (e.g., ketorolac) may also be useful but are expensive and of limited efficacy. Topical vasoconstrictor/antihistamine combinations (e.g., Vasocon-A or Naphcon-A) work well and are now OTC. However, they can cause rebound hyperemia with prolonged use.

II. Iritis.

A. Symptoms. Photophobia and ciliary injection of straight deep vessels radiating from the limbus (ciliary flush). The pupil is variable in size (usually small) and poorly reactive, and it may be irregularly shaped; distant vision may be impaired. On slit lamp examination, inflammatory cells in the anterior chamber appear as "dust particles," and white keratitic precipitates can be seen on the posterior surface of the cornea. Topical anesthetic does not relieve pain.

B. Etiology. Often the cause is not found. The most common etiology is trauma, but history should include questions about the presence of collagen vascular and autoimmune diseases. Diseases commonly associated with iritis include ankylosing spondylitis, sarcoidosis, juvenile rheumatoid arthritis, lupus, Reiter's syndrome, Wegener's granulomatosis, brucellosis, leptospirosis, tuberculosis, syphilis, and Behçet's syndrome, among others.

C. **Treatment.** Blocking pupillary sphincter and ciliary body action with a cycloplegic agent (such as 0.25% scopolamine, 2% homatropine, or 1% cyclopentolate) reduces pain and photophobia. Topical corticosteroids are indicated to suppress inflammation, but **patients need to be seen by an ophthalmologist if this diagnosis is considered.**

III. **Acute Closed-Angle Glaucoma.**

A. **General. Ocular emergency requiring immediate diagnosis and treatment** as even hours of increased ocular pressure can lead to permanent visual loss. Caused by the closure of an already narrow anterior chamber angle. It is more common in women, Asians, those with hypermetropia, and the elderly (physiologically enlarged lens).

B. **Symptoms.** Expect greatly decreased visual acuity, colored halos around lights, aching orbital pain, headache, mid-dilated nonreactive pupil, diffuse conjunctival hyperemia, steamy cornea, and elevated intraocular pressures. Precipitants include being in a dark room (dilates pupil), stress, and certain drugs (e.g., sympathomimetics or anticholinergics). **Acute glaucoma can manifest as abdominal pain or nausea and vomiting, and this diagnosis should not be overlooked in those with a GI presentation. An ophthalmologist should be consulted immediately upon making the diagnosis.**

C. **Diagnosis** is clinical along with the demonstration of an elevated intraocular pressure.

D. **Treatment.** Treat with acetazolamide 500 mg PO or IV followed by 250 mg q6h with or without topical β-adrenergic antagonists (timolol maleate 0.5% 1 drop) to decrease aqueous humor production. Constrict pupil with topical pilocarpine 2%, one drop every 5 minutes for the first 2 hours. Vitreous humor volume can be decreased with systemic hyperosmotic agents such as mannitol 1 g/kg IV. Sedate the patient, provide adequate analgesia, and **refer immediately to an ophthalmologist.** Definitive treatment involves laser iridotomy/iridoplasty or peripheral iridectomy.

IV. **Corneal Abrasion.**

A. **General.** A localized loss of epithelium from the cornea typically caused by foreign bodies, fingernails, or contact lenses (i.e., direct trauma).

B. **Symptoms.** Sudden pain and foreign-body sensation in the eye; this is generally relieved by topical anesthetics. There may be associated injection of the conjunctival vessels, tearing, blepharospasm, and photophobia.

C. **Diagnosis.** Made by fluorescein staining. Carefully search for any remaining foreign bodies by using the slit lamp and by everting the lids. Foreign bodies can be removed using a cotton swab or needle. Always evaluate for a rust ring when the foreign body is metallic.

D. Treatment.

1. Most heal in 24 to 48 hours, but **refer to ophthalmologist if ulceration is present.**

2. Topical analgesics (diclofenac 0.1%, ketorolac 0.5%) can be used but are expensive and of only modest benefit. Avoid prescribing topical anesthetics as they retard healing and may lead to corneal epithelial breakdown. Oral pain medications are more effective but may be less well tolerated.

3. Topical antibiotics are generally prescribed (erythromycin, sulfacetamide, gentamicin). Aminoglycosides may reduce the rate of reepithelialization. **Use an agent with anti-pseudomonal coverage in contact lens wearers:** ofloxacin, ciprofloxacin, or gentamicin/tobramycin with piperacillin ticarcillin. Topical steroids also retard healing and increase infection risk. Tetanus status should be ascertained and updated, if needed.

4. **Patching is optional and should be used for patient comfort only, although patches often *increase* pain.** Patching may actually delay healing.

5. Cycloplegics can be used if the injury is particularly severe. Apply two drops of 0.25% scopolamine, 2% homatropine, or 1% cyclopentolate for cycloplegia into the affected eye or eyes if indicated by severity of injury. This will prevent spasm of the pupil, which can cause pain.

6. Patients should be advised to avoid reading, watching TV, and other "eye-intensive" activities. Re-evaluate the patient in 24 hours, and again in 3 to 4 days if not healed. If no improvement at each visit, refer to an ophthalmologist.

V. Subconjunctival Hemorrhage.

A. Sharply demarcated area of injection resulting from the rupture of small subconjunctival vessels. Hemorrhages can result from trauma, bleeding diathesis, coughing, vomiting, straining, or viral hemorrhagic conjunctivitis (adenovirus, enterovirus, and Coxsackievirus). Excessive rubbing from dry eyes may contribute.

B. Subconjunctival hemorrhage alone is self-limited and requires no treatment. The presence of blood in the anterior chamber indicates a hyphema and requires immediate ophthalmologic referral.

TRAUMA

I. Blunt Trauma.

A. Orbital wall fracture, including **blow-out fracture,** should be considered after any blunt eye trauma. Signs and symptoms may include diplopia, epistaxis, ecchymosis, crepitus, hypesthesia in the infraorbital nerve distribution, and restricted upward gaze secondary to inferior rectus entrapment. Plain facial films are often inadequate, although fluid in the sinus or fat protruding from the orbital floor are presumptive evidence of a fracture. A CT scan with axial and coronal cuts is necessary for definitive diagnosis. Visual impairment or globe injury warrants immediate referral.

Otherwise, repair is often delayed for 7 to 10 days even with diplopia. Discussion with your ophthalmologist or otolaryngologist is recommended.

B. Hyphema is presence of blood in the anterior chamber and is typically easily visualized. Symptoms include pain, photophobia, and blurring of vision. Elevated intraocular pressure is a possible side effect and should be treated like acute angle closure glaucoma if it occurs. Bedrest with elevation of the head may prevent the frequent complication of rebleeding, but the data are unclear. Immediate ophthalmologic consultation should be obtained to determine need for surgical evacuation.

C. Periorbital contusions are treated with ice, head elevation, and reassurance that symptoms will resolve in 2 to 3 weeks.

D. Air bag trauma. Most common injuries are to the eyelids, conjunctiva, and cornea. Hyphemas often occur. Less commonly seen are retinal detachment, scleral rupture, and lens dislocation. Injuries are bilateral in 27%. All patients should get complete ophthalmologic exam because of this high-velocity trauma. Alkaline chemical keratitis can develop from the NaOH produced during the chemical reaction that inflates the bag.

II. Penetrating Trauma.

A. Corneal laceration, scleral laceration, intraocular foreign body, or globe rupture. Any high-velocity injury should be treated as a penetrating trauma. Treatment includes placement of a shield (an inverted paper or Styrofoam cup will do) without applying pressure to the globe, initiation of systemic antibiotics to cover both gram-positive and gram-negative organisms (such as vancomycin and gentamicin), tetanus prophylaxis, sedation, analgesia, and urgent referral.

B. Chemical exposure (especially alkali). Expect to find lacrimation, blepharospasm, painful red sclera, and photophobia.

1. Direct lavage should be done at the scene for at least 15 minutes with any water or saline solution available. To irrigate in the ED, instill a topical anesthetic (Pontocaine, tetracaine, and others). Irrigate and sweep under lids and in conjunctival cul-de-sacs to remove particulate matter. Hang IV solution bags of normal saline connected through IV tubing to an 18-gauge plastic IV catheter or a continuous-flow contact lens. For patients who cannot tolerate saline, balanced salt solution is a good, although expensive, alternative. **Lavage should be continued for at least 20 minutes by the clock.**

2. When eye is adequately lavaged, use litmus paper to ensure that eye pH is neutral immediately after the lavage is completed and again 10 minutes later. **This is especially crucial to document in alkali injuries. Continue to irrigate until the pH is neutral (pH of 7.4 to 7.6).**

3. Once pH is normal, use fluorescein stain to evaluate for damage or residual abrasions. Reapply ophthalmic anesthetic and apply two drops of 0.25% scopolamine, 2% homatropine, or 1% cyclopentolate for cycloplegia into the affected eye or eyes if indicated by severity of injury. This will prevent spasm of the pupil, which can cause pain.

OPHTHALMOLOGY 19

4. Use an antibiotic ointment. Erythromycin is a good choice. Gentamicin and other aminoglycosides inhibit corneal repair. **Provide adequate oral analgesia and follow-up within 24 hours.**

5. Contact lenses should not be worn for 2 weeks. Refer immediately for acid or alkali burn of significance (that is, corneal epithelial damage, any haziness of cornea) or for subnormal visual acuity, severe conjunctival swelling. See all others back in 24 hours.

ORBITS, EYELIDS, AND LACRIMAL APPARATUS

I. Orbital Cellulitis.

A. Orbital cellulitis is infection of tissues posterior to the orbital septum. Rarely seen, it is typically caused by extension of sinusitis (usually maxillary and ethmoid) or periorbital cellulitis. It is more likely to be seen in children than adults.

B. Presentation includes dull aching periorbital pain, conjunctival injection, fever, URI symptoms, violaceous swelling and tenderness of upper and lower lids, impaired vision, and limited ocular movement. CT or MRI is necessary for diagnosis and to rule out orbital subperiosteal abscess and tumor.

C. Complications include orbital abscess, cavernous sinus thrombosis, brain abscess, and meningitis. *S. aureus, Strep.* spp., *Enterobacteriaceae*, and rarely *H. influenzae* are bacterial pathogens. Consider viruses, fungi, and parasites in the immunocompromised. In diabetics, think of mucormycosis.

D. Treatment includes IV antibiotics such as ampicillin/sulbactam or a second- or third-generation cephalosporin (cefuroxime, cefoxitin, or cefotetan) for 7 to 10 days before switching to an oral agent to complete a 21-day course. Other options include ticarcillin/clavulanate or piperacillin/tazobactam. Add vancomycin if resistant staphylococcus is prevalent. Appropriate surgical consultation is necessary.

II. Periorbital Cellulitis.

A. Infection is confined to structures anterior to orbital septum. The possibility of orbital extension must always be considered. Vision is normal, and ocular movements are intact.

B. Adults may be managed as outpatients with penicillinase-resistant antibiotics (such as amoxicillin-clavulanate) and daily examinations. Children should be hospitalized because of a strong association with bacteremia, septicemia, and meningitis, and treated with a second- or third-generation cephalosporin.

III. Dacryocystitis and dacryostenosis are inflammations of the lacrimal sac, which are usually unilateral and secondary to nasolacrimal duct obstruction.

A. Congenital. Usually manifests by 3 to 12 weeks of age and generally resolves by 6 months. It can be treated by bid massaging of the lacrimal duct area, although this is of questionable efficacy. Antibiotics are used if infection develops (see below). Occasionally requires surgical probing to open the duct.

B. Infectious. Mucopurulent discharge, excessive tearing, erythema, and tender swelling of the medial lower lid are seen. Because infection can be polymicrobial, the purulent material expressed from the lacrimal punctum should be cultured to help in choosing an antibiotic. Usual organisms include *S. pneumoniae, S. aureus, H. influenzae*, and *S. pyogenes*. Use oral first-generation cephalosporin, erythromycin, or penicillinase-resistant penicillin. Daily examinations are necessary because orbital cellulitis is a possible complication. Adults can develop infection secondary to chronic sinusitis, trauma, or neoplasia, and referral may be necessary for dacryocystorhinostomy. Surgery may be indicated if abscess develops.

IV. Hordeolum is an acute infection of anterior lid margin usually related to staphylococci.

A. Acute external hordeolum (stye). A stye is an infection of the Zeiss or Moll glands along the lash line. Exam reveals a tender focal mounding of one eyelid that develops over days, often with a pustule. Treatment includes warm compresses bid to qid as well as topical or oral antibiotics depending on severity. Pulling the affected lash may promote drainage. Expect spontaneous drainage within one week. Rarely, if the stye does not drain, I&D is required along with systemic antibiotics. Usually this can be done in the office with an 18-G needle once the abscess is "pointing."

B. Acute internal hordeolum (chalazion). A chalazion is a chronic granulomatous inflammation in the meibomian gland. It can become secondarily infected, resulting in an acute internal hordeolum. Acute chalazion is treated with oral antibiotics and warm compresses. The chronic chalazion will continue to grow, and excision or steroid injection is required for cosmetic reasons or when vision is affected.

V. Blepharitis is eyelid inflammation caused by chemicals, seborrhea, rosacea, or staphylococci.

A. Anterior blepharitis is chronic bilateral inflammation of the skin, cilium follicles, or accessory glands of the eyelids. Recurrent conjunctivitis, burning, and itching of the eyelids are common complaints. The lid margins are erythematous, with dry crusted areas. Treatment involves removing crusts and cleaning the lid margins with diluted baby shampoo daily. Antistaphylococcal antibiotic ointment (bacitracin or erythromycin) should be applied to the lid margins bid to qid for 2 weeks, then nightly.

B. Posterior blepharitis is chronic bilateral inflammation of the eyelids caused by inflammation and plugging of the meibomian glands. Persons with rosacea or seborrheic dermatitis of the scalp and face are especially vulnerable to this posterior form. Treatment involves warm compresses, expression of the meibomian gland secretions, and long-term therapy with tetracycline 250 mg qid for 1 month then daily, or doxycycline 50 to 100 mg once or twice daily (for effects on lipid metabolism to thin secretions, not as an antibiotic).

CORNEA AND LENS

I. **Corneal Ulcers** are the result of an epithelial defect with stromal infiltration. Ulcers of the cornea appear as whitish, infiltrated areas surrounding a corneal epithelial defect. Ulcer is usually a complication of conjunctivitis, contact lens use, or a corneal abrasion. Soft contact and extended-wear lenses are up to 19 times more likely than daily-wear rigid lenses to cause ulceration. Fluorescein examination reveals the lesion. Apply topical gentamicin or tobramycin hourly and obtain immediate ophthalmology consultation.

II. **Optic photalgia (flash burns, "welder's burns")** occurs as a result of exposure to ultraviolet radiation (welding, sun exposure, snow blindness) and generally manifests several hours after the insult. Fluorescein shows an epithelial keratitis with diffuse uptake in the cornea. Treatment is similar to that for corneal abrasion, including strong oral analgesia and sedation if necessary. If no reduction of symptoms is noted after 24 hours, refer. Topical analgesics produce slow healing and can lead to additional injury.

III. **Corneal Abrasions.** See section on Red Eye.

IV. **Corneal transplantation** is a successful procedure for restoring sight in corneal disease. The most common indication is edema after cataract extraction. Rejection is a life-long risk, and topical steroids are used to reduce risk.

V. **Cataracts.**

A. **Cataracts are the most common cause of blindness worldwide** and a common cause of vision loss in the elderly. They can be congenital but most are acquired. Some medications (e.g., steroids, including inhaled) and systemic diseases (e.g., diabetes) can contribute. Prevalence increases with age: 5% prior to age 65 years, to up to 50% at 75 years. UV light can accelerate progression but cataracts generally progress over months to years. Symptoms include blurred vision, glare, and monocular diplopia.

B. **Treatment is surgical and done only when vision loss interferes with everyday life.** The most common technique is phacoemulsification (ultrasound fragmentation of lens with aspiration). Artificial lens implants are placed. Posterior lens capsule opacification occurs in up to 50% within 3 to 5 years, but incidence is decreasing with newer techniques. Treat with laser capsulotomy. Overall, 90% derive visual improvement with surgery. Potential complications include glaucoma, vitreous loss, retinal detachment and loss of vision, but complications occur in less than 1%.

RETINA

I. **Retinal Detachment.**
A. Retinal detachment is separation of the neurosensory retinal layer from its underlying pigmented epithelium. Patients experience some degree of vision loss and complain of cloudy vision, floaters, flashes of light, or a black curtain across their vision.
B. Risk factors include aging, myopia, eye surgery, inflammation, trauma, a prior retinal detachment, or a family history of retinal detachment. Fundoscopic exam reveals a gray or opaque retina instead of the normal pink retina. The arterioles and venules may appear dark, and floaters may be visualized.
C. Retinal detachment is an ocular emergency, and prompt surgical intervention is necessary.
II. **Retinal vascular occlusion** can involve either retinal arterial occlusions (resulting from embolism or thrombosis) or venous occlusions (resulting from thrombosis). Both manifest as painless monocular vision loss, with arterial occlusion occurring suddenly and venous occlusion causing vision to decrease over hours. The patient may experience transient episodes of blindness before the final event.
A. **Retinal arterial occlusion.** On ophthalmoscopic exam, a small occlusion produces a flame-shaped hemorrhage or a cotton-wool spot; a large occlusion produces a pale retina and a cherry red spot in the area of the macula. Intermittent digital pressure should be applied to the globe in an attempt to dislodge the embolus. Increasing the Pco_2 to dilate the artery can be attempted if one has the patient breathe into a paper bag or inhale carbogen (95% oxygen, 5% carbon dioxide). Urgent consultation should be obtained.
B. **Retinal vein occlusion.** Ophthalmoscopic exam reveals a blood-and-thunder optic fundus: massive hemorrhage covering the retinal surface and dilated veins. There is no immediate treatment for retinal vein occlusion, and the deficits are often reversible. Look for a cause including hyperviscosity, hypertension, glaucoma, or diabetes. These patients need to be followed by an ophthalmologist, because many will develop neovascularization of the iris or retina.
III. **Diabetic Retinopathy.**
A. This is the most common cause of blindness in middle adulthood. Prevalence increases with duration of diabetes. Symptoms include blurred vision, floaters, field loss, and poor night vision. **Nonproliferative retinopathy** includes microaneurysms, hemorrhages, cotton-wool spots, lipid exudate, and macular edema. **Proliferative retinopathy** involves neovascularization from the optic disc, retina, or iris secondary to retinal ischemia. These new vessels require laser photocoagulation.
B. Tight glucose control reduces the development and progression of this problem. Early detection/treatment is best to reduce vision loss: all diabetic

19

OPHTHALMOLOGY

patients should see an ophthalmologist at least annually and at the time of initial diagnosis.

IV. Age-Related Macular Degeneration.

A. Background. Macular degeneration is the most common cause of vision loss in persons older than 65 years. Prevalence increases with age: 8% of persons age 55 to 74 years and 30% of persons older than 75 years. The macula serves central vision but symptoms can include blurred vision, image distortion (metamorphopsia), central scotoma, and trouble reading. Risk factors include age, family history, cardiovascular disease, smoking, UV light exposure, blue eyes, and antioxidant vitamin deficiency.

B. Two types exist: nonexudative ("dry") and exudative ("wet"). About 90% have the dry form, but this accounts for only 10% to 20% of severe vision loss. The **dry form** is characterized by drusen (deposits of extracellular debris that appear yellow on exam) and geographic atrophy (patches of dead retinal layers). The **wet form** is characterized by choroidal neovascularization secondary to retinal injury. These vessels leak fluid and blood. Fibrosis develops months to years later, leaving a macular scar.

C. Treatment

1. **Laser photocoagulation** can reduce severe vision loss in wet macular degeneration, but only 10% to 15% of patients are candidates. Recurrence is high (at least 50%), and laser can worsen vision. Low vision aids help.

2. **Verteporfin, a light-activated drug administered IV,** concentrates in new vessels, sclerosing them, and can be used in wet macular degeneration. Pegaptanib sodium (Macugen) is an antivascular endothelial growth factor that is injected intraocularly every 6 weeks (NNT = 10 to maintain or increase visual acuity; NNT = 6 to lose fewer than 15 letters of vision on visual chart).

3. **Experimental treatments** include surgery, radiation, retinal transplantation, and antiangiogenic drugs (e.g., interferon-α-2a and thalidomide).

4. **Prevention.** Data suggest that antioxidant supplements (vitamins C and E, beta carotene) plus zinc may help prevent macular degeneration. Patients older than 65 years should see an eye doctor annually and use an Amsler grid periodically to self-check for vision problems.

OPTIC NERVE AND VISUAL PATHWAY

I. Overview.

A. *Strabismus* refers to an ocular misalignment. Strabismus affects 4% of children and may result in amblyopia (a vision loss that is uncorrectable by refractive lenses), reduced stereovision, and a deformed appearance. It is described according to the direction of the misalignment: *esotropia* refers to an in-turning of the eye; *exotropia*, an outward turning of the eye; and *hypertropia*, an upturning of the eye.

B. Strabismus may also be categorized as paralytic or nonparalytic depending on whether the involved eye moves at all. **Paralytic strabismus is suggestive of the possibility of a brainstem lesion and requires immediate evaluation.**

C. **Amblyopia secondary to strabismus** is correctable if treatment is begun by 3 to 4 years of age. Once the child reaches 6 or 7 years, vision loss is generally permanent.

II. **Examination. To determine misalignment,** look at the corneal light reflex when the patient looks in all directions. The light should be reflected on the same portion of the cornea bilaterally (i.e., light reflects off center of cornea bilaterally when child looks forward). Alternatively, use the cover test. In those with strabismus, the uncovered eye will move to focus properly on the object being looked at.

III. **Etiology. Predominant causes of strabismus** in adulthood include cranial nerve palsies, ocular myopathies, and myasthenia gravis. Consider MS, diabetes, etc.

IV. **Four Common Childhood Forms.**

A. **Strabismus of visual deprivation** often develops when clear vision is interrupted in one or both eyes. The most serious underlying causes are retinoblastoma and optic nerve or chiasmal tumors. Any strabismus in which there is visual loss at the onset of strabismus must be investigated immediately.

B. **Pseudostrabismus.** Eyes are functioning well, but the infant appears to have strabismus because of prominent epicanthal folds, flattened nasal bridge, or close-set eyes. No treatment is needed.

C. **Esotropia**

1. **Infantile esotropia** (about 20%) is an idiopathic form that is present at birth or develops in the first months of life. If it is intermittent, it should resolve by 6 months of age and does not need to be investigated before this age.

2. **Accommodative esotropia** (about 50%) occurs in children who have a hyperopic refractive error and must therefore accommodate to see clearly. It begins as intermittent and then becomes permanent as vision gets worse. As part of this accommodative effort, convergence is triggered, and esotropia may develop. This usually first appears between 6 months and 7 years of age (2 years average) but can appear as early as 2 months of age. Treat with refractive lenses.

3. **Congenital esotropia.** Children have no refractive errors beyond those of normal peers. Etiology is unknown and debated. Child needs an ophthalmologic exam to rule out other causes such as congenital VI nerve palsy, retinoblastoma, and accommodative esotropia. Early treatment results in better vision; treatment is surgical.

D. **Exotropia** can be intermittent, occurring with distant vision initially; may be noted more often when child is ill or tired. Usually, deviation becomes more severe and more frequent over time.

OPHTHALMOLOGY 19

V. Treatment.

A. Referral is recommended for initiation of treatment.

B. For those with refractive errors, correct refractive errors. Try to prevent amblyopia by patching the good eye or blurring the vision in the good eye with atropine (less effective). This forces the "bad" eye to strengthen.

C. For those with normal vision and congenital esotropia or exotropia, treatment is generally surgery.

BIBLIOGRAPHY

Age-Related Eye Disease Study Research Group: A randomized, placebo-controlled, clinical trial of high-dose supplementation with vitamins C and E, beta carotene, and zinc for age-related macular degeneration and vision loss: AREDS report no. 8. *Arch Ophthalmol* 119:1417-1436, 2001.

Akpek EK, Merchant A, Pinar V, Foster CS: Ocular rosacea: Patient characteristics and follow-up. *Ophthalmology* 104:1863-1867, 1997.

Block SL, Hedrick J, Tyler R, et al: Increasing bacterial resistance in pediatric acute conjunctivitis (1997-1998). *Antimicrob Agents Chemother* 44:1650-1654, 2000.

Douglas M, Strelnick A: Corneal abrasions need not be patched. *J Fam Pract* 48: 8-9, 1999.

Frank RN: Diabetic retinopathy. *N Engl J Med* 350:48-58, 2004.

Gariano RF, Kim CH: Evaluation and management of suspected retinal detachment. *Am Fam Physician* 69:1691-1698, 2004.

Khaw PT, Shah P, Elkington AR: Glaucoma-1: Diagnosis. *BMJ* 328:97-99, 2004.

Khaw PT, Shah P, Elkington AR: Glaucoma-2: Treatment. *BMJ* 328:156-158, 2004.

Khaw PT, Shah P, Elkington AR: Injury to the eye. *BMJ* 328:36-38, 2004.

Morrow GL, Abbott RL: Conjunctivitis. *Am Fam Physician* 57:735-746, 1998.

Nishimoto JY: Iritis: How to recognize and manage a potentially sight-threatening disease. *Postgrad Med* 99:255-257, 261-262, 1996.

Olitsky SE, Nelson LB: Common ophthalmologic concerns in infants and children. *Pediatr Clin North Am* 45:993-1012, 1998.

Pasternak A, Irish B: Ophthalmologic infections in primary care. *Clin Fam Prac* 6:19-31, 2004.

Quillen DA: Common causes of vision loss in elderly patients. *Am Fam Physician* 60:99-107, 1999.

Retveld RP, ter Riet G, Bindels PJ, et al: Predicting bacterial cause in infectious conjunctivitis: Cohort study on informativeness of combinations of signs and symptoms. *BMJ* 329:206-210, 2004.

Rubin GS, Bressler NM; Treatment of Age-Related Macular Degeneration with Photodynamic Therapy (TAP) Study Group: Effects of verteporfin therapy on contrast on sensitivity. *Retina* 22:536-544, 2002.

Sheikh A, Hurwitz B, Cave J: Antibiotics versus placebo for acute bacterial conjunctivitis. *Cochrane Database Syst Rev* 2:CD001211, 2000.

Shields SR: Managing eye disease in primary care. Part 3: When to refer for ophthalmologic care. *Postgrad Med* 108:99-106, 2000.

Solomon R, Donnenfeld ED: Recent advances and future frontiers in treating age-related cataracts. *JAMA* 290:248-251, 2003.

Tintinalli JE, Kelen GD, Stapczynski S (eds): *Emergency medicine: A comprehensive study guide*. New York, McGraw-Hill, 2000.

Wilson SA, Last A: Management of corneal abrasions. *Am Fam Phys* 70:123-128, 2004.

Fine SL, Berger JW, Maguire MG, Ho AC: Age-related macular degeneration. *N Engl J Med* 342:483-492, 2000.

Young JD, MacEwen CJ: Managing congenital lacrimal obstruction in general practice. *BMJ* 315:293-296, 1997.

Otorhinolaryngology

Mark A. Graber

EAR

Hearing Loss

I. **General.** Hearing loss can develop over time or acutely.

A. **Chronic hearing loss** has a prevalence of about 46% in adults aged 48 to 92 years and is more common in men.

B. **Conductive hearing loss** is caused by traumatic disruption of the ossicle, perforation of the tympanic membrane from cotton swabs or from noise, etc., cerumen in the canal, otitis media, and barotrauma.

C. **Sensorineural hearing loss** is caused by CVA (including sickle cell disease, polycythemia, hypercoagulable states, thrombocytosis), tumor, Ménière's disease, infection (syphilis, CMV, influenza, herpes zoster [may see vesicles, etc.], collagen-vascular disease), and ototoxic drugs (e.g., salicylates, aminoglycosides). An isolated vascular event causing unilateral hearing loss is not uncommon in young adults.

II. **Presentation.** Decrease in auditory acuity. Audiometry can be especially useful if readily available.

III. **To Differentiate between Conductive and Sensorineural Hearing Loss.**

A. **Rinne's test** measures air conduction versus bone conduction. In a conductive hearing loss (e.g., otosclerosis, perforated TM), bone conduction is greater than air conduction. The opposite is true for sensorineural hearing loss.

B. **Weber's test** checks lateralization of sound. The sound is louder on the side with a conductive problem. The sound is softer on the side with a sensorineural problem.

C. **Use these two tests together to determine the type of hearing loss.**

IV. **Approach.** Treat cause if found. If no obvious cause is found and serious illness has been ruled out by a complete history and physical (especially neurologic exam and perhaps CT scan), patient may be discharged with a follow-up appointment with ENT or audiology for further evaluation.

V. **Neonatal Screening.** Universal screening with automated auditory brainstem response can optimize language development in those with hearing loss. Test failure rate is about 4%, and incidence of bilateral loss needing aids is 1.4:1000. False positive rate is 3.5%. However, there is not enough evidence to recommend routine screening of the normal newborn at this time.

Ear Trauma

The exposed and prominent auricle makes it susceptible to trauma.

 I. Auricular Hematoma.
 A. Auricular hematoma is a subperichondrial collection of blood typically caused by blunt trauma to the pinna. The hematoma separates the perichondrium from the cartilage, predisposing the cartilage to avascular necrosis, infection, and "cauliflower-ear" deformity (blood stimulates overlying perichondrium, causing asymmetric new cartilage formation, which results in a deformed auricle).
 B. The hematoma must be evacuated by needle or an incision. A compressive dressing (e.g., a dental roll trimmed to fit over undermined skin on both sides of ear and held in place with a through-and-through suture) is then placed to prevent re-collection of the hematoma. The ear should be examined daily for signs of infection or recurrence of the hematoma. Use oral prophylactic antibiotics in immunocompromised or diabetic patients. If the patient presents 10 days or more after injury, the ear usually has fibrosis and needs open otoplasty.
 II. Lacerations involving cartilage should be thoroughly cleaned, sutured (carefully realign to maintain auricular contour), covered with antibiotic ointment, and reevaluated daily for signs of infection or hematoma collection.

Ear Pathology

 I. Box 20-1 lists the **differential diagnosis of earache** (otalgia).
 II. Otitis externa is inflammation or infection of the external auditory canal and auricle.
 A. Examination. Expect to find maceration of the canal (looks pale and boggy), erythema, edema (may cause hearing loss or aural fullness), perhaps fungal colonization, ulceration, and pain with manipulation of the pinna or with mastication. Fever and lymphadenitis may be seen in severe cases.
 B. Predisposing conditions include lack of cerumen, which is antimicrobial, and active removal of cerumen. Removal can cause breaks in the skin and exposure to water, which macerates the skin and raises pH, allowing growth of pathogens. *Pseudomonas aeruginosa* and *Staphylococcus aureus* are the most common pathogens in acute otitis externa.
 C. Treatment
 1. **The canal can be anesthetized** with 4 drops of ophthalmic tetracaine for 5 minutes. Lidocaine aerosol 10% and lidocaine 4% topical suspension have also been shown to be very effective at providing local analgesia, but lidocaine 5% solution has not.
 2. **Clean debris from the canal.** Depending on severity of disease, insert a wick (cotton or Merocel sponge packs) into the canal and then moisten

---

BOX 20-1

DIFFERENTIAL DIAGNOSIS OF EARACHE (OTALGIA)

- Auricular disease
- Canal disease
- Otitis externa
  - Foreign body (including wax)
  - Trauma (e.g., from cotton swab)
  - Ear eczema
- Middle ear disease
  - Otitis media
  - Mastoiditis
  - Other middle ear disease
  - Menière's disease (pressure sensation)
- Referred pain
  - Dental problems including abscess, impacted molar and caries
  - TMJ syndrome
  - Pharyngeal disorders including pharyngitis, malignancy, foreign body, etc.
  - Carotidynia
  - Cervical spine problems including osteoarthritis and spondylolysis
  - Neurologic problems including herpes zoster, glossopharyngeal neuralgia, trigeminal neuralgia
  - Bell's palsy (frequently starts with retroauricular headache)
  - Any **cranial** nerve V, VII, IX, or X lesion
  - Upper **cervical** nerve lesions

---

the wick with 4 or 5 drops of either polymyxin B–neomycin otic suspension (e.g., Cortisporin otic suspension) or a drying, acidic agent (e.g., Vosol-HC) every 4 hours for 2 or 3 days. Other options, such as ciprofloxacin drops, are more expensive but can be used in the patient allergic to neomycin.

3. **If cotton-like fibers of otomycosis are seen** (especially in warm, moist climates), add topical clotrimazole 1% solution. *Aspergillus* accounts for 80% to 90% and *Candida* 10% to 20%. Frequent removal of debris from the ear is crucial; the wick will help. Alternatives include amphotericin B (Fungizone), nystatin (Mycostatin), acetic acid (otic Domeboro), or gentian violet (2% in 95% alcohol).

4. **Change the wick or wicks daily in all cases.** Use oral antibiotics if auricular/facial cellulitis or lymphadenitis is present. Generally, use antistaphylococcal drugs or extended-spectrum fluoroquinolones such as levofloxacin. *Note:* This is not for malignant external otitis. See below for the treatment and diagnosis of malignant external otitis.

D. **Preventive measures** include waterproof earplugs for swimming. Do not use cotton swabs; dry the canal with a blow dryer on cool or use 70% ethanol mixed 50/50 with vinegar following swimming or other water exposure.

III. Malignant otitis externa is a progressive, necrotizing *Pseudomonas* infection typically occurring in elderly diabetic patients. The infection may extend to involve the parotid gland, cartilage, bone, nerves, and blood vessels. Potential complications include osteomyelitis of the temporal bone, facial nerve paralysis, meningitis, and brain abscess. Prolonged IV antibiotics with an aminoglycoside and third-generation cephalosporin or anti-pseudomonal penicillin (ticarcillin, piperacillin) can result in complete resolution. CT scan is necessary to evaluate bone involvement. Hyperbaric oxygen and surgical debridement may be necessary for more advanced cases.

IV. Otitis Media.

A. General. Otitis media is the most common reason for prescribing outpatient antibiotics and accounts for more than 25 million office visits per year. Many episodes are viral in origin, and recent research suggests RSV is the primary virus. The most common bacterial pathogens are *Pneumococcus* (40%-50% and least likely to resolve without treatment), *Haemophilus influenzae* (20%-30%), and *Moraxella catarrhalis* (10%-15%). To reduce antibiotic resistance, it is critical to distinguish acute otitis from otitis media with effusion and to prescribe antibiotics only for the latter.

B. Definitions

1. **Acute otitis media** is fluid in the middle ear demonstrated by insufflation or tympanometry with signs of infection. **The presence or absence of fever, vomiting, diarrhea, ear pain, irritability, and pulling at the ear are not helpful in making the diagnosis of AOM. The diagnosis must be made by strict criteria.** Table 20-1 gives diagnostic criteria for otitis media.

2. **Otitis media with effusion** is fluid in the middle ear without evidence of infection (e.g., lack of systemic manifestations). Antibiotics are not recommended for this group. Effusion may be present in 10% of patients for up to 3 months after an episode of acute otitis media or a URI.

TABLE 20-1
CRITERIA FOR TREATMENT OF ACUTE OTITIS MEDIA

Age	Certain Diagnosis*	Uncertain Diagnosis
<6 mo	Treat	Treat
6 mo to 2 y	Treat	Treat if severe illness, otherwise observation an option
>2 y	Treat only if severe disease	Observation an option

Note: To withhold antibiotics: Ability to follow up patient, temperature <39° C over past 24 h, mild otalgia.

*Sudden onset of symptoms, signs of middle ear effusion (e.g., bulging TM, immobility of TM [use pneumatoscopy or tympanometry], air-fluid level, otorrhea), signs/symptoms of middle ear inflammation.

C. Diagnosis. Overdiagnosis and unnecessary prescribing has contributed to spread of antimicrobial resistance. Hyperemia of the TM is an early sign of otitis media, but "red ear" alone does not establish the diagnosis.

D. Treatment of acute otitis media. It is necessary to treat seven patients to affect the outcome in one patient (NNT = 7). Eighty percent of untreated cases resolve in 1 or 2 weeks, versus 95% treated. It is difficult if not impossible to demonstrate the superiority of one antibiotic over another. Few controlled data support the traditional 10-day course. If there is evidence of TM rupture, add Cortisporin otic **suspension** qid. The **solution** is acidic and tends to sting when administered.

1. **Guidelines for treating otitis media**
   a. **Pain control** with topical solutions (such as Auralgan) or systemic agents such as acetaminophen, ibuprofen, or acetaminophen with codeine or hydrocodone may be required for patient comfort.
   b. **A 5-day course of antibiotics** is effective but should be reserved for those older than 2 years and those not at high risk for failure (e.g., no history of chronic and recurrent otitis).
   c. **Recent guidelines suggest withholding antibiotics from some patients** with acute otitis media. (See Table 20-1.)
   d. **Drug of choice is amoxicillin** 80 mg/kg per day divided bid-tid (125 mg/5 mL or 250 mg/5 mL suspension) for 10 days. High dose amoxicillin now recommended for all otitis media. **If the child has a penicillin "allergy" and not a type 1 hypersensitivity reaction,** use cefuroxime 30 mg/kg divided bid, cefdinir 14 mg/kg qd or divided bid, or cefpodoxime 10 mg/kg qd.
   e. **Second-line drugs.**
      (1) Amoxicillin–clavulanate dosed as 40 mg amoxicillin per kg/d divided tid for increased β-lactamase activity.
      (2) Trimethoprim–sulfamethoxazole oral suspension 1 ml/kg per day divided bid (8 mg/kg trimethoprim and 40 mg/kg sulfamethoxazole per day) for 10 days. Avoid in children younger than 2 months.
      (3) Erythromycin–sulfisoxazole dosed as 50 mg erythromycin per kg/d divided qid (suspension is 200 mg erythromycin per 5 mL) for 10 days. See above note in 1b.
      (4) Clarithromycin 500 mg PO bid or 7.5 mg/kg PO bid for children.
      (5) Azithromycin 10 mg/kg once, then 5 mg/kg for 4 additional days.
      (6) Ceftriaxone 50 mg/kg IM has been shown to be almost as effective as a traditional 10-day course of antibiotics. However, it is expensive and, because of emerging resistant bacteria, it should be reserved for cases in which compliance is questionable or as an alternative when treatment failure is apparent at 3 days of therapy.

OTORHINOLARYNGOLOGY 20

f. **When to change antibiotics.** If treatment failure occurs in 3 days, consider changing antibiotic to amoxicillin–clavulanate, cefuroxime axetil, or IM ceftriaxone.

E. **Treatment of otitis media with effusion.** Persistent middle ear effusion is expected at the end of acute otitis: 70% at 2 weeks, 50% at 1 month, 20% at 2 months, and 10% at 3 months. Overall, the benefit of antibiotics is marginal and increases the chance of drug-resistant *S. pneumoniae* carriage. See below for criteria for antibiotic prophylaxis and tympanostomy tubes.

F. **Follow-up.** Although traditional, a follow-up exam is not necessary in the asymptomatic patient who is older than 15 months to 2 years. If, however, the patient is still symptomatic or the parent does not believe the otitis is resolved, follow-up exam can be done at 2 weeks.

1. In adults, complete resolution of symptoms such as ear fullness may take 6 weeks.

2. **Decongestants play no role in the resolution of acute otitis media, although they may be needed for associated conditions.**

G. **For recurrent acute otitis**

1. **Antibiotic prophylaxis** (erythromycin, amoxicillin, TMP–SMX qd) use should be based on strict criteria. Prophylaxis should be reserved for those with more than three episodes of acute otitis in 6 months or more than four in 12 months. High-risk patients are those younger than 2 years and children in daycare. Don't use antibiotic prophylaxis for more than 6 months because longer courses are no more effective and resistance is more likely. TMP–SMX is the most effective first-line drug.

2. **Tympanostomy tubes.** Referral for discussion of tympanostomy tube placement should be considered if there is chronic bilateral effusion lasting longer than 3 months and with bilateral hearing loss, language-development delay, hearing loss of more than 20 dB, or failure of antibiotic prophylaxis to prevent recurrent otitis.

3. **Other preventive measures** include xylitol gum or syrup, avoiding smoke, reducing daycare attendance and use of pacifiers, giving influenza/pneumococcal vaccines, and encouraging breastfeeding.

FACIAL NERVE PARALYSIS

I. Bell's palsy (idiopathic) is the most frequent diagnosis but is a diagnosis of exclusion. **Bell's palsy (a peripheral VII cranial nerve lesion) can be differentiated from a central VII nerve lesion by exam.** In Bell's palsy, the motor fibers of all three branches are involved, including the ophthalmic branch (forehead weakness). In a central VII nerve lesion, the forehead is partially spared because of crossed nerve fibers.

II. **Symptoms include** preceding retroauricular headache, numbness of middle and lower areas of the face (which might not be demonstrable on exam) otalgia, hyperacusis, decreased tearing, altered taste (anterior $2/3$ of tongue), and facial weakness with equal weakness in all branches of the VII cranial nerve. Annual incidence is about 25:100,000.

III. **Onset is rapid** over 24 to 48 hours, with maximum paralysis within 5 days. Up to 16% develop sequelae after Bell's palsy.

IV. **Differential Diagnosis and Possible Causes.** Herpes simplex, Lyme disease (bilateral in 30%), *Mycoplasma*, sarcoid, vasculitis, diabetes, rickettsial disease, intracranial pathologic condition (e.g., acoustic neuroma), complication of otologic surgery, HIV, otitis media, multiple sclerosis, and trauma. Herpes zoster oticus (Ramsay–Hunt syndrome) manifests with vesicular eruptions. Intracranial pathology (tumor, meningitis, CVA) should be ruled out by history, physical exam, and testing as indicated. History of facial twitching, slowly progressing weakness, hearing loss, or additional cranial nerve involvement is suggestive of tumor and should be evaluated with CT or MRI. **Influenza-like symptoms and erythema chronicum migrans suggest Lyme disease.** See Chapter 10 for further information.

V. **Treatment.** Even without treatment, up to 85% improve in 3 weeks. Many others improve up to 6 months out.

A. **If the patient is unable to close the eye,** tape or patch the eye and prescribe lubricating ointment (such as Lacri-Lube at night and artificial tears during the day) to prevent drying and injury of the cornea. In severe cases a surgeon can put a gold weight in the upper eyelid or do a tarsorrhaphy.

B. **Steroids** continue to be widely used; however their use is controversial and there is contradictory evidence of their effect on the course of the illness. If you choose to use steroids, a reasonable course is 60 mg PO qd for 5 days, with a taper over 7 to 10 days.

C. **Acyclovir** has been used, but again the evidence is contradictory. Many would use this while recognizing the lack of good efficacy data.

D. **Some evidence suggests a benefit with a prednisone–acyclovir combination,** but this needs further trials to confirm.

E. **Those with a dense paralysis or with evidence of complete muscle denervation** by EMG have a worse prognosis. An EMG can be checked during the second week of disease if there is no evidence of improvement. Some recommend surgical decompression of the nerve at this point.

NOSE

I. **Rhinitis.**

A. **General.** Rhinitis is inflammation of the nasal membranes resulting in sneezing, itching, rhinorrhea, postnasal drip, and nasal congestion. Examination of a smear of nasal mucus stained with Wright stain can often make the diagnosis.

1. **The presence of eosinophils** suggests an allergic rhinitis or, in the absence of other allergic symptoms, a nonallergic eosinophilic rhinitis.

OTORHINOLARYNGOLOGY 20

Risk factors for allergic rhinitis include a family history of atopy, higher socioeconomic class, and exposure to indoor allergens.

2. **The presence of many PMNs** suggests an infectious cause (e.g., bacterial or viral).

3. If cells area not present, **vasomotor rhinitis (also known as idiopathic rhinitis)** is likely.

B. **Allergic rhinitis** affects 20 million to 40 million people. It often has a seasonal component or specific inciting agents such as animals or dust. Exam often reveals excessive tearing and pale mucous membranes.

1. **Antihistamines** help itching, sneezing, and rhinorrhea but have little effect on nasal congestion. For the latter symptom use decongestants like pseudoephedrine. Antihistamines also help the commonly associated allergic conjunctivitis. Chlorpheniramine is the most cost effective. Other options include the nonsedating antihistamines such as cetirizine (Zyrtec), loratadine (Claritin), and fexofenadine (Allegra). Antihistamines have class characteristics. If a patient does not respond to an antihistamine in one class, consider changing classes.

2. **Nasal steroids** such as aqueous beclomethasone or flunisolide are more effective than oral antihistamines for isolated nasal symptoms.

3. Non-steroid nasal sprays are available. These include cromolyn (Nasalcrom), ipratropium nasal spray, and azelastine (H_1 and mast cell stabilizer).

4. **Oral steroids.** Consider a short course of oral steroids for very severe symptoms or for those with concomitant nasal polyps.

5. **Leukotriene inhibitors** are modestly better than placebo and should be reserved for patients who do not respond to other therapy.

6. **Consider referral to allergy or ENT** if symptoms are recalcitrant because allergen immunotherapy or surgery (e.g., for septal deviation) may be useful.

C. **Vasomotor rhinitis (also known as idiopathic rhinitis)** is characterized by swelling of the nasal mucosa and rhinorrhea secondary to nonspecific, nonallergic causes such as recumbency, cold, and humidity. Oral decongestants, topical decongestants (such as oxymetazoline), and nasal steroids and ipratropium nasal spray (0.06%) may be helpful. Do not use oxymetazoline or any other topical decongestant (e.g., phenylephrine) more than 3 or 4 days because of the risk of rhinitis medicamentosa.

D. **Nonspecific eosinophilic rhinitis** might respond to the same measures as vasomotor rhinitis, especially the topical steroids.

E. **Hormonal rhinitis** is seen mainly in hypothyroidism and pregnancy (second month to term). Treatment is the same as for allergic rhinitis.

II. **Acute Sinusitis.**

A. **General**

1. Acute sinusitis accounts for 16 million visits annually. Sinusitis is the fifth most common diagnosis for which antibiotics are used. However, only 0.5% of URIs in adults develop into sinusitis.

2. Sinusitis can occur in any age group and often involves the maxillary and ethmoid sinuses in children. Children have 6 to 12 URIs per year,

and about 5% to 10% are sinusitis. Children are also prone to mucopurulent rhinitis.

3. A CT scan or MRI can radiographically evaluate the sinuses. **However, abnormal radiographic findings are seen in most children and adults with URI and in many asymptomatic children (i.e., high false-positive rate), so a positive CT does not always indicate sinusitis.**

4. **The majority of sinusitis is viral.** Of cases that are bacterial, *Pneumococcus* and *H. influenzae* are responsible for 70%; most other cases are secondary to *M. catarrhalis*. *Staphylococcus* and anaerobes may be involved in those with chronic and recurrent disease. Fungi (usually *Aspergillus*) can be causative in diabetic and immunocompromised patients. Some evidence suggests fungi may be involved in severe/chronic cases.

5. **Risk factors for sinusitis** include URI, allergic rhinitis, abnormal nasal anatomy, iatrogenic issues (e.g., NG tube), and immunocompromise.

B. **Clinically,** a history of a recent URI with biphasic symptoms—initial improvement followed by worsening—facial fullness, purulent nasal drainage, dental pain (especially with maxillary infection), and failure of OTC preparations to resolve the symptoms in 7 to 10 days are all predictive of sinusitis. About 25% of patients with a URI are still symptomatic at 14 days, so persistence of symptoms alone is not diagnostic of sinusitis. Other clinical findings can include fever, facial headache with pain worsened with bending over, malaise, and failure of the sinus to be transilluminated (indicating a fluid-filled sinus).

C. **Positive history and clinical findings are sufficient to treat.** Although many cases of sinusitis resolve spontaneously (self-limited in 40%-50%), antibiotics do shorten the time course and provide symptomatic relief. Note that most URIs are associated with viral sinusitis, however, which does *not* respond to antibiotics. Use the criteria above when determining whom to treat.

D. **Treatment** is topical decongestants (oxymetazoline [Afrin] 2 inhalations each nostril bid for 3 days or phenylephrine nasal spray 2 sprays q4h), rinsing the nose several times a day with saline solution, oral decongestants, increased clear liquid intake, occasional shower or sauna steamy air inhalation, and antibiotics. Antihistamines dry the mucous membranes and can cause crusts that block the sinus ostia. Traditionally, a 10- to 14-day course of antibiotics has been prescribed for initial episodes, although a 3-day course of TMP–SMX given with a topical decongestant (oxymetazoline or phenylephrine) may be effective in acute uncomplicated sinusitis. Those who fail a 3-day course can be treated with a 10- to 14-day course. Multiple studies suggest that broad-spectrum antibiotics have no superior outcome. For recurrent disease, 4 to 6 weeks of antibiotics may be needed.

1. **First-line regimen** (by far the most cost effective) is amoxicillin 500 to 1000 mg PO tid, trimethoprim–sulfamethoxazole DS PO bid, or doxycycline 100 mg PO bid.

OTORHINOLARYNGOLOGY **20**

2. **Second line** if initial treatment fails to reduce symptoms is amoxicillin–clavulanate 500 mg PO tid, cefuroxime axetil 500 mg PO bid, azithromycin, cefixime, cefuroxime, clarithromycin, clindamycin, or a fluoroquinolone.

E. **If a second-line regimen is deemed necessary to treat refractory acute sinusitis,** it is often necessary to treat for 4 to 6 weeks with antibiotics. Refer for possible surgical intervention if a pathologic condition is discovered or sinusitis becomes recurrent, chronic, or refractory to treatment. Sinus CT may be helpful prior to referral. Functional endoscopic sinus surgery (FESS) restores normal sinus ventilation, improves symptoms in up to 90%, and is more effective than adenoidectomy.

III. **Epistaxis.**

A. **Causes include** nose picking, external trauma, dry nasal mucosa with vascular fragility, foreign bodies, blood dyscrasias, neoplasms, infections, vitamin deficiencies, toxic metal exposures, septal deformities, telangiectasias, angiofibromas, and aneurysm ruptures.

B. **Determining the source of bleeding is often the most difficult part of the examination.** The posterior area of the nose is supplied by the ethmoid arteries (from the superior internal carotids) and the sphenopalatine arteries (from the external carotids); bleeding from these vessels is often difficult to control. Kiesselbach's arterial plexus supplies the anterior nasal mucosa and is easier to tamponade with a pack.

C. **If the bleeding has been prolonged,** check the patient's Hb and Hct. A PT/INR, PTT, and platelet count may also be indicated depending on the clinical situation.

1. If bleeding is easily seen and is coming from the septum, **direct pressure to the site** after generously spraying the area with a vasoconstrictor–anesthetic solution may be sufficient (pinch nose for 10-15 min).

2. If this doesn't work, try **silver nitrate for small bleeders or electrocautery** for the larger vessels on a well-anesthetized septum. Although there is no clear advantage to electrocautery, it may be effective in a patient who fails chemical cautery.

3. If this is ineffective, or if the bleeding is from under the turbinates, **insert the dry Merocel pack entirely into the nostril** (using a lubricant such as K-Y Jelly) and moisten it with phenylephrine, oxymetazoline, or saline until it has completely formed to the convoluted nasal passage, leaving it in for at least 24 hours. Alternatively, pack with petrolatum gauze soaked with phenylephrine or other commercial pack.

4. **Prescribe broad-spectrum antibiotics to all patients requiring nasal packing** while they are packed, because there is a high risk of sinusitis; TMP–SMX, amoxicillin–clavulanate, or clarithromycin are good choices.

5. **Examine the uvula.** If it is still dripping blood, hemostasis is inadequate and posterior packing may be required. Temporizing measures: Insert one of several commercially available posterior nasal packs or a Foley

catheter into the posterior nasal area and inflate. Anyone requiring posterior packing should also have an anterior pack. Obtain an ENT consultation and hospitalize any patient with a posterior nose bleed for observation or vascular intervention.

6. **Surgical treatment** includes arterial ligation, endoscopic cauterization, and angiographic embolization.

IV. Trauma.

A. Septal hematoma

1. **Diagnosis** requires a high index of suspicion and direct inspection of the septum after any nasal trauma. The main symptom is progressive posttraumatic nasal obstruction. The nostril may be obstructed by a large, soft, red or bluish mass. Its appearance can be confused with a polyp, a deviated septum, or enlarged turbinates. Septal hematomas can be easily missed unless the entire septum is observed visually and palpated with a blunt instrument.

2. **Treatment** is evacuation of the hematoma as soon as possible to avoid avascular necrosis of the cartilage, abscess formation, or saddle deformity of the nose. Any finding of a boggy, fluctuant septum that is tender out of proportion to other findings warrants treatment.

B. Nasal fracture.
Palpate dorsum of nose for deformity, instability, crepitus, and tenderness after any blunt injury causing bleeding from the nose. Diagnosis is confirmed by radiographs. However, treatment is based on the presence of deformity when swelling is resolved, and so deferring radiographs until swelling is resolved is acceptable; this should be discussed with the patient. Early reduction is possible if the injury is acute and swelling is insignificant. Closed reduction should occur within 3 to 7 days for children and 5 to 10 days for adults.

TONGUE AND MOUTH

I. Aphthous Ulcers, "Canker Sores."

A. **General.** Aphthous ulcers are recurrent painful lesions of nonkeratinized mucosa that vary in size and may appear as solitary lesions or in clusters (herpetiform ulcerations). The typical appearance is of an erythematous periphery with a white or yellow depressed center. Healing within 10 to 14 days is the rule.

B. **Causes.** Viral (Coxsackievirus, herpesvirus), systemic illness (Crohn's disease, lupus, Behçet's disease, erythema multiforme, gluten sensitive enteropathy), toothpaste (sodium lauryl sulfate), stress, food hypersensitivity, and smoking. Dental trauma, vitamin B_{12}, folate, and iron deficiency have also been implicated in some cases.

C. **Treatment**

1. **Symptomatic relief** can be obtained with diphenhydramine elixir used as a mouth rinse that is not swallowed. Alternatively, viscous lidocaine 2% can be used in adults. This can suppress the gag reflex, however, and may result in systemic toxicity in children. Application of a topical

steroid (triamcinolone as 0.1% in Orabase) or steroid mouth rinse (betamethasone syrup) may accelerate recovery. Herpetiform ulcerations may respond to tetracycline syrup, which is used as a mouth rinse and then swallowed. A burst of oral prednisone may be required in some cases.

2. The use of **multiple other drugs** including cyclosporin A, colchicine, thalidomide, and dapsone attest to the stubborn nature of these lesions. A mixture of nystatin 12,500 U, diphenhydramine 1.25 mg, and hydrocortisone 0.25 mg/mL has been used as a "shotgun" solution. Some also include tetracycline syrup in the mixture. **Amlexanox (Aphthasol) 5% oral paste markedly accelerates healing. In one study, healing at 3 days was 21% versus 8% with placebo. Complete resolution of pain after 3 days was reported for 44% and 20% of patients, respectively.**

D. **Prevention.** Using a toothpaste free of sodium lauryl sulfate or changing toothpaste is helpful in some cases. Topical use of steroids and mouth rinses can decrease recurrence. Avoid smoking and make sure there are no nutritional deficiencies.

E. **Herpes simplex virus** infrequently causes recurrent intraoral herpes. The lesions occur as a cluster of vesicles that rupture, leaving superficial ulcerations that remain for 3 to 10 days. Keratinized tissues, attached gingiva, and the hard palate are often involved, and such features distinguish herpes from aphthous ulcers. Treatment with acyclovir may decrease healing time.

II. Xerostomia (Dry Mouth).

A. **Causes** include Sjögren's syndrome, anticholinergics, radiation changes, diuretics, dehydration, surgical changes, infection (e.g., by CMV), mouth breathing, and diabetes mellitus. Xerostomia can lead to problems with eating, speaking, swallowing, dentures, and sometimes taste. Lack of saliva can increase risk of infection, thrush, and cavities.

B. **Treatment** includes artificial saliva, mouth washes, or hard candy; pilocarpine (saliva stimulant) tablets 5 mg PO tid; pilocarpine solution 1% 15 gtt in 4 oz of water, swish and spit. Pilocarpine solution can also be swallowed and will provide 5 mg of pilocarpine. Another option is cevimeline (Evoxac) or pilocarpine pills. However, swish-and-spit pilocarpine has fewer cholinergic side effects.

THROAT

I. Pharyngitis and Tonsillitis.

A. **General.** Most sore throats are caused by viruses and thus don't require antibiotics. Acute tonsillitis and pharyngitis manifest with throat pain, which can radiate to the ears, and dysphagia. Fever is more commonly associated with group A β-hemolytic streptococci (*Streptococcus pyogenes*), which accounts for about 15% of all cases. The proportion of pharyngitis and tonsillitis that is caused by group A streptococci is related to the patient's age. About 50% of children 6 to 15 years of age presenting with pharyngitis have streptococcal infection. The primary reason to diagnose and treat strep throat is to decrease acute renal failure from poststreptococcal glomerulonephritis (incidence 0.2-2:100,000) and rheumatic fever (which is already virtually nonexistent in the United States). **Table 20-2** shows partial differential diagnosis of sore throat.

1. **Classic strep symptoms** include sore throat, dysphagia, fever, malaise, and headache in the absence of other URI symptoms. Occasional patients have abdominal pain and vomiting. Signs include exudative erythema, palatal petechiae, and tender anterior cervical adenopathy.

2. **Other causes of exudative pharyngitis** include *Mycoplasma*, Epstein–Barr virus, adenovirus, influenza virus, *Arcanobacterium hemolyticum*, gonococcal pharyngitis, etc.

3. **Noninfectious causes of pharyngitis** include mouth breathing secondary to nasal obstruction (as with a URI). Mouth breathing classically manifests as a sore throat that is worse in the morning and abates as the day progresses. Viral thyroiditis can manifest as a "sore throat" as may carotidynia, an ill-defined entity characterized by tenderness over the carotid artery, painful swallowing, and pain radiating to the ears. Carotidynia responds to NSAIDs; antibiotic treatment is not indicated. Consider adult epiglottitis in the febrile adult with severe sore throat, trouble in swallowing, and anterior neck tenderness. Also consider peritonsillar abscess.

B. **Testing for streptococci.** Rapid streptococcal tests demonstrate a sensitivity of approximately 95%. Avoid false negatives with proper sampling technique (vigorous samples of both tonsils and posterior pharynx while avoiding the uvula and soft palate because they dilute the sample). The newer tests have a concordance of 91% to 95% with those of a culture.

C. **Whom to treat.** The central question in pharyngitis is deciding which patients require antibiotics and doing so in a cost-effective manner, keeping in mind antibiotic resistance. The treatment and approach to pharyngitis is mired in controversy **(Table 20-3).** Note that Table 20-3 applies to immunocompetent patients in the absence of rheumatic fever in the community.

D. **Treatment.** Strep throat is a self-limited disease that resolves in 2 to 5 days without treatment. Treatment may be delayed up to 9 days after onset of symptoms and still be effective at preventing poststreptococcal glomerulonephritis and rheumatic fever.

1. **Analgesics** should be offered to all patients.

2. **Treat for the entire 10-day course.** Clinical/bacteriologic cure is more than 90% (shorter courses are less effective).

3. **Group A β-hemolytic streptococci are essentially uniformly sensitive to penicillin.** However, some isolates are resistant to macrolides (>3.5%, with higher rates in Japan).

OTORHINOLARYNGOLOGY **20**

TABLE 20-2

PARTIAL DIFFERENTIAL OF SORE THROAT WITH SOME DISTINGUISHING FEATURES

Cause	Oral Examination	Skin Examination	Systemic Symptoms	Adenopathy	Age Group
Adenovirus	Exudative pharyngitis	No rash	Conjunctivitis, cough, bronchitis		Primarily children but also adults
Arcanobacterium hemolyticus	Injected pharynx with exudate	May have morbilliform rash			Young adults
Carotidynia	Throat exam normal	No rash	None	Tender over carotid bulb, no adenopathy. *Note:* may have pain radiating to ear when swallowing	Adults
Mononucleosis-like illnesses (EBV, CMV)	Injected pharynx, exudate	Rash in response to amoxicillin	Fatigue, fever	Posterior cervical adenopathy, axillary adenopathy, perhaps splenomegaly	Young adults
Streptococcal pharyngitis	Beefy red pharynx, palatal petechiae	Sandpaper-like rash with scarlet fever only	Fever, absent URI symptoms	Tender anterior cervical adenopathy	Children
Viral pharyngitis	Mild injection, pain out of proportion to exam	No rash	URI symptoms may be present	Rare	All

TABLE 20-3
DIAGNOSIS AND TREATMENT OF STREPTOCOCCAL PHARYNGITIS:
Symptoms suggestive of strep: fever, adenopathy, exudate, absence of URI symptoms

Patients	Number of Symptoms Present			
	0	1	2	3-4
Adults	Do not treat, no rapid strep	Do not treat, no rapid strep	Rapid strep, treat if positive	Treat, no rapid strep
Children*	Do not treat, no rapid strep	Do not treat, no rapid strep	Rapid strep, treat if positive	Treat, no rapid strep

*Some physicians would do a rapid strep test on all children and follow that up with a culture if negative. *But do not give antibiotics unless the patient has a positive strep test or meets clinical criteria for strep.*

4. **Some resistance to treatment may be noted** if the patient is simultaneously colonized with β-lactamase–producing *H. influenzae*.
5. **Drugs of choice** are penicillin (Pen-VK 500 mg PO bid or tid or penicillin G benzathine 1.2 million U IM in adults, 600,000 U IM in children) and erythromycin 250 to 500 mg PO q6h for 10 days. Consider amoxicillin for young children because it is more palatable and just as inexpensive. **If these fail,** a first-generation cephalosporin (such as cephalexin 250 mg PO qid or 500 mg PO bid) may be used. Alternatives include amoxicillin–clavulanate, azithromycin, clarithromycin, cefixime, cefuroxime, and clindamycin.
6. **Children may return to school after 24 hours of therapy.** Suggest that patients obtain a new toothbrush because strep can be harbored on toothbrushes and lead to reinfection.
7. **Proof of cure need not be documented.**
8. **Treating family members.** About 25% of family members of those with strep throat will be colonized. Guidelines suggest that there is no need to test or treat these persons unless they become symptomatic.
9. **Carriers.** Eradication need not be undertaken in asymptomatic carriers unless the patient or someone in the family had rheumatic fever; the patient works in nursing homes, hospitals, other chronic care facility; there is rheumatic fever in the community; or recurrent cases in a family are likely secondary to the carrier.
E. **Indications for tonsillectomy** include history of peritonsillar abscess and history of airway obstruction (sleep apnea) secondary to tonsil hypertrophy. Some suggest four or five episodes of streptococcal pharyngitis in a 1-year period; "chronic sore throat" with adenopathy for 6 months that is unresponsive to treatment is another indication. However, there is little evidence to support this and it is only a relative indication. Tonsillectomy will not prevent recurrent otitis media, although adenoidectomy might.
F. **Scarlet fever** is a self-limited systemic manifestation of streptococcal pharyngitis. Symptoms include "strawberry tongue" (a red tongue with

red or whitish papillae) and a fine "sandpaper" rash that appears as a diffuse erythema beginning and concentrating in the skin folds (especially axillary) but spares the palms and soles. Often there is circumoral pallor. A fine desquamation that begins on the fingers and toes may occur. The differential diagnosis includes Kawasaki's disease.

G. **For recurrent streptococcal disease,** attempt to identify a carrier in the family with throat and nasal cultures. Treat any identified carriers. Consider IM treatment to rule out noncompliance as a reason for treatment failure. Change all toothbrushes.

II. **Peritonsillar Abscess (Quinsy).**

A. **General.** Quinsy is a localized abscess that is typically unilateral and occurs in patients with tonsillitis.

B. **Cause.** Depending on the series, the most common organism is *Streptococcus* followed by anaerobes.

C. **Clinically,** symptoms include severe throat pain with radiation to the ear, drooling from inability to swallow saliva, trismus, and fever. Almost pathognomonic of a peritonsillar abscess is a muffled "hot potato" voice. On exam there is unilateral swelling of the palate and anterior pillar, with displacement of the tonsil downward and medially and deviation of the uvula away from the involved side.

D. **Treatment.** Clindamycin or amoxicillin–clavulanate and tonsillectomy. Several series have documented good results using oral antibiotics and needle drainage, which may need to be done many times. The major concern is the possibility of airway obstruction, although this is very rare. ENT consultation is recommended.

III. **Mononucleosis.**

A. **General.** Classically, the term *mononucleosis* has referred to the syndrome caused by the Epstein–Barr virus, which is characterized by an exudative pharyngitis, diffuse lymphadenopathy (including splenomegaly in 50%), malaise, fever, and fatigue. "Heterophil-negative mononucleosis," with the same symptoms, may be caused by other organisms including CMV, *Toxoplasma*, acute HIV infection, or leptospirosis. Mononucleosis is most common in young adults, and most of the adult population has had clinically inapparent EBV disease as evidenced by antibody titers. If patients with mononucleosis are treated with ampicillin or similar drug, they will almost uniformly develop a morbilliform rash. Rarely EBV causes genital ulcerations.

B. **Diagnosis.** Diagnosis is by CBC revealing a lymphocytosis with atypical lymphocytes. This is present in most of the mono syndromes. A positive heterophil antibody (monospot test) may or may not be present in the early stages of the disease (only 60% by 2 weeks) but eventually becomes positive in 90% of young adults. The heterophil test rarely becomes positive in those younger than 5 years. If there is any doubt, perform an EBV antibody titer. IgM antibodies against the EBV capsid (IgM-VCA) are produced acutely and can be used to diagnose acute EBV infection. Generally, they persist for 2 to 4 weeks. This is followed by

IgG against the capsid (IgG-VCA), which persists for life. Antibodies against EBV nuclear antigen are detectable at 2 to 4 weeks following infection. Liver enzymes are almost uniformly elevated.

C. Complications: CNS complications including encephalitis and aseptic meningitis, hematologic complications including hemolytic anemia and splenic rupture, hepatitis, and airway obstruction secondary to paratracheal lymphadenopathy. Rarely there is acute renal failure secondary to interstitial nephritis.

D. Treatment is symptomatic, and the illness generally resolves within 2 weeks. However, prednisone has been shown to reduce the length of the illness. A steroid burst of 30 to 60 mg of prednisone PO per day for 3 days or 4 mg of methylprednisolone PO tid for a week may be used but should be reserved for treating the complications of mononucleosis, including respiratory obstruction, myocarditis–pericarditis, aseptic meningitis, and hemolysis–thrombocytopenia. Contact sports or activities producing other forms of trauma should be avoided because of the risk of splenic rupture. Spontaneous rupture can occur in 0.1% to 0.5% of patients with documented mononucleosis.

E. Contacts. EBV is spread primarily via saliva and is not particularly contagious. For example, the college roommate of a patient with EBV is no more likely to contract the illness than is the general public. Ten percent to 20% of the population are chronic shedders of the virus. Despite this, there are no epidemics.

IV. Hoarseness (Dysphonia).

A. Hoarseness results from various pathologic processes affecting the vocal cords. Voice quality may be described as breathy, weak, strained, or tremulous. Descriptions can suggest certain diagnoses **(Box 20-2).**

B. Causes. Infectious laryngitis is the most likely cause in primary care practice. However, the history should elicit information regarding smoking and alcohol (risk factors for laryngeal cancer), voice abuse (risk factors for singers' nodules), and trauma. Hypothyroidism can cause a gradual and progressive hoarseness that resolves with treatment. Gastroesophageal reflux disease and tumor should also be considered (including HPV papillomatosis). Other causes include neurologic disease (stroke, Eaton–Lambert syndrome, myasthenia gravis, Parkinson's, essential tremor), lung malignancy, and other pulmonary processes (Wegener's granulomatosis, sarcoid), especially with hilar involvement, inhalation injury (e.g., smoke). Also consider recurrent laryngeal nerve injury from surgery or trauma.

C. Therapy. Hydration and voice rest are the primary therapy of suspected infectious laryngitis. Address the underlying cause. Treatment may include vocal hygiene, voice therapy, GERD treatment, speech therapy, surgery, or radiation. If symptoms persist beyond 2 weeks in the absence of URI, perform nasopharyngoscopy or refer for evaluation.

20

OTORHINOLARYNGOLOGY

BOX 20-2

DIFFERENTIAL DIAGNOSIS OF HOARSENESS

- **Breathy:** Vocal cord paralysis, abductor spasmodic dysphonia, functional dysphonia
- **Hoarse:** Vocal cord lesion, muscle tension dysphonia, reflux laryngitis
- **Low pitched:** Reinke's edema, voice abuse, reflux laryngitis, vocal cord paralysis, muscle tension dysphonia
- **Strained:** Adductor spasmodic dysphonia, muscle tension dysphonia, reflux laryngitis
- **Tremor:** Parkinson's disease, essential tremor of the head and neck, spasmodic dysphonia, muscle tension dysphonia
- **Vocal fatigue:** Muscle tension dysphonia, vocal cord paralysis, reflux laryngitis, voice abuse

Adapted from Rosen CA, Anderson D, Murry T: *Am Fam Physician* 57:2775-2780, 1998. Used with permission.

TEMPOROMANDIBULAR JOINT

I. **General.** TMJ disorders include arthritis of the joint, anterior cartilage (meniscus) displacement, and pain in the muscles of mastication (myofascial pain dysfunction).

II. **Symptoms** can include ear pain, headache, pain on chewing or opening the mouth wide with pain radiating to the ear, limited jaw mobility, clicking or crepitance, and tenderness on palpation of the joint.

III. **Treatment.** The balance of the data does not favor one treatment as best for initial management. True efficacy of most therapies for TMJ are unknown because they have not been adequately evaluated in long-term studies. Avoid clenching and grinding the teeth (bruxism). Eat a soft diet and use moist heat, massage, and NSAIDs. Avoid gum chewing. Some patients benefit from the use of muscle relaxants, bite appliances worn at night, or physical therapy. Relaxation and cognitive behavior therapy are effective for chronic pain. Referral to otolaryngology, oral surgery, or TMJ centers should be considered for refractory pain.

BIBLIOGRAPHY

Bisno AL, Gerber MA, Gwaltney JM, et al: Practice guidelines for the diagnosis and management of group A streptococcal pharyngitis. *Clin Infect Dis* 35:113-125, 2002.

Gilden DH: Clinical practice. Bell's palsy. *N Engl J Med* 351:1323-1331, 2004.

Lee D, Sperling N: Initial management of auricular trauma. *Am Fam Physician* 53:2339-2344, 1996.

Piccirillo JF: Clinical practice. Acute bacterial sinusitis. *N Engl J Med* 351:902-910, 2004.

Rosen CA, Anderson D, Murry T: Evaluating hoarseness: Keeping your patient's voice healthy. *Am Fam Physician* 57:2775-2780, 1998.

Sharp JF, Denholm S: Routine x-rays in nasal trauma: The influence of audit on clinical practice. *J R Soc Med* 87:153-154, 1994.

Slack R, Bates G: Functional endoscopic sinus surgery. *Am Fam Physician* 58:707-718, 1998.

American Academy of Pediatrics Subcommittee on Management of Acute Otitis Media: Diagnosis and management of acute otitis media. *Pediatrics* 113:1451-1465, 2004.

Williams JW Jr, Simel DL: Does this patient have sinusitis? Diagnosing acute sinusitis by history and physical examination. *JAMA* 270:1242-1246, 1993.

Long-Term Care

Jason K. Wilbur

GENERAL CONSIDERATIONS IN LONG-TERM CARE

I. The terms *long-term care facility* (LTCF), *nursing home*, and *intermediate care facility* (ICF) are used interchangeably in the literature.

II. **Providers should maintain a high index of suspicion for mistreatment in LTCFs.** Residents are at increased risk due to institutionalization and the specific characteristics (e.g., functional dependence, physical disability, dementia) that resulted in placement in the LTCF. Types of mistreatment include physical, psychological, and sexual abuse; neglect; and financial exploitation. Perpetrators may be employees, family members, or other residents.

DEMENTIA BEHAVIOR PROBLEMS

I. The Omnibus Budget Reconciliation Act of 1987 (OBRA) set forth **regulations regarding the use of antipsychotic medication in LTCFs.**

A. **Indications for appropriate use of antipsychotic medications** per OBRA:

1. **Agitated psychotic symptoms** (e.g., physical or sexual aggressiveness) presenting a danger to the patient or others or interfering with necessary care.

2. **Psychotic symptoms** (hallucinations, delusions, paranoia).

3. **Continuous crying out or screaming** (>24 hours).

B. **Inappropriate reasons that antipsychotic therapy is initiated** (and therefore should be avoided) include:

1. Repetitive, bothersome behavior

2. Isolated, withdrawn behavior

3. Apathy

4. Restlessness

5. Poor self-care

C. **Attempts at dose reduction are required within 6 months** of starting an antipsychotic unless there are legitimate reasons not to do so and these reasons are well documented. Identifying and monitoring target benign behavioral and psychological symptoms of dementia (BPSD) are essential to this requirement.

II. **BPSD are common in all types of dementia.** BPSD are due to disturbances in cognition, mood, perception, and sleep and include agitation, aggressive behavior (physical, sexual, other), apathy, depression, hallucinations, delusions, nighttime insomnia, and daytime somnolence. Symptoms tend to worsen as the dementia becomes more severe until eventually end-stage dementia causes the symptoms to lessen.

A. Nursing assessment. The staff at the LTCF should closely monitor BPSD and record what problems occur and when. Close attention should be paid to associated events (e.g., is the behavior related to transfers, bathing, or eating?). This is required by law if the patient is on anti-psychotic medications for treatment of BPSD.

B. Physician assessment

1. **Think of delirium** because the differential diagnosis is the same (see Chapter 9 for details about delirium).

2. BPSD may be the result of **progression of dementia** or may occur in response to acute or chronic pain, infection, metabolic disturbances, drug interactions and side effects (e.g., TCAs, digoxin, narcotics; see below for more), poor nutrition and dehydration, constipation, urinary retention, sensory deprivation, environmental changes, etc.

3. **Treat underlying causes.** Empiric therapy, such as scheduled doses of acetaminophen for suspected pain, should be considered as well.

4. **For the demented patient with BPSD** (symptoms not related to another underlying condition besides dementia), the first interventions are nonpharmacologic. Even severe problems may respond to redirection. Caregiver and patient education are key. Orienting stimuli (e.g., clocks, signs, family pictures) and continuous reorientation are proven to reduce BPSD. Patients tend to respond well to structure and socialization.

5. **Pharmacologic treatment**

a. **Antipsychotics.** These represent the mainstay of pharmacotherapy for BPSD despite lack of strong evidence. A systematic review in 2004 found little evidence to support the use of antipsychotics for any BPSD other than aggression, but several trials are ongoing. New atypical antipsychotics such as quetiapine, risperidone, and olanzapine may also be used but are no more effective and do not have fewer side effects in this group than haloperidol. All antipsychotics likely increase adverse outcomes in these patients!

b. **If an antipsychotic is started for BPSD,** use low-dose risperidone (0.25-1 mg/d) or olanzapine (5-10 mg/d) for most patients. Remember that risperidone is associated with a slight increase in stroke risk.

c. **Low-dose haloperidol** (0.5-2 mg/d) may be effective for patients who require more sedation.

d. **Frail elderly are more sensitive to the adverse effects** (e.g., sedation, extrapyramidal symptoms) of antipsychotics.

e. **Nursing staff must monitor and record** patient behavior and adverse effects while on these medications, and periodic trials of dose reduction and discontinuation should be made.

f. Generally, **antipsychotics should be avoided in patients with Lewy body dementia** because they worsen extrapyramidal and psychotic symptoms. Olanzapine and clozapine may be safer than other antipsychotics. Consider psychiatry or neurology assistance with these patients.

6. See Chapter 9 for a discussion of drug treatment of dementia.

7. **Antidepressants** have a role in treating patients with evidence of mood disorders and/or anxiety disorders. They are not used to treat primary BPSD.

8. **Others**

a. **Trazodone** may be effective in patients with sundowning (nighttime agitation, wandering, etc.). Use low doses, 25 to 50 mg hs to start. Trazodone has no anticholinergic effect, so it is considered safer than other options.

b. **Benzodiazepines** are used for short durations in patients with sundowning, insomnia, or severe anxiety. Lorazepam (0.5 mg hs) and oxazepam (10 mg hs) are preferred in elderly patients (half-lives are less affected by aging and they are less commonly associated with adverse effects compared with other benzodiazepines).

c. The antiepileptics carbamazepine and valproate have shown small clinical benefits, but risk of harm may outweigh benefit (valproate in particular).

INFECTIONS

I. **Infection Control.** The average resident of a LTCF will have at least one serious infection per year.

II. **All residents should be up to date on pneumococcal, influenza, and tetanus-diphtheria vaccinations.**

III. **Residents who are colonized with resistant pathogens** (e.g., MRSA, vancomycin resistant enterococcus) should not be denied entry into a LTCF, isolated, or kept from group activities. Decolonization of such patients is not effective.

IV. In general, **hospitalized patients have no better outcome than those treated in the nursing facility.** This is because of nosocomial infections, increased injury from delirium, etc.

V. **Evaluation of Fever or Suspected Infection.**

A. **Many of the typical signs and symptoms of infection are absent in the elderly.** Infection can be manifested as falling, confusion, delirium, fatigue, weakness, and other nonspecific signs and symptoms.

B. **Consider a lower criterion for "fever"** in LTCF residents. In this population, a temperature of 100° F (37.8° C) has a sensitivity of 70% and a specificity of 90% for predicting infection.

C. At a minimum, **assess the most frequent sources of infection:** upper and lower respiratory tract, skin, urinary tract, and gastrointestinal tract. The presence of tachypnea may be useful. One study of LTCF residents showed that the sensitivity and specificity of tachypnea for pneumonia was 90% and 95%, respectively.

D. **Diagnostic tests depend on the situation.** In a patient with no localizing symptoms, the minimum evaluation includes CBC with differential, urinalysis, and pulse oximetry. Chest x-ray and other studies should be ordered if indicated. Blood cultures are recommended only if the patient will be transferred to an acute care facility.

21

LONG-TERM CARE

> **BOX 21-1**
>
> **DIAGNOSTIC CRITERIA FOR UTI IN PATIENTS IN A LONG-TERM CARE FACILITY**
>
> Positive urine culture* *plus* three or more of the following:
> - Fever
> - Suprapubic tenderness
> - Flank pain
> - Decrease in mental status
> - Change in character of the urine

*A urine specimen obtained by clean catch or catheterization should have $\geq 10^5$ CFU/mL of a pathogenic organism to be considered positive. 10%-25% of residents are infected with multiple organisms, so a culture with more than one isolated organism should not be dismissed as contaminated.

VI. Urinary tract infection (UTI) is the most common source of bacterial infection in LTCFs and the most frequent cause of sepsis.

A. Asymptomatic bacteriuria is extremely common in LTCF residents. Up to 30% of men and 50% of women with no urinary symptoms or signs of infection have $>10^5$ CFU/mL of bacteria upon urine culture. Treatment of asymptomatic bacteriuria in LTCF residents does not reduce morbidity or mortality.

B. Diagnosis of UTI is not based solely on culture but rather on the presence of symptoms and laboratory evidence of UTI. **Box 21-1** lists criteria for diagnosis of UTI in patients in LTCFs. Chronic urinary incontinence and genitourinary symptoms, common in LTCF residents, do not improve with treatment of acute UTI.

D. Although outcome data are lacking, **a longer course of antibiotics, generally 7 to 14 days, is recommended in geriatric patients,** especially residents of LTCFs. For specific antibiotic regimens, see Chapter 8.

VII. Influenza. See Chapter 10.

VIII. Tuberculosis. LTCF residents should undergo a two-step Mantoux test, with 1 to 2 weeks between applications, to identify booster phenomena. Most often, a positive PPD in the LTCF represents past exposure rather than a new infection.

PRESSURE ULCERS

I. Definitions, Epidemiology, and Pathophysiology.

A. The terms *decubitus ulcer* **and** *bedsore* **are often used, but** *pressure ulcer* **is most appropriate.** The mechanism of injury involves pressure in any position. Pressure ulcers are staged based on thickness **(Box 21-2).** Stage I ulcers are only of clinical consequence because they are associated with a 10-fold increased risk of developing a higher stage ulcer.

BOX 21-2

STAGING OF PRESSURE ULCERS

Stage I

Nonblanchable erythema

Intact skin

Changes in skin temperature, consistency, or sensation

Stage II

- Partial thickness skin loss
- Epidermis and/or dermis
- Manifests as abrasion, blister, or shallow crater

Stage III

Full-thickness skin loss

Damage or necrosis of subcutaneous tissues, extending to underlying fascia

Manifests as deep crater

Stage IV

Full-thickness skin loss

Extensive destruction, tissue necrosis, or damage to muscle, bone or supporting structures

---

B. The **incidence** of pressure ulcer during hospitalization or LTCF admission ranges from 8% to 30%.

C. **Important factors in the development of pressure ulcers** include age older than 70 years (50% occur in this population), pressure, friction, shearing force, and moisture. Prolonged pressure between an external surface and a bony prominence (e.g., occiput, sacrum, ischial tuberosities, and heels) results in tissue ischemia. Shearing force has a similar effect. Direct mechanical injury does not contribute much to pressure ulcer formation; ulcers are mostly a result of pressure-induced tissue ischemia.

D. **Risk factors** include poor nutrition, incontinence, immobility or limited activity, altered mental status, advanced age, dry skin, hyperthermia, hypotension. Consider mistreatment or self-neglect as potential causes.

II. Assessment.

A. **Stage and measure the ulcer.** Ulcers cannot be staged accurately unless overlying eschar is first débrided. Evaluate surrounding skin. Explore the wound to assess for sinus tracts and undermining. Repeat the assessment periodically.

B. **Assess nutritional status.** Weight loss, poor oral intake, hypoalbuminemia, lymphopenia, and depleted triceps skin fold have been associated with the development of pressure ulcers.

C. **Assess for pain.**

D. Assess for infection by examination. *Do not* swab ulcers for culture. If culture is needed, use tissue biopsy or needle aspiration. Swabs are misleading and usually reflect polymicrobial contamination, not infection.

E. Assess for complications. The diagnosis of osteomyelitis can be difficult because radiographic changes due to pressure can mimic changes associated with osteomyelitis. Bone biopsy may be necessary.

III. Management. Institute prevention strategies listed below:

A. Pressure relief. For large ulcers and those not responding to usual therapy, consider an air-fluidized or low–air loss mattress, which increases the odds of pressure ulcer healing.

B. Débridement. Necrotic tissue must be débrided. One or more methods may be used: sharp débridement, wet-to-dry dressings, hydrotherapy, enzymatic agents (collagenase), and autolytic débridement (*not* for infected wounds).

C. Moist wound healing. Once débrided, the wound should be kept moist. Wet-to-dry dressings have no place in wound healing (although as noted above they can be used for débridement). A variety of dressings are available:

1. Transparent film (OpSite, Tegaderm) is good for superficial wounds with minimal exudate. It is waterproof but gas permeable. Change weekly and prn.

2. Hydrogel (ClearSite, FlexiGel) is good for minimal exuding wounds and helps in autolysis; change every 3 to 4 days and more frequently if needed.

3. Hydrocolloid (DuoDerm, RepliCare) is good for light to moderate amounts of exudates; occlusive gel-like covering protects the wound bed. Change every 3 to 4 days and prn.

4. Foam dressing (Allevyn, Nu-Derm) is good for heavily exuding and deep wounds; generally requires a waterproof covering. Change every 3 to 4 days and prn.

5. Alginate (SORBSAN, AlgiSite) is good for moderately to heavily exuding wounds. These dressings are antibacterial, require secondary dressing, might dry out minimally exuding wounds, and are expensive. Change every 1 or 2 days.

6. Gauze kept moist (not wet-to-dry dressings) with saline. This is good for various wound types and economical; it is usually changed daily or several times per day.

D. Nutrition. For malnourished patients with pressure ulcers, aim to provide 30 to 35 kcal/kg per day and 1.25 to 1.5 g protein/kg per day. Consider vitamin supplementation in patients with suspected deficiency.

E. Adjuvant therapies. Minimal evidence for any of these, but there is some suggestion that electrical stimulation of the wound after 4 weeks of conventional treatment may be beneficial. There is less evidence for radiant heat therapy, vacuum devices, hyperbaric oxygen, ultrasound, or platelet-derived growth factor.

F. Antibiotics. Topical and systemic antibiotics are not needed for most pressure ulcers. Consider a topical antibiotic (e.g., silver sulfadiazine) for ulcers that appear to have local infection or for clean ulcers that are not improving with usual therapy. Avoid iodine products, sodium hypochlorite, and hydrogen peroxide; these are toxic to fibroblasts and impair wound healing. Systemic antibiotics are indicated for patients with cellulitis, osteomyelitis, and bacteremia and for patients with cardiac valve disease (subacute bacterial endocarditis prophylaxis). See appropriate sections in this book.

G. Surgery. When a prolonged trial of wound closure using many methods has failed, surgery may be considered. Numerous types of surgery are available (e.g., skin graft, myocutaneous flap closure). The success rate approaches 70%, but the rate of complications and recurrence is high.

IV. Prevention.

A. For at-risk patients, maintain good skin care. Inspect skin daily; minimize xerosis (dry, cracked skin is a poor barrier); maintain good hygiene; minimize moisture caused by incontinence, sweating, and wound drainage; and use topical barrier creams as appropriate. Use transfer and turning techniques that minimize shearing force and friction. Ensure adequate nutrition. Document interventions and outcomes.

B. Frequent repositioning. Turn high-risk patients every 2 to 3 hours.

C. Pressure-relief surfaces. High-specification foam, water mattresses, and alternating–air pressure mattresses may reduce the risk of pressure ulcers.

D. An interdisciplinary team (physician, nursing staff, therapists, nutritionist, wound care specialist) increases the success of prevention and treatment efforts.

E. *Avoid* **massaging bony prominences** and using donut-shaped devices (they increase the risk of pressure ulcer development).

V. Complications include pain, local soft tissue infection, osteomyelitis, sepsis, prolonged hospitalization, and increased incidence of death in patients with stage II or higher pressure ulcers.

APPROPRIATE PRESCRIBING

I. The average LTCF resident takes six medications, and 20% take 10 or more. This high rate of medication use places these patients at greater risk for adverse effects and drug interactions. However, LTC may be ideal for slowly withdrawing drugs in a controlled setting and to optimize drug therapy.

II. To make appropriate decisions regarding pharmacotherapy in LTCFs, ask the following questions:

A. What is the problem being treated?

B. Is the drug necessary and is it effective for this problem?

C. Is the lowest effective dose being used?

D. Are there symptoms potentially attributable to the drug?

E. Are there significant drug–drug or drug–disease interactions?

F. Is there a more cost-effective alternative?

G. How often and by what criteria will the need for the drug be reassessed?

III. Inappropriate Prescribing. Due to narrow therapeutic indices and the possibility of severe adverse reactions, certain drugs are generally thought to be inappropriate in LTC. Some examples are given here (below and **Table 21-1**). Medications from the updated Beers criteria (Fick et al, 2003) are listed at http://www.dcri.duke.edu/ccge/curtis/beers.html.

A. NSAIDs. Potential adverse effects include GI bleeding, dyspepsia, renal failure, hypertension, and liver toxicity. For pain, including osteoarthritis, acetaminophen is better tolerated and often as effective as NSAIDs. COX-2 inhibitors cannot be recommended because of an increased risk of stroke and MI. Further, the GI safety data in this population are not convincing; acetaminophen is still first line. If NSAIDs are deemed necessary, use the lowest effective dose for the shortest possible duration, and use NSAIDs that have fewer GI side effects (e.g., ibuprofen, etodolac, diclofenac, nonacetylated salicylates [salsalate, Trilisate]). Avoid indomethacin; safer NSAIDs may be used for gout.

B. Benzodiazepines. Adverse reactions include paradoxical agitation, excessive sedation, and falls. benzodiazepines are potentially fatal when combined with other CNS depressants. Long-acting benzodiazepines should be avoided. Preferred are intermediate half-life benzodiazepines (e.g., oxazepam, lorazepam), which are inactivated by direct conjugation in the liver (therefore less affected by aging). Short-term use (30-60 days) is recommended.

TABLE 21-1
DRUGS CONSIDERED HIGH SEVERITY

Drug/Class	Comment
Amitriptyline	May be used for neurogenic pain if an evaluation of risk vs. benefit of the drug is documented, including consideration of alternative therapies.
Chlorpropamide	
Digoxin in doses >0.125 mg	Acceptable if an atrial arrhythmia is being treated; considered high severity if started in the last month.
Disopyramide	
GI antispasmodics (e.g., belladonna)	Using for short terms (max 7 d) on an intermittent basis (every 3 mo) does not require review by the surveyor.
Meperidine, oral	If started within the last month.
Methyldopa	If started within the last month.
Pentazocine	
Ticlopidine	*Not* considered high-severity *if* patient has previous stroke or TIA and cannot tolerate aspirin.

IV. **Drugs Often Underprescribed in LTCFs.**

A. **Vitamins and minerals** should be given to *all* patients (high rate of subclinical deficiencies). LTCF resident often do not receive adequate calcium and vitamin D. Most of these patients should have supplemental calcium (1500 mg/d) and vitamin D (800 IU/d).

B. **Opioids.** Studies have documented underuse of opioids in elderly patients with cancer pain; up to 60% of older cancer patients have substantial and undertreated pain. Nonmalignant chronic pain (e.g., osteoarthritis) may be treated with opioids if other modalities have failed and the addition of an opioid represents the safest alternative.

C. **Drugs for osteoporosis.** See the point about calcium and vitamin D above. Bisphosphonates are underused in this group. In most studies, bisphosphonates start to show a significant difference in fracture reduction at 6 to 12 months. Even given the decreased longevity in LTCF residents, bisphosphonate therapy for osteoporosis may still make sense.

MALNUTRITION AND WEIGHT LOSS

I. **Physiologic changes affect weight loss in older persons,** including a decrease in the resting metabolic rate and diminished taste and olfaction. **Causes of weight loss and malnutrition in the LTCF may differ from those in the community and include:**

A. **Medications.** Digoxin, antipsychotics, SSRIs, NSAIDs, narcotics, theophylline, clonidine, excessive doses of L-thyroxine.

B. **Depression and other psychiatric illness,** including anorexia tardive (nervosa).

C. **Swallowing disorders.**

D. **Inability to feed oneself** and insufficient staff to properly assist patients.

E. **Wandering and other dementia behavior.**

F. **Malabsorption.**

G. **Limited diet choices:** unpalatable foods, low-salt/low-cholesterol diets, monotonous diets.

H. **Metabolic disorders:** hyperthyroidism, hyperparathyroidism, hypoadrenalism.

I. **Other medical illnesses:** cancer, ischemic bowel disease, chronic and acute infections, tuberculosis, congestive heart failure, COPD, Parkinson's disease.

II. **Evaluation** depends on the clinical scenario. At a minimum, all patients should be evaluated for depression (consider using the Geriatric Depression Scale) and adverse effects of medication. Otherwise, consider the causes listed above when initiating an evaluation.

III. **Management.**

A. **Conservative management strategies**

1. Monitor weights periodically for early detection and intervention.

2. Eliminate anorexigenic drugs.

21

LONG-TERM CARE

3. Avoid restrictive diets (e.g., diabetic diets, low-cholesterol, etc.) when possible.
4. Maximize the taste and smell of foods.
5. Assess self-feeding and assist with feeding if necessary.
6. Consider bedside swallow evaluation by a speech pathologist.
7. Add concentrated feeding formulas (e.g., Ensure, Boost) between meals and with medication administration. Note that the beneficial effect of these formulas in LTC residents is in question.

B. **In general, tube feedings do not help and do not increase life expectancy.** A small subset of LTC residents may benefit from tube feeding. Residents who are thought more likely to benefit are generally younger, are less functionally impaired, and have tube feeding started for dysphagia or aspiration risk. Studies have shown that cognitively impaired and demented LTC residents gain neither mortality benefit nor improvement in their quality of life from tube feeding. The major risk of tube feeding is aspiration pneumonia. The decision to institute tube feeding should depend as much on the values and desires of the family and patient as on the medical evidence. If tube feeding is started, most LTC patients require 1.2 to 1.5 g/kg per day of protein, 30 to 35 kcal/kg per day of total calories, 30% of calories from fat, and 30 to 35 mL/kg per day of free water. Remember that tube feedings can be discontinued at any time by the patient or appropriate surrogate decision maker if so desired.

C. **Pharmacologic treatment** (note that there is no FDA-approved drug to treat weight loss in older patients).

1. **Megesterol acetate (Megace).** Recommended dose is 400 to 800 mg/d. There is definite, but only slight, weight gain in patients with AIDS and cancer cachexia; results are weaker in LTC patients, but some small studies demonstrate a benefit. Side effects include edema, hypoadrenalism, and vaginal bleeding.

2. **Mirtazapine.** Recommended initial dose is 7.5 to 15 mg qhs, with a maximum of 45 mg. It is effective for increasing appetite and weight in patients with depression. The most common side effects are somnolence and dry mouth. Note that other antidepressants may be effective in promoting weight gain in patients with depression.

3. **Dronabinol, human growth hormone, and testosterone** have not been shown in randomized, controlled trials to have any efficacy in promoting weight gain in older patients with weight loss and malnutrition.

END-OF-LIFE CARE

I. **General Considerations.**

A. The **principles of end-of-life care** focus on the overall comfort and quality of life of the patient. Symptom management rather than disease cure is the goal. Assess and support the family members.

B. **Attend to quality of life.** Help patients focus on life affairs beyond illness, taking "one day at a time," and completing unfinished business.

C. **Discuss advance directives (ADs) early.** Usually, LTCF residents have ADs in place. Properly verified oral statements are equivalent to those in writing, and patients may alter their ADs at any time. Communicate with the next of kin and check durable power of attorney (DPOA); ensure that DPOA is in writing.

D. **Remember to offer hospice referral early.** Hospice services are available in LTCFs and offer additional care to the dying patient. Patients must have a life expectancy of 6 months or less to qualify for the Medicare hospice benefit. Consider hospice for patients with any illness in its terminal stage (e.g., Alzheimer's disease, CHF, metastatic cancer, etc.)

E. **It may be appropriate to withdraw or withhold certain treatments** that do not fulfill the goal of improving quality of life (e.g., withdrawing lipid-lowering drugs, withholding antibiotics for dying patients who develop pneumonia). There is no ethical or legal difference between withholding and withdrawing treatment; a life-sustaining treatment (e.g., tube feeds) once begun can be stopped at any time, and discontinuation should rely on the patient and family preferences and values rather than perceived "medical necessity."

F. **Pain control.** (Refer to section on "Postoperative Care" in Chapter 15 for further information on acute pain control with opioid analgesics.)

1. **Freedom from or control of pain** is consistently ranked as one of the most important attributes of a "good death" by patients and physicians. The goal is to eliminate pain. If the primary goal is to relieve pain, the risk that sufficient medication will produce an unintended effect (e.g., hastening death) is ethically acceptable (principle of double effect).

2. **Assess pain regularly** to determine if it is present and if your therapy is effective. Standardize: Use visual analog and/or number scales. In demented patients, pain may be subtle and hard to assess: look for facial expressions of pain (e.g., grimacing, frowning), decline in function, change in behavior, change in sleep patterns.

3. **Tips for pain control in LTC.** Encourage frequent, consistent assessment by nurses; **use scheduled analgesics** for continuous or frequent pain; give clear parameters and dosing instructions for prn analgesia; anticipate the need for prn analgesics for PT, transfers, wound care, etc.

4. **If the oral route is not available** for medications or fluids, consider SL, PR, IV, and SQ routes. The SQ route is used increasingly in palliation because of its ease of application and because most medications that are given IV can be given SQ. Up to 1500 mL of isotonic fluid can be given SQ per day. Narcotics and benzodiazepines can be given SQ: Start with the same dose that would be given IV. Due to decreased muscle mass, the IM route is less preferable in the elderly.

II. **Pain Control.** The goal is to have good pain control on long-acting narcotics with a minimal use of breakthrough medication. Follow the

21

LONG-TERM CARE

scheme below for optimal patient analgesia. **Calcitonin is an excellent analgesic that works by increasing endogenous CNS opioids.** *Note:* The steps below apply not only to palliative care situations but also to pain management in general.

A. **Step 1.** Schedule a nonopioid analgesic. Acetaminophen is preferable because of safety. Other options include NSAIDs or adjunctive therapy **(Table 21-2).**

B. **Step 2.** Start a short-acting opioid (e.g., immediate-release morphine, oxycodone) on a prn basis to establish the dose needed.

C. **Step 3.** Once the dose is known, switch to longer-acting preparations (e.g., MS Contin, OxyContin, methadone, fentanyl patches). Methadone is particularly useful as a long-acting agent. Fentanyl patches can be very useful but they are expensive ($900 per month minimum and up to $2500 per month), can be erratically absorbed, and do not reach peak serum levels for 12 to 24 hours.

D. **Step 4.** Have a short-acting narcotic available for prn use for breakthrough pain.

E. **Step 5.** Increase long-duration opiate in response to the need for breakthrough narcotics. The goal is to have good pain control on long-acting narcotics with a minimal use of breakthrough medication.

F. **Start a bowel regimen with the initiation of frequent opioid dosing.** Give both a stool softener and a stimulant laxative. Some commonly used medications include docusate, senna, bisacodyl, sorbitol, and lactulose. Other common adverse effects of opioids include constipation, nausea, dry mouth, pruritus, sedation, and respiratory depression. All of these tend to resolve with continued opioid use except for constipation.

G. *Avoid* **meperidine in the elderly** due to increased risk of neurotoxicity.

TABLE 21-2
PHARMACOTHERAPY FOR PAIN CONTROL

Category	Adjuvant Analgesics*
Metastatic bone pain	Bisphosphonates, calcitonin, NSAIDs, acetaminophen
Musculoskeletal pain (not metastatic)	NSAIDs, corticosteroids (inflammatory conditions), muscle relaxants, acetaminophen, topical analgesics (capsaicin)
Increased intracranial pressure	Corticosteroids, acetaminophen
Neuropathic pain	Anticonvulsants (including gabapentin), tricyclic antidepressants, acetaminophen, topical analgesics (capsaicin), methadone, calcitonin, tocainide
Visceral pain	Acetaminophen

Note: NSAIDs, including COX-2 inhibitors, carry increased risk in LTCF residents but may be appropriate for adjuvant analgesia in terminal illness. Narcotics are effective for all types of pain but less so for neuropathic pain.
*Not in order of priority or efficacy.

H. **Propoxyphene/acetaminophen combination** is no more effective than acetaminophen alone and carries greater risk. **The authors avoid tramadol because of marginal if any effectiveness and high risk of CNS side effects.** Butorphanol, nalbuphine, and pentazocine are not recommended for LTCF residents.

I. When possible, in any given patient, **use a single opioid** (e.g., MS Contin and immediate-release morphine) rather than different opioids (e.g., hydrocodone and oxycodone). Exception: Methadone may provide additional benefit to an ongoing pain regimen with other opioids.

J. **When changing opioids,** use equianalgesic tables and reduce the dose slightly (due to incomplete cross-tolerance).

K. As a general rule, increase the dose of an opioid by a maximum of 100% (e.g., oxycodone 10 mg q6h increased to oxycodone 20 mg q6h).

L. **In case of a significant adverse effect** of an opioid (excessive sedation or respiratory depression), first try holding the drug. Then consider administering low dose naloxone 20 to 80 μg IV prn (about 1/10th the usual dose made by mixing a 0.4 mg/mL vial with 9 mL of normal saline to achieve a concentration of 40 μg/mL). Because naloxone has a shorter half-life than most opioids, monitor patients closely.

III. **Nonpain Symptoms.**

A. **Dyspnea** is common in the terminal phase of many diseases; it has multiple causes. Therapy may be directed at the underlying cause or may be nonspecific.

1. **Nonspecific therapy.** Elevate head of bed, provide suction, humidify air, teach relaxation techniques, and give supplemental O_2 for hypoxemia.

2. **Morphine** 5 to 10 mg PO/SL q15min or 1 to 2 mg IV/SQ 110 min, titrated to effect. Equivalent doses of other opioids may be used.

3. **Lorazepam** PO/SL/SQ/IV 0.5 to 1 mg every hour, titrated to effect. Equivalent doses of other anxiolytics may be used.

4. **For suspected small airway obstruction:** nebulized albuterol 2.5 mg inhaled every hour (or continuous), nebulized ipratropium 0.5 mg inhaled every hour (or continuous), or albuterol/ipratropium combined.

5. **For volume overload** see CHF in Chapters 2 and 3.

B. **Excessive oropharyngeal secretions** may be manifested by gurgling noises with breathing, which can be upsetting to the family. Place patient in upright seated or lateral decubitus position. Apply 1 to 3 1.5-mg scopolamine patches behind the ear every 72 hours. Other options include glycopyrrolate 0.1 to 0.4 mg q4h prn; atropine eye drops 1 gt sublingual q4h prn.

C. **Nausea and vomiting.** Seek a cause (the long list includes many drugs, intracranial tumors, bowel obstruction, infections, radiation therapy, metabolic conditions, etc.) and treat appropriately if one is found. Nonspecific therapy includes:

1. **Treat dehydration and electrolyte disturbances.**

2. **Antiemetics.** In palliative care, no antiemetic has been shown to be more effective than any other. Route of drug may be very important for

patient comfort: consider PR, SQ, IV dosing. In no particular order, try the following: prochlorperazine 10 mg PO/PR/IV q6h, promethazine 25 mg PO/PR/IV q6h, metoclopramide 10 mg PO/IV/SQ q4h, ondansetron 4 mg PO/IV q4h, haloperidol 1 to 5 mg PO/IV q6h, hydroxyzine 50 mg PO/IV q6h, dexamethasone 4 mg PO/IV/SQ q4h, scopolamine (see dosing above).

3. **Constipation and bowel obstruction.** May need a radiograph to differentiate constipation from bowel obstruction. Obviate constipation with stool softeners and stimulant laxatives in appropriate patients (see discussion of constipation in Chapter 5). Bowel obstruction is very common in colon and ovarian cancer; it may be best treated surgically, even late in the disease. Give scopolamine and/or opioids (see above) for spasm/cramping. Octreotide 0.1 to 0.3 mg SQ q12h or dexamethasone 4 mg PO/SQ qid may help to relieve obstruction. Percutaneous venting gastrostomy or NG suction may help patients who do not respond to other therapies.

BIBLIOGRAPHY

Quigley EM, Hasler WL, Parkman HP: AGA technical review on nausea and vomiting. *Gastroenterology* 120:263-286, 2001.

Besdine RW, Rubenstein LZ, Snyder L: *Medical Care of the Nursing Home Resident.* Philadelphia, American College of Physicians, 1996.

Medical College of Wisconsin: End-of-Life/Palliative Education Resource Center. Available at http://www.eperc.mcw.edu (accessed January 4, 2005).

Fabiny AR, Kiel DP: Assessing and treating weight loss in nursing home patients. *Clin Geriatr Med* 13:737-752, 1997.

Fick DM, Cooper JW, Wade WE, et al: Updating the Beers criteria for potentially inappropriate medication use in older adults. *Arch Intern Med* 163:2716-2724, 2003. Available at http://archinte.ama-assn.org/cgi/content/full/163/22/2716 (accessed January 6, 2005).

Thomas DR, Hosam KK, Morley JE: Management of protein energy malnutrition and dehydration. *Ann Long-Term Care* 6:250-258, 1998.

Tinetti ME: Preventing falls in elderly persons. *N Engl J Med* 348:42-49, 2003.

Office and Hospital Procedures

Mark A. Graber

TYMPANOMETRY

I. Indications. Tympanometry is useful for detecting fluid in the middle ear and for checking negative middle ear pressure, tympanic membrane perforation, ossicular chain disruption, or the patency of ventilation tubes.

II. Procedures.

A. Examine the ear canal and remove any occluding cerumen or exudate. Inspect the tympanic membrane. Select the appropriate tip for the tympanometer.

B. Grasp the helix and straighten the ear canal. Position the probe. When the probe is positioned properly, the automatic recording device will be triggered.

C. Leave the probe in position until the tympanometer signals the conclusion of the test. Repeat in the contralateral ear. **Figure 22-1** shows interpretation.

CHEST TUBE PLACEMENT

I. Indications: pneumothorax, hemothorax, or drainage of pleural effusion.

II. Contraindications. There are no contraindications to chest tube placement in patients symptomatic from the listed indications. However, care should be used in patients with a potential for serious bleeding.

III. Materials.

A. Iodine and alcohol swabs for preparing skin.

B. Sterile drapes and gloves.

C. No. 11 scalpel blade and handle.

D. Mayo clamp and Kelly clamp.

E. Silk suture (size 0).

F. Needle holder.

G. Petrolatum-impregnated gauze and sterile gauze.

H. Tape.

I. Suction apparatus.

J. Chest tube (size 32-40 Fr, depending upon clinical setting).

K. 1% lidocaine with epinephrine, 10 mL syringe, 25- and 22-gauge needles.

IV. Technique (Fig. 22-2).

A. Prepare the site. Position the patient with affected side up. Identify the insertion site, which is generally at the anterior axillary line just behind the lateral edge of the pectoralis major at the level of the nipple. Prep and drape the insertion site. Generously anesthetize the insertion site along the insertion tract to the pleura. The appropriate position can be

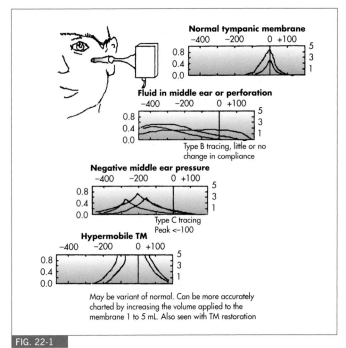

Normal tympanic membrane
-400   -200   0 +100
0.8   5
0.4   3
0.0   1

Fluid in middle ear or perforation
-400   -200   0 +100
0.8   5
0.4   3
0.0   1
Type B tracing, little or no
change in compliance

Negative middle ear pressure
-400   -200   0 +100
0.8   5
0.4   3
0.0   1
Type C tracing
Peak <-100

Hypermobile TM
-400   -200   0 +100
0.8   5
0.4   3
0.0   1
May be variant of normal. Can be more accurately
charted by increasing the volume applied to the
membrane 1 to 5 mL. Also seen with TM restoration

FIG. 22-1
Tympanometry. TM, tympanic membrane.

checked by aspirating through the needle used for instilling the local anesthetic.

B. Prepare the insertion tract. Incise the skin directly over the body of the rib; the incision length should be 1½ times the diameter of the chest tube to be used. Use the Kelly or Mayo clamp to bluntly dissect superiorly over the superior margin of the next higher rib. Then push the Mayo clamp, with tips closed, through the parietal pleura with slow, steady pressure. Once the pleura is penetrated, open the clamps wide to enlarge the insertion tract; then remove the clamps. You can insert your index finger along the tract to further enlarge the opening, if needed.

C. Insert the tube. Use the Mayo clamp to grasp chest tube near the end to be inserted; hold the jaws of the clamp parallel to the length of the tube. Advance the tube into the pleural space. Once the tube is inserted so that all drainage ports are inside the thoracic cavity, connect the tube to suction and suture it in place with silk suture by closing the skin edges of the incision around the tube and tying the suture ends up around the tube. Dress the area with petrolatum-impregnated gauze and sterile gauze sponges. Obtain a chest x-ray to confirm proper placement.

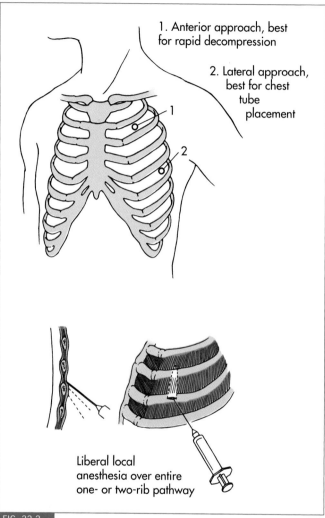

FIG. 22-2

Chest tube placement.

(Continued)

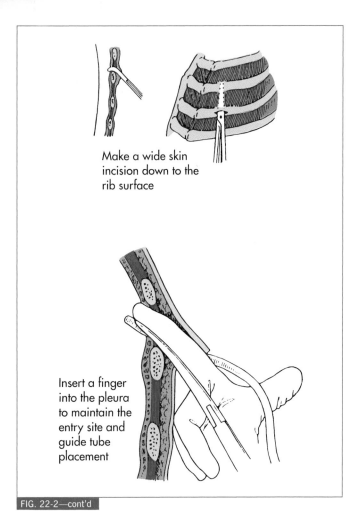

Make a wide skin incision down to the rib surface

Insert a finger into the pleura to maintain the entry site and guide tube placement

FIG. 22-2—cont'd

D. **Remove the tube.** Have the patient inhale fully and hold the breath. Pull the tube out swiftly. Cover the site with antibiotic-impregnated gauze.

V. **Complications** can include:

A. Hemorrhage at the site of insertion.

B. Infection.

C. Hematoma.

D. Lung laceration.

E. Laceration of intra-abdominal organs if the tube is inadvertently inserted into the abdominal cavity.

INTRAOSSEOUS INFUSION

Intraosseous infusion can provide a very rapid and dependable route of vascular access in children and adults (where vascular access is likely to be difficult in settings where it is most urgent). Almost any infusate can be instilled at a rapid rate through an intraosseous line, including blood and blood products, plasma protein fraction (Plasmanate), glucose, crystalloids, and pressor agents (including epinephrine, dopamine and dobutamine, and atropine).

I. **Indications.**

A. Emergency fluid infusion, especially in the setting of circulatory collapse where rapid IV access is essential.

B. Difficult IV access.

C. Burn or other injury preventing access to the venous system at other sites.

II. **Contraindications.**

A. Overlying cellulitis.

B. Bone lesion at site.

C. Osteomyelitis.

III. **Materials.**

A. Material for preparing the area (alcohol and iodine prep solutions).

B. 1% lidocaine if local anesthesia is appropriate.

C. 3-mL syringe with 25-gauge needle for infiltration of local anesthetic.

D. Sterile gloves and drape.

E. IV infusion set.

F. 18- or 20-gauge short spinal needle or bone marrow needle.

IV. **Technique (Fig. 22-3).**

A. Identify landmarks and prepare the insertion site with iodine or alcohol solution. Sites for insertion:

1. Proximal tibia 2 to 5 cm below the tibial tuberosity in the midline in children.

2. Distal tibia in the midline 2 to 5 cm above the medial malleolus in adults.

B. Infiltrate the overlying skin to the periosteum if the patient is sensitive to pain.

C. For insertion in the proximal tibia, direct the spinal needle inferiorly at a 45-degree angle from the perpendicular. If the insertion site is the distal tibia, angle the needle 45 degrees superiorly. In both instances the goal is to angle away from the region of the growth plate and/or joint.

D. Using a rotary motion, advance needle (with stylet in place) through skin, subcutaneous tissue, and cortex of bone into the marrow space.

E. Remove the stylet and confirm placement by aspirating marrow. Try infusing 5-mL saline with a syringe.

F. Detach the syringe and connect IV tubing to begin the infusion. Secure the tubing in position with tape.

OFFICE AND HOSPITAL PROCEDURES 22

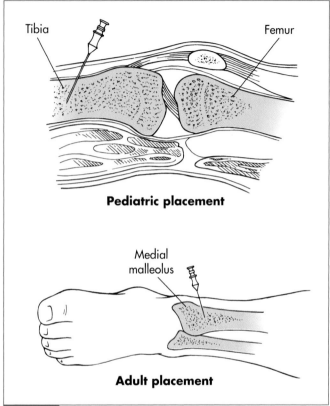

Tibia

Femur

Pediatric placement

Medial
malleolus

Adult placement

FIG. 22-3

Intraosseous infusion.

V. Complications.
A. Local abscess or cellulitis.
B. Osteomyelitis.
C. Injury to growth plate has not been identified as a complication that occurs with any significant frequency.

REGIONAL BLOCKS

I. Prep Skin and Draw up Anesthetic. Always raise a skin wheal before advancing the needle, and always inject slowly and aspirate to prevent intravascular administration.

II. **Digital Block.** Use a digital block to give complete finger anesthesia for reductions or for repair of lacerations **(Fig. 22-4).**

A. Raise a skin wheal using 1% lidocaine without epinephrine at the base of the digit at the level of the interphalangeal skin creases.

B. Use a 1.5-cm (⅝-inch) 25-gauge needle. Angle the needle 45 degrees from the finger in the horizontal and vertical planes and advance until the bone is reached.

C. Butt the needle tip against the bone of the proximal phalanx. Periodically aspirate for blood and inject local anesthetic while walking the needle (through the same puncture site) over the dorsal and volar aspects of the phalanx to leave a complete "half-ring" of anesthetized tissue on both sides of the digit. Use no more than 1 to 2 mL through either puncture site. Set the syringe aside for further use if needed. Gently massage the zone of anesthesia to ensure that an adequate block occurs after 5 to 10 minutes. If a distal pinprick sensation is still present by 10 minutes, you may repeat the procedure through the same puncture sites using another milliliter of lidocaine on either side.

III. **Femoral Nerve Block (Fig. 22-5).**

A. **Indications.** Pain management in patients with hip fracture. Bupivacaine should provide 6 to 10 hours of pain relief.

B. **Technique.**

1. Identify the femoral artery and the inguinal ligament. Use a 3.75-cm (1½-inch) 25-gauge needle.

2. Keeping a finger over the femoral artery, insert the needle 1 cm lateral to the femoral artery at or just below the level of the inguinal ligament and angled slightly cranially. The nerve is 2 to 3 cm deep. You may feel a double pop.

3. Aspirate to ensure you are not in a vessel, and inject 15 to 20 mL bupivacaine 0.5% *without* epinephrine.

C. **Complications** include intraarterial or intravenous injection of bupivacaine.

THORACENTESIS

I. **Indications.** Evaluation of a pulmonary effusion or relief of respiratory distress caused by a large effusion.

II. **Contraindications** include severe coagulopathies, small stable effusions, patients who are unable to cooperate, and patients responding to medical therapy.

III. **Materials.**

A. Povidone–iodine solution and swabs.

B. Gauze.

C. Alcohol pads.

D. Sterile drape and gloves.

E. 1.5-cm (⅝-inch) 25-gauge needle and 1% lidocaine.

F. 5-cm (2-inch) 22-gauge needle.

G. Three-way stopcock.

22

OFFICE AND HOSPITAL PROCEDURES

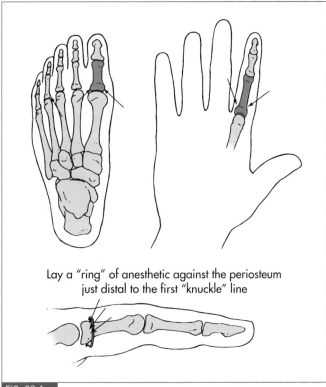

Lay a "ring" of anesthetic against the periosteum
just distal to the first "knuckle" line

FIG. 22-4

Digital nerve block techniques.

H. 5-mL syringe and 50-mL syringe.
 I. Three specimen tubes with stoppers.
 J. Adhesive tape.
 K. Optional: vacuum bottle, to attach to 15-gauge needle clamp.
IV. Technique.
 A. Determine puncture site by CXR and percussion. Have patient sit
     leaning forward. Put on sterile gloves. Prep and drape area.
 B. Choose entry site below the air–fluid interface and at the upper edge of
     the rib. Raise skin wheal with a 25-gauge needle and carry anesthesia
     down through the chest wall. Use a 22-gauge 5-cm (2-inch) needle to
     anesthetize the pleural surface. "Pop" the needle into the pleural space
     and confirm location with aspiration of fluid.

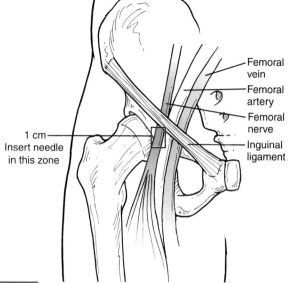

Femoral vein
Femoral artery
Femoral nerve
Inguinal ligament

1 cm
Insert needle in this zone

FIG. 22-5

Femoral nerve block.

C. Remove the needle and attach it to the three-way stopcock and 50-mL syringe. Reinsert the needle and withdraw enough fluid to fill the specimen tubes.

D. To remove a large volume of fluid, fill a 50-mL syringe and turn the stopcock to permit emptying. Repeat if necessary. If you will be emptying up to 1 L of fluid, attach a vacuum bottle by rubber tubing to a 15-gauge needle clamp tubing, and insert the needle in the clamp and allow the vacuum to aspirate the fluid.

E. When you have finished aspirating, withdraw the needle and apply pressure over the site for a few minutes and dress with a pressure dressing. Observe for dyspnea. Send fluid for cell count and differential, protein, glucose, LDH, culture, Gram stain, specific gravity, cytology, AFB, and fungal cultures. Obtain post-tap CXR.

V. Interpretation. See Chapter 4.

VI. Complications include pneumothorax, hematoma, hemothorax, and infection.

NASAL FOREIGN BODY REMOVAL

I. Indications. Nasal foreign bodies are common in young children and mentally retarded adults. Suspect nasal foreign body with sudden onset of respiratory distress, nasal flaring, unilateral mucopurulent discharge, and foul smell.

II. **Contraindications.** Few contraindications exist. ABCs take precedence over any procedures.

III. **Materials.** None.

IV. **Technique.**

A. Reassure and calm the patient and instruct the caregiver or parent to give the patient a breath "mouth-to-mouth" while occluding the unobstructed naris.

B. Place the child supine in the Trendelenburg position. Then place the child's head in the sniffing position with his or her mouth open wide.

C. The parent may obtain full cooperation by telling the child that he or she is going to give the child a big kiss. Then the parent delivers a breath with a tight seal. Subsequently, the obstructing object is dislodged, often onto the cheek of the caregiver.

D. Reattempts may be required with minor adjustments. Alternatively, an Ambu bag may be used to deliver a "breath." A drop of local vasoconstrictor may also be used prior to the procedure to minimize mucosal edema.

V. **Complications.** For sharp objects or objects not dislodged with this technique, refer the patient to ENT.

VI. **Other techniques,** such as using a Foley catheter or Fogarty biliary balloon catheter, positive-pressure ventilation or high-frequency ventilation, and bronchoscopic removal, are not discussed here.

Herbs and Supplements Formulary

Michael E. Ernst and Jennifer J. G. Steffensmeier

BOX 23-1

UNSAFE HERBS

CARCINOGENIC

Borage
Calamus
Coltsfoot
Comfrey
Life root
Sassafras

HEPATOTOXIC

Chaparral
Germander
Life root

MISCELLANEOUS TOXICITY

Licorice
Ma huang
Pokeroot

TABLE 23-1

HERBAL FORMULARY

Herb/Supplement	Indication	Efficacy	Contraindication	Drug Interactions	Side Effects
Androstenedione	To enhance athletic performance, increase energy, heighten sexual function	Probably ineffective	Should not be used by children or pregnant women or by patients with hepatic disease or prostate cancer	Can increase effects of exogenous administered steroids (estrogen, testosterone)	Decreased endogenous testosterone, increased levels of estrogen, reduced HDL, masculinization of women, testicular atrophy, gynecomastia, decreased spermatogenesis; possible increase in risk of prostate cancer and heart disease
Bilberry dried ripe fruit	Enhance vision; treat nonspecific diarrhea, mild inflammation of mucous membranes of the mouth and throat	Possibly effective for treating inflammation of the mouth and throat, improving retinal lesions	Hypersensitivity to bilberry	Anticoagulants, antiplatelets, LMW heparin, thrombolytics (may increase bleeding risk)	Well tolerated; nausea has been occasionally reported
Black cohosh	Premenstrual symptoms, painful or difficult menstruation, and neurovegetative symptoms (hot flushes) caused by menopause	Probably effective and comparable to estriol, conjugated estrogens, and estrogen–progesterone therapy	Pregnancy Unknown if suitable when HRT is contraindicated, such as estrogen receptor-positive breast cancer Duration of use should not exceed 6 months	None known	Occasional intestinal problems, possible weight gain Large doses can cause dizziness, nausea, severe headaches, stiffness, and trembling limbs

	Indications	Effectiveness	Contraindications	Interactions	Adverse effects
Chaste tree berry	Menstrual cycle disorders, premenstrual syndrome, mastodynia	Probably effective	Not for women who are pregnant, lactating, receiving HRT	None reported; however, dopamine-receptor antagonists, such as haloperidol, might weaken or block the effects	Gastrointestinal and lower abdominal complaints, allergic reactions (itching and rash), headache, menorrhagia
Chondroitin	Nonapproved indications: as viscoelastic agent in ophthalmic procedures and treatment of osteoarthritis	Probably effective for osteoarthritis; can take 2-4 mo	Previous hypersensitivity to chondroitin sulfate	None reported	Nausea and epigastric pain
Chromium picolinate	To improve glycemic control in T1DM and T2DM; to enhance weight loss, athletic performance; to increase energy	Possibly effective for T2DM Probably ineffective for weight loss and other indications	None known	Antacids, H_2 blockers, proton-pump inhibitors (can decrease chromium levels); insulin (can potentiate hypoglycemia); NSAIDs (can increase chromium levels); corticosteroids (chromium can decrease corticosteroid-induced increases in blood sugar)	Well-tolerated; cognitive, perceptual, and motor dysfunction has been occasionally reported; weight gain; headache, insomnia, sleep disturbance, irritability, mood changes

(Continued)

TABLE 23-1

HERBAL FORMULARY—cont'd

Herb/Supplement	Indication	Efficacy	Contraindication	Drug Interactions	Side Effects
Coenzyme Q10	Nonapproved indications: CHF, hypertension, stable angina, ventricular arrhythmias, cancer, heart surgery, periodontal disease *Orphan drug for mitochondrial diseases*	Possibly effective for CHF; efficacy for other indications not yet proven, except benefit shown for mitochondrial diseases	Biliary obstruction, diabetes (hypoglycemia), hepatic insufficiency, renal insufficiency	Hypolipidemic agents lower plasma concentrations of CoQ10; oral hypoglycemic agents potentially inhibit effects of exogenous administration	Rash and gastrointestinal disturbances such as nausea, anorexia, epigastric pain, diarrhea Elevations of serum aminotransferases have occurred with relatively high oral doses
Cranberry	To prevent and treat urinary tract infections	Possibly effective for preventing UTIs	Nephrolithiasis	Proton-pump inhibitors (can increase absorption of vitamin B_{12})	Well tolerated; consumption of large amounts and over an extended period of time can lead to GI upset and an increased risk of uric acid kidney stone formation

	Uses	Effectiveness	Contraindications	Interactions	Adverse Effects
Creatine	To improve exercise performance and increase muscle mass; to treat CHF, muscular dystrophies, rheumatoid arthritis	Possibly effective for enhancing muscle performance during brief, high-intensity exercise; might improve exercise tolerance in patients with CHF; might improve muscle strength in various muscular dystrophies; probably ineffective for RA	Pregnancy, renal dysfunction	Avoid concurrent use with nephrotoxic drugs	GI pain, nausea, diarrhea; muscle cramps; weight gain (with prolonged supplementation); renal dysfunction (rare in patients with normal renal function)
Dong quai	Menstrual disorders, anemia, constipation, insomnia, rheumatism, neuralgia, and hypertension	Probably not effective	Pregnancy (uterine stimulant) and lactation; hypermenorrhea; diarrhea; hemorrhagic disease; colds or flu; allergy to parsley	Unknown	Photodermatitis can occur in persons collecting the plant Safrole, found in the oil of dong quai, is carcinogenic and not recommended for ingestion

(Continued)

TABLE 23-1

HERBAL FORMULARY—cont'd

Herb/Supplement	Indication	Efficacy	Contraindication	Drug Interactions	Side Effects
Echinacea	Internal use: supportive therapy for infections of the upper respiratory tract (colds) and lower urinary tract. External use: local application to treat hard-to-heal superficial wounds and ulcers	Probably mildly effective for common cold. Insufficient evidence for influenza	Infectious and autoimmune diseases (tuberculosis, leukosis, collagenosis, multiple sclerosis, AIDS, HIV, lupus). Use caution in patients who are allergic to members of the sunflower family. The effects of echinacea in children and in pregnant and lactating women are unknown	None known	None known
Feverfew	Prophylaxis for migraine headaches	Probably effective	Pregnancy and lactation. Do not use in children younger than 2 years	Might interact with anticoagulants, increasing the risk of bleeding	Gastric discomfort; minor ulcerations of oral mucosa, irritation of tongue, and swelling of lips can occur when fresh leaves are chewed

Fish oil	Hypercholesterolemia and CAD	Likely effective for treating hypertriglyceridemia Possibly effective for reducing mortality risk from coronary artery disease, hypercholesterolemia	Cirrhosis	Anticoagulant and antiplatelet medications (increased risk of bleeding); hypoglycemic medications (may interfere with blood glucose control); antihypertensives (may have an additive effect at lowering blood pressure)	Should not take continuously for >4 mo without medical advice Belching, heartburn, nausea, loose stools At doses >3 g, potential for increased bleeding from inhibition of platelets; can interfere with immune system
Garlic	To support dietary measures treating hyperlipoproteinemia and to prevent age-related changes in the blood vessels (arteriosclerosis)	Proven to reduce blood pressure and cholesterol, but data are not the best Possibly effective in colorectal and prostate cancer prevention (aged garlic)	Caution in diabetic patients Caution in pregnant women (emmenagogue and abortifacient)	Anticoagulants (increased bleeding)	Gastrointestinal discomfort (heartburn, flatulence), sweating, lightheadedness, allergic reactions, menorrhagia

(Continued)

HERBS AND SUPPLEMENTS FORMULARY 23

TABLE 23-1
HERBAL FORMULARY—cont'd

Herb/Supplement	Indication	Efficacy	Contraindication	Drug Interactions	Side Effects
Ginger	To treat dyspepsia; as prophylaxis for symptoms of travel sickness	No benefit overall for motion sickness Possibly effective for chemotherapy-related nausea, morning sickness, perioperative nausea and vomiting, vertigo	Postoperative nausea (may prolong bleeding time); gallstone pain Avoid in pregnancy (uterine relaxant [low doses]; uterine stimulant [high doses])	None known	None reported
Ginkgo (leaf extract; ginkgo fruit likely ineffective)	Cerebral circulatory disturbances resulting in reduced functional capacity and vigilance (vertigo, tinnitus, weakened memory, and mood swings accompanied by anxiety); peripheral arterial circulatory disturbance such as intermittent claudication	Minor effects for improving CNS function (including in Alzheimer's disease) Possible benefit in claudication	None known	Antiplatelet drugs: spontaneous hyphema (bleeding from iris into the anterior chamber) from ginkgo and aspirin	Gastric disturbances, headache, dizziness, vertigo Toxic ingestion can produce tonic–clonic seizures and loss of consciousness

Herb				
Ginseng (Asian, *Panax*)	Feelings of lassitude and debility, lack of energy and ability to concentrate, and during convalescence	Possible benefit for fatigue, cognitive function, diabetes	Pregnancy Do not use in children Avoid in patients with hypertension, emotional or psychological imbalances, headaches, heart palpitations, insomnia, asthma, inflammation, or infections with high fever	Phenelzine (hallucinations and psychosis) Warfarin (can decrease INR)	Nervousness and excitation; inability to concentrate with long-term use Hypertension, euphoria, restlessness, nervousness, insomnia, skin eruptions, edema, and diarrhea have been reported with long-term ginseng use with an average daily dose of 3 g ginseng root
Ginseng (Siberian)	Fatigue, convalescence, decreased work capacity, difficulty concentrating	No benefit in randomized, placebo-controlled study	Hypertension, febrile states, hypertonic crisis, myocardial infarction	Increases sleep latency and duration; can increase serum levels of digoxin	Mild, transient diarrhea and insomnia Can lower blood glucose
Glucosamine	Nonapproved indications: osteoarthritis	Likely effective; may be comparable to NSAIDs or not quite as good as ibuprofen; not all studies positive	Hypersensitivity to glucosamine Might impair insulin secretion in diabetic persons	Fluoxetine can increase serum concentrations of glucosamine	Gastrointestinal side effects, e.g., epigastric pain and tenderness, heartburn, diarrhea, nausea Central nervous system side effects, e.g., drowsiness, headache, insomnia Long-term side effects are unknown

(Continued)

HERBS AND SUPPLEMENTS FORMULARY　23

TABLE 23-1

HERBAL FORMULARY—cont'd

Herb/Supplement	Indication	Efficacy	Contraindication	Drug Interactions	Side Effects
Grapefruit	Primarily consumed as fruit or juice; no specific health conditions treated	Might reduce cholesterol, reduce risk of cancer	None known	Inhibits cytochrome (CYP) activity; avoid concurrent ingestion primarily with drugs metabolized by CYP3A4 (calcium channel blockers, HMG-CoA reductase inhibitors, warfarin, benzodiazepines, carbamazepine, cyclosporine, itraconazole, losartan, quinidine, saquinavir, fexofenadine)	Consumption of one half to one grapefruit per day can reduce hematocrit levels
Grape seed extract	To prevent and treat vascular disorders	Possibly effective for treating venous insufficiency	Unknown	Warfarin (increased risk of bleeding)	None known

Hawthorn	Mild cardiac conditions such as congestive heart failure, NYHA stages I or II, "uneasiness and oppressed feeling of the heart," not yet digitalized heart, and light forms of bradycardic arrhythmia	Possibly effective in providing symptomatic relief of CHF	Pregnancy, lactation Not for self-treatment	Interaction unknown with other cardiovascular drugs, e.g., digoxin, calcium channel blockers, β-blockers, antiarrhythmics	Large doses can induce hypotension, arrhythmias, sedation
Horse chestnut seed	Venous conditions, eczema, leg pains, hemorrhoids, phlebitis, menstrual cramps	Likely effective	Renal and hepatic insufficiency	Anticoagulants	Gastrointestinal irritation, pruritus, giddiness
Kava	Insomnia, nervousness, benzodiazepine withdrawal	Possibly effective	Depression (increased risk of suicide) Operating machinery or motor vehicles Should not be taken longer than 3 mo without doctor's supervision Pregnancy, lactation Not for children	Sedatives, anxiolytics, MAO inhibitors, antidepressants, alcohol, antiplatelets Levodopa (decreased levels)	Yellowing skin, nails, hair; allergic skin reactions; gastrointestinal complaints; pupil dilation; disorders of oculomotor equilibrium; morning fatigue; neurologic choreoathetosis; dystonic reactions; dyskinesia

(Continued)

HERBS AND SUPPLEMENTS FORMULARY 23

TABLE 23-1

HERBAL FORMULARY—cont'd

Herb/Supplement	Indication	Efficacy	Contraindication	Drug Interactions	Side Effects
Lactobacillus	To treat and prevent diarrhea; for general digestive problems	Possibly effective for treating and preventing diarrhea (infectious types, travelers', antibiotic-associated) Possibly ineffective when used for general digestive problems (inflammatory bowel syndrome and lactose intolerance)	Pregnancy, lactation, immunocompromise	Antibiotics (may decrease effectiveness of lactobacillus)	Well tolerated; flatulence is the most common side effect
Licorice	Expectorant; to treat ulcers	Negative human evidence or insufficient evidence to rate	Liver cirrhosis, cholestatic liver disorders, hypertonia, kidney diseases, cardiovascular diseases (especially hypertension), hypokalemia, and pregnancy	Potassium loss may be increased in the presence of other drugs, e.g., thiazide and loop diuretics; with loss of potassium, sensitivity to digitalis glycosides increases	Prolongation of P-R and Q-T intervals With long-term use or acute toxic ingestion, pseudoaldosteronism (headache, lethargy, sodium and water retention, hypokalemia, high blood pressure, heart failure and cardiac arrest)

		German Commission E stipulates duration of use no longer than 4-6 wk		
Lutein	Macular degeneration	Possibly effective when consumed as part of a healthy diet; might reduce risk of age-related macular degeneration	None known	None known
Lycopene	Prevention of cancer	When consumed as part of a healthy diet, possibly effective in preventing prostate, lung, and ovarian cancers	None known	None known
Ma huang	CNS stimulant (derivative of ephedrine)	Dangerous; should not be used	Heart conditions, hypertension, diabetes, thyroid disease	Similar to those of ephedrine and pseudoephedrine; avoid consumption with caffeine	Nervousness, headache, insomnia, dizziness, palpitations, skin flushing, tingling, vomiting, hypertension, myocardial infarction

(Continued)

HERBS AND SUPPLEMENTS FORMULARY 23

TABLE 23-1
HERBAL FORMULARY—cont'd

Herb/Supplement	Indication	Efficacy	Contraindication	Drug Interactions	Side Effects
Melatonin	Circadian rhythm sleep disorders in blind people with no light perception Nonapproved indications: jet lag, insomnia, depression, cancer *Orphan drug*	Likely effective in circadian rhythm disturbances; possibly effective for jet lag Likely ineffective in preventing fatigue in shift workers	Depression (can aggravate depressive symptoms)	Vitamin B$_{12}$ influences melatonin secretion: Low levels of vitamin B$_{12}$ produce low levels of melatonin MAO inhibitors and SSRIs can increase serum concentrations β-Blockers can decrease nocturnal secretion of melatonin	Heavy head, headache, transient depression; long-term side effects unknown
Milk thistle	Supportive treatment for chronic inflammatory liver conditions and cirrhosis	Insufficient evidence to rate, but early data are promising	Safety not established in pregnancy	None reported	Rare mild transient diarrhea and rash

Red clover	Symptoms of menopause; prevention of cancer, indigestion, bronchitis, asthma	Insufficient evidence to rate effectiveness for osteoporosis or benign prostatic hyperplasia, but early data are promising	Pregnancy, lactation, coagulation disorders, hormone-sensitive cancers	Anticoagulant drugs (increase risk of bleeding); oral contraceptives (may compete for the same estrogen-receptor sites); may inhibit CPY4503A4 (avoid concurrent administration with drugs also metabolized by CPY4503A4)	Rash, estrogen-like side effects
S-adenosylmethionine (SAM-e)	Depression; heart disease; fibromyalgia; osteoarthritis and other musculoskeletal disorders; aging	Likely effective for relief of osteoarthritis; possibly effective for short-term treatment of depression	Pregnancy	Antidepressants (theoretical risk of serotonin syndrome–like effects)	Flatulence, vomiting, diarrhea, headache, nausea
Saw palmetto	Micturition difficulties associated with benign prostatic hyperplasia	Likely ineffective	Avoid in children and pregnant women	None reported	Headache, stomach upset

(Continued)

HERBS AND SUPPLEMENTS FORMULARY 23

TABLE 23-1

HERBAL FORMULARY—cont'd

Herb/Supplement	Indication	Efficacy	Contraindication	Drug Interactions	Side Effects
Shark cartilage	Prevention and treatment of cancer; arthritis	Probably ineffective for cancer treatment; no information for other indications	Pregnancy	None known	Taste perversion, nausea, vomiting, dyspepsia, constipation, hypotension, dizziness, hyperglycemia, decreased sensation
Soy	Hyperlipidemia; menstrual symptoms; prevention of osteoporosis and breast cancer	Likely effective for hyperlipidemia Possibly effective in treating symptoms related to menopause (hot flushes) and reducing risk of osteoporosis	Pregnancy, breast cancer, cystic fibrosis, nephrolithiasis, milk allergy	Estrogen and tamoxifen	Constipation, bloating, nausea, potential for allergic reactions

| St. John's wort | Anxiety and depression | Proven as effective as low-dose tricyclics in placebo-controlled studies | Caution in pregnant women and in fair-skinned persons when exposed to bright sunlight | Drug interactions: possibly similar to MAO inhibitors (anesthetics, antidepressants, antidiabetic agents, β-blockers, dextromethorphan, guanethidine, levodopa, meperidine, SSRIs, sympathomimetics, L-tryptophan), SSRIs, benzodiazepines Markedly reduces levels of protease inhibitors Food interactions: possibly similar to MAO inhibitors (tyramine-containing foods: cheeses, beer, wine, herring, and yeast) | Photodermatitis, gastrointestinal irritations, allergic reactions, fatigue, restlessness |

(Continued)

TABLE 23-1

HERBAL FORMULARY—cont'd

Herb/Supplement	Indication	Efficacy	Contraindication	Drug Interactions	Side Effects
Valerian	Restlessness and nervous disturbance of sleep	Possibly effective	Caution while driving or performing other tasks requiring alertness and coordination	Can potentiate sedative effect of barbiturates, benzodiazepines, opiates, alcohol	Headache, hangover, excitability, insomnia, uneasiness, cardiac disturbances Toxicity includes ataxia, decreased sensibility, hypothermia, hallucinations, increased muscle relaxation
Yohimbe	Used as an aphrodisiac and for impotence and general sexual dysfunction in men and women	Possibly effective for impotence; may improve sexual dysfunction associated with SSRIs	Pregnancy Not for children	Avoid concurrent use with antihypertensives and other hypotensive medications, MAO inhibitors, and other sympathomimetic drugs	Excitation, tremor, insomnia, hypertension, tachycardia, dizziness; high doses can lead to cardiac conduction disorders, hypotension

BIBLIOGRAPHY

German Federal Institute for Drugs and Medical Devices Commission E; American Botanical Council: *The Compete German Commission E Monographs: Therapeutic Guide to Herbal Medicines*. Philadelphia: Lippincott Williams & Wilkins, 1998.

Therapeutic Research Center: Natural Medicines Comprehensive Database. Available at http://www.naturaldatabase.com (accessed December 10, 2005).

Reference Materials

Mark A. Graber

PEDIATRIC SEDATION

I. **Sedation can facilitate procedures in the ED** and minimize the psychologic trauma to the child as well as to the ED staff and the parents.

II. **Sedation Requirements.**

A. Good monitoring including O_2 saturation, pulse, BP if possible, level of consciousness, and respirations is required. The child should be closely monitored until he or she has returned to functional baseline value.

B. **Sedation does not equal pain relief.** Give medications that relax the child and medications that provide pain relief.

C. The traditional DPT (Demerol, Phenergan, and Thorazine), aka Kiddy Cocktail or Lytic Cocktail, is fraught with problems and cannot be recommended.

D. Benzodiazepines, especially midazolam, have the advantage of causing amnesia.

E. Despite drug company marketing, there is no significant difference in the recovery times from a single dose of diazepam or midazolam when used for sedation in the ED. In fact, the recovery time was faster with diazepam in most studies.

F. Postsedation discharge requires return to baseline verbal skills if appropriate, return to baseline muscular control, return to baseline mental status, and a parent or responsible person who can understand instructions.

III. **Drugs for sedation and pain control in children** are shown in Table 24-1. *Note:* **Sedative doses are for conscious sedation, which requires constant monitoring. Be familiar with these agents and their side effects before using!**

TABLE 24-1
MEDICATIONS FOR SEDATION AND PAIN CONTROL IN CHILDREN

Medication	Route	Dose (mg/kg)	Maximum Dose	Side Effects and Comments
PAIN MEDICATIONS				
Fentanyl	IV	2-3 µg/kg	0.0 5mg	Rapidly effective IV (1-2 min) and short acting (20-30 min); causes respiratory depression
Meperidine (Demerol)	IV/IM	0.5-1.0 mg/kg	100 mg	Reversible with naloxone. Watch for respiratory depression. Can cause hypotension
Morphine	IV/IM	0.1-0.2 mg/kg	10 mg	Same as for meperidine
Codeine	PO	1.0 mg/kg	60 mg	Same as for meperidine
SEDATIVES				
Diazepam (Valium and others)	IV	0.05-0.2 mg/kg	10 mg	Watch for respiratory depression. Reversible with flumazenil
	PR	0.5 mg/kg		
Midazolam (Versed)	IV/IM	0.01-0.08 mg/kg (some have used ≤0.2 mg/kg)	4 mg	Titrate to effect; precautions as for diazepam
	PO/IN/PR	0.3-0.7 mg/kg		As for diazepam
Chloral hydrate	PR	25-100 mg/kg PO or PR	1000 mg, though some will go to 2000 mg	Cannot reverse. Less likely to be effective in head-injured or neurologically impaired pts

DISSOCIATIVE AGENT

Ketamine	IM/IV	0.5-2.0 mg/kg IV up to 4 mg/kg IM	100 mg IV	Onset 1 min; duration 15 min. IM use prolongs ED stay. Excellent drug, few adverse reactions, but raises intracranial and intraocular pressure. Airway reactivity and respirations generally maintained. Do not use if pt is <3 mo old or has respiratory infection. Use with glycopyrrolate or atropine to dry secretions

TO REVERSE

Naloxone (Narcan)	IV or IM 0.01 mg/kg/dose	0.01 mg/kg/dose	2 mg/dose; may repeat	Watch for narcotic withdrawal
Flumazenil (Romazicon)	IV or IM	0.01 mg/kg/dose	1 mg; may repeat	Do not use flumazenil for those with chronic benzodiazepine use!

REFERENCE MATERIALS 24

TABLE 24-2
PEDIATRIC VITAL SIGNS

Age	Heart Rate		Blood Pressure		Respiratory Rate
	Awake	*Sleeping*	*Systolic*	*Diastolic*	
Neonate	100-180	80-160	70-100	50-65	30-60
6 mo	120-160	80-180	87-105	53-66	25-50
2 y	80-150	70-120	90-106	55-67	18-35
5 y	80-110	60-90	94-109	56-69	17-27
10 y	70-110	60-90	102-117	62-75	15-23
>10 y	55-100	50-90	105-128	66-80	10-23

TABLE 24-3
FAHRENHEIT/CELSIUS CONVERSION

Fahrenheit	Celsius	Fahrenheit	Celsius
104.0	40.0	100.2	37.9
103.8	39.9	100.0	37.8
103.6	39.8	99.9	37.7
103.5	39.7	99.7	37.6
103.3	39.6	99.5	37.5
103.1	39.5	99.3	37.4
102.8	39.4	99.1	37.3
102.7	39.3	99.0	37.2
102.6	39.2	98.8	37.1
102.4	39.1	98.6	37.0
102.2	39.0	98.4	36.9
102.0	38.9	98.2	36.8
101.8	38.8	98.0	36.7
101.6	38.7	97.9	36.6
101.5	38.6	97.7	36.5
101.3	38.5	97.5	36.4
101.1	38.4	97.3	36.3
100.9	38.3	97.2	36.2
100.8	38.2	97.0	36.1
100.6	38.1	96.8	36.0
100.4	38.0		

Note: To convert degree *intervals:* 1° C = 1.8° F; 1° F = 0.6° C.

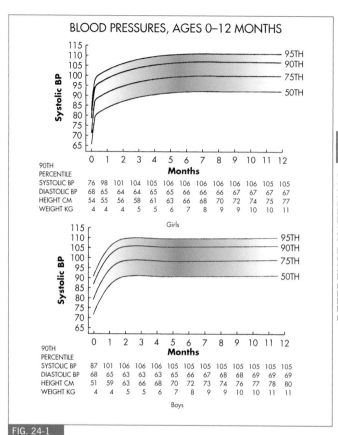

BLOOD PRESSURES, AGES 0–12 MONTHS

Girls

90TH PERCENTILE												
SYSTOLIC BP	76	98	101	104	105	106	106	106	106	106	105	105
DIASTOLIC BP	68	65	64	64	65	65	66	66	66	67	67	67
HEIGHT CM	54	55	56	58	61	63	66	68	70	72	74	75	77
WEIGHT KG	4	4	4	5	5	6	7	8	9	9	10	10	11

Boys

90TH PERCENTILE												
SYSTOLIC BP	87	101	106	106	106	105	105	105	105	105	105	105	105
DIASTOLIC BP	68	65	63	63	63	65	66	67	68	68	69	69	69
HEIGHT CM	51	59	63	66	68	70	72	73	74	76	77	78	80
WEIGHT KG	4	4	5	5	6	7	8	9	9	10	10	11	11

FIG. 24-1

Blood pressures for infants ages birth to 12 months. From Task Force on Blood Pressure Control in Children: *Pediatrics* 79:1, 1987.

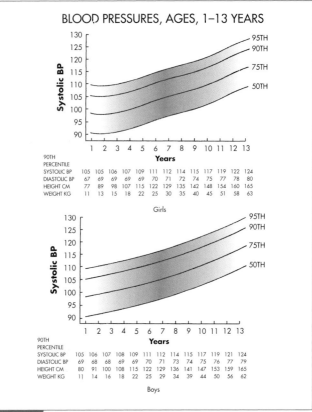

FIG. 24-2

Blood pressures for children ages 1 to 13 years. From Task Force on Blood Pressure Control in Children: *Pediatrics* 79:1, 1987.

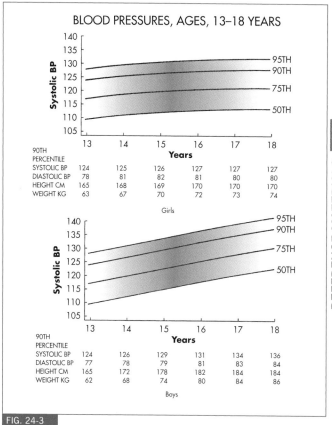

FIG. 24-3

Blood pressures for adolescents ages 13 to 18 years. From Task Force on Blood Pressure Control in Children: *Pediatrics* 79:1, 1987.

24

REFERENCE MATERIALS

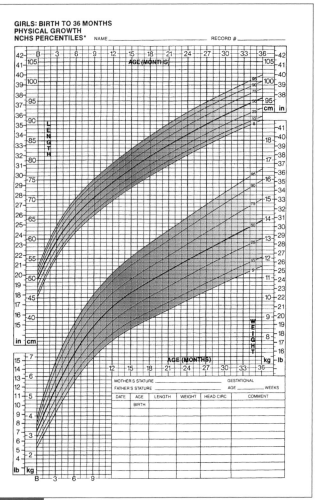

GIRLS: BIRTH TO 36 MONTHS
PHYSICAL GROWTH
NCHS PERCENTILES*   NAME _____   RECORD # _____

FIG. 24-4

Length and weight of girls from birth to 23 months. Adapted from Hamill PV, Johnson CL, Reed RB, et al: *Am J Clin Nutr* 32:607-629, 1979. Data from the Fels Longitudinal Study, Wright University School of Medicine, Yellow Springs, Colo.

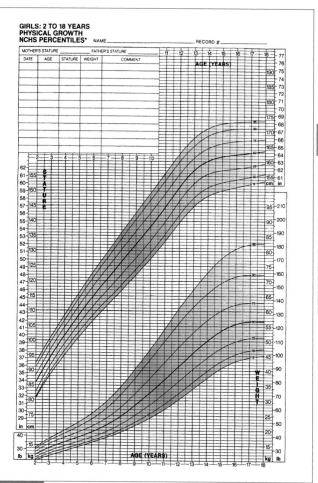

FIG. 24-5

Height and weight of girls from 2 to 18 years. Adapted from Hamill PV, Johnson CL, Reed RB, et al: *Am J Clin Nutr* 32:607-629, 1979. Data from the Fels Longitudinal Study, Wright University School of Medicine, Yellow Springs, Colo.

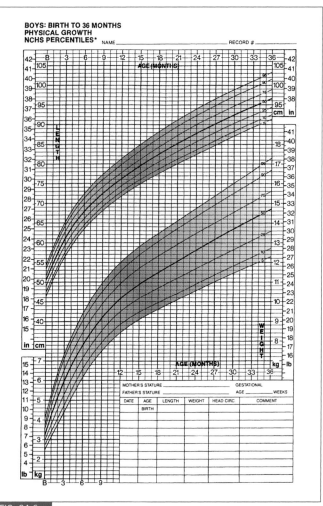

FIG. 24-6

Length and weight of boys from birth to 23 months. Adapted from Hamill PV, Johnson CL, Reed RB, et al: *Am J Clin Nutr* 32:607-629, 1979. Data from the Fels Longitudinal Study, Wright University School of Medicine, Yellow Springs, Colo.

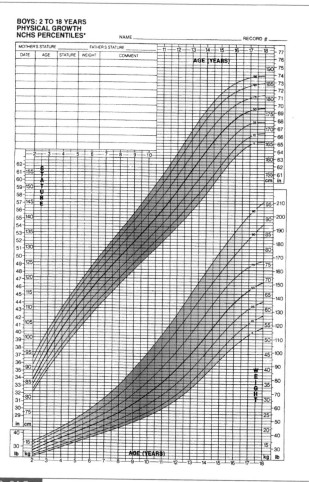

FIG. 24-7

Height and weight of boys from 2 to 18 years. Adapted from Hamill PV, Johnson CL, Reed RB, et al: *Am J Clin Nutr* 32:607-629, 1979. Data from the Fels Longitudinal Study, Wright University School of Medicine, Yellow Springs, Colo.

TABLE 24-4
DEVELOPMENTAL MILESTONES

Age	Gross Motor	Visual Motor	Language	Social
1 mo	Raises head slightly from prone, makes crawling movements, lifts chin up	Has tight grasp, follows to midline	Alert to sound (e.g., by blinking, moving, startling)	Regards face
2 mo	Holds head in midline, lifts chest off table	No longer clenches fist tightly, follows object past midline	Smiles after being stroked or talked to	Recognizes parent
3 mo	Supports on forearms in prone, holds head up steadily	Holds hands open at rest, follows in circular fashion	Coos (produces long vowel sounds in musical fashion)	Reaches for familiar people or objects, anticipates feeding
4-5 mo	Rolls front to back and back to front, sits well when propped, supports on wrists, and shifts weight	Moves arms in unison to grasp, touches cube placed on table	Orients to voice; 5 mo: orients to bell (localized laterally), says "ahgoo," razzes	Enjoys looking around environment
6 mo	Sits well unsupported, puts feet in mouth in supine position	Reaches with either hand, transfers, uses raking grasp	Babbles; 7 mo: orients to bell (localizes indirectly); 8 mo: "dada/mama" indiscriminately	Recognizes strangers
9 mo	Creeps, crawls, cruises, pulls to stand, pivots when sitting	Uses pincer grasp, probes with forefinger, holds bottle, finger-feeds	Understands "no," waves bye-bye; 10 mo: "dada/mama" discriminantly; 11 mo: one word other than "dada/mama"	Starts to explore environment, plays pat-a-cake
12 mo	Walks alone	Throws objects, lets go of toys, hand release, uses mature pincer grasp	Follows one-step command with gesture, uses 2 words other than "dada/mama"; 14 mo: uses 3 words	Imitates actions, comes when called, cooperates with dressing
15 mo	Creeps upstairs, walks backward	Builds tower of 2 blocks in imitation of examiner,	Follows one-step command without gesture, uses 4 to 6 words and	Indicates some simple needs by pointing, hugs parents

		scribbles in imitation	immature jargon (runs several unintelligible words together)	Copies parent in tasks (e.g., sweeping, dusting), plays in company of other children
18 mo	Runs, throws toy from standing without falling		Knows 7 to 20 words, knows 1 body part, uses mature jargon (includes intelligible words in jargon)	Copies parent in tasks (e.g., sweeping, dusting), plays in company of other children
21 mo	Squats in play, goes up steps	Turns 2 or 3 pages at a time, fills spoon and feeds self	Points to 3 body parts, uses 2-word combinations, has 20 word vocabulary	Asks to have food and to go to toilet
24 mo	Walks up and down steps without help	Builds tower of 5 blocks, drinks well from cup	Uses 50 words, 2-word sentences, uses pronouns (I, you, me) inappropriately, points to 5 body parts, understands 2-step command	Parallel play
30 mo	Jumps with both feet off floor, throws ball overhand	Turns pages one at a time, removes shoes, pants, etc., imitates behavior of others	Uses pronouns (I, you, me) appropriately, understands concept of "one," repeats 2 digits forward	Tells first and last names when asked, gets drink without help
3 yr	Pedals tricycle, can alternate feet when going up steps	Unbuttons, holds pencil in adult fashion, differentiates horizontal and vertical line	Uses 3-word sentences, plurals, and past tense. Knows all pronouns. Minimum of 250 words, understands concept of "two"	Group play, shares toys, takes turns, plays well with others, knows full name, age, sex
4 yr	Hops, skips, alternates feet going downstairs	Dresses and undresses partially, dries hands if reminded, draws a circle	Knows colors, says song or poem from memory, asks questions	Tells "tall tales," plays cooperatively with a group of children
5 y	Skips, alternating feet, jumps over low obstacles	Buttons clothing fully, catches ball	Prints first name, asks what a word means	Plays competitive games, abides by rules, likes to help in household tasks
		Ties shoes, spreads with knife		

REFERENCE MATERIALS 24

TABLE 24-5

NORMAL HEMATOLOGY VALUES

Age	Hb (g/dL), mean (±2 SD)	Hct (%), mean (±2 SD)	MCV (fL), mean (±2 SD)	MCHC, mean (±2 SD)	Reticulocytes (%)	WBC/mm² × 100, mean (±2 SD)	Platelets (10³/mm³), mean (± 2 SD)
WEEKS OF GESTATION*							
26-30	13.4 (11)	41.5 (34.9)	118.2 (106.7)	37.9 (30.6)	—	4.4 (2.7)	254 (180-327)
28	14.5	45	120	31	5-10	—	275
32	15.0	47	118	32	3-10	—	290
Term†							
Cord	16.5 (13.5)	51 (42)	108 (98)	33 (30)	3-7	18.1(9-30)‡	290
1-3 d	18.5 (14.5)	56 (45)	108 (95)	33 (30)	3-7	18.1(9-30)‡	290
2 wk	16.6 (13.4)	53 (41)	105 (88)	31.4 (28.1)		11.4 (5-20)	252
1 mo	13.9 (10.7)	44 (33)	101 (91)	31.8 (28.1)	0.1-1.7	10.8 (5-19.5)	
2 mo	11.2 (9.4)	34 (28)	95 (84)	31.8 (28.3)			
6 mo	12.6 (11.1)	36 (31)	76 (68)	35 (32.7)	0.7-2.3	11.9 (6-17.5)	
6 mo-2 y	12 (10.5)	36 (33)	78 (70)	33 (30)		10.6 (6-17)	150-350
2-6 y	12.5 (11.5)	37 (34)	81 (75)	34 (31)	0.5-1.0	8.5 (5-15.5)	150-350
6-12 y	13.5 (11.5)	40 (35)	86 (77)	34 (31)	0.5-1.0	8.1 (4.5-13.5)	150-350
12-18 YEARS							
Male	14.5 (13)	43 (36)	88 (78)	34 (31)	0.5-1.0	7.8 (4.5-13.5)	150-350
Female	13 (12)	41 (37)	90 (78)	34 (31)	0.5-1.0	7.8 (4.5-13.5)	150-350
ADULT							
Male	15.5 (13.5)	47 (41)	90 (80)	34 (31)	0.8-2.5	7.4 (4.5-11)	150-350
Female	14 (12)	41 (36)	90 (80)	34 (31)	0.8-4.1	7.4 (4.5-11)	150-350

*Values are from fetal samplings.

†Under 1 month, capillary hemoglobin exceeds venous: 1 hour, 3.6 g difference; 5 days, 2.2 g difference; 3 weeks, 1 g difference.

‡Mean (95%) confidence limits.

MCHC, mean corpuscular hemoglobin concentration; MCV, mean corpuscular volume.

TABLE 24-6
DENTAL DEVELOPMENT

| | Deciduous Teeth | | | | Permanent Teeth | |
| | Eruption | | Shedding | | Eruption | |
Teeth	Maxillary	Mandibular	Maxillary	Mandibular	Maxillary	Mandibular
Central incisors	6-8 mo	5-7 mo	7-8 y	6-7 y	7-8 y	6-7 y
Lateral incisors	8-11 mo	7-10 mo	8-9 y	7-8 y	8-9 y	7-8 y
Cuspids	16-20 mo	16-20 mo	11-12 y	9-11 y	11-12 y	9-11 y
First premolar	—	—	—	—	10-11 y	10-12 y
Second premolar	—	—	—	—	10-12 y	11-13 y
First molars	10-16 mo	10-16 mo	10-11 y	10-12 y	6-7 y	6-7 y
Second molars	20-30 mo	20-30 mo	10-12 y	11-13 y	12-13 y	12-13 y
Third molars	—	—	—	—	17-22 y	12-22 y

Note: Sexes are combined although girls tend to be slightly more advanced than boys. Averages are approximate values derived from various studies.
Adapted from Driscoll CE, Bope ET, Smith CW, Carter BL: The Family Practice Desk Reference, 3rd ed. St. Louis, Mosby, 1996.

REFERENCE MATERIALS 24

TABLE 24-7
CEREBROSPINAL FLUID IN TERM AND PRETERM INFANTS AND CHILDREN

Component	Normal Values
CELL COUNT (WBCs/mm^3)	
Preterm mean	9.0 (0-25.4), 57% PMNs
Term mean	8.2 (0-22.4), 61% PMNs
>1 mo	0-7, 0% PMNs
GLUCOSE (mg/dL)	
Preterm	24-63 (mean, 50)
Term	34-119 (mean, 52)
Child	40-80
CSF GLUCOSE/BLOOD GLUCOSE (%)	
Preterm	55-105
Term	44-128
Child	50
PRESSURE AT INITIAL LP (mm H$_2$O)	
Newborn	80-110 (<110)
Infant/child	<200 (lateral recumbent position)
PROTEIN (mg/dL)	
Preterm	65-150 (mean, 115)
Term	20-170 (mean, 90)
Child	5-15, ventricular
	5-25, cisternal
	5-40, lumbar
OTHER	
Myelin basic protein	<4 ng/mL
Lactic acid dehydrogenase	20 U/mL (mean; range, 5-30 U/mL)

TABLE 24-8
RECOMMENDATIONS FOR PARTICIPATION IN COMPETITIVE SPORTS

Factor	Contact/ Collision	Limited Contact/ Impact	Noncontact Strenuous	Moderately Strenuous	Not Strenuous
CARDIOVASCULAR					
Carditis	No	No	No	No	No
Congenital heart disease	1	1	1	1	1
Hypertension					
Mild	Yes	Yes	Yes	Yes	Yes
Moderate	2	2	2	2	2
Severe	2	2	2	2	2
EYES*					
Absence or loss of function of one eye	2	2	2	2	2
Detached retina	1	1	1	1	1
NEUROLOGIC					
History of serious head or spine trauma, repeated concussion, or craniotomy	2	2	Yes	Yes	Yes
Convulsive disorder†					
Well controlled	Yes	Yes	Yes	Yes	Yes
Poorly controlled	No	No	Yes	Yes	Yes
RESPIRATORY‡					
Asthma	Yes	Yes	Yes	Yes	Yes
Pulmonary insufficiency	2	2	2	2	2
VISCERAL AND REPRODUCTIVE ORGANS					
Inguinal hernia	Yes	Yes	Yes	Yes	Yes
Kidney: absence of one	No	Yes	Yes	Yes	Yes
Liver: enlarged	No	No	Yes	Yes	Yes
Ovary: absence of one	Yes	Yes	Yes	Yes	Yes
Spleen: enlarged	No	No	No	Yes	Yes
Testicle: absent or undescended	Yes	Yes	Yes	Yes	Yes
OTHER					
Acute illness§	2	2	2	2	2
Atlantoaxial instability‖	No	No	Yes	Yes	Yes
Musculoskeletal disorders	2	2	2	2	2
Sickle cell trait	Yes	Yes	Yes	Yes	Yes

(Continued)

TABLE 24-8

RECOMMENDATIONS FOR PARTICIPATION IN COMPETITIVE SPORTS—cont'd

			Noncontact		
Factor	Contact/ Collision	Limited Contact/ Impact	Strenuous	Moderately Strenuous	Not Strenuous
OTHER—cont'd					
Skin: boils, herpes, impetigo, scabies[¶]	2	2	Yes	Yes	Yes

Note: Certain sports may require a protective cup.

[1]Patients with mild forms can be allowed a full range of activities; patients with moderate or severe forms or those who are postoperative need evaluation by a cardiologist before athletic participation.

[2]Needs individual assessment.

[*]Availability of eye guards approved by the American Society for Testing and Materials (ASTM) may allow a competitor to participate in most sports, but this must be judged on an individual basis. Consult an ophthalmologist.

[†]Needs individual assessment; no swimming or weight lifting; no archery or riflery.

[‡]May be allowed to compete if oxygenation remains satisfactory during a graded stress test.

[§]Needs individual assessment, such as contagiousness to others, risk of worsening illness.

[‖]Swimming: no butterfly, breaststroke, or diving starts.

[¶]No gymnastics with mats, martial arts, wrestling, or contact sports until not contagious.

Adapted from American Academy of Pediatrics: Sports Medicine: Health Care For Young Athletes. Elk Grove Village, Ill, American Academy of Pediatrics, 1991.

TABLE 24-9

NORMAL PREDICTED AVERAGE PEAK EXPIRATORY FLOW FOR CHILDREN

Height (in)	Peak Flow (mL/min)	Height (in)	Peak Flow (mL/min)	Height (in)	Peak Flow (mL/min)
43	147	51	254	59	360
44	160	52	267	60	373
45	173	53	280	61	387
46	187	54	293	62	400
47	200	55	307	63	413
48	214	56	320	64	427
49	227	57	334	65	440
50	240	58	347	66	454

Adapted from iVillage Pregnancy and Parenting: Asthma: Normal peak flow meter readings. Available at http://parenting.ivillage.com/tweens/twhealth/0,3qk5,00.html (accessed January 2, 2005). Used by permission.

TABLE 24-10

NORMAL PREDICTED AVERAGE PEAK EXPIRATORY FLOW (AFTER PUBERTY)

Males		Females	
Height (in)	Peak Flow (mL/min)	Height (in)	Peak Flow (mL/min)
60	554	55	390
65	602	60	423
70	649	65	460
75	693	70	496
80	740	75	529

Adapted from iVillage Pregnancy and Parenting: Asthma: Normal peak flow meter readings. Available at http://parenting.ivillage.com/tweens/twhealth/0,3qk5,00.html (accessed January 2, 2005). Used by permission.

REFERENCE MATERIALS 24

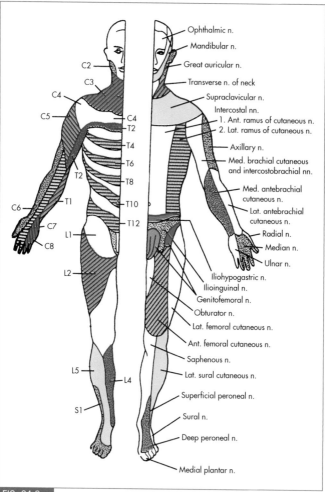

FIG. 24-8

Anterior view of dermatomes *(left)* and cutaneous areas supplied by individual peripheral nerves *(right)*. Modified from Carpenter MB, Sutin J: *Human Neuroanatomy*, 8th ed. Baltimore, Williams & Wilkins, 1983; Isselbacher KJ, Braunwald E, Wilson JD, et al (eds): *Harrison's Principles of Internal Medicine*, 13th ed. New York, McGraw–Hill, 1987.

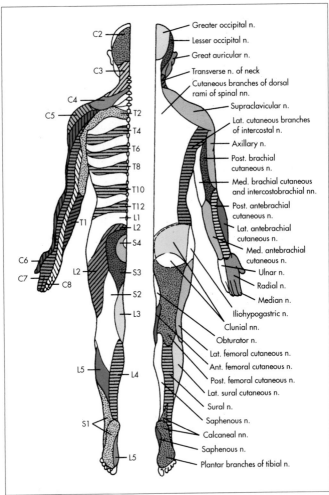

FIG. 24-9

Posterior view of dermatomes *(left)* and cutaneous areas supplied by individual peripheral nerves *(right)*. Modified from Carpenter MB, Sutin J: *Human Neuroanatomy,* 8th ed. Baltimore, Williams & Wilkins, 1983; Isselbacher KJ, Braunwald E, Wilson JD, et al (eds): *Harrison's Principles of Internal Medicine,* 13th ed. New York, McGraw–Hill, 1987.

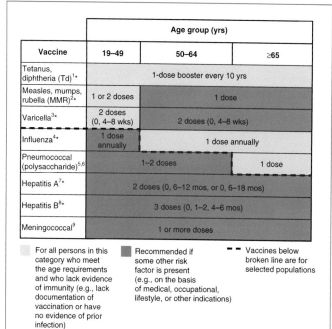

	Age group (yrs)		
Vaccine	**19–49**	**50–64**	**≥65**
Tetanus, diphtheria (Td)[1]*	1-dose booster every 10 yrs		
Measles, mumps, rubella (MMR)[2]*	1 or 2 doses	1 dose	
Varicella[3]*	2 doses (0, 4–8 wks)	2 doses (0, 4–8 wks)	
Influenza[4]*	1 dose annually	1 dose annually	
Pneumococcal (polysaccharide)[5,6]	1–2 doses		1 dose
Hepatitis A[7]*	2 doses (0, 6–12 mos, or 0, 6–18 mos)		
Hepatitis B[8]*	3 doses (0, 1–2, 4–6 mos)		
Meningococcal[9]	1 or more doses		

> For all persons in this category who meet the age requirements and who lack evidence of immunity (e.g., lack documentation of vaccination or have no evidence of prior infection)

> Recommended if some other risk factor is present (e.g., on the basis of medical, occupational, lifestyle, or other indications)

> - - Vaccines below broken line are for selected populations

FIG. 24-10

Recommended adult immunization schedule, by vaccine and age group—United States. From Centers for Disease Control and Prevention: *MMWR* 54:Q1-Q4, 2005.

[1]**Tetanus and diphtheria (Td) vaccination.** Adults with uncertain histories of a complete primary vaccination series with diphtheria and tetanus toxoid–containing vaccines should receive a primary series using combined Td toxoid. A primary series for adults is 3 doses; administer the first 2 doses at least 4 weeks apart and the third dose 6–12 months after the second. Administer 1 dose if the person received the primary series and if the last vaccination was received ≥ 10 years previously. Consult the Advisory Committee on Immunization Practices statement for recommendations for administering Td as prophylaxis in wound management (http://www.cdc.gov/mmwr/preview/mmwrhtml/00041645.htm). The American College of Physicians Task Force on Adult Immunization supports a second option for Td use in adults: a single Td booster at age 50 years for persons who have completed the full pediatric series, including the teenage/young adult booster. A newly licensed tetanus-diptheria-acellular–pertussis vaccine is available for adults. ACIP recommendations for its use will be published.

[2]**Measles, mumps, rubella (MMR) vaccination.** *Measles component:* adults born before 1957 can be considered immune to measles. Adults born during or after 1957 should receive ≥ 1 dose of MMR unless they have a medical contraindication, documentation of ≥ 1 dose, history of measles based on health-care provider

(Continued)

FIG. 24-10—cont'd

diagnosis, or laboratory evidence of immunity. A second dose of MMR is recommended for adults who (1) were recently exposed to measles or in an outbreak setting; (2) were previously vaccinated with killed measles vaccine; (3) were vaccinated with an unknown type of measles vaccine during 1963–1967; (4) are students in postsecondary educational institutions; (5) work in a health-care facility; or (6) plan to travel internationally. Withhold MMR or other measles-containing vaccines from HIV-infected persons with severe immunosuppression. *Mumps component:* 1 dose of MMR vaccine should be adequate for protection for those born during or after 1957 who lack a history of mumps based on health-care provider diagnosis or who lack laboratory evidence of immunity. *Rubella component:* administer 1 dose of MMR vaccine to women whose rubella vaccination history is unreliable or who lack laboratory evidence of immunity. For women of childbearing age, regardless of birth year, routinely determine rubella immunity and counsel women regarding congenital rubella syndrome. Do not vaccinate women who are pregnant or who might become pregnant within 4 weeks of receiving vaccine. Women who do not have evidence of immunity should receive MMR vaccine upon completion or termination of pregnancy and before discharge from the health-care facility.

[3]**Varicella vaccination.** Varicella vaccination is recommended for all adults without evidence of immunity to varicella. Special consideration should be given to those who (1) have close contact with persons at high risk for severe disease (health-care workers and family contacts of immunocompromised persons) or (2) are at high risk for exposure or transmission (e.g., teachers of young children; child care employees; residents and staff members of institutional settings, including correctional institutions; college students; military personnel; adolescents and adults living in households with children; nonpregnant women of childbearing age; and international travelers). Evidence of immunity to varicella in adults includes any of the following: (1) documented age-appropriate varicella vaccination (i.e., receipt of 1 dose before age 13 years or receipt of 2 doses [administered at least 4 weeks apart] after age 13 years); (2) U. S.-born before 1996 or history of varicella disease before 1966 for non-U.S.–born persons; (3) history of varicella based on health-care provider diagnosis or parental or self-report of typical varicella disease for persons born during 1966–1997 (for a patient reporting a history of an atypical, mild case, health-care providers should seek either an epidemiologic link with a typical varicella case or evidence of laboratory confirmation, if it was performed at the time of acute disease); (4) history of herpes zoster based on health-care provider diagnosis; or (5) laboratory evidence of immunity. Do not vaccinate women who are pregnant or who might become pregnant within 4 weeks of receiving the vaccine. Assess pregnant women for evidence of varicella immunity. Women who do not have evidence of immunity should receive dose 1 of varicella vaccine upon completion or termination of pregnancy and before discharge from the health-care facility. Dose 2 should be administered 4–8 weeks after dose 1.

[4]**Influenza vaccination.** *Medical indications:* chronic disorders of the cardiovascular or pulmonary systems, including asthma; chronic metabolic diseases, including diabetes mellitus, renal dysfunction, hemoglobinopathies, or immunosuppresion (including immunosuppresion caused by medications or HIV); any condition (e.g., cognitive

FIG. 24-10—cont'd

dysfunction, spinal cord injury, seizure disorder, or other neuromuscular disorder) that compromises respiratory function or the handling of respiratory secretions or that can increase the risk for aspiration; and pregnancy during the influenza season. No data exist on the risk for severe or complicated influenza disease among persons with asplenia; however, influenza is a risk factor for secondary bacterial infections that can cause severe disease among persons with asplenia. *Occupational indications:* health-care workers and employees of long-term–care and assisted living facilities. *Other indications:* residents of nursing homes and other long-term–care and assisted living facilities; persons likely to transmit influenza to persons at high risk (i.e., in-home household contacts and caregivers of children aged 0–23 months, or persons of all ages with high-risk conditions), and anyone who wishes to be vaccinated. For healthy, nonpregnant persons aged 5–49 years without high-risk conditions who are not contacts of severely immunocompromised persons in special care units, intranasally administered influenza vaccine (FluMist) may be administered in lieu of inactivated vaccine.

[5]**Pneumococcal polysaccharide vaccination.** *Medical indications:* chronic disorders of the pulmonary system (excluding asthma); cardiovascular diseases; diabetes mellitus; chronic liver diseases, including liver disease as a result of alcohol abuse (e.g., cirrhosis); chronic renal failure or nephrotic syndrome; functional or anatomic asplenia (e.g., sickle cell disease or splenectomy [if elective splenectomy is planned, vaccinate at least 2 weeks before surgery]); immunosuppressive conditions (e.g., congenital immunodeficiency, HIV infection [vaccinate as close to diagnosis as possible when CD4 cell counts are highest], leukemia, lymphoma, multiple myeloma, Hodgkin disease, generalized malignancy, or organ or bone marrow transplantation); or chemotherapy with alkylating agents, antimetabolites, or long-term systemic corticosteroids; and cochlear implants. *Other indications:* Alaska Natives and certain American Indian populations; residents of nursing homes and other long-term–care facilities.

[6]**Revaccination with pneumococcal polysaccharide vaccine.** One-time revaccination after 5 years for persons with chronic renal failure or nephritic syndrome; functional or anatomic asplenia (e.g., sickle cell disease or splenectomy); immunosuppressive conditions (e.g., congenital immunodeficiency, HIV infection, leukemia, lymphoma, multiple myeloma, Hodgkin disease, generalized malignancy or organ or bone marrow transplantation); or chemotherapy with alkylating agents antimetabolites, or long-term systemic corticosteroids. For persons aged ≥65 years, one-time revaccination if they were vaccinated ≥5 years previously and were aged <65 years at the time of primary vaccination.

[7]**Hepatitis A vaccination.** *Medical indications:* persons with clotting-factor disorders or chronic liver disease. *Behavioral indications:* men who have sex with men or users of illegal drugs. *Occupational indications:* Persons working with hepatitis A virus (HAV)–infected primates or with HAV in a research laboratory setting. *Other indications:* persons traveling to or working in countries that have high or intermediate endemicity of hepatitis A (for list of countries, see http://www.cdc.gov/travel/diseases.htm#hepa) as well as any person wishing to obtain immunity. Current vaccines should be administered in a 2-dose series at either 0 and 6–12 months or 0 and 6–18 months. If the combined hepatitis A and hepatitis B vaccine is used, administer 3 doses at 0, 1, and 6 months.

(Continued)

REFERENCE MATERIALS 24

FIG. 24-10—cont'd

[8]**Hepatitis B vaccination.** *Medical indications:* hemodialysis patients (use special formulation [40μg/mL] or two 20-μg/mL doses) or patients who receive clotting-factor concentrates. *Occupational indications:* health-care workers and public-safety workers who have exposure to blood in the workplace and persons in training in schools of medicine, dentistry, nursing, laboratory technology, and other allied health professions. *Behavioral indications:* injection-drug users; persons with more than one sex partner during the previous 6 months; persons with a recently acquired sexually transmitted disease (STD); and men who have sex with men. *Other indications:* household contacts and sex partners of persons with chronic hepatitis B virus (HBV) infection; clients and staff members of institutions for developmentally disabled persons; all clients of STD clinics; inmates of correctional facilities; and international travelers who will be in countries with high or intermediate prevalence of chronic HBV infection for more than 6 months (for list of countries, see http://www.cdc.gov/travel/diseases.htm#hepa).

[9]**Meningococcal vaccination.** *Medical indications:* adults with anatomic or functional asplenia or terminal complement component deficiencies. *Other indications:* first-year college students living in dormitories; microbiologists who are routinely exposed to isolates of *Neisseria meningitidis*; military recruits; and persons who travel to or reside in countries in which meningococcal disease is hyperendemic or epidemic (e.g., the "meningitis belt" of sub-saharan Africa during the dry season [December–June]), particularly if contact with local populations will be prolonged. Vaccination is required by the government of Saudi Arabia for all travelers to Mecca during the annual Hajj. Meningococcal conjugate vaccine is preferred for adults meeting any of the above indications who are aged ≤55 years, although meningococcal polysaccharide vaccine (MPSV4) is an acceptable alternative. Revaccination after 5 years might be indicated for adult previously vaccinated with MPSV4 who remain at high risk for infection (e.g., persons residing in areas in which disease is epidemic).

Vaccine	Pregnancy	Indication					
		Congenital immunodeficiency, leukemia[10] lymphoma, generalized malignancy, therapy with alkylating agents, antimetabolites, radiation, or large amounts of corticosteroids	Diabetes, heart disease, chronic pulmonary disease, or chronic liver disease, including chronic alcoholism	Asplenia[10] (including elective splenectomy and terminal complement component deficiencies)	Kidney failure, end-stage renal disease, recipients of hemodialysis, or clotting factor concentrates	Human immunodeficiency virus (HIV) infection[2,10]	Health-care workers
Tetanus, diphtheria (Td)[1]*		1-dose booster every 10 yrs					
Measles, mumps, rubella (MMR)[2]*			1 or 2 doses				
Varicella[3]*			2 doses (0, 4–8 wks)				2 doses
Influenza[4]*		1 dose annually		1 dose annually		1 dose annually	
Pneumococcal (polysaccharide)[5,6]	1–2 doses	1–2 doses					
Hepatitis A[7]*		2 doses (0, 6–12 mos, or 0, 6–18 mos)					
Hepatitis B[8]*		3 doses (0, 1–2, 4–6 mos)			3 doses (0, 1–2, 4–6 mos)		
Meningococcal[9]		1 dose		1 dose	1 dose		1–2 doses

For all persons in this category who meet the age requirements and who lack evidence of immunity (e.g., lack documentation of vaccination or have no evidence of prior infection)

■ Recommended if some other risk factor is present (e.g., on the basis of medical, occupational, lifestyle, or other indications)

■ Contraindicated

REFERENCE MATERIALS 24

FIG. 24-11

Adult immunizations for patients with underlying illness or condition—United States. From Centers for Disease Control and Prevention: *MMWR* 54:Q1-Q4, 2005.

(Continued)

FIG. 24-11—cont'd

[1-9]For numbered footnotes, see legend for Fig. 24-10.

[10]**Selected conditions for which *Haemophilus influenzae* type b (Hib) vaccine may be used.** Hib conjugate vaccines are licensed for children aged 6 weeks – 71 months. No efficacy data are available on which to base a recommendation concerning use of Hib vaccine for older children and adults with the chronic conditions associated with an increased risks for Hib disease. However, studies suggest good immunogenicity in patients who have sickle cell disease, leukemia, or HIV infection or who have had splenectomies; administering vaccine to these patients is not contraindicated.

Vaccine	Birth	1 month	2 months	4 months	6 months	12 months	15 months	18 months	24 months	4–6 years	11–12 years	13–14 years	15 years	16–18 years
Hepatitis B [1]	HepB	HepB	HepB[1]	HepB[1]		HepB					HepB series			
Diphtheria, tetanus, pertussis[2]			DTaP	DTaP	DTaP		DTaP	DTaP		DTaP	Tdap		Tdap	
Haemophilus influenzae type b [3]			Hib	Hib	Hib[3]	Hib								
Inactivated Poliovirus			IPV	IPV		IPV				IPV				
Measles, mumps, rubella[4]						MMR				MMR	MMR			
Varicella[5]						Varicella					Varicella			
Meningococcal[6]									MPSV4		MCV4	MCV4	MCV4	MCV4
Pneumococcal[7]			PCV	PCV	PCV	PCV			PCV	PCV	PPV			
Influenza[8]					Influenza (yearly)					Influenza (yearly)				
Hepatitis A[9]						HepA series					HepA series			

Range of recommended ages ▓ Catch-up immunization ▓ Assessment at age 11–12 years - - - Vaccines within broken line are for selected populations

This schedule indicates the recommended ages for routine administration of currently licensed childhood vaccines, as of December 1, 2005, for children through age 18 years. Any dose not administered at the recommended age should be administered at any subsequent visit, when indicated and feasible. ▓ Indicates age groups that warrant special effort to administer those vaccines not previously administered. Additional vaccines may be licensed and recommended during the year. Licensed combination vaccines may be used whenever any components of the combination are indicated and other components of the vaccine are not contraindicated and if approved by the Food and Drug Administration for that dose of the series. Providers should consult respective Advisory Committee on Immunization Practices (ACIP) statements for detailed recommendations. Clinically significant adverse events that follow vaccination should be reported through the Vaccine Adverse Event Reporting System (VAERS). Guidance about how to obtain and complete a VAERS form is available at http://www.vaers.hhs.gov or by telephone, 800-822-7967.

REFERENCE MATERIALS 24

FIG. 24-12

Recommended childhood and adolescent immunization schedule, United States, 2006. From CDC: *MMWR* 54 (Nos. 51 & 52):Q1-4, 2005.

(Continued)

FIG. 24-12—cont'd

[1]**Hepatitis B vaccine (HepB).** *At birth: All newborns* should receive monovalent HepB soon after birth and before hospital discharge. *Infants born to mothers who are hepatitis B surface antigen (HBsAg)-positive* should receive HepB and 0.5 mL of hepatitis B immune globulin (HBIG) within 12 hours of birth. *Infants born to mothers whose HBsAg status is is unknown* should receive HepB within 12 hours of birth. The mother should have blood drawn as soon as possible to determine her HBsAg status; if HBsAg-positive, the infant should receive HBIG as soon as possible (no later than age 1 week). *For infants born to HBsAg-negative mothers,* the birth dose can be delayed in rare circumstances but only if a physician's order to withhold the vaccine and a copy of the mother's original HBsAg-negative laboratory report are documented in the infant's medical record. *Following the birth dose:* The HepB series should be completed with either monovalent HepB or a combination vaccine containing HepB. The second dose should be administered at age 1–2 months. The final dose should be administered at age ≥24 weeks. Administering four doses of HepB is permissible (e.g., when combination vaccines are administered after the birth dose); however, if monovalent HepB is used, a dose at age 4 months is not needed. *Infants born to HBsAg-positive mothers* should be tested for HBsAg and antibody to HBsAg after completion of the HepB series at age 9–18 months (generally at the next well-child visit after completion of the vaccine series).

[2]**Diphtheria and tetanus toxoids and acellualar pertussis vaccine (DTaP).** The fourth dose of DTaP may be administered as early as age 12 months, provided 6 months have elapsed since the third dose and the child is unlikely to return at age 15–18 months. The final dose in the series should be administered at age ≥4 years. *Tetanus toxoid, reduced diphtheria toxoid, and acellular pertussis vaccine (Tdap adolescent preparation)* is recommended at age 11–12 years for those who have completed the recommended childhood DTP/DtaP vaccination series and have not received a tetanus and diphtheria toxoids (Td) booster dose. Adolescents aged 13–18 years who missed the age 11–12-year Td/Tdap booster dose should also receive a single dose of Tdap if they have completed the recommended childhood DTP/DtaP vaccination series. *Subsequent Td boosters are recommended every 10 years.*

[3]***Haemophilus influenzae* type b conjugate vaccine (Hib).** Three Hib conjugate vaccines are licensed for infant use. If PRP-OMP (PedvaxHIB or ComVax [Merck]) is administered at ages 2 and 4 months, a dose at age 6 months is not required. DTaP/Hib combination products should not be used for primary immunization in infants at ages 2, 4, or 6 months but may be used as boosters after any Hib vaccine. The final dose in the series should be administered at age ≥12 months.

[4]**Measles, mumps, and rubella vaccine (MMR).** The second dose of MMR is recommended routinely at age 4–6 years but may be administered during any visit, provided at least 4 weeks have elapsed since the first dose and both doses are administered at or after age 12 months. Children who have not previously received the second dose should complete the schedule by age 11–12 years.

[5]**Varicella vaccine.** Varicella vaccine is recommended at any visit at or after age 12 months for susceptible children (i.e., those who lack a reliable history of varicella). Susceptible persons aged ≥ 13 years should receive 2 doses administered at least 4 weeks apart.

FIG. 24-12—cont'd

[6]**Meningococcal vaccine (MCV4).** Meningococcal conjugate vaccine (MCV4) should be administered to all children at age 11–12 years as well as to unvaccinated adolescents at high school entry (age 15 years). Other adolescents who wish to decrease their risk for meningococcal disease may also be vaccinated. All college freshmen living in dormitories should also be vaccinated, preferably with MCV4, although *meningococcal polysaccharide vaccine (MPSV4)* is an acceptable alternative. Vaccination against invasive meningococcal disease is recommended for children and adolescents aged ≥2 years with terminal complement deficiencies or anatomic or functional asplenia and for certain other high risk groups (see *MMWR* 2005;54[No. RR-7]); use MPSV4 for children aged 2–10 years and MCV4 for older children, although MPSV4 is an acceptable alternative.

[7]**Pneumococcal vaccine.** The heptavalent *pneunococcal conjugate vaccine (PCV)* is recommended for all children aged 2–23 months and for certain children aged 24–59 months. The final dose in the series should be administered at age ≥ 12 months. *Pneumococcal polysaccharide vaccine (PPV)* is recommended in addition to PCV for certain high-risk groups. See *MMWR* 2000; 49(No. RR-9).

[8]**Influenza vaccine.** Influenza vaccine is recommended annually for children aged ≥6 months with certain risk factors (including, but not limited to, asthma, cardiac disease, sickle cell disease, human immunodeficiency virus infection, diabetes, and conditions that can compromise respiratory function or handling of respiratory secretions or that can increase the risk for aspiration), health-care workers, and other persons (including household members) in close contact with persons in groups at high risk (see *MMWR* 2005;54[No. RR-8]). In addition, healthy children aged 6–23 months and close contacts of healthy children aged 0–5 months are recommended to receive influenza vaccine because children in this age group are at substantially increased risk for influenza-related hospitalizations. For healthy, nonpregnant persons aged 5–49 years, the intranasally administered, live, attenuated influenza vaccine (LAIV) is an acceptable alternative to the intramuscular trivalent inactivated influenza vaccine (TIV). See *MMWR* 2005;54(No. RR-8).Children receiving TIV should be administered an age-appropriate dosage (0.25 mL for children aged 6–35 months or 0.5 mL for children aged ≥3 years). Children aged ≤8 years who are receiving influenza vaccine for the first time should receive 2 doses (separated by at least 4 weeks for TIV and at least 6 weeks for LAIV).

[9]**Hepatitis A vaccine (HepA).** HepA is recommended for all children at age 1 year (i.e., 12–23 months). The 2 doses in the series should be administered at least 6 months apart. States, counties, and communities with existing HepA vaccination programs for children aged 2–18 years are encouraged to maintain these programs. In these areas, new efforts focused on routine vaccination of children aged 1 year should enhance, not replace, ongoing programs directed at a broader population of children. HepA is also recommended for certain high risk groups (see *MMWR* 1999;48[No. RR-12]).

24

REFERENCE MATERIALS

Catch-up schedule for children aged 4 months–6 years

Vaccine	Minimum age for dose 1	Minimum interval between doses			
		Dose 1 to dose 2	Dose 2 to dose 3	Dose 3 to dose 4	Dose 4 to dose 5
Diphtheria, tetanus, pertussis	6 wks	4 weeks	4 weeks	6 months	6 mos[1]
Inactivated Poliovirus	6 wks	4 weeks	4 weeks	4 weeks[2]	
Hepatitis B[3]	Birth	4 weeks	8 weeks (and 16 weeks after first dose)		
Measles, mumps, rubella	12 mos	4 weeks[4]			
Varicella	12 mos				
Haemophilus influenzae type b[5]	6 wks	4 weeks: if first dose administered at age <12 months 8 weeks (as final dose): if first dose administered at age 12–14 months No further doses needed if first dose administered at age ≥15 months	4 weeks[6]: if current age <12 months 8 weeks (as final dose)[6]: if current age ≥12 months and second dose administered at age <15 months No further doses needed if previous dose administered at age ≥15 months	8 weeks (as final dose): This dose only necessary for children aged 12 months–5 years who received 3 doses before age 12 months	
Pneumococcal[7]	6 wks	4 weeks: if first dose administered at age ≥12 months and current age <24 months 8 weeks (as final dose): if first dose administered at age ≥12 months or current age 24–59 months No further doses needed for healthy children if first dose administered at age ≥24 months	4 weeks: if current age <12 months 8 weeks (as final dose): if current age ≥12 months No further doses needed for healthy children if previous dose administered at age ≥24 months	8 weeks (as final dose): This dose only necessary for children aged 12 months–5 years who received 3 doses before age 12 months	

FIG. 24-13

Catch-up immunization schedule for children ages 4 months to 6 years. From Centers for Disease Control and Prevention: *MMWR* 54 (Nos. 51 & 52):Q1-4, 2005.

FIG. 24-13—cont'd

[1]**DTaP.** The fifth dose is not necessary if the fourth dose was administered after the fourth birthday.

[2]**IPV.** For children who received an all-IPV or all-oral poliovirus (OPV) series, a fourth dose is not necessary if the third dose was administered at age ≥years. If both OPV and IPV were administered as part of a series, a total of 4 doses should be administrated, regardless of the child's current age.

[3]**HepB.** Administer the 3-dose series to all persons aged <19 years if they were not previously vaccinated.

[4]**MMR.** The second dose of MMR is recommended routinely at age 4-6 years but may be administered earlier if desired.

[5]**Hib.** Vaccine is not generally recommended for children ages ≥5 years

[6]**Hib.** If current age is >12 months and the first 2 doses were **PRP-OMP** (PedvaxHIB or ComVax [Merck]), the third (and final) dose should be administered at age 12-15 months and at least 8 weeks after the second dose.

[7]**PCV.** Vaccine is not generally recommended for children aged ≥5 years.

Catch-up schedule for children aged 7–18 years

Vaccine	Minimum interval between doses		
	Dose 1 to dose 2	Dose 2 to dose 3	Dose 3 to booster dose
Tetanus, diphtheria[1]	4 weeks	6 months	6 months: if first dose administered at age <12 months and current age <11 years; otherwise 5 years
Inactivated Poliovirus[3]	4 weeks	4 weeks	IPV[2,3]
Hepatitis B	4 weeks	8 weeks (and 16 weeks after first dose)	
Measles, mumps, rubella	4 weeks		
Varicella[4]	4 weeks		

FIG. 24-14

Catch-up immunization schedule for children ages 6 to 18 years. From Centers for Disease Control and Prevention: *MMWR* 54 (Nos. 51 & 52):Q1-4, 2005.

[1]**Td.** Tdap adolescent preparation may be substituted for any dose in a primary catch-up series or as a booster if age appropriate for Tdap. A 5-years interval from the last Td dose is encouraged when Tdap is used as a booster dose.

[2]**IPV.** For children who received an all-IPV or all-oral poliovirus (OPV) series, a fourth dose is not necessary if the third dose was administered at age ≥years. If both OPV and IPV were administered as part of a series, a total of 4 doses should be administered, regardless of the child's current age.

[3]**IPV.** Vaccine is not generally recommended for persons aged ≥18 years.

[4]**Varicella.** Administer the 2-dose series to all susceptible adolescents aged ≥13 years.

24

REFERENCE MATERIALS

METABOLIC FORMULAS

Electrolyte Formulas

I. Hyperglycemia Effect on Serum Na+.

Corrected serum Na+
= Measured Na+ + 1.6 × ([Measured serum glucose − 100] / 100)

for serum glucose over 100 mg/dL. *Note:* Correction may be up to 2.4 mg/dL.

II. Hyperlipidemia or Hyperproteinemia Effect on Na+.

Correct serum Na+ = Measured Na+ × (93/% of serum H_2O)

% Serum H_2O = 99 − (1.03 × Lipids) − (0.73 × Protein)

Lipids and protein are in g/dL.

III. Fractional Excretion of Na+ (FE_{Na}).

% FE_{Na} = (Urine Na+/Serum Na+) / (Urine Cr/Serum Cr) × 100

IV. Serum Na+ Requirement in Hyponatremia.

Desired Na+ mEq/L = (Desired serum Na+ − Measured Na+) × TBW

TBW = 0.6 × Body weight

TBW is total body water in liters; body weight is in kilograms.

V. Body Water Deficit in Hypernatremia.

Deficit = Desired TBW − Current TBW

Desired TBW = Measured Na+ × (Current TBW/normal serum Na+)

Current TBW = 0.6 × Current body weight

or

Deficit = 0.6 × (Current weight) × ([Serum Na+/140] − 1)

TBW is total body water in liters; body weight is in kilograms.

VI. Creatinine Clearance.

Creatinine clearance = [(140 − Age) × (Weight)] / (72 × Serum Cr)

where body weight is in kilograms and serum creatinine is in mg/dL. Normal male = 125 mL/min; normal female = 105 mL/min.

VII. Serum Osmolarity.

Serum osmolarity = 2(Na+ + K+) + (BUN/2.8) + (Glucose/18)

A. Normal value is 280 to 296 mOsm/kg of water.

B. A difference between the measured and calculated osmolarity (osmolar gap) can indicate a circulating osmotically active substance such as ethanol, methanol, or ethylene glycol (antifreeze).

VIII. Anion gap.

$$\text{Anion gap} = Na^+ - (Cl^- + HCO_3^-)$$

Normal is up to 15. Greater than this in presence of acidosis indicates an anion gap acidosis (see Chapter 6 for discussion).

IX. Alveolar–arterial Gradient.

$$\text{A-a gradient} = P_{AO_2} - Pa_{O_2}$$

$$P_{AO_2} = 150 - (1.2 \times Pa_{CO_2})$$

P_{AO_2} is the partial pressure of alveolar oxygen; Pa_{O_2} is partial pressure of arterial oxygen. Pa_{CO_2} is partial pressure of carbon dioxide. These equations assume the patient is breathing room air (F_{iO_2} 21%). Normal A-a gradient is 5 to 20 and increases with age.

X. Mean Arterial Pressure.

$$MAP = [SBP + (2 \times DBP)]/3$$

XI. Relationship between P_{CO_2} and pH.

If uncompensated, a change in P_{CO_2} of 10 results in a pH change of 0.08.

Index

Note: Page numbers followed by the letter b refer to boxed material; those followed by the letter f refer to figures, and those followed by t refer to tables.

INDEX

INDEX

INDEX

INDEX

INDEX